Clinical Periodontology and Implant Dentistry

Fifth Edition

Edited by

Jan Lindhe
Niklaus P. Lang
Thorkild Karring

Associate Editors
Tord Berglundh
William V. Giannobile
Mariano Sanz

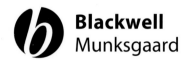
Blackwell
Munksgaard

Volume 1
BASIC CONCEPTS

Edited by

Jan Lindhe
Niklaus P. Lang
Thorkild Karring

© 2008 by Blackwell Munksgaard, a Blackwell Publishing company

Blackwell Publishing editorial offices:
Blackwell Publishing Ltd, 9600 Garsington Road, Oxford OX4 2DQ, UK
Tel: +44 (0)1865 776868
Blackwell Publishing Professional, 2121 State Avenue, Ames, Iowa 50014-8300, USA
Tel: +1 515 292 0140
Blackwell Publishing Asia Pty Ltd, 550 Swanston Street, Carlton, Victoria 3053, Australia
Tel: +61 (0)3 8359 1011

First published 1983 by Munksgaard
Second edition published 1989
Third edition published 1997
Fourth edition published by Blackwell Munksgaard 2003
Reprinted 2003, 2005, 2006
Fifth edition 2008 by Blackwell Publishing Ltd
6 2012

ISBN: 978-1-4051-6099-5

Library of Congress Cataloging-in-Publication Data
Clinical periodontology and implant dentistry / edited by Jan Lindhe,
Niklaus P. Lang, Thorkild Karring. — 5th ed.
p. ; cm.
Includes bibliographical references and index.
ISBN: 978-1-4051-6099-5 (hardback : alk. paper)
1. Periodontics. 2. Periodontal disease. 3. Dental implants. I. Lindhe, Jan.
II. Lang, Niklaus Peter. III. Karring, Thorkild.
[DNLM: 1. Periodontal Diseases. 2. Dental Implantation. 3. Dental Implants.
WU 240 C6415 2008]
RK361.C54 2008
617.6′32—dc22

2007037124

A catalogue record for this title is available from the British Library

Set in 9.5/12 pt Palatino by SNP Best-set Typesetter Ltd., Hong Kong
Printed and bound in Singapore by Fabulous Printers Pte Ltd

For further information on Blackwell Publishing, visit our website:
www.blackwellmunksgaard.com

Contents

Volume 1: BASIC CONCEPTS
Editors: Jan Lindhe, Niklaus P. Lang, and Thorkild Karring

Volume 2: CLINICAL CONCEPTS
Editors: Niklaus P. Lang and Jan Lindhe

Contributors

Martin Addy
Division of Restorative Dentistry (Periodontology)
Department of Oral and Dental Science
Bristol Dental School and Hospital
Bristol
UK

Maurício Araújo
Department of Dentistry
State University of Maringá
Maringá
Paraná
Brazil

Gary C. Armitage
Division of Periodontology
School of Dentistry
University of California San Francisco
San Francisco
CA
USA

Rolf Attström
Department of Periodontology
Centre for Oral Health Sciences
Malmö University
Malmö
Sweden

Robert A. Bagramian
Department of Periodontics and Oral Medicine
University of Michigan School of Dentistry
Ann Arbor
MI
USA

Hans-Rudolf Baur
Department of Internal Medicine
Spital Bern Tiefenau
Berne
Switzerland

Urs C. Belser
Department of Prosthetic Dentistry
School of Dental Medicine
University of Geneva
Geneva
Switzerland

Gunnar Bergenholtz
Department of Endodontology
Institute of Odontology
The Sahlgrenska Academy at Göteborg University
Göteborg
Sweden

Tord Berglundh
Department of Periodontology
Institute of Odontology
The Sahlgrenska Academy at Göteborg University
Göteborg
Sweden

Jean-Pierre Bernard
Department of Oral Surgery and Stomatology
School of Dental Medicine
University of Geneva
Geneva
Switzerland

Urs Brägger
Department of Periodontology and Fixed
    Prosthodontics
School of Dental Medicine
University of Berne
Berne
Switzerland

Rino Burkhardt
Private Practice
Zürich
Switzerland

Daniel Buser
Department of Oral Surgery and Stomatology
School of Dental Medicine
University of Berne
Berne
Switzerland

Gianfranco Carnevale
Private Practice
Rome
Italy

Delwyn Catley
Department of Psychology
University of Missouri – Kansas City
Kansas City
MO
USA

Noel Claffey
Dublin Dental School and Hospital
Trinity College
Dublin
Ireland

Lyndon F. Cooper
Department of Prosthodontics
University of North Carolina
Chapel Hill
NC
USA

Pierpaolo Cortellini
Private Practice
Florence
Italy

José J. Echeverría
Department of Periodontics
School of Dentistry
University of Barcelona
Barcelona
Spain

Ingvar Ericsson
Department of Prosthetic Dentistry
Faculty of Odontology
Malmö University
Malmö
Sweden

William V. Giannobile
Michigan Center for Oral Health Research
University of Michigan Clinical Center
Ann Arbor
MI
USA

Hans-Göran Gröndahl
Department of Oral and Maxillofacial Radiology
Institute of Odontology
The Sahlgrenska Academy at Göteborg University
Göteborg
Sweden

Kerstin Gröndahl
Department of Oral and Maxillofacial Radiology
Institute of Odontology
The Sahlgrenska Academy at Göteborg University
Göteborg
Sweden

Anne D. Haffajee
Department of Periodontology
The Forsyth Institute
Boston
MA
USA

Christoph H.F. Hämmerle
Clinic for Fixed and Removable Prosthodontics
Center for Dental and Oral Medicine and Cranio-
   Maxillofacial Surgery
University of Zürich
Zürich
Switzerland

Gunnar Hasselgren
Division of Endodontics
School of Dental and Oral Surgery
Columbia University College of Dental Medicine
New York
NY
USA

Lars Heijl
Department of Periodontology
Institute of Odontology
The Sahlgrenska Academy at Göteborg University
Göteborg
Sweden

David Herrera
Faculty of Odontology
University Complutense
Madrid
Spain

Palle Holmstrup
Department of Periodontology
School of Dentistry
University of Copenhagen
Copenhagen
Denmark

Reinhilde Jacobs
Oral Imaging Center
School of Dentistry, Oral Pathology and Maxillofacial
   Surgery
Catholic University of Leuven
Leuven
Belgium

Ronald E. Jung
Clinic for Fixed and Removable Prosthodontics
Center for Dental and Oral Medicine and Cranio-
   Maxillofacial Surgery
University of Zürich
Zürich
Switzerland

Thorkild Karring
Department of Periodontology and Oral Gerontology
Royal Dental College
University of Aarhus
Aarhus
Denmark

Denis F. Kinane
Oral Health and Systemic Disease Research Facility
School of Dentistry
University of Louisville
Louisville
KY
USA

Y. Joon Ko
Department of Prosthodontics
University of Iowa
Iowa City
IA
USA

Susan Krigel
Department of Psychology
University of Missouri – Kansas City
Kansas City
MO
USA

Marja L. Laine
Department of Oral Microbiology
Academic Centre for Dentistry Amsterdam (ACTA)
Amsterdam
The Netherlands

Niklaus P. Lang
Department of Periodontology and Fixed
    Prosthodontics
School of Dental Medicine
University of Berne
Berne
Switzerland

Ulf Lekholm
Department of Oral and Maxillofacial Surgery
Institute of Odontology
The Sahlgrenska Academy at Göteborg University
Göteborg
Sweden

Jan Lindhe
Department of Periodontology
Institute of Odontology
The Sahlgrenska Academy at Göteborg University
Göteborg
Sweden

Bruno G. Loos
Department of Periodontology
Academic Centre for Dentistry Amsterdam (ACTA)
Amsterdam
The Netherlands

Tord Lundgren
Department of Periodontics
School of Dentistry
Loma Linda University
Loma Linda
CA
USA

Angelo Mariotti
Section of Periodontology
Ohio State University College of Dentistry
Columbus
OH
USA

Andrea Mombelli
Department of Periodontology and Oral
    Pathophysiology
School of Dental Medicine
University of Geneva
Geneva
Switzerland

John Moran
Division of Restorative Dentistry (Periodontology)
Department of Oral and Dental Science
Bristol Dental School and Hospital
Bristol
UK

Sture Nyman
Deceased

Richard Palmer
Restorative Dentistry
King's College London Dental Institute
Guy's, King's and St Thomas' Hospitals
London
UK

Panos N. Papapanou
Division of Periodontics
Section of Oral and Diagnostic Sciences
Columbia University College of Dental Medicine
New York
NY
USA

David W. Paquette
Department of Periodontology
University of North Carolina School of Dentistry
Chapel Hill
NC
USA

Giovan P. Pini Prato
Department of Periodontology
University of Florence
Florence
Italy

Bjarni E. Pjetursson
Department of Periodontology and Fixed
    Prosthodontics
School of Dental Medicine
University of Berne
Berne
Switzerland

Ioannis Polyzois
Dublin Dental School and Hospital
Trinity College
Dublin
Ireland

Roberto Pontoriero
Private Practice
Milan
Italy

Marc Quirynen
Department of Periodontology
School of Dentistry
Catholic University of Leuven
Leuven
Belgium

Christoph A. Ramseier
Michigan Center for Oral Health Research
Department of Periodontics and Oral Medicine
University of Michigan School of Dentistry
Ann Arbor
MI
USA

Domenico Ricucci
Private Practice
Rome
Italy

Hector F. Rios
Department of Periodontics and Oral Medicine
University of Michigan School of Dentistry
Ann Arbor
MI
USA

Giovanni E. Salvi
Department of Periodontology
School of Dental Medicine
University of Berne
Berne
Switzerland

Mariano Sanz
Faculty of Odontology
University Complutense
Madrid
Spain

Marc A. Schätzle
Department of Orthodontics and Pediatric Dentistry
University of Zürich
Zürich
Switzerland

Sigmund S. Socransky
Department of Periodontology
The Forsyth Institute
Boston
MA
USA

Mena Soory
Restorative Dentistry
King's College London Dental Institute
Guy's, King's and St Thomas' Hospitals
London
UK

Clark M. Stanford
Dows Institute for Dental Research
University of Iowa
Iowa City
IA
USA

Ricardo P. Teles
Department of Periodontology
The Forsyth Institute
Boston
MA
USA

Maurizio S. Tonetti
Private Practice
Genoa
Italy

Leonardo Trombelli
Research Center for the Study of Periodontal
  Diseases
University of Ferrara
Ferrara
Italy

Ubele van der Velden
Department of Periodontology
Academic Centre for Dentistry Amsterdam (ACTA)
Amsterdam
The Netherlands

Fridus van der Weijden
Department of Periodontology
Academic Centre for Dentistry Amsterdam (ACTA)
Amsterdam
The Netherlands

Arie J. van Winkelhoff
Department of Oral Microbiology
Academic Centre for Dentistry Amsterdam (ACTA)
Amsterdam
The Netherlands

Hans-Peter Weber
Department of Restorative Dentistry and Biomaterials
  Science
Harvard School of Dental Medicine
Boston
MA
USA

Jan L. Wennström
Department of Periodontology
Institute of Odontology
The Sahlgrenska Academy at Göteborg University
Göteborg
Sweden

Jytte Westergaard
Department of Periodontology
School of Dentistry
University of Copenhagen
Copenhagen
Denmark

Ray C. Williams
Department of Periodontology
University of North Carolina School of Dentistry
Chapel Hill
NC
USA

Edwin G. Winkel
Department of Periodontology
Academic Centre for Oral Health
University Medical Centre Groningen
Groningen
The Netherlands

Björn U. Zachrisson
Department of Orthodontics
Dental Faculty
University of Oslo
Oslo
Norway

Giovanni Zucchelli
Department of Periodontology
Bologna University
Bologna
Italy

Preface

When the groundwork for the fifth edition of *Clinical Periodontology and Implant Dentistry* began in early 2007, it became clear that we had reached a fork in the road. It has always been my intention that each successive edition of this work should reflect the state of the art of clinical periodontology and, in doing such, should run the gamut of topics within this subject area. However, thorough coverage of an already large and now rapidly expanding specialty has resulted in a book of commensurate size and therefore for the fifth edition, the decision was taken to divide the book into two volumes: basic concepts and clinical concepts. The decision to make the split a purely physical one, and not an intellectual one, reflects the realization that over the past decade, implant dentistry has become a basic part of periodontology. The integrated structure of this latest edition of the textbook mirrors this merger.

In order for the student of dentistry, whatever his or her level, to learn how teeth and implants may function together as separate or connected units in the same dentition, a sound knowledge of the tissues that surround the natural tooth and the dental implant, as well as an understanding of the various lesions that may occur in the supporting tissues, is imperative. Hence, in both volumes of the textbook, chapters dealing with traditional periodontal issues, such as anatomy, pathology and treatment, are followed by similar topics related to tissues surrounding dental implants. In the first volume of the fifth edition, "basic concepts" as they relate to anatomy, microbiology and pathology, for example, are presented, while in the second volume ("clinical concepts"), various aspects of often evidence-based periodontal and restorative examination and treatment procedures are outlined.

It is my hope that the fifth edition of *Clinical Periodontology and Implant Dentistry* will challenge the reader intellectually, provide elucidation and clarity of information, and also impart an understanding of how the information presented in the text can, and should, be used in the practice of contemporary dentistry.

Jan Lindhe

Part 1: Anatomy

Chapter 1

The Anatomy of Periodontal Tissues

Jan Lindhe, Thorkild Karring, and Maurício Araújo

Introduction

This chapter includes a brief description of the characteristics of the normal periodontium. It is assumed that the reader has prior knowledge of oral embryology and histology. The periodontium (peri = around, odontos = tooth) comprises the following tissues (Fig. 1-1): (1) the *gingiva* (G), (2) the *periodontal ligament* (PL), (3) the *root cementum* (RC), and (4) the *alveolar bone* (AP). The alveolar bone consists of two components, the *alveolar bone proper* (ABP) and the alveolar process. The alveolar bone proper, also called "bundle bone", is continuous with the alveolar process and forms the thin bone plate that lines the alveolus of the tooth.

The main function of the periodontium is to attach the tooth to the bone tissue of the jaws and to maintain the integrity of the surface of the masticatory mucosa of the oral cavity. The periodontium, also called "the attachment apparatus" or "the supporting tissues of the teeth", constitutes a developmental, biologic, and functional unit which undergoes certain changes with age and is, in addition, subjected to morphologic changes related to functional alterations and alterations in the oral environment.

The development of the periodontal tissues occurs during the development and formation of teeth. This process starts early in the embryonic phase when cells from the neural crest (from the neural tube of the embryo) migrate into the first branchial arch. In this position the neural crest cells form a band of *ectomesenchyme* beneath the epithelium of the stomatodeum (the primitive oral cavity). After the uncommitted neural crest cells have reached their location in the jaw space, the epithelium of the stomatodeum releases factors which initiate epithelial–ectomesen-

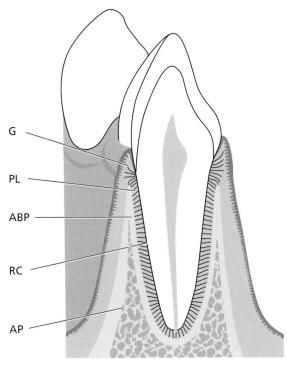

Fig. 1-1

chymal interactions. Once these interactions have occurred, the ectomesenchyme takes the dominant role in the further development. Following the formation of the *dental lamina*, a series of processes are initiated (bud stage, cap stage, bell stage with root development) which result in the formation of a tooth and its surrounding periodontal tissues, including the alveolar bone proper. During the cap stage, condensation of ectomesenchymal cells appears in relation to the dental epithelium (the dental organ (DO)),

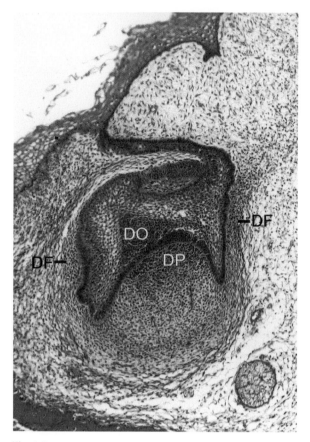

Fig. 1-2

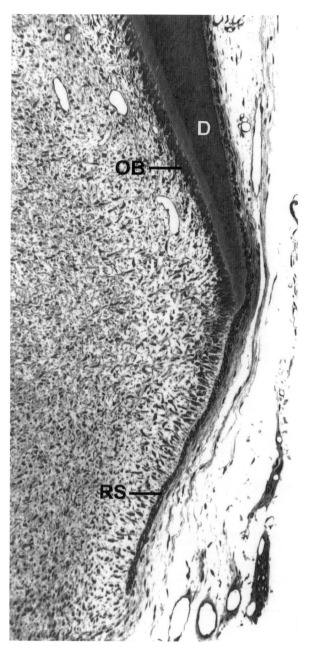

Fig. 1-3

forming the *dental papilla* (DP) that gives rise to the dentin and the pulp, and the *dental follicle* (DF) that gives rise to the periodontal supporting tissues (Fig. 1-2). The decisive role played by the ectomesenchyme in this process is further established by the fact that the tissue of the dental papilla apparently also determines the shape and form of the tooth.

If a tooth germ in the bell stage of development is dissected and transplanted to an ectopic site (e.g. the connective tissue or the anterior chamber of the eye), the tooth formation process continues. The crown and the root are formed, and the supporting structures, i.e. cementum, periodontal ligament, and a thin lamina of alveolar bone proper, also develop. Such experiments document that all information necessary for the formation of a tooth and its attachment apparatus obviously resides within the tissues of the dental organ and the surrounding ectomesenchyme. The dental organ is the formative organ of enamel, the dental papilla is the formative organ of the dentin–pulp complex, and the dental follicle is the formative organ of the attachment apparatus (the cementum, the periodontal ligament, and the alveolar bone proper).

The development of the root and the periodontal supporting tissues follows that of the crown. Epithelial cells of the external and internal dental epithelium (the dental organ) proliferate in an apical direction forming a double layer of cells named *Hertwig's epithelial root sheath* (RS). The odontoblasts (OB) forming the dentin of the root differentiate from ecto-

mesenchymal cells in the dental papilla under inductive influence of the inner epithelial cells (Fig. 1-3). The dentin (D) continues to form in an apical direction producing the framework of the root. During formation of the root, the periodontal supporting tissues, including acellular cementum, develop. Some of the events in the cementogenesis are still unclear, but the following concept is gradually emerging.

At the start of dentin formation, the inner cells of Hertwig's epithelial root sheath synthesize and secrete enamel-related proteins, probably belonging to the amelogenin family. At the end of this period, the epithelial root sheath becomes fenestrated and ectomesenchymal cells from the dental follicle penetrate through these fenestrations and contact the root surface. The ectomesenchymal cells in contact with the enamel-related proteins differentiate into cementoblasts and start to form cementoid. This cementoid

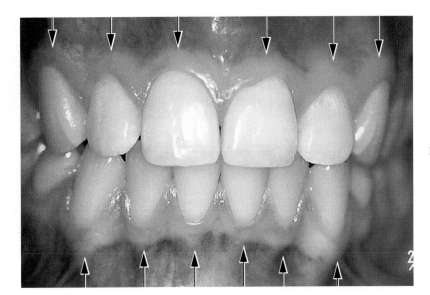

Fig. 1-4

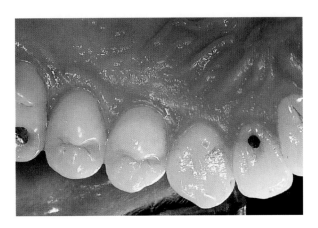

Fig. 1-5

represents the organic matrix of the cementum and consists of a ground substance and collagen fibers, which intermingle with collagen fibers in the not yet fully mineralized outer layer of the dentin. It is assumed that the cementum becomes firmly attached to the dentin through these fiber interactions. The formation of the cellular cementum, which covers the apical third of the dental roots, differs from that of acellular cementum in that some of the cementoblasts become embedded in the cementum.

The remaining parts of the periodontium are formed by ectomesenchymal cells from the dental follicle lateral to the cementum. Some of them differentiate into periodontal fibroblasts and form the fibers of the periodontal ligament while others become osteoblasts producing the alveolar bone proper in which the periodontal fibers are anchored. In other words, the primary alveolar wall is also an ectomesenchymal product. It is likely, but still not conclusively documented, that ectomesenchymal cells remain in the mature periodontium and take part in the turnover of this tissue.

Gingiva

Macroscopic anatomy

The oral mucosa (mucous membrane) is continuous with the skin of the lips and the mucosa of the soft palate and pharynx. The oral mucosa consists of (1) the *masticatory mucosa*, which includes the gingiva and the covering of the hard palate, (2) the *specialized mucosa*, which covers the dorsum of the tongue, and (3) the remaining part, called the *lining mucosa*.

Fig. 1-4 The gingiva is that part of the masticatory mucosa which covers the alveolar process and surrounds the cervical portion of the teeth. It consists of an epithelial layer and an underlying connective tissue layer called the *lamina propria*. The gingiva obtains its final shape and texture in conjunction with eruption of the teeth.

In the coronal direction the coral pink gingiva terminates in the *free gingival margin*, which has a scalloped outline. In the apical direction the gingiva is continuous with the loose, darker red *alveolar mucosa* (lining mucosa) from which the gingiva is separated by a usually easily recognizable borderline called

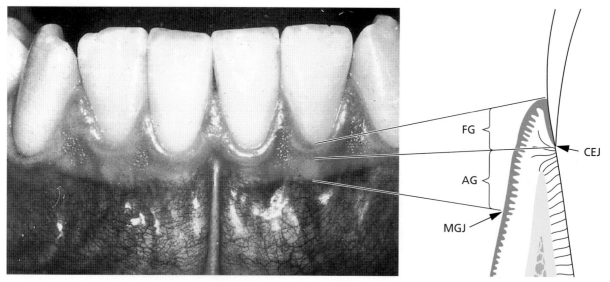

Fig. 1-6

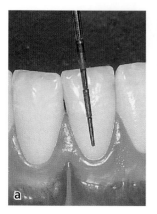
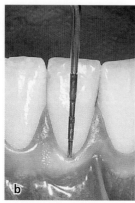

Fig. 1-7

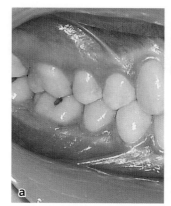
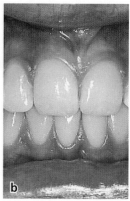

Fig. 1-8

either the mucogingival junction (arrows) or the mucogingival line.

Fig. 1-5 There is no mucogingival line present in the palate since the hard palate and the maxillary alveolar process are covered by the same type of masticatory mucosa.

Fig. 1-6 Two parts of the gingiva can be differentiated:

1. The free gingiva (FG)
2. The attached gingiva (AG).

The free gingiva is coral pink, has a dull surface and firm consistency. It comprises the gingival tissue at the vestibular and lingual/palatal aspects of the teeth, and the *interdental gingiva* or the *interdental papillae*. On the vestibular and lingual side of the teeth, the free gingiva extends from the gingival margin in apical direction to the *free gingival groove* which is positioned at a level corresponding to the level of the *cemento-enamel junction* (CEJ). The attached gingiva is demarcated by the mucogingival junction (MGJ) in the apical direction.

Fig. 1-7 The free gingival margin is often rounded in such a way that a small invagination or sulcus is formed between the tooth and the gingiva (Fig. 1-7a).

When a periodontal probe is inserted into this invagination and, further apically, towards the cemento-enamel junction, the gingival tissue is separated from the tooth, and a "*gingival pocket*" or "*gingival crevice*" is artificially opened. Thus, in normal or clinically healthy gingiva there is in fact no "gingival pocket" or "gingival crevice" present but the gingiva is in close contact with the enamel surface. In the illustration to the right (Fig. 1-7b), a periodontal probe has been inserted in the tooth/gingiva interface and a "gingival crevice" artificially opened approximately to the level of the cemento-enamel junction.

After completed tooth eruption, the free gingival margin is located on the enamel surface approximately 1.5–2 mm coronal to the cemento-enamel junction.

Fig. 1-8 The shape of the interdental gingiva (the interdental papilla) is determined by the contact relationships between the teeth, the width of the approximal tooth surfaces, and the course of the cemento-enamel junction. In anterior regions of the

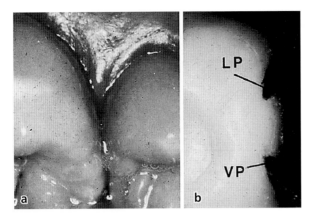

Fig. 1-9

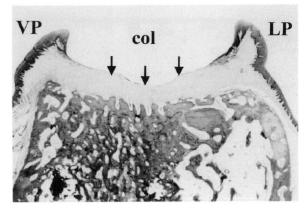

Fig. 1-9c

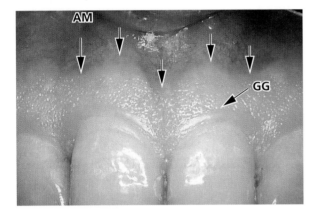

Fig. 1-10

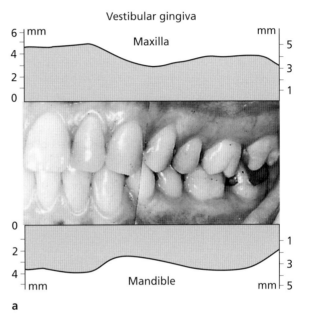

Vestibular gingiva

a

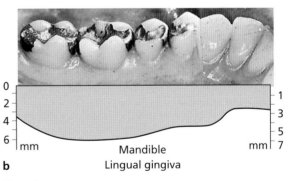

b

Fig. 1-11

dentition, the interdental papilla is of pyramidal form (Fig. 1-8b) while in the molar regions, the papillae are more flattened in the buccolingual direction (Fig. 1-8a). Due to the presence of interdental papillae, the free gingival margin follows a more or less accentuated, scalloped course through the dentition.

Fig. 1-9 In the premolar/molar regions of the dentition, the teeth have approximal contact surfaces (Fig. 1-9a) rather than contact points. Since the interdental papilla has a shape in conformity with the outline of the interdental contact surfaces, a concavity – *a col* – is established in the premolar and molar regions, as demonstrated in Fig. 1-9b, where the distal tooth has been removed. Thus, the interdental papillae in these areas often have one vestibular (VP) and one lingual/palatal portion (LP) separated by the col region. The col region, as demonstrated in the histological section (Fig. 1-9c), is covered by a thin non-keratinized epithelium (arrows). This epithelium has many features in common with the junctional epithelium (see Fig. 1-34).

Fig. 1-10 The attached gingiva is demarcated in the coronal direction, by the free gingival groove (GG) or, when such a groove is not present, by a horizontal plane placed at the level of the cemento-enamel junction. In clinical examinations it was observed that a free gingival groove is only present in about 30–40% of adults.

The free gingival groove is often most pronounced on the vestibular aspect of the teeth, occurring most frequently in the incisor and premolar regions of the mandible, and least frequently in the mandibular molar and maxillary premolar regions.

The attached gingiva extends in the apical direction to the mucogingival junction (arrows), where it becomes continuous with the alveolar (lining) mucosa (AM). It is of firm texture, coral pink in color, and often shows small depressions on the surface. The depressions, named "stippling", give the appearance

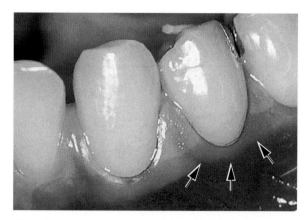

Fig. 1-12

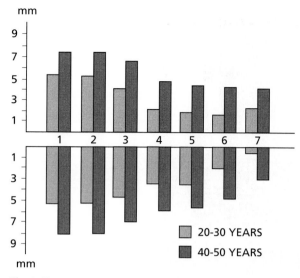

Fig. 1-13

of orange peel. It is firmly attached to the underlying alveolar bone and cementum by connective tissue fibers, and is, therefore, comparatively immobile in relation to the underlying tissue. The darker red alveolar mucosa (AM) located apical to the mucogingival junction, on the other hand, is loosely bound to the underlying bone. Therefore, in contrast to the attached gingiva, the alveolar mucosa is mobile in relation to the underlying tissue.

Fig. 1-11 describes how the width of the gingiva varies in different parts of the mouth. In the maxilla (Fig. 1-11a) the vestibular gingiva is generally widest in the area of the incisors and most narrow adjacent to the premolars. In the mandible (Fig. 1-11b) the gingiva on the lingual aspect is particularly narrow in the area of the incisors and wide in the molar region. The range of variation is 1–9 mm.

Fig. 1-12 illustrates an area in the mandibular premolar region where the gingiva is extremely narrow. The arrows indicate the location of the mucogingival junction. The mucosa has been stained with an iodine solution in order to distinguish more accurately between the gingiva and the alveolar mucosa.

Fig. 1-13 depicts the result of a study in which the width of the attached gingiva was assessed and related to the age of the patients examined. It was found that the gingiva in 40–50-year-olds was significantly wider than that in 20–30-year-olds. This observation indicates that the width of the gingiva tends to increase with age. Since the mucogingival junction remains stable throughout life in relation to the lower border of the mandible, the increasing width of the gingiva may suggest that the teeth, as a result of occlusal wear, erupt slowly throughout life.

Microscopic anatomy

Oral epithelium

Fig. 1-14a A schematic drawing of a histologic section (see Fig. 1-14b) describing the composition of the

gingiva and the contact area between the gingiva and the enamel (E).

Fig 1-14b The free gingiva comprises all epithelial and connective tissue structures (CT) located coronal to a horizontal line placed at the level of the cemento-enamel junction (CEJ). The epithelium covering the free gingiva may be differentiated as follows:

- *Oral epithelium* (OE), which faces the oral cavity
- *Oral sulcular epithelium* (OSE), which faces the tooth without being in contact with the tooth surface
- *Junctional epithelium* (JE), which provides the contact between the gingiva and the tooth.

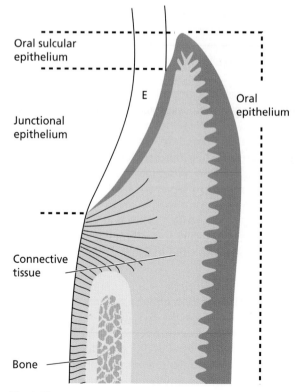

Fig. 1-14a

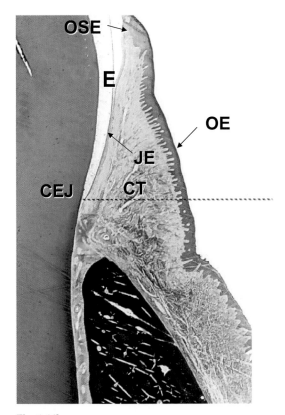

Fig. 1-14b

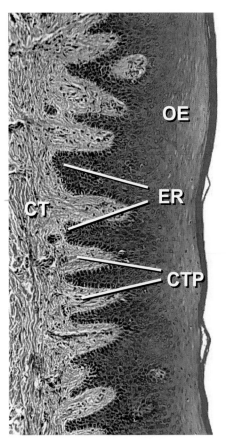

Fig. 1-14c

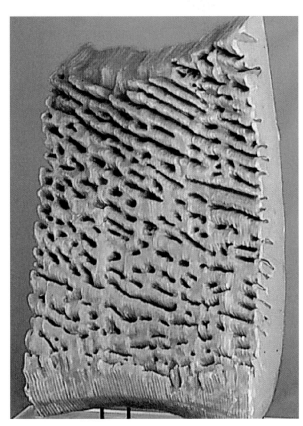

Fig. 1-15

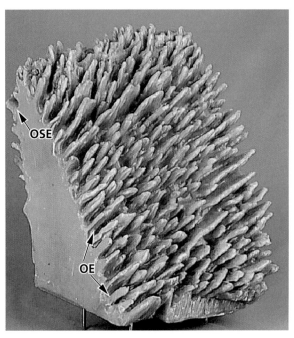

Fig. 1-16

Fig. 1-14c The boundary between the oral epithelium (OE) and underlying connective tissue (CT) has a wavy course. The connective tissue portions which project into the epithelium are called *connective tissue papillae* (CTP) and are separated from each other by

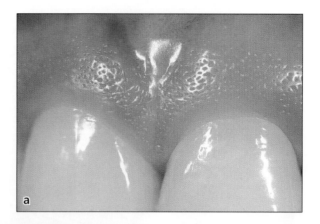

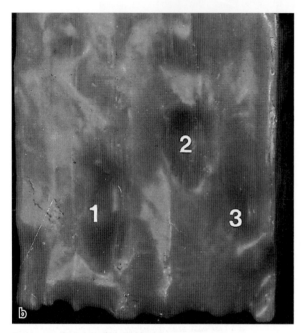

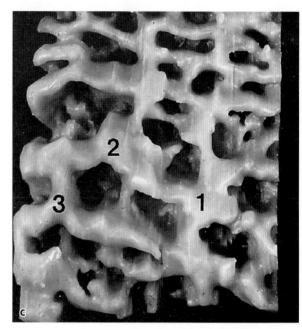

Fig. 1-17

epithelial ridges – so-called *rete pegs* (ER). In normal, non-inflamed gingiva, rete pegs and connective tissue papillae are lacking at the boundary between the junctional epithelium and its underlying connective tissue (Fig. 1-14b). Thus, a characteristic morphologic feature of the oral epithelium and the oral sulcular epithelium is the presence of rete pegs, while these structures are lacking in the junctional epithelium.

Fig. 1-15 presents a model, constructed on the basis of magnified serial histologic sections, showing the subsurface of the oral epithelium of the gingiva after the connective tissue has been removed. The subsurface of the oral epithelium (i.e. the surface of the epithelium facing the connective tissue) exhibits several depressions corresponding to the connective tissue papillae (in Fig. 1-16) which project into the epithelium. It can be seen that the epithelial projections,

which in histologic sections separate the connective tissue papillae, constitute a continuous system of epithelial ridges.

Fig. 1-16 presents a model of the connective tissue, corresponding to the model of the epithelium shown in Fig. 1-15. The epithelium has been removed, thereby making the vestibular aspect of the gingival connective tissue visible. Notice the connective tissue papillae which project into the space that was occupied by the oral epithelium (OE) in Fig. 1-15 and by the oral sulcular epithelium (OSE) on the back of the model.

Fig. 1-17a In 40% of adults the attached gingiva shows a stippling on the surface. The photograph shows a case where this stippling is conspicuous (see also Fig. 1-10).

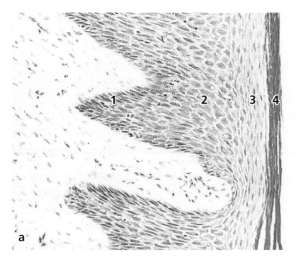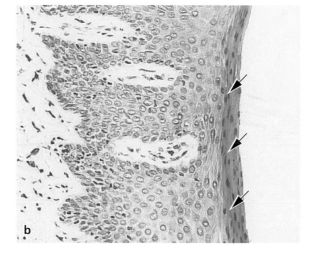

Fig. 1-18

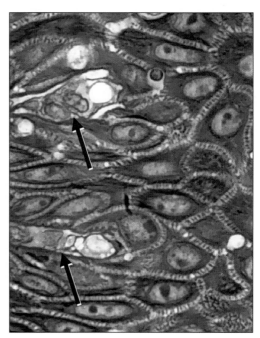

Fig. 1-19

Fig. 1-17b presents a magnified model of the outer surface of the oral epithelium of the attached gingiva. The surface exhibits the minute depressions (1–3) which, when present, give the gingiva its characteristic stippled appearance.

Fig. 1-17c shows a photograph of the subsurface (i.e. the surface of the epithelium facing the connective tissue) of the same model as that shown in Fig. 1-17b. The subsurface of the epithelium is characterized by the presence of epithelial ridges which merge at various locations (1–3). The depressions (1–3) seen on the outer surface of the epithelium (shown in Fig. 1-17b) correspond with the fusion sites (1–3) between epithelial ridges. Thus, the depressions on the surface of the gingiva occur in the areas of fusion between various epithelial ridges.

Fig. 1-18 (a) A portion of the oral epithelium covering the free gingiva is illustrated in this photomicrograph. The oral epithelium is a *keratinized, stratified, squamous epithelium* which, on the basis of the degree to which the keratin-producing cells are differentiated, can be divided into the following cell layers:

1. *Basal layer* (stratum basale or stratum germinativum)
2. *Prickle cell layer* (stratum spinosum)
3. *Granular cell layer* (stratum granulosum)
4. *Keratinized cell layer* (stratum corneum).

It should be observed that in this section, cell nuclei are lacking in the outer cell layers. Such an epithelium is denoted *orthokeratinized*. Often, however, the cells of the stratum corneum of the epithelium of human gingiva contain remnants of the nuclei (arrows) as seen in Fig. 1-18b. In such a case, the epithelium is denoted *parakeratinized*.

Fig. 1-19 In addition to the keratin-producing cells which comprise about 90% of the total cell popula-

tion, the oral epithelium contains the following types of cell:

• *Melanocytes*
• *Langerhans cells*
• *Merkel's cells*
• *Inflammatory cells.*

These cell types are often stellate and have cytoplasmic extensions of various size and appearance. They are also called "clear cells" since in histologic sections, the zone around their nuclei appears lighter than that in the surrounding keratin-producing cells.

The photomicrograph shows "clear cells" (arrows) located in or near the stratum basale of the oral epithelium. Except the Merkel's cells, these "clear cells", which do not produce keratin, lack desmosomal attachment to adjacent cells. The melanocytes are

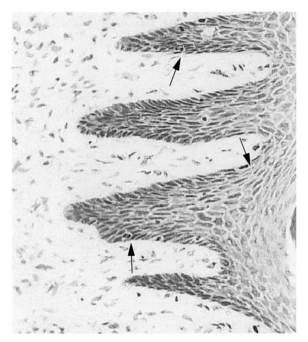

Fig. 1-20

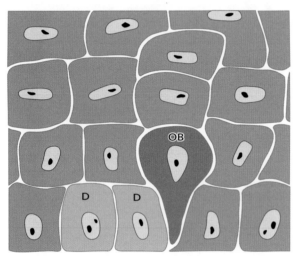

Fig. 1-21

pigment-synthesizing cells and are responsible for the melanin pigmentation occasionally seen on the gingiva. However, both lightly and darkly pigmented individuals present melanocytes in the epithelium.

The Langerhans cells are believed to play a role in the defense mechanism of the oral mucosa. It has been suggested that the Langerhans cells react with antigens which are in the process of penetrating the epithelium. An early immunologic response is thereby initiated, inhibiting or preventing further antigen penetration of the tissue. The Merkel's cells have been suggested to have a sensory function.

Fig. 1-20 The cells in the basal layer are either cylindric or cuboid, and are in contact with the *basement membrane* that separates the epithelium and the connective tissue. The basal cells possess the ability to divide, i.e. undergo mitotic cell division. The cells

marked with arrows in the photomicrograph are in the process of dividing. It is in the basal layer that the epithelium is renewed. Therefore, this layer is also termed *stratum germinativum*, and can be considered the *progenitor cell compartment* of the epithelium.

Fig. 1-21 When two daughter cells (D) have been formed by cell division, an adjacent "older" basal cell (OB) is pushed into the spinous cell layer and starts, as a *keratinocyte*, to traverse the epithelium. It takes approximately 1 month for a keratinocyte to reach the outer epithelial surface, where it becomes shed from the stratum corneum. Within a given time, the number of cells which divide in the basal layer equals the number of cells which become shed from the surface. Thus, under normal conditions there is complete equilibrium between cell renewal and cell loss so that the epithelium maintains a constant thickness. As the basal cell migrates through the epithelium, it becomes flattened with its long axis parallel to the epithelial surface.

Fig. 1-22 The basal cells are found immediately adjacent to the connective tissue and are separated from this tissue by the basement membrane, probably produced by the basal cells. Under the light microscope this membrane appears as a structureless zone approximately 1–2 μm wide (arrows) which reacts positively to a PAS stain (periodic acid-Schiff stain). This positive reaction demonstrates that the basement membrane contains carbohydrate (glycoproteins). The epithelial cells are surrounded by an extracellular substance which also contains protein–polysaccharide complexes. At the ultrastructural level, the basement membrane has a complex composition.

Fig. 1-23 is an electronmicrograph (magnification ×70 000) of an area including part of a basal cell, the basement membrane, and part of the adjacent connective tissue. The basal cell (BC) occupies the upper portion of the picture. Immediately beneath the basal cell an approximately 400 Å wide electron-lucent zone can be seen which is called *lamina lucida* (LL). Beneath the lamina lucida an electron-dense zone of approximately the same thickness can be observed. This zone is called *lamina densa* (LD). From the lamina densa so-called *anchoring fibers* (AF) project in a fan-shaped fashion into the connective tissue. The anchoring fibers are approximately 1 μm in length and terminate freely in the connective tissue. The basement membrane, which appeared as an entity under the light microscope, thus, in the electronmicrograph, appears to comprise one lamina lucida and one lamina densa with adjacent connective tissue fibers (anchoring fibers). The cell membrane of the epithelial cells facing the lamina lucida harbors a number of electron-dense, thicker zones appearing at various intervals along the cell membrane. These structures are called *hemidesmosomes* (HD). The cytoplasmic

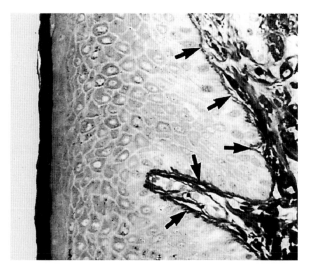

Fig. 1-22

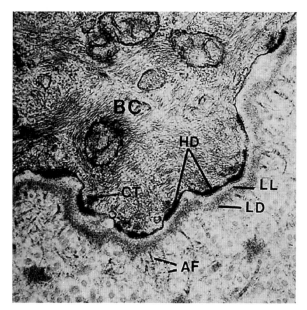

Fig. 1-23

tonofilaments (CT) in the cell converge towards the hemidesmosomes. The hemidesmosomes are involved in the attachment of the epithelium to the underlying basement membrane.

Fig. 1-24 illustrates an area of stratum spinosum in the gingival oral epithelium. Stratum spinosum consists of 10–20 layers of relatively large, polyhedral cells, equipped with short cytoplasmic processes resembling spines. The cytoplasmic processes (arrows) occur at regular intervals and give the cells a prickly appearance. Together with intercellular protein–carbohydrate complexes, cohesion between the cells is provided by numerous "desmosomes" (pairs of hemidesmosomes) which are located between the cytoplasmic processes of adjacent cells.

Fig. 1-25 shows an area of stratum spinosum in an electronmicrograph. The dark-stained structures between the individual epithelial cells represent the *desmosomes* (arrows). A desmosome may be considered to be two hemidesmosomes facing one another. The presence of a large number of desmosomes indicates that the cohesion between the epithelial cells is solid. The light cell (LC) in the center of the illustration harbors no hemidesmosomes and is, therefore, not a keratinocyte but rather a "clear cell" (see also Fig. 1-19).

Fig. 1-26 is a schematic drawing describing the composition of a desmosome. A desmosome can be

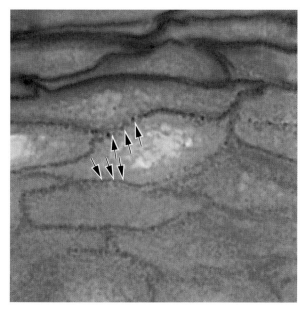

Fig. 1-24

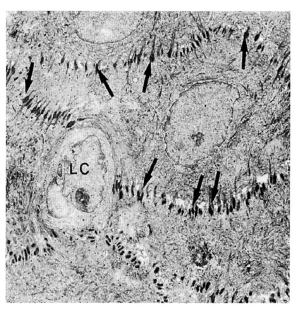

Fig. 1-25

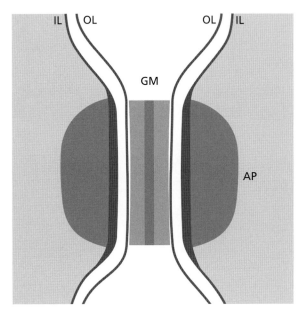

Fig. 1-26

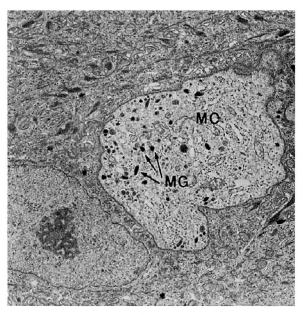

Fig. 1-27

considered to consist of two adjoining hemidesmosomes separated by a zone containing electron-dense granulated material (GM). Thus, a desmosome comprises the following structural components: (1) the *outer leaflets* (OL) of the cell membrane of two adjoining cells, (2) the thick *inner leaflets* (IL) of the cell membranes and (3) the *attachment plaques* (AP), which represent granular and fibrillar material in the cytoplasm.

Fig. 1-27 As mentioned previously, the oral epithelium also contains melanocytes, which are responsible for the production of the pigment melanin. Melanocytes are present in individuals with marked pigmentation of the oral mucosa as well as in individuals where no clinical signs of pigmentation can be seen. In this electronmicrograph a melanocyte (MC) is present in the lower portion of the stratum spinosum. In contrast to the keratinocytes, this cell contains melanin granules (MG) and has no tonofilaments or hemidesmosomes. Note the large amount of tonofilaments in the cytoplasm of the adjacent keratinocytes.

Fig. 1-28 When traversing the epithelium from the basal layer to the epithelial surface, the keratinocytes undergo continuous differentiation and specialization. The many changes which occur during this process are indicated in this diagram of a keratinized stratified squamous epithelium. From the basal layer (stratum basale) to the granular layer (stratum granulosum) both the number of tonofilaments (F) in the cytoplasm and the number of desmosomes (D) increase. In contrast, the number of organelles, such as mitochondria (M), lamellae of rough endoplasmic reticulum (E) and Golgi complexes (G), decrease in the keratinocytes on their way from the basal layer towards the surface. In the stratum granulosum, electron-dense *keratohyalin bodies* (K) and clusters of

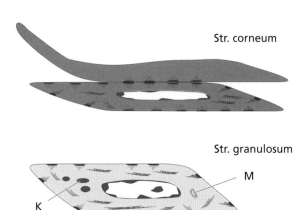

Str. corneum

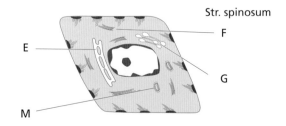

Str. granulosum

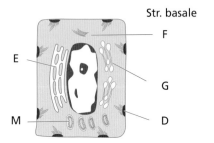

Str. spinosum

Str. basale

Fig. 1-28

glycogen-containing granules start to occur. Such granules are believed to be related to the synthesis of keratin.

Fig. 1-29 is a photomicrograph of the stratum granulosum and stratum corneum. Keratohyalin granules (arrows) are seen in the stratum granulosum. There is an abrupt transition of the cells from the stratum granulosum to the stratum corneum. This is indicative of a very sudden keratinization of the cytoplasm of the keratinocyte and its conversion into a horny squame. The cytoplasm of the cells in the stratum corneum (SC) is filled with keratin and the entire apparatus for protein synthesis and energy production, i.e. the nucleus, the mitochondria, the endoplasmic reticulum, and the Golgi complex, is lost. In a parakeratinized epithelium, however, the cells of the stratum corneum contain remnants of nuclei. Keratinization is considered a process of differentiation rather than degeneration. It is a process of protein synthesis which requires energy and is dependent on functional cells, i.e. cells containing a nucleus and a normal set of organelles.

Summary: The keratinocyte undergoes continuous differentiation on its way from the basal layer to the surface of the epithelium. Thus, once the keratinocyte has left the basement membrane it can no longer divide but maintains a capacity for production of protein (tonofilaments and keratohyalin granules). In the granular layer, the keratinocyte is deprived of its energy- and protein-producing apparatus (probably by enzymatic breakdown) and is abruptly converted into a keratin-filled cell which, via the stratum corneum, is shed from the epithelial surface.

Fig. 1-30 illustrates a portion of the epithelium of the alveolar (lining) mucosa. In contrast to the epithelium of the gingiva, the lining mucosa has no stratum corneum. Notice that cells containing nuclei can be identified in all layers, from the basal layer to the surface of the epithelium.

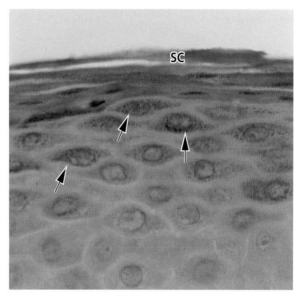

Fig. 1-29

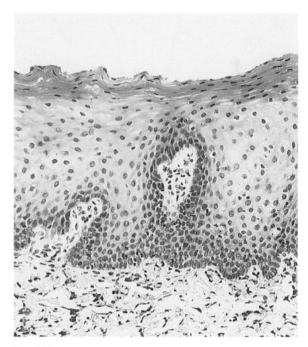

Fig. 1-30

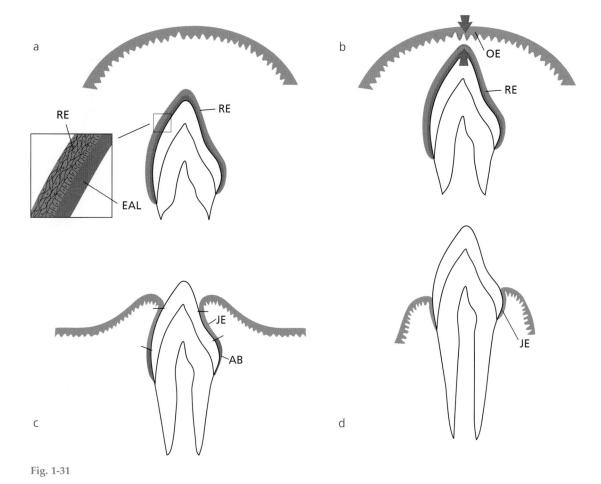

Fig. 1-31

Dento-gingival epithelium

The tissue components of the dento-gingival region achieve their final structural characteristics in conjunction with the eruption of the teeth. This is illustrated in Fig. 1-31a–d.

Fig. 1-31a When the enamel of the tooth is fully developed, the enamel-producing cells (ameloblasts) become reduced in height, produce a basal lamina and form, together with cells from the outer enamel epithelium, the so-called reduced dental epithelium (RE). The basal lamina (epithelial attachment lamina: EAL) lies in direct contact with the enamel. The contact between this lamina and the epithelial cells is maintained by hemidesmosomes. The reduced enamel epithelium surrounds the crown of the tooth from the moment the enamel is properly mineralized until the tooth starts to erupt.

Fig. 1-31b As the erupting tooth approaches the oral epithelium, the cells of the outer layer of the reduced dental epithelium (RE), as well as the cells of the basal layer of the oral epithelium (OE), show increased mitotic activity (arrows) and start to migrate into the underlying connective tissue. The migrating epithelium produces an epithelial mass between the oral epithelium and the reduced dental epithelium so that the tooth can erupt without bleeding. The former ameloblasts do not divide.

Fig. 1-31c When the tooth has penetrated into the oral cavity, large portions immediately apical to the incisal area of the enamel are covered by a junctional epithelium (JE) containing only a few layers of cells. The cervical region of the enamel, however, is still covered by ameloblasts (AB) and outer cells of the reduced dental epithelium.

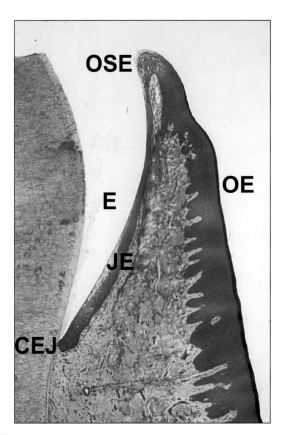

Fig. 1-32

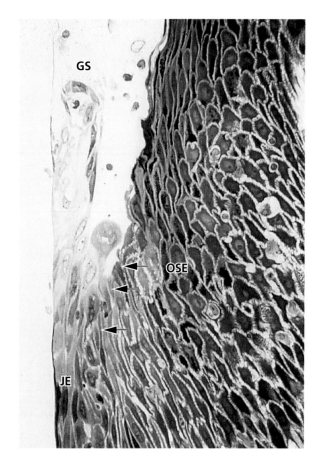

Fig. 1-33

Fig. 1-31d During the later phases of tooth eruption, all cells of the reduced enamel epithelium are replaced by a junctional epithelium. This epithelium is continuous with the oral epithelium and provides the attachment between the tooth and the gingiva. If the free gingiva is excised after the tooth has fully erupted, a new junctional epithelium, indistinguishable from that found following tooth eruption, will develop during healing. The fact that this new junctional epithelium has developed from the oral epithelium indicates that the cells of the oral epithelium possess the ability to differentiate into cells of junctional epithelium.

Fig. 1-32 is a histologic section cut through the border area between the tooth and the gingiva, i.e. the *dento-gingival region*. The enamel (E) is to the left. To the right are the *junctional epithelium* (JE), the *oral sulcular epithelium* (OSE), and the *oral epithelium* (OE). The oral sulcular epithelium covers the shallow groove, the gingival sulcus, located between the enamel and the top of the free gingiva. The junctional epithelium

differs morphologically from the oral sulcular epithelium and oral epithelium, while the two latter are structurally very similar. Although individual variation may occur, the junctional epithelium is usually widest in its coronal portion (about 15–20 cell layers), but becomes thinner (3–4 cells) towards the cemento-enamel junction (CEJ). The borderline between the junctional epithelium and the underlying connective tissue does not present epithelial rete pegs except when inflamed.

Fig. 1-33 The junctional epithelium has a free surface at the bottom of the *gingival sulcus* (GS). Like the oral sulcular epithelium and the oral epithelium, the junctional epithelium is continuously renewed through cell division in the basal layer. The cells migrate to the base of the gingival sulcus from where they are shed. The border between the junctional epithelium (JE) and the oral sulcular epithelium (OSE) is indicated by arrows. The cells of the oral sulcular epithelium are cuboidal and the surface of this epithelium is keratinized.

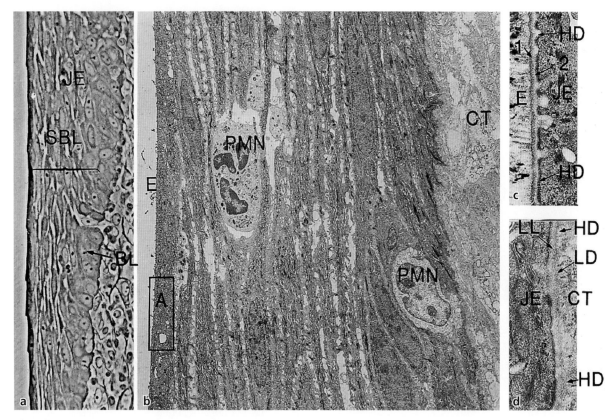

Fig. 1-34

Fig. 1-34 illustrates different characteristics of the junctional epithelium. As can be seen in Fig. 1-34a, the cells of the junctional epithelium (JE) are arranged into one basal layer (BL) and several suprabasal layers (SBL). Fig. 1-34b demonstrates that the basal cells as well as the suprabasal cells are flattened with their long axis parallel to the tooth surface. (CT = connective tissue, E = enamel space.)

There are distinct differences between the oral sulcular epithelium, the oral epithelium and the junctional epithelium:

1. The size of the cells in the junctional epithelium is, relative to the tissue volume, larger than in the oral epithelium.
2. The intercellular space in the junctional epithelium is, relative to the tissue volume, comparatively wider than in the oral epithelium.
3. The number of desmosomes is smaller in the junctional epithelium than in the oral epithelium.

Note the comparatively wide intercellular spaces between the oblong cells of the junctional epithelium, and the presence of two neutrophilic granulocytes (PMN) which are traversing the epithelium.

The framed area (A) is shown in a higher magnification in Fig. 1-34c, from which it can be seen that the basal cells of the junctional epithelium are not in direct contact with the enamel (E). Between the enamel and the epithelium (JE) one electron-dense zone (1) and one electron-lucent zone (2) can be seen. The electron-lucent zone is in contact with the cells

of the junctional epithelium (JE). These two zones have a structure very similar to that of the lamina densa (LD) and lamina lucida (LL) in the basement membrane area (i.e. the epithelium (JE)–connective tissue (CT) interface) described in Fig. 1-23. Furthermore, as seen in Fig. 1-34d, the cell membrane of the junctional epithelial cells harbors hemidesmosomes (HD) towards the enamel as it does towards the connective tissue. Thus, the interface between the enamel and the junctional epithelium is similar to the interface between the epithelium and the connective tissue.

Fig. 1-35 is a schematic drawing of the most apically positioned cell in the junctional epithelium. The enamel (E) is depicted to the left in the drawing. It can be seen that the electron-dense zone (1) between the junctional epithelium and the enamel can be considered a continuation of the lamina densa (LD) in the basement membrane of the connective tissue side. Similarly, the electron-lucent zone (2) can be considered a continuation of the lamina lucida (LL). It should be noted, however, that at variance with the epithelium–connective tissue interface, there are no anchoring fibers (AF) attached to the lamina densa-like structure (1) adjacent to the enamel. On the other hand, like the basal cells adjacent to the basement membrane (at the connective tissue interface), the cells of the junctional epithelium facing the lamina lucida-like structure (2) harbor hemidesmosomes. Thus, the interface between the junctional epithelium and the enamel is structurally very similar to the

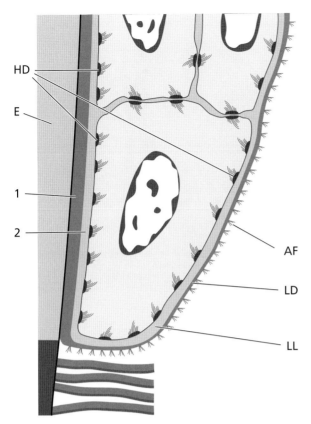

Fig. 1-35

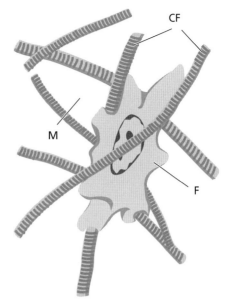

Fig. 1-36

epithelium–connective tissue interface, which means that the junctional epithelium is not only in contact with the enamel but is actually physically attached to the tooth via hemidesmosomes.

Lamina propria

The predominant tissue component of the gingiva is the connective tissue (lamina propria). The major components of the connective tissue are *collagen fibers* (around 60% of connective tissue volume), *fibroblasts* (around 5%), *vessels and nerves* (around 35%) which are embedded in an amorphous ground substance (matrix).

Fig. 1-36 The drawing illustrates a fibroblast (F) residing in a network of connective tissue fibers (CF). The intervening space is filled with matrix (M), which constitutes the "environment" for the cell.

Cells
The different types of cell present in the connective tissue are: (1) *fibroblasts*, (2) *mast cells*, (3) *macrophages*, and (4) *inflammatory cells*.

Fig. 1-37 The *fibroblast* is the predominant connective tissue cell (65% of the total cell population). The fibroblast is engaged in the production of various types of fibers found in the connective tissue, but is also instrumental in the synthesis of the connective tissue matrix. The fibroblast is a spindle-shaped or stellate cell with an oval-shaped nucleus containing one or

more nucleoli. A part of a fibroblast is shown in electron microscopic magnification. The cytoplasm contains a well developed granular endoplasmic reticulum (E) with ribosomes. The Golgi complex (G) is usually of considerable size and the mitochondria (M) are large and numerous. Furthermore, the cytoplasm contains many fine tonofilaments (F). Adjacent to the cell membrane, all along the periphery of the cell, a large number of vesicles (V) can be found.

Fig. 1-38 The *mast cell* is responsible for the production of certain components of the matrix. This cell also produces vasoactive substances, which can affect the function of the microvascular system and control the flow of blood through the tissue. A mast cell is presented in electron microscopic magnification. The cytoplasm is characterized by the presence of a large number of vesicles (V) of varying size. These vesicles

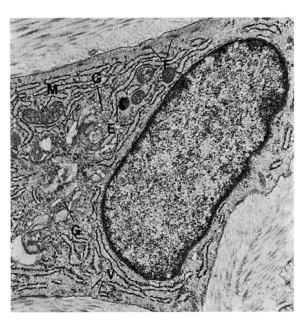

Fig. 1-37

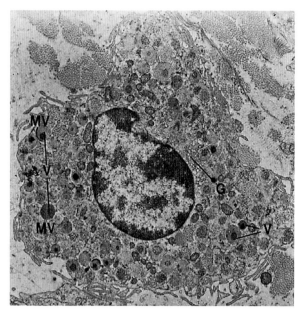

Fig. 1-38

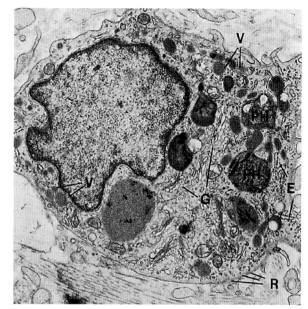

Fig. 1-39

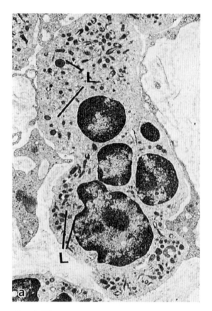
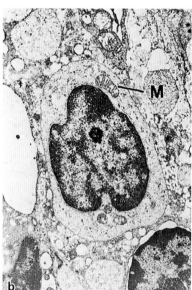
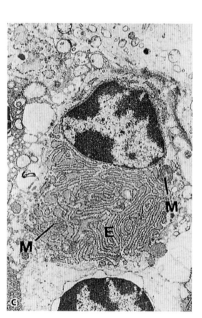

Fig. 1-40

contain biologically active substances such as proteolytic enzymes, histamine and heparin. The Golgi complex (G) is well developed, while granular endoplasmic reticulum structures are scarce. A large number of small cytoplasmic projections, i.e. microvilli (MV), can be seen along the periphery of the cell.

Fig. 1-39 The *macrophage* has a number of different phagocytic and synthetic functions in the tissue. A macrophage is shown in electron microscopic magnification. The nucleus is characterized by numerous invaginations of varying size. A zone of electron-

dense chromatin condensations can be seen along the periphery of the nucleus. The Golgi complex (G) is well developed and numerous vesicles (V) of varying size are present in the cytoplasm. Granular endoplasmic reticulum (E) is scarce, but a certain number of free ribosomes (R) are evenly distributed in the cytoplasm. Remnants of phagocytosed material are often found in lysosomal vesicles: phagosomes (PH). In the periphery of the cell, a large number of microvilli of varying size can be seen. Macrophages are particularly numerous in inflamed tissue. They are derived from circulating blood monocytes which migrate into the tissue.

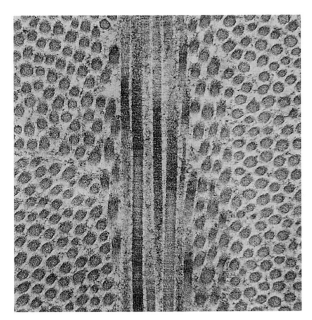

Fig. 1-41

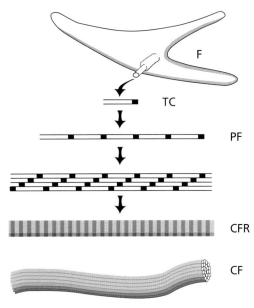

Fig. 1-42

Fig. 1-40 Besides fibroblasts, mast cells and macrophages, the connective tissue also harbors *inflammatory cells* of various types, for example neutrophilic granulocytes, lymphocytes, and plasma cells.

The *neutrophilic granulocytes*, also called *polymorphonuclear leukocytes*, have a characteristic appearance (Fig. 1-40a). The nucleus is lobulate and numerous lysosomes (L), containing lysosomal enzymes, are found in the cytoplasm.

The *lymphocytes* (Fig. 1-40b) are characterized by an oval to spherical nucleus containing localized areas of electron-dense chromatin. The narrow border of cytoplasm surrounding the nucleus contains numerous free ribosomes, a few mitochondria (M), and, in localized areas, endoplasmic reticulum with fixed ribosomes. Lysosomes are also present in the cytoplasm.

The *plasma cells* (Fig. 1-40c) contain an eccentrically located spherical nucleus with radially deployed electron-dense chromatin. Endoplasmic reticulum (E) with numerous ribosomes is found randomly distributed in the cytoplasm. In addition, the cytoplasm contains numerous mitochondria (M) and a well developed Golgi complex.

Fibers

The connective tissue fibers are produced by the fibroblasts and can be divided into: (1) *collagen fibers*, (2) *reticulin fibers*, (3) *oxytalan fibers*, and (4) *elastic fibers*.

Fig. 1-41 The *collagen fibers* predominate in the gingival connective tissue and constitute the most essential components of the periodontium. The electronmicrograph shows cross sections and longitudinal sections of collagen fibers. The collagen fibers have a characteristic cross-banding with a periodicity of 700 Å between the individual dark bands.

Fig. 1-42 illustrates some important features of the synthesis and the composition of collagen fibers produced by fibroblasts (F). The smallest unit, the collagen molecule, is often referred to as *tropocollagen*. A tropocollagen molecule (TC) which is seen in the upper portion of the drawing is approximately 3000 Å long and has a diameter of 15 Å. It consists of three polypeptide chains intertwined to form a helix. Each chain contains about 1000 amino acids. One third of these are glycine and about 20% proline and hydroxyproline, the latter being found practically only in collagen. Tropocollagen synthesis takes place inside the fibroblast from which the tropocollagen molecule is secreted into the extracellular space. Thus, the polymerization of tropocollagen molecules to collagen fibers takes place in the extracellular compartment. First, tropocollagen molecules are aggregated longitudinally to *protofibrils* (PF), which are subsequently laterally aggregated parallel to *collagen fibrils* (CFR), with an overlapping of the tropocollagen molecules by about 25% of their length. Due to the fact that special refraction conditions develop after staining at the sites where the tropocollagen molecules adjoin, a cross-banding with a periodicity of approximately 700 Å occurs under light microscopy. The *collagen fibers* (CF) are bundles of collagen fibrils, aligned in such a way that the fibers also exhibit a cross-banding with a periodicity of 700 Å. In the tissue, the fibers are usually arranged in bundles. As the collagen fibers mature, covalent crosslinks are formed between the tropocollagen molecules, resulting in an age-related reduction in collagen solubility.

Cementoblasts and *osteoblasts* are cells which also possess the ability to produce collagen.

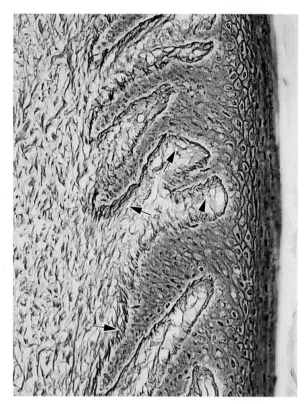

Fig. 1-43

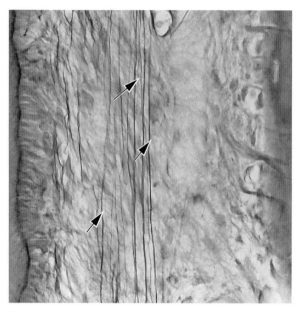

Fig. 1-44

Fig. 1-43 *Reticulin fibers*, as seen in this photomicrograph, exhibit argyrophilic staining properties and are numerous in the tissue adjacent to the basement membrane (arrows). However, reticulin fibers also occur in large numbers in the loose connective tissue surrounding the blood vessels. Thus, reticulin fibers are present at the epithelium–connective tissue and the endothelium–connective tissue interfaces.

Fig 1-44 *Oxytalan fibers* are scarce in the gingiva but numerous in the periodontal ligament. They are composed of long thin fibrils with a diameter of approximately 150 Å. These connective tissue fibers can be demonstrated light microscopically only after previous oxidation with peracetic acid. The photomicrograph illustrates oxytalan fibers (arrows) in the periodontal ligament, where they have a course mainly parallel to the long axis of the tooth. The function of these fibers is as yet unknown. The cementum is seen to the left and the alveolar bone to the right.

Fig. 1-45 *Elastic fibers* in the connective tissue of the gingiva and periodontal ligament are only present in association with blood vessels. However, as seen in this photomicrograph, the lamina propria and submucosa of the alveolar (lining) mucosa contain numerous elastic fibers (arrows). The gingiva (G) seen coronal to the mucogingival junction (MGJ) contains no elastic fibers except in association with the blood vessels.

Fig. 1-46 Although many of the collagen fibers in the gingiva and the periodontal ligament are irregularly or randomly distributed, most tend to be arranged in groups of bundles with a distinct orientation. According to their insertion and course in the tissue, the oriented bundles in the gingiva can be divided into the following groups:

1. *Circular fibers* (CF) are fiber bundles which run their course in the free gingiva and encircle the tooth in a cuff- or ring-like fashion.
2. *Dento-gingival fibers* (DGF) are embedded in the cementum of the supra-alveolar portion of the root and project from the cementum in a fan-like configuration out into the free gingival tissue of the facial, lingual and interproximal surfaces.
3. *Dento-periosteal fibers* (DPF) are embedded in the same portion of the cementum as the dento-gingival fibers, but run their course apically over the vestibular and lingual bone crest and terminate in the tissue of the attached gingiva. In the border area between the free and attached gingiva, the epithelium often lacks support by underlying oriented collagen fiber bundles. In this area the free gingival groove (GG) is often present.
4. *Trans-septal fibers* (TF), seen on the drawing to the right, extend between the supra-alveolar cementum of approximating teeth. The trans-septal fibers run straight across the interdental septum and are embedded in the cementum of adjacent teeth.

Fig. 1-47 illustrates in a histologic section the orientation of the trans-septal fiber bundles (arrows) in the supra-alveolar portion of the interdental area. It should be observed that, besides connecting the cementum (C) of adjacent teeth, the trans-septal fibers also connect the supra-alveolar cementum (C) with the crest of the alveolar bone (AB). The four groups

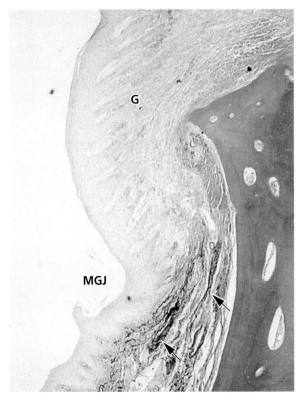

Fig. 1-45

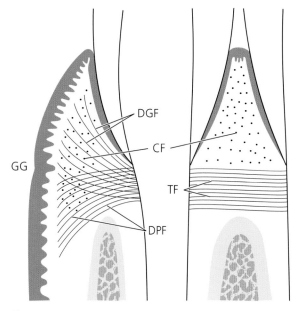

Fig. 1-46

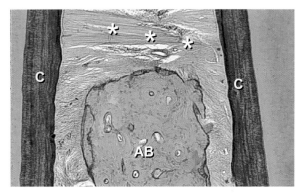

Fig. 1-47

of collagen fiber bundles presented in Fig. 1-46 reinforce the gingiva and provide the resilience and tone which is necessary for maintaining its architectural form and the integrity of the dento-gingival attachment.

Matrix

The *matrix* of the connective tissue is produced mainly by the fibroblasts, although some constituents are produced by mast cells, and other components are derived from the blood. The matrix is the medium in which the connective tissue cells are embedded and it is essential for the maintenance of the normal function of the connective tissue. Thus, the transportation of water, electrolytes, nutrients, metabolites, etc., to and from the individual connective tissue cells occurs within the matrix. The main constituents of the connective tissue matrix are protein–carbohydrate macromolecules. These complexes are normally divided into *proteoglycans* and *glycoproteins*. The proteoglycans contain *glycosaminoglycans* as the carbohydrate units (hyaluronan sulfate, heparan sulfate, etc.), which are attached to one or more protein chains via

covalent bonds. The carbohydrate component is always predominant in the proteoglycans. The glycosaminoglycan called hyaluronan or "hyaluronic acid" is probably not bound to protein. The glycoproteins (fibronectin, osteonectin, etc.) also contain polysaccharides, but these macromolecules are different from glycosaminoglycans. The protein component is predominating in glycoproteins. In the macromolecules, mono- or oligosaccharides are connected to one or more protein chains via covalent bonds.

Fig. 1-48 Normal function of the connective tissue depends on the presence of proteoglycans and gly-

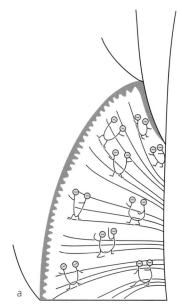 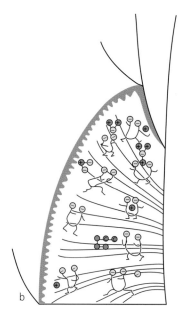 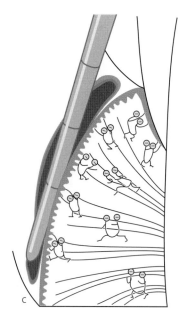

Fig. 1-48

cosaminoglycans. The carbohydrate moiety of the proteoglycans, the glycosaminoglycans (), are large, flexible, chain formed, negatively charged molecules, each of which occupies a rather large space (Fig. 1-48a). In such a space, smaller molecules, e.g. water and electrolytes, can be incorporated while larger molecules are prevented from entering (Fig. 1-48b). The proteoglycans thereby regulate diffusion and fluid flow through the matrix and are important determinants for the fluid content of the tissue and the maintenance of the osmotic pressure. In other words, the proteoglycans act as a molecule filter and, in addition, play an important role in the regulation of cell migration (movements) in the tissue. Due to their structure and hydration, the macromolecules exert resistance towards deformation, thereby serving as regulators of the consistency of the connective tissue (Fig. 1-48c). If the gingiva is suppressed, the macromolecules become deformed. When the pressure is eliminated, the macromolecules regain their original form. Thus, the macromolecules are important for the resilience of the gingiva.

Epithelial mesenchymal interaction

There are many examples of the fact that during the embryonic development of various organs, a mutual inductive influence occurs between the epithelium and the connective tissue. The development of the teeth is a characteristic example of such phenomena. The connective tissue is, on the one hand, a determining factor for normal development of the tooth bud while, on the other, the enamel epithelia exert a definite influence on the development of the mesenchymal components of the teeth.

It has been suggested that tissue differentiation in the adult organism can be influenced by environmental factors. The skin and mucous membranes, for instance, often display increased keratinization and hyperplasia of the epithelium in areas which are exposed to mechanical stimulation. Thus, the tissues seem to adapt to environmental stimuli. The presence of keratinized epithelium on the masticatory mucosa has been considered to represent an adaptation to mechanical irritation released by mastication. However, research has demonstrated that the char-

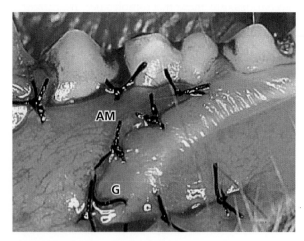

Fig. 1-49

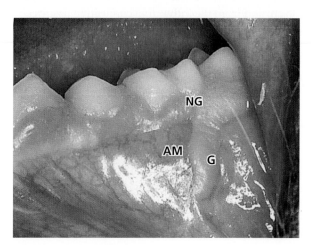

Fig. 1-50

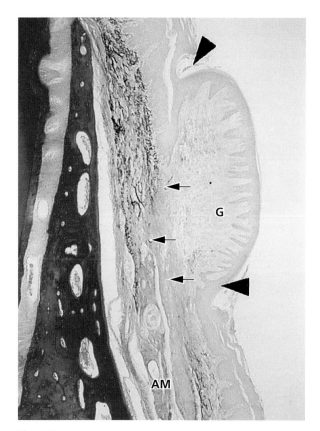

Fig. 1-51

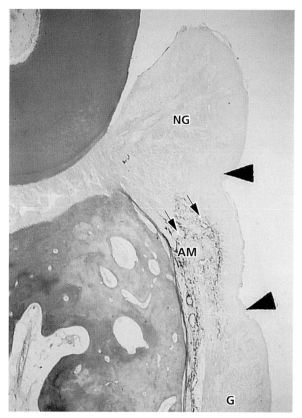

Fig. 1-52

acteristic features of the epithelium in such areas are genetically determined. Some pertinent observations are reported in the following:

Fig. 1-49 shows an area in a monkey where the gingiva (G) and the alveolar mucosa (AM) have been transposed by a surgical procedure. The alveolar mucosa is placed in close contact with the teeth while the gingiva is positioned in the area of the alveolar mucosa.

Fig. 1-50 shows the same area, as seen in Fig. 1-49, 4 months later. Despite the fact that the transplanted gingiva (G) is mobile in relation to the underlying bone, like the alveolar mucosa, it has retained its characteristic, morphologic features of a masticatory mucosa. However, a narrow zone of new keratinized gingiva (NG) has regenerated between the transplanted alveolar mucosa (AM) and the teeth.

Fig. 1-51 presents a histologic section cut through the transplanted gingiva seen in Fig. 1-50. Since elastic fibers are lacking in the gingival connective tissue (G), but are numerous (small arrows) in the connective tissue of the alveolar mucosa (AM), the transplanted gingival tissue can readily be identified. The epithelium covering the transplanted gingival tissue exhibits a distinct keratin layer (between large arrows) on the surface, and also the configuration of the epithelium–connective tissue interface (i.e. rete pegs and connective tissue papillae) is similar to that of normal non-transplanted gingiva. Thus, the heterotopically located gingival tissue has maintained

its original specificity. This observation demonstrates that the characteristics of the gingiva are genetically determined rather than being the result of functional adaptation to environmental stimuli.

Fig. 1-52 shows a histologic section cut through the coronal portion of the area of transplantation (shown in Fig. 1-50). The transplanted gingival tissue (G) shown in Fig. 1-51 can be seen in the lower portion of the photomicrograph. The alveolar mucosa transplant (AM) is seen between the large arrows in the middle of the illustration. After surgery, the alveolar mucosa transplant was positioned in close contact with the teeth as seen in Fig. 1-49. After healing, a narrow zone of keratinized gingiva (NG) developed coronal to the alveolar mucosa transplant (see Fig. 1-50). This new zone of gingiva (NG), which can be seen in the upper portion of the histologic section, is covered by keratinized epithelium and the connective tissue contains no purple-stained elastic fibers. In addition, it is important to notice that the junction between keratinized and non-keratinized epithelium (large arrows) corresponds exactly to the junction between "elastic" and "inelastic" connective tissue (small arrows). The connective tissue of the new gingiva has regenerated from the connective tissue of the supra-alveolar and periodontal ligament compartments and has separated the alveolar mucosal transplant (AM) from the tooth (see Fig. 1-53). However, it is most likely that the epithelium which covers the new gingiva has migrated from the adjacent epithelium of the alveolar mucosa.

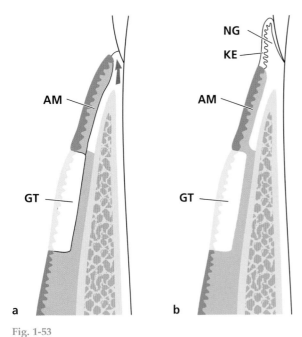

Fig. 1-53

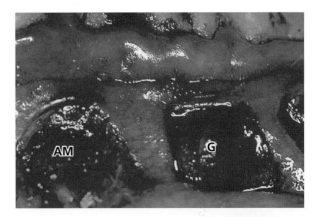

Fig. 1-54

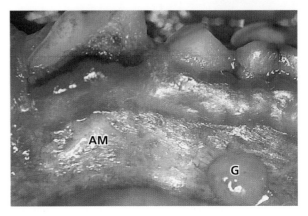

Fig. 1-55

Fig. 1-53 presents a schematic drawing of the development of the new, narrow zone of keratinized gingiva (NG) seen in Figs. 1-50 and 1-52.

Fig. 1-53a Granulation tissue has proliferated coronally along the root surface (arrow) and has separated the alveolar mucosa transplant (AM) from its original contact with the tooth surface.

Fig. 1-53b Epithelial cells have migrated from the alveolar mucosal transplant (AM) on to the newly formed gingival connective tissue (NG). Thus, the newly formed gingiva has become covered with a keratinized epithelium (KE) which originated from the non-keratinized epithelium of the alveolar mucosa (AM). This implies that the newly formed gingival connective tissue (NG) possesses the ability to induce changes in the differentiation of the epithelium originating from the alveolar mucosa. This epithelium, which is normally non-keratinized, apparently differentiates to keratinized epithelium because of stimuli arising from the newly formed gingival connective tissue (NG). (GT: gingival transplant.)

Fig. 1-54 illustrates a portion of gingival connective tissue (G) and alveolar mucosal connective tissue (AM) which, after transplantation, has healed into wound areas in the alveolar mucosa. Epithelialization of these transplants can only occur through migration of epithelial cells from the surrounding alveolar mucosa.

Fig. 1-55 shows the transplanted gingival connective tissue (G) after re-epithelialization. This tissue portion has attained an appearance similar to that of the normal gingiva, indicating that this connective tissue is now covered by keratinized epithelium. The trans-

planted connective tissue from the alveolar mucosa (AM) is covered by non-keratinized epithelium, and has the same appearance as the surrounding alveolar mucosa.

Fig. 1-56 presents two histologic sections through the area of the transplanted gingival connective tissue. The section shown in Fig. 1-56a is stained for elastic fibers (arrows). The tissue in the middle without elastic fibers is the transplanted gingival connective tissue (G). Fig. 1-56b shows an adjacent section stained with hematoxylin and eosin. By comparing Figs. 1-56a and 1-56b it can be seen that:

1. The transplanted gingival connective tissue is covered by keratinized epithelium (between arrowheads)
2. The epithelium–connective tissue interface has the same wavy course (i.e. rete pegs and connective tissue papillae) as seen in normal gingiva.

The photomicrographs seen in Figs. 1-56c and 1-56d illustrate, at a higher magnification, the border area between the alveolar mucosa (AM) and the transplanted gingival connective tissue (G). Note the distinct relationship between keratinized epithelium (arrow) and "inelastic" connective tissue (arrowheads), and between non-keratinized epithelium and

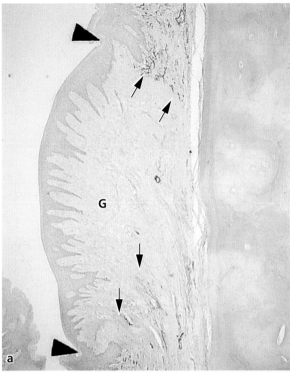
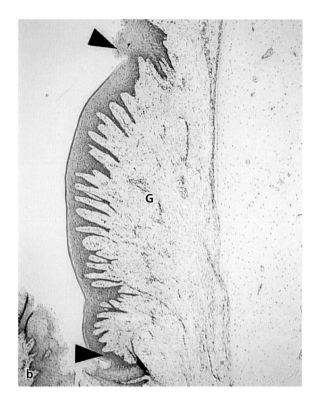
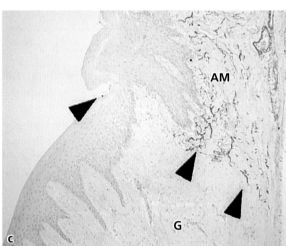
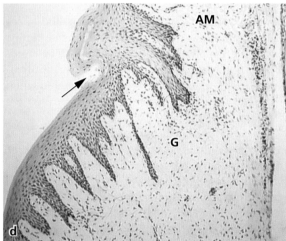

Fig. 1-56

"elastic" connective tissue. The establishment of such a close relationship during healing implies that the transplanted gingival connective tissue possesses the ability to alter the differentiation of epithelial cells as previously suggested (Fig. 1-53). From being non-keratinizing cells, the cells of the epithelium of the alveolar mucosa have evidently become keratinizing cells. This means that the specificity of the gingival epithelium is determined by genetic factors inherent in the connective tissue.

Periodontal ligament

The periodontal ligament is the soft, richly vascular and cellular connective tissue which surrounds the roots of the teeth and joins the root cementum with the socket wall. In the coronal direction, the periodontal ligament is continuous with the lamina propria of the gingiva and is demarcated from the gingiva by the collagen fiber bundles which connect the alveolar bone crest with the root (the alveolar crest fibers).

Fig. 1-57 is a radiograph of a mandibular premolar–molar region. In radiographs two types of alveolar bone can be distinguished:

1. The part of the alveolar bone which covers the alveolus, called "lamina dura" (arrows)
2. The portion of the alveolar process which, in the radiograph, has the appearance of a meshwork. This is called the "spongy bone".

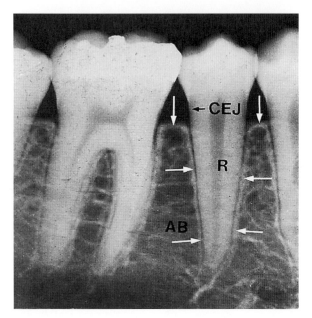

Fig. 1-57

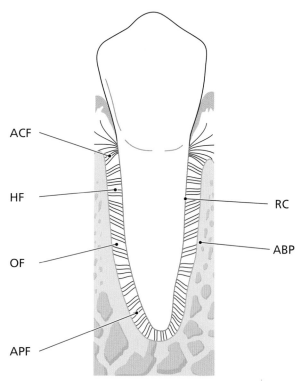

Fig. 1-58

The periodontal ligament is situated in the space between the roots (R) of the teeth and the lamina dura or the alveolar bone proper (arrows). The alveolar bone (AB) surrounds the tooth to a level approximately 1 mm apical to the cemento-enamel junction (CEJ). The coronal border of the bone is called the *alveolar crest* (arrows).

The periodontal ligament space has the shape of an hourglass and is narrowest at the mid-root level. The width of the periodontal ligament is approximately 0.25 mm (range 0.2–0.4 mm). The presence of a periodontal ligament permits forces, elicited during masticatory function and other tooth contacts, to be distributed to and resorbed by the alveolar process via the alveolar bone proper. The periodontal ligament is also essential for the mobility of the teeth. Tooth mobility is to a large extent determined by the width, height, and quality of the periodontal ligament (see Chapters 14 and 51).

Fig. 1-58 illustrates in a schematic drawing how the periodontal ligament is situated between the alveolar bone proper (ABP) and the root cementum (RC). The tooth is joined to the bone by bundles of collagen fibers which can be divided into the following main groups according to their arrangement:

1. *Alveolar crest fibers* (ACF)
2. *Horizontal fibers* (HF)
3. *Oblique fibers* (OF)
4. *Apical fibers* (APF).

Fig. 1-59 The periodontal ligament and the root cementum develop from the loose connective tissue

(the follicle) which surrounds the tooth bud. The schematic drawing depicts the various stages in the organization of the periodontal ligament which forms concomitantly with the development of the root and the eruption of the tooth.

Fig. 1-59a The tooth bud is formed in a crypt of the bone. The collagen fibers produced by the fibroblasts in the loose connective tissue around the tooth bud are embedded, during the process of their maturation, into the newly formed cementum immediately apical to the cemento-enamel junction (CEJ). These fiber bundles oriented towards the coronal portion of the bone crypt will later form the dento-gingival fiber group, the dento-periosteal fiber group and the transseptal fiber group which belong to the oriented fibers of the gingiva (see Fig. 1-46).

Fig. 1-59b The true periodontal ligament fibers, the *principal fibers*, develop in conjunction with the eruption of the tooth. First, fibers can be identified entering the most marginal portion of the alveolar bone.

Fig. 1-59c Later, more apically positioned bundles of oriented collagen fibers are seen.

Fig. 1-59d The orientation of the collagen fiber bundles alters continuously during the phase of tooth eruption. First, when the tooth has reached contact in occlusion and is functioning properly, the fibers of the periodontal ligament associate into groups of

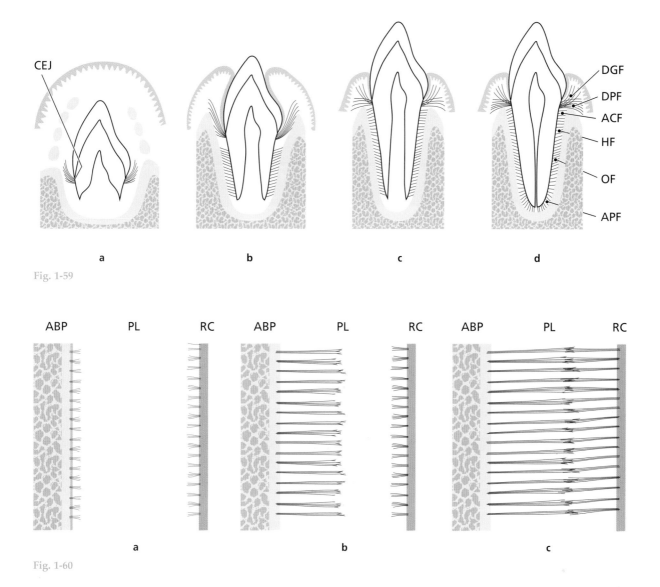

Fig. 1-59

Fig. 1-60

well oriented dentoalveolar collagen fibers demonstrated in Fig. 1-58. These collagen structures undergo constant remodeling (i.e. resorption of old fibers and formation of new ones).

Fig. 1-60 This schematic drawing illustrates the development of the principal fibers of the periodontal ligament. The alveolar bone proper (ABP) is seen to the left, the periodontal ligament (PL) is depicted in the center and the root cementum (RC) is seen to the right.

Fig. 1-60a First, small, fine, brush-like fibrils are detected arising from the root cementum and projecting into the PL space. At this stage the surface of the bone is covered by osteoblasts. From the surface of the bone only a small number of radiating, thin collagen fibrils can be seen.

Fig. 1-60b Later on, the number and thickness of fibers entering the bone increase. These fibers radiate towards the loose connective tissue in the mid-portion of the periodontal ligament area (PL), which contains more or less randomly oriented collagen fibrils. The fibers originating from the cementum are still short while those entering the bone gradually become longer. The terminal portions of these fibers carry finger-like projections.

Fig. 1-60c The fibers originating from the cementum subsequently increase in length and thickness and fuse in the periodontal ligament space with the fibers originating from the alveolar bone. When the tooth, following eruption, reaches contact in occlusion and starts to function, the principal fibers become organized in bundles and run continuously from the bone to the cementum.

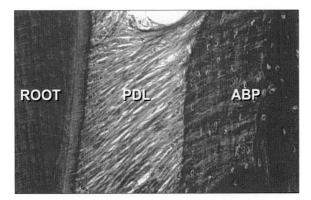

Fig. 1-61a

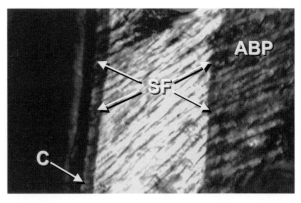

Fig. 1-61b

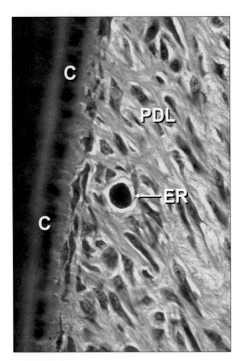

Fig. 1-62a

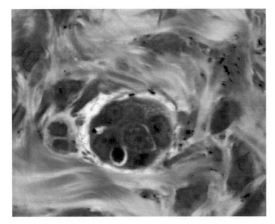

Fig. 1-62b

Fig. 1-61a illustrates how the principal fibers of the periodontal ligament (PDL) run continuously from the root cementum to the alveolar bone proper (ABP). The principal fibers embedded in the cementum

(Sharpey's fibers) have a smaller diameter but are more numerous than those embedded in the alveolar bone proper (Sharpey's fibers).

Fig. 1-61b presents a polarized version of Fig. 1-61a. In this illustration the Sharpey's fibers (SF) can be seen penetrating not only the cementum (C) but also the entire width of the alveolar bone proper (ABP). The periodontal ligament also contains a few elastic fibers associated with the blood vessels. Oxytalan fibers (see Fig. 1-44) are also present in the periodontal ligament. They have a mainly apico-occlusal orientation and are located in the ligament closer to the tooth than to the alveolar bone. Very often they insert into the cementum. Their function has not been determined.

The cells of the periodontal ligament are: *fibroblasts, osteoblasts, cementoblasts, osteoclasts,* as well as *epithelial cells* and *nerve fibers*. The fibroblasts are aligned along the principal fibers, while cementoblasts line the surface of the cementum, and the osteoblasts line the bone surface.

Fig. 1-62a shows the presence of clusters of epithelial cells (ER) in the periodontal ligament (PDL). These cells, called the *epithelial cell rests of Mallassez*, represent remnants of the Hertwig's epithelial root sheath. The epithelial cell rests are situated in the periodontal ligament at a distance of 15–75 μm from the cementum (C) on the root surface. A group of such epithelial cell rests is seen in a higher magnification in Fig. 1-62b.

Fig. 1-63 Electron microscopically it can be seen that the epithelial cell rests are surrounded by a basement membrane (BM) and that the cell membranes of the epithelial cells exhibit the presence of desmosomes (D) as well as hemidesmosomes (HD). The epithelial cells contain only few mitochondria and have a poorly developed endoplasmic reticulum. This means that they are vital, but resting, cells with minute metabolism.

Fig. 1-64 is a photomicrograph of a periodontal ligament removed from an extracted tooth. This

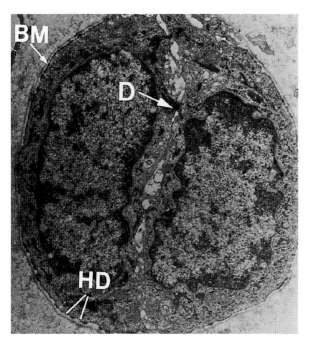

Fig. 1-63

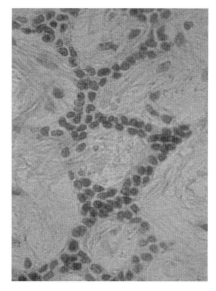

Fig. 1-64

specimen, prepared tangential to the root surface, shows that the epithelial cell rests of Mallassez, which in ordinary histologic sections appear as isolated groups of epithelial cells, in fact form a continuous network of epithelial cells surrounding the root. Their function is unknown at present.

Root cementum

The cementum is a specialized mineralized tissue covering the root surfaces and, occasionally, small portions of the crown of the teeth. It has many features in common with bone tissue. However, the cementum contains no blood or lymph vessels, has no innervation, does not undergo physiologic resorption or remodeling, but is characterized by continuing deposition throughout life. Like other mineralized tissues, it contains collagen fibers embedded in an organic matrix. Its mineral content, which is mainly hydroxyapatite, is about 65% by weight; a little more than that of bone (i.e. 60%). Cementum serves different functions. It attaches the periodontal ligament fibers to the root and contributes to the process of repair after damage to the root surface.

Different forms of cementum have been described:

1. *Acellular, extrinsic fiber cementum* (AEFC) is found in the coronal and middle portions of the root and contains mainly bundles of Sharpey's fibers. This type of cementum is an important part of the attachment apparatus and connects the tooth with the alveolar bone proper.
2. *Cellular, mixed stratified cementum* (CMSC) occurs in the apical third of the roots and in the furcations. It contains both extrinsic and intrinsic fibers as well as cementocytes.
3. *Cellular, intrinsic fiber cementum* (CIFC) is found mainly in resorption lacunae and it contains intrinsic fibers and cementocytes.

Fig. 1-65a shows a portion of a root with adjacent periodontal ligament (PDL). A thin layer of acellular, extrinsic fiber cementum (AEFC) with densely packed extrinsic fibers covers the peripheral dentin. Cementoblasts and fibroblasts can be observed adjacent to the cementum.

Fig. 1-65b represents a scanning electron micrograph of AEFC. Note that the extrinsic fibers attach to the dentin (left) and are continous with the collagen fiber

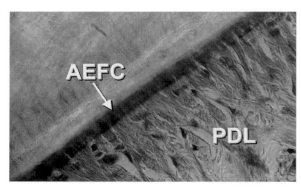

Fig. 1-65a

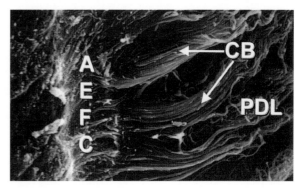

Fig. 1-65b

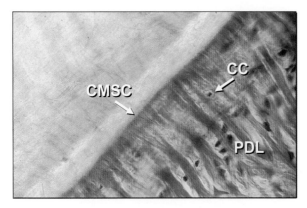

Fig. 1-66

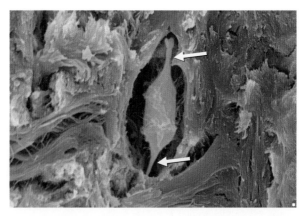

Fig. 1-67

bundles (CB) of the periodontal ligament (PDL). The AEFC is formed concomitantly with the formation of the root dentin. At a certain stage during tooth formation, the epithelial sheath of Hertwig, which lines the newly formed predentin, is fragmented. Cells from the dental follicle then penetrate the epithelial sheath of Hertwig and occupy the area next to the predentin. In this position, the ectomesenchymal cells from the dental follicle differentiate into cementoblasts and begin to produce collagen fibers at right angles to the surface. The first cementum is deposited on the highly mineralized superficial layer of the mantle dentin called the "hyaline layer" which contains enamel matrix proteins and the initial collagen fibers of the cementum. Subsequently, cementoblasts drift away from the surface resulting in increased thickness of the cementum and incorporation of principal fibers.

Fig. 1-66 demonstrates the structure of cellular, mixed stratified cementum (CMSC) which, in contrast to AEFC, contains cells and intrinsic fibers. The CMSC is laid down throughout the functional period of the tooth. The various types of cementum are produced by cementoblasts or periodontal ligament (PDL) cells lining the cementum surface. Some of these cells become incorporated into the cementoid, which subsequently mineralizes to form cementum. The cells which are incorporated in the cementum are called *cementocytes* (CC).

Fig. 1-67 illustrates how cementocytes (blue cell) reside in lacunae in CMSC or CIFC. They communicate with each other through a network of cytoplasmic processes (arrows) running in canaliculi in the cementum. The cementocytes also communicate with

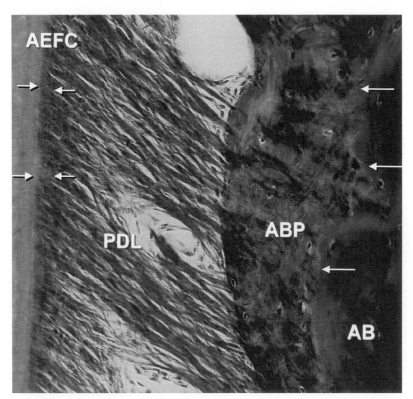

Fig. 1-68a

the cementoblasts on the surface through cytoplasmic processes. The presence of cementocytes allows transportation of nutrients through the cementum, and contributes to the maintenance of the vitality of this mineralized tissue.

Fig. 1-68a is a photomicrograph of a section through the periodontal ligament (PDL) in an area where the root is covered with acellular, extrinsic fiber cementum (AEFC). The portions of the principal fibers of the periodontal ligament which are embedded in the root cementum (arrows) and in the alveolar bone proper (ABP) are called *Sharpey's fibers*. The arrows to the right indicate the border between ABP and the alveolar bone (AB). In AEFC the Sharpey's fibers have a smaller diameter and are more densely packed than their counterparts in the alveolar bone. During the continuous formation of AEFC, portions of the periodontal ligament fibers (principal fibers) adjacent to the root become embedded in the mineralized tissue. Thus, the Sharpey's fibers in the cementum are a direct continuation of the principal fibers in the periodontal ligament and the supra-alveolar connective tissue.

Fig. 1-68b The Sharpey's fibers constitute the *extrinsic fiber system* (E) of the cementum and are produced by fibroblasts in the periodontal ligament. The *intrinsic fiber system* (I) is produced by cementoblasts and is composed of fibers oriented more or less parallel to the long axis of the root.

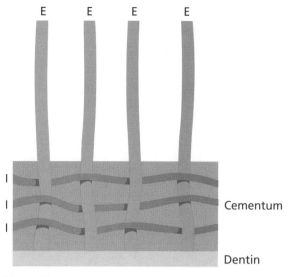
Fig. 1-68b

Fig. 1-69 shows extrinsic fibers penetrating acellular, extrinsic fiber cementum (AEFC). The characteristic cross-banding of the collagen fibers is masked in the cementum because apatite crystals have become deposited in the fiber bundles during the process of mineralization.

Fig. 1-70 In contrast to the bone, the cementum (C) does not exhibit alternating periods of resorption and apposition, but increases in thickness throughout life by deposition of successive new layers. During this

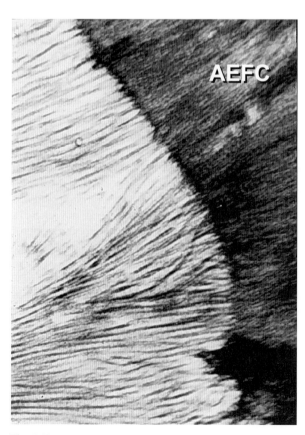
Fig. 1-69

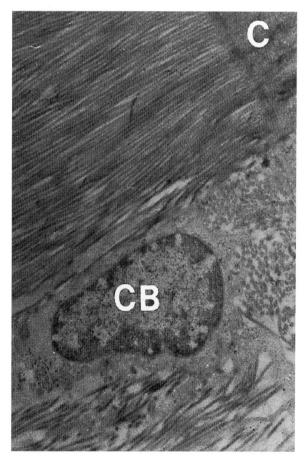
Fig. 1-70

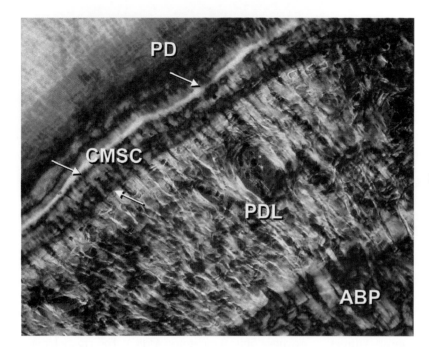

Fig. 1-71

process of gradual apposition, the particular portion of the principal fibers which resides immediately adjacent to the root surface becomes mineralized. Mineralization occurs by the deposition of hydroxyapatite crystals, first within the collagen fibers, later upon the fiber surface, and finally in the interfibrillar matrix. The electronphotomicrograph shows a cementoblast (CB) located near the surface of the cementum (C) and between two inserting principal fiber bundles. Generally, the AEFC is more mineralized than CMSC and CIFC. Sometimes only the periphery of the Sharpey's fibers of the CMSC is mineralized, leaving an unmineralized core within the fiber.

Fig. 1-71 is a photomicrograph of the periodontal ligament (PDL) which resides between the cementum (CMSC) and the alveolar bone proper (ABP). The CMSC is densely packed with collagen fibers oriented parallel to the root surface (intrinsic fibers) and Sharpey's fibers (extrinsic fibers), oriented more or less perpendicularly to the cementum–dentin junction (predentin (PD)). The various types of cementum increase in thickness by gradual apposition throughout life. The cementum becomes considerably wider in the apical portion of the root than in the cervical portion, where the thickness is only 20–50 µm. In the apical root portion the cementum is often 150–250 µm wide. The cementum often contains incremental lines indicating alternating periods of formation. The CMSC is formed after the termination of tooth eruption, and after a response to functional demands.

Alveolar bone

The alveolar process is defined as the parts of the maxilla and the mandible that form and support the sockets of the teeth. The alveolar process develops in conjunction with the development and eruption of the teeth. The alveolar process consists of bone which is formed both by cells from the dental follicle (alveolar bone proper) and cells which are independent of tooth development. Together with the root cementum and the periodontal membrane, the alveolar bone constitutes the attachment apparatus of the teeth, the main function of which is to distribute and resorb forces generated by, for example, mastication and other tooth contacts.

Fig. 1-72 illustrates a cross section through the alveolar process (pars alveolaris) of the maxilla at the midroot level of the teeth. Note that the bone which covers the root surfaces is considerably thicker at the palatal than at the buccal aspect of the jaw. The walls of the sockets are lined by *cortical bone* (arrows), and the area between the sockets and between the compact jaw bone walls is occupied by *cancellous bone*. The cancellous bone occupies most of the interdental septa but only a relatively small portion of the buccal and palatal bone plates. The cancellous bone contains *bone trabeculae*, the architecture and size of which are partly genetically determined and partly the result of the forces to which the teeth are exposed during function. Note how the bone on the buccal and palatal aspects of the alveolar process varies in thickness from one region to another. The bone plate is thick at the palatal aspect and on the buccal aspect of the molars but thin in the buccal anterior region.

Fig. 1-73 shows cross sections through the mandibular alveolar process at levels corresponding to the coronal (Fig. 1-73a) and apical (Fig. 1-73b) thirds of the roots. The bone lining the wall of the sockets (alveolar bone proper) is often continuous with the compact or cortical bone at the lingual (L) and buccal

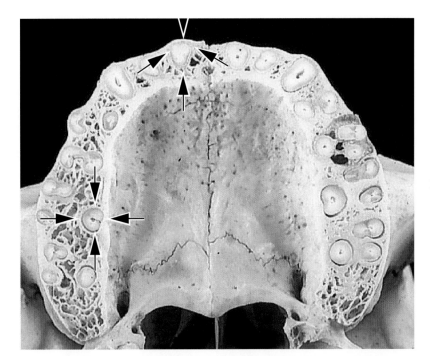

Fig. 1-72

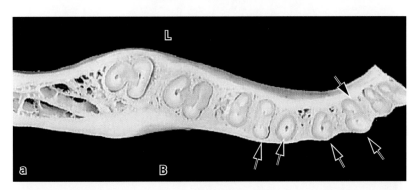

Fig. 1-73

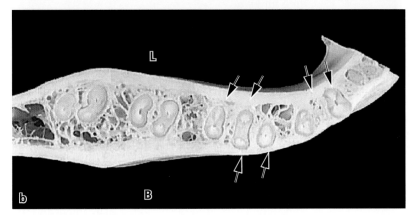

(B) aspects of the alveolar process (arrows). Note how the bone on the buccal and lingual aspects of the alveolar process varies in thickness from one region to another. In the incisor and premolar regions, the bone plate at the buccal aspects of the teeth is considerably thinner than at the lingual aspect. In the molar region, the bone is thicker at the buccal than at the lingual surfaces.

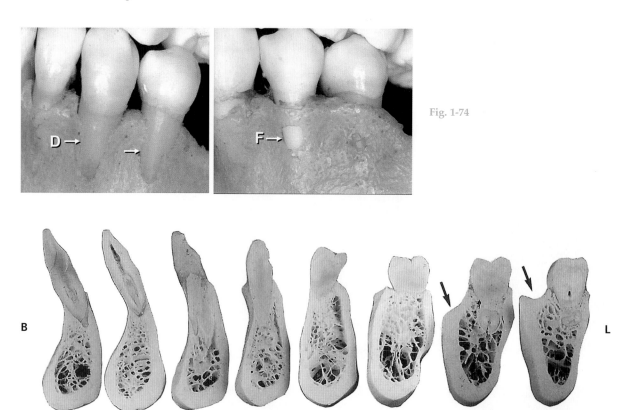

Fig. 1-74

Incisors   Premolars   Molars

Fig. 1-75

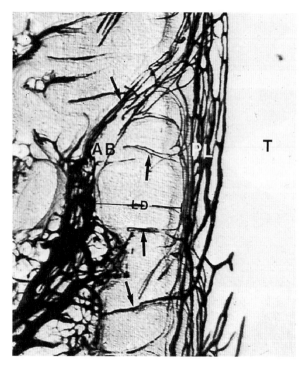

Fig. 1-76

Fig. 1-74 At the buccal aspect of the jaws, the bone coverage is sometimes missing at the coronal portion of the roots, forming a so-called *dehiscence* (D). If some bone is present in the most coronal portion of such an area the defect is called a *fenestration* (F).

These defects often occur where a tooth is displaced out of the arch and are more frequent over anterior than posterior teeth. The root in such defects is covered only by periodontal ligament and the overlying gingiva.

Fig. 1-75 presents vertical sections through various regions of the mandibular dentition. The bone wall at the buccal (B) and lingual (L) aspects of the teeth varies considerably in thickness, e.g. from the premolar to the molar region. Note, for instance, how the presence of the oblique line (*linea obliqua*) results in a shelf-like bone process (arrows) at the buccal aspect of the second and third molars.

Fig. 1-76 shows a section through the periodontal ligament (PL), tooth (T), and the alveolar bone (AB). The blood vessels in the periodontal ligament and the alveolar bone appear black because the blood system was perfused with ink. The compact bone (alveolar bone proper) which lines the tooth socket, and in a radiograph (Fig. 1-57) appears as "lamina dura" (LD), is perforated by numerous *Volkmann's canals* (arrows) through which blood vessels, lymphatics, and nerve fibers pass from the alveolar bone (AB) to the periodontal ligament (PL). This layer of bone into which the principal fibers are inserted (Sharpey's fibers) is sometimes called "bundle bone". From a functional and structural point of view, this "bundle bone" has many features in common with the cementum layer on the root surfaces.

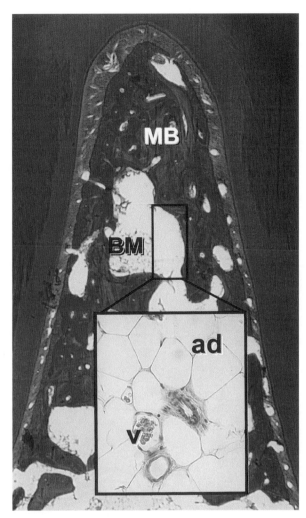

Fig. 1-77

Fig. 1-77 The alveolar process starts to form early in fetal life, with mineral deposition at small foci in the mesenchymal matrix surrounding the tooth buds. These small mineralized areas increase in size, fuse, and become resorbed and remodeled until a continuous mass of bone has formed around the fully erupted teeth. The mineral content of bone, which is mainly hydroxyapatite, is about 60% on a weight basis. The photomicrograph illustrates the bone tissue within the furcation area of a mandibular molar. The bone tissue can be divided into two compartments: mineralized bone (MB) and bone marrow (BM). The mineralized bone is made up of lamellae – lamellar bone – while the bone marrow contains adipocytes (ad), vascular structures (v), and undifferentiated mesenchymal cells (see insertion).

Fig. 1-78 The mineralized, lamellar bone includes two types of bone tissue: the bone of the alveolar process (AB) and the alveolar bone proper (ABP), which covers the alveolus. The ABP or the bundle bone has a varying width and is indicated with white arrows. The alveolar bone (AB) is a tissue of mesenchymal origin and it is not considered as part of the genuine attachment apparatus. The alveolar bone proper (ABP), on the other hand, together with the periodontal ligament (PDL) and the cementum (C), is responsible for the attachment between the tooth and the skeleton. AB and ABP may, as a result of altered functional demands, undergo adaptive changes.

Fig. 1-79 describes a portion of lamellar bone. The lamellar bone at this site contains *osteons* (white

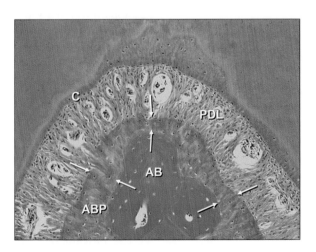

Fig. 1-78

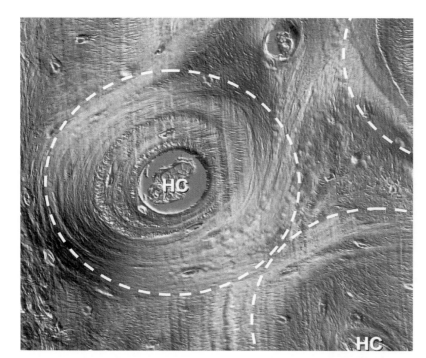

Fig. 1-79

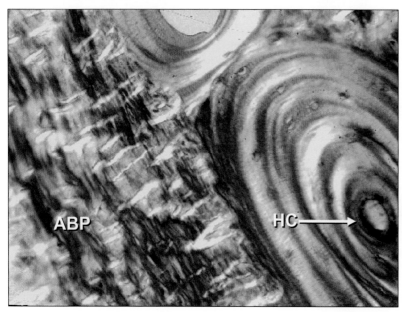

Fig. 1-80a

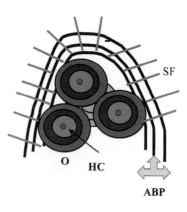

Fig. 1-80b

circles) each of which harbors a blood vessel located in a Haversian canal (HC). The blood vessel is surrounded by concentric, mineralized lamellae to form the osteon. The space between the different osteons is filled with so-called interstitial lamellae. The osteons in the lamellar bone are not only structural units but also metabolic units. Thus, the nutrition of the bone is secured by the blood vessels in the Haversian canals and connecting vessels in the Volkmann canals.

Fig. 1-80 The histologic section (Fig. 1-80a) shows the borderline between the alveolar bone proper (ABP) and lamellar bone with an osteon. Note the presence of the Haversian canal (HC) in the center of the

osteon. The alveolar bone proper (ABP) includes circumferential lamellae and contains Sharpey's fibers which extend into the periodontal ligament. The schematic drawing (Fig. 1-80b) is illustrating three active osteons (brown) with a blood vessel (red) in the Haversian canal (HC). Interstitial lamella (green) is located between the osteons (O) and represents an old and partly remodelled osteon. The alveolar bone proper (ABP) is presented by the dark lines into which the Sharpey's fibers (SF) insert.

Fig. 1-81 illustrates an osteon with osteocytes (OC) residing in osteocyte lacunae in the lamellar bone. The osteocytes connect via canaliculi (can) which

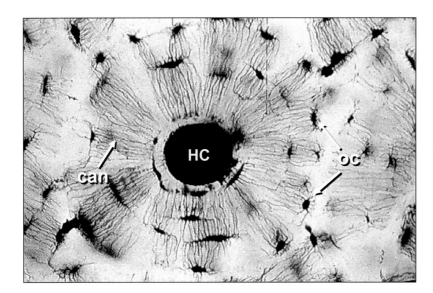

Fig. 1-81

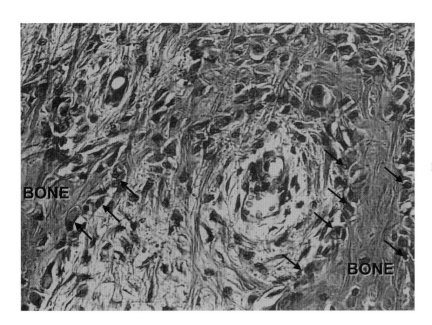

Fig. 1-82

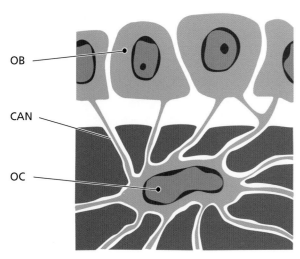

Fig. 1-83

contain cytoplasmatic projections of the osteocytes. A Haversian canal (HC) is seen in the middle of the osteon.

Fig. 1-82 illustrates an area of the alveolar bone in which bone formation occurs. The osteoblasts (arrows), the bone-forming cells, are producing bone matrix (osteoid) consisting of collagen fibers, glycoproteins, and proteoglycans. The bone matrix or the osteoid undergoes mineralization by the deposition of minerals such as calcium and phosphate, which are subsequently transformed into hydroxyapatite.

Fig. 1-83 The drawing illustrates how osteocytes, present in the mineralized bone, communicate with osteoblasts on the bone surface through canaliculi.

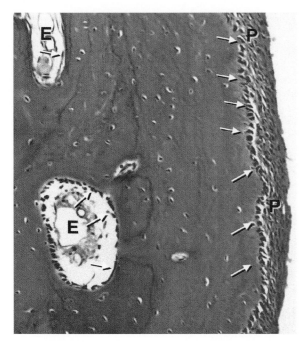

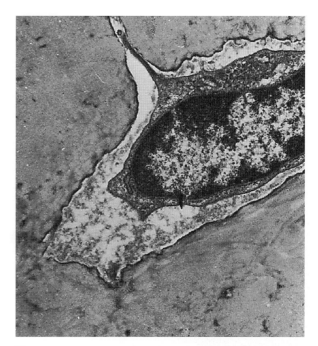

Fig. 1-84

Fig. 1-85

Fig. 1-84 All active bone-forming sites harbor osteoblasts. The outer surface of the bone is lined by a layer of such osteoblasts which, in turn, are organized in a periosteum (P) that contains densely packed collagen fibers. On the "inner surface" of the bone, i.e. in the bone marrow space, there is an endosteum (E), which presents similar features as the periosteum.

Fig. 1-85 illustrates an osteocyte residing in a lacuna in the bone. It can be seen that cytoplasmic processes radiate in different directions.

Fig. 1-86 illustrates osteocytes (OC) and how their long and delicate cytoplasmic processes communicate through the canaliculi (CAN) in the bone. The resulting canalicular–lacunar system is essential for cell metabolism by allowing diffusion of nutrients and waste products. The surface between the osteocytes with their cytoplasmic processes on the one

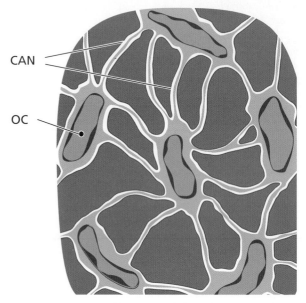

Fig. 1-86

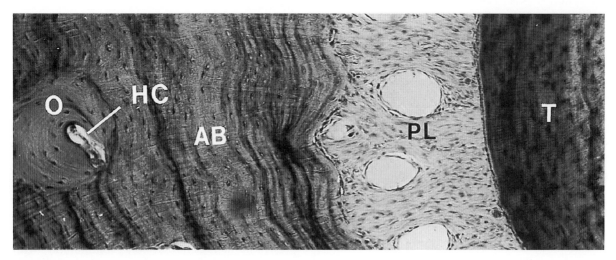

Fig. 1-87

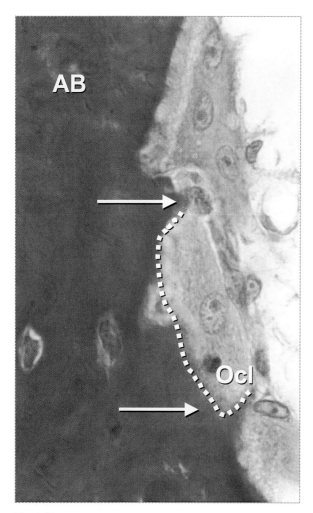

Fig. 1-88

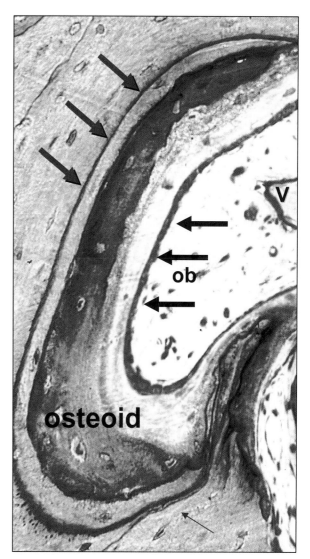

Fig. 1-89

side, and the mineralized matrix on the other, is very large. It has been calculated that the interface between cells and matrix in a cube of bone, $10 \times 10 \times 10$ cm, amounts to approximately 250 m^2. This enormous surface of exchange serves as a regulator, e.g. for serum calcium and serum phosphate levels via hormonal control mechanisms.

Fig. 1-87 The alveolar bone is constantly renewed in response to functional demands. The teeth erupt and migrate in a mesial direction throughout life to compensate for attrition. Such movement of the teeth implies remodeling of the alveolar bone. During the process of remodeling, the bone trabeculae are continuously resorbed and reformed and the cortical bone mass is dissolved and replaced by new bone. During breakdown of the cortical bone, resorption canals are formed by proliferating blood vessels. Such canals, which contain a blood vessel in the center, are subsequently refilled with new bone by the formation of lamellae arranged in concentric layers around the blood vessel. A new Haversian system (O) is seen in the photomicrograph of a horizontal section through the alveolar bone (AB), periodontal ligament (PL), and tooth (T).

Fig. 1-88 The resorption of bone is always associated with *osteoclasts* (Ocl). These cells are giant cells special-

ized in the breakdown of mineralized matrix (bone, dentin, cementum) and are probably developed from blood monocytes. The resorption occurs by the release of acid substances (lactic acid, etc.) which form an acidic environment in which the mineral salts of the bone tissue become dissolved. Remaining organic substances are eliminated by enzymes and osteoclastic phagocytosis. Actively resorbing osteoclasts adhere to the bone surface and produce lacunar pits called *Howship's lacunae* (dotted line). They are mobile and capable of migrating over the bone surface. The photomicrograph demonstrates osteoclastic activity at the surface of alveolar bone (AB).

Fig. 1-89 illustrates a so-called bone multicellular unit (BMU), which is present in bone tissue undergoing active remodeling. The reversal line, indicated by red arrows, demonstrates the level to which bone resorption has occurred. From the reversal line new bone has started to form and has the character of osteoid. Note the presence of osteoblasts (ob) and vascular structures (v). The osteoclasts resorb organic as well as inorganic substances.

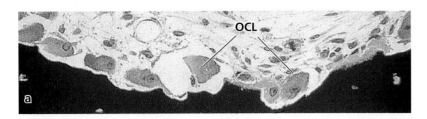

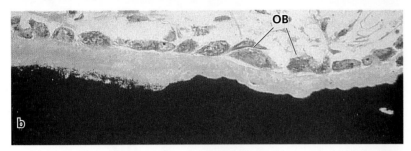

Fig. 1-90

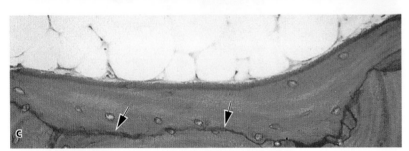

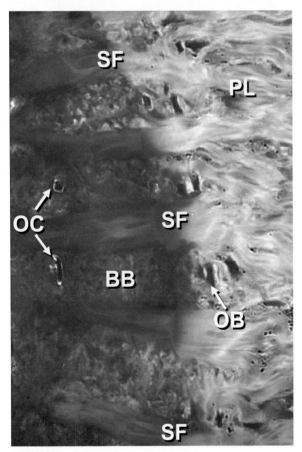

Fig. 1-91

tooth drifting and changes in functional forces acting on the teeth. Remodeling of the trabecular bone starts with resorption of the bone surface by osteoclasts (OCL) as seen in Fig. 1-90a. After a short period, osteoblasts (OB) start depositing new bone (Fig. 1-90b) and finally a new bone multicellular unit is formed, clearly delineated by a reversal line (arrows) as seen in Fig. 1-90c.

Fig. 1-91 Collagen fibers of the periodontal ligament (PL) insert in the mineralized bone which lines the wall of the tooth socket. This bone, called alveolar bone proper or bundle bone (BB), has a high turnover rate. The portions of the collagen fibers which are inserted inside the bundle bone are called Sharpey's fibers (SF). These fibers are mineralized at their periphery, but often have a non-mineralized central core. The collagen fiber bundles inserting in the bundle bone generally have a larger diameter and are less numerous than the corresponding fiber bundles in the cementum on the opposite side of the periodontal ligament. Individual bundles of fibers can be followed all the way from the alveolar bone to the cementum. However, despite being in the same bundle of fibers, the collagen adjacent to the bone is always less mature than that adjacent to the cementum. The collagen on the tooth side has a low turnover rate. Thus, while the collagen adjacent to the bone is renewed relatively rapidly, the collagen adjacent to the root surface is renewed slowly or not at all. Note the occurrence of osteoblasts (OB) and osteocytes (OC).

Fig. 1-90 Both the cortical and cancellous alveolar bone are constantly undergoing remodeling (i.e. resorption followed by formation) in response to

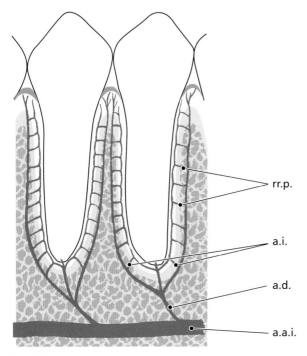

Fig. 1-92

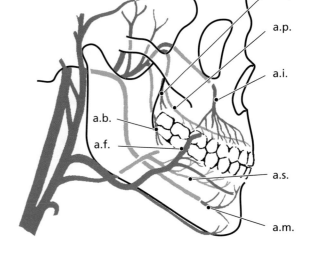

Fig. 1-93

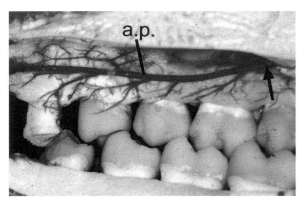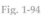

Fig. 1-94

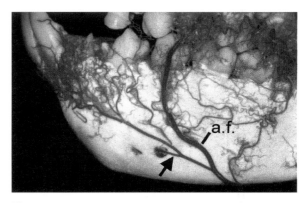

Fig. 1-95

Blood supply of the periodontium

Fig. 1-92 The schematic drawing depicts the blood supply to the teeth and the periodontal tissues. The *dental artery* (a.d.), which is a branch of the *superior* or *inferior* alveolar artery (a.a.i.), dismisses the *intraseptal artery* (a.i.) before it enters the tooth socket. The terminal branches of the *intraseptal artery* (*rami perforantes*, rr.p.) penetrate the alveolar bone proper in canals at all levels of the socket (see Fig. 1-76). They anastomose in the periodontal ligament space, together with blood vessels originating from the apical portion of the periodontal ligament and with other terminal branches, from the intraseptal artery (a.i.). Before the dental artery (a.d.) enters the root canal it puts out branches which supply the apical portion of the periodontal ligament.

Fig. 1-93 The gingiva receives its blood supply mainly through *supraperiosteal* blood vessels which

are terminal branches of the *sublingual artery* (a.s.), the *mental artery* (a.m.), the *buccal artery* (a.b.), the *facial artery* (a.f.), the *greater palatine artery* (a.p.), the *infra orbital artery* (a.i.), and the *posterior superior dental artery* (a.ap.).

Fig. 1-94 depicts the course of the greater palatine artery (a.p.) in a specimen of a monkey which was perfused with plastic at sacrifice. Subsequently, the soft tissue was dissolved. The greater palatine artery (a.p.), which is a terminal branch of the *ascending palatine artery* (from the *maxillary*, "internal maxillary", artery), runs through the *greater palatine canal* (arrow) to the palate. As this artery runs in a frontal direction it puts out branches which supply the gingiva and the masticatory mucosa of the palate.

Fig. 1-95 The various arteries are often considered to supply certain well defined regions of the dentition. In reality, however, there are numerous anastomoses

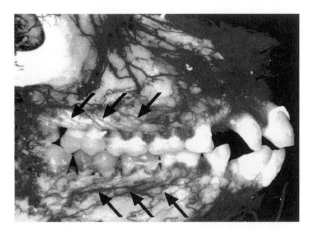

Fig. 1-96

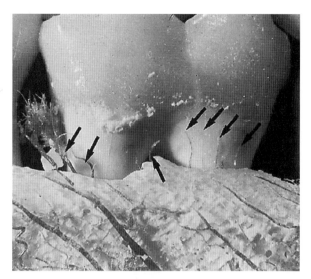

Fig. 1-97

present between the different arteries. Thus, the *entire system of blood vessels*, rather than individual groups of vessels, should be regarded as the unit supplying the soft and hard tissue of the maxilla and the mandible, e.g. in this figure there is an anastomosis (arrow) between the *facial artery* (a.f.) and the blood vessels of the mandible.

Fig. 1-96 illustrates a vestibular segment of the maxilla and mandible from a monkey which was perfused with plastic at sacrifice. Notice that the vestibular gingiva is supplied with blood mainly through *supraperiosteal* blood vessels (arrows).

Fig. 1-97 As can be seen, blood vessels (arrows) originating from vessels in the periodontal ligament pass the alveolar bone crest and contribute to the blood supply of the free gingiva.

Fig. 1-98 shows a specimen from a monkey which was perfused with ink at the time of sacrifice. Subsequently, the specimen was treated to make the tissue transparent (cleared specimen). To the right, the supraperiosteal blood vessels (sv) can be seen. During

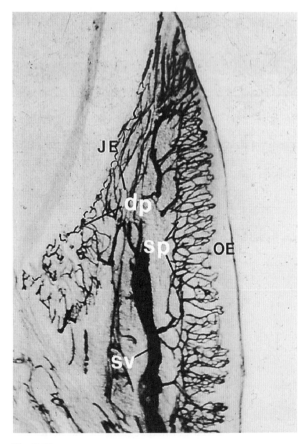

Fig. 1-98

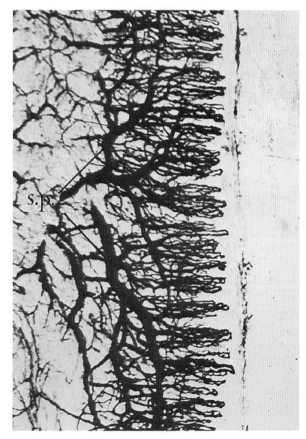

Fig. 1-99

their course towards the free gingiva they put forth numerous branches to the *subepithelial plexus* (sp), located immediately beneath the oral epithelium of the free and attached gingiva. This subepithelial plexus in turn yields thin *capillary loops* to each of the connective tissue papillae projecting into the oral epithelium (OE). The number of such capillary loops is constant over a very long time and is not altered by application of epinephrine or histamine to the gingival margin. This implies that the blood vessels of the lateral portions of the gingiva, even under normal circumstances, are fully utilized and that the blood flow to the free gingiva is regulated entirely by velocity alterations. In the free gingiva, the supraperiosteal blood vessels (sv) anastomose with blood vessels from the periodontal ligament and the bone. Beneath the junctional epithelium (JE) seen to the left, is a plexus of blood vessels termed the *dento-gingival plexus* (dp). The blood vessels in this plexus have a thickness of approximately 40 µm, which means that they are mainly venules. In healthy gingiva, no capillary loops occur in the dento-gingival plexus.

Fig. 1-99 This specimen illustrates how the subepithelial plexus (sp), beneath the oral epithelium of the free and attached gingiva, yields thin capillary loops to each connective tissue papilla. These capillary loops have a diameter of approximately 7 µm, which means they are the size of true capillaries.

Fig. 1-100 illustrates the dento-gingival plexus in a section cut parallel to the subsurface of the junctional epithelium. As can be seen, the dento-gingival plexus consists of a fine-meshed network of blood vessels. In the upper portion of the picture, capillary loops can be detected belonging to the subepithelial plexus beneath the oral sulcular epithelium.

Fig. 1-101 is a schematic drawing of the blood supply to the free gingiva. As stated above, the main blood supply of the free gingiva derives from the *supraperiosteal* blood vessels (SV) which, in the gingiva, anastomose with blood vessels from the *alveolar bone* (ab) and *periodontal ligament* (pl). To the right in the drawing, the oral epithelium (OE) is depicted with its underlying subepithelial plexus of vessels (sp). To the left beneath the junctional epithelium (JE), the dento-gingival plexus (dp) can be seen, which, under normal conditions, comprises a fine-meshed network without capillary loops.

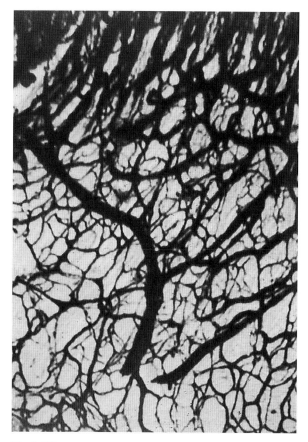
Fig. 1-100

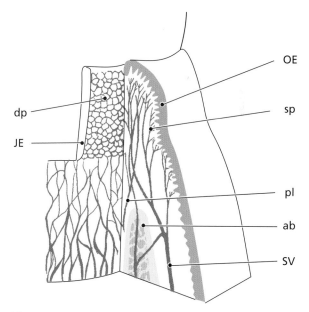
Fig. 1-101

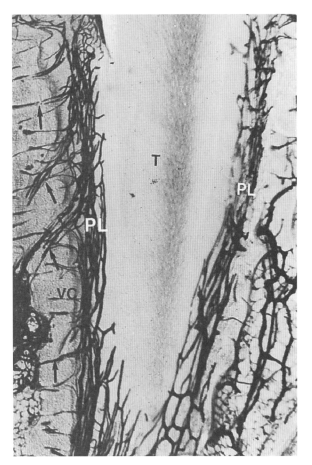

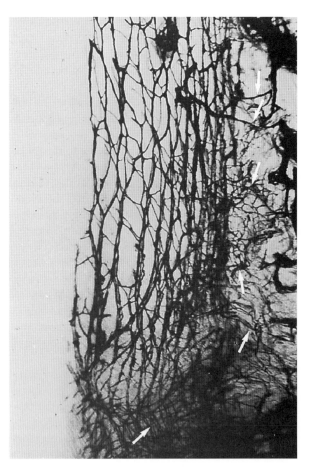

Fig. 1-102

Fig. 1-103

Fig. 1-102 shows a section prepared through a tooth (T) with its periodontium. Blood vessels (perforating rami; arrows) arising from the intraseptal artery in the alveolar bone run through canals (Volkmann's canals) in the socket wall (VC) into the periodontal ligament (PL), where they anastomose.

Fig. 1-103 shows blood vessels in the periodontal ligament in a section cut parallel to the root surface. After entering the periodontal ligament, the blood vessels (perforating rami; arrows) anastomose and form a polyhedral network which surrounds the root like a stocking. The majority of the blood vessels in the periodontal ligament are found close to the alveolar bone. In the coronal portion of the periodontal ligament, blood vessels run in coronal direction, passing the alveolar bone crest, into the free gingiva (see Fig. 1-97).

Fig. 1-104 is a schematic drawing of the blood supply of the periodontium. The blood vessels in the periodontal ligament form a polyhedral network surrounding the root. Note that the free gingiva receives its blood supply from (1) supraperiosteal blood vessels, (2) the blood vessels of the periodontal ligament, and (3) the blood vessels of the alveolar bone.

Fig. 1-105 illustrates schematically the so-called *extravascular* circulation through which nutrients and other substances are carried to the individual cells and metabolic waste products are removed from the tissue. In the arterial (A) end of the capillary, to the left in the drawing, a hydraulic pressure of approximately 35 mmHg is maintained as a result of the pumping function of the heart. Since the hydraulic pressure is higher than the osmotic pressure (OP) in the tissue (which is approximately 30 mmHg), transportation of substances will occur from the blood vessels to the extravascular space (ES). In the venous (V) end of the capillary system, to the right in the drawing, the hydraulic pressure has decreased to approximately 25 mmHg (i.e. 5 mmHg lower than the osmotic pressure in the tissue). This allows transportation of substances from the extravascular space to the blood vessels. Thus, the difference between the hydraulic pressure and the osmotic pressure (OP) results in transportation of substances from the blood vessels to the extravascular space in the arterial part of the capillary while, in the venous part, transportation of substances occurs from the extravascular space to the blood vessels. An extravascular circulation is hereby established (small arrows).

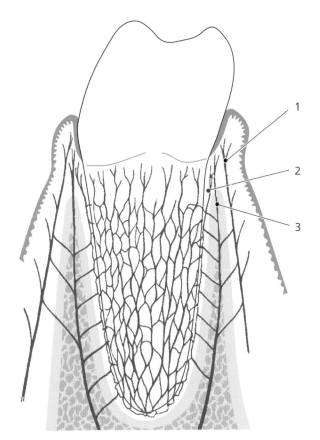

Fig. 1-104

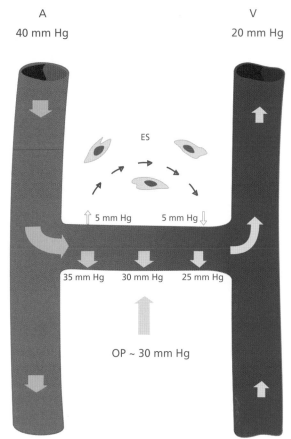

Fig. 1-105

Lymphatic system of the periodontium

Fig. 1-106 The smallest lymph vessels, the *lymph capillaries*, form an extensive network in the connective tissue. The wall of the lymph capillary consists of a single layer of endothelial cells. For this reason such capillaries are difficult to identify in an ordinary histologic section. The lymph is absorbed from the tissue fluid through the thin walls into the lymph capillaries. From the capillaries, the lymph passes into larger lymph vessels which are often in the vicinity of corresponding blood vessels. Before the lymph enters the blood stream it passes through one or more *lymph nodes* in which the lymph is filtered and supplied with lymphocytes. The lymph vessels are like veins provided with valves. The lymph from the periodontal tissues drains to the lymph nodes of the head and the neck. The labial and lingual gingiva of the mandibular incisor region is drained to the *submental lymph nodes* (sme). The palatal gingiva of the maxilla is drained to the *deep cervical lymph nodes* (cp). The buccal gingiva of the maxilla and the buccal and lingual gingiva in the mandibular premolar–molar region are drained to *submandibular lymph nodes* (sma). Except for the third molars and mandibular incisors, all teeth with their adjacent periodontal tissues are drained to the submandibular lymph

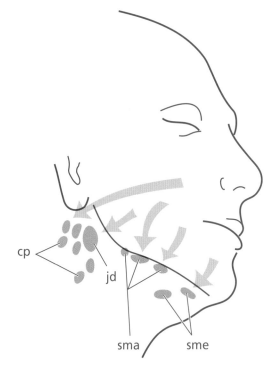

Fig. 1-106

nodes (sma). The third molars are drained to the *jugulodigastric lymph node* (jd) and the mandibular incisors to the *submental lymph nodes* (sme).

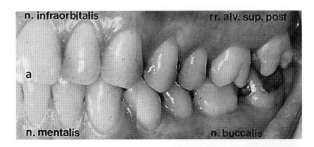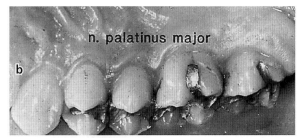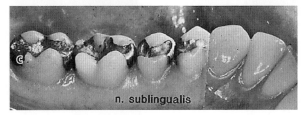

Fig. 1-107

Nerves of the periodontium

Like other tissues in the body, the periodontium contains receptors which record pain, touch, and pressure (*nociceptors* and *mechanoreceptors*). In addition to the different types of sensory receptors, nerve components are found innervating the blood vessels of the periodontium. Nerves recording pain, touch, and pressure have their trophic center in the *semilunar ganglion* and are brought to the periodontium via the *trigeminal nerve* and its end branches. Owing to the presence of receptors in the periodontal ligament, small forces applied on the teeth may be identified. For example, the presence of a very thin (10–30 µm) metal foil strip placed between the teeth during occlusion can readily be identified. It is also well known that a movement which brings the teeth of the mandible in contact with the occlusal surfaces of the maxillary teeth is arrested reflexively and altered into an opening movement if a hard object is detected in the chew. Thus, the receptors in the periodontal ligament, together with the proprioceptors in muscles and tendons, play an essential role in the regulation of chewing movements and chewing forces.

Fig. 1-107 shows the various regions of the gingiva which are innervated by end branches of the trigeminal nerve. The gingiva on the labial aspect of maxillary incisors, canines, and premolars is innervated by *superior labial branches* from the *infraorbital nerve* (n. infraorbitalis) (Fig. 1-107a). The buccal gingiva in the maxillary molar region is innervated by branches from the *posterior superior dental nerve* (rr. alv. sup. post) (Fig. 1-107a). The palatal gingiva is innervated by the *greater palatal nerve* (n. palatinus major) (Fig. 1-107b), except for the area of the incisors, which is innervated by the *long sphenopalatine nerve* (n. pterygopalatini). The lingual gingiva in the mandible is innervated by the *sublingual nerve* (n. sublingualis) (Fig. 1-107c), which is an end branch of the *lingual nerve*. The gingiva at the labial aspect of mandibular

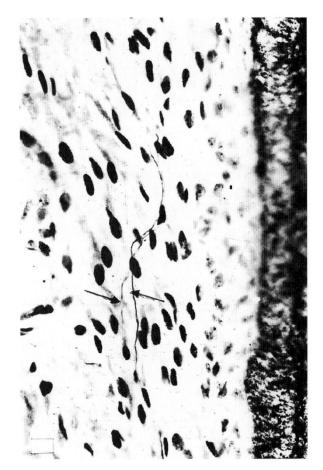

Fig. 1-108

incisors and canines is innervated by the *mental nerve* (n. mentalis), and the gingiva at the buccal aspect of the molars by the *buccal nerve* (n. buccalis) (Fig. 1-107a). The innervation areas of these two nerves frequently overlap in the premolar region. The teeth in the mandible, including their periodontal ligament, are innervated by the *inferior alveolar nerve* (n. alveolaris inf.), while the teeth in the maxilla are innervated by the *superior alveolar plexus* (n. alveolares sup).

Fig. 1-108 The small nerves of the periodontium follow almost the same course as the blood vessels. The nerves to the gingiva run in the tissue superficial to the periosteum and put out several branches to the oral epithelium on their way towards the free gingiva. The nerves enter the periodontal ligament through the perforations (Volkmann's canals) in the socket wall (see Fig. 1-102). In the periodontal ligament, the nerves join larger bundles which take a course parallel to the long axis of the tooth. The photomicrograph illustrates small nerves (arrows) which have emerged from larger bundles of ascending nerves in order to supply certain parts of the periodontal ligament tissue. Various types of neural terminations such as free nerve endings and Ruffini's corpuscles have been identified in the periodontal ligament.

Acknowledgment

We thank the following for contributing to the illustrations in Chapter 1: M. Listgarten, R.K. Schenk, H.E. Schroeder, K.A. Selvig, and K. Josephsen.

References

Ainamo, J. & Talari, A. (1976). The increase with age of the width of attached gingiva. *Journal of Periodontal Research* **11**, 182–188.

Anderson, D.T., Hannam, A.G. & Matthews, G. (1970). Sensory mechanisms in mammalian teeth and their supporting structures. *Physiological Review* **50**, 171–195.

Bartold, P.M. (1995). Turnover in periodontal connective tissue: dynamic homeostasis of cells, collagen and ground substances. *Oral Diseases* **1**, 238–253.

Beertsen, W., McCulloch, C.A.G. & Sodek, J. (1997). The periodontal ligament: a unique, multifunctional connective tissue. *Periodontology 2000* **13**, 20–40.

Bosshardt, D.D. & Schroeder, H.E. (1991). Establishment of acellular extrinsic fiber cementum on human teeth. A light- and electron-microscopic study. *Cell Tissue Research* **263**, 325–336.

Bosshardt, D.D. & Selvig, K.A. (1997). Dental cementum: the dynamic tissue covering of the root. *Periodontology 2000* **13**, 41–75.

Carranza, E.A., Itoiz, M.E., Cabrini, R.L. & Dotto, C.A. (1966). A study of periodontal vascularization in different laboratory animals. *Journal of Periodontal Research* **1**, 120–128.

Egelberg, J. (1966). The blood vessels of the dentogingival junction. *Journal of Periodontal Research* **1**, 163–179.

Fullmer, H.M., Sheetz, J.H. & Narkates, A.J. (1974). Oxytalan connective tissue fibers. A review. *Journal of Oral Pathology* **3**, 291–316.

Hammarström, L. (1997). Enamel matrix, cementum development and regeneration. *Journal of Clinical Periodontology* **24**, 658–677.

Karring, T. (1973). Mitotic activity in the oral epithelium. *Journal of Periodontal Research, Suppl.* **13**, 1–47.

Karring, T. & Löe, H. (1970). The three-dimensional concept of the epithelium-connective tissue boundary of gingiva. *Acta Odontologica Scandinavia* **28**, 917–933.

Karring, T., Lang, N.R. & Löe, H. (1974). The role of gingival connective tissue in determining epithelial differentiation. *Journal of Periodontal Research* **10**, 1–11.

Karring, T., Ostergaard, E. & Löe, H. (1971). Conservation of tissue specificity after heterotopic transplantation of gingiva and alveolar mucosa. *Journal of Periodontal Research* **6**, 282–293.

Kvam, E. (1973). Topography of principal fibers. *Scandinavian Journal of Dental Research* **81**, 553–557.

Lambrichts, I., Creemers, J. & van Steenberghe, D. (1992). Morphology of neural endings in the human periodontal ligament: an electron microscopic study. *Journal of Periodontal Research* **27**, 191–196.

Listgarten, M.A. (1966). Electron microscopic study of the gingivo-dental junction of man. *American Journal of Anatomy* **119**, 147–178.

Listgarten, M.A. (1972). Normal development, structure, physiology and repair of gingival epithelium. *Oral Science Review* **1**, 3–67.

Lozdan, J. & Squier, C.A. (1969). The histology of the mucogingival junction. *Journal of Periodontal Research* **4**, 83–93.

Melcher, A.H. (1976). Biological processes in resorption, deposition and regeneration of bone. In: Stahl, S.S., ed. *Periodontal Surgery, Biologic Basis and Technique*. Springfield: C.C. Thomas, pp. 99–120.

Page, R.C., Ammons, W.F., Schectman, L.R. & Dillingham, L.A. (1974). Collagen fiber bundles of the normal marginal gingiva in the marmoset. *Archives of Oral Biology* **19**, 1039–1043.

Palmer, R.M. & Lubbock, M.J. (1995). The soft connective tissue of the gingiva and periodontal ligament: are they unique? *Oral Diseases* **1**, 230–237.

Saffar, J.L., Lasfargues, J.J. & Cherruah, M. (1997). Alveolar bone and the alveolar process: the socket that is never stable. *Periodontology 2000* **13**, 76–90.

Schenk, R.K. (1994). Bone regeneration: Biologic basis. In: Buser, D., Dahlin, C. & Schenk, R. K., eds. *Guided Bone Regeneration in Implant Dentistry*. Berlin: Quintessence Publishing Co.

Schroeder, H.E. (1986). The periodontium. In: Schroeder, H. E., ed. *Handbook of Microscopic Anatomy*. Berlin: Springer, pp. 47–64.

Schroeder, H.E. & Listgarten, M.A. (1971). *Fine Structure of the Developing Epithelial Attachment of Human Teeth*, 2nd edn. Basel: Karger, p. 146.

Schroeder, H.E. & Listgarten, M.A. (1997). The gingival tissues: the architecture of periodontal protection. *Periodontology 2000* **13**, 91–120.

Schroeder, H.E. & Münzel-Pedrazzoli, S. (1973). Correlated morphometric and biochemical analysis of gingival tissue. Morphometric model, tissue sampling and test of stereologic procedure. *Journal of Microscopy* **99**, 301–329.

Schroeder, H.E. & Theilade, J. (1966). Electron microscopy of normal human gingival epithelium. *Journal of Periodontal Research* **1**, 95–119.

Selvig, K.A. (1965). The fine structure of human cementum. *Acta Odontologica Scandinavica* **23**, 423–441.

Valderhaug, J.R. & Nylen, M.U. (1966). Function of epithelial rests as suggested by their ultrastructure. *Journal of Periodontal Research* **1**, 67–78.

Chapter 2

The Edentulous Alveolar Ridge

Maurício Araújo and Jan Lindhe

Clinical considerations

The alveolar process forms in harmony with the development and eruption of the teeth and it gradually regresses when the teeth are lost. In other words, the formation as well as the continued preservation of the alveolar process is dependent on the continued presence of teeth. Furthermore, the morphologic characteristics of the alveolar process are related to the size and shape of the teeth, events occurring during tooth eruption as well as the inclination of the erupted teeth. Thus, subjects with long and narrow teeth, compared with subjects who have short and wide teeth, appear to have a more delicate alveolar process and, in particular, a thin, sometimes fenestrated buccal bone plate (Fig. 2-1).

The tooth and its surrounding attachment tissues – the root cementum, the periodontal ligament and the bundle bone – establish a functional unit (Fig. 2-2). Hence, forces elicited, for example during mastication, are transmitted from the crown of the tooth via the root and the attachment tissues to the load-carrying hard tissue structures in the alveolar process, where they are dispersed. The loss of teeth, and the loss or change of function within and around the socket will result in a series of adaptive alterations of the now edentulous portion of the ridge. Thus, it is well documented that following *multiple tooth* extractions and the subsequent restoration with removable dentures, the size of the alveolar ridge will become markedly reduced, not only in the horizontal but also in the vertical dimension (Figs. 2-3, 2-4); in addition, the arch will be shortened (Atwood 1962, 1963; Johnson 1963, 1969; Carlsson *et al.* 1967).

Also following the removal of *single* teeth the alveolar ridge will be markedly diminished (Fig. 2-5). The magnitude of this change was studied and reported

in a publication by Pietrokovski and Massler (1967). The authors had access to 149 dental cast models (72 maxillary and 77 mandibular) in which one tooth was missing (and not replaced) on one side of the jaw. The outer contours of the buccal and lingual (palatal) portions of the ridge at a tooth site and at

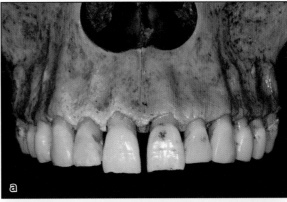

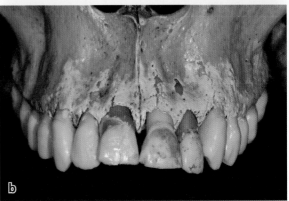

Fig. 2-1 Buccal aspect of adult skull preparations illustrating a dentate maxilla of one subject with a thick (a) and another subject with a thin (b) periodontal biotype.

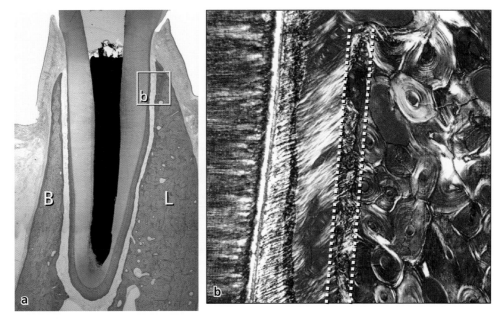

Fig. 2-2 Buccal–lingual section of a dentate portion of the alveolar process. B = buccal aspect; L = lingual aspect. (a) The tooth is surrounded by its attachment tissues. (b) Larger magnification of the attachment tissues. Note that the dentin is connected to the alveolar bone via the root cementum, the periodontal ligament and the alveolar bone. The inner portion of the alveolar bone (dotted line) is called the alveolar bone proper or the bundle bone.

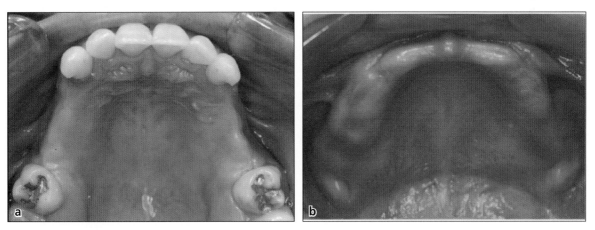

Fig. 2-3 (a) Clinical view of a partially edentulous maxilla. Note that the crest of the edentulous portions of the ridge is narrow in the buccal–palatal direction. (b) Clinical view of a fully edentulous and markedly resorbed maxilla. Note that *papilla incisiva* is located in the center of the ridge. This indicates that the entire buccal but also a substantial portion of the palatal ridge are missing.

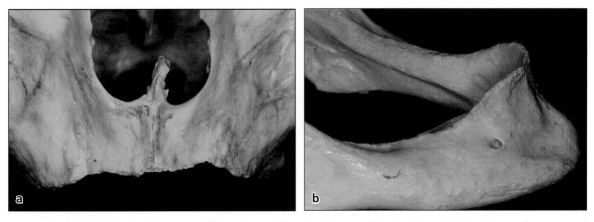

Fig. 2-4 Buccal aspect of a skull preparation illustrating a fully edentulous maxilla (a) and mandible (b). The small segments of the alveolar ridge that still remain are extremely thin in the buccal–palatal/lingual direction.

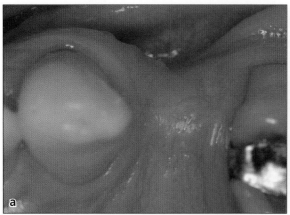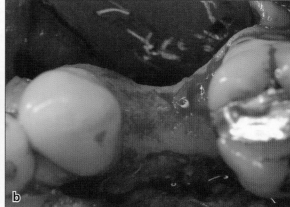

Fig. 2-5 Clinical view of an edentulous ridge in the maxillary premolar region. The premolar was extracted several years before the clinical documentation was made. (a) Note the presence of a buccal invagination of the ridge. (b) Following flap elevation, the crest region of the severely resorbed buccal portion of alveolar process is disclosed.

the contralateral edentulous site were determined by the use of a profile stylus and an imaging technique. Their findings are reported in Table 2-1.

It was concluded that the amount of tissue resorption (hard and soft tissues combined) following the loss of a single tooth was substantial and that the reduction of the ridge was greater along the buccal surface than along the lingual and palatal surfaces in every specimen examined, although the absolute amounts and differences varied from one group of teeth to the next. As a result of this tissue modeling, the center of the edentulous site shifted toward the lingual or palatal aspect of the ridge. The observations made by Pietrokovski and Massler (1967) were supported by recent findings presented by Schropp *et al.* (2003). They studied bone and soft tissue volume changes that took place during a 12-month period following the extraction of single premolars and molars. Clinical as well as cast model measurements were made immediately after tooth extraction and subsequently after 3, 6, and 12 months of healing. It was observed that the buccal–lingual/palatal dimension during the first 3 months was reduced about 30%, and after 12 months the edentulous site had lost at least 50% of its original width. Furthermore, the height of the buccal bone plate was reduced and after 12 months of healing the buccal prominence was located 1.2 mm apical of its lingual/palatal counterpart.

Conclusion: The extraction of single as well as multiple teeth induces a series of adaptive changes in the soft and hard tissues that result in an overall regress of the edentulous site(s). Resorption appears to be more pronounced at the buccal than at lingual/palatal aspects of the ridge.

In this context it should be observed that the alveolar process might also undergo change as the result of tooth-related disease processes, such as aggressive, chronic and necrotizing forms of marginal periodontitis as well as periapical periodontitis. Furthermore, traumatic injuries may cause marked alter-

Table 2-1 Average amount of resorption of tooth extraction in different tooth areas*

Tooth	Average amount of resorption (mm)		Difference
	Buccal surface	Lingual/ palatal surface	
Mandibular teeth			
Central incisor	2.08	0.91	1.17
Lateral incisor	3.54	1.41	2.13
Canine	3.25	1.59	1.66
First premolar	3.45	1.40	2.05
Second premolar	3.28	0.75	2.53
First molar	4.69	2.79	1.90
Second molar	4.30	3.00	1.30
Maxillary teeth			
Central incisor	3.03	1.46	1.57
Lateral incisor	3.47	0.86	2.61
Canine	3.33	1.91	1.42
First premolar	3.33	2.04	1.29
Second premolar	2.58	1.62	0.96
First molar	5.25	3.12	2.13

* "The amount of resorption was greater along the buccal surface than along the lingual or palatal surface in every specimen examined, although the absolute amounts and differences varied very widely. This caused a shift in the center of the edentulous ridge toward the lingual or palatal side of the ridge with a concomitant *decrease* in arch length in the mandible as well as the maxillae." (Pietrokovski & Massler 1967)

ations of the maxilla and mandible including their alveolar processes.

Remaining bone in the edentulous ridge

In the publication by Schropp *et al.* (2003) bone tissue formation in extraction sockets was studied by means of subtraction radiography. Thus, radiographs of the study sites were obtained using a standardized technique immediately after tooth extraction and then

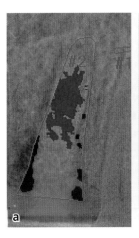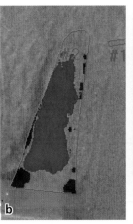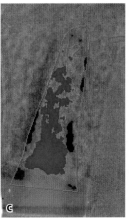

Fig. 2-6 Radiographic (subtraction radiography) images of an extraction site obtained after (a) 3 months, (b) 6 months, and (c) 12 months of healing. The blue color represents areas of new bone formation. During the first 6 months, the deposition of new bone was intense. Between 6 and 12 months, some of the newly formed bone was remodeled. (Courtesy of Dr. L. Schropp.)

after 3, 6, and 12 months of healing (Fig. 2-6). It was observed that in the first few months some bone loss (height) took place in the alveolar crest region. Most of the bone gain in the socket occurred in the first 3 months. There was additional gain of bone in the socket between 3 and 6 months. In the interval between 6 and 12 months, the newly formed bone obviously remodeled and the amount of mineralized tissue was reduced. In other words, towards the end of socket healing small amounts of mineralized tissue may have remained in the center of the edentulous site.

Classification of remaining bone

Based on the volume of remaining mineralized bone, the edentulous sites may, according to Lekhom and Zarb (1985), be classified into five different groups (Fig. 2-7). In groups A and B substantial amounts of the alveolar process still remain, whereas in groups C, D, and E, there are only minute remnants of the alveolar process present. Lekholm and Zarb (1985) also classified the "quality" of the bone in the edentulous site. Class 1 and class 2 characterized a location in which the walls – the cortical plates – of the site are thick and the volume of bone marrow is small. Sites that belong to class 3 and class 4, however, are bordered by relatively thin walls of cortical bone, while the amount of cancellous bone (spongiosa), including trabeculae of lamellar bone and marrow, is large.

Topography of the alveolar process

The dentate alveolar process is defined as the portion of the mandible or maxilla that contains the sockets of the teeth (Fig. 2-8). There is, however, no distinct boundary between the alveolar process and the basal bone of the jaws.

The alveolar process (Fig. 2-9) is comprised of the outer walls – buccal and lingual/palatal cortical plates – and a central portion of spongy bone (anatomic term) – or trabecular bone (radiographic term) or cancellous bone (histologic term) – that contains

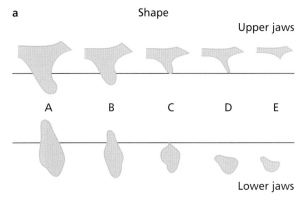
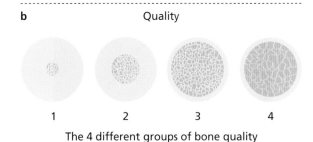

Fig. 2-7 Schematic drawings showing (a) a classification of residual jaw shape, and (b) jaw bone quality, according to Lekholm and Zarb (1985).

bone trabeculae as well as marrow. The cortical plates are continuous with the bone that lines the sockets, i.e. the alveolar bone proper (Fig. 2-10). The alveolar bone proper can also be identified as the cribriform plate (anatomic term; Fig. 2-11), or the lamina dura dentes (radiographic term; Fig. 2-12) or the bundle bone (histologic term; Fig. 2-2b). The bundle bone is the tissue in which the extrinsic collagen fiber bundles of the periodontal ligament are embedded.

The cortical plates (the outer walls) of the alveolar process meet the alveolar bone proper at the crest of the interdental septum (Fig. 2-10); at sites with a normal periodontium this is located about 1–2 mm apical of the cemento-enamel junction of adjacent teeth. In some portions of the anterior dentition, the spongy bone of the alveolar process may be absent.

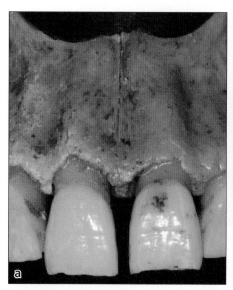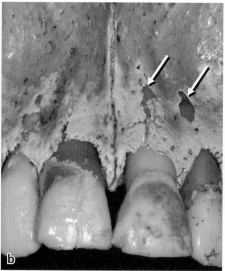

Fig. 2-8 Buccal aspect of the maxillary incisor region of a skull preparation illustrating one subject with a thick (a) and another subject with a thin (b) periodontal biotype. Arrows indicate the presence of fenestrations in the buccal bone.

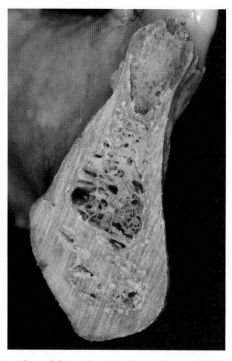

Fig. 2-9 A buccal–lingual section from a human skull preparation illustrating the outer buccal and lingual cortical plates of the alveolar process, as well as the spongy bone in the center of the ridge.

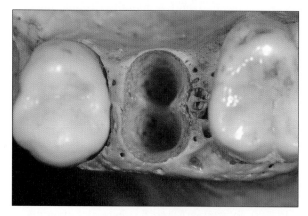

Fig. 2-10 The empty alveolus of a second maxillary premolar is illustrated in the skull preparation. The buccal and palatal cortical plates are continuous with the alveolar bone proper and the bone tissue of the interdental septum. The perforations in the crest region represent the Volkman's canals.

The trabeculae of the spongy bone are orientated in directions that allow them to take up and distribute stress that occurs during mastication and other tooth contacts.

Alterations of the alveolar process following tooth extraction

The alterations that occur in the alveolar ridge following the extraction of single teeth can, for didactic reasons, be divided in two interrelated series of events, namely *intra-alveolar processes* and *extra-alveolar processes*.

Intra-alveolar processes

The healing of extraction sockets in human volunteers was studied by e.g. Amler (1969) and Evian

The cortical plates in such locations are continuous with the alveolar bone proper of the socket.

The cortical plate is made up of lamellar bone. Lamellar bone contains both concentric and interstitial lamellae (see Chapter 1). The spongy bone contains trabeculae of lamellar bone; in the adult these are surrounded by a marrow that is rich in adipocytes and pluripotent, mesenchymal stroma cells (Fig. 2-13). Such cells may be induced to form bone, but also to support the differentiation of hemapoietic cells and thereby the differentiation of osteoclasts.

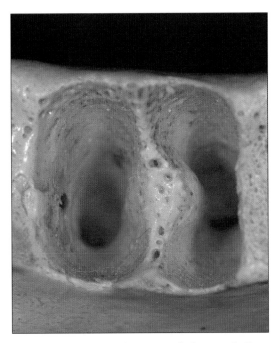

Fig. 2-11 A mandibular molar region of a human skull preparation. The second molar was removed in the skull preparation. In such an anatomic section, the alveolar bone proper (on the inside of the alveolus) is often termed the *cribriform plate*. This is due to the numerous perforations (Volkman's canals) that are present on the bone surface.

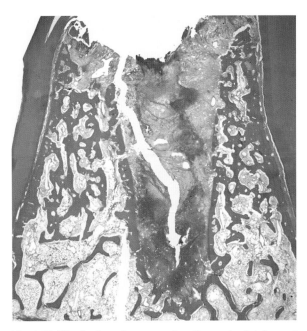

Fig. 2-13 Histologic section presenting the mesio-distal aspect of a fresh extraction socket bordered by two neighboring roots. Note that the alveolar bone from the tooth sites is continuous with the walls of the empty socket. The interdental septum contains cancellous bone including trabeculae of lamellar bone and marrow.

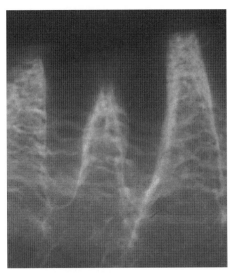

Fig. 2-12 Radiograph obtained from the specimen illustrated in Fig. 2-11. In the radiograph the alveolar bone proper is often identified as lamina dura (dentes).

et al. (1982). Although the biopsy technique used by Amler only allowed the study of healing in the marginal portions of the empty socket, his findings are often referred to. A copy of the drawing included in Amler's publication "The time sequence of tissue regeneration in human extraction wounds" is presented in Fig. 2-14.

Amler stated that following tooth extraction, the first 24 hours are characterized by the formation of a

blood clot in the socket. Within 2–3 days the blood clot is gradually being replaced with *granulation tissue*. After 4–5 days, the *epithelium* from the margins of the soft tissue starts to proliferate to cover the granulation tissue in the socket. One week after extraction, the socket contains granulation tissue, *young connective tissue*, and *osteoid* formation is ongoing in the apical portion of the socket. After 3 weeks, the socket contains connective tissue and there are signs of mineralization of the osteoid. The *epithelium* covers the wound. After 6 weeks of healing, bone formation in the socket is pronounced and trabeculae of newly formed bone can be seen.

Amler's study was of short duration, so it could only evaluate events that took place in the marginal portion of the healing socket. His experimental data did not include the important later phase of socket healing that involves the processes of modeling and remodeling of the newly formed tissue in various parts of the alveolus. Thus, the tissue composition of the fully healed extraction site was not documented in the study.

The results from a recent, long-term experiment in the dog (Cardaropoli *et al.* 2003) will therefore be used to describe more in detail the various phases of socket healing including processes of both modeling and remodeling. Following the elevation of buccal and lingual full-thickness flaps, the distal roots of mandibular premolars were extracted (Fig. 2-15a). The mucosal flaps were managed to provide soft tissue coverage of the fresh extraction wound (Fig. 2-15b). Healing of the extraction sites was monitored

Tooth extraction

Hemorrhagia,
Bleeding,
Blood clot

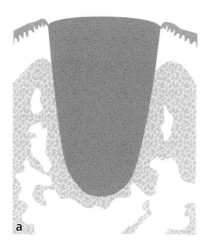

48-72 h after extraction

Blood clot,
Beginning of
granulation tissue formation

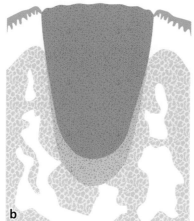

96 h after extraction

Residual blood clot,
Granulation tissue,
Epithelial proliferation

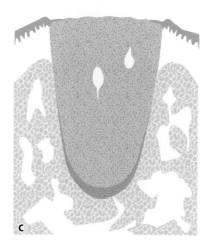

7 days after extraction

Young connective tissue,
Primary osteoid formation,
Epithelial proliferation

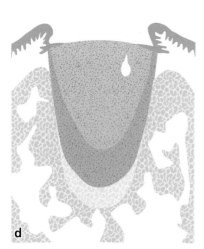

21 days after extraction

Connective tissue,
Osteoid start of mineralization,
Reepithelialization

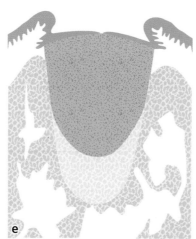

6 weeks after extraction

Connective tissue,
Woven bone, trabeculae,
Reepithelialization

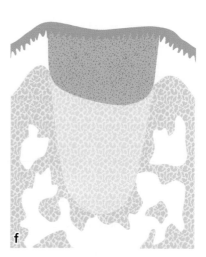

Fig. 2-14 Healing of the alveolar socket after tooth extraction according to Amler (1969). (a) Bleeding and formation of a blood clot immediately after tooth extraction. Blood vessels are closed by trombi and a fibrin network is formed. (b) Already, during the first 48 hours, neutrophilic granulocytes, monocytes and fibroblasts begin to migrate within the fibrin network. (c) The blood clot is slowly replaced by granulation tissue. (d) Granulation tissue forms predominantly in the apical third of the alveolus. There is increased density of fibroblasts. After 4 days, contraction of the clot and proliferation of the oral epithelium is seen. Osteoclasts are visible at the margin of the alveolus. Osteoblasts and osteoids seem to appear in the bottom of the alveolus. (e) Reorganization of the granulation tissue through formation of osteoid trabeculae. Epithelial proliferation from the wound margins on the top of the young connective tissue. Again, the formation of osteoid trabeculae is evident from the wall of the alveolus in a coronal direction. After 3 weeks some of the trabeculae start to mineralize. (f) Radiographically, bone formation may be visible. The soft tissue wound is closed and epithelialized after 6 weeks. However, bone fill in the alveolus takes up to 4 months and does not seem to reach the level of the neighboring teeth.

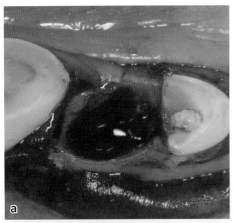
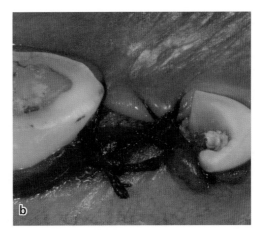
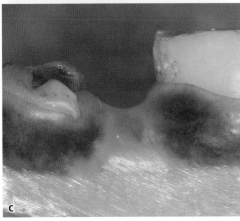

Fig. 2-15 (a) Photograph illustrating a mandibular premolar site (from a dog experiment) from which the distal root of the 4th premolar was removed. (b) The mucosal, full-thickness flaps were replaced and sutured to close the entrance of the socket. (c) The site after 6 months of healing. Note the saddle-shaped outline (loss of tissue) of the alveolar crest region.

in biopsy specimens obtained at time intervals between 1 day and 6 months (Fig. 2-15c).

Overall pattern of socket healing

Figure 2-13 presents a mesio-distal section of a fresh extraction socket bordered by adjacent roots. The socket is filled with a coagulum. The socket walls are continuous with the alveolar bone proper of the neighboring teeth. The tissue inside the interdental (inter-radicular) septa is made up of cancellous bone and includes trabeculae of lamellar bone within bone marrow.

The empty socket is first filled with blood and a *coagulum* (clot) forms (Fig. 2-16a). Inflammatory cells (polymorphonuclear leukocytes and monocytes/ macrophages) migrate into the coagulum and start to phagocytose elements of necrotic tissue. The process of wound cleansing is initiated (Fig. 2-16b). Sprouts of newly formed vessels and mesenchymal cells (from the severed periodontal ligament) enter the coagulum and *granulation tissue* is formed. The granulation tissue is gradually replaced with *provisional connective tissue* (Fig. 2-16c) and subsequently immature bone (*woven bone*) is laid down (Fig. 2-16d). The hard tissue walls of the socket – the alveolar bone proper or the bundle bone – are resorbed and the socket wound becomes filled with woven bone (Fig. 2-16e). The initial phases of the healing process are now completed. In subsequent phases the woven

bone in the socket is gradually remodeled into lamellar bone and marrow (Fig. 2-16f, g, h).

Important events in socket healing

Blood clotting

Immediately after tooth extraction, blood from the severed blood vessels will fill the cavity. Proteins derived from vessels and damaged cells initiate a series of events that lead to the formation of a fibrin network (Fig. 2-17). *Platelets* form aggregates and interact with the fibrin network to produce a *blood clot* (a coagulum) that effectively plugs the severed vessels and stops bleeding. The blood clot acts as a physical matrix that directs cellular movements and it contains substances that are of importance for the forthcoming healing process. Thus, the clot contains substances that (1) influence mesenchymal cells (i.e. *growth factors*) and (2) enhance the activity of inflammatory cells. Such substances will thus induce and amplify the migration of various types of cells into the socket wound, as well as their proliferation, differentiation and synthetic activity within the coagulum.

Although the blood clot is crucial in the initial phase of wound healing, its removal is mandatory to allow the formation of new tissue. Thus, within a few days after the tooth extraction, the blood clot will start to break down, i.e. the process of "fibrinolysis" is initiated (Fig. 2-18).

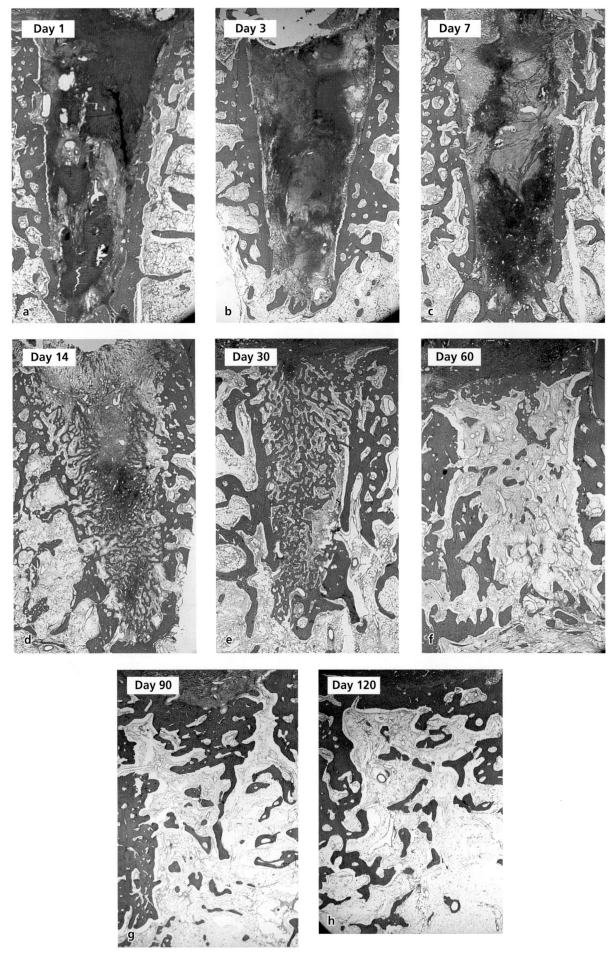

Fig. 2-16 Overall pattern of bone formation in an extraction socket. For details see text.

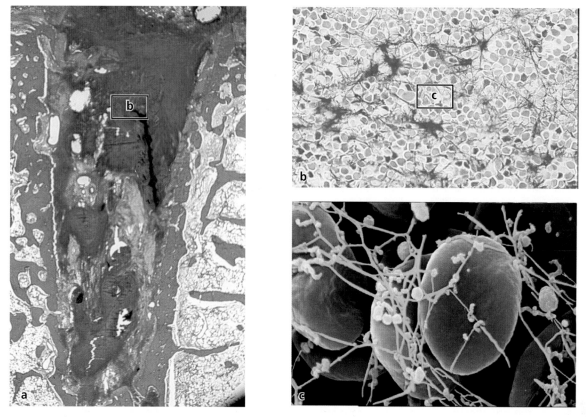

Fig. 2-17 Histologic section (mesio-distal aspect) representing 1 day of healing (a). The socket is occupied with a blood clot that contains large numbers of erythrocytes (b) entrapped in a fibrin network, as well as platelets (blue in (c)).

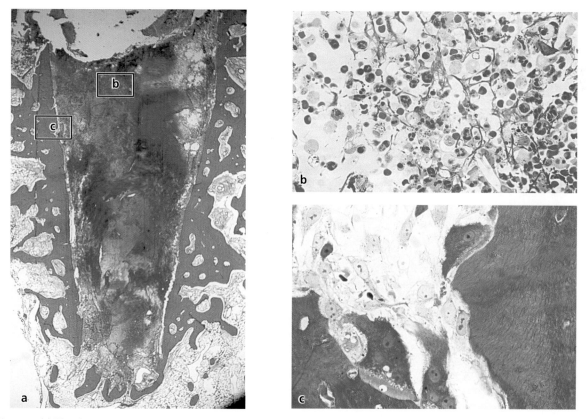

Fig. 2-18 (a) Histologic section (mesio-distal aspect) representing 3 days of healing. (b) Note the presence of neutrophils and macrophages that are engaged in wound cleansing and the break down of the blood clot. (c) Osteoclastic activity occurs on the surface of the old bone in the socket walls.

Wound cleansing

Neutrophils and macrophages migrate into the wound, engulf bacteria and damaged tissue (Fig. 2-18) and clean the site before the formation of new tissue can start. The neutrophils enter the wound early while macrophages appear somewhat later. The macrophages are not only involved in the cleaning of the wound but they also release growth factors and cytokines that further promote the migration, proliferation and differentiation of mesenchymal cells. Once the debris has been removed and the wound has become "sterilized", the neutrophils undergo a programmed cell death (*apoptosis*) and are removed from the site through the action of macrophages. The macrophages subsequently withdraw from the wound.

Tissue formation

Sprouts of vascular structures (from the severed periodontal ligament) as well as mesenchymal, fibroblast-like cells (from the periodontal ligament and from adjacent bone marrow regions) enter the socket. The mesenchymal cells start to proliferate and deposit matrix components in an extracellular location (Fig. 2-19a,b,c); a new tissue, i.e. *granulation tissue*, will gradually replace the blood clot. The granulation tissue eventually contains macrophages, and a large number of fibroblast-like cells as well as numerous newly formed blood vessels. The fibroblast-like cells continue (1) to release growth factors, (2) to prolifer-

ate, and (3) to deposit a new extra cellular matrix that guides the ingrowth of additional cells and allows the further differentiation of the tissue. The newly formed vessels provide the oxygen and nutrients that are needed for the increasing number of cells that occur in the new tissue. The intense synthesis of matrix components exhibited by the mesenchymal cells is called *fibroplasia*, while the formation of new vessels is called *angiogenesis*. A *provisional connective tissue* is established through the combination of fibroplasia and angiogenesis (Fig. 2-20).

The transition of the provisional connective tissue into bone tissue occurs along the vascular structures. Thus, osteoprogenitor cells (e.g. pericytes) migrate and gather in the vicinity of the vessels. They differentiate into osteoblasts that produce a matrix of collagen fibers, which takes on a woven pattern. The *osteoid* is formed. The process of mineralization is initiated within the osteoid. The osteoblasts continue to lay down osteoid and occasionally such cells are trapped in the matrix and become osteocytes. This newly formed bone is called *woven bone* (Fig. 2-21).

The woven bone is the first type of bone to be formed and is characterized by (1) its rapid deposition as fingerlike projections along the route of vessels, (2) the poorly organized collagen matrix, (3) the large number of osteoblasts that are trapped in its mineralized matrix, and (4) its low load-bearing capacity. Trabeculae of woven bone are shaped around and encircle the vessel. The trabeculae become

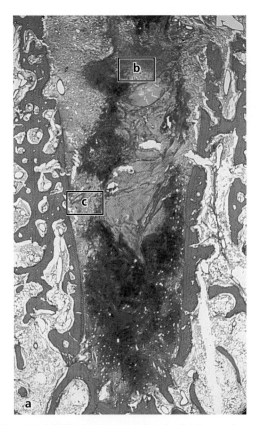

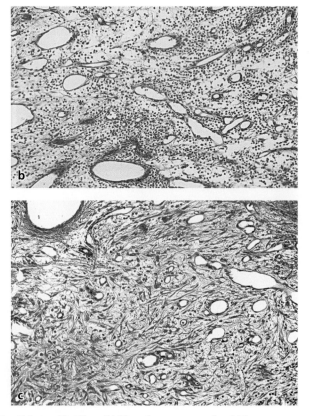

Fig. 2-19 (a) Histologic section (mesio-distal aspect) representing 7 days of healing. (b) Note the presence of a richly vascularized early granulation tissue with large numbers of inflammatory cells in the upper portion of the socket. (c) In more apical areas, a tissue including large numbers of fibroblast-like cells is present, i.e. late granulation tissue.

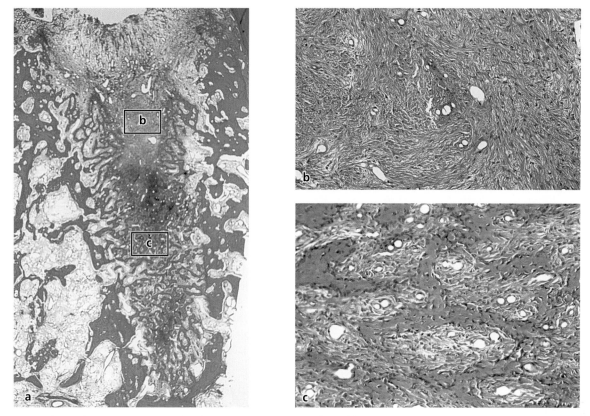

Fig. 2-20 (a) Histologic section (mesio-distal aspect) representing 14 days of healing. (b) In the marginal portion of the wound, a provisional connective tissue rich in fibroblast-like cells is present. (c) The formation of woven bone has at this time interval already begun in apical and lateral regions of the socket.

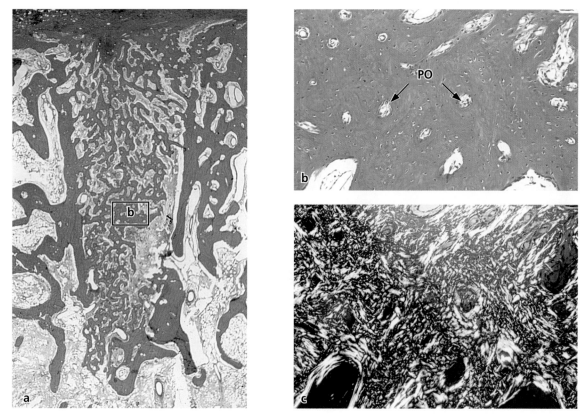

Fig. 2-21 (a) Histologic section (mesio-distal aspect) representing 30 days of healing. The socket is filled with woven bone. (b) This woven bone contains a large number of cells and primary osteons (PO). (c) The woven pattern of the collagen fibers of this type of bone is illustrated (polarized light).

thicker through the deposition of additional woven bone. Cells (osteocytes) become entrapped in the bone tissue and the first set of osteons, the *primary osteons*, are organized. The woven bone is occasionally reinforced by the deposition of so called *parallel-fibered bone*, that has its collagen fibers organized not in a woven but in a concentric pattern.

It is important to realize that during this early phase of healing the bone tissue in the walls of the socket (the bundle bone) is removed and replaced with woven bone.

Tissue modeling and remodeling

The initial bone formation is a fast process. Within a few weeks, the entire extraction socket will become filled with woven bone or, as this tissue is also called, *primary bone spongiosa*. The woven bone offers (1) a stable scaffold, (2) a solid surface, (3) a source of osteoprogenitor cells, and (4) ample blood supply for cell function and matrix mineralization.

The woven bone with its primary osteons is gradually replaced with lamellar bone and bone marrow (Fig. 2-22). In this process, the primary osteons are replaced with *secondary osteons*. The woven bone is first resorbed to a certain level. This level of the resorption front will establish a so-called *reversal line*, which is also the level from which new bone with secondary osteons will form (Fig. 2-23). Although

this remodeling may start early during socket healing it will take several months until all woven bone in the extraction socket has been replaced with lamellar bone and marrow.

An important part of socket healing involves the formation of a *hard tissue cap* that will close the marginal entrance to the socket. This cap is initially comprised of woven bone (Fig. 2-24a) but is subsequently remodeled and replaced with lamellar bone that becomes continuous with the cortical plate at the periphery of the edentulous site (Fig. 2-24b). This process is called corticalization.

The wound is now healed, but the tissues in the site will continue to adapt to functional demands. Since there is no stress from forces elicited during mastication and other occlusal contacts there is no demand on mineralized bone in the areas previously occupied by the tooth. Thus, the socket apical of the hard tissue cap will remodel mainly into marrow. Indeed, in many edentulous patients the entire alveolar ridge will regress as a result of continuous adaptation to lack of function.

Extra-alveolar processes

In an experiment in the dog (Araújo & Lindhe 2005) alterations in the profile of the edentulous ridge that occurred following tooth extraction were carefully examined. In this study the 3rd and 4th mandibular

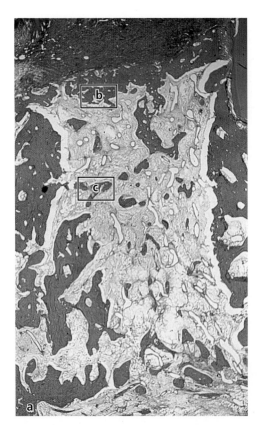
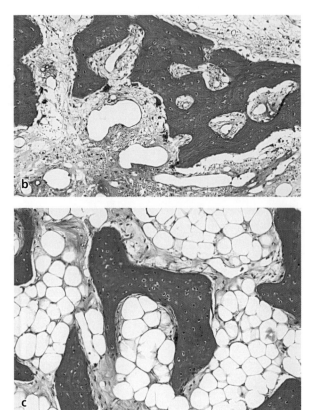

Fig. 2-22 (a) Histologic section (mesio-distal aspect) representing 60 days of healing. (b) A large portion of the woven bone has been replaced with bone marrow. (c) Note the presence of a large number of adipocytes residing in a tissue that still contains woven bone.

Woven bone   BMU   Lamellar bone

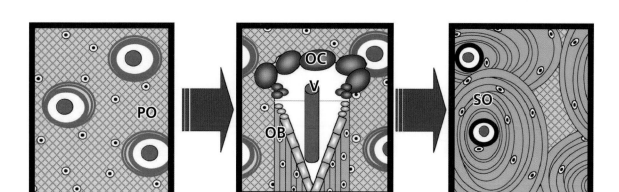

Fig. 2-23 Schematic drawing that describes how woven bone is replaced by lamellar bone. Woven bone with primary osteons is substituted by lamellar bone in a process that involves the presence of bone multicellular units (BMUs). The BMU contains osteoclasts (OC), as well as vascular structures (V) and osteoblasts (OB). Thus, the osteoblasts in the BMU produce bone tissue in a concentric fashion around the vessel, and lamellar bone with secondary osteons is formed.

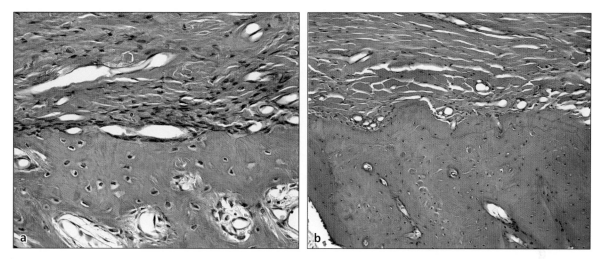

Fig. 2-24 Histologic sections (mesio-distal aspect) describing the hard tissue that has formed at the entrance of a healing extraction socket and the process of corticalization. (a) Woven bone with primary osteons occupies the socket entrance after 60 days of healing. (b) After 180 days the woven bone has been replaced with mainly lamellar bone.

premolars were hemi-sected. Buccal and lingual full-thickness flaps were raised; the distal roots were carefully removed. The flaps were replaced and sutured to cover the fresh extraction socket (Fig. 2-25). Biopsy specimens, including an individual extraction socket and adjacent roots, were obtained after 1, 2, 4, and 8 weeks of healing. The blocks were sectioned in the *buccal–lingual* plane.

Figure 2-26 illustrates a buccal–lingual section of the distal root of an intact 3rd premolar with surrounding soft and hard tissues. The lingual hard tissue wall is substantially wider than its buccal counterpart. The marginal portion of the lingual wall is presented in a higher magnification in Fig. 2-26a. A layer of bundle bone occupies the inner portion of the lingual bone wall. A thin layer of bundle bone is also present at the top of the ridge. Figure 2-26b illustrates the corresponding portion of the buccal bone wall. Note that all the mineralized tissue in the mar-

ginal 1–2 mm of the buccal ridge is comprised of bundle bone. In this context, it must be remembered that bundle bone is part of the attachment tissues for the tooth; this tissue has no obvious function following the removal of the tooth and will thus eventually be resorbed and disappear.

- *1 week after tooth extraction* (Fig. 2-27). At this interval the socket is occupied by a coagulum. Furthermore, a large number of osteoclasts can be seen on the outside as well as on the inside of the buccal and lingual bone walls. The presence of osteoclasts on the inner surface of the socket walls indicates that the bundle bone is being resorbed.
- *2 weeks after tooth extraction* (Fig. 2-28). Newly formed immature bone (woven bone) resides in the apical and lateral parts of the socket, while more central and marginal portions are occupied by a provisional connective tissue. In the marginal

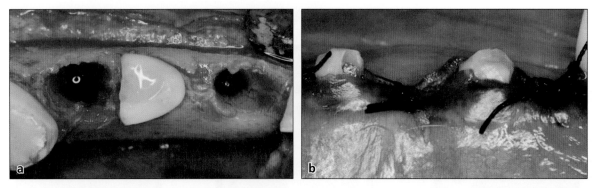

Fig. 2-25 (a) Photograph illustrating mandibular premolar sites (from a dog experiment) from which the distal roots of the 4th and 3rd premolars were extracted. (b) The mucosal, full-thickness flaps were replaced and sutured to close the entrance of the socket.

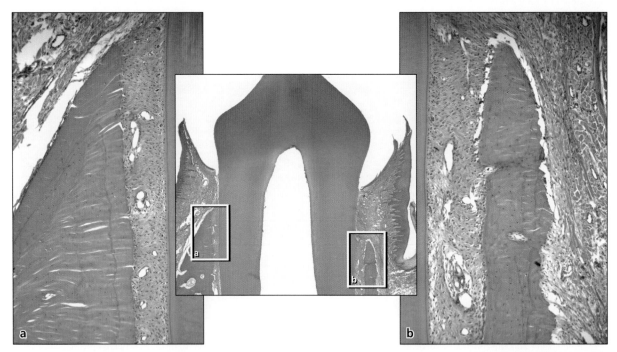

Fig. 2-26 Histologic section (buccal–lingual aspect) of the distal root of an intact 3rd premolar in the dog. Note the wide lingual and thinner buccal bone wall. Higher magnification of the crestal bone of the lingual wall (a) and buccal wall (b). B = buccal bone; L = lingual bone.

and outer portions of the socket walls numerous osteoclasts can be seen. In several parts of the socket walls the bundle bone has been replaced with woven bone.

• *4 weeks after tooth extraction* (Fig. 2-29). The entire socket is occupied with woven bone at this stage of healing. Large numbers of osteoclasts are present in the outer and marginal portions of the hard tissue walls. Osteoclasts also line the trabeculae of woven bone present in the central and lateral aspects of the socket. In other words the newly formed woven bone is being replaced with a more mature type of bone.

• *8 weeks after tooth extraction* (Fig. 2-30). A layer of cortical bone covers the entrance to the extraction site. Corticalization has occurred. The woven bone that was present in the socket at the 4-week interval is replaced with bone marrow and some

trabeculae of lamellar bone in the 8-week specimens. On the outside and on the top of the buccal and lingual bone wall there are signs of ongoing hard tissue resorption. The crest of the buccal bone wall is located apical of its lingual counterpart.

The relative change in the location of the crest of the buccal and lingual bone walls that took place during the 8 weeks of healing is illustrated in Fig. 2-31. While the level of the margin of the lingual wall remained reasonably unchanged, the margin of the buccal wall shifted several millimeters in an apical direction.

There are at least two reasons why, in this animal model, more bone loss occurred in the buccal than in the lingual wall during socket healing. First, prior to tooth extraction, the marginal 1–2 mm

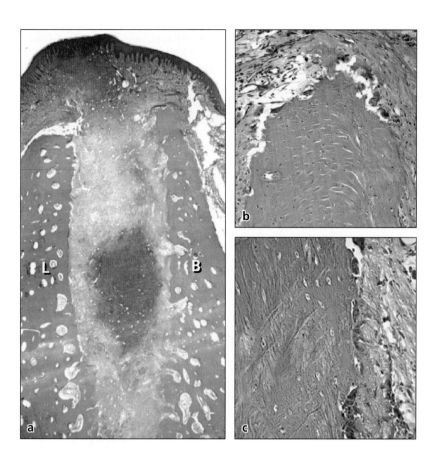

Fig. 2-27 (a) Histologic section (buccal–lingual aspect) of the socket after 1 week of healing. Note the presence of a large number of osteoclasts on the crestal portion (b) and inner portion (c) of the buccal wall. B = buccal bone; L = lingual bone.

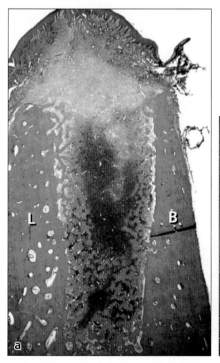

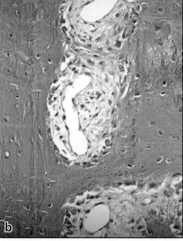

Fig. 2-28 (a) Histologic section (buccal–lingual aspect) of the socket after 2 weeks of healing. (b) Note that the bundle bone in the lingual aspect of the socket is being replaced with woven bone. B = buccal bone; L = lingual bone.

of the crest of the buccal bone wall was occupied by bundle bone. Only a minor fraction of the crest of the lingual wall contained bundle bone. Bundle bone, as stated above, is a tooth-dependent tissue and will gradually disappear after tooth extraction. Thus, since there is relatively more bundle bone in the crest region of the buccal than of the lingual wall,

hard tissue loss will become most pronounced in the buccal wall. Secondly, the lingual bone wall of the socket is markedly wider than that of the buccal wall. It is well known from the periodontal literature (e.g. Wilderman *et al.* 1960; Wilderman 1963; Tavtigian 1970; Wood *et al.* 1972; Araújo *et al.* 2005) that flap elevation and the separation of the periosteum from the bone tissue will result in surface resorption; this will result in more vertical height reduction of the thin buccal than of the wider lingual bone wall.

Topography of the edentulous ridge

As described previously in this chapter, the processes of modeling and remodeling that occur following tooth extraction (loss) result in pronounced resorp-

tion of the various components of the alveolar ridge. The resorption of the buccal bone wall is more pronounced than the resorption of the lingual/palatal wall and hence the center of the ridge will move in lingual/palatal direction. In the extreme case, the entire alveolar process may be lost following tooth loss and in such situations only the bone of the base of the mandible and the base of the maxilla remains.

Figure 2-32 presents a buccal–lingual section of an edentulous site prepared from a biopsy of a dog obtained 2–3 years after tooth extraction. The ridge

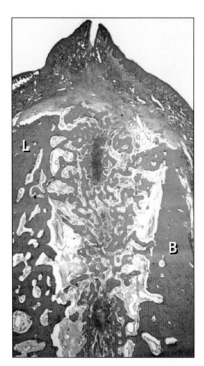

Fig. 2-29 Histologic section (buccal–lingual aspect) of the socket after 4 weeks of healing. The extraction socket is filled with woven bone. On the top of the buccal wall the old bone in the crest region is being resorbed and replaced with either connective tissue or woven bone. B = buccal bone; L = lingual bone.

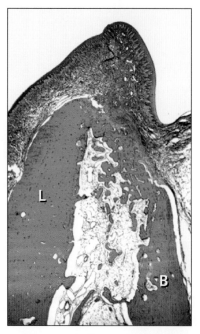

Fig. 2-30 Histologic section (buccal–lingual aspect) of the socket after 8 weeks of healing. The entrance of the socket is sealed with a cap of newly formed mineralized bone. Note that the crest of the buccal wall is located apical of the crest of the lingual wall. B = buccal bone; L = lingual bone.

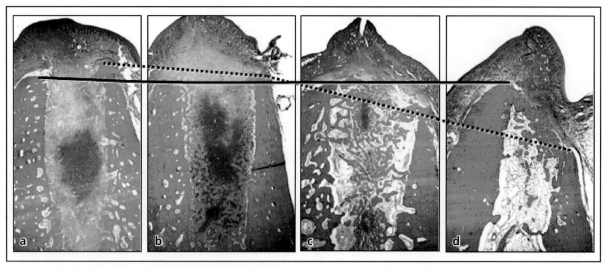

Fig. 2-31 Histologic sections (buccal–lingual aspects) describing the profile of the edentulous region in the dog after (a) 1, (b) 2, (c) 4, and (d) 8 weeks of healing following tooth extraction. While the marginal level of the lingual wall was maintained during the process of healing (solid line), the crest of the buccal wall was replaced >2 mm in the apical direction (dotted line).

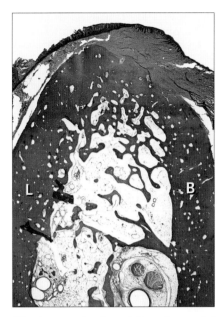

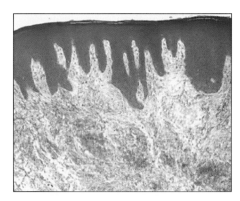

Fig. 2-33 Histologic section illustrating the mucosa residing over the bone crest. The mucosa has a well keratinized epithelium and a connective tissue densely packed with collagen fibers.

Fig. 2-32 Histologic section (buccal–lingual aspect) describing an edentulous mandibular site (from a dog experiment) 2 years after the extraction of the tooth. Note that the crest is higher at the lingual than at the buccal aspect of the site. B = buccal bone; L = lingual bone.

is covered by a mucosa (Fig. 2-33) that in this particular case is about 2–3 mm high and is comprised of keratinized epithelium and dense connective tissue that is attached via the periosteum to the cortical bone. Depending on factors such as the biotype, the jaw (maxilla or mandible), the location (anterior, posterior) in the jaw, location of the muco-gingival junction, depth of the buccal and lingual vestibule, and the amount of hard tissue resorption, the edentulous site may be lined with either masticatory, keratinized mucosa or lining, non-keratinized mucosa.

The outer walls of the remaining portion of the alveolar process are comprised of lamellar bone. The buccal bone plate is comparatively thin and the lingual/palatal plate comparatively thick. The cortical plates enclose the cancellous bone that harbors trabeculae of lamellar bone and marrow. The bone marrow contains numerous vascular structures as well as adipocytes and pluripotent mesenchymal cells. As a rule the ridge of the edentulous site in the maxilla contains comparatively more cancellous bone than a site in the mandible.

References

Amler, M.H. (1969). The time sequence of tissue regeneration in human extraction wounds. *Oral Surgery, Oral Medicine and Oral Pathology* **27**, 309–318.

Araújo, M.G. & Lindhe, J. (2005). Dimensional ridge alterations following tooth extraction. An experimental study in the dog. *Journal of Clinical Periodontology* **32**, 212–218.

Araújo, M.G., Sukekava, F., Wennström, J.L. & Lindhe, J. (2005). Ridge alterations following implant placement in fresh extraction sockets; an experimental study in the dog. *Journal of Clinical Periodontology* **32**, 645–652.

Atwood, D.A. (1962). Some clinical factors related to the rate of resorption of residual ridges. *Journal of Prosthetic Dentistry* **12**, 441–450.

Atwood, D.A. (1963). Postextraction changes in the adult mandible as illustrated by microradiographs of midsagittal section and serial cephalometric roentgenograms. *Journal of Prosthetic Dentistry* **13**, 810–816.

Cardaropoli, G., Araújo, M. & Lindhe, J. (2003). Dynamics of bone tissue formation in tooth extraction sites. An experimental study in dogs. *Journal of Clinical Periodontology* **30**, 809–818.

Carlsson, G.E., Thilander, H. & Hedegård, B. (1967). Histological changes in the upper alveolar process after extraction with or without insertion of an immediate full denture. *Acta Odontologica Scandinavica* **25**, 21–43.

Evian, C.I., Rosenberg, E.S., Cosslet, J.G. & Corn, H. (1982). The osteogenic activity of bone removed from healing extraction sockets in human. *Journal of Periodontology* **53**, 81–85.

Friedenstein, A.G. (1973). Determined and inducible osteogenic precursor cells. In: *Hand Tissue Growth Repair and Remineralization*. Aba Foundation Symposium 11, pp. 169–181.

Johnson, K. (1963). A study of the dimensional changes occurring in the maxilla after tooth extraction. Part I. Normal healing. *Australian Dental Journal* **8**, 241–244.

Johnson, K. (1969). A study of the dimensional changes occurring in the maxilla following tooth extraction. *Australian Dental Journal* **14**, 428–433.

Lekholm, U. & Zarb, G.A. (1985). Patient selection. In: Brånemark, P-I., Zarb, G.A. & Albreksson, T., eds. *Tissue Integrated Prostheses. Osseointegrationin Clinical Dentistry*. Chicago: Quintessence, pp. 199–209.

Pietrokovski, J. & Massler, M. (1967). Alveolar ridge resorption following tooth extraction. *Journal of Prosthetic Dentistry* **17**, 21–27.

Schropp, L., Wenzel, A., Kostopoulos, L. & Karring, T. (2003). Bone healing and soft tissue contour changes following single-tooth extraction: a clinical and radiograhic 12-month prospective study. *International Journal of Periodontics & Restorative Dentistry* **23**, 313–323.

Tavtigian, R. (1970). The height of the facial radicular alveolar crest following apically positioned flap operations. *Journal of Periodontology* **41**, 412–418.

Wilderman, M.N. (1963). Repair after a periosteal retention procedure. *Journal of Periodontology* **34**, 487–503.

Wilderman, M.N., Wentz, F. & Orban, B.J. (1960). Histogenesis of repair after mucogingival surgery. *Journal of Periodontology* **31**, 283–299.

Wood, D.L., Hoag, P.M., Donnenfeld, W.O. & Rosenfeld, L.D. (1972). Alveolar crest reduction following full and partial thickness flaps. *Journal of Periodontology* **42**, 141–144.

Chapter 3

The Mucosa at Teeth and Implants

Jan Lindhe, Jan L. Wennström, and Tord Berglundh

The gingiva

Biologic width

A term frequently used to describe the dimensions of the soft tissues that face the teeth is *the biologic width of the soft tissue attachment*. The development of the *biologic width concept* was based on studies and analyses by, among others, Gottlieb (1921), Orban and Köhler (1924), and Sicher (1959), who documented that the soft tissue attached to the teeth was comprised of two parts, one fibrous tissue and one attachment of epithelium. In a publication by Gargiulo *et al.* (1961) called "Dimensions and relations of the dentogingival junction in humans", sections from autopsy block specimens that exhibited different degree of "passive tooth eruption" (i.e. periodontal tissue breakdown) were examined. Histometric assessments were made to describe the length of the sulcus (not part of the attachment), the epithelial attachment (today called junctional epithelium), and of the connective tissue attachment (Fig. 3-1). It was observed that the length of the connective tissue attachment varied within narrow limits (1.06–1.08 mm) while the length of the attached epithelium was about 1.4 mm at sites with normal periodontium, 0.8 mm at sites with moderate and 0.7 mm at sites with advanced periodontal tissue breakdown. In other words, (1) the biologic width of the attachment varied between about 2.5 mm in the normal case and 1.8 mm in the advanced disease case, and (2) the most variable part of the attachment was the length of the epithelial attachment (junctional epithelium).

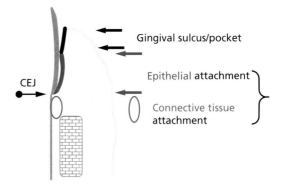

Fig. 3-1 Drawing describing the "biologic width" of the soft tissue attachment at the buccal surface of a tooth with healthy periodontium. The combined length of the junctional epithelium (epithelial attachment) and the connective tissue attachment is considered to represent the "biologic width" of the soft tissue attachment. Note the gingival sulcus is NOT part of the attachment.

Dimensions of the buccal tissue

The morphologic characteristics of the gingiva are related to the dimension of the alveolar process, the form (anatomy) of the teeth, events that occur during tooth eruption, and the eventual inclination and position of the fully erupted teeth (Wheeler 1961; O'Connor & Biggs 1964; Weisgold 1977). Ochenbein

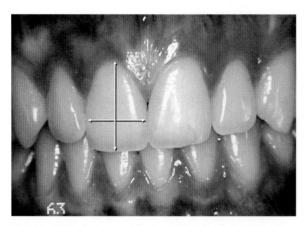

Fig. 3-2 Clinical photograph of a subject that belongs to the "pronounced scalloped" gingival biotype. The crowns of the teeth are comparatively long and slender. The papillae are comparatively long, the gingival margin is thin and the zone of attached gingiva is short.

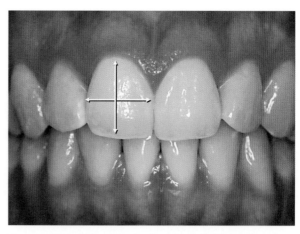

Fig. 3-3 Clinical photograph of a subject that belongs to the "flat" gingival biotype. The crowns of the teeth are comparatively short but wide. The papillae are comparatively short but voluminous and the zone of attached gingiva is wide.

and Ross (1969) and Becker *et al.* (1997) proposed (1) that the anatomy of the gingiva is related to the contour of the osseous crest, and (2) that two basic types of gingival architecture may exist, namely the "*pronounced scalloped*" and the "*flat*" biotype.

Subjects who belong to the "*pronounced scalloped*" biotype have long and slender teeth with tapered crown form, delicate cervical convexity and minute interdental contact areas that are located close to the incisal edge (Fig. 3-2). The maxillary front teeth of such individuals are surrounded with a thin free gingiva, the buccal margin of which is located at or apical of the cemento-enamel junction. The zone of gingiva is narrow, and the outline of the gingival margin is highly scalloped (Olsson *et al.* 1993). On the other hand, subjects who belong to the "*flat*" gingival biotype have incisors with squared crown form with pronounced cervical convexity (Fig. 3-3). The gingiva of such individuals is wider and more voluminous, the contact areas between the teeth are large and more apically located, and the interdental papillae are short. It was reported that subjects with pronounced scalloped gingiva often exhibited more advanced soft tissue recession in the anterior maxilla than subjects with a flat gingiva (Olsson & Lindhe 1991).

Kan *et al.* (2003) measured the dimension of the gingiva – as determined by bone sounding – at the buccal-mesial and buccal-distal aspects of maxillary anterior teeth. Bone sounding determines the distance between the soft tissue margin and the crest of the bone and, hence, provides an estimate that is about 1 mm greater than that obtained in a regular probing pocket depth measurement. The authors reported that the thickness of the gingiva varied between subjects of different gingival biotypes. Thus, the height of the gingiva at the buccal-approximal

surfaces in subjects who belonged to the flat biotype was, on average, 4.5 mm, while in subjects belonging to the pronounced scalloped biotype the corresponding dimension (3.8 mm) was significantly smaller. This indicates that subjects who belong to the flat biotype have more voluminous soft buccal/approximal tissues than subjects who belong to the pronounced scalloped biotype.

Pontoriero and Carnevale (2001) performed evaluations of the reformation of the gingival unit at the buccal aspect of teeth exposed to crown lengthening procedures using a denudation technique. At the 1-year follow-up examination after surgery the regain of soft tissue – measured from the level of the denuded osseous crest – was greater in patients with a thick (flat) biotype than in those with a thin (pronounced scalloped) biotype (3.1 mm versus 2.5 mm). No assessment was made of the bone level change that had occurred between the baseline and the follow-up examination. It must, however, be anticipated that some bone resorption had taken place during healing and that the biologic width of the new connective tissue attachment had been re-established coronal to the level of the resected osseous crest.

The dimensions of the buccal gingiva may also be affected by the buccal–lingual position of the tooth within the alveolar process. A change of the tooth position in buccal direction results in reduced dimensions of the buccal gingiva, while an increase is observed following a lingual tooth movement (Coatoam *et al.* 1981; Andlin-Sobocki & Brodin 1993). In fact, Müller and Könönen (2005) demonstrated in a study of the variability of the thickness of the buccal gingiva of young adults that most of the variation in gingival thickness was due to the tooth position and that the contribution of subject variability (i.e. flat and pronounced scalloped) was minimal.

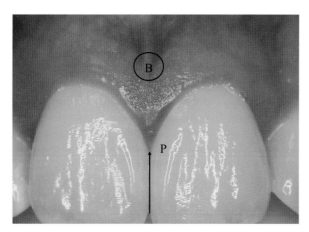

Fig. 3-4 Tarnow *et al.* (1992) measured the distance between the contact point (P) between the crowns of the teeth and the bone crest (B) using sounding (transgingival probing).

Dimensions of the interdental papilla

The interdental papilla in a normal, healthy dentition has one buccal and one lingual/palatal component that are joined in the col region (Chapter 1; Figs. 1-1–1-9). Experiments performed in the 1960s (Kohl & Zander 1961; Matherson & Zander 1963) revealed that the shape of the papilla in the col region was not determined by the outline of the bone crest but by the shape of the contact relationship that existed between adjacent teeth.

Tarnow *et al.* (1992) studied whether the distance between the contact point (area) between teeth and the crest of the corresponding inter-proximal bone could influence the degree of papilla fill that occurred at the site. Presence or absence of a papilla was determined visually in periodontally healthy subjects. If there was no space visible apical of the contact point, the papilla was considered complete. If a "black space" was visible at the site, the papilla was considered incomplete. The distance between the facial level of the contact point and the bone crest (Fig. 3-4) was measured by sounding. The measurement thus included not only the epithelium and connective tissue of the papilla but in addition the entire supra-alveolar connective tissue in the inter-proximal area (Fig. 3-5). The authors reported that the papilla was always complete when the distance from the contact point to the crest of the bone was ≤5 mm. When this distance was 6 mm, papilla fill occurred in about 50% of cases and at sites where the distance was ≥7 mm, the papilla fill was incomplete in about 75% of cases. Considering that the supracrestal connective tissue attachment is about 1 mm high, the above data indicate that the papilla height may be limited to about 4 mm in most cases. Interestingly, papillae of similar height (3.2–4.3 mm) were found to reform following surgical denudation procedures (van der Velden 1982; Pontoriero & Carnevale 2001), but to a greater

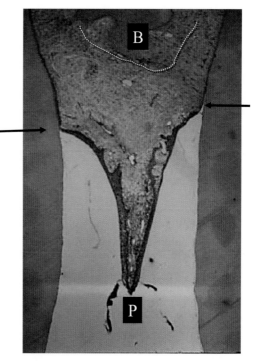

Fig. 3-5 Mesio-distal section of the interproximal area between the two central incisors. Arrows indicate the location of the cemento-enamel junction. Dotted line indicates the outline of the marginal bone crest. The distance between the contact point (P) between the crowns of the teeth and the bone crest (B) indicates the height of the papilla.

height in patients with a thick (flat) than in those with a thin (pronounced scalloped) biotype.

Summary

- *Flat gingival (periodontal) biotype*: the buccal marginal gingiva is comparatively thick, the papillae are often short, the bone of the buccal cortical wall is thick, and the vertical distance between the interdental bone crest and the buccal bone is short (about 2 mm).
- *Pronounced scalloped gingival (periodontal) biotype*: the buccal marginal gingiva is delicate and may often be located apical of the cemento-enamel junction (receded), the papillae are high and slender, the buccal bone wall is often thin and the vertical distance between the interdental bone crest and the buccal bone is long (>4 mm).

The peri-implant mucosa

The soft tissue that surrounds dental implants is termed *peri-implant mucosa*. Features of the peri-implant mucosa are established during the process of wound healing that occurs subsequent to the closure of mucoperiosteal flaps following implant installation (one-stage procedure) or following abutment connection (two-stage procedure) surgery. Healing of the mucosa results in the establishment of a soft tissue attachment (transmucosal attachment) to the implant. This attachment serves as a seal that prevents products from the oral cavity reaching the bone tissue, and thus ensures osseointegration and the rigid fixation of the implant.

The peri-implant mucosa and the gingiva have several clinical and histological characteristics in common. Some important differences, however, also exist between the gingiva and the peri-implant mucosa.

Biologic width

The structure of the mucosa that surrounds implants made of titanium has been examined in man and several animal models (for review see Berglundh 1999). In an early study in the dog, Berglundh *et al.* (1991) compared some anatomic features of the gingiva (at teeth) and the mucosa at implants. Since the research protocol from this study was used in subsequent experiments that will be described in this chapter, details regarding the protocol are briefly outlined here.

The mandibular premolars in one side of the mandible were extracted, leaving the corresponding teeth in the contralateral jaw quadrant. After 3 months of healing following tooth extraction (Fig. 3-6) the fixture part of implants (Brånemark system®, Nobel

Biocare, Gothenburg, Sweden) were installed (Fig. 3-7) and submerged according to the guidelines given in the manual for the system. Another 3 months later, abutment connection was performed (Fig. 3-8) in a second-stage procedure, and the animals were placed in a carefully monitored plaque-control program. Four months subsequent to abutment connection, the dogs were exposed to a clinical examination following which biopsy specimens of several tooth and all implant sites were harvested.

The clinically healthy gingiva and peri-implant mucosa had a pink color and a firm consistency (Fig. 3-9). In radiographs obtained from the tooth sites it

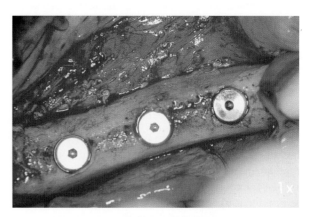

Fig. 3-7 Three titanium implants (i.e. the fixture part and cover screw; Brånemark System®) are installed.

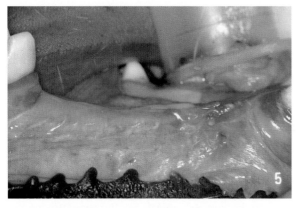

Fig. 3-6 The edentulous mandibular right premolar region 3 months following tooth extraction (from Berglundh *et al.* 1991).

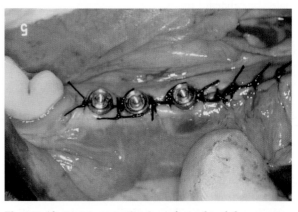

Fig. 3-8 Abutment connection is performed and the mucosa sutured with interrupted sutures.

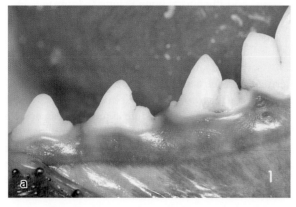

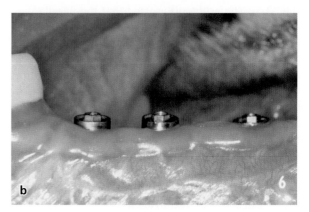

Fig. 3-9 After 4 months of careful plaque control the gingiva (a) and the peri-implant mucosa (b) are clinically healthy.

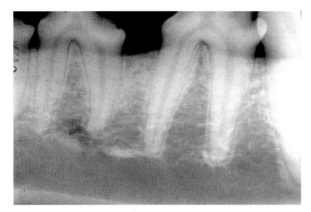

Fig. 3-10 Radiograph obtained from the premolars in the left side of the mandible.

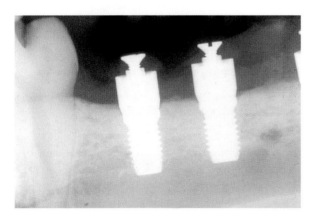

Fig. 3-11 Radiograph obtained from the implants in the right side of the mandible.

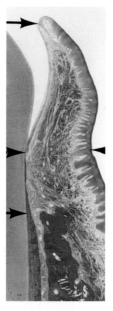

Fig. 3-12 Microphotograph of a cross section of the buccal and coronal part of the periodontium of a mandibular premolar. Note the position of the soft tissue margin (top arrow), the apical cells of the junctional epithelium (center arrow) and the crest of the alveolar bone (bottom arrow). The junctional epithelium is about 2 mm long and the supracrestal connective tissue portion about 1 mm high.

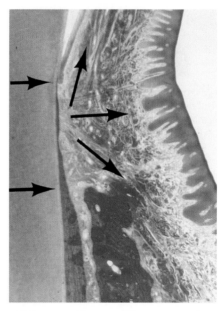

Fig. 3-13 Higher magnification of the supracrestal connective tissue portion seen in Fig. 3-12. Note the direction of the principal fibers (arrows).

was observed that the alveolar bone crest was located about 1 mm apical of a line connecting the cemento-enamel junction of neighboring premolars (Fig. 3-10). The radiographs from the implant sites disclosed that the bone crest was close to the junction between the abutment and the fixture part of the implant (Fig. 3-11).

Histological examination of the sections revealed that the two soft tissue units, the gingiva and the peri-implant mucosa, had several features in common. The oral epithelium of the gingiva was well keratinized and continuous with the thin junctional epithelium that faced the enamel and that ended at the cemento-enamel junction (Fig. 3-12). The supra-alveolar connective tissue was about 1 mm high and the periodontal ligament about 0.2–0.3 mm wide. The principal fibers were observed to extend from the root cementum in a fan-shaped pattern into the soft and hard tissues of the marginal periodontium (Fig. 3-13).

The outer surface of the peri-implant mucosa was also covered by a keratinized oral epithelium, which in the marginal border connected with a thin barrier epithelium (similar to the junctional epithelium at the teeth) that faced the abutment part of the implant (Fig. 3-14). It was observed that the barrier epithelium was only a few cell layers thick (Fig. 3-15) and

that the epithelial structure terminated about 2 mm apical of the soft tissue margin (Fig. 3-14) and 1–1.5 mm from the bone crest. The connective tissue in the compartment above the bone appeared to be in direct contact with the surface (TiO_2) of the implant (Figs. 3-14, 3-15, 3-16). The collagen fibers in this connective tissue apparently originated from the periosteum of the bone crest and extend towards the margin of the soft tissue in directions parallel to the surface of the abutment.

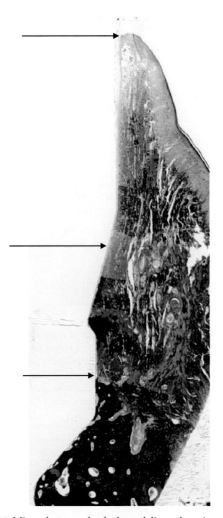

Fig. 3-14 Microphotograph of a buccal–lingual section of the peri-implant mucosa. Note the position of the soft tissue margin (top arrow), the apical cells of the junctional epithelium (center arrow), and the crest of the marginal bone (bottom arrow). The junctional epithelium is about 2 mm long and the implant–connective tissue interface about 1.5 mm high.

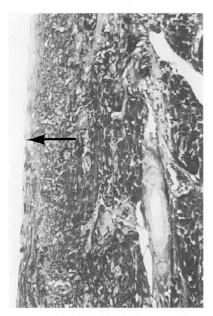

Fig. 3-15 Higher magnification of the apical portion of the barrier epithelium (arrow) in Fig. 3-14.

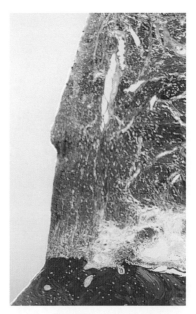

Fig. 3-16 Microphotograph of a section (buccal–lingual) of the implant–connective tissue interface of the peri-implant mucosa. The collagen fibers invest in the periosteum of the bone and project in directions parallel to the implant surface towards the margin of the soft tissue.

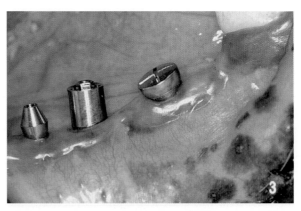

Fig. 3-17 Implants of three systems installed in the mandible of a beagle dog. Astra Tech Implants® Dental System (left), Brånemark System® (center) and ITI® Dental Implant System (right).

The observation that the barrier epithelium of the healthy mucosa consistently ended at a certain distance (1–1.5 mm) from the bone is important. During healing following implant installation surgery, fibroblasts of the connective tissue of the mucosa apparently formed a biological attachment to the TiO_2 layer of the "apical" portion of the abutment portion of the implant. This attachment zone was evidently not recognized as a wound and was therefore not covered with an epithelial lining.

In further dog experiments (Abrahamsson *et al.* 1996, 2002) it was observed that a similar mucosal attachment formed when different types of implant systems were used (e.g. Astra Tech Implant System, Astra Tech Dental, Mölndal, Sweden; Brånemark System®, Nobel Biocare, Göteborg, Sweden; Strau-

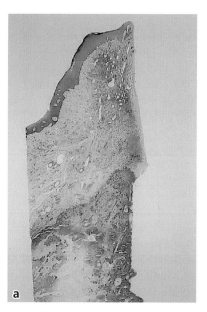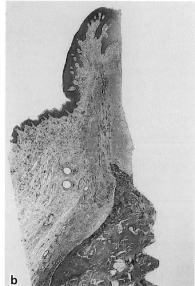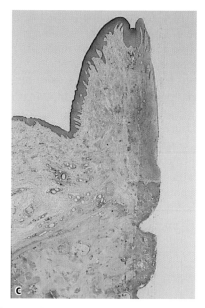

Fig. 3-18 Microphotographs illustrating the mucosa (buccal–lingual view) facing the three implant systems. (a) Astra. (b) Brånemark. (c) ITI.

mann® Dental Implant System, Straumann AG, Basel, Switzerland; 3i® Implant System, Implant Innovation Inc., West Palm Beach, FL, USA). In addition, the formation of the attachment appeared to be independent of whether the implants were initially submerged or not (Figs. 3-17, 3-18).

In another study (Abrahamsson *et al.* 1998), it was demonstrated that the material used in the abutment part of the implant was of decisive importance for the location of the connective tissue portion of the transmucosal attachment. Abutments made of aluminum-based sintered ceramic (Al_2O_3) allowed for the establishment of a mucosal attachment similar to that which occurred at titanium abutments. Abutments made of a gold alloy or dental porcelain, however, provided conditions for inferior mucosal healing. When such materials were used, the connective tissue attachment failed to develop at the abutment level. Instead, the connective tissue attachment occurred in a more apical location. Thus, during healing following the abutment connection surgery, some resorption of the marginal peri-implant bone took place to expose the titanium portion of the fixture (Brånemark System®) to which the connective tissue attachment was eventually formed.

The location and dimensions of the transmucosal attachment were examined in a dog experiment by Berglundh and Lindhe (1996). Implants (fixtures) of the Brånemark System® were installed in edentulous premolar sites and submerged. After 3 months of healing, abutment connection was performed. In the left side of the mandible the volume of the ridge mucosa was maintained while in the right side the vertical dimension of the mucosa was reduced to ≤2 mm (Fig. 3.19) before the flaps were replaced and sutured. In biopsy specimens obtained after another 6 months, it was observed that the transmucosal

Flap adaptation and suturing

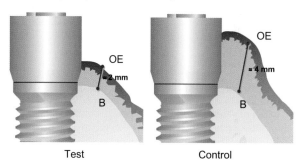

Test   Control

Fig. 3-19 Schematic drawing illustrating that the mucosa at the test site was reduced to about 2 mm. From Berglundh & Lindhe (1996).

attachment at all implants included one barrier epithelium that was about 2 mm long and one zone of connective tissue attachment that was about 1.3–1.8 mm high.

A further examination disclosed that at sites with a thin mucosa, wound healing consistently had included marginal bone resorption to establish space for a mucosa that eventually could harbor both the epithelial and the connective tissue components of the transmucosal attachment (Figs. 3-20, 3-21).

The dimensions of the epithelial and connective tissue components of the transmucosal attachment at implants are established during wound healing following implant surgery. As is the case for bone healing after implant placement (see Chapter 5), the wound healing in the mucosa around implants is a delicate process that requires several weeks of tissue remodeling.

In a recent animal experiment, Berglundh *et al.* (2007) described the morphogenesis of the mucosa attachment to implants made of c.p. titanium. A non-submerged implant installation technique was used and the mucosal tissues were secured to the conical marginal portion of the implants (Straumann® Dental Implant System) with interrupted sutures. The sutures were removed after 2 weeks and a plaque-control program was initiated. Biopsies were performed at various intervals to provide healing periods extending from day 0 (2 hours) to 12 weeks. It was reported that large numbers of neutrophils infiltrated and degraded the coagulum that occupied the compartment between the mucosa and the implant during the initial phase of healing. The first signs of epithelial proliferation were observed in specimens representing 1–2 weeks of healing and a mature barrier epithelium was seen after 6–8 weeks. It was also demonstrated that the collagen fibers of the mucosa were organized after 4–6 weeks of healing. Thus, prior to this time interval, the connective tissue is not properly arranged.

Conclusion

The junctional and barrier epithelia are about 2 mm long and the zones of supra-alveolar connective tissue are between 1 and 1.5 mm high. Both epithelia are attached via hemi-desmosomes to the tooth/implant surface (Gould *et al.* 1984). The main attachment fibers (the principal fibers) invest in the root cementum of the tooth, but at the implant site the equivalent fibers run in a direction parallel with the implant and fail to attach to the metal body. The soft tissue attachment to implants is properly established several weeks following surgery.

Quality

The quality of the connective tissue in the supra-alveolar compartments at teeth and implants was examined by Berglundh *et al.* (1991). The authors observed that the main difference between the mesenchymal tissue present at a tooth and at an implant site was the occurrence of a cementum on the root surface. From this cementum (Fig. 3-22), coarse dento-gingival and dento-alveolar collagen fiber bundles projected in lateral, coronal, and apical

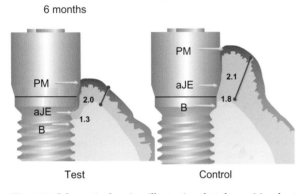

Fig. 3-20 Schematic drawing illustrating that the peri-implant mucosa at both control and test sites contained a 2 mm long barrier epithelium and a zone of connective tissue that was about 1.3–1.8 mm high. Bone resorption occurred in order to accommodate the soft tissue attachment at sites with a thin mucosa. From Berglundh & Lindhe (1996).

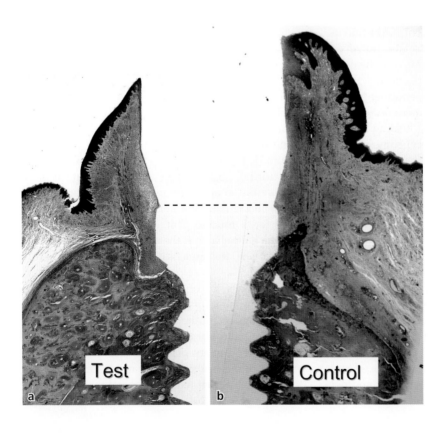

Fig. 3-21 Microphotograph illustrating the peri-implant mucosa of a normal dimension (left) and reduced dimension (right). Note the angular bone loss that had occurred at the site with the thin mucosa.

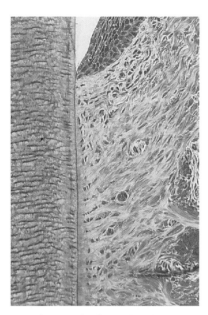

Fig. 3-22 Microphotograph of a tooth with marginal periodontal tissues (buccal–lingual section). Note on the tooth side the presence of an acellular root cementum with inserting collagen fibers. The fibers are orientated more or less perpendicular to the root surface.

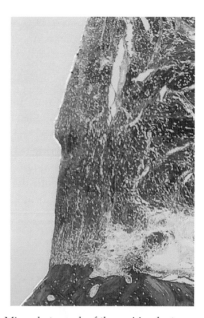

Fig. 3-23 Microphotograph of the peri-implant mucosa and the bone at the tissue/titanium interface. Note that the orientation of the collagen fibers is more or less parallel (not perpendicular) to the titanium surface.

directions (Fig. 3-13). At the implant site, the collagen fiber bundles were orientated in an entirely different manner. Thus, the fibers invested in the periosteum at the bone crest and projected in directions parallel with the implant surface (Fig. 3-23). Some of the fibers became aligned as coarse bundles in areas distant from the implant (Buser *et al.* 1992).

The connective tissue in the supra-crestal area at implants was found to contain more collagen fibers, but fewer fibroblasts and vascular structures, than the tissue in the corresponding location at teeth. Moon *et al.* (1999), in a dog experiment, reported that the attachment tissue close to the implant (Fig. 3-24) contained only few blood vessels but a large number of fibroblasts that were orientated with their long axes parallel with the implant surface (Fig. 3-25). In more lateral compartments, there were fewer fibroblasts but more collagen fibers and more vascular structures. From these and other similar findings it may be concluded that the connective tissue attachment between the titanium surface and the connective tissue is established and maintained by fibroblasts.

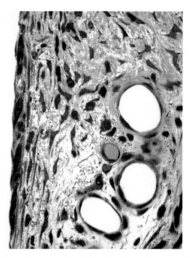

Fig. 3-24 Microphotograph of the implant/connective tissue interface of the peri-implant mucosa. A large number of fibroblasts reside in the tissue next to the implant.

Vascular supply

The vascular supply to the gingiva comes from two different sources (Fig. 3-26). The first source is represented by the large *supraperiosteal blood vessels*, that put forth branches to form (1) the capillaries of the connective tissue papillae under the oral epithelium and (2) the vascular plexus lateral to the junctional epithelium. The second source is the *vascular plexus of the periodontal ligament*, from which branches run in a coronal direction and terminate in the supra-

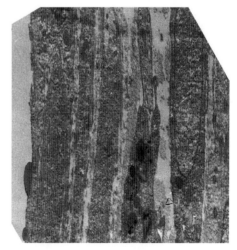

Fig. 3-25 Electron micrograph of the implant–connective tissue interface. Elongated fibroblasts are interposed between thin collagen fibrils (magnification ×24 000).

alveolar portion of the free gingiva. Thus, the blood supply to the zone of supra-alveolar connective tissue attachment in the periodontium is derived from two apparently independent sources (see also Chapter 1).

Berglundh *et al.* (1994) observed that the vascular system of the peri-implant mucosa of dogs (Fig. 3-27) originated *solely* from the large *supra-periosteal blood vessel* on the outside of the alveolar ridge. This vessel that gave off branches to the supra-alveolar mucosa and formed (1) the capillaries beneath the oral epithelium and (2) the vascular plexus located immedi-

ately lateral to the barrier epithelium. The connective tissue part of the transmucosal attachment to titanium implants contained only few vessels, all of which could be identified as terminal branches of the *supra-periosteal blood vessels.*

Summary

The gingiva at teeth and the mucosa at dental implants have some characteristics in common, but differ in the composition of the connective tissue, the alignment of the collagen fiber bundles, and the distribution of vascular structures in the compartment apical of the barrier epithelium.

Probing gingiva and peri-implant mucosa

It was assumed for many years that the tip of the probe in a pocket depth measurement identified the most apical cells of the junctional (pocket) epithelium or the marginal level of the connective tissue attachment. This assumption was based on findings by, for example, Waerhaug (1952), who reported that the "epithelial attachment" (e.g. Gottlieb 1921; Orban & Köhler 1924) offered no resistance to probing. Waerhaug (1952) inserted, "with the greatest caution", thin blades of steel or acrylic in the gingival pocket of various teeth of >100 young subjects without signs of periodontal pathology. In several sites the blades were placed in approximal pockets, "in which position radiograms were taken of them". It was concluded that the insertion of the blades could be performed without a resulting bleeding and that the device consistently reached to the cemento-enamel junction (Fig. 3.28). Thus, the epithelium or the epithelial attachment offered no resistance to the insertion of the device.

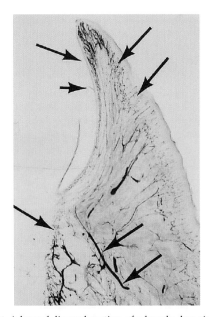

Fig. 3-26 A buccal–lingual section of a beagle dog gingiva. Cleared section. The vessels have been filled with carbon. Note the presence of a supraperiosteal vessel on the outside of the alveolar bone, the presence of a plexus of vessels within the periodontal ligament, as well as vascular structures in the very marginal portion of the gingiva.

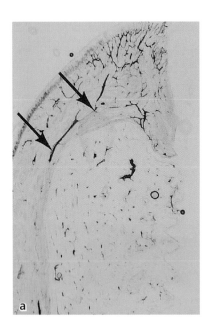
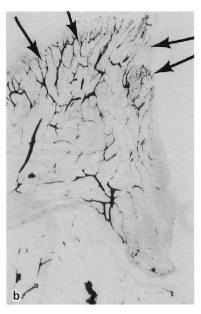

Fig. 3-27 (a) A buccal–lingual cleared section of a beagle dog mucosa facing an implant (the implant was positioned to the right). Note the presence of a supraperiosteal vessel on the outside of the alveolar bone, but also that there is no vasculature that corresponds to the periodontal ligament plexus. (b) Higher magnification (of a) of the peri-implant soft tissue and the bone implant interface. Note the presence of a vascular plexus lateral to the junctional epithelium, but the absence of vessels in the more apical portions of the soft tissue facing the implant and the bone.

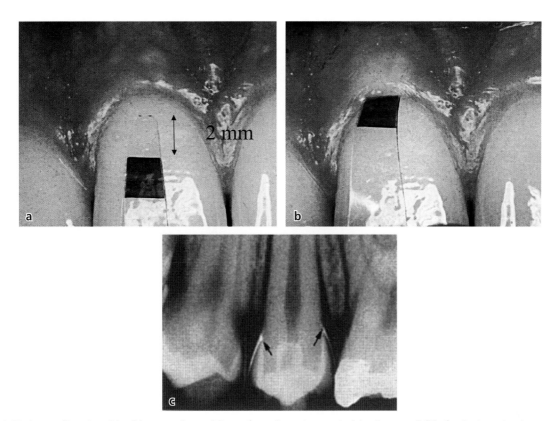

Fig. 3-28 An acrylic strip with a blue zone located 2 mm from the strip margin (a) prior to and (b) after its insertion into a buccal "pocket". The strip could with a light force be inserted 2 mm into the "pocket". (c) Thin blades of steel were inserted in pockets at approximal sites of teeth with healthy periodontal conditions. In radiographs, Waerhaug (1952) could observe that the blades consistently reached the cemento-enamel junction.

In subsequent studies it was observed, however, that the tip of a periodontal probe in a pocket depth measurement only identified the base of the dento-gingival epithelium by chance. In the absence of an inflammatory lesion the probe frequently failed to reach the apical part of the junctional epithelium (e.g. Armitage *et al.* 1977; Magnusson & Listgarten 1980). If an inflammatory lesion, rich in leukocytes and poor in collagen, was present in the gingival connective tissue, however, the probe penetrated beyond the epithelium to reach the apical–lateral border of the infiltrate.

The outcome of probing depth measurements at *implant sites* was examined in various animal models. Ericsson and Lindhe (1993) used the model by Berglundh *et al.* (1991) referred to above and, hence, had both teeth and implants available for examination. The gingiva at mandibular premolars and the mucosa at correspondingly positioned implants (Brånemark System®) were, after extended periods of plaque control, considered clinically healthy. A probe with a tip diameter of 0.5 mm was inserted into the buccal "pocket" using a standardized force of 0.5 N. The probe was anchored to the tooth or to the implant and biopsies from the various sites were performed. The histologic examination of the biopsy material revealed that probing the dento-gingival interface had resulted in a slight compression of the gingival

tissue. The tip of the probe was located coronal to the apical cells of the junctional epithelium. At the implant sites, probing caused both compression and a lateral dislocation of the peri-implant mucosa, and the average "histologic" probing depth was markedly deeper than at the tooth site: 2.0 mm versus 0.7 mm. The tip of the probe was consistently positioned deep in the connective tissue/abutment interface and apical of the barrier epithelium. The distance between the probe tip and the bone crest at the tooth sites was about 1.2 mm. The corresponding distance at the implant site was 0.2 mm. The findings presented by Ericsson and Lindhe (1993) regarding the difference in probe penetration in healthy gingiva and peri-implant mucosa are not in agreement with data reported in subsequent animal experiments.

Lang *et al.* (1994) used beagle dogs and prepared the implant (Straumann® Dental Implant System) sites in such a way that at probing some regions were healthy, a few sites exhibited signs of mucositis, and some sites exhibited peri-implantitis. Probes with different geometry were inserted into the pockets using a standardized probing procedure and a force of only 0.2 N. The probes were anchored and block biopsy specimens were harvested. The probe locations were studied in histologic ground sections. The authors reported that the mean "histologic" probing depth at healthy sites was about 1.8 mm, i.e. similar to the depth (about 2 mm) recorded by Ericsson and Lindhe (1993). The corresponding depth at sites with mucositis and peri-implantitis was about 1.6 mm and 3.8 mm respectively. Lang *et al.* (1994) further stated that at healthy and mucositis sites, the probe tip identified "the connective tissue adhesion level" (i.e. the base of the barrier epithelium) while at peri-implantitis sites, the probe exceeded the base of the ulcerated pocket epithelium by a mean distance of 0.5 mm. At such peri-implantitis sites the probe reached the base of the inflammatory cell infiltrate.

Schou *et al.* (2002) compared probing measurements at implants and teeth in eight cynomolgus monkeys. Ground sections were produced from tooth and implant sites that were (1) clinically healthy, (2) slightly inflamed (mucositis/gingivitis), and (3) severely inflamed (peri-implantitis/periodontitis) and in which probes had been inserted. An electronic probe (Peri-Probe®) with a tip diameter 0.5 mm and a standardized probing force of 0.3–0.4 N was used. It was demonstrated that the probe tip was located at a similar distance from the bone in healthy tooth sites and implant sites. On the other hand, at implants exhibiting mucositis and peri-implantitis, the probe tip was consistently identified at a more apical position than at corresponding sites at teeth (gingivitis and periodontitis). The authors concluded that (1) probing depth measurements at implant and teeth yielded different information, and (2) small alterations in probing depth at implants may reflect changes in soft tissue inflammation rather than loss of supporting tissues.

Recently, Abrahamsson and Soldini (2006) evaluated the location of the probe tip in healthy periodontal and peri-implant tissues in dogs. It was reported that probing with a force of 0.2 N resulted in a probe penetration that was similar at implants and teeth. Furthermore, the tip of the probe was often at or close to the apical cells of the junctional/barrier epithelium. The distance between the tip of the probe and the bone crest was about 1 mm at both teeth and implants (Figs. 3-29, 3-30). Similar observations were reported from clinical studies in which different implant systems were used (Buser *et al.* 1990; Quirynen *et al.* 1991; Mombelli *et al.* 1997). In these studies the distance between the probe tip and the bone was assessed in radiographs and was found to vary between 0.75 and 1.4 mm when a probing force of 0.25–0.45 N was used.

By comparing the findings from the studies reported above, it becomes apparent that probing depth and probing attachment level measurements are also meaningful at implant sites. When a "normal" probing force is applied in healthy tissues the probe seems to reach similar levels at implant and tooth sites. Probing inflamed tissues both at tooth and implant sites will, however, result in a more advanced probe penetration and the tip of the probe may come closer to the bone crest.

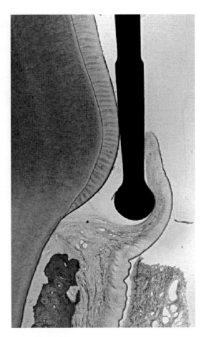

Fig. 3-29 Buccal–lingual ground section from a tooth site illustrating the probe tip position in relation to the bone crest (from Abrahamsson & Soldini 2006).

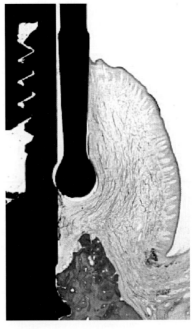

Fig. 3-30 Buccal–lingual ground section from an implant site illustrating the probe tip position in relation to the bone crest (from Abrahamsson & Soldini 2006).

Dimensions of the buccal soft tissue at implants

Chang *et al.* (1999) compared the dimensions of the periodontal and peri-implant soft tissues of 20 subjects who had been treated with an implant-supported single-tooth restoration in the esthetic zone of the maxilla and had a non-restored natural tooth in the contralateral position (Fig. 3-31). In

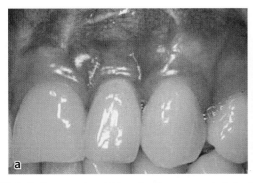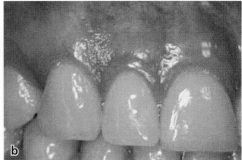

Fig. 3-31 Clinical photographs of (a) an implant-supported single tooth replacement in position 12 and (b) the natural tooth in the contralateral position (from Chang *et al.* 1999).

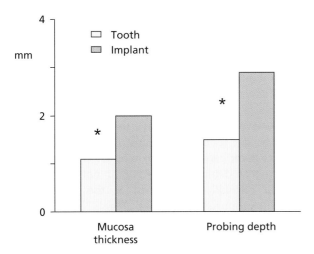

Fig. 3-32 Comparison of mucosa thickness and probing depth at the facial aspect of single-implant restorations and the natural tooth in the contralateral position (from Chang *et al.* 1999).

comparison to the natural tooth, the implant-supported crown was bordered by a thicker buccal mucosa (2.0 mm versus 1.1 mm), as assessed at a level corresponding to the bottom of the probeable pocket, and had a greater probing pocket depth (2.9 mm versus 2.5 mm) (Fig. 3-32). It was further observed that the soft tissue margin at the implant was more apically located (about 1 mm) than the gingival margin at the contralateral tooth.

Kan *et al.* (2003) studied the dimensions of the peri-implant mucosa at 45 single implants placed in the anterior maxilla that had been in function for an average of 33 months. Bone sounding measurements performed at the buccal aspect of the implants showed that the height of the mucosa was 3–4 mm in the majority of the cases. Less than 3 mm of mucosa height was found at only 9% of the implants. It was suggested that implants in this category were (1) found in subjects that belonged to a *thin periodontal biotype*, (2) had been placed too labially, and/or (3) had an overcontoured facial prosthetic emergence. A peri-implant soft tissue dimension of >4 mm was usually associated with a *thick periodontal biotype*.

Dimensions of the papilla between teeth and implants

In a study by Schropp *et al.* (2003) it was demonstrated that following single tooth extraction the height of the papilla at the adjacent teeth was reduced about 1 mm. Concomitant with this reduction (recession) of the papilla height the pocket depth was reduced and some loss of clinical attachment occurred.

Following single tooth extraction and subsequent implant installation, the height of the papilla in the tooth–implant site will be dependent on the attachment level of the tooth. Choquet *et al.* (2001) studied the papilla level adjacent to single-tooth dental implants in 26 patients and in total 27 implant sites. The distance between the apical extension of the contact point between the crowns and the bone crest, as well as the distance between the soft tissue level and the bone crest, was measured in radiographs. The examinations were made 6–75 months after the insertion of the crown restoration. The authors observed that the papilla height consistently was about 4 mm, and, depending on the location of the contact point between adjacent crowns papilla, fill was either complete or incomplete (Fig. 3-33). The closer the contact point was located to the incisal edge of the crowns (restorations) the less complete was the papilla fill.

Chang *et al.* (1999) studied the dimensions of the papillae at implant-supported single-tooth restorations in the anterior region of the maxilla and at non-restored contralateral natural teeth. They found that the papilla height at the implant-supported crown was significantly shorter and showed less fill of the embrasure space than the papillae at the natural tooth (Fig. 3-34). This was particularly evident for the distal papilla of implant-supported restorations in the central incisor position, both in comparison to the distal papilla at the contralateral tooth and to the papilla at the mesial aspect of the implant crown. This indicates that the anatomy of the adjacent natural teeth (e.g. the diameter of the root, the proximal outline/curvature of the cemento-enamel junction/connective tissue attachment

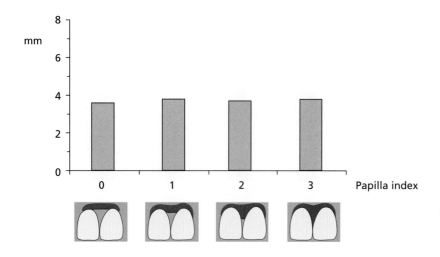

Fig. 3-33 Soft tissue height adjacent to single-tooth dental implants in relation to the degree of papilla fill (from Choquet *et al.* 2001).

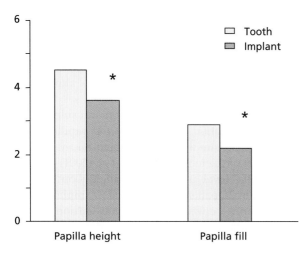

Fig. 3-34 Comparison of papilla height and papilla fill adjacent to single-implant restorations and the natural tooth in the contralateral position (from Chang *et al.* 1999).

level) may have a profound influence on the dimension of the papilla lateral to an implant. Hence, the wider facial–lingual root diameter and the higher proximal curvature of the cemento-enamel junction of the maxillary central incisor – in comparison to corresponding dimensions of the lateral incisor (Wheeler 1966) – may favor the maintenance of the height of the mesial papilla at the single-implant supported restoration.

Kan *et al.* (2003) assessed the dimensions of the peri-implant mucosa lateral to 45 single implants placed in the anterior maxilla and the 90 adjacent teeth using bone sounding measurements. The bone sounding measurements were performed at the mesial and distal aspects of the implants and at the mesial and distal aspects of the teeth. The authors reported that the thickness of the mucosa at the mesial/distal surfaces of the implant sites was on the average 6 mm while the corresponding dimension at the adjacent tooth sites was about 4 mm. It was further observed that the dimensions of the peri-

implant mucosa of subjects who belonged to the *thick periodontal biotype* were significantly greater than that of subjects of a *thin biotype*.

The level of the connective tissue attachment on the adjacent tooth surface and the position of the contact point between the crowns are obviously key factors that determine whether or not a complete papilla fill will be obtained at the single-tooth implant-supported restoration (Fig. 3.35). Although there are indications that the dimensions of the approximal soft tissue may vary between individuals having thin and thick periodontal biotypes, the height of the papilla at the single-implant restoration seems to have a biological limit of about 4 mm (compare the dimension of the interdental papilla). Hence, to achieve a complete papilla fill of the embrasure space, a proper location of the contact area between the implant crown and the tooth crown is mandatory. In this respect it must also be recognized that the papilla fill at single-tooth implant restorations is unrelated to whether the implant is inserted according to a one- or two-stage protocol and whether a crown restoration is inserted immediately following surgery or delayed until the soft tissues have healed (Jemt 1999; Ryser *et al.* 2005).

Dimensions of the "papilla" between adjacent implants

When two neighboring teeth are extracted, the papilla at the site will be lost (Fig. 3-36). Hence, at replacement of the extracted teeth with implant-supported restorations the topography of the bone crest and the thickness of the supracrestal soft tissue portion are the factors that determine the position of the soft tissue margin in the inter-implant area ("implant papilla"). Tarnow *et al.* (2003) assessed the height above the bone crest of the inter-implant soft tissue ("implant papilla") by transmucosal probing at 136 anterior and posterior sites in 33 patients who had maintained implant-supported prostheses for at least

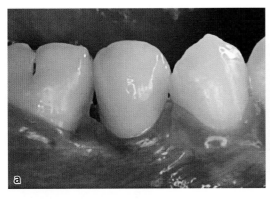
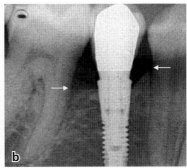

Fig. 3-35 See text for details.

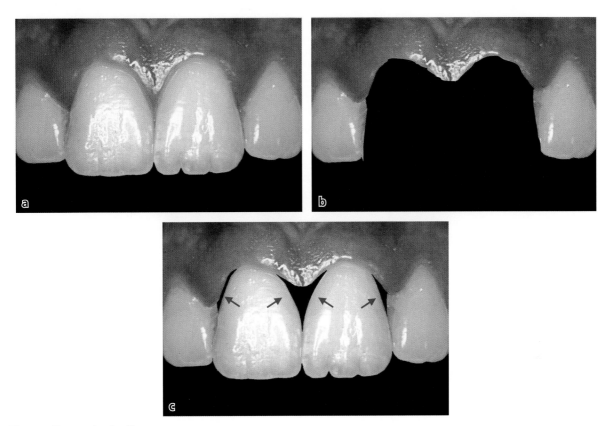

Fig. 3-36 See text for details.

2 months. It was found that the mean height of the "papillae" was 3.4 mm, with 90% of the measurements in the range of 2–4 mm.

The dimension of the soft tissues between adjacent implants seems to be independent of the implant design. Lee *et al.* (2006) examined the soft tissue height between implants of two different systems (Brånemark Implant® and Astra Tech Implant® systems) as well as the potential influence of the horizontal distance between implants. The height of the inter-implant "papilla", i.e. the height of soft tissue coronal to the bone crest measured in radiographs, was about 3.1 mm for both implant systems. No difference was found regarding the "papilla" height for any of the implant systems with regard to sites with

<3 mm and ≥3 mm in horizontal distance between the implants. Gastaldo *et al.* (2004) evaluated the presence or absence of "papilla" at 96 inter-implant sites in 58 patients. It was reported that the "papilla" filled the entire space between the implants only when the distance from the bone crest to the base of the contact point between the crown restorations, assessed by sounding, was <4 mm. Thus, taken together these observations indicate that the soft tissue between two implants will have a maximum height of 3–4 mm, and that the location of the contact point between the crown restorations in relation to the bone crest level determines whether a complete soft tissue fill will be obtained in the embrasure space between two implants (Fig. 3-37).

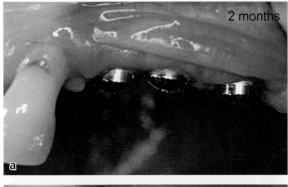

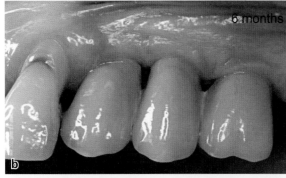

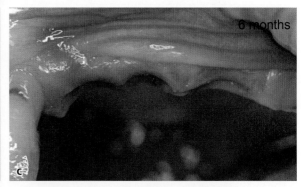

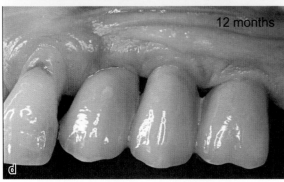

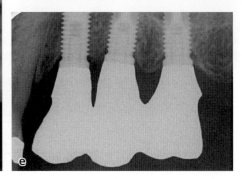

Fig. 3-37 See text for details.

References

Abrahamsson, I., Berglundh, T., Glantz, P.O. & Lindhe, J. (1998). The mucosal attachment at different abutments. An experimental study in dogs. *Journal of Clinical Periodontology* **25**, 721–727.

Abrahamsson, I., Berglundh, T., Wennström, J. & Lindhe, J. (1996). The peri-implant hard and soft tissues at different implant systems. A comparative study in the dog. *Clinical Oral Implants Research* **7**, 212–219.

Abrahamsson, I., Zitzmann, N.U., Berglundh, T., Linder, E., Wennerberg, A. & Lindhe, J. (2002). The mucosal attachment to titanium implants with different surface characteristics: an experimental study in dogs. *Journal of Clinical Periodontology* **29**, 448–455.

Abrahamsson, I. & Soldini, C. (2006). Probe penetration in periodontal and peri-implant tissues: an experimental study in the beagle dog. *Clinical Oral Implants Research* **17**, 601–605.

Andlin-Sobocki, A. & Bodin, L. (1993). Dimensional alterations of the gingiva related to changes of facial/lingual tooth position in permanent anterior teeth of children. A 2-year longitudinal study. *Journal of Clinical Periodontology* **20**, 219–224.

Armitage, G.C., Svanberg, G.K. & Löe, H. (1977). Microscopic evaluation of clinical measurements of connective tissue attachment levels. *Journal of Clinical Periodontology* **4**, 173–190.

Becker, W., Ochenbein, C., Tibbets, L. & Becker, B.E. (1997). Alveolar bone anatomic profiles as measured from dry skulls. *Journal of Clinical Periodontology* **24**, 727–731.

Berglundh, T. (1999). Soft tissue interface and response to microbial challenge. In: Lang, N.P., Lindhe, J. & Karring, T., eds. *Implant Dentistry. Proceedings from 3rd European Workshop on Periodontology.* Berlin: Quintessence, pp. 153–174.

Berglundh, T. & Lindhe, J. (1996). Dimensions of the peri-implant mucosa. Biological width revisited. *Journal of Clinical Periodontology* **23**, 971–973.

Berglundh, T., Lindhe, J., Ericsson, I., Marinello, C.P., Liljenberg, B. & Thomsen, P. (1991). The soft tissue barrier at implants and teeth. *Clinical Oral Implants Research* **2**, 81–90.

Berglundh, T., Lindhe, J., Jonsson, K. & Ericsson, I. (1994). The topography of the vascular systems in the periodontal and peri-implant tissues dog. *Journal of Clinical Periodontology* **21**, 189–193.

Berglundh, T., Abrahamsson, I., Welander, M., Lang, N.P. & Lindhe, J. (2007). Morphogenesis of the periimplant mucosa. An experimental study in dogs. *Clinical Oral Implants Research* (in press).

Buser, D., Weber, H.P. & Lang, N.P. (1990). Tissue integration of non-submerged implants. 1-year results of a prospective study on 100 ITI-hollow-cylinder and hollow-screw implants. *Clinical Oral Implants Research* **1**, 225–235.

Buser, D., Weber, H.P., Donath, K., Fiorellini, J.P., Paquette, D.W. & Williams, R.C. (1992). Soft tissue reactions to non-submerged unloaded titanium implants in beagle dogs. *Journal of Periodontology* **63**, 226–236.

Chang, M., Wennström, J., Ödman, P. & Andersson, B. (1999). Implant supported single-tooth replacements compared to contralateral natural teeth. *Clinical Oral Implants Research* **10**, 185–194.

Choquet, V., Hermans, M., Adriaenssens, P., Daelemans, P., Tarnow, D. & Malevez, C. (2001). Clincal and radiographic evaluation of the papilla level adjacent to single-tooth dental implants. A retrospective study in the maxillary anterior region. *Journal of Periodontology* **72**, 1364–1371.

Coatoam, G.W., Behrents, R.G. & Bissada, N.F. (1981). The width of keratinized gingiva during orthodontic treatment: its significance and impact on periodontal status. *Journal of Periodontology* **52**, 307–313.

Ericsson, I. & Lindhe, J. (1993). Probing depth at implants and teeth. *Journal of Clinical Periodontology* **20**, 623–627.

Gargiulo, A.W., Wentz, F.M. & Orban, B. (1961). Dimensions and relations of the dentogingival junction in humans. *Journal of Periodontology* **32**, 261–267.

Gastaldo, J.F., Cury, P.R. & Sendyk, W.R. (2004). Effect of the vertical and horizontal distances between adjacent implants and between a tooth and an implant on the incidence of interproximal papilla. *Journal of Periodontology* **75**, 1242–1246.

Gottlieb, B. (1921). Der Epithelansatz am Zahne. *Deutsche monatschrift führ Zahnheilkunde* **39**, 142–147.

Gould, T.R.L., Westbury, L. & Brunette, D.M. (1984). Ultrastructural study of the attachment of human gingiva to titanium in vivo. *Journal of Prosthetic Dentistry* **52**, 418–420.

Jemt, T. (1999). Restoring the gingival contour by means of provisional resin crowns after single-implant treatment. *International Journal of Periodontics and Restorative Dentistry* **19**, 21–29.

Kan, J., Rungcharassaeng, K., Umezu, K. & Kois, J. (2003). Dimensions of the periimplant mucosa: An evaluation of maxillary anterior single implants in humans. *Journal of Periodontology* **74**, 557–562.

Kohl, J. & Zander, H. (1961). Morphology of interdental gingival tissue. *Oral Surgery, Oral Medicine and Oral Pathology* **60**, 287–295.

Lang, N.P., Wetzel, A.C., Stich, H. & Caffesse, R.G. (1994). Histologic probe penetration in healthy and inflamed peri-implant tissues. *Clinical Oral Implants Research* **5**, 191–201.

Lee, D-W., Park, K-H. & Moon, I-S. (2006). Dimension of interproximal soft tissue between adjacent implants in two distinctive implant systems. *Journal of Periodontology* **77**, 1080–1084.

Magnusson, I. & Listgarten, M.A. (1980). Histological evaluation of probing depth following periodontal treatment. *Journal of Clinical Periodontology* **7**, 26–31.

Matherson, D. & Zander, H. (1963). Evaluation of osseous surgery in monkeys. *Journal of Dental Research* **42**, 116.

Mombelli, A., Mühle, T., Brägger, U., Lang, N.P. & Bürgin, W.B. (1997). Comparison of periodontal and peri-implant probing by depth-force pattern analysis. *Clinical Oral Implants Research* **8**, 448–454.

Moon, I-S., Berglundh, T., Abrahamsson, I., Linder, E. & Lindhe, J. (1999). The barrier between the keratinized mucosa and the dental implant. An experimental study in the dog. *Journal of Clinical Periodontology* **26**, 658–663.

Müller, H.P. & Könönen, E. (2005). Variance components of gingival thickness. *Journal of Periodontal Research* **40**, 239–244.

O'Connor, T.W. & Biggs, N. (1964). Interproximal craters. *Journal of Periodontology* **35**, 326–330.

Olsson, M. & Lindhe, J. (1991). Periodontal characteristics in individuals with varying forms of upper central incisors. *Journal of Clinical Periodontology* **18**, 78–82.

Olsson, M., Lindhe, J. & Marinello, C. (1993). On the relationship between crown form and clinical features of the gingiva in adolescents. *Journal of Clinical Periodontology* **20**, 570–577.

Orban, B & Köhler, J. (1924). Die physiologische Zanhfleischetasche, Epithelansatz und Epitheltiefenwucherung. *Zeitschrift für Stomatologie* **22**, 353.

Oschenbein, C. & Ross, S. (1969). A reevaluation of osseous surgery. In: *Dental Clinics of North America.* Philadelphia, PA: W.B. Saunders, pp. 87–102.

Pontoriero, R. & Carnevale, G. (2001). Surgical crown lengthening: A 12-month clinical wound healing study. *Journal of Periodontology* **72**, 841–848.

Quirynen, M., van Steenberge, D., Jacobs, R., Schotte, A. & Darius, P. (1991). The reliability of pocket probing around screw-type implants. *Clinical Oral Implants Research* **2**, 186–192.

Ryser, M.R., Block, M.S. & Mercante, D.E. (2005). Correlation of papilla to crestal bone levels around single tooth implants in immediate or delayed crown protocols. *Journal of Maxillofacial Surgery* **63**, 1184–1195.

Schou, S., Holmstrup, P., Stolze, K., Hjørting-Hansen, E., Fien, N.E. & Skovgaard, L.T. (2002). Probing around implants and teeth with healthy or inflamed marginal tissues. A histologic comparison in cynomolgus monkeys (*Macaca fascicularis*). *Clinical Oral Implants Research* **13**, 113–126.

Schropp, L., Wenzel, A., Kostopoulos, L. & Karring, T. (2003). Bone healing and soft tissue contour changes following singe-tooth extraction: A clinical and radiographic 12-month prospective study. *International Journal of Periodontics and Restorative Dentistry* **23**, 313–323.

Sicher, H. (1959). Changing concepts of the Supporting Dental Structure. *Oral Surgery, Oral Medicine and Oral Pathology* **12**, 31–35.

Tarnow, D., Elian, N., Fletcher, P., Froum, S., Magner, A., Cho, S-C., Salama, M., Salama, H. & Garber, D.A. (2003). Vertical distance from the crest of bone to the height of the interproximal papilla between adjacent implants. *Journal of Periodontology* **74**, 1785–1788.

Tarnow, D., Magner, A. & Fletcher, P. (1992). The effect of the distance from the contact point to the crest of bone on the presence or absence of the interproximal dental papilla. *Journal of Periodontology* **63**, 995–996.

van der Velden, U. (1982). Regeneration of the interdental soft tissues following denudation procedures. *Journal of Clinical Periodontology* **9**, 455–459.

Weisgold, A. (1977). Contours of the full crown restoration. *Alpha Omegan* **7**, 77–89.

Waerhaug, J. (1952). Gingival pocket: anatomy, pathology, deepening and elimination. *Odontologisk Tidskrift* **60** (Suppl 1).

Wheeler, R.C. (1961). Complete crown form and the periodontium. *Journal of Prosthetic Dentistry* **11**, 722–734.

Wheeler, R. C. (1966). *An Atlas of Tooth Form.* Philadelphia: W.B. Saunders Co, pp. 24–25.

Chapter 4

Bone as a Tissue

William V. Giannobile, Hector F. Rios, and Niklaus P. Lang

During embryogenesis, in the alveolar process of the maxilla and the mandible, bone is formed within a primary connective tissue. This process is termed *intramembranous* bone formation and also occurs at the cranial vault and in the midshaft or diaphysis of the long bones. In contrast, bone formation in the remaining parts of the skeleton occurs via an initial deposition of a cartilage template that is subsequently replaced by bone. This process is called *endochondral* bone formation.

Alveolar bone lost as a result of disease, trauma or extensive post-extraction bone modeling may pose therapeutic problems in periodontal reconstructive and/or implant dentistry. Thus, implant placement both in the maxilla and in the mandible may be hampered by the lack of sufficient volume of alveolar bone at the recipient sites. *De novo* formation of alveolar bone in such compromised sites may be necessary and different regenerative therapies need to be considered to promote new bone. They all, however, have one aspect in common: the compliance with the principles of bone biology. There are several reconstructive modalities for restoration of the alveolar process, such as bone graft replacements and guided bone regeneration (GBR).

Basic bone biology

Bone is a specialized connective tissue that is mainly characterized by its mineralized organic matrix. The bone organic matrix is comprised of collagenous and non-collagenous proteins. Within this matrix, ions of calcium and phosphate are laid down in the ultimate form of hydroxyapatite. This composition allows the bone tissue to: (1) resist load, (2) protect highly sensitive organs (e.g. the central nervous system) from external forces, and (3) participate as a reservoir of minerals that contribute to systemic homeostasis of the body.

Bone cells

Osteoblasts are the primary cells responsible for the formation of bone; they synthesize the organic extracellular matrix (ECM) components and control the mineralization of the matrix. Osteoblasts are located on bone surfaces exhibiting active matrix deposition and may eventually differentiate into two different types of cells: *bone lining cells* and *osteocytes*. Bone lining cells are elongated cells that cover a surface of bone tissue and exhibit no synthetic activity. Osteocytes are stellate-shaped cells that are trapped within the mineralized bone matrix but remain in contact with other bone cells by thin cellular processes. The osteocytes are organized as a syncytium that provides a very large contact area between the cells (and their processes) and the noncellular part of the bone tissue. This arrangement allows osteocytes to: (1) participate in the regulation of the blood-calcium homeostasis, and (2) sense mechanical loading and to signal this information to other cells within the bone.

The osteoblasts are fully differentiated cells and lack the capacity for migration and proliferation. Thus, in order to allow bone formation to occur at a given site, undifferentiated mesenchymal progenitor cells (*osteoprogenitor cells*) must migrate to the site and proliferate to become osteoblasts. Friedenstein (1973) divided osteoprogenitor cells into *determined* and *inducible osteogenic precursor cells*. The determined osteoprogenitor cells are present in the bone marrow, in the endosteum and in the periosteum that covers the bone surface. Such cells possess an intrinsic capacity to proliferate and differentiate into osteoblasts. Inducible osteogenic precursor cells, on the other hand, represent mesenchymal cells present in other organs and tissues (e.g. myoblasts or adipocytes) that may differentiate into bone-forming cells when exposed to specific stimuli. As osteogenesis is generally closely related to the ingrowth of vascular tissue,

Table 4-1 Effects of growth factors in bone wound healing

Wound healing phase	Growth factor	Cell of origin	Functions
Inflammatory	PDGF	Platelets	Increases chemotaxis of neutrophils and monocytes
	TGF-β	Platelets, leukocytes, fibroblasts	Increases chemotaxis of neutrophils and monocytes Autocrine expression – generation of additional cytokines (TNFα, IL-1β, PDGF, and chemokines)
	VEGF	Platelets, leukocytes, fibroblasts	Increases vascular permeability
Proliferative	EGF	Macrophages, mesenchymal cells, platelets	Stimulates epithelial proliferation and migration
	FGF-2	Macrophages, endothelial cells	Stimulates fibroblast proliferation and ECM synthesis Increases chemotaxis, proliferation, and differentiation of endothelial cells
	KGF (FGF-7)	Keratinocytes, fibroblasts	Stimulates epithelial proliferation and migration
	PDGF	Macrophages, endothelial cells	Stimulates fibroblast proliferation and ECM synthesis Increases chemotaxis, proliferation, and differentiation of endothelial cells
	TGF-β	Macrophages, leukocytes, fibroblast	Stimulates epithelial proliferation and migration Stimulates fibroblasts proliferation and ECM synthesis Inhibits proteases and enhances inhibitor production
	VEGF	Macrophages	Increases chemotaxis of endothelial progenitor cells Stimulates endothelial cell proliferation
Bone remodeling, matrix synthesis	BMPs 2–4	Osteoblasts	Stimulates mesenchymal progenitor cell migration
	BMP-7	Osteoblasts	Stimulates osteoblast and chondroblast differentiation
	FGF-2	Macrophages, endothelial cells	Stimulates mesenchymal progenitor cell migration
	IGF-II	Macrophages, fibroblasts	Stimulates osteoblast proliferation and bone matrix synthesis
	PDGF	Macrophages, osteoblasts	Stimulates differentiation of fibroblasts into myofibroblasts Stimulates proliferation of mesenchymal progenitor cells
	TGF-β	Fibroblasts, osteoblasts	Induces endothelial cell and fibroblast apoptosis Induces differentiation of fibroblasts into myofibroblasts Stimulates chemotaxis and survival of osteoblasts
	VEGF	Macrophages	Chemotaxis of mesenchymal stem cells, antiapoptotic effect on the bone forming cells, angiogenesis promotion

Adapted from: Kaigler, D., Cirelli, J.A. & Giannobile, W.V. (2006). Growth factor delivery for oral and periodontal tissue engineering. *Expert Opinion on Drug Delivery* **3**, 647–662, with permission.
PDGF = platelet-derived growth factor; TGF = transforming growth factor; VEGF = vascular endothelial growth factor; EGF = epidermal growth factor; FGF = fibroblast growth factor; KGF = keratinocyte growth factor; BMP = bone morphogenetic protein; IGF = insulin-like growth factor; TNFα = tumor necrosis factor alpha.

the stellate-shaped perivascular cell (the *pericyte*) is considered to be the main osteoprogenitor cell. The differentiation and development of osteoblasts from osteoprogenitor cells are dependent on the release of osteoinductive or osteopromotive growth factors (GFs) such as bone morphogenetic proteins (BMP) and other growth factors such as insulin-like growth factor (IGF), platelet-derived growth factor (PDGF) and fibroblast growth factor (FGF) (Table 4-1).

The bone formation activity is consistently coupled to bone resorption that is initiated and maintained by *osteoclasts*. Osteoclasts are multinucleated cells that originate from hematopoietic precursor cells.

Modeling and remodeling

Once bone has formed, the new mineralized tissue starts to be reshaped and renewed by processes of resorption and apposition, i.e. through *modeling* and *remodeling*. Modeling represents a process that allows a change in the initial bone architecture. It has been suggested that external demands (such as load) on bone tissue may initiate modeling. Remodeling, on the other hand, represents a change that occurs within the mineralized bone without a concomitant alteration of the architecture of the tissue. The process of remodeling is important (1) during bone formation, and (2) when old bone is replaced with new bone. During bone formation, remodeling enables the substitution of the primary bone (woven bone), which has low load-bearing capacity, with lamellar bone that is more resistant to load.

The bone remodeling that occurs in order to allow replacement of old bone with new bone involves two processes: bone resorption and bone apposition (formation). These processes are coupled in time and are

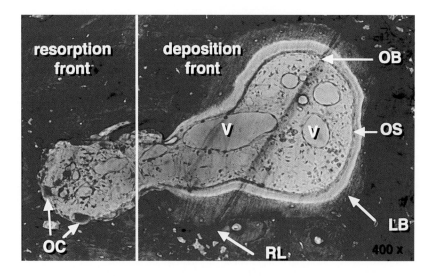

Fig. 4-1 Histological section illustrating a bone multicellular unit (BMU). Note the presence of a resorption front with osteoclast (OC) and a deposition front that contains osteoblasts (OB), and osteoid (OS). Vascular structures (V) occupy the central area of the BMU. RL = reversal line; LB = lamellar bone.

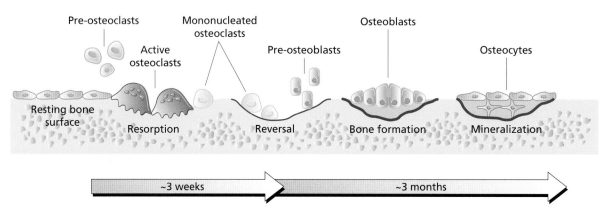

Fig. 4-2 The bone remodeling cycle. Preosteoblasts are recruited to sites of resorption, induced to differentiate into active osteoclasts, and form resoption pits. After their period of active resorption, transient mononuclear cells replace them. Through the process of coupling, preosteoblasts are recruited, differentiate into active matrix-secreting cells, and form bone. Some osteoblasts become entrapped in the matrix and become osteocytes. Adapted from McCauley, L.K. & Nohutcu, R.M. (2002) Mediators of periodontal osseous destruction and remodeling: principles and implications for diagnosis and therapy. *Journal of Periodontology* **73**, 1377–1391, with permission.

characterized by the presence of so called *bone multicellular units* (BMUs). A BMU (Fig. 4-1) is comprised of (1) a front osteoclast residing on a surface of newly resorbed bone (the resorption front), (2) a compartment containing vessels and pericytes, and (3) a layer of osteoblasts present on a newly formed organic matrix (the deposition front). The process of the bone remodeling cycle is shown in Figs. 4-2 and 4-3. Local stimuli and release of hormones, such as parathyroid hormone (PTH), growth hormone, leptin, and calcitonin, are involved in the control of bone remodeling. Modeling and remodeling occur throughout life to allow bone to adapt to external and internal demands.

Growth factors and alveolar bone healing

Understanding the complex processes of wound healing has been a challenge for researchers for many years. Recently, advances in the areas of cellular and molecular biology have allowed the elucidation of functions of GFs and their participation in the different phases of wound healing. Restoration of normal form and function is the ultimate goal of regenerative approaches of alveolar bone disrupted by trauma, surgical resection or infectious disease. However, if the functional integrity of the tissue is not achieved, the process of repair will take place and a fibrous tissue will replace the original tissue (Le *et al.* 2005). Recent studies have confirmed that GFs can improve the capacity of alveolar bone to regenerate, improving cellular chemoattraction, differentiation, and proliferation. GFs are natural biological mediators that regulate important cellular events involved in tissue repair by binding to specific cell surface receptors (Giannobile 1996). After reaching specific target cells, GFs induce intracellular signaling pathways, which result in the activation of genes that change cellular activity and phenotype (Anusaksathien & Giannobile 2002). However, the effect of each GF is regulated through a complex system of feedback loops, which involve other GFs, enzymes, and binding proteins (Schilephake 2002; Ripamonti *et al.* 2005). Recent studies have taken place with the target of defining the proper application for therapeutic purposes of many different growth factors and other cytokines,

Woven bone   BMU   Lamellar bone

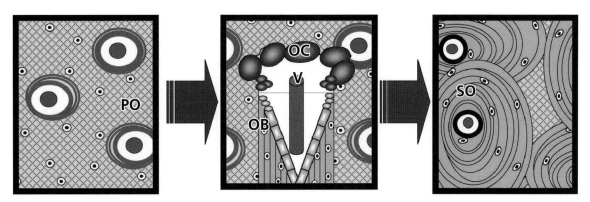

Fig. 4-3 Schematic drawing describing the transition between woven bone and lamellar bone, i.e. remodeling. Woven bone with primary osteons (PO) is transformed into lamellar bone in a process that involves the presence of BMUs. The BMU contains osteoclasts (OC), as well as vascular structures (V) and osteoblasts (OB). Thus, the osteoblasts in the BMU produce bone tissue that has a concentric orientation around the vessel, and secondary osteons (SO) are formed within lamellar bone.

each of which has several functions during the different phases of wound healing (Schilephake 2002; Ripamonti *et al.* 2005).

Healing of osseous tissue is regulated by GFs and other cytokines in a sequence of overlapping events similar to cutaneous wound repair. In ideal circumstances, this process mimics embryonic bone development allowing replacement of damaged bone with new bone, rather than with fibrous scar tissue. This process is driven by cellular and molecular mechanisms controlled by the TGF-β superfamily of genes, which encode a large number of extracellular signaling molecules (Blair *et al.* 2002). Bone morphogenetic proteins (BMPs) are a well studied group of these GFs involved in the processes of bone healing; the human genome encodes at least 20 of these multifunctional polypeptides (Blumenthal *et al.* 2002). Among several functions, BMPs induce the formation of both bone and cartilage by stimulating the cellular events of mesenchymal progenitor cells. However, only a subset of BMPs, most notably BMP-2, -4, -6, -7, and -9, has osteoinductive activity, a property of inducing *de novo* bone formation by themselves (Cheng *et al.* 2003). Studies involving mutations of BMP ligands, receptors, and signaling proteins have shown important roles of BMPs in embryonic and postnatal development. Severe skeletal deformation, development of osteoporosis, reduction in bone mineral density and bone volume are all aberrations associated with disrupted and dysregulated BMP signaling (Chen *et al.* 2004).

Several other GFs produced by osteogenic cells, platelets and inflammatory cells participate in bone healing, including IGF-I and -II, TGFβ-1, PDGF, and FGF-2 (Sykaras & Opperman, 2003). The bone matrix serves as a reservoir for these GFs and BMPs and they are activated during matrix resorption by matrix metalloproteinases (Baylink *et al.* 1993; Janssens *et al.* 2005). Additionally, the acidic environment that develops during the inflammatory process leads to activation of latent GFs (Linkhart *et al.* 1996), which

assist in the chemoattraction, migration, proliferation, and differentiation of mesenchymal cells into osteoblasts (Linkhart *et al.* 1996). All of these functions are driven by a complex mechanism of interaction among GFs and other cytokines, which is influenced by several regulatory factors (King & Cochran, 2002).

Local and systemic factors affecting bone volume and healing

Metabolic disorders affecting bone metabolism

A variety of systemic situations can affect local bone density, ultimately influencing tooth support or available bone volume for dental implant installation. Such diseases affecting bone mass include osteopenia, osteoporosis, and diabetes mellitus. The later two will be discussed in detail given their overall prevalence and implications to alveolar bone reconstruction.

Osteoporosis

Osteoporosis is a systemic skeletal disease characterized by low bone mass and microarchitectural deterioration of the bone scaffold that result in increased bone fragility and susceptibility to fracture. In osteoporosis, the *bone mineral density* (BMD) is reduced, bone microarchitecture is disrupted, and the amount and variety of non-collagenous proteins in bone is altered. *Dual energy X-ray absorptiometry* (DXA, formerly DEXA) is considered the gold standard for diagnosis of osteoporosis. Diagnosis is made when the BMD is less than or equal to 2.5 standard deviations below that of a young adult reference population. This is translated as a T-score. The World Health Organization has established diagnostic guidelines as T-score −1.0 or greater is "normal", T-score between −1.0 and −2.5 is osteopenia, and −2.5 or below as osteoporosis (WHO Study Group 1994).

Oral bone loss has been shown to be associated with osteoporosis and low skeletal BMD. In their search for oral radiographic changes associated with osteoporosis, most investigators have focused on measures of jaw bone mass or morphology. The commonly used assessment of oral bone status include radiographic measures of loss of alveolar crestal height (ACH), measures of resorption of the residual ridge after tooth loss (RRR), and assessment of oral BMD. Tools used to measure bone mass include single and dual photon absorptiometry, DXA, quantitative computed tomography (QCT), and film densitometry.

Periodontitis results from pathogenic bacterial infection, which produces factors that destroy collagenous support of the tooth, as well as loss of alveolar bone. Systemic factors can lead to loss of BMD throughout the body, including bone loss in the maxilla and mandible. The resulting local reduction of BMD in the jaw bones could set the stage for more rapid ACH loss because a comparable challenge of bacterial bone-resorbing factors could be expected to result in greater alveolar crestal bone loss than in an individual with good bone mass. In addition to this, there are systemic risk factors such as smoking, diabetes, diet, and hormone levels that affect systemic bone level and may also affect periodontitis (discussed in Chapters 12 and 13). Although periodontal disease has historically been thought to be the result of a local infectious process, others have suggested that periodontal disease may be an early manifestation of generalized osteopenia (Whalen & Krook 1996), which would classify osteoporosis as a risk indicator, rather than a risk factor, for periodontal disease.

Mandibular mineral content is reduced in subjects with osteoporotic fractures (von Wowern et al. 1994). Further, the BMD of buccal mandibular bone correlates with osteoporosis (low skeletal BMD) (Klemetti et al. 1993; Taguchi et al. 1996). Mandibular density also correlates with skeletal BMD (Horner et al. 1996). Using film densitometry, the optical density of the mandible has been found to be increased in subjects with osteoporosis compared with controls. Further, mandibular radiographic optical density correlates with vertebral BMD in osteoporotic women (Kribbs 1990), control women (Kribbs 1990), and in women with a history of vertebral fracture (Kribbs et al. 1990; Law et al. 1996). Reduction in cortical and subcortical alveolar bone density has also been reported to correlate with osteoporosis in longitudinal studies (Payne et al. 1997, 1999; Civitelli et al. 2002). As concluded by Hildebolt (1997), the preponderance of the evidence indicates that the jaws of subjects with osteoporosis show reduced bone mass with potential implications on dental implant installation.

Several potential mechanisms by which osteoporosis or systemic bone loss may be associated with periodontal attachment loss, loss of alveolar bone height or density, and tooth loss have been proposed.

One of these mechanisms states that low BMD or loss of BMD may lead to more rapid resorption of alveolar bone after insult by periodontal bacteria. With less dense oral bone to start with, loss of bone surrounding the teeth may occur more rapidly. Another mechanism proposes that systemic factors affecting bone remodeling may also modify local tissue response to periodontal infection. Persons with systemic bone loss are known to have increased production of cytokines (i.e. interleukin-1, interleukin-6) that may have effects on bone throughout the body, including the bones of the oral cavity. Periodontal infection has been shown to increase local cytokine production that, in turn, increases local osteoclast activity resulting in increased bone resorption. A third mechanism would be related to genetic factors that predispose an individual to systemic bone loss and also influence or predispose an individual to periodontal destruction. Also, certain lifestyle factors such as cigarette smoking and suboptimal calcium intake, among others, may put individuals at risk for development of both systemic osteopenia and oral bone loss (Oh et al. 2007).

Recently, long-term use of bone anti-resorptive agents, specifically bisphosphonates, has been associated with osteonecrosis of the jaw (ONJ) (Marx 2003; Ruggiero et al. 2004). According to a web-based survey conducted by the International Myeloma Foundation (Durie et al. 2005), an increased incidence of ONJ has been observed after 36 months from the start of therapy in patients receiving zoledronic acid or pamidronate for the treatment of myeloma or breast cancer. This data also indicated that patients with prior dental problems might have a higher risk of ONJ. As the bisphosphonates are potent osteoclast inhibitors, their long-term use may suppress bone turnover and compromise healing of even physiological micro-injuries within bone (Odvina et al. 2005). Despite the encouraging therapeutic results, further long-term studies are warranted to determine the relative risk : benefit ratio of bisphosphonate therapy. See Fig. 4-4 for therapies used to treat bone loss.

With regard to osseointegration, preclinical animal studies note the influence of osteoporosis on bone–implant contact as suggesting a negative effect (Mori et al. 1997; Duarte et al. 2003; Cho et al. 2004). For instance, Cho et al. (2004), using an osteoporotic animal model, found a bone contact reduction of 50%. Lugero et al. (2000), using an induced osteoporosis rabbit model, also found that integration was impaired, although they pointed out that cortical thickness was decreased as well.

Some early clinical reports have difficulties demonstrating an increased loss of implants during early stages of implant therapy (Becker et al. 2000; Friberg et al. 2001), mostly because osteopenia is treated at the time of placement. Yet early implant failure is often correlated with local lack of bone density or volume (van Steenberghe et al. 2002). For instance, Esposito et al. (2005) in a recent systematic review,

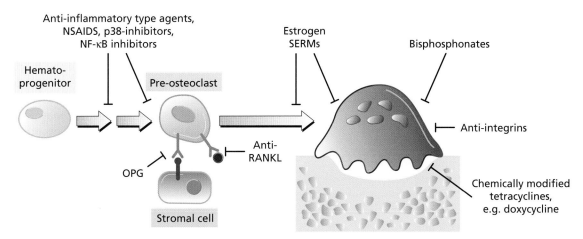

Fig. 4-4 Potential therapeutic strategies to treat bone resorption: agents that block the differentiation or activity of osteoclasts are potential therapeutic agents. Osteoprotegrin (OPG) inhibits the differentiation of osteoclasts through its action as a decoy receptor that blocks RANK (receptor activator of nuclear factor-kappa beta) and RANKL (RANK ligand) juxtacrine interaction. Non-steroidal anti-inflammatory drugs (NSAIDs) and other anti-inflammatory type molecules can inhibit the formation of hematoprogenitor cells to pre-osteoclasts. Antibodies to RANKL can also block this interaction. Estrogen and selective estrogen receptor modulators (SERMs) may inhibit the activity of osteoclasts but also promote apoptosis of osteoclasts, thus reducing their active lifespan. Bisphosphonates also promote osteoclast apoptosis. Chemically modified tetracylines reduce the protease degradation of the organic matrix, and anti-integrins block the initial osteoclast adhesion to the matrix. Adapted with permission from Kirkwood, K.L., Taba, M. Jr., Rossa, C., Preshaw, P. & Giannobile, W.V. (2006). Molecular biology concepts in host-microbe interaction in periodontal diseases. In: Newman M.G. *et al.* (eds). *Carranza's Clinical Periodontology*, 10th Edn. Elsevier Publishing, St. Louis, MO, pp. 259–274.

reported that implant failure is three times greater in the posterior maxilla, where bone density is less, than in the mandible. On the other hand, clinical evaluation or resistance during surgical osteotomy creation for implant installation may be indicative of osteopenia or osteoporosis (Friberg *et al.* 2001). It has also been reported that dental radiography and clinical evaluation at the time of surgery can suggest the presence of osteopenia, but early implant survival is not affected (Becker *et al.* 2000). Although the influence of bone density on early failure is unclear, mostly because bone volume is often a confounding factor, this suggests that it is more critical to study long-term consequences. There is, however, little information available on long-term maintenance of implants in the presence of osteoporosis. Thus, based on the available data, there is evidence to interpret an association between osteoporosis and bone density that exists around teeth and dental implant fixtures. There is also some information to suggest that decreased bone mass may place dental implants at a greater risk to failure or to decreased ability to handle load over the long term.

Diabetes mellitus

Diabetes mellitus is associated with a variety of metabolic sequalae including effects on bone maintenance and healing. There are three main types of diabetes mellitus. Type 1 is caused by damage or destruction of the beta cells of the pancreas which leads to production of insufficient amounts of insulin. Type 2 is caused by resistance to insulin with failure to produce

enough additional insulin to compensate for the insulin resistance (see also Chapter 12). Type 2 diabetes constitutes 90–95% of the individuals suffering from diabetes mellitus in the US (Kahn & Flier 2000). There is a third type of diabetes that is gestational and occurs when there is a glucose intolerance of variable severity that starts or is first recognized during pregnancy (Novak *et al.* 2006).

The liver, the skeletal muscles, and the adipose tissue are the main insulin-responsive tissues, yet insulin also influences the physiology of other tissues, including bone and cartilage. In conditions of hypo-insulinemia (e.g. type 1 diabetes) or hyperinsulinemia with or without glucose intolerance or fasting hyperglycemia (type 2 diabetes), endochondral bone growth and bone remodeling show significant alterations.

Type 1 diabetes
Although bone histomorphometry data are lacking, results from biochemical markers of bone formation studies reveal unequivocal evidence that bone formation is decreased in diabetes mellitus. Serum osteocalcin concentrations are about 25% lower in diabetic children, adolescents and adults (Bouillon *et al.* 1995). Several relatively small studies that have investigated the effect of type 1 diabetes on axial bone density have found that the BMD Z score (age-matched BMD) from the lumbar spine or the femoral neck of diabetic patients is either not significantly different from that of the control groups or that there is a small decrease in cortical bone density but no difference in trabecular bone density (Roe *et al.* 1991; Ponder *et al.* 1992;

Gallacher *et al.* 1993; Olmos *et al.* 1994). The conclusion from these studies is that type 1 diabetic subjects have a mean Z score below, but generally within 1 SD of, reference values (Lunt *et al.* 1998; Miazgowski & Czekalski 1998; Rix *et al.* 1999). This effect can be seen within a few years after diagnosis and is not progressive.

Type 2 diabetes

Bone formation and bone mineralization are also decreased in type 2 diabetes. Histomorphometry results showed a significant decrease in the osteoid thickness and in the dynamic bone formation rate of a human bone biopsy specimen of a type 2 diabetic patient with a low BMD Z score at the radius. However, low bone turnover in type 2 diabetes does not cause bone loss (Krakauer *et al.* 1995).

In support of these data, hyperinsulinemia, which is a marker of insulin resistance and the central mechanism in the pathogenesis of type 2 diabetes, has been found to be linked with higher cortical thickness and a small but significant increase in BMD (Wakasugi *et al.* 1993; Rishaug *et al.* 1995; Bauer *et al.* 2002).

Insulin stimulates endochondral bone growth and osteoblast proliferation and function *in vitro* and *in vivo* at physiological concentrations. Severe diabetes in animal models typically induces reduction in bone blood flow, bone growth, periosteal bone apposition, and bone remodeling (both resorption and formation). Consequently, bone size and bone mass are reduced. However, no effect on bone mineral density has been identified when adjusted for bone size. Less apparent changes are observed in (insulin-treated) human type 1 diabetes, although many studies report a mild reduction in growth velocity in pubertal children with this condition, a mild deficit in BMD area (maximum 10%) which does not deteriorate with longer diabetes duration, and significantly reduced bone remodeling parameters. On the other hand, individuals with hyperinsulinemia and/or type 2 diabetes have a mild increase (3–5%) in BMD area.

Apart from insulin deficiency, there are likely to be other causative factors in the development of diabetes bone disease such as alterations in the IGF-IGFBP system and hypercorticolism. The cellular and molecular mechanisms by which diabetes affects chondrocyte, (pre)osteoblast, and (pre)-osteoclast proliferation and function still need to be elucidated.

In conclusion, diabetes is associated with an increased risk of periodontitis and progressive bone loss of the alveolus; however, this risk may vary depending on differences in susceptibility to periodontitis among populations (Kinane *et al.* 2006).

Diabetes as a risk factor for alveolar bone loss around implants

Studies investigating dental implants in the presence of diabetes mellitus are limited, but there is evidence that this disease is not a contra-indication for placement (Shernoff *et al.* 1994). In fact, there is evidence that early implant survival in well controlled patients is similar to that in non-diabetic patients. It is also noticeable that this may be true for all indications (Abdulwassie & Dhanrajani 2002), as well as for more advanced surgical techniques, such as bone grafting (Farzad *et al.* 2002). However, animal experiments have shown that bone–implant contact is affected (Nevins *et al.* 1998), suggesting that clinical consequences in long-term maintenance may arise. In a large prospective 5-year clinical study, Olson *et al.* (2000) found that duration of diabetes was an important factor in implant survival. Other retrospective or observational studies have also concluded that diabetes contributes to an increase in failure rates (Moy *et al.* 2005). In a 4-year retrospective clinical analysis of 215 implants of controlled diabetes mellitus patients, Fiorellini *et al.* (2000) reported an overall success rate of 85.6%, with some variation with regard to implant location and cumulative time in function. They concluded that the implant failure rate was significantly greater than in non-diabetic patients. However, there is controversy as to whether this is due to initial failure (Fiorellini *et al.* 2000).

In contrast to the previous studies where early implant loss was greater in diagnosed patients, Peled *et al.* (2003), in a clinical evaluation of well controlled edentulous patients who had received two implants, found that there was no difference in initial osseointegration. Van Steenberghe *et al.* (2002), in a large clinical evaluation exploring various systemic parameters, found that diabetes was not a detrimental factor during initial phases of integration and prosthesis fabrication, again supporting the importance of long-term studies. The influence of underlying elevated glucose levels on osseointegration is also supported by animal studies (Ottoni & Chopard 2004). For instance, using a diabetic rat model, Siqueira *et al.* (2003) reported a 50% decrease of osseointegration when animals did not receive insulin therapy, suggesting that an association exists. Kopman *et al.* (2005), using a similar model, also reported that bone–implant contact was significantly reduced. Interestingly, these previous studies also found that treatment of the condition did not improve osseointegration, when compared to uncontrolled diabetic animals, suggesting that treated individuals may have impaired implant healing regardless of their disease stability. Furthermore, there are suggestions that poorly controlled conditions could lead to loss of bone–implant contact, resulting in a weaker bone–implant interface (Kwon *et al.* 1997). Therefore, it is likely that long-term risks for complications are greater in the presence of diabetes mellitus. This hypothesis can only be reinforced when diabetes is poorly controlled or undiagnosed.

Diabetes has been reported to adversely affect bone repair by decreasing expression of genes that induce osteoblast differentiation, and diminishing growth factor and ECM production (Bouillon 1991; Kawaguchi *et al.* 1994; Lu *et al.* 2003). One proposed mechanism for these adverse effects is through the contribution of advanced glycation end-products (AGEs) to decreased extracellular matrix production and inhibition of osteoblast differentiation (McCarthy *et al.* 2001; Cortizo *et al.* 2003; Santana *et al.* 2003). AGEs may also delay wound healing by inducing apoptosis of ECM-producing cells. This enhanced apoptosis would reduce the number of osteoblastic and fibroblastic cells available for the repair of resorbed alveolar bone (Graves *et al.* 2006). In addition to promoting apoptosis, AGEs could affect oral tissue healing by reducing expression of collagen and promoting inflammation. The mechanisms suggested for AGE-enhanced apoptosis include the direct activation of caspase activity, and indirect pathways that increase oxidative stress or the expression of pro-apoptotic genes that regulate apoptosis (Graves *et al.* 2006).

Bone healing

Healing of an injured tissue usually leads to the formation of a tissue that differs in morphology or function from the original tissue. This type of healing is termed *repair*. Tissue *regeneration*, on the other hand, is a term used to describe a healing that leads to complete restoration of morphology and function.

The healing of bone tissue includes both regeneration and repair phenomena depending on the nature of the injury. For example, a properly stabililized, narrow bone fracture (e.g. greenstick fracture) will heal by regeneration, while a larger defect (e.g. segmental bone defect) will often heal with repair. There are certain factors that may interfere with the bone tissue formation following injury, such as:

1. Failure of vessels to proliferate into the wound
2. Improper stabilization of the coagulum and granulation tissue in the defect
3. Ingrowth of "non-osseous" or fibrous tissues with a high proliferative activity
4. Bacterial contamination.

The healing of a wound includes four phases:

1. Blood clotting
2. Wound cleansing
3. Tissue formation
4. Tissue modeling and remodeling.

These phases occur in an orderly sequence but, in a given site, may overlap in such a way that in some areas of the wound, tissue formation may be in progress, while in other areas tissue modeling is the dominating event. Examples of bone remodeling can be also seen in Chapter 2 on the edentulous ridge and Chapter 49 on ridge augmentation procedures.

Bone grafting

Although bone tissue exhibits a large regeneration potential and may restore its original structure and function completely, bony defects may often fail to heal with bone tissue. In order to facilitate and/or promote healing, bone grafting materials have been placed into bony defects. It is generally accepted that the biologic mechanisms forming the basis for bone grafting include three basic processes: *osteogenesis, osteoconduction*, and *osteoinduction*.

Osteogenesis occurs when viable osteoblasts and precursor osteoblasts are transplanted with the grafting material into the defects, where they may establish centers of bone formation. Autogenous iliac bone and marrow grafts are examples of transplants with osteogenic properties (see Chapter 49).

Osteoconduction occurs when non-vital implant material serves as a scaffold for the ingrowth of precursor osteoblasts into the defect. This process is usually followed by a gradual resorption of the implant material. Autogenous cortical bone or banked bone allografts may be examples of grafting materials with osteoconductive properties (Fig. 4-5). Such grafting materials, as well as bone-derived or synthetic bone substitutes, have similar osteoconductive properties. However, degradation and substitution by viable bone is often poor. If the implanted material is not resorbable, which is the case for most porous hydroxylapatite implants, the incorporation is restricted to bone apposition to the material surface, but no substitution occurs during the remodeling phase.

Osteoinduction involves new bone formation by the differentiation of local uncommitted connective tissue cells into bone-forming cells under the influence of one or more inducing agents. *Demineralized bone matrix* (DMB) or *bone morphogenetic proteins* (BMP) are examples of such grafting materials (Giannobile & Somerman 2003; Reynolds *et al.* 2003).

It often occurs that all three basic bone-forming mechanisms are involved in bone regeneration. In fact, osteogenesis without osteoconduction and osteoinduction is unlikely to occur, since almost none of the transmitted cells of autogenous cancellous bone grafts survive the transplantation. Thus, the grafting material predominantly functions as a scaffold for invading cells of the host. In addition, the osteoblasts and osteocytes of the surrounding bone lack the ability to migrate and divide which, in turn, means that the transplant is invaded by uncommitted mesenchymal cells that later differentiate into osteoblasts.

On that basis, it is appropriate to define three basic conditions as prerequisites for bone regeneration:

1. The *supply of bone-forming cells* or cells with the capacity to differentiate into bone-forming cells

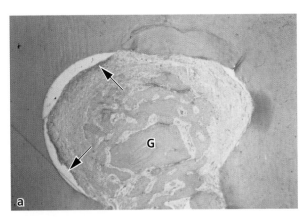
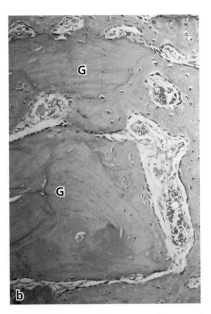

Fig. 4-5 (a) Microphotograph demonstrating bifurcation defect 3 weeks after grafting with autogenous cancellous jaw bone (G). New bone has invaded the defect, and the bone grafts have exerted an osteoconductive function. Epithelium (arrows) has migrated into one side of the defect. (b) Higher magnification of (a) showing that new bone has formed around the bone grafts (G), which have lost their vitality, indicated by the empty osteocyte lacunae.

2. The presence of *osteoinductive stimuli* to initiate the differentiation of mesenchymal cells into osteoblasts
3. The presence of an *osteoconductive environment* forming a scaffold upon which invading tissue can proliferate and in which the stimulated osteoprogenitor cells can differentiate into osteoblasts and form bone.

The placement of bone-grafting materials to favor healing in osseous defects or to augment atrophic alveolar ridges has been evaluated in a number of experimental and clinical studies (Boyne 1970; Thompson & Casson 1970; Steinhauser & Hardt 1977; Fazili *et al.* 1978; Baker *et al.* 1979; Mulliken & Glowacki 1980; Swart & Allard 1985; Block *et al.* 1987; Cullum *et al.* 1988; Hupp & McKenna 1988) (also see Chapter 49). However, there are several reports indicating that this type of treatment fails predictably to produce bone fill and augment alveolar ridges (Korlof *et al.* 1973; Curtis & Ware 1977; Steinhauser & Hardt 1977; Taylor 1983; Davis *et al.* 1984; Jackson *et al.* 1986; Hupp & McKenna 1988). Often the bone grafts do not attach to the graft site through bony attachment and there is bone resorption and bone loss associated with grafting procedures. As a consequence, much of the intended volume is lost, and frequently the defects heal with a fibrous connective tissue instead of bone.

Human experimental studies on alveolar bone repair

At present, most of the information regarding the biologic events which lead to new bone formation is derived from animal studies. Results regarding bone formation collected in animal studies have to be applied with proper caution in humans. In particular, the time sequence of the various steps ultimately leading to the formation of mineralized mature bone in man is different from that in all experimental animal systems known. A few human specimens, often harvested under poorly controlled conditions, contribute relatively little to the understanding of the biologic events of bone regeneration in humans.

A model system was designed to obtain human specimens of regenerated and also newly generated alveolar bone for the study of the biologic events under a variety of conditions (Hämmerle *et al.* 1996). A mucoperiosteal flap was raised in the retromolar area of the mandible of nine healthy volunteers. Following flap reflection, a standardized hole was drilled through the cortical bone into the bone marrow. Congruent test cylinders were firmly placed into the prepared bony bed, yielding primary stability; 1.5–2 mm of the test device were submerged below the level of the surrounding bone, leaving 2–3 mm above the bone surface. The bone-facing end of the cylinder was left open, while the coronal soft tissue-facing end was closed by an expanded polytetrafluoroethylene (ePTFE) membrane. The flap was sutured to obtain primary wound closure. In order to prevent infection, penicillin was prescribed systemically and oral rinses of chlorhexidine were administered. After 2, 7, and 12 weeks, one test device, including the regenerated tissue, was surgically harvested, while after 16, 24, and 36 weeks, respectively, two devices were harvested and processed for soft or hard tissue histology or immunohistochemistry. The tissue generated after 2 and 7 weeks (Fig. 4-6) presented with a cylindrical shape, whereas the specimens harvested at 12 weeks and thereafter resembled the form of an hourglass.

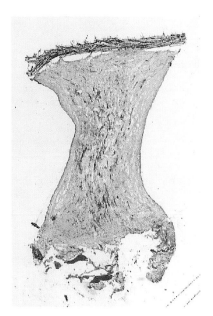

Fig. 4-6 Histological section of a 7-week specimen, comprising non-mineralized connective tissue in the shape of an hourglass. Note the covering e-PTFE membrane.

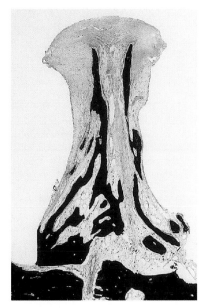

Fig. 4-7 Histological section of a 9-month specimen. The height of the mineralized tissue has reached the top 20% of the cylinder space area.

Specimens of 12 weeks and less regeneration time were almost entirely composed of soft tissue, while specimens with a regeneration time of 4 months and more were composed of both soft and increasing amounts of mineralized tissue (Fig. 4-7). It was concluded that the model system is suitable for studying temporal dynamics and tissue physiology of bone regeneration in humans with minimal risk of complications or adverse effects for the volunteers.

In a retrospective re-entry study (Lang *et al.* 1994), the bone volume regenerated using non-bioresorbable membrane barriers was assessed. Nineteen patients with jaw bone defects of various sizes and configurations were included. Combined split-thickness/full-thickness mucosal flaps were elevated in the area of missing bone. The size of the defects was assessed geometrically. Following the placement of Gore-Tex® augmentation material as a barrier, the maximum possible volume for bone regeneration was calculated. At the time of membrane removal (3–8 months later), the same measurements were performed and the percentages of regenerated bone in relation to the possible volume for regeneration determined. In six patients in whom the membranes had to be removed early, between 3 and 5 months, due to an increased risk of infection, bone regeneration varied between 0 and 60%. In 13 patients in whom the membranes were left for 6–8 months, regenerated bone filled 90–100% of the possible volume. It was concluded that successful bone regeneration consistently occurred with an undisturbed healing period of at least 6 months.

Conclusion: In summary, the bone of the alveolar process is of critical importance to maintain the structure and function of the jaws and subsequently the housing of teeth or tooth replacements. The physiological and biomechanical influences on bone by local and systemic mediators of bone homeostasis are important in the maintenance of alveolus. Reconstructive modalities aimed at the repair of bone tissues as a result of disease or injury utilize fundamental principles of bone biology. These regenerative biology approaches have been exploited in implant dentistry and periodontology with the use of bone grafting biomaterials, guided bone regeneration approaches, and more recently with polypeptide growth factors. Future work in this area will focus on the implications of systemic disease on bone maintenance during function as well as more predictable modalities for alveolar bone reconstruction.

References

Abdulwassie, H. & Dhanrajani, P.J. (2002). Diabetes mellitus and dental implants: a clinical study. *Implant Dentistry* **11**, 83–86.

Anusaksathien, O. & Giannobile, W.V. (2002). Growth factor delivery to re-engineer periodontal tissues. *Current Pharmaceutical Biotechnology* **3**, 129–139.

Baker, R.D., Terry, B.C., Davis, W.H. & Connole, P.W. (1979). Long-term results of alveolar ridge augmentation. *Journal of Oral Surgery* **37**, 486–489.

Bauer, D.C., Bauer, D.C., Palermo, L., Black, D. & Cauley, J.A. (2002). Quantitative ultrasound and mortality: a prospective study. *Osteoporosis International* **13**, 606–612.

Baylink, D.J., Finkelman, R.D. & Mohan, S. (1993). Growth factors to stimulate bone formation. *Journal of Bone and Mineral Research* **8** (Suppl 2), S565–572.

Becker, W., Hujoel, P.P., Becker, B.E. & Willingham, H. (2000). Osteoporosis and implant failure: an exploratory case-control study. *Journal of Periodontology* **71**, 625–631.

Blair, H.C., Zaidi, M. & Schlesinger, P.H. (2002). Mechanisms balancing skeletal matrix synthesis and degradation. *Biochemical Journal* **364**, 329–341.

Block, M.S., Kent, J.N., Ardoin, R.C. & Davenport, W. (1987). Mandibular augmentation in dogs with hydroxylapatite combined with demineralized bone. *Journal of Oral and Maxillofacial Surgery* **45**, 414–420.

Blumenthal, N.M., Koh-Kunst, G., Alves, M.E., Miranda, D., Sorensen, R.G., Wozney, J.M. & Wikesjo, U. M. (2002). Effect of surgical implantation of recombinant human bone morphogenetic protein-2 in a bioabsorbable collagen sponge or calcium phosphate putty carrier in intrabony periodontal defects in the baboon. *Journal of Periodontology* **73**, 1494–1506.

Bouillon, R. (1991). Diabetic bone disease. *Calcified Tissue International* **49**, 155–160.

Bouillon, R., Bex, M., Van Herck, E., Laureys, J., Dooms, L., Lesaffre, E. & Ravussin, E. (1995). Influence of age, sex, and insulin on osteoblast function: osteoblast dysfunction in diabetes mellitus. *Journal of Clinical Endocrinology and Metabolism* **80**, 1194–1202.

Boyne, P.J. (1970). Autogenous cancellous bone and marrow transplants. *Clinical Orthopaedics and Related Research* **73**, 199–209.

Chen, D., Zhao, M. & Mundy, G.R. (2004). Bone morphogenetic proteins. *Growth Factors* **22**, 233–241.

Cheng, H., Jiang, W., Phillips, F.M., Haydon, R.C., Peng, Y., Zhou, L., Luu, H.H., An, N., Breyer, B., Vanichakarn, P., Szatkowski, J.P., Park, J.Y. & He, T.C. (2003). Osteogenic activity of the fourteen types of human bone morphogenetic proteins (BMPs). *Journal of Bone and Joint Surgery. American Volume* **85-A**, 1544–1552.

Cho, P., Schneider, G.B., Krizan, K. & Keller, J.C. (2004). Examination of the bone-implant interface in experimentally induced osteoporotic bone. *Implant Dentistry*, **13**, 79–87.

Civitelli, R., Pilgram, T.K., Dotson, M., Muckerman, J., Lewandowski, N., Armamento-Villareal, R., Yokoyama-Crothers, N., Kardaris, E.E., Hauser, J., Cohen, S. & Hildebolt, C.F. (2002). Alveolar and postcranial bone density in postmenopausal women receiving hormone/estrogen replacement therapy: a randomized, double-blind, placebo-controlled trial. *Archives of Internal Medicine* **162**, 1409–1415.

Cortizo, A.M., Lettieri, M.G., Barrio, D.A., Mercer, N., Etcheverry, S.B. & McCarthy, A.D. (2003). Advanced glycation end-products (AGEs) induce concerted changes in the osteoblastic expression of their receptor RAGE and in the activation of extracellular signal-regulated kinases (ERK). *Molecular and Cellular Biochemistry* **250**, 1–10.

Cullum, P.E., Frost, D.E., Newland, T.B., Keane, T.M. & Ehler, W.J. (1988). Evaluation of hydroxylapatite particles in repair of alveolar clefts in dogs. *Journal of Oral and Maxillofacial Surgery* **46**, 290–296.

Curtis, T.A. & Ware, W.H. (1977). Autogenous bone graft procedures for atrophic edentulous mandibles. *Journal of Prosthetic Dentistry* **38**, 366–379.

Davis, W.H., Martinoff, J.T. & Kaminishi, R.M. (1984). Long-term follow up of transoral rib grafts for mandibular atrophy. *Journal of Oral and Maxillofacial Surgery* **42**, 606–609.

Duarte, P.M., Cesar Neto, J.B., Goncalves, P.F., Sallum, E.A. & Nociti, F.H. (2003). Estrogen deficiency affects bone healing around titanium implants: a histometric study in rats. *Implant Dentistry* **12**, 340–346.

Durie, B.G., Katz, M. & Crowley, J. (2005). Osteonecrosis of the jaw and bisphosphonates. *New England Journal of Medicine* **353**, 99–102.

Esposito, M., Coulthard, P., Thomsen, P. & Worthington, H. V. (2005). The role of implant surface modifications, shape and material on the success of osseointegrated dental implants. A Cochrane systematic review. *European Journal of Prosthodontics & Restorative Dentistry* **13**, 15–31.

Farzad, P., Andersson, L. & Nyberg, J. (2002). Dental implant treatment in diabetic patients. *Implant Dentistry* **11**, 262–267.

Fazili, M., von Overvest-Eerdmans, G.R., Vernooy, A.M., Visser, W.J. & von Waas, M.A. (1978). Follow-up investigation of reconstruction of the alveolar process in the atrophic mandible. *International Journal of Oral Surgery* **7**, 400–404.

Fiorellini, J.P., Chen, P.K., Nevins, M. & Nevins, M.L. (2000). A retrospective study of dental implants in diabetic patients. *International Journal of Periodontics and Restorative Dentistry* **20**, 366–373.

Friberg, B., Ekestubbe, A., Mellstrom, D. & Sennerby, L. (2001). Branemark implants and osteoporosis: a clinical exploratory study. *Clinical Implant Dentistry & Related Research* **3**, 50–56.

Friedenstein, A.J. (1973). Determined and inducible osteogenic precursor cells. In: *Hand Tissue Growth Repair and Remineralisation. Ciba Foundation Symposium. New series* **11**, 169–181.

Gallacher, S.J., Fenner, J.A., Fisher, B.M., Quin, J.D., Fraser, W.D., Logue, F.C., Cowan, R.A., Boyle, I.T. & MacCuish, A.C. (1993). An evaluation of bone density and turnover in premenopausal women with type 1 diabetes mellitus. *Diabetic Medicine* **10**, 129–133.

Giannobile, W.V. (1996). Periodontal tissue engineering by growth factors. *Bone* **19**, 23S-37S.

Giannobile, W.V. & Somerman, M.J. (2003). Growth and amelogenin-like factors in periodontal wound healing. A systematic review. *Annals of Periodontology* **8**, 193–204.

Graves, D.T., Liu, R., Alikhani, M., Al-Mashat, H. & Trackman, P.C. (2006). Diabetes-enhanced inflammation and apoptosis–impact on periodontal pathology. *Journal of Dental Research* **85**, 15–21.

Hämmerle, C.H., Schmid, J., Olah, A.J. & Lang, N.P. (1996). A novel model system for the study of experimental guided bone formation in humans. *Clinical Oral Implants Research* **7**, 38–47.

Hildebolt, C.F. (1997). Osteoporosis and oral bone loss. *Dentomaxillofacial Radiology* **26**, 3–15.

Horner, K., Devlin, H., Alsop, C.W., Hodgkinson, I.M. & Adams, J.E. (1996). Mandibular bone mineral density as a predictor of skeletal osteoporosis. *British Journal of Radiology* **69**, 1019–1025.

Hupp, J.R. & McKenna, S.J. (1988). Use of porous hydroxylapatite blocks for augmentation of atrophic mandibles. *Journal of Oral and Maxillofacial Surgery* **46**, 538–545.

Jackson, I.T., Helden, G. & Marx, R. (1986). Skull bone grafts in maxillofacial and craniofacial surgery. *Journal of Oral and Maxillofacial Surgery* **44**, 949–955.

Janssens, K., ten Dijke, P., Janssens, S. & Van Hul, W. (2005). Transforming growth factor-beta1 to the bone. *Endocrine Reviews* **26**, 743–774.

Kahn, B.B. & Flier, J.S. (2000). Obesity and insulin resistance. *Journal of Clinical Investigation* **106**, 473–481.

Kawaguchi, H., Kurokawa, T., Hanada, K., Hiyama, Y., Tamura, M., Ogata, E. & Matsumoto, T. (1994). Stimulation of fracture repair by recombinant human basic fibroblast growth factor in normal and streptozotocin-diabetic rats. *Endocrinology*, **135**, 774–781.

Kinane, D.F., Peterson, M. & Stathopoulou, P.G. (2006). Environmental and other modifying factors of the periodontal diseases. *Periodontology 2000* **40**, 107–119.

King, G.N. & Cochran, D.L. (2002). Factors that modulate the effects of bone morphogenetic protein-induced periodontal regeneration: a critical review. *Journal of Periodontology* **73**, 925–936.

Klemetti, E., Vainio, P., Lassila, V. & Alhava, E. (1993). Cortical bone mineral density in the mandible and osteoporosis status in postmenopausal women. *Scandinavian Journal of Dental Research* **101**, 219–223.

Kopman, J.A., Kim, D.M., Rahman, S.S., Arandia, J.A., Karimbux, N.Y. & Fiorellini, J.P. (2005). Modulating the effects of diabetes on osseointegration with aminoguanidine and doxycycline. *Journal of Periodontology* **76**, 614–620.

Korlof, B., Nylen, B. & Rietz, K.A. (1973). Bone grafting of skull defects. A report on 55 cases. *Plastic and Reconstructive Surgery* **52**, 378–383.

Krakauer, J.C., McKenna, M.J., Buderer, N.F., Rao, D.S., Whitehouse, F.W. & Parfitt, A.M. (1995). Bone loss and bone turnover in diabetes. *Diabetes* **44**, 775–782.

Kribbs, P.J. (1990). Comparison of mandibular bone in normal and osteoporotic women. *Journal of Prosthetic Dentistry* **63**, 218–222.

Kribbs, P.J., Chesnut, C.H., 3rd, Ott, S.M. & Kilcoyne, R.F. (1990). Relationships between mandibular and skeletal bone in a population of normal women. *Journal of Prosthetic Dentistry* **63**, 86–89.

Kwon, Y.K., Bhattacharyya, A., Alberta, J.A., Giannobile, W.V., Cheon, K., Stiles, C.D. & Pomeroy, S.L. (1997). Activation of ErbB2 during wallerian degeneration of sciatic nerve. *Journal of Neuroscience* **17**, 8293–8299.

Lang, N.P., Hammerle, C.H., Bragger, U., Lehmann, B. & Nyman, S.R. (1994). Guided tissue regeneration in jawbone defects prior to implant placement. *Clinical Oral Implants Research* **5**, 92–97.

Law, A.N., Bollen, A.M. & Chen, S.K. (1996). Detecting osteoporosis using dental radiographs: a comparison of four methods. *Journal of the American Dental Association* **127**, 1734–1742.

Le, A.D., Basi, D.L. & Abubaker, A.O. (2005). Wound healing: findings of the 2005 AAOMS Research Summit. *Journal of Oral and Maxillofacial Surgery* **63**, 1426–1435.

Linkhart, T.A., Mohan, S. & Baylink, D.J. (1996). Growth factors for bone growth and repair: IGF, TGF beta and BMP. *Bone* **19**, 1S-12S.

Lu, H., Kraut, D., Gerstenfeld, L.C. & Graves, D.T. (2003). Diabetes interferes with the bone formation by affecting the expression of transcription factors that regulate osteoblast differentiation. *Endocrinology* **144**, 346–352.

Lugero, G.G., de Falco Caparbo, V., Guzzo, M.L., Konig, B., Jr. & Jorgetti, V. (2000). Histomorphometric evaluation of titanium implants in osteoporotic rabbits. *Implant Dentistry* **9**, 303–309.

Lunt, H., Florkowski, C.M., Cundy, T., Kendall, D., Brown, L. J., Elliot, J.R., Wells, J.E. & Turner, J.G. (1998). A population-based study of bone mineral density in women with long-standing type 1 (insulin dependent) diabetes. *Diabetes Research and Clinical Practice* **40**, 31–38.

Marx, R.E. (2003). Pamidronate (Aredia) and zoledronate (Zometa) induced avascular necrosis of the jaws: a growing epidemic. *Journal of Oral and Maxillofacial Surgery* **61**, 1115–1117.

McCarthy, A.D., Etcheverry, S.B. & Cortizo, A.M. (2001). Effect of advanced glycation endproducts on the secretion of insulin-like growth factor-I and its binding proteins: role in osteoblast development. *Acta Diabetologica* **38**, 113–122.

Miazgowski, T. & Czekalski, S. (1998). A 2-year follow-up study on bone mineral density and markers of bone turnover in patients with long-standing insulin-dependent diabetes mellitus. *Osteoporosis International* **8**, 399–403.

Mori, H., Manabe, M., Kurachi, Y. & Nagumo, M. (1997). Osseointegration of dental implants in rabbit bone with low mineral density. *Journal of Oral & Maxillofacial Surgery* **55**, 351–361; discussion 362.

Moy, P.K., Medina, D., Shetty, V. & Aghaloo, T.L. (2005). Dental implant failure rates and associated risk factors. *International Journal of Oral & Maxillofacial Implants* **20**, 569–577.

Mulliken, J.B. & Glowacki, J. (1980). Induced osteogenesis for repair and construction in the craniofacial region. *Plastic and Reconstructive Surgery* **65**, 553–560.

Nevins, M.L., Karimbux, N.Y., Weber, H.P., Giannobile, W.V. & Fiorellini, J.P. (1998). Wound healing around endosseous implants in experimental diabetes. *International Journal of Oral & Maxillofacial Implants* **13**, 620–629.

Novak, K.F., Taylor, G.W., Dawson, D.R., Ferguson, J.E., 2nd & Novak, M.J. (2006). Periodontitis and gestational diabetes mellitus: exploring the link in NHANES III. *Journal of Public Health Dentistry* **66**, 163–168.

Odvina, C.V., Zerwekh, J.E., Rao, D.S., Maalouf, N., Gottschalk, F.A. & Pak, C.Y. (2005). Severely suppressed bone turnover: a potential complication of alendronate therapy. *Journal of Clinical Endocrinology and Metabolism* **90**, 1294–1301.

Oh, T.J., Bashutski, J. & Giannobile, W.V. (2007). Inter-relationship between osteoporosis and oral bone loss. *Grand Rounds in Oral Systemic Medicine*, **2**, 10–21.

Olmos, J.M., Perez-Castrillon, J.L., Garcia, M.T., Garrido, J.C., Amado, J.A. & Gonzalez-Macias, J. (1994). Bone densitometry and biochemical bone remodeling markers in type 1 diabetes mellitus. *Bone and Mineral* **26**, 1–8.

Olson, J.W., Shernoff, A.F., Tarlow, J.L., Colwell, J.A., Scheetz, J.P. & Bingham, S.F. (2000). Dental endosseous implant assessments in a type 2 diabetic population: a prospective study. *International Journal of Oral & Maxillofacial Implants* **15**, 811–818.

Ottoni, C.E. & Chopard, R.P. (2004). Histomorphometric evaluation of new bone formation in diabetic rats submitted to insertion of temporary implants. *Brazilian Dental Journal* **15**, 87–92.

Payne, J.B., Reinhardt, R.A., Nummikoski, P.V. & Patil, K.D. (1999). Longitudinal alveolar bone loss in postmenopausal osteoporotic/osteopenic women. *Osteoporosis International* **10**, 34–40.

Payne, J.B., Zachs, N.R., Reinhardt, R.A., Nummikoski, P.V. & Patil, K. (1997). The association between estrogen status and alveolar bone density changes in postmenopausal women with a history of periodontitis. *Journal of Periodontology* **68**, 24–31.

Peled, M., Ardekian, L., Tagger-Green, N., Gutmacher, Z. & Machtei, E.E. (2003). Dental implants in patients with type 2 diabetes mellitus: a clinical study. *Implant Dentistry* **12**, 116–122.

Ponder, S.W., McCormick, D.P., Fawcett, H.D., Tran, A.D., Ogelsby, G.W., Brouhard, B.H. & Travis, L.B. (1992). Bone mineral density of the lumbar vertebrae in children and adolescents with insulin-dependent diabetes mellitus. *Journal of Pediatrics* **120**, 541–545.

Reynolds, M.A., Aichelmann-Reidy, M.E., Branch-Mays, G.L. & Gunsolley, J.C. (2003). The efficacy of bone replacement grafts in the treatment of periodontal osseous defects. A systematic review. *Annals of Periodontology* **8**, 227–265.

Ripamonti, U., Herbst, N.N. & Ramoshebi, L.N. (2005). Bone morphogenetic proteins in craniofacial and periodontal tissue engineering: experimental studies in the non-human primate Papio ursinus. *Cytokine and Growth Factor Review* **16**, 357–368.

Rishaug, U., Birkeland, K.I., Falch, J.A. & Vaaler, S. (1995). Bone mass in non-insulin-dependent diabetes mellitus. *Scandinavian Journal of Clinical and Laboratory Investigation* **55**, 257–262.

Rix, M., Andreassen, H. & Eskildsen, P. (1999). Impact of peripheral neuropathy on bone density in patients with type 1 diabetes. *Diabetes Care* **22**, 827–831.

Roe, T.F., Mora, S., Costin, G., Kaufman, F., Carlson, M.E. & Gilsanz, V. (1991). Vertebral bone density in insulin-dependent diabetic children. *Metabolism* **40**, 967–971.

Ruggiero, S.L., Mehrotra, B., Rosenberg, T.J. & Engroff, S.L. (2004). Osteonecrosis of the jaws associated with the use of bisphosphonates: a review of 63 cases. *Journal of Oral and Maxillofacial Surgery* **62**, 527–534.

Santana, R.B., Xu, L., Chase, H.B., Amar, S., Graves, D.T. & Trackman, P.C. (2003). A role for advanced glycation end products in diminished bone healing in type 1 diabetes. *Diabetes* **52**, 1502–1510.

Schilephake, H. (2002). Bone growth factors in maxillofacial skeletal reconstruction. *International Journal of Oral & Maxillofacial Surgery* **31**, 469–484.

Shernoff, A.F., Colwell, J.A. & Bingham, S.F. (1994). Implants for type II diabetic patients: interim report. VA Implants in Diabetes Study Group. *Implant Dentistry* **3**, 183–185.

Siqueira, J.T., Cavalher-Machado, S.C., Arana-Chavez, V.E. & Sannomiya, P. (2003). Bone formation around titanium implants in the rat tibia: role of insulin. *Implant Dentistry* **12**, 242–251.

Steinhauser, E.W. & Hardt, N. (1977). Secondary reconstruction of cranial defects. *Journal of Maxillofacial Surgery* **5**, 192–198.

Swart, J.G. & Allard, R.H. (1985). Subperiosteal onlay augmentation of the mandible: a clinical and radiographic survey. *Journal of Oral and Maxillofacial Surgery* **43**, 183–187.

Sykaras, N. & Opperman, L.A. (2003). Bone morphogenetic proteins (BMPs): how do they function and what can they offer the clinician? *Journal of Oral Science* **45**, 57–73.

Taguchi, A., Tanimoto, K., Suei, Y., Ohama, K. & Wada, T. (1996). Relationship between the mandibular and lumbar vertebral bone mineral density at different postmenopausal stages. *Dentomaxillofacial Radiology* **25**, 130–135.

Taylor, G.I. (1983). The current status of free vascularized bone grafts. *Clinical Plastic Surgery* **10**, 185–209.

Thompson, N. & Casson, J.A. (1970). Experimental onlay bone grafts to the jaws. A preliminary study in dogs. *Plastic and Reconstructive Surgery* **46**, 341–349.

van Steenberghe, D., Jacobs, R., Desnyder, M., Maffei, G. & Quirynen, M. (2002). The relative impact of local and endogenous patient-related factors on implant failure up to the abutment stage. *Clinical Oral Implants Research* **13**, 617–622.

von Wowern, N., Klausen, B. & Kollerup, G. (1994). Osteoporosis: a risk factor in periodontal disease. *Journal of Periodontology* **65**, 1134–1138.

Wakasugi, M., Wakao, R., Tawata, M., Gan, N., Koizumi, K. & Onaya, T. (1993). Bone mineral density measured by dual energy x-ray absorptiometry in patients with non-insulin-dependent diabetes mellitus. *Bone* **14**, 29–33.

Whalen, J.P. & Krook, L. (1996). Periodontal disease as the early manifestation of osteoporosis. *Nutrition* **12**, 53–54.

Chapter 5

Osseointegration

Jan Lindhe, Tord Berglundh, and Niklaus P. Lang

The edentulous site

The fully healed, edentulous site of the alveolar ridge (see Fig. 2-23 and Chapter 2) is most often covered by a masticatory mucosa that is about 2–3 mm thick. This type of mucosa is covered by a keratinized epithelium and includes a connective tissue, rich in collagen fibers and fibroblasts, that is firmly attached to the bone via the periosteum. The outer walls of the alveolar process, the cortical plates, are comprised of lamellar bone and enclose the spongy or cancellous bone that contains bone trabeculae (lamellar bone) embedded in marrow. The bone marrow contains numerous vascular structures as well as adipocytes and pluripotent mesenchymal cells.

Osseointegration

Different types of implant systems have been used to replace missing teeth, including subperiosteal implants, endosseous implants with fibrous encapsulation, and endosseous implants with direct bone contact (*osseointegrated*). One definition of *osseointegration* (a term originally proposed by Brånemark *et al.* 1969) was provided by Albrektsson *et al.* (1981) who suggested that this was "a direct functional and structural connection between living bone and the surface of a load carrying implant". Another, clinical definition was provided by Zarb and Albrektsson (1991) who proposed that *osseointegration* was "a process whereby clinically asymptomatic rigid fixation of alloplastic materials is achieved and maintained in bone during functional loading".

Schroeder *et al.* (1976, 1981, 1995) used the term *"functional ankylosis"* to describe the rigid fixation of the implant to the jaw bone, and stated that "new bone is laid down directly upon the implant surface, provided that the rules for atraumatic implant placement are followed (rotation of the cutting instrument and less than 800 rpm, cooling with sterile physio-

logic saline solution) and the implant exhibits primary stability".

Thus, in order to acquire proper conditions for osseointegration (or functional ankylosis), the implant must exhibit proper initial fixation (stability) following installation in the recipient site. This initial (primary) stability is the result of the contact relationship or friction that is established following insertion of the implant, between mineralized bone (often the cortical bone) at the recipient site and the metal device.

Implant installation

Tissue injury

Basic rule: the less traumatic the surgical procedure is and the smaller the tissue injury (the damage) becomes in the recipient site during implant installation, the more expeditious is the process through which new bone is formed and laid down on the implant surface.

The various steps used in the implant installation procedure, such as (1) *incision* of the mucosa, often but not always followed by (2) the elevation of *mucosal flaps* and the separation of the periosteum from the cortical plates, (3) the preparation of the *canal* in the cortical and spongy bone of the recipient site, and (4) the insertion of the titanium device (the implant) in this canal, bring to bear a series of mechanical insults and injury to both the mucosa and the bone tissue. The host responds to this injury with an inflammatory reaction, the main objective of which is to eliminate the damaged portions of the tissues and prepare the site for regeneration or repair. To the above described hard tissue injury must be added the effect of the so-called "press fit", i.e. when the inserted implant is slightly wider than the canal prepared in the host bone at the recipient site. In such situations, (1) the mineralized bone tissue in the periphery of the implant is compressed, (2) the blood vessels particularly in the cortical portion of the canal are collapsed, (3) the nutrition to this portion of the bone compromised, and (4) the affected tissues most often become non-vital.

The damage or injury to the soft and hard tissues of the recipient site initiates the process of wound healing that ultimately ensures that (1) the implant becomes "ankylotic" with the bone, i.e. osseointegrated, and (2) a delicate mucosal attachment (see Chapter 3) is established and a soft tissue seal formed that protects the bone tissue from substances in the oral cavity.

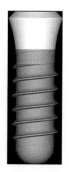

Fig. 5-1 A "non-cutting" implant (solid screw: Straumann® Implant System).

Wound healing

The healing of the severed bone following implant installation is a complex process that apparently involves different events in the cortical and in the spongy (cancellous) compartments of the surgical site.

In the *cortical bone compartment*, the non-vital mineralized tissue must first be removed (resorbed) before new bone can form. In the *spongy compartment* of the recipient site, on the other hand, the surgically inflicted damage (preparation of the canal and the installation of the implant) results mainly in soft tissue (marrow) injury that initially is characterized by localized bleeding and clot (coagulum) formation. The coagulum is gradually resorbed and the compartment thus becomes occupied by proliferating blood vessels and mesenchymal cells; granulation tissue. As result of the continuous migration of mesenchymal cells from the surrounding marrow, the young granulation tissue becomes replaced with provisional connective tissue and eventually with osteoid. In the osteoid, deposition of hydroxyapatite will occur around the newly formed vascular structures. Hereby, immature bone, most often woven bone, is formed (for detail see Chapter 2) and sequentially osseointegration, a direct connection between the newly formed bone and the metal device, takes place.

In summary: in the initial phase of the process that results in osseointegration, the non-vital lamellar bone in the cortical compartment is of importance for the initial fixation of the implant. Osseointegration, however, is often first established in areas occupied by cancellous bone.

Cutting and non-cutting implants

In this chapter only screw-shaped implants made of c.p. titanium will be discussed. The design of the metal device and the installation protocol followed may influence the speed of the process that leads to osseointegration.

"Non-cutting" implants (Fig. 5-1) require meticulous handling of the recipient site including the preparation of a standardized track (thread) on the inside

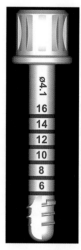

Fig. 5-2 A thread-tap (Straumann® Implant System) that is used to cut a track in the walls of the hard tissue canal. Following this preparation the cavity in the host tissue and the implant are congruent.

of the hard tissue canal. This preparation (precutting) of the track (thread) is made by the use of a thread-tap that is fitted with cutting edges (Fig. 5-2).

Figure 5.1 illustrates a "non-cutting" implant (solid screw, 4.1 mm: Straumann® implant system) that is designed as a cylinder with a rounded "apical" base. The diameter of the cylinder is 3.5 mm. Pilot and twist drills of gradually increasing dimension are used to prepare the hard tissue canal of the recipient site to a final diameter of 3.5 mm. On the surface of the cylinder the implant is designed with a helix-shaped pitch that is 0.3 mm high. The diameter of the entire screw shaped device therefore becomes 4.1 mm.

In sites with a high bone density a thread-tap (Fig. 5-2) is used to cut a 4.1 mm wide helix-shaped track in the walls of the hard tissue canal. The implant and the cavity prepared in the hard tissues of the recipient site are now congruent. When the implant is installed, the pitch on the device will capture and follow the helix-shaped track on the walls of the hard tissue canal and hereby guide the implant with a minimum of force into the pre-prepared position (Fig. 5-3).

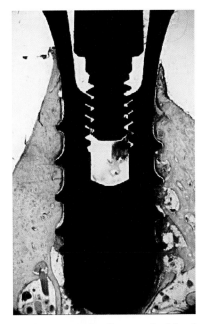

Fig. 5-3 Ground section with a "non-cutting" implant and surrounding tissues obtained from a biopsy performed 24 hours after implant installation.

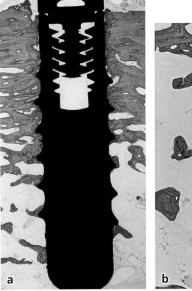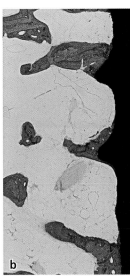

Fig. 5-5 (a) Ground section illustrating a "non-cutting" implant and surrounding bone after 16 weeks of healing. In the cortical portion of the recipient site, the bone density is high. (b) Detail of (a). In more apical areas a thin coat of bone is present on the implant surface. Note also the presence of trabeculae of lamellar bone that extend from the implant into the bone marrow.

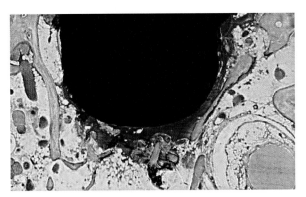

Fig. 5-4 Detail from the apical region of the implant described in Fig. 5-3. Note the presence of a coagulum in the bone marrow.

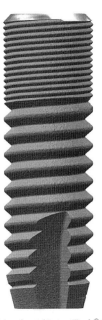

Fig. 5-6 A "cutting" implant (Astra Tech® Implant System). Note the presence of cutting edges in the "apical" portion of the implant. During insertion this implant will cut a 0.3 mm wide chip from the lateral border of the canal prepared in the recipient site.

Figure 5-3 illustrates a "non-cutting" Straumann® solid screw with surrounding tissues in a biopsy sampled 24 hours after implant installation. The implant had proper initial fixation (stability) obtained by the large contact area that was achieved between the metal screw and the buccal and lingual bone walls in the cortical compartment of the recipient site. During site preparation and placement of the implant, bone trabeculae in the spongy compartment of the site were obviously dislocated into the bone marrow. Blood vessels in the marrow compartment were severed, bleeding provoked and a coagulum formed (Fig. 5-4).

After 16 weeks of healing (Fig. 5-5) the marginal portions of the "non-cutting" implant are surrounded by dense lamellar bone that is in direct contact with the rough surface of the metal device. Also in the apical portion of the implant, a thin coat of mature bone can be seen to contact the implant surface and

to separate the titanium screw from the bone marrow.

Cutting or self-tapping implants (e.g. Astra Tech® implants, diameter 4.0 mm) (Fig. 5-6) are designed with cutting edges placed in the "apical" portion of the screw-shaped device. The threads of the screw are prepared during manufacturing by cutting a continuous groove into the body of the titanium

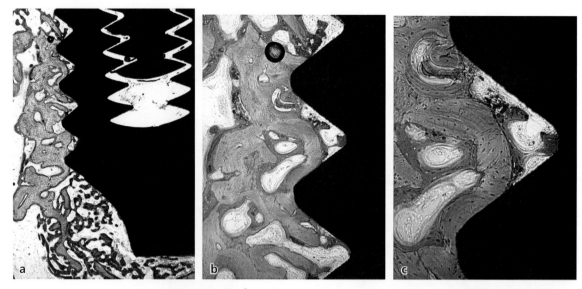

Fig. 5-7 (a) Ground section of an implant (Astra Tech®) site from a biopsy sampled after 2 weeks of healing. In the apical area large amounts of woven bone has formed. (b) Detail of (a). In the threaded region, newly formed bone can be seen to reach contact with the implant surface. (c) Higher magnification of (b). Newly formed bone extends from the old bone and reaches the titanium surface in the invagination between two consecutive "threads".

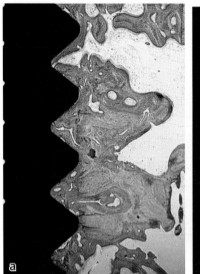
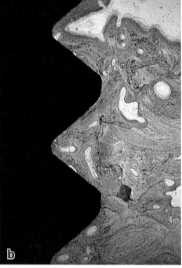

Fig. 5-8 Ground section of an implant site (Astra Tech® self-tapping implant) from a biopsy specimen obtained after 6 weeks of healing. (a) In the marginal area a continuous layer of bone covers most of the TiOblast® surface. (b) Higher magnification. Note the zone of newly formed (darker stained) bone that is in direct contact with the implant surface.

cylinder. When a self-tapping 4.0 mm wide implant is to be placed, the recipient site is first prepared with pilot and twist drills to establish a hard tissue canal that most often has a final diameter of 3.7 mm. During the insertion the cutting edges in the "apical" portion of the implant create a 0.15 mm wide track in the walls of the canal and thereby establish the final 4.0 mm dimension. When the implant has reached its insertion depth, contact has been established between the outer portions of the threads and the mineralized bone in the cortical compartment (initial or primary fixation is hereby secured) and with the severed bone marrow tissue in the spongy compartment.

Figure 5-7 illustrates a recipient site with a self-tapping implant (Astra Tech® implant). This implant is designed with a TiOblast® surface modification. The biopsy was harvested 2 weeks after installation

surgery. The outer portion of the thread is in contact with the parent "old" bone, while bone formation is the dominant feature in the invaginations between the threads and in areas lateral to the "apical" portions of the implant. Thus, discrete areas of newly formed bone can be seen also in direct contact with the implant surface. In sections representing 6 weeks of healing (Fig. 5-8), it was observed that a continuous layer of newly formed bone covers most of the TiOblast® surface. This newly formed bone is also in contact with the old, mature bone that is present in the periphery of the recipient site. After 16 months of healing (Fig. 5-9), the bone tissue in the zone of osseointegration has remodeled and the entire hard tissue bed for the implant is comprised of lamellar bone including both concentric and interstitial lamella.

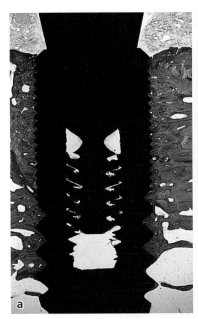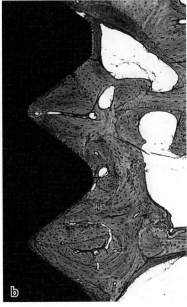

Fig. 5-9 Ground section of an implant site representing 16 months of healing. (a) The implant is surrounded by dense lamellar bone. (b) Higher magnification.

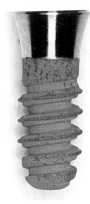

Fig. 5-10 The device used in the dog experiment. The implant is a modification of a solid screw (Straumann® Implant System). The distance between two consecutive threads is 1.25 mm. The depth of the trough is 0.4 mm.

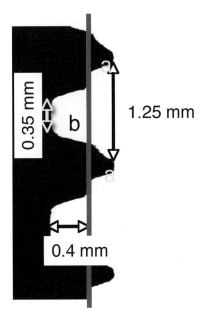

Fig. 5-11 The device. Schematic drawing illustrating the dimensions of the "wound chamber".

The process of osseointegration

De novo bone formation in the severed alveolar ridge following implant placement was studied in experiments in various experimental animal models (for review see Schroeder *et al.* 1995).

Recently Berglundh *et al.* (2003) and Abrahamsson *et al.* (2004) described various steps involved in bone formation and osseointegration to implants placed in the mandible of dogs.

The device: Custom-made implants that had the shape of a solid screw (Straumann® implant), that were made of c.p. titanium and configured with a rough surface topography (SLA®; Straumann) were utilized (Fig. 5-10). In the implant device the distance between two consecutive profiles of the pitch (i.e. the threads in a vertical cross section) was 1.25 mm. A 0.4 mm deep U-shaped circumferential trough had been prepared within the thread region during manufacturing (Fig. 5-11). The tip of the pitch was left untouched. Following the installation of the non-

cutting device (Fig. 5-12) the pitch was engaged in the hard tissue walls prepared by the cutting tapping device. This provided intitial or primary fixation of the device. The void between the pitch and the body of the implant established a geometrically well defined wound chamber (Fig. 5-13). Biopsies were performed to provide healing periods extending from 2 hours following implant insertion to 12 weeks of healing. The biopsy specimens were prepared for ground sectioning as well as for decalcification and embedding in epon.

The wound chamber: Figure 5.13 illustrates a cross section (ground section) of an implant with surrounding soft and hard tissues from a biopsy specimen sampled 2 hours after installation of the metal device. The peripheral portions of the pitch were in contact with the invaginations of the track prepared by the tap in the cortical bone. The wound chambers (Fig. 5-14a) were occupied with a blood clot in which erythrocytes, neutrophils, and monocytes/macrophages occurred in a network of fibrin (Fig. 5-14b). The leukocytes were apparently engaged in the wound cleansing process.

Fibroplasia: Figure 5-15a illustrates a device with surrounding tissues after 4 days of healing. The coagulum had in part been replaced with granulation tissue that contained numerous mesenchymal cells, matrix components, and newly formed vascular structures (angiogenesis) (Fig. 5-15b). A *provisional connective tissue* had been established.

Bone modeling: After 1 week of healing the wound chambers were occupied by a provisional connective tissue that was rich in vascular structures and contained numerous mesenchymal cells (Fig 5-16a). The number of remaining inflammatory cells was relatively small. In large compartments of the chamber, a cell-rich immature bone (woven bone) was seen in the mesenchymal tissues that surrounded the blood vessels. Such areas of woven bone formation occurred in the center of the chamber as well as in discrete locations that apparently were in direct contact with the surface of the titanium device (Fig. 5-16b). This

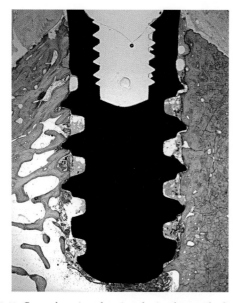

Fig. 5-12 Ground section showing the implant and adjacent tissues immediately after implant installation. The pitch region is engaged in the hard tissue walls. The void between two consecutive pitch profiles includes the wound chamber.

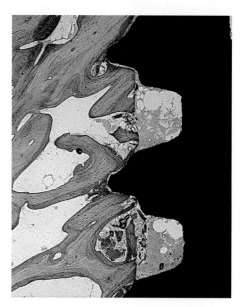

Fig. 5-13 Detail of Fig. 5-12. The wound chamber was filled with blood and a coagulum has formed.

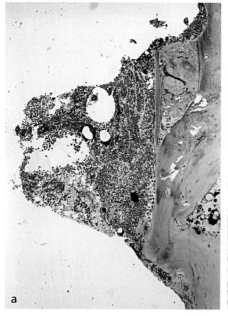
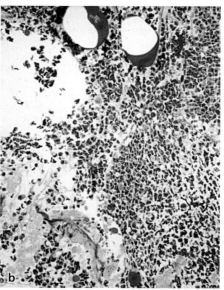

Fig. 5-14 The wound chamber 2 hours after implant installation. Decalcified sections. (a) The wound chamber is filled with blood. (b) Erythrocytes, neutrophils, and macrophages are trapped in a fibrin network.

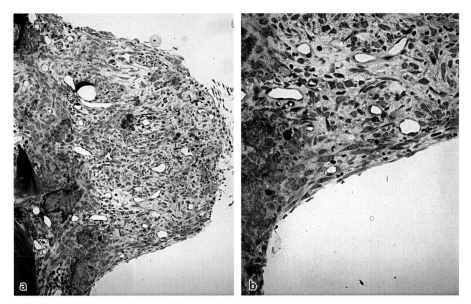

Fig. 5-15 The wound chamber after 4 days of healing (decalcified sctions). (a) Most portions of the wound chamber are occupied by granulation tissue (fibroplasia). (b) In some areas of the chamber provisional connective tissue (matrix) is present. This tissue includes large numbers of mesenchymal cells.

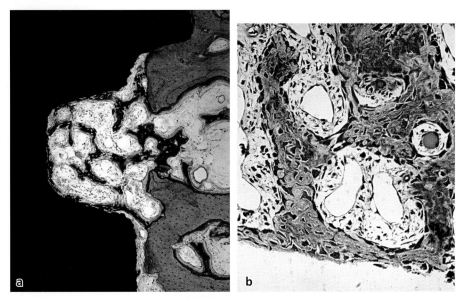

Fig. 5-16 (a) Ground section representing 1 week of healing. Note the presence of newly formed woven bone in the wound chamber. (b) Decalcified section. The woven bone is in direct contact with the implant surface.

was considered to represent the very first phase of osseointegration; contact between the implant surface and newly formed woven bone.

After 2 weeks of healing, woven bone formation appeared to be pronounced in all compartments, apical as well as lateral, surrounding the implant (Fig. 5-17a). Large areas of woven bone were found in the bone marrow regions "apical" of the implant. In the wound chamber, portions of the newly formed woven bone apparently extended from the parent bone into the provisional connective tissue (Fig. 5-17b) and had in many regions reached the surface of the titanium device. At this interval most of the implant surface was occupied by newly formed bone

and a more comprehensive and mature osseointegration had been established (Fig. 5-17c). In the pitch regions there were signs of ongoing new bone formation (Fig. 5-17d). Thus, areas of the recipient site located lateral to the device, that were in direct contact with the host bone immediately following installation surgery and provided initial fixation for the implant, had undergone tissue resorption and were also involved in new bone formation after 2 weeks of healing.

At 4 weeks (Fig. 5-18a), the newly formed mineralized bone extended from the cut bone surface into the chamber and a continuous layer of cell-rich, woven bone covered most of the titanium wall of the

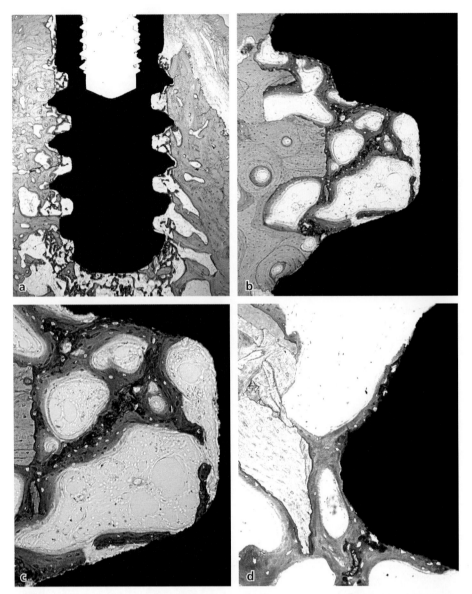

Fig. 5-17 Ground sections illustrating, in various magnifications, the tissues in the wound chamber after 2 weeks of healing. (a) Darker stained woven bone is observed in the apical area of the metal device. (b, c, d) Most portions of the implant surface are coated with bone.

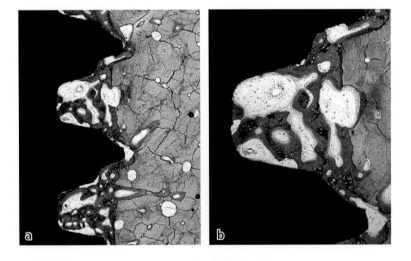

Fig. 5-18 Ground sections representing 4 weeks of healing. (a) The newly formed bone (dark blue) extends from the "old" bone into the wound chamber. (b) Appositional growth. Note the presence of primary osteons.

chamber. The central portion of the chamber was filled with a primary spongiosa (Fig. 5-18b), rich in vascular structures and a multitude of mesenchymal cells.

Remodeling: After 6–12 weeks of healing most of the wound chambers were filled with mineralized bone (Fig. 5-19). Bone tissue, including primary and secondary osteons, could be seen in the newly formed tissue and in the mineralized bone that made contact with the implant surface. Bone marrow that contained blood vessels, adipocytes, and mesenchymal cells was observed to surround the trabeculae of mineralized bone.

Summary: The wound chambers were first occupied with a coagulum. With the ingrowth of vessels and migration of leukocytes and mesenchymal cells, the coagulum was replaced with granulation tissue. The migration of mesenchymal cells continued and the granulation tissue was replaced with a provisional matrix, rich in vessels, mesenchymal cells, and fibers. The process of *fibroplasia* and angiogenesis had started. Formations of newly formed bone could be recognized already during the first week of healing; the newly formed woven bone projected from the lateral wall of the cut bony bed (appositional bone formation; distance osteogenesis) (Davies 1998) but *de novo* formation of new bone could also be seen on the implant surface, i.e. at a distance from the parent

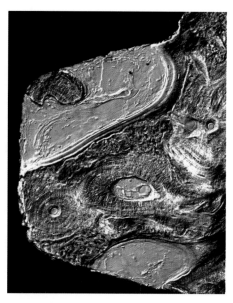

Fig. 5-19 Ground section representing 12 weeks of healing. The woven bone is being replaced with lamellar bone and marrow. Note the formation of secondary osteons.

bone (contact osteogenesis) (Davies 1998). During subsequent weeks the trabeculae of woven bone were replaced with mature bone, i.e. lamellar bone and marrow (bone remodeling).

References

Abrahamsson, I., Berglundh, T., Linder, E., Lang, N.P. & Lindhe, J. (2004). Early bone formation adjacent to rough and turned endosseous implant surfaces. An experimental study in the dog. *Clinical Oral Implants Research* **15**, 381–392.

Albrektsson, T., Brånemark, P-I., Hansson, H-A. & Lindström, J. (1981). Osseointegrated titanium implants. Requirements for ensuring a long-lasting, direct bone anchorage in man. *Acta Orthopaedica Scandinavica* **52**, 155–170.

Berglundh, T., Abrahamsson, I., Lang, N.P. & Lindhe, J. (2003). De novo alveolar bone formation adjacent to endosseous implants. a model study in the dog. *Clinical Oral Implants Research* **14**, 251–262.

Brånemark, P.I., Adell, R., Breine, U., Hansson, B.O., Lindström, J. & Ohlsson, Å. (1969). Intra-osseous anchorage of dental prostheses I. Experimental studies. *Scandinavian Journal of Plastic Reconstructive Surgery* **3**, 81–100.

Davies, J.E. (1998). Mechanisms of endosseous integration. *International Journal of Prosthodontics* **11**, 391–401.

Schroeder, A., Pohler, O. & Sutter, F. (1976). Gewebsreaktion auf ein Titan-Hohlzylinderimplant mit Titan-Spritzschichtoberfläche. *Schweizerisches Monatsschrift für Zahnheilkunde* **86**, 713–727.

Schroeder, A., van der Zypen, E., Stich, H. & Sutter, F. (1981). The reactions of bone, connective tissue, and epithelium to endosteal implants with titanium-sprayed surfaces. *Journal of Maxillofacial Surgery* **9**, 15–25.

Schroeder, A., Buser, D. & Stich, H. (1995) Tissue response. In: Schroeder, A., Sutter, F., Buser, D. & Krekeler, G., eds. *Oral Implantology. Basics, ITI Hollow Cylinder System*. New York: Thieme, pp. 80–111.

Zarb, G.A. & Albrektsson, T. (1991). Osseointegration – a requiem for the periodontal ligament? Editorial. *International Journal of Periodontology and Restorative Dentistry* **11**, 88–91.

Chapter 6

Periodontal Tactile Perception and Peri-implant Osseoperception

Reinhilde Jacobs

Introduction

Perception is the ability to detect external stimuli. In man, several kinds of sensory systems enable perception (vision, audition, balance, somatic function, taste, and smell) (Martin 1991). In all sensory systems, the initial contact with the external world is made through special neural structures called sensory receptors, endings or organs. A distinction is needed between nociceptors, chemo-, photo-, thermo-, and mechanoreceptors, each responding to a particular stimulus. In the oral cavity, taste and somatic sensory systems predominate. The former are sensitive to chemical stimuli while the latter respond to mechanical, thermal, and nociceptive stimuli. In this chapter, only the somatic sensory system is explored. The preponderance of the oral somatosensory system is illustrated by its major representation, besides that of the hand, on the sensory homunculus proposed by

Penfield (Penfield and Rasmussen 1950). In general, the somatosensory function is essential for fine-tuning of limb movements. In analogy with the rest of the skeleton, the tactile function of teeth plays a crucial role in refinement of jaw motor control. Periodontal mechanoreceptors, especially those located in the periodontal ligament, are extremely sensitive to external mechanical stimuli. The periodontal ligament can thus be considered as a keystone for masticatory and other oral motor behaviours. Any condition that may influence periodontal mechanoreceptors, may alter the sensory feedback pathway and thus affect tactile function and fine-tuning of jaw motor control (e.g. periodontal breakdown, bruxism, re-implantation, anesthesia).

The most dramatic change may occur after extraction of teeth, as this eliminates all periodontal ligament receptors. This condition may persist after implant placement as functional re-innervation has not yet been proven in humans. Surprisingly enough, patients with implant-supported prostheses often seem to function quite well. The underlying mechanism of this so-called "osseoperception" phenomenon remains a matter of debate, but the response of assumed peri-implant receptors might help to restore the proper peripheral feedback pathway. This hypothesized physiological integration might thus lead to better acceptance, improved psychological integration, and more natural functioning.

This chapter will unravel periodontal tactile function and guide the reader through the mysteries of peri-implant osseoperception in order to find neuro-anatomical, histological, physiological, and psycho-physical evidence to confirm the hypothesis.

Neurophysiological background

Afferent nerve fibres and receptors

When considering the human somatic sensory system, four types of afferent nerve fibers can be distinguished in association with sensation: Aα, Aβ, Aδ and C. Some types of afferent nerve fibers exist in specific tissues only, while others are widely distributed throughout the body. Based on the structure or signalling properties, receptors may be divided into several classes or categories (Birder & Perl 1994). Three different groups of receptors are associated with thermal and (vibro)tactile sensation: thermo-receptors, nociceptors and mechanoreceptors.

Thermoreceptors and nociceptors

Thermal sensations are divided into warm and cold and are perceived by specific receptors. There are indeed separate spots on skin and mucosal surface where thermal stimulation elicits either warm or cold sensation. Cold-sensitive spots are more numerous than warm-sensitive with the highest density of both cold and warm spots on the face (Bradley 1995). Unmyelinated neurite complexes are responsible for cold sensation and some free nerve endings for warm sensation (Bradley 1995). Receptors which can induce pain feeling are referred to as nociceptors and mostly supplied by Aδ and C fibers. In the periodontal ligament, one can identify free nerve endings which may be responsive to pain, but not thermal receptors. The majority of the receptors located within the periodontal ligament are of the mechanoreceptive type.

Mechanoreceptors

Mechanoreceptors are responsive to mechanical stimuli. These can be classified on the basis of their morphology, receptive field, and adaptation characteristics. In man, four receptor structures have been associated with mechanoperception: Meissner corpuscles, Pacinian corpuscles, Merkel cells, and Ruffini endings (Martin & Jessell 1991). These structural ele-

ments do determine, to some extent, the physiological characteristics of the peripheral receptors. On the basis of their receptive field, two subgroups of mechanoreceptors have been identified: receptors with small and distinct receptive fields (type I) and receptors with large and diffuse receptive fields (type II). Mechanoreceptors can also be subdivided based on their adaptation properties: rapidly adapting (RA) and slowly adapting (SA) receptors. The RA receptors, also called fast adapting receptors, only respond during the dynamic phase of stimulus application. In contrast, the SA receptors respond to both dynamic and static force applications (Iggo 1985). A relationship has been established between the aforementioned receptor morphologies and their adaptation characteristics. Rapidly adapting receptors include Meissner corpuscles (RA I) and Pacinian corpuscles (RA II) while SA receptors include Merkel cells (SA I) and Ruffini endings (SA II).

Trigeminal neurophysiology

Trigeminal neurosensory pathway

The trigeminal nerve is the largest cranial nerve, including a motor root supplying the masticatory muscles, and a predominant sensory root supplying the oral cavity, head, and face. The trigeminal nerve has three divisions (ophthalmic, maxillary, mandibular). The ophthalmic nerve is a sensory nerve and the smallest division. The maxillary nerve is a sensory nerve and intermediate, both in position and size, between ophthalmic and mandibular divisions. The mandibular nerve is the largest and made up of two roots: a large, sensory root and a small motor root.

The sensory inputs of the oral region are carried by the mandibular and maxillary divisions of the trigeminal nerve via the trigeminal ganglion to the brainstem. This is part of an important sensory feedback pathway, involved in refinement of jaw movements. The afferent signals are transmitted either to the main sensory nucleus of the trigeminal nerve (responsive to discriminate tactile senses, light touch and pressure) or to the descending spinal tract nuclei, including: (1) nucleus oralis, responsive to cutaneous sensation of oral mucosa; (2) nucleus interpolaris, responsive to tooth pulp pain; and (3) nucleus caudalis, responsive to pain, temperature, and crude touch.

From there, signals are transferred across the midline and sent to the thalamus and, via thalamo-cortical projections, to the respective cortical areas involved in orofacial sensation where they can result in conscious perception.

Neurovascularization of the jaw bones

The jaws are richly supplied by neurovascular structures, and it is thus of utmost important to identify vital anatomic structures before carrying out a

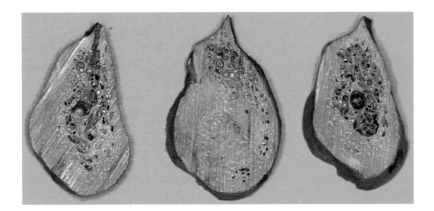

Fig. 6-1 These human dry mandibular bone sections illustrate the presence and dimensional importance of the mandibular incisive nerve, even in edentulism. The middle section is actually visualizing the mandibular midline, confirming that there is no true connection between the left and right sections.

surgical procedure. During a radiographic preoperative planning procedure, neurovascular structures need to be precisely localized to attempt avoiding interference. Particular attention should be paid to the anterior jaw bones, which are often considered as relatively safe surgical areas. The increasing rate of surgical interventions in the anterior jaw bone, such as oral implant placement and bone grafting, has indeed highlighted potential risks and raised the number of reported complications. Recent studies reveal that edentulous and dentate anterior jaws present significant variation in the occurrence of the mandibular incisive canal and genial spinal foramina as well as the maxillary nasopalatine canal (for review see Jacobs *et al.* 2007). All these canal structures contain a neurovascular bundle, whose diameter may be large enough to cause clinically significant trauma. While surgeons need to avoid the nervous structures, these critical structures may afterwards become essential to potentially reinnervate peri-implant bone. Indeed, the existence of remaining neurovascular bundles in the edentulous jaw bone may support the idea that nerves may regenerate after tooth extraction and implant placement. This particular assumption is the basis of the so-called osseoperception phenomenon and will be further outlined below.

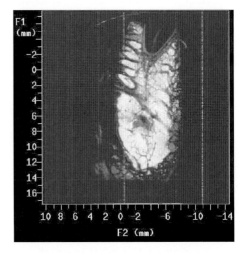

Fig. 6-2 Single cross-sectional slice of an high resolution MRI dataset localized at the incisor region of a dentate anterior human mandible, with the fatty marrow colored white. A black root-form structure corresponds to the root of an incisor tooth. It is surrounded by a small band of intermediate signal intensity, representing the periodontal ligament. The dental neurovascular supply is seen as a line of intermediate signal intensity in the middle of the root. The latter descends to the level of a larger structure of intermediate signal intensity (incisive nerve) with a black oval area on top (vascular structure). (Reprinted from Jacobs *et al.* 2007, Copyright 2006, with permission from Elsevier.)

Mandibular neuroanatomy

The mandibular nerve is the largest of the three divisions of the fifth cranial nerve and gives off the inferior alveolar nerve. The latter enters the mandible through the mandibular foramen and continues to run forward through the mandibular canal. At the mental foramen it gives off an important branch, called the mental nerve. It should not be considered as the only terminal branch of the inferior alveolar nerve. The mandibular incisive nerve is often detected as a second terminal branch with an intraosseous course in a so-called mandibular incisive canal, located anterior to the mental foramen (Mraiwa *et al.* 2003a,b) (Fig. 6-1). Conventional intraoral and panoramic radiographs often fail to show this canal (Jacobs *et al.* 2004). Cross-sectional imaging may

however be used to locate the canal and as such avoid any risk for neurovascular damage (Jacobs *et al.* 2002a) The mandibular incisive canal contains a true neurovascular bundle with nervous sensory structures (Fig. 6-2). Its existence in edentulous patients is underlined by reported surgical complications. Indeed, sensory disturbances, caused by direct trauma to the mandibular incisive canal bundle have been reported after implant placement in the interforaminal region (Jacobs & van Steenberghe 2006; Jacobs *et al.* 2007) (Fig. 6-3).

A sensory disorder might also be related to indirect trauma caused by a hematoma in the canal, which acts as a closed chamber; this will affect the mandibular incisive canal bundle and spread to the main mental branch (Mraiwa *et al.* 2003b).

Other anatomic landmarks to be noted are superior and inferior genial spinal foramina and their bony canals, situated in the midline of the mandible in 85–99% of people (Liang *et al.* 2005a,b; Jacobs *et al.* 2007). The superior one is at the level of, or superior to, the genial spine; the inferior one is below the genial spine (Fig. 6-4). The superior genial spinal foramen has been found to contain a branch of the lingual artery, vein and nerve. Furthermore, a branch of the mylohyoid nerve together with branches or anastomoses of sublingual and/or submental arteries and veins have been identified upon entering the inferior genial spinal foramen. This artery could be of sufficient size to provoke hemorrhage intraosseously or in the connective soft tissue, which might be difficult to control (Darriba & Mendonca-Cardad 1997; Liang *et al.* 2005a,b) (Fig. 6-5).

The observation that immediate loading of implants in the anterior mandible results in a significant reduction of tactile function using the Bråne-mark Novum® concept rather than a conventional implant-supported overdenture might be explained by contact with the aforementioned neurovascular bundles in the anterior mandible (Abarca *et al.* 2006).

Maxillary neuroanatomy

The maxillary nerve is a sensory nerve, with its superior nasal and alveolar branches supplying the maxilla, including the palate, nasal and maxillary sinus mucosa, upper teeth and their periodontium. One of the superior nasal branches is named the nasopalatine nerve. It descends to the roof of the mouth through the nasopalatine canal and communicates with the corresponding nerve of the opposite side and with the anterior palatine nerve. The nasopalatine foramen and canals are situated at the maxillary midline, posterior to the central incisor teeth (Mraiwa *et al.* 2004). Typically, it has been described as having a Y-shape with the orifices of two lateral canals, terminating at the nasal floor level in the foramina of Stenson (Fig. 6-6). The nasopalatine nerve and the terminal branch of the descending palatine artery pass through these canals. Occasionally, two additional minor canals are seen (foramina of Scarpa), which may carry the nasopalatine nerves (Fig. 6-7). Mraiwa *et al.* (2004) point out a significant variability both regarding dimensions and morphological appearance of the nasopalatine canal.

To avoid disturbing neurovascular bundles and further complications, this important variability should be taken into account when dealing with surgical procedures such as implant placement in the maxillary incisor region.

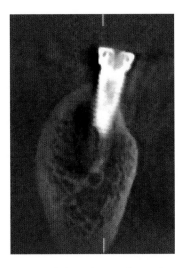

Fig. 6-3 Cross-sectional slice of a cone beam dataset showing an osseointegrated implant placed in an edentulous lateral incisor region, on top of a prominent incisive canal lumen. Chronic pressure on the incisive nerve resulted in a neuropathic pain problem. (Reprinted from Jacobs & van Steenberghe 2006, Copyright 2006, with permission from Blackwell Publishing.)

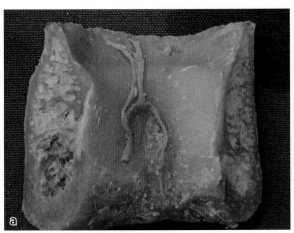
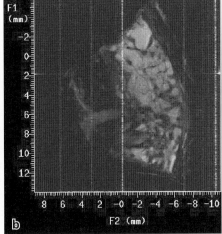

Fig. 6-4 (a) A macroanatomical view of a human anterior mandible showing a clear neurovascular bundle entering the superior genial spinal foramen. (b) A matching horizontal slice acquired through high-resolution MRI confirms the entry of a neurovascular bundle into the superior genial spinal foramen. (Courtesy of Professor I. Lambrichts, University of Hasselt.)

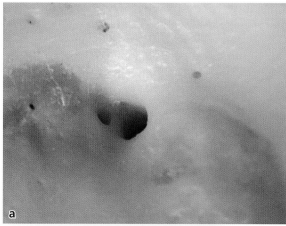

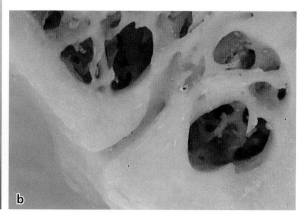

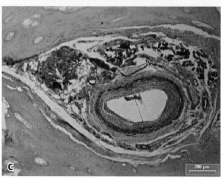

Fig. 6-5 Stereomicroscopic images. (a) A single genial spinal foramen. (b) A section of the canal. (c) The neurovascular content of the canal is confirmed histologically. In this particular image, the artery has a width of about 0.5 mm (red and green lines for inner and outer wall dimensions).

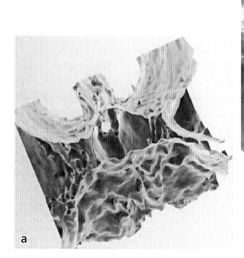

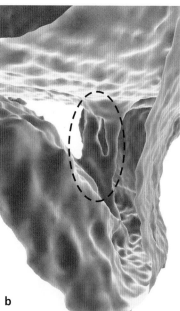

Fig. 6-6 Outline of the common Y-morphology of the nasopalatine canal (seen in black oval) on a three-dimensional reconstruction of the palate and the floor of the nose, seen from a posterior viewing angle (a) and a side view (b).

Periodontal innervation

Periodontal receptors are located within the gingiva, jaw bone, periosteum, and periodontal ligament. Most receptors seem to have mechanoreceptive characteristics, contributing to a sophisticated exteroceptive tactile function. This tactile information is not primarily used for protective purposes, but rather applied by the human brain to improve oral motor behavior and fine-tuning of biting and chewing (Trulsson 2006).

It is clear that the periodontal ligament plays a predominant role in this dedicated mechanoreceptive function. It has an extremely rich sensory nerve supply, especially in those locations that are more prone to displacement (peri-apical, buccal, and lingual periodontal ligament). It contains three types of nerve endings: free nerve endings, Ruffini-like endings, and lamellated corpuscles (Lambrichts et al. 1992). Free nerve endings stem from both unmyelinated and myelinated nerve fibers. Lamellated corpuscles are found in close contact to each other. Most

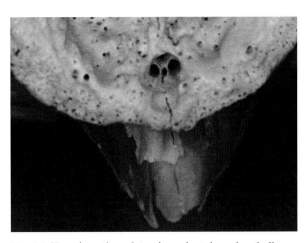

Fig. 6-7 View from the palate of an edentulous dry skull, showing the nasopalatine foramen, formed at the articulation of both maxillae, behind the incisor teeth. In the depth of the canal, the orifices of two lateral canals are seen. As an anatomic variant, two minor canals can be observed on the midline, one anterior and one posterior to the major nasopalatine canals.

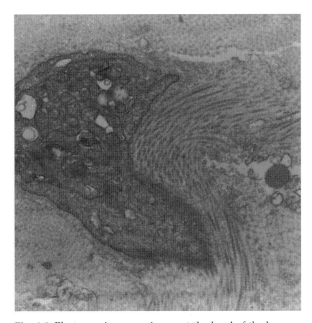

Fig. 6-8 Electron microscope image at the level of the human periodontal ligament, showing collagen fibrils inserted into the basal lamina of an ensheating cell in a Ruffini-like receptor. (Reprinted from Lambrichts *et al.* 1992, Copyright 2006, with permission from Ivo Lambrichts, University of Hasselt and Blackwell Publishing.)

mechanoreceptive endings are, however, Ruffini-like, and are predominantly present in the apical part of the periodontal ligament. Morphologic studies indicate that these endings are in close contact with collagen fibres of the surrounding tissues (Lambrichts *et al.* 1992) (Fig. 6-8). This particular association may explain their extremely high sensitivity upon loading a tooth. This results in low threshold levels for periodontal tactile function, and is considered as the basis of an elaborate sensory apparatus that may be linked to a number of clinical phenomena.

Recordings from the inferior alveolar nerve reveal that human periodontal mechanoreceptors discharge continuously during sustained loading of teeth (Trulsson *et al.*, 1992). Like the slowly adapting type II receptors in the human skin, most periodontal ligament mechanoreceptors are spontaneously active with a regular discharge in response to forces applied to teeth.

The mechanoreceptive function of the periodontal ligament allows it to signal differential information about the mechanical events that occur when manipulating and biting food with anterior teeth and chewing food with the posterior teeth (Trulsson 2006). The detailed differential signalling allows the brain to analyze and characterize the specific mechanical events enabling further processing for fine-tuning, resulting in an optimized masticatory sequence (Trulsson 2006). Considering this crucial role, it is clear that some sensory–motor interactions are impaired or even lost when altering or damaging the periodontal ligament. When teeth are extracted and thus ligament receptors eliminated, tactile functioning may be hampered. Indeed, Haraldson (1983) describes a similar muscle activity during the entire masticatory sequence in patients with implant-supported fixed prosthesis. This finding contrasts to subjects with natural teeth, having a chewing pattern that gradually changes with altering food bolus properties. Jacobs and van Steenberghe (1994) identify a silent period in muscle activity (reflex response) when tapping teeth or implanting neighboring teeth. A reflex response remains absent, however, when tapping implants in a fully edentulous jaw bone. Both findings may illustrate the modulatory role of periodontal ligament input in jaw muscle activity.

Testing tactile function

Neurophysiological assessment

Information on the exteroceptive function can be examined by neurophysiological as well as psychophysical methods. Neurophysiological investigations on the sensory function of the human trigeminal system are scarce. Afferent nerve recordings of the human trigeminal nerve require skilful performance. Only few studies have been performed so far (Johansson *et al.* 1988a,b; Trulsson *et al.* 1992). Alternatively, non-invasive approaches may be considered to evaluate oral tactile function. The first approach is the recording of the so-called trigeminal somatosensory evoked potentials (TSEP) after stimulation of receptors in the oral cavity (Van Loven *et al.* 2000, 2001). This set-up has the advantage of obtaining information on the cortical response of the trigeminal afferent system upon non-invasive stimulation of oral receptors. Unfortunately, SEPs from the trigeminal branches are, in contrast to those recorded from limbs, weak and difficult to discriminate from the background noise; advanced signal analysis is required to gain reliable information (Swinnen *et al.* 2000; van Loven *et al.* 2000, 2001). Another non-invasive method to assess sensory function is to visualize brain activity by functional magnetic resonance imaging (fMRI) (Borsook *et al.* 2004, 2006). This is a complex but most promising method, which has received hardly any attention in relation to tactile function of teeth and implants (Lundborg *et al.* 2006; Miyamoto *et al.* 2006).

The main drawbacks of fMRI include complexity of the signal, relatively long imaging time, potential hazard imposed by the presence of ferromagnetic material in the vicinity of the imaging magnet, potential risk for claustrophobia, and costs. The technique is most promising, however. When combined with other techniques, such as psychophysics and TSEPs, it may offer a new non-invasive approach to evaluate how the human oral somatosensory system functions (Ducreux *et al.* 2006; Lundborg *et al.* 2006).

Psychophysical assessment

Sensory function can also be evaluated by psychophysical testing, relying on the patient's response. This technique has often been applied for testing oral tactile function (Jacobs & van Steenberghe 1994; Jacobs *et al.* 2002b,c,d). When carried out in a strictly standardized condition, the psychophysical response can be directly linked to the neural receptor activation (Vallbo & Johansson 1984).

Psychophysical studies on the oral sensory function are numerous. A major advantage of this type of study is that they are simple non-invasive techniques that can be performed in a clinical environment. Psychophysics include a series of well defined methodologies to help determine the threshold level of sensory receptors in man. Psychophysical methods allow connection between the psychological response of the patient to the physiological functions of the receptors involved. The methods should be carried out in a standardized and accurate manner, to enable one to draw conclusions about their outcome with regard to sensory function (Jacobs *et al.* 2002b,c,d).

Regardless of the tests used, one must keep in mind that many variables contribute to the subjective nature of psychophysical sensory testing. Some variables are manageable, others are more difficult to deal with. Influencing factors exist in various components of the experiment set-up (environmental influence, psychophysical approach, patient-related factors) (Jacobs *et al.* 2002b).

Environmental factors should be well controlled, as background noise is distracting to patient and examiner. To minimize the effect of noise, testing should be done in a quiet room with stable background illumination.

Patient-related variables may contribute greatly to the outcome of the testing. Psychological and/or physical factors may lead to an inter- and intra-subject variability, making the expression of a threshold level more obvious than assessment of an absolute value. Psychological factors include motivation, level of concentration, and anxiety level. The psychophysical approach may attempt to control such variability.

Different psychophysical procedures have been described in order to assess tactile function reliably (Falmagne 1985). Adaptive methods are generally recommended for threshold level determination, as these seem very effective and consistent. Such approaches are termed adaptive, as the subsequent stimulus value depends on the subject's response in preceding trials. In the staircase method, the stimulus value is changed by a constant amount. When the response shifts from one answer to another, the stimulus direction is reversed. Afterwards, the threshold is determined by averaging peaks and valleys throughout all runs. Some patients may imagine a stimulus when there is none. Others admit feeling a sensation, only if they are absolutely positive that it was felt. The inclusion of false alarms (implying that no stimulus is presented in the specified time interval) may exclude response bias and a guessing strategy of the subject. A thorough and standardized instruction to all subjects is important in this respect.

Other patient-related factors that should be considered are of physical origin and include age, gender, dental status and dexterity. Age is an important variable with respect to implant physiology, considering the fact that edentulous patients are usually found amongst the elderly. Age-related impairment is seen, both of motor function and most sensory modalities in the extremities (Masoro 1986). A decline in oral sensory function is also established. After the age of 80, the ability to differentiate tactile and vibratory stimuli on the lip decreases and two-point discrimination deteriorates on the upper lip, on the cheeks, and on the lower lip, but not on the tongue and the palate (Calhoun *et al.* 1992). Stereognostic ability also declines with age (Müller *et al.* 1995). It is clear that this age effect should be considered in experimental studies.

In contrast to age, the influence of gender on tactile function remains a matter of debate. Taking into account the important inter-individual variability, clear-cut gender differences are not easily discerned with regard to oral sensory function. There is no marked gender effect on stereognostic ability or vibrotactile function (Jacobs *et al.* 1992, 2002b). The tactile sensory systems of men and women seem to operate similarly at both threshold and suprathreshold levels of stimulation (Chen *et al.* 1995). However, females seem to have greater ability to discern subtle changes in lip, cheek, and chin position than males (Chen *et al.* 1995). Dexterity is another patient-related variable. Although there is some relation between masticatory performance and dexterity (Hoogmartens & Caubergh 1987), this is not the case for either tactile function or stereognosis (Jacobs *et al.* 1992, 2002b).

Periodontal tactile function

A variety of psychophysical tests has been used to evaluate oral exteroceptive function by assessment of threshold levels. Although some of the methods designed for functional psychophysical testing are unable to identify the specific receptor groups involved in the mechanisms of oral sensation, the tests may clearly reflect periodontal tactile function. Assessing light touch or the tactile function of teeth is performed by determination of the threshold levels for active and passive detection and discrimination tasks (Jacobs *et al.* 1992, 2002b,d). The distinction between detection and discrimination is based on the fact that, in a detection task, the subject has to indicate the presence or absence of a stimulus ("yes" or "no" strategy) while in a discrimination task, the subject has to compare two stimuli ("smaller" or "larger" strategy). A further division is made between active and passive tasks. In the passive task, forces are applied to a tooth in the upper jaw. The active tactile function of teeth is evaluated by inserting an object, mostly a foil of a certain thickness, in between two antagonistic teeth. The latter rather reflects daily functioning and automatically involves other than periodontal receptors (e.g. joint, muscle and inner ear receptors), while the passive test involves solely activation of periodontal ligament mechanoreceptors.

Active threshold determination

The active absolute threshold level is determined by the interocclusal detection of small objects such as foils of varying thicknesses (Fig. 6-9). This may involve the activation of mechanoreceptors, mainly originating from the periodontium but also from the muscles, inner ear, and temporomandibular joints (TMJs). It should, however, be realized that the foil materials used may have different thermal and

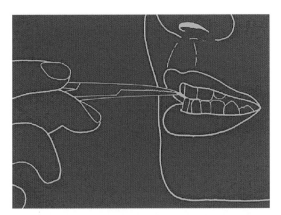

Fig. 6-9 Active threshold determination by interocclusal thickness perception yields superior results for teeth than for implant-supported prostheses, with fixed prostheses being more sensitive than removable ones.

mechanical properties, resulting in conflicting results (Jacobs *et al.* 1992). Foil materials with high thermal conductivity (e.g. steel, aluminium) may lower the threshold level by activation of thermal receptors.

Another factor that may affect the active tactile function is chewing activity, because this involves progressive intrusion of the tooth after each chewing cycle. The latter leads to adaptation of the periodontal mechanoreceptive inputs. Chewing or bruxism may thus lead to an increase in threshold levels up to 60 times the normal values (Kiliaridis *et al.* 1990). An interocclusal discrimination task of small objects determines the differential threshold level. The active threshold level varies according to the experiment set-up, but the most important variable is test stick dimension (Jacobs & van Steenberghe 1994). For size discrimination with a mouth opening of less than 5 mm, periodontal mechanoreceptive input plays the primary role. For increased mouth opening, the response of muscle spindles predominates.

Passive threshold determination

The most common device used in clinical neurology to measure light touch sensation is a set of Semmes-Weinstein monofilaments (Semmes-Weinstein Aesthesiometer®, Stoelting, Illinois, USA). The original idea dates back from the nineteenth century when von Frey suggested testing cutaneous light touch by using calibrated hairs of different stiffness by changing their length and hardness. Later on, the so-called von Frey hairs were replaced by nylon monofilaments mounted into a plastic handle (Fig. 6-10). This technique has also been applied intraorally for assessment of light touch thresholds for teeth, implants or oral mucosa (Jacobs & van Steenberghe 1994; Jacobs *et al.* 2002d). The drawback remains the variation caused by the hand-held and thus variable nature of stimulation application. Other stimulators have therefore been developed, enabling a controlled force level under more standardized stimulation conditions for measuring both manual and oral light touch (Jacobs *et al.* 2002b,d).

The passive discrimination task allows testing of the ability to differentiate between intensities of forces applied to a tooth. It depends on the force characteristics such as the rate of force application and the range of forces presented. When comparing teeth and implants, passive threshold levels are much lower for teeth but at suprathreshold force levels, implants and teeth become equally sensitive. For the passive detection of forces applied to a tooth, different stimulating devices have been developed. In order to avoid tapping and subsequent transmission of the waves through the jaw bone with activation of other receptors, such as in the inner ear, pushing forces are recommended (Fig. 6-11). This is done by placement of the stimulating rod in contact with the tissue under investigation (Jacobs & van Steenberghe 1993).

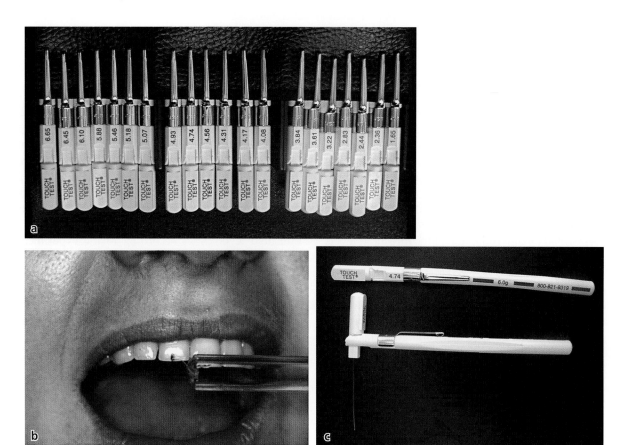

Fig. 6-10 Passive threshold determination. (a) Using a kit of pressure esthesiometers of increasing loads. (b) From determination of the absolute detection threshold upon tooth loading. (c) Using the individual hand-held stimulation rod.

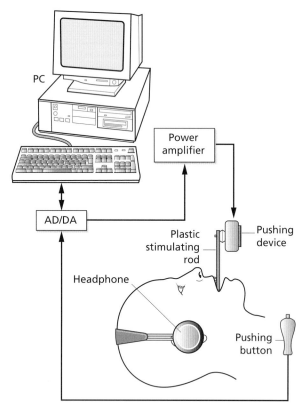

Fig. 6-11 Set-up of passive threshold determination of a maxillary front tooth by applying axial pushing forces against the tooth.

Influence of dental status on tactile function

From several psychophysical studies, it has been established that the oral tactile function is influenced by tooth position and dental status (Jacobs *et al.* 2002b). The tactile function of teeth is primarily determined by the presence of periodontal ligament receptors. Vital or non-vital teeth may show a comparable tactile function. However, when periodontal ligament receptors are reduced or eliminated (e.g. periodontitis, bruxism, chewing, extraction, anesthesia, etc.), tactile function is impaired (Table 6-1). This clinically implies that a patient's ability to detect occlusal inaccuracies (e.g. induced by restorative treatment) is decreased in these situations. Indeed, exteroceptors inform the nervous system on the characteristics of the stimulus, which then allows modulation of the motoneuron pool to optimize jaw motor activity and avoid overloading. Elimination of these exteroceptors by tooth extraction may reduce the tactile function to an important extent (Jacobs *et al.* 2001; Jacobs & van Steenberghe 1991, 1994, 2006; Mericske-Stern 1994; Mericske-Stern *et al.* 1995; Jacobs 1998). Even after rehabilitation with a prosthesis, tactile function remains impaired and inappropriate exteroceptive feedback may thus present a risk for overloading the prosthesis (Jacobs & van Steenberghe 2006). In comparison to the tactile function of a natural dentition, the active threshold is seven to

Table 6-1 Factors influencing the tactile function of teeth (for review see Jacobs *et al.* 2002b; Jacobs & van Steenberghe 2006)

Influencing factors	Active threshold (thickness detection)	Passive threshold (force detection)
Vital tooth	20 µm	2 g
Non-vital tooth	20 µm	2 g
Anesthesia	↑	↑
Periodontitis	↑	↑ (> 5 g)
Chewing	↑	↑
Bruxism	↑	↑
Extraction	↑	↑
Reimplantation	↑	↑
Denture	150 µm	150 g
Implant-supported prosthesis	50 µm	100 g
Ageing	↑	↑
Polyneuropathy	↑	↑

↑: increase in threshold level implying a decrease in tactile function and hampered feedback.

eight times higher for dentures but only three to five times higher for implants (see Table 6-1). For the passive detection of forces applied to upper teeth, thresholds are increased 75 times for dentures and 50 times for implants (see Table 6-1). The large discrepancies between active and passive thresholds can be explained by the fact that several receptor groups may respond to active testing, while the passive method selectively activates periodontal ligament receptors. The latter are eliminated after extraction, which may explain the reduced tactile function in edentulous patients.

After rehabilitation with a bone-anchored prosthesis, however, edentulous patients seem to function quite well. These patients perceive mechanical stimuli exerted on osseointegrated implants in the jaw bone. Some of them even note a special sensory awareness with the bone-anchored prosthesis, coined "osseoperception". It can be defined as a perception of external stimuli transmitted via the implant through the bone by activation of receptors located in peri-implant environment, periosteum, skin, muscles, and/or joints (Jacobs 1998). The existence of this phenomenon could imply that the feedback pathway to the sensory cortex is partly restored with a hypothetical representation of the prosthesis in the sensory cortex; this may allow an adjusted modulation of the motoneuron pool leading to more natural functioning and avoiding overload.

Activation of oral mechanoreceptors during oral tactile function

When performing psychophysical testing, various types of oral mechanoreceptors may be activated. Mechanoreceptors in the oral region may be located in the periodontal ligament, oral mucosa, gingiva, bone, periosteum, and tongue. Mechanoreceptors in the periodontal ligament contribute to the very high sensitivity of teeth to mechanical stimuli (Jacobs & van Steenberghe 1994). The periodontal ligament is richly supplied with mechanoreceptors, with the majority being identified histologically as Ruffini-like endings (Lambrichts *et al.* 1992). During passive threshold determination, these receptors will be activated. The assessment of the active tactile threshold level is, however, not solely based on activation of periodontal mechanoreceptors. Temporomandibular joint receptors are found to only play a minor role, but muscular receptors are important in the discriminatory ability for mouth openings of 5 mm and more (Broekhuijsen & Van Willigen 1983).

Considering that mechanoreceptors in the periodontal ligament largely contribute to tactile function, one can question what happens after tooth extraction. It can be assumed that remaining receptors in the peri-implant environment (gingiva, alveolar mucosa, periosteum, and bone) may take over part of the normal exteroceptive function.

In the oral mucosa, different types of mechanoreceptors can be identified including lamellar organs, Ruffini-like endings, and free nerve endings (Lambrichts *et al.* 1992). The number of nerve fibers per unit area is greater in the anterior areas of the oral cavity, making this region the most sensitive part of the oral mucosa (Mason 1967).

The gingiva contains round and oval lamellar corpuscles. These receptors respond to mechanical stimuli for coordination of the lip and buccal muscles during mastication (Johansson *et al.* 1988a,b). Cutaneous mechanoreceptors in the facial skin are activated by skin stretching or contraction of facial muscles and may operate as proprioceptors involved in facial kinesthesia and motor control (Nordin & Hagbarth 1989).

The periosteum contains free nerve endings, complex unencapsulated, and encapsulated endings. The free nerve endings are activated by pressure or stretching of the periosteum through the action of masticatory muscles and the skin (Sakada 1974). Periosteal innervation has been suggested to play a role in peri-implant tactile function (Jacobs 1998). Indeed, when applying forces to osseointegrated implants in the jaw bone, pressure build-up in the bone is sometimes large enough to allow deformation of the bone and its surrounding periosteum (Jacobs 1998). The involvement of bone innervation in mechanoreception and peri-implant osseoperception remains a matter of debate, however (Jacobs & van Steenberghe 2006).

Functional testing of the oral somatosensory system

Functional testing of the oral somatosensory system may include two-point and size discrimination as well as stereognosis. Two-point discrimination is the ability to differentiate between two points of simultaneous contact. A traditional disk for two-point discrimination is divided into equal triangles containing two points placed at standard distances, usually between 2 and 25 mm (Fig. 6-12). This kind of test can be applied on different areas of the skin or the oral mucosa (Jacobs *et al.* 2002b,c,d). Size discrimination consists in holding a stick between two antagonistic teeth or fingers. This discriminatory ability is better for antagonistic teeth than for fingers (Morimoto 1990). The most documented and relevant test for the oral cavity is, however, stereognosis, which is considered as a complex functional test, evaluating the ability to recognize and discriminate different forms (Jacobs *et al.* 1997).

Oral stereognosis

While touch may obtain information on the mechanoreceptors activated by simple detection or discrimination of mechanical stimuli, stereognosis is a more complex process. It is a function of both peripheral

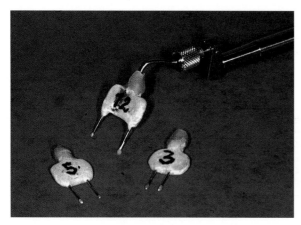

Fig. 6-12 Intraoral two-point discrimination testing device based on a constant pressure probe to compensate for the variability induced by hand-held equipment.

receptors (touch and kinesthetic) and central integrating processes (Jacobs *et al.* 1998). It may give an idea on daily functioning and may be applied to measure sensory impairment due to the presence of general or local pathology (speech pathology, blindness, deafness, cleft lip and palate, temporary sensory ablations, etc.).

Influence of dental status on stereognostic ability

A change in the oral cavity by means of partial or complete loss of the dentition certainly creates certain changes to the oral sensory function. The roles of periodontal neural receptors and of the tongue seem essential in dentate subjects. After bilateral mandibular block, the stereognostic ability decreases by about 20% (Mason 1967). When comparing teeth with full dentures, a far better stereognostic ability is noted for natural teeth when freely manipulating the test pieces (Litvak *et al.* 1971). When removing the denture(s) in complete denture wearers, a considerable reduction in stereognostic ability is noted (Jacobs *et al.* 1998).

Lundqvist (1993) demonstrated that stereognostic ability improved after rehabilitation with oral implants. Jacobs *et al.* (1997) compared different prosthetic superstructures and noted no significantly different stereognostic ability with implant-supported fixed or removable prostheses, even when eliminating the involvement of tongue and lip receptors (Fig. 6-13).

Other compromising factors for oral stereognosis

Stutterers and speakers with articulation problems have an impaired stereognostic ability in comparison to normal speakers (Moser *et al.* 1967). They require more time to identify objects than normal speakers. Speakers with cerebral palsy also have an impaired stereognostic ability (Moser *et al.* 1967). Hemiplegic

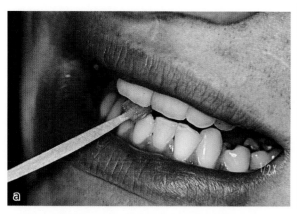
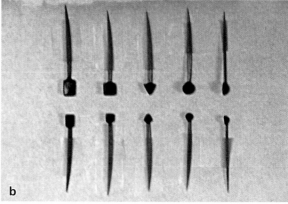

Fig. 6-13 (a) Stereognostic detection of objects in between teeth is better than for implant-supported prostheses. (b) The use of toothpicks to which the forms are attached and manipulated may avoid direct lip and tongue contact.

subjects make approximately three times as many errors as normal subjects in oral stereognosis tests. A surgical reduction of the tongue in case of macroglossia has a minor influence on the subject's performance in the test for oral stereognosis (Ingervall & Schmoker 1990). Other pathological conditions in the perioral area have no direct influence on the stereognostic ability (Jacobs *et al.* 1998). Cleft lip and palate is not accompanied by a sensory deficit of the oral area. There is also no overall sensory impairment following tissue manipulation in cleft lip and palate surgery. Furthermore, the stereognostic ability and oral size perception of patients with burning mouth syndrome is not significantly different from normal subjects (Jacobs *et al.* 1998).

Receptor activation during oral stereognosis

To assess the stereognostic ability, test pieces are inserted in the oral cavity and in most experimental set-ups, free manipulation of the test pieces is allowed. The latter implies activation of a large number of receptor groups (periodontal, mucosal, muscular, articular, etc.). Since the tip of the tongue is one of the most densely innervated areas of the human body, it plays an important role in stereognosis of objects inserted in the mouth (Jacobs *et al.* 1998). Based on studies involving anesthesia of the tongue, the palate or the absence of teeth, it could be stated that oral stereognostic ability is determined mostly by receptors in the tongue mucosa, the palate, and to a lesser extent the periodontal ligament (Jacobs *et al.* 1998). A major modification to the experimental set-up is the insertion of a toothpick in each test piece to eliminate the involvement of lip and tongue receptors, to allow easy handling and standardized placement in between two antagonistic teeth (Jacobs *et al.* 1997) (see Fig. 6-13).

The role of the TMJ receptors is less clear. In fact, in studies on tactile function, an interocclusal thickness of 5 mm and more seems able to activate receptors in the TMJ and the jaw muscles (Jacobs *et al.* 1998, 2002b). In the stereognostic ability tests, pieces are mostly manipulated inside the mouth and seldom kept between two antagonistic teeth, which frequently excludes the need for a mouth opening of 5 mm or even more.

Stereognostic ability testing is not designed to detect specific receptor groups, it rather reflects an overall sensory ability. A good result in a stereognosis test should indicate that the subject receives full and accurate information about what is going on in the mouth. Even if manipulation is allowed to identify the test piece, identification itself is a sensory rather than a motor accomplishment (Jacobs *et al.* 1998). It is an indicator of functional sensibility including synthesis of numerous sensory inputs in higher brain centers.

From periodontal tactile function to peri-implant osseoperception

Tooth extraction considered as sensory amputation

Sensory feedback plays an essential role in fine tuning of limb motor control. Thus, it is clear that amputation of a limb will not only involve destruction of an important part of the peripheral feedback pathways, but also hamper fine motor control. Conventional socket prostheses do not carry enough sensory information to restore the necessary natural feedback pathways for motor function (Jacobs *et al.* 2000). Comparable observations can be made after extraction of teeth. The periodontal ligament harbors a very rich innervation, carrying refined mechanoreceptive properties by an intimate contact between collagen fibres and Ruffini-like endings (Lambrichts *et al.* 1992) (see Fig. 6-8). The role of periodontal neural feedback is well known (Jacobs & van Steenberghe 1994, 2006). After extraction of teeth, however, the periodontal neural feedback pathway may be damaged as periodontal ligament receptors are eliminated. Dentures can be compared to socket prostheses and are not able to fully compensate for normal tooth loading and force transfer. The peripheral feedback mechanisms are more limited since the mucosal mechanoreceptor function is less efficient than the periodontal ligament function. Consequently, oral function remains impaired (Jacobs & van Steenberghe 1991, 1994, 2006; Jacobs *et al.* 1992; Mericske-Stern 1994; Mericske-Stern *et al.* 1995).

It has been assumed that by anchoring prosthetic limbs directly to the bone via osseointegrated implants, partial sensory substitution can be realized (Jacobs 1998; Jacobs *et al.* 2000). If the feedback pathway can be restored, such concept of bone-anchored limb prostheses would signify an important step towards global integration of a prosthesis in the body. Amputees and edentulous patients, rehabilitated with a bone-anchored prosthesis, report a specific feeling around endosseous implants. Psychophysical threshold determination studies confirm that patients may perceive mechanical stimuli exerted on osseointegrated implants in the bone. This phenomenon introduces discussion of which receptor groups are responsible for this perception phenomenon. New insights and more objective non-invasive approaches may help to clarify this question. It seems attractive to explain the observed tactile sensitivity of endosseous implants, coined osseoperception, by the surrounding endosseous and periosteal neural endings. Neurophysiological evidence can be found in some experiments evoking TSEPs upon implant stimulation. By triggering sweeps in the electroencephalogram by means of an implant-stimulation device and by cumulating and advanced analysis of the sweeps, one can observe significant waves (Fig. 6-14). The experiments indicate that endosseous

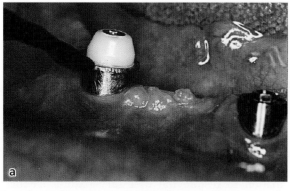
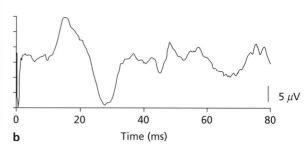

Fig. 6-14 (a) Electrical stimulation of an osseointegrated implant using a ring-shaped stimulation electrode fixed by a coverscrew. (b) Trigeminal evoked potential elicited by electrical stimulation of an osseointegrated implant in the mandible. A similar potential could be maintained after topical anesthesia of the peri-implant soft tissues indicating that the trigeminal potentials originated from other peri-implant structures such as bone and periosteal receptors.

and/or periosteal receptors around the implants convey the sensation (Van Loven *et al.* 2000). These mechanisms could be the basis of implant-mediated sensory–motor control, which may have important clinical implications, because more natural functioning with implant-supported prostheses can be attempted. It may thus open the gate for global integration of implants in the human body.

Histological background of peri-implant osseoperception

Tooth extraction results in damage to a large number of sensory nerve fibres and corresponds to an amputation, where the target organ and peripheral nervous structures have been destroyed (Mason & Holland 1993). After extraction of teeth, the myelinated fibre content of the inferior alveolar nerve is reduced by 20% (Heasman 1984). This finding indicates that fibers originally innervating the tooth and periodontal ligament are still present in the inferior alveolar nerve. Linden and Scott (1989) succeeded in stimulating nerves of periodontal origin in healed extraction sockets, which implies that some nerve endings remain functional. Nevertheless, most of the surviving mechanoreceptive neurons represented in the mesencephalic nucleus may lose some functionality (Linden & Scott 1989). These experiments have been the basis for a further and long-lasting debate on the presence and potential function of sensory nerve fibers in the bone and peri-implant environment. Histologic evidence indicates that there may be some re-innervation around osseointegrated implants (Wang *et al.* 1998; Lambrichts 1998) (Figs. 6-15, 6-16). Indeed, it has been shown that endosseous implants may lead to degeneration of surrounding neural fibers by surgical trauma. Soon however, sprouting of new fibers is observed and the number of free nerve endings close to the bone–implant interface gradually increases during the first weeks of healing (Wada *et al.* 2001). A more recent study in the dog has succeeded in partially regenerating the

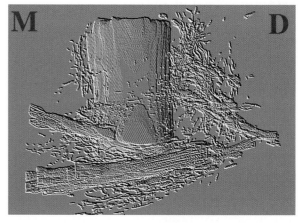

Fig. 6-15 A reconstruction of histologic slices indicating the regeneration of nerve tissue 3 months after implantation of a cylindrical oral implant in a dog's jaw bone. M = mesial; D = distal. (Reprinted from Wang *et al.* 1998, Copyright 2006, with permission from R. Jacobs, editor-publisher of *Osseoperception*, Dept of Periodontology, KU Leuven.)

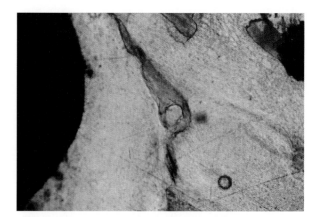

Fig. 6-16 Bone–implant specimen, obtained from a cat model, subjected to a light microscopic and immunohistochemical detection of neural structures. Elaborate neural structures in the bone trabeculae are seen surrounding the titanium implant. This histologic slice visualizes the titanium implant–bone tissue, with a bundle of myelinated nerve fibers in the bone trabeculum. (Reprinted from Lambrichts *et al.* 1998, Copyright 2006, with permission from Ivo Lambrichts, University of Hasselt and R. Jacobs, editor-publisher of *Osseoperception*, Dept of Periodontology, KU Leuven.)

periodontal ligament on an implant surface (Jahangiri *et al.* 2005). Whether such regeneration might also induce restoration of the peripheral feedback pathway needs further verification.

On the other hand, existing mechanoreceptors in the periosteum may also play a role in tactile function upon implant stimulation. It is evident that oral implants offer another type of loading and force transfer than teeth, considering an intimate bone–implant contact with elastic bone properties instead of the characteristic viscoelasticity of the periodontal ligament. Thus, forces applied to osseointegrated implants are directly transferred to the bone and bone deformation may lead to receptor activation in the peri-implant bone and the neighboring periosteum.

Cortical plasticity after tooth extraction

The cortex of the brain reveals a somatotopically ordered representational map with the teeth, gingiva, and jaws (Penfield & Rasmussen 1950). In this so-called sensory homunculus by Penfield, the representation of teeth in the postcentral gyrus of the primary somatosensory cortex is located superior to that of the tongue and inferior to that of the lip. This could be confirmed in a recent fMRI study, although this clear distinction between representation of tongue, lip, and teeth disappeared in the more caudal portions of the postcentral gyrus (Miyamoto *et al.* 2006). This established overlap of sensory representations might assume converging input from various oral structures including teeth. This finding could be relevant to the dedicated but intricate sensory information processing for modulation and coordination of oral motor function.

Recent findings on neuroplasticity of somatosensory and motor processes are also applicable in the orofacial region (Sessle 2006). After limb amputation or extraction, the regions of the cortex deprived of a target acquire new targets. Remodeling takes place at a (sub)cortical level. The potential cortical adaptation and/or plasticity that might occur after tooth extraction and implant placement has not yet been fully explored. A most interesting study was recently carried out on mole-rats, in which lower incisors were extracted (Henry *et al.* 2005). Five to eight months afterwards, functional MRI analysis yielded that the orofacial representation in S1 was considerably reorganized. Neurons in the cortical lower tooth representation were responsive to tactile inputs from surrounding orofacial structures. This study may indicate that cortical representation of teeth may significantly restructure after tooth loss. Unfortunately, until now, similar evidence in humans has not yet been produced. However, a very recent fMRI study by Lundborg *et al.* (2006) demonstrates that upon tactile stimulation of an osseointegrated prosthetic thumb, the primary somatosensory cortex is bilaterally activated in an area corresponding to that of the

hand. As one would only expect activation of the contralateral cortex for healthy thumb stimulation, the presence of bilateral cortical activation may be explained by some compensatory mechanism, recruiting additional sensory areas after amputation (Lundborg *et al.* 2006). This recent finding confirms once more that osseoperception and cortical plasticity may truly exist. At present, the central neural pathways and neural characteristics contributing to implant-mediated sensory motor control remain unclear. Future research should therefore try to visualize cortical plasticity after tooth extraction and further functional rehabilitation with implants in man. It should be considered that an immediate extraction and implant rehabilitation protocol might induce different cortical remodeling than a traditional two-stage implant rehabilitation protocol. An interesting phenomenon with respect to sensory–motor integration of osseointegrated implants, may be the so-called phantom tooth (after extraction) or phantom limb (after amputation), allowing perception of lost body parts (Jacobs *et al.* 2002c). In fact, it could be assumed that such a phantom feeling of the lost limb may overlap with or enforce the feeling of a bone-anchored prosthetic limb (Jacobs 1998). In this way, phantom sensations might contribute to physiological integration of a bone-anchored prosthesis in the human body.

If neuroplasticity after amputation and osseointegration could be fully unravelled, it might be considered during treatment to optimize adaptation to oral rehabilitation and implant placement (Feine *et al.* 2006).

From osseoperception to implant-mediated sensory motor interactions

During the last few decades, millions of patients have been rehabilitated by means of osseointegrated implants. Even though part of the peripheral feedback mechanism is lost after tooth extraction, edentulous patients seem to function quite well, especially when rehabilitated with a prosthesis retained by or anchored to osseointegrated implants (Jacobs 1998). These findings correspond well to the observation in amputees rehabilitated with a bone-anchored prosthesis rather than a socket prosthesis. During skeletal reconstruction, psychophysical testing reveals an improved tactile and vibrotactile capacity with an osseointegrated implant and a bone-anchored prosthetic limb (Fig. 6-17). Furthermore, both edentulous patients and amputees seem to report an improved awareness and special feeling with the implant-supported prosthesis, allowing a partial restoration of the peripheral feedback pathway with a hypothesized potential representation of the artificial limb feeling in the sensory cortex (Lundborg *et al.* 2006). If that could be confirmed, osseointegrated implants in the jaw or other skeletal bones might contribute to implant-mediated sensory–motor control allowing

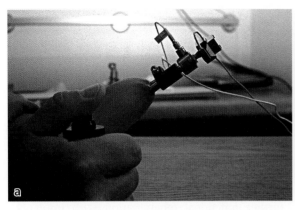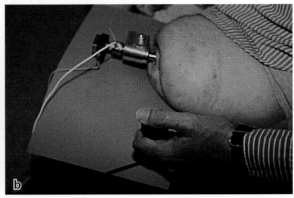

Fig. 6-17 Psychophysical test set-up using a patient-controlled remote control for a vibrotactile stimulator fixed to a radial (a) and femoral (b) osseointegrated implant. This particular test set-up yields superior perception for implants and bone-anchored prosthetic limbs compared to socket prostheses (Jacobs *et al.* 2000).

physiological integration of the implant in the human body, resulting in more natural functioning (Jacobs & van Steenberghe 2006).

Clinical implications of implant-deviated sensory motor interaction

Psychophysical testing on various bone-anchored prostheses confirms an improved tactile function leading to a better physiological integration of the limb. If perception upon implant stimulation is working well, peripheral feedback mechanisms may be restored and help fine tuning of motor control. This implant-mediated sensory–motor interaction may thus help to achieve a more natural function with the bone-anchored prosthesis (Jacobs 1998; Jacobs *et al.* 2000). Osseointegrated thumb prostheses even allow patients to perform the activities of daily life without any problem, which can be attributed to bone anchorage and bilateral cortical representation after prosthesis stimulation (Lundborg *et al.* 1996, 2006).

Considering the increased tactile threshold level for oral implant stimulation, one should, however, consider a few clinical implications. During rehabilitation by means of implant-supported prostheses, dentists should not rely on the patient's perception of occlusion. In this respect, one should also be aware of gradually increasing tactile function during the healing period after implant placement. This may be of particular importance when dealing with immediate loading protocols. To avoid any overloading related to suboptimal feedback mechanisms, patients should be encouraged to limit chewing forces by soft food intake during the healing period. Furthermore, parafunctional habits, such as grinding or clenching, might have a negative impact during the implant healing phase, but more research is needed to confirm this assumption (Lobbezoo *et al.* 2006). Until further evidence is collected, bruxism may be considered as a relative contraindication for immediate loading protocols (Glauser *et al.* 2001).

Conclusions

Sensory feedback plays an essential role in fine tuning of jaw and limb motor control. Periodontal mechanoreceptors, and more specifically those located in the periodontal ligament, are extremely sensitive to external mechanical stimuli. These receptors play the key role in tactile function of teeth, yielding detection thresholds of about 20 µm of thickness in between antagonistic teeth and 1–2 g upon tooth loading. Their sensory characteristics and the related peripheral feedback make the periodontal ligament receptors dedicated for fine tuning of masticatory and other oral motor behaviors.

It is clear that any condition that influences periodontal mechanoreceptors may also alter the sensory feedback pathway, and thus influence tactile function and modulation of jaw motor control (e.g. periodontal breakdown, bruxism, re-implantation, anesthesia). After extraction of teeth, the periodontal ligament has disappeared and so have its mechanoreceptors. After placement of oral implants, detection thresholds are increased to at least 50–100 µm of thickness and 50–100 g upon tooth loading.

Surprisingly enough, patients rehabilitated by means of osseointegrated implants seem to function quite well and/or sense better. In accordance with this, amputees rehabilitated with a lower limb prosthesis anchored to the bone by means of an osseointegrated implant, have reported that they could recognize the type of soil they were walking on, while patients with a bone-anchored thumb prosthesis have a cortical representation and thus conscious perception of their digit.

The underlying mechanism of this so-called "osseoperception" phenomenon remains a matter of debate, but is assumed that mechanoreceptors in the peri-implant bone and neighboring periosteum may be activated upon implant loading. Histological, neurophysiological and psychophysical evidence of osseoperception has been collected, making the assumption more likely that a proper peripheral feedback pathway can be restored when using osseointegrated implants. This implant-mediated sensory–motor control may have important clinical implications, because a more natural func-

tioning with implant-supported prostheses can be attempted. It may open doors for physiological and psychophysical integration of implants in the human body.

References

Abarca, M., van Steenberghe, D., Malevez, C., De Ridder, J. & Jacobs, R. (2006). Neurosensory disturbances after immediate loading of implants in the anterior mandible: an initial questionnaire approach followed by a psychophysical assessment. *Clinical Oral Investigations* **10**, 269–277.

Birder, L.A. & Perl, E.R. (1994). Cutaneous sensory receptors. *Journal of Clinical Neurophysiology* **11**, 534–552.

Borsook, D., Burstein, R. & Becerra, L. (2004). Functional imaging of the human trigeminal system: opportunities for new insights into pain processing in health and disease. *Journal of Neurobiology* **61**, 107–125.

Borsook, D., Burstein, R., Moulton, E. & Becerra, L. (2006). Functional imaging of the trigeminal system: applications to migraine pathophysiology. *Headache* **46** (suppl 1), S32–S38.

Bradley, R.M. (1995). *Essentials of Oral Physiology*, 2nd edn. Missouri, Mosby, pp. 145–160.

Broekhuijsen, M.L. & Van Willigen, J.D. (1983). Factors influencing jaw position sense in man. *Archives of Oral Biology* **28**, 387–391.

Calhoun, K., Gibson, B., Hartley, L., Minton, J. & Hokanson, J. (1992). Age-related changes in oral sensation. *Laryngoscope* **102**, 109–116.

Chen, C.C., Essick, G.K., Kelly, M.G., Nestor, J.M. & Masse, B. (1995). Gender-, side- and site-dependent variations in human perioral spatial resolution. *Archives of Oral Biology* **40**, 539–548.

Darriba, M.A. & Mendonca-Cardad, J.J. (1997). Profuse bleeding and life-threatening airway obstruction after placement of mandibular dental implants. *Journal of Oral and Maxillofacial Surgery* **55**, 1328–1330.

Ducreux, D., Attal, N., Parker, F. & Bouhassira D. (2006). Mechanisms of central neuropathic pain a combined psychophysical and fMRI study in syringomyelia. *Brain* **129**, 936–976.

Falmagne, J.C. (1985). *Elements of psychophysical theory*, 1st edn. Oxford: Oxford Clarendon Press.

Feine, J., Jacobs, R., Lobbezoo, F., Sessle, B.J., van Steenberghe, D., Trulsson, M., Fejerskov, O. & Svensson, P. (2006). A functional perspective on oral implants – state-of-the-science and future recommendations. *Journal of Oral Rehabilitation* **33**, 309–312.

Glauser, R., Ree, A., Lundgren, A., Gottlow, J., Hämmerle, C.H. & Schärer, P. (2001). Immediate occlusal loading of Brånemark implants applied in various jawbone regions: a prospective, 1-year clinical study. *Clinical Implant Dentistry and Related Research* **3**, 204–213.

Haraldson, T. (1983). Comparisons of chewing patterns in patients with bridges supported on osseointegrated implants and subjects with natural dentitions. *Acta Odontologica Scandinavica* **41**, 203–208.

Heasman, P.A. (1984). The myelinated fibre content of human inferior alveolar nerves from dentate and edentulous subjects. *Journal of Dentistry* **12**, 283–286.

Henry, E.C., Marasco, P.D. & Catania, K.C. (2005). Plasticity of the cortical dentition representation after tooth extraction in naked mole-rats. *Journal of Comparative Neurology* **485**, 64–74.

Hoogmartens, M.J. & Caubergh, M.A. (1987). Chewing side preference in man correlated with handedness, footedness, eyedness and earedness. *Electromyography and Clinical Neurophysiology* **27**, 293–300.

Iggo, A. (1985). Sensory receptors in the skin of mammals and their sensory functions. *Revue Neurologique (Paris)* **141**, 599–613.

Ingervall, B. & Schmoker, R. (1990). Effect of surgical reduction of the tongue on oral stereognosis, oral motor ability, and the rest position of the tongue and mandible. *American Journal of Orthodontics and Dentofacial Orthopedics* **97**, 58–65.

Jacobs, R. (1998). *Osseoperception*, 1st edn. Leuven: Department of Periodontology, Catholic University Leuven.

Jacobs, R., Bou Serhal, S. & van Steenberghe, D. (1997). Stereognosis with teeth and implants: a comparison between natural dentition, implant-supported fixed prostheses and overdentures on implants. *Clinical Oral Investigations* **1**, 89–94.

Jacobs, R., Bou Serhal, S. & van Steenberghe, D. (1998). Oral stereognosis: a review of the literature. *Clinical Oral Investigations* **2**, 3–10.

Jacobs, R., Brånemark, R., Olmarker, K., Rydevik, B., van Steenberghe, D. & Brånemark, P-I. (2000). Evaluation of the psychophysical detection threshold level for vibrotactile and pressure stimulation of prosthetic limbs using bone anchorage or soft tissue support. *Prosthetics and Orthotics International* **24**, 133–142.

Jacobs, R., Lambrichts, I., Liang, X., Martens, W., Mraiwa, N., Adriaensens, P. & Gelan, J. (2007). Neurovascularisation of the anterior jaw bones revisited using high resolution magnetic resonance imaging. *Oral Surgery Oral Medicine Oral Pathology Oral Radiology and Endodontics* **103**, 683–693.

Jacobs, R., Mraiwa, N., van Steenberghe, D., Gijbels, F. & Quirynen, M. (2002a). Appearance, location, course, and morphology of the mandibular incisive canal: an assessment on spiral CT scan. *Dentomaxillofacial Radiology* **31**, 322–327.

Jacobs, R., Mraiwa, N., van Steenberghe, D., Sanderink, G. & Quirynen, M. (2004). Appearance of the mandibular incisive canal on panoramic radiographs. *Surgical and Radiologic Anatomy* **26**, 329–333.

Jacobs, R., Schotte, A. & van Steenberghe, D. (1992). Influence of temperature and hardness of foils on interocclusal tactile threshold. *Journal of Periodontal Research* **27**, 581–587.

Jacobs, R. & van Steenberghe, D. (1991). Comparative evaluation of the oral tactile function by means of teeth or implant-supported prostheses. *Clinical Oral Implants Research* **2**, 75–80.

Jacobs, R. & van Steenberghe, D. (1993). Comparison between implant-supported prostheses and teeth regarding the passive threshold level. *The International Journal of Oral and Maxillofacial Implants* **8**, 549–554.

Jacobs, R. & van Steenberghe, D. (1994). Role of periodontal ligament receptors in the tactile function of teeth: a review. *Journal of Periodontal Research* **29**, 153–167.

Jacobs, R. & van Steenberghe, D. (2006). From osseoperception to implant-mediated sensory-motor interactions and related clinical implications. *Journal of Oral Rehabilitation* **33**, 282–292.

Jacobs, R., Wu, C-H., Desnyder, M., Kolenaar, B. & van Steenberghe, D. (2002d). Methodologies of oral sensory tests. *Journal of Oral Rehabilitation* **29**, 720–730.

Jacobs, R., Wu, C-H., Goossens, K., De Laat, A., Van Loven, K., Antonis, Y., Lambrechts, P. & van Steenberghe, D. (2002c). A case-control study on the psychophysical and psychological characteristics of the phantom tooth phenomenon. *Clinical Oral Investigations* **6**, 58–64.

Jacobs, R., Wu, C-H., Goossens, K., Van Loven, K, Van Hees, J & van Steenberghe, D. (2002b). Oral versus cutaneous sensory testing: a review of the literature. *Journal of Oral Rehabilitation* **29**, 923–950.

Jacobs, R., Wu, C-H., Goossens, K., Van Loven, K. & van Steenberghe, D. (2001). Perceptual changes in the anterior maxilla after placement of endosseous implants. *Clinical Implant Dentistry and Related Research* **3**, 148–155.

Jahangiri, L., Hessamfar, R. & Ricci, J.L. (2005). Partial generation of periodontal ligament on endosseous dental implants in dogs. *Clinical Oral Implant Research* **16**, 396–401.

Johansson, R.S., Trullson, M., Olsson, K.Å. & Abbs, J.H. (1988b). Mechanoreceptive afferent activity in the infraorbital nerve in man during speech and chewing movements. *Experimental Brain Research* **72**, 209–214.

Johansson, R.S., Trulsson, M., Olsson, K.Å. & Westberg, K-G. (1988a). Mechanoreceptor activity from the human face and oral mucosa. *Experimental Brain Research* **72**, 204–208.

Kiliaridis, S., Tzakis, M.G. & Carlsson, G.E. (1990). Short-term and long-term effects of chewing training on occlusal perception of thickness. *Scandinavian Journal of Dental Research* **98**, 159–166.

Lambrichts, I. (1998). Histological and ultrastructural aspects of bone innervation. In: Jacobs, R., ed. *Osseoperception*. Leuven: Department of Periodontology, KU Leuven.

Lambrichts, I., Creemers, J. & van Steenberghe, D. (1992). Morphology of neural endings in the human periodontal ligament: an electronmicroscopic study. *Journal of Periodontal Research* **27**, 191–196.

Liang, X, Jacobs, R. & Lambrichts, I. (2005b). Appearance, location, course and morphology of the superior and inferior genial spinal foramina and their bony canals: an assessment on spiral CT scan. *Surgical and Radiologic Anatomy* **9**, 1–7.

Liang, X., Jacobs, R., Lambrichts, I., Vandewalle, G., van Oostveldt, D., Schepers, E., Adriaensens, P. & Gelan, J. (2005a). Microanatomical and histological assessment of the content of superior genial spinal foramen and its bony canal. *Dentomaxillofacial Radiology* **34**, 362–368.

Linden, R.W. & Scott, B.J. (1989). The effect of tooth extraction on periodontal ligament mechanoreceptors represented in the mesencephalic nucleus of the cat. *Archives of Oral Biology* **34**, 937–941.

Litvak, H., Silverman, S.I. & Garfinkel, L. (1971). Oral stereognosis in dentulous and edentulous subjects. *Journal of Prosthetic Dentistry* **25**, 139–151.

Lobbezoo, F., Van Der Zaag, J. & Naeije, M. (2006). Bruxism: its multiple causes and its effects on dental implants – an updated review. *Journal of Oral Rehabilitation* **33**, 293–300.

Lundborg, G., Brånemark, P-I. & Rosén, B. (1996). Osseointegrated thumb prostheses: a concept for fixation of digit prosthetic devices. *Journal of Hand Surgery (America)* **21**, 216–221.

Lundborg, G., Waites, A., Björkman, A., Rosén, B. & Larsson, E-M. (2006). Functional magnetic resonance imaging shows cortical activation on sensory stimulation of an osseointegrated prosthetic thumb. *Scandinavian Journal of Plastic and Reconstructive Surgery and Hand Surgery* **40**, 234–239.

Lundqvist, S. (1993). Speech and other oral functions. *Swedish Dental Journal (Suppl)* **91**, 1–39.

Martin, J.H. (1991). Coding and processing of sensory information. In: Kandel, E.R., Schwartz, J.H., Jessel, T.M., eds. *Principles of Neural Science*, 3rd edn. Norwalk, CT: Appleton & Lange, pp. 329–340.

Martin, J.H. & Jessell, T.M. (1991). Modality coding in the somatosensory system. In: Kandel, E.R., Schwartz, J.H., Jessel, T.M., eds. *Principles of Neural Science*, 3rd edn. Norwalk, CT: Appleton & Lange, pp. 341–352.

Mason, A.G. & Holland, G.R. (1993). The reinnervation of healing extraction sockets in the ferret. *Journal of Dental Research* **72**, 1215–1221.

Mason, R. (1967). Studies on oral perception involving subjects with alterations in anatomy and physiology. In: Bosma, J.F., ed. *Second Symposium on Oral Sensation and Perception*. Springfield, Ill: Charles C Thomas Publisher, pp. 295–301.

Masoro, E.J. (1986). Physiology of aging. In: Holm-Pederson, P., Löe, H. eds. *Geriatric Dentistry*. Copenhagen: Munksgaard, pp. 34–55.

Mericske-Stern, R. (1994). Oral tactile sensibility recorded in overdenture wearers with implants or natural roots: a comparative study. Part 2. *The International Journal of Oral and Maxillofacial Implants* **9**, 63–70.

Mericske-Stern, R., Assal, P., Mericske, E. & Burgin, W-I. (1995). Occlusal force and oral tactile sensibility measured in partially edentulous patients with ITI implants. *International Journal of Oral and Maxillofacial Implants* **10**, 345–354.

Miyamoto, J.J., Honda, M., Saito, D.N., Okada, T., Ono, T., Ohyama, K. & Sadato, N. (2006). The representation of the human oral area in the somatosensory cortex: a functional MRI study. *Cerebral Cortex* **16**, 669–675.

Morimoto, T. (1990). Perception of intraoral stimulation. In: Taylor, A. ed. *Neurophysiology of the Jaws and Teeth*. Houndmills: The Macmillan Press Ltd, pp. 369–390.

Moser, H., LaGourgue J. & Class, L. (1967). Studies of oral stereognosis in normal, blind and deaf subjects. In: Bosma, J.F. ed. *Second Symposium on Oral Sensation and Perception*. Springfield, Ill: Charles C Thomas Publisher, pp. 245–286.

Mraiwa, N., Jacobs, R., Moerman, P., Lambrichts, I., van Steenberghe, D. & Quirynen, M. (2003a). Presence and course of the incisive canal in the human mandibular interforaminal region: two-dimensional imaging versus anatomical observations. *Surgical and Radiologic Anatomy* **25**, 416–423.

Mraiwa, N., Jacobs, R., van Steenberghe, D. & Quirynen, M. (2003b). Clinical assessment and surgical implications of anatomic challenges in the anterior mandible. *Clinical Implant Dentistry and Related Research* **5**, 219–225.

Mraiwa, N., Jacobs, R., Van Cleynenbreugel, J., Sanderink, G., Schutyser, F., Suetens, P., van Steenberghe, D. & Quirynen, M. (2004). The nasopalatine canal revisited using 2D and 3D CT imaging. *Dentomaxillofacial Radiology* **33**, 396–402.

Müller, F., Link, I., Fuhr, K. & Utz, K-H. (1995). Studies on adaptation to complete dentures. Part II: Oral stereognosis and tactile sensibility. *Journal of Oral Rehabilitation* **22**, 759–767.

Nordin, M. & Hagbarth, K.E. (1989). Mechanoreceptive units in the human infra-orbital nerve. *Acta Physiologica Scandinavica* **135**, 149–161.

Penfield, W. & Rasmussen, T. (1950). *The Cerebral Cortex of Man: a Clinical Study of Localization of Function*. New York: Macmillan.

Sakada, S. (1974). Mechanoreceptors in fascia, periosteum and periodontal ligament. *Bulletin of the Tokyo Medical and Dental University* **21** (Suppl), 11–13.

Sessle, B.J. (2006). Mechanisms of oral somatosensory and motor functions and their clinical correlates. *Journal of Oral Rehabilitation* **33**, 243–261.

Swinnen, A., Van Huffel, S., Van Loven, K. & Jacobs, R. (2000). Detection and multichannel SVD based filtering of trigeminal somatosensory evoked potentials. *Medical and Biological Engineering and Computing* **38**, 297–305.

Trulsson, M., Johansson, R.S. & Olsson, K.Å. (1992). Directional sensitivity of human periodontal mechanoreceptive afferents to forces applied to the teeth. *Journal of Physiology (London)* **447**, 373–389.

Trulsson, M. (2006). Sensory-motor function of periodontal mechanoreceptors. *Journal of Oral Rehabilitation* **33**, 262–273.

Vallbo, Å.B. & Johansson, R.S. (1984). Properties of cutaneous mechanoreceptors in the human hand related to touch sensation. *Human Neurobiology* **3**, 3–14.

Van Loven, K., Jacobs, R., Swinnen, A., van Huffel, S., Van Hees, J. & van Steenberghe, D. (2000) Sensations and trigeminal somatosensory-evoked potentials elicited by electrical stimulation of endosseous oral implants in humans. *Archives of Oral Biology* **45**, 1083–1090.

Van Loven K, Jacobs, R., Van Hees, J., Van Huffel, S. & van Steenberghe, D. (2001). Trigeminal somatosensory evoked potentials in humans. *Electromyography and Clinical Neurophysiology* **41**, 357–375.

Wada, S., Kojo, T., Wang, Y.H., Ando, H., Nakanishi, E., Zhang, M., Fukuyama, H. & Uchida, Y. (2001). Effect of loading on the development of nerve fibers around oral implants in the dog mandible. *Clinical Oral Implants Research* **12**, 219–224.

Wang, Y.-H., Kojo, T., Ando, H., Nakanishi, E., Yoshizawa. H., Zhang, M., Fukuyama, H., Wada, S. & Uchida, Y. (1998). Nerve regeneration after implantation in peri-implant area: a histological study on different implant materials in dogs. In: Jacobs, R., ed. *Osseoperception*. Leuven: Dept of Periodontology, Catholic University Leuven, pp. 3–11.

Part 2: Epidemiology

Chapter 7

Epidemiology of Periodontal Diseases

Panos N. Papapanou and Jan Lindhe

Introduction

The term epidemiology is of Hellenic origin; it consists of the preposition "epi", which means "among" or "against", and the noun "demos" which means "people". As denoted by its etymology, epidemiology is defined as "the study of the distribution of disease or a physiological condition in human populations and of the factors that influence this distribution" (Lilienfeld 1978). A more inclusive description by Frost (1941) emphasizes that "epidemiology is essentially an inductive science, concerned not merely with describing the distribution of disease, but equally or more with fitting it into a consistent philosophy". Thus, the information obtained from an epidemiologic investigation should extend beyond a mere description of the distribution of the disease in different populations (*descriptive* epidemiology). It should be further expanded to (1) elucidate the etiology of a specific disease by combining epidemiologic data with information from other disciplines such as genetics, biochemistry, microbiology, sociology, etc. (*etiologic* epidemiology); (2) evaluate the consistency of epidemiologic data with hypotheses developed clinically or experimentally (*analytical* epidemiology); and (3) provide the basis for developing and evaluating preventive procedures and public health practices (*experimental/intervention* epidemiology).

Based on the above, epidemiological research in periodontology must (1) fulfill the task of providing data on the *prevalence* of periodontal diseases in different populations, i.e. the frequency of their occur-

rence, as well as on the *severity* of such conditions, i.e. the level of occurring pathologic changes; (2) elucidate aspects related to the *etiology* and the *determinants of development* of these diseases (*causative* and *risk* factors); and (3) provide documentation concerning the effectiveness of preventive and therapeutic measures aimed against these diseases on a population basis.

Methodological issues

Examination methods – index systems

Examination of the periodontal status of a given individual includes clinical assessments of inflammation in the periodontal tissues, recording of probing depths and clinical attachment levels and radiographic assessments of supporting alveolar bone. A variety of index systems for the scoring of these parameters has been developed over the years. Some of these systems were designed exclusively for examination of patients in a dental practice set-up, while others were developed in order to be utilized in epidemiologic research. The design of the index systems and the definition of the various scores inevitably reflects the knowledge of the etiology and pathogenesis of periodontal disease at the time these systems were introduced, as well as concepts related to the current therapeutic approaches and strategies. This section will not provide a complete list of all available scoring systems, but rather give a brief description of a limited number of indices that are either currently used or are likely to be encountered in the recent literature. For description of earlier scoring systems and a historical perspective of their development, the reader is referred to Ainamo (1989).

Assessment of inflammation of the periodontal tissues

Presence of inflammation in the marginal portion of the gingiva is usually recorded by means of probing assessments, according to the principles of the Gingival Index outlined in the publication by Löe (1967). According to this system, entire absence of visual signs of inflammation in the gingival unit is scored as 0, while a slight change in color and texture is scored as 1. Visual inflammation and bleeding tendency from the gingival margin right after a periodontal probe is briefly run along the gingival margin is scored as 2, while overt inflammation with tendency for spontaneous bleeding is scored as 3. A parallel index for scoring plaque deposits (Plaque Index) in a scale from 0 to 3 (Silness & Löe 1964) was introduced, according to which absence of plaque deposits is scored as 0, plaque disclosed after running the periodontal probe along the gingival margin as 1, visible plaque as 2 and abundant plaque as 3. Simplified variants of both the Gingival and the Plaque Index (Ainamo & Bay 1975) have been extensively used, assessing presence/absence of inflammation or plaque, respectively, in a binomial fashion (dichotomous scoring). In such systems, bleeding from the gingival margin and visible plaque score 1, while absence of bleeding and no visible plaque score 0.

Bleeding after probing to the base of the probeable pocket (Gingival Sulcus Bleeding Index) has been a common way of assessing presence of subgingival inflammation (Mühlemann & Son 1971). In this dichotomous registration, 1 is scored in cases where bleeding emerges within 15 seconds after probing. Presence/absence of bleeding on probing to the base of the pocket is increasingly tending to substitute the use of the Gingival Index in epidemiologic studies.

Assessment of loss of periodontal tissue support

One of the early indices providing indirect information on the loss of periodontal tissue support was the Periodontal Index (PI) developed in the 1950s by Russell (1956), and until the 1980s it was the most widely used index in epidemiologic studies of periodontal disease. Its criteria are applied to each tooth and the scoring is as follows: a tooth with healthy periodontium scores 0, a tooth with gingivitis around only part of the tooth circumference scores 1, a tooth with gingivitis encircling the tooth scores 2, pocket formation scores 6, and loss of function due to excessive tooth mobility scores 8. Due to the nature of the

criteria used, the PI is a reversible scoring system, i.e. after treatment a tooth or an individual can have the score lowered or reduced to 0.

In contrast to the PI system, the Periodontal Disease Index (PDI), developed by Ramfjord (1959), is a system designed to assess destructive disease; it measures loss of attachment instead of pocket depth and is, therefore, an irreversible index. The scores, ranging from 0–6, denote periodontal health or gingivitis (scores 0–3) and various levels of attachment loss (scores 4–6).

In contemporary epidemiologic studies, loss of periodontal tissue support is assessed by measurements of pocket depth and attachment level. Probing pocket depth (PPD) is defined as the distance from the gingival margin to the location of the tip of a periodontal probe inserted in the pocket with moderate probing force. Likewise, probing attachment level (PAL) or clinical attachment level (CAL) is defined as the distance from the cemento-enamel junction (CEJ) to the location of the inserted probe tip. Probing assessments may be carried out at different locations of the tooth circumference (buccal, lingual, mesial or distal sites). The number of probing assessments per tooth has varied in epidemiologic studies from two to six, while the examination may either include all present teeth (full-mouth) or a subset of index teeth (partial-mouth examination).

Carlos et al. (1986) proposed an index system which records loss of periodontal tissue support. The index was denoted the Extent and Severity Index (ESI) and consists of two components (bivariate index): (1) the Extent, describing the proportion of tooth sites of a subject examined showing signs of destructive periodontitis, and (2) the Severity, describing the amount of attachment loss at the diseased sites, expressed as a mean value. An attachment loss threshold of >1 mm was set as the criterion for a tooth site to qualify as affected by the disease. Although arbitrary, the introduction of a threshold value serves a dual purpose: (1) it readily distinguishes the fraction of the dentition affected by disease at levels exceeding the error inherent in the clinical measurement of attachment loss, and (2) it prevents unaffected tooth sites from contributing to the individual subject's mean attachment loss value. In order to limit the assessments to be performed, a partial examination comprising the mid-buccal and mesio-buccal aspects of the upper right and lower left quadrants was recommended. It has to be emphasized that the system was designed to assess the cumulative effect of destructive periodontal disease rather than the presence of the disease itself. The bivariate nature of the index facilitates a rather detailed description of attachment loss patterns: for example an ESI of (90, 2.5) suggests a generalized but rather mild form of destructive disease, in which 90% of the tooth sites are affected by an average attachment loss of 2.5 mm. In contrast, an ESI of (20, 7.0) describes a severe, localized form of disease. Validation of various partial extent and severity scoring systems against the full-mouth estimates has been also performed (Papapanou *et al.* 1993).

Radiographic assessment of alveolar bone loss

The potential and limitations of intraoral radiography to describe loss of supporting periodontal tissues were reviewed by Lang and Hill (1977) and Benn (1990). Radiographs have been commonly employed in cross-sectional epidemiologic studies to evaluate the result of periodontal disease on the supporting tissues rather than the presence of the disease itself and are thought to provide valid estimates of the extent and severity of destructive periodontitis (Pitiphat *et al.* 2004). Radiographic assessments have been particularly common as screening methods for detecting subjects suffering from juvenile periodontitis as well as a means for monitoring periodontal disease progression in longitudinal studies. Assessments of bone loss in intraoral radiographs are usually performed by evaluating a multitude of qualitative and quantitative features of the visualized interproximal bone, e.g. (1) presence of an intact lamina dura, (2) the width of the periodontal ligament space, (3) the morphology of the bone crest ("even" or "angular" appearance), and (4) the distance between the CEJ and the most coronal level at which the periodontal ligament space is considered to retain a normal width. The threshold for bone loss, i.e. the CEJ – bone crest distance considered to indicate that bone loss has occurred, varies between 1 and 3 mm in different studies. Radiographic data are usually presented as (1) mean bone loss scores per subject (or group of subjects), and (2) number or percentage of tooth surfaces per subject (or group of subjects) exhibiting bone loss exceeding certain thresholds. In early studies, bone loss was frequently recorded using "ruler" devices, describing the amount of lost or remaining bone as a percentage of the length of the root or the tooth (Schei *et al.* 1959; Lavstedt *et al.* 1975).

Assessment of periodontal treatment needs

An index system aimed at assessing the need for periodontal treatment in large population groups was developed, at the initiative of the World Health Organization (WHO), by Ainamo *et al.* (1982). The principles of the Community Periodontal Index for Treatment Needs (CPITN) can be summarized as follows:

1. The dentition is divided into six *sextants* (one anterior and two posterior tooth regions in each dental arch). The treatment need in a sextant is recorded when two or more teeth, not intended for extraction, are present. If only one tooth remains in the sextant, the tooth is included in the adjoining sextant.

2. Probing assessments are performed either around all teeth in a sextant or around certain index teeth (the latter approach has been recommended for epidemiologic surveys). However, only the most severe measure in the sextant is chosen to represent the sextant.

3. The periodontal conditions are scored as follows:
   - *Code 1* is given to a sextant with no pockets, calculus or overhangs of fillings but in which bleeding occurs after gentle probing in one or several gingival units.
   - *Code 2* is assigned to a sextant if there are no pockets exceeding 3 mm, but in which dental calculus and plaque-retaining factors are seen or recognized subgingivally.
   - *Code 3* is given to a sextant that harbors 4–5 mm deep pockets.
   - *Code 4* is given to a sextant that harbors pockets 6 mm deep or deeper.

4. The treatment needs are scores based on the most severe code in the dentition as TN 0, in case of gingival health, TN 1 indicating need for improved oral hygiene if code 1 has been recorded, TN 2 indicating need for scaling, removal of overhangs, and improved oral hygiene (codes 2 + 3) and TN 3 indicating complex treatment (code 4).

Although not designed for epidemiological purposes, this index system has been extensively used worldwide, and CPITN-based studies have often been the exclusive source of epidemiologic information on periodontal conditions, particularly from developing countries. A later modification of the index, termed Community Periodontal Index (CPI; WHO 1997), places more emphasis on the assessment of periodontal conditions rather than the assessment of periodontal treatment needs. A substantial amount of data generated by the use of CPITN/CPI have been accumulated in the WHO Global Oral Data Bank (Miyazaki *et al.* 1992; Pilot & Miyazaki 1994 Petersen *et al.* 2005; Petersen & Ogawa 2005) and are accessible electronically through servers maintained at the Niigata University, Japan (WHO Collaborating Centre) and University of Malmö, Sweden (WHO Collaborating Centre).

Critical evaluation

A fundamental prerequisite for any meaningful comparative assessment of prevalence is a valid and accurate definition of the disease under investigation. Unfortunately, no uniform criteria have been established in periodontal research for this purpose. Epidemiologic studies have employed a wide array of symptoms, including gingivitis, probing depth, clinical attachment level, and radiographically assessed alveolar bone loss, in an inconsistent manner. Considerable variation characterizes the threshold values employed for defining periodontal pockets as "deep" or "pathologic", or the clinical attachment level and alveolar bone scores required for assuming that "true" loss of periodontal tissue support has, in fact, occurred. In addition, the number of "affected" tooth surfaces required for assigning an individual subject as a "case", i.e. as suffering from periodontal disease, has varied. These inconsistencies in the definitions inevitably affect the figures describing the distribution of the disease (Papapanou 1996; Kingman & Albandar 2002) and, consequently, the identification of risk factors (Borrell & Papapanou 2005). A review of the literature charged with the task of comparing disease prevalence or incidence in different populations or at different time periods must first be confronted with the interpretation of the figures reported and literally "decode" the published data in order to extract relevant information that is amenable to inter-study comparisons. These problems have been addressed in the literature and two specific aspects have attracted special attention, namely (1) the ability of partial recording methodologies to reflect full-mouth conditions, and (2) the use of the CPITN system in epidemiological studies of periodontal disease.

There is little doubt that an optimal examination of periodontal conditions should include circumferential probing assessments around all teeth. Nevertheless, the majority of epidemiological studies have, for practical reasons, employed partial recording methodologies. The rationale for the use of partial examinations has been the assumption that (1) the time required for the performance of a partial survey, and consequently its cost, is significantly decreased, and (2) the amount of information lost is kept to a minimum, provided that the examined segments adequately reflect the periodontal condition of the entire dentition. However, attempts to quantify accurately the amount of information lost through the different partial recording systems made by several investigators (Hunt 1987; Kingman et al. 1988; Hunt & Fann 1991; Stoltenberg et al. 1993a; Diamanti-Kipioti et al. 1993; Eaton et al. 2001; Susin et al. 2005a) have revealed that the discrepancy between the findings obtained by means of partial and full-mouth surveys may be substantial. These studies have typically employed full-mouth data for a series of periodontal parameters and compared them with the values obtained by assessments performed at a subset of teeth or tooth surfaces. Their results suggest that:

1. High correlations between full-mouth and half-mouth attachment loss scores should be expected in adult populations, due to the apparent symmetry of periodontal conditions around the midline.
2. The performance of a partial recording system is directly dependent on the actual prevalence of periodontal disease in the population in question and, consequently, on the age of the subjects examined; the less frequent the disease in the population and the lower the number of sites that are

affected in each individual mouth, the more difficult it becomes for the partial examination to detect the periodontal lesions.
3. A full-mouth examination provides the best means of accurately assessing the prevalence and severity of periodontal disease in a population.

The use of the CPITN system in epidemiological studies of periodontal disease was critically evaluated in a number of publications (Grytten & Mubarak 1989; Holmgren & Corbet 1990; Schürch et al. 1990; Butterworth & Sheiham 1991; Baelum et al. 1993a,b, 1995; Benigeri et al. 2000). At the time the system was designed, the conversion of periodontal health to disease was thought to include a continuum of conditions, ranging from an inflammation-free state developing through gingivitis (bleeding), calculus deposition, shallow and deep pocket formation to progressive, destructive disease. The treatment concepts were based on the assumption that probing depths determined the choice between non-surgical and more complicated, surgical periodontal therapy. It should also be remembered that this particular index was clearly intended for screening large population groups in order to determine treatment needs and to facilitate preventive and therapeutic strategies and not for describing prevalence and severity of periodontal disease. In view of the revised, contemporary views on the pathogenesis and treatment of the periodontal diseases, studies have questioned the suitability of the CPITN for such purposes. For example, Butterworth and Sheiham (1991) addressed the suitability of CPITN to record changes in periodontal conditions and examined patients of a general dental practice before and after periodontal therapy. Despite a substantial improvement in the state of health of the periodontal tissues, assessed through gingivitis, calculus, and pocketing scores, the CPITN scores were only marginally improved. In a rural Kenyan subject sample, Baelum et al. (1993b) examined and refuted the validity of the hierarchical principle of the CPITN, i.e. the assumptions that a tooth with calculus is assumed to be positive also for bleeding on probing, and that a tooth with moderately deep or deep pockets is assumed to be positive for both calculus and bleeding. In a companion paper, results from a full-mouth examination were compared with those generated by the use of the ten index teeth recommended by the WHO for surveys of adults (Baelum et al. 1993a). The study revealed that the partial CPITN methodology seriously underestimates the more severe periodontal conditions both in terms of prevalence and severity, since it fails to detect a substantial proportion of subjects with periodontal pockets. Finally, an examination of the relationship between CPITN findings and the prevalence and severity of clinical attachment loss, demonstrated that the CPITN scores do not consistently correlate with attachment loss measures, but tend to overestimate prevalence and severity among younger subjects while they underestimate such parameters in elderly populations (Baelum *et al.* 1995). The above data call for caution in the interpretation of epidemiologic studies based on the CPITN/CPI systems.

Prevalence of periodontal diseases

Introduction

The currently used classification of periodontal diseases was introduced by the 1999 International Workshop for a Classification of Periodontal Diseases and Conditions (Anon 1999) and encompasses eight main categories, namely:

I   Gingival diseases
II   Chronic periodontitis
III   Aggressive periodontitis
IV   Periodontitis as a manifestation of systemic diseases
V   Necrotizing periodontal diseases
VI   Abscesses of the periodontium
VII   Periodontitis associated with endodontic lesions
VIII   Developmental or acquired deformities and conditions.

Since the current nomenclature has been in use for less than a decade, a substantial part of the existing literature on the prevalence and extent of periodontal diseases in various populations is still based on earlier classification systems. Inevitably, the following review of epidemiologic studies uses data stemming from publications employing both the earlier and the current diagnostic systems. Although the current classification no longer employs the individual subject's age as a primary determinant of diagnosis, the descriptive epidemiologic findings have still been grouped in the text below according to age, in order to facilitate data extraction from studies using inconsistent terminologies.

Periodontitis in adults

An epidemiologic survey performed during the 1950s in India used assessments of alveolar bone height to distinguish between gingivitis and destructive periodontal disease in a sample involving 1187 dentate subjects (Marshall-Day *et al.* 1955). The authors reported (1) a decrease in the percentage of subjects with "gingival disease without any bone involvement" with increasing age concomitant with an increase in the percentage of subjects with "chronic, destructive periodontal disease", and (2) a 100% occurrence of destructive periodontitis after the age of 40 years. Findings from other epidemiologic studies from the same period verified a high prevalence of destructive periodontal disease in the adult population in general, and a clear increase in disease prevalence with age. In the 1960s, Scherp (1964)

reviewed the available literature on the epidemiology of periodontal disease and concluded that (1) periodontal disease appears to be a major, global public health problem affecting the majority of the adult population after the age of 35–40 years, (2) the disease starts as gingivitis in youth, which, if left untreated, leads to progressive destructive periodontitis, and (3) more than 90% of the variance of the periodontal disease severity in the population can be explained by age and oral hygiene. These notions, based on established concepts on the pathogenesis of periodontal disease of that time, dominated the periodontal literature until the late 1970s.

Studies performed during the 1980s provided a more thorough description of the site-specific features of periodontal disease and the high variation in periodontal conditions between and within different populations. Contrary to what was customary until then, the prevalence issue was no longer addressed through a mere assignment of individuals to a "periodontitis-affected" or a "disease-free" group, based on presence or absence of attachment or alveolar bone loss. Instead, studies began to unravel details concerning the *extent* to which the dentition was affected by destructive disease (i.e. the percentage of tooth sites involved), and the *severity* of the defects (expressed through the magnitude of the tissue support lost due to the disease). The traditional description of pocket depth and attachment loss scores through *subject mean values* was soon complemented by *frequency distributions*, revealing percentages of tooth sites exhibiting probing depth or attachment level of varying severity. Such an additional analysis appeared necessary after it became clear that mean values offer a crude description of periodontal conditions and fail to reflect the variability in the severity of periodontal disease within and between individuals. In an article presenting different methods of evaluating periodontal disease data in epidemiological research, Okamoto *et al.* (1988) proposed the use of *percentile plots* in the graphic illustration of attachment loss data. As exemplified by Fig. 7-1, such plots make it possible to illustrate simultaneously both the proportion of subjects exhibiting attachment loss of different levels and the severity of the loss within the subjects. Similar plots may be produced for other parameters, such as gingivitis, probing depths and gingival recession, and may provide a comprehensive description of both the prevalence and the severity of periodontal disease in a given sample.

Pioneering research by a Danish research group made significant contributions to our current understanding of epidemiologic issues in periodontal research. Baelum *et al.* (1986) described cross-sectional findings on dental plaque, calculus, gingivitis, loss of attachment, periodontal pockets, and tooth loss in a sample of adult Tanzanians aged 30–69 years. Despite the fact that the subjects examined exhibited large amounts of plaque and calculus,

% of sites

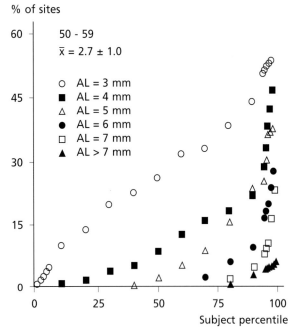

% of individuals

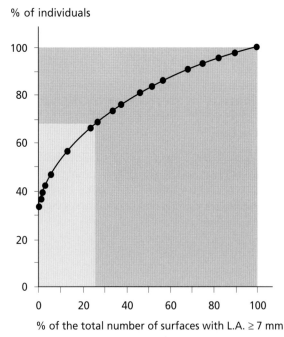

Fig. 7-1 Attachment loss in a group of Japanese subjects 50–59 years of age. The mean value of attachment level and the standard deviation are shown in the top of the figure. The x-axis represents the subject percentile and the y-axis represents the percentage of sites in the subjects showing attachment loss of 3, 4, 5, 6, 7, and >7 mm (represented by 8). Subjects with no or only minor signs of attachment loss are reported to the left and subjects with increasing amounts of periodontal destruction are reported to the right of the graph. For example, the median subject (50th percentile), exhibited 5 mm attachment loss at 2%, 4 mm loss at 8%, and 3 mm attachment loss at 25% of its sites. From Okamoto *et al.* (1988), reproduced with permission.

Fig. 7-2 Cumulative distribution of individuals aged ≥50 years according to the cumulated proportion of surfaces with loss of attachment (L.A.) ≥7 mm. All individuals are arranged according to increasing number of surfaces with L.A. ≥7 mm present in each individual. Thus, individuals with few such surfaces are represented by the dots in the left side of the diagram and those with many such surfaces by dots in the right side. It is seen that 31% (100%–69%) of the individuals account for 75% (100%–25%) of the total number of surfaces with L.A. ≥7 mm present (shaded area). From Baelum *et al.* (1986), reproduced with permission.

pockets deeper than 3 mm and attachment loss of >6 mm occurred at less than 10% of the tooth surfaces. Edentulousness was virtually non-existent, and a very small percentage of subjects had experienced major tooth loss. Of particular interest was the analysis of the distribution of sites within subjects (Fig. 7-2). This analysis revealed that 75% of the tooth sites with attachment loss of ≥7 mm were found in 31% of the subjects, indicating that a subfraction of the sample was responsible for the major part of the observed periodontal breakdown. In other words, advanced periodontal disease was not evenly distributed in the population and not readily correlated to supragingival plaque levels; instead, the majority of the subjects examined exhibited negligible periodontal problems while a limited group was affected by advanced disease.

In a study of similar design performed in Kenya, the same investigators analyzed data from 1131 subjects aged 15–65 years and confirmed their earlier observations (Baelum *et al.* 1988a). Poor oral hygiene in the sample was reflected by high plaque, calculus, and gingivitis scores. However, pockets ≥4 mm deep were found in less than 20% of the surfaces and the proportion of sites per individual with deep pockets and advanced loss of attachment revealed a pronounced skewed distribution. The authors suggested

that "destructive periodontal disease should not be perceived as an inevitable consequence of gingivitis which ultimately leads to considerable tooth loss" and called for a more specific characterization of the features of periodontal breakdown in those individuals who seem particularly susceptible.

At approximately the same time, Löe *et al.* (1986) published their landmark paper that showed that the *progression* of untreated periodontitis also shared similar features. In a population never exposed to any preventive or therapeutic intervention related to oral diseases in Sri Lanka, an original cohort of 480 male tea-plantation laborers, aged 14–31 years, was initially recruited in 1970, and underwent subsequent follow-up examinations. A total of 161 of subjects were re-examined at the final examination in 1985, essentially generating data on the natural history of periodontal disease between the age of 14 and 46 years. Despite poor plaque control and virtually ubiquitous gingival inflammation in the entire sample, three distinct patterns of progression of periodontitis were observed over the follow-up period, based on interproximal longitudinal attachment loss and tooth mortality rates: one group, comprising approximately 8% of the total, with rapid progression of periodontal disease (RP); another group (approximately 11%) who exhibited no progression

(NP) of periodontal disease beyond gingivitis; and a third group between the two extremes (approximately 81%) with moderate progression (MP). The mean loss of attachment in the RP group was 9 mm and 13 mm, at the age of 35 and 45 years, respectively, as opposed to 1 mm and 1.5 mm in the NP group, and 4 mm and 7 mm in the MP group. As a result, the annual rate of longitudinal attachment loss in the RP group varied between 0.1 and 1.0 mm, in the MP group between 0.05 and 0.5 mm, and in the NP group between 0.05 and 0.09 mm. Thus, what this study clearly demonstrated is the huge variability in progression of periodontitis in a seemingly homogeneous population, and suggested that variables other than age, plaque, and gingival inflammatory status are important determinants of periodontal deterioration over time.

Several epidemiological studies have been published in the last two decades, verifying the above principals. In these studies, periodontal disease has been assessed by means of clinical examination of the periodontal tissues (Brown et al. 1989, 1990; McFall et al. 1989; Stuck et al. 1989; Beck et al. 1990; Horning et al. 1990; Hunt et al. 1990; Matthesen et al. 1990; Gilbert & Heft 1992; Löe et al. 1992; Bagramian et al. 1993; Douglass et al. 1993; Kiyak et al. 1993; Locker & Leake 1993; Slade et al. 1993; Weyant et al. 1993; Querna et al. 1994; Söder et al. 1994; Anagnou Vareltzides et al. 1996; Oliver et al. 1998; Albandar et al. 1999; Albandar & Kingman 1999; Schürch & Lang 2004; Susin et al. 2004a; Krustrup & Erik Petersen 2006; Thomson et al. 2006); radiographic assessments of alveolar bone loss (Papapanou et al. 1988; Jenkins & Kinane 1989; Wouters et al. 1989; Salonen et al. 1991; Diamanti-Kipioti et al. 1995); or a combination of clinical and radiographic means (Hugoson et al. 1998a, 1992, 2005; Papapanou et al. 1990).

Table 7-1 summarizes the design and main findings from a number of cross-sectional studies in adults from geographically divergent areas that involve samples of a relatively large size. Most of the studies focus on assessments of prevalence of "advanced periodontitis", the definition of which is, however, far from identical among the studies, rendering comparisons difficult. Nevertheless, it appears that severe forms of periodontitis affect a minority of the subjects in the industrialized countries, at proportions usually not exceeding 10–15% of the population. The percentage of such subjects increases considerably with age and appears to reach its peak at the age of 50–60 years. The increased tooth loss occurring after this age appears to account for the subsequent decline in prevalence. It is worth pointing out that, among the studies reviewed in Table 7-1, the study employing probing assessments at six sites per tooth around all teeth (Susin et al. 2004a) reported the highest prevalence of advanced disease, suggesting that the impact of the methodology used may have been decisive. The interesting issue of disparities in the severity of periodontitis was brought up

by Baelum et al. (1996). The authors recalculated their own data from a Kenyan (Baelum et al. 1988a) and a Chinese (Baelum et al. 1988b) adult population to conform with the methods of examination and data presentation utilized in each of six other surveys (from Japan (Yoneyama et al. 1988); Norway (Löe et al. 1978); New Mexico (Ismail et al. 1987); Sri Lanka (Löe et al. 1978); and two South Pacific islands (Cutress et al. 1982)). Among the samples included in this analysis, only the Sri Lankan and the South Pacific subjects appeared to suffer a severe periodontal tissue breakdown, while the distribution of advanced disease was strikingly similar in six out of the eight samples, despite marked differences in oral hygiene conditions. Hence, the data failed to corroborate the traditional generalization that the prevalence and severity of periodontitis is markedly increased in African and Asian populations. On the other hand, data from the Third National Health and Nutrition Study (NHANES III; Albandar et al. 1999) which examined a large nationally representative, stratified, multistage probability sample in the USA clearly showed that the prevalence of deep pockets and advanced attachment loss was more pronounced in non-Hispanic black people and Hispanics than in non-Hispanic white subjects. This observation was consistent even when several alternative thresholds defining advanced disease were employed. Thus, current evidence suggests that the prevalence of severe periodontitis is not uniformly distributed among various races, ethnicities, or socioeconomic groups (Hobdell 2001).

Table 7-2 summarizes a number of prevalence studies of periodontal disease in elderly subjects. In five studies (Beck et al. 1990; Hunt et al. 1990; Gilbert & Heft 1992; Locker & Leake 1993; Weyant et al. 1993) data on attachment loss have been used to calculate extent and severity index scores (ESI) which appear to be relatively consistent between the surveys. It is evident that attachment loss of moderate magnitude was frequent and widespread in these subject samples; however, severe disease was again found to affect relatively limited proportions of the samples and generally only a limited proportion of teeth per subject. Similar findings were reported in more recent studies carried out in Iowa, USA (Levy et al. 2003), Pomerania, Germany (Mack et al. 2004), Japan (Hirotomi et al. 2002), and Sweden (Holm-Pedersen et al. 2006). Interestingly, a significant relationship was reported between advanced periodontitis and other co-morbidities in both institutionalized (Maupome et al. 2003) and home-dwelling elderly individuals (Ajwani et al. 2003).

The limitations of the findings from studies using the CPITN system were discussed above. However, a substantial part of the available information from the developing countries has been collected by the use of this index. An article providing a summary of almost 100 CPITN surveys from more than 50 countries performed over the period 1981–89 for the age

Table 7-1 Selected prevalence studies of periodontitis in adults

Authors/country	Sample/methodology	Findings
Löe et al. (1978) Norway/Sri Lanka	Two samples, one comprising 565 Norwegian students and academicians and the other 480 Sri Lankan tea laborers, of ages 16–30+ yrs; assessments of plaque, gingivitis, calculus, PD and AL at the mesial and facial aspects of all teeth	Norwegian group: excellent oral hygiene, negligible amounts of plaque and gingivitis, virtually no deep pockets and minimal attachment loss; mean AL at the age of 30 < 1 mm. Sri Lankan group: poor oral hygiene, abundant plaque and calculus, attachment loss present at the age of 16, increasing with age; mean AL at the age of 30 ≈ 3 mm, a substantial number of teeth with AL of > 10 mm
Baelum et al. (1988a) Kenya	A stratified random sample of 1131 subjects, 15–65 yrs; full-mouth assessments of tooth mobility, plaque, calculus, bleeding on probing (BoP), PD and AL	Plaque in 75–95% and calculus in 10–85% of all surfaces; PD ≥ 4 mm in < 20% of the sites; AL of ≥ 1 mm in 10–85% of the sites; the percentage of sites/subject with PD or AL of ≥ 4 mm or ≥ 7 mm conspicuously skewed
Yoneyama et al. (1988) Japan	A random sample of 319 subjects, 20–79 years old; full-mouth probing assessments of PD, AL, and gingival recession	0.2% of the sites in subjects 30–39 years and 1.2% of the sites in subjects 70–79 years had a PD of > 6 mm; AL > 5 mm affected 1% of the sites in the youngest group and 12.4% of the sites in the oldest group; skewed distribution of advanced AL; advanced disease more prevalent and widespread in older ages
Brown et al. (1990) USA	A sample of 15 132 subjects, stratified by geographic region, representing 100 million employed adults aged 18–64 years; probing assessments at mesial and buccal sites in one upper and one lower quadrant; mesial assessments performed from the buccal aspect of the teeth; assessments of gingivitis, PD, AL, and gingival recession	44% of all subjects had gingivitis at an average of 2.7 sites/subject and at < 6% of all sites assessed; pockets 4–6 mm were observed in 13.4% of the subjects at an average of 0.6 sites/person and at 1.3% of all sites assessed; corresponding figures for pockets ≥ 7 mm were 0.6%, 0.01 and 0.03%; AL ≥ 3 mm was prevalent in 44% of the subjects (increasing with age from 16% to 80%) affecting an average of 3.4 sites/subject; corresponding figures for AL ≥ 5 mm were 13% (2–35%) and 0.7 sites/subject
Salonen et al. (1991) Sweden	A random sample of 732 subjects, 20–80+ yrs, representing 0.8% of the population a southern geographic region; full-mouth radiographic examination; alveolar bone level expressed as a percentage of the root length (B/R ratio); B/R of ≥ 80% represents intact periodontal bone support	Age group of 20–29 yrs: 38% of the subjects had no sites with B/R < 80% and 8% of the subjects had five or more sites below this threshold; corresponding figures for the age group 50–59 years were 5% and 75%; after the age of 40, women displayed more favorable B/R ratios than men
Hugoson et al. (1998a) Sweden	Three random samples of 600, 597, and 584 subjects aged 20–70 years, examined in 1973, 1983, and 1993, respectively; full-mouth clinical and radiographic examination; based on clinical and radiographic findings, the subjects were classified according to severity of periodontal disease in five groups, where group 1 included subjects with close to faultless periodontal tissues and group 5 subjects with severe disease	Edentulism decreased over the 20-year period from 11% to 8% to 5%; percentage distribution of the subjects in the five groups in 1973, 1983, and 1993 respectively, was as follows: G1: 8%/23%/22%, G2: 41%/22%/38%, G3: 47%/41%/27%, G4: 2%/11%/10%, G5: 1%/2%/3%; the increase in the prevalence of subjects with severe disease was apparently due to increase of dentate subjects in older ages
Albandar et al. (1999) USA	A nationally representative, multi-stage probability sample comprising 9689 subjects, 30–90 years old (NHANES III study); probing assessments at mesial and buccal sites in one upper and one lower quadrant; mesial assessments performed from the buccal aspect of the teeth; assessments of gingivitis, PD, and location of the gingival margin in relation to the CEJ	Pockets ≥ 5 mm were found in 8.9% of all subjects (7.6% in non-Hispanic white subjects, 18.4% in non-Hispanic black subjects, and 14.4% in Mexican Americans); AL ≥ 5 mm occurred in 19.9% of all subjects (19.9% in non-Hispanic white subjects, 27.9% in non-Hispanic black subjects, and 28.34% in Mexican Americans)
Schürch & Lang (2004) Switzerland	A total of 1318 subjects, randomly selected based on community rosters in seven regions, aged 20–89 years; probing assessments of PD and AL at all present teeth; assessments of plaque and gingivitis at index teeth	7.1% of the subjects were edentulous; the mean number of present teeth in dentate subjects was 21.6; mean values of probing depth reached a plateau of 3 mm in the age of 49 years; however, but attachment levels increased dramatically after the age of 50 years and paralleled a marked loss of teeth
Susin et al. (2004a) Brazil	A sample of 853 dentate individuals, selected by multi-stage probability sampling, aged 30–103 years; full-mouth examination of AL at six sites per tooth	Moderate AL (≥ 5 mm) and advanced AL (≥ 7 mm) occurred in 70% and 52% of the subjects, affecting an average of 36% and 16% of their teeth, respectively; in comparison to 30–39-year-olds, 40–49-year-olds had three-fold increased risk for moderate and 7.4-fold increased risk for advanced AL; corresponding figures for ≥ 50 year olds were 5.9-fold and 25.4-fold, respectively

PD = probing depth; AL = attachment level; CEJ = cemento-enamel junction.

Table 7-2 Selected prevalence studies of periodontitis in elderly subjects

Authors/country	Sample/methodology	Findings
Baelum et al. (1988b) China	544 persons, aged 60+, from two urban and one rural area of Beijing area; assessments of plaque, calculus, gingivitis, loss of attachment, pocket depth, and tooth mobility	0–29% edentulous; mean number of teeth 6.9–23.9, depending on age and sex; ≈ 50% of all surfaces with plaque and calculus; 50% of all sites with AL of ≥ 4 mm, < 15% with PD ≥ 4 mm; conspicuously skewed percentage of sites/person with AL of ≥ 7 mm and PD ≥ 4 mm
Locker & Leake (1993) Canada	907 subjects, aged 50–75+ years, living independently in four communities; probing assessments at mesio-buccal and mid-buccal aspects of all teeth; mid-palatal and mesio-palatal probing assessments in upper molars; 23% of the subjects edentulous; calculation of extent and severity index (ESI) with AL threshold set at ≥ 2 mm; "severe disease": more than four sites with AL ≥ 5 mm and PD ≥ 4 mm at one or more of those sites	59% of the subjects with PD of ≥ 4 mm, 16% with ≥ 6 mm and 3% with ≥ 8 mm; 86% of the subjects with AL of ≥ 4 mm, 42% with ≥ 6 mm and 16% with ≥ 8 mm; 20% of the subjects with a mean AL of ≥ 4 mm; severe disease at 22% of the subjects; mean ESI: 77, 2.44
Beck et al. (1990) USA	690 community-dwelling adults, age 65+; probing assessments at mesio- and mid-buccal surfaces, all teeth; "advanced disease": four or more sites with AL of ≥ 5 mm and one or more of these sites with PD of ≥ 4 mm	Mean ESI in black people: 78, 4; in white people: 65, 3.1; advanced disease in 46% of the black people and 16% of the white people
Gilbert & Heft (1992) USA	671 dentate subjects, 65–97 years old, attending senior activity centers; probing assessments at mesial and buccal surfaces of one upper and one lower quadrant; questionnaire data; calculation of ESI	An average of 17.0 teeth/subject; 50.7% of the subjects with most severe mesial pocket of 4–6 mm and 3.4% with pockets ≥ 7 mm; 61.6% with most severe AL of 4.6 mm and 24.2% with AL of ≥ 7 mm; ESI increased with age: 84.8, 3.6 (65–69 years); 88.7, 3.8 (75–79 years); 91.2, 3.9 (85+ years)
Douglass et al. (1993) USA	1151 community-dwelling elders, age 70+ yrs; probing assessments at three or more sites/tooth, all teeth; 57% of the sample female, predominantly white (95%); 37.6% edentulous; mean no. of teeth present between 21.5 and 17.9, depending on age	85% of the subjects with BOP; 66% with 4–6 mm deep pockets affecting an average of 5.3 teeth/subject; 21% with pockets of > 6 mm affecting an average of 2.2 teeth; 39% with AL of 4–6 mm at 6.7 sites/subject and 56% AL of > 6 mm at 2.7 teeth/subject
Kiyak et al. (1993) USA	1063 residents in 31 nursing homes, 72–98 years old; visual inspection of the oral cavity; periodontal status assessed indirectly through registration of intraoral swelling or suppuration, sore or bleeding gums, increased tooth mobility, and poor oral hygiene	42% of the subjects with remaining natural teeth; 43% of those with sore or bleeding gums, 18% with significant tooth mobility, 6% with intraoral swelling or suppuration and 72% with poor oral hygiene
Weyant et al. (1993) USA	650 long-term residents of nursing home care units, mean age 72 years; probing assessments at mesial and buccal surfaces, all teeth; demographic, oral, and general health data recorded; sample predominantly male and white; calculation of ESI scores	42% of the sample edentulous; 60% of the subjects with PD of mm at an average of 5.8 sites/person; 3.7% with PD of ≥ 6 mm at < 1 site/person; overall mean mesial ESI: 74, 2.91
Bourgeois et al. (1999) France	603 non-institutionalized elderly, 65–74 years old; stratified sample with respect to gender, place of residence and socioeconomic group; periodontal conditions assessed by means of the CPITN	16.3% of the sample edentulous; 31.5% of the subjects had pockets ≥ 4 mm; 2.3% had pockets ≥ 6 mm
Pajukoski et al. (1999) Finland	181 hospitalized patients (mean age 81.9 yrs) and 254 home-living patients (mean age 76.9 yrs); periodontal conditions assessed by means of the CPITN	66.3% of the hospitalized and 42.1% of the non-hospitalized subjects were edentulous; 26% of both the hospitalized and the non-hospitalized subjects had pockets ≥ 6 mm
Levy et al. (2003) USA	From a sample of 449 community-dwelling elders, mean age 85 years, 342 (76%) were dentate and 236 were examined with respect to PD and AL at four sites per tooth in all present teeth	91% of the subjects had one or more site with ≥ 4 mm AL, 45% had one or more site with ≥ 6 mm AL, and 15% one or more site with ≥ 8 mm AL
Mack et al. (2004) Germany	1446 randomly selected subjects aged 60–79 years; per tooth; plaque calculus and BoP were assessed at half-mouth examination of PD and AL at four sites index teeth	16% of the 60–65 year olds and 30% of the 75–79 year olds were edentulous; among 70–79 year olds, the median BoP was 37.5% in men and 50% in women, the prevalence of PD ≥ 6 mm was 31.8% and 28.5%, and the prevalence of AL ≥ 5 mm 71.9% and 66.9%, respectively

PD = probing depth; AL = attachment level; BoP = bleeding on probing; CEJ = cemento-enamel junction; ESI = Extent and Severity Index; CPITN = Community Periodontal Index of Treatment Needs.

group of 35–44 years was published by Miyazaki *et al.* (1991b). These studies indicate a huge variation in the percentage of subjects with one or several deep (≥6 mm) pockets both between and within different geographic areas. Hence, the percentage of subjects with such pockets ranged between 1 and 74% in Africa (data from 17 surveys), 8 and 22% in North and South America (4 surveys), 2 and 36% in the eastern Mediterranean (6 surveys), 2 and 40% in Europe (38 surveys), 2 and 64% in South-East Asia, and between 1 and 22% in the western Pacific area (17 surveys). The average number of sextants per subject with ≥6 mm deep pockets varied also considerably and ranged between 0 and 2.1 in Africa, 0.1 and 0.4 in America, 0.1 and 0.6 in the eastern Mediterranean, 0.1 and 0.8 in Europe, 0.1 and 2.1 in South-East Asia and between 0 and 0.4 in the western Pacific area. However, it is difficult to assess the extent at which these values reflect true differences in the periodontal conditions given the methodological limitations of the CPITN system.

Periodontal disease in children and adolescents

The form of periodontal disease that affects the *primary* dentition, the condition formerly termed *prepubertal periodontitis*, has been reported to appear in both a generalized and a localized form (Page *et al.* 1983). Information about this disease was mainly provided by clinical case reports and no data related to the prevalence and the distribution of the disease in the general population are available. However, a few studies involving samples of children have provided limited data on the frequency with which deciduous teeth may be affected by loss of periodontal tissue support. The criteria used in these studies are by no means uniform, hence the prevalence data vary significantly. In an early study, Jamison (1963) examined by the use of the Periodontal Disease Index the "prevalence of destructive periodontal disease" (indicated by PDI scores >3) in a sample of 159 children in Michigan, USA and reported figures of 27% for 5–7-year-old children, 25% for 8–10-year-olds and 21% for 11–14-year-olds. Shlossman *et al.* (1986) used an attachment level value of ≥2 mm as a cut-off point and reported a prevalence of 7.7% in 5–9-year-olds and 6.1% in 10–14-year-olds in a sample of Pima Indians. Sweeney *et al.* (1987) examined radiographs obtained from 2264 children, aged 5–11 years, who were referred to a University Clinic for routine dental treatment and reported that a distinct radiographic bone loss was evident at one or more primary molars in 19 children (0.8%), 16 of whom were black, 2 Caucasian and 1 Asian.

In contrast, relatively uniform criteria have been used in epidemiologic studies of *aggressive periodontitis* in young subjects, the condition formerly termed *juvenile periodontitis* (JP), and particularly the *localized* form, formerly termed *localized juvenile periodontitis*

(LJP). Typically, a two-stage approach has been adopted in these studies: first, bite-wing radiographs are used to screen for bone lesions adjacent to molars and incisors and then a clinical examination is performed to verify the diagnosis. As illustrated by the data in Table 7-3, the prevalence of localized aggressive periodontitis (LAP) varies in geographically and/or racially different populations. In Caucasians, the disease appears to affect females more frequently than males and the prevalence is low (approximately 0.1%). In other races, and in particular in black subjects, the disease is more prevalent, probably at levels over 1%, and the sex ratio appears to be reversed, since males are affected more frequently than females. Smoking and low socioeconomic status have been confirmed to be associated with aggressive periodontitis in various populations (Lopez *et al.* 2001; Susin & Albandar 2005; Levin *et al.* 2006).

Epidemiological studies of periodontal conditions in adolescents have been also carried out by means of the CPITN system. Miyazaki *et al.* (1991a) presented an overview of 103 CPITN surveys of subjects aged 15–19 years from over 60 countries. The most frequent finding in these groups was the presence of calculus which was much more prevalent in subjects from non-industrialized than industrialized countries. Probing pocket depths of 4–5 mm were present in about two thirds of the populations examined. However, deep pockets (≥6 mm) were relatively infrequent: score 4 quadrants were reported to occur in only ten of the examined populations (in 4 out of 9 examined American samples, 1 out of 16 African, 1 out of 10 eastern Mediterranean, 2 out of 35 European, 2 out of 15 South-East Asian and in none out of 18 western Pacific samples).

The progression pattern of periodontitis in a sample of 167 adolescents in the UK was studied in a 5-year longitudinal study by Clerehugh *et al.* (1990). In this study, 3% of the initially 14-year-olds had loss of attachment of ≥1 mm affecting <1% of their sites. However, at age 19 years, 77% showed a similar level of attachment loss and 31% of their sites were affected. Presence of subgingival calculus at baseline was significantly linked to disease progression. In a study involving a larger sample size in the US, Brown *et al.* (1996) studied a nationally representative sample comprising 14 013 adolescents with respect to the pattern of progression of the disease entity formerly termed *early-onset periodontitis*, i.e. the kind of periodontitis that occurs in individuals of a young age. Subjects were diagnosed at baseline as free from periodontitis, or suffering from localized aggressive periodontitis (LAP), generalized aggressive periodontitis (GAP), or incidental attachment loss (IAL). Of the individuals diagnosed with localized aggressive periodontitis at baseline, 62% continued to display localized periodontitis lesions 6 years later, but 35% developed a generalized disease pattern. Among the group initially diagnosed as suffering

Table 7-3 Selected prevalence studies of localized and generalized aggressive periodontitis (LAP and GAP) in adolescents and young adults

Authors/country	Sample/methodology	Findings
Saxén (1980) Finland	A random sample of 8096 16-year olds; radiographic and clinical criteria (bone loss adjacent to first molars without any obvious iatrogenic factors and presence of pathologic pockets)	Prevalence of LAP 0.1% (eight subjects, five of which were females)
Kronauer et al. (1986) Switzerland	A representative sample of 7604 16-year olds; two-step examination (radiographic detection of bone lesion on bite-wing radiographs, clinical verification of presence of pathological pockets)	Prevalence of LAP of 0.1%; 1 : 1 sex ratio
Saxby (1987) UK	A sample of 7266 schoolchildren; initial screening by probing assessments around incisors and first molars; LAP cases diagnosed definitively by full-mouth clinical and radiographic examination	Overall prevalence of LAP of 0.1%, 1 : 1 sex ratio; however, prevalence varied in different ethnic groups (0.02% in Caucasians, 0.2% in Asians and 0.8% in Afro-Caribbeans)
Neely (1992) USA	1038 schoolchildren 10–12 years old, volunteers in a dentifrice trial; three-stage examination including radiographic and clinical assessments; bite-wing radiographs screened for possible cases; bone loss measurements of the CEJ–bone crest distance of ≥ 2 mm used to identify probable cases; LAP diagnosed clinically as PD of ≥ 3 mm at one or more first permanent molars in absence of local irritants	117 possible and 103 probable cases identified in step 1 and 2, respectively; out of 99 probable cases contacted, 43 were examined clinically; two cases of LAP could be confirmed in stage 3, yielding a prevalence rate of 0.46%
Cogen et al. (1992) USA	4757 children, age < 15 yrs, from the pool of a children's hospital; retrospective radiographic examination of two sets of bite-wings; LAP diagnosed in case of arc-shaped alveolar bone loss in molars and/or incisors	White people: LAP prevalence 0.3%, female:male ratio 4 : 1; black people: LAP prevalence 1.5%, female : male ratio ≈ 1 : 1; among black LAP cases with available radiographs from earlier examinations, 85.7% showed evidence of bone loss in the mixed dentition and 71.4% in the deciduous dentition
Löe & Brown (1991) USA	National Survey of US children, multi-stage probability sampling representing 45 million schoolchildren; 40 694 subjects, 14–17 years old examined; probing assessments at mesial and buccal sites, all teeth; LAP: ≥ 1 first molar and ≥ 1 incisor or second molar and ≤ 2 cuspids or premolars with ≥ 3 mm AL; GAP: if LAP criteria not met and four or more teeth (of which two or more were second molars, cuspids or premolars) with ≥ 3 mm attachment loss (AL); incidental loss of attachment (ILA): if neither LAP nor GAP criteria met but one or more teeth with ≥ 3 mm AL; bivariate and multi-variate analysis	Population estimates: LAP 0.53%; GAP 0.13%; ILA 1.61%; altogether 2.27% representing almost 300 000 adolescents; black people at much higher risk for all forms of early-onset disease than whites; males more likely (4.3 : 1) to have GAP than females, after adjusting for other variables; black males 2.9 times as likely to have LAP than black females; white females more likely to have LAP than white males by the same odds
Bhat (1991) USA	A sample of 11 111 schoolchildren, 14–17 years old; probing assessments at mesial and buccal surfaces of all teeth; multi-stage cluster sampling stratified by age, sex, seven geographic regions, and rural or urban residence; not stratified by race or ethnicity	22% of the children with one or more site with AL of ≥ 2 mm, 0.72% of ≥ 4 mm and 0.04% of ≥ 6 mm; supra- and subgingival calculus in 34% and 23% of the children, respectively
van der Velden et al. (1989) The Netherlands	4565 subjects 14–17 years old examined; randomization among high school students; probing assessments at the mesio- and distofacial surfaces of first molars and incisors; one bacterial sample from the dorsum of the tongue and one subgingival plaque sample from the site with maximal attachment loss obtained from 103 out of the 230 subjects with AL and cultured for identification of A. actinomycetemcomitans	Overall, AL occurred in 5% of the sample and was more frequent in males; 16 subjects (0.3%) had one or more site with AL of 5–8 mm; female : male ratio in this group 1.3 : 1; A. actinomycetemcomitans was identified in 17% of the sampled subjects with AL
Lopez et al. (1991) Chile	2500 schoolchildren in Santiago (1318 male, 1182 female), 15–19 years of age; clinical and radiographic assessments; three stage screening: (1) clinical assessments of probing depth at incisors and molars, (2) children with two or more teeth with PD of ≥ 5.5 mm subjected to a limited radiographic	After screening, 27 subjects had a tentative diagnosis of LAP out of which eight were confirmed (seven female, one male); overall prevalence of LAP 0.32%, 95% confidence limits between 0.22% and 0.42%; LAP significantly more frequent in the low socioeconomic group

(Continued)

Table 7-3 *Continued*

Authors/country	Sample/methodology	Findings
	examination, and (3) children with alveolar bone loss of ≥ 2 mm invited for a full-mouth clinical and radiographic examination	
Ben Yehouda et al. (1991) Israel	1160 male Israeli army recruits, aged 18–19 years; panoramic radiography; juvenile periodontitis diagnosed on the basis of bone loss involving ≥ 30% of the root length adjacent to first molars or incisors	Ten recruits (0.86%, 95% CI 0.84–0.88%) had a bone loss pattern consistent with localized juvenile periodontitis
Melvin et al. (1991) USA	5013 military recruits, 17–26 years old; panoramic radiography followed by full-mouth clinical examination; diagnosis of JP if bone loss and attachment loss was greater at first molars and/or incisors than at other teeth	Overall prevalence of JP 0.76%, female : male ratio 1.1 : 1; prevalence in black subjects 2.1%, female: male ratio 0.52 : 1; prevalence in white subjects 0.09%, female : male ratio 4.3 : 1
Tinoco et al. (1997) Brazil	7843 schoolchildren, 12–19 years old; two-stage screening: (1) clinical assessment of PD at first molars, (2) children with one or more tooth with PF ≥ 5 mm examined further; LAP diagnosed if a person with no systemic disease presented with AL > 2 mm at one or more sites with radiographic evidence of bone loss and one or more infrabony defects at molars/incisors	119 subjects identified at initial screening; 25 confirmed cases of LAP; overall prevalence 0.3%; ethnic origins and gender ratios not reported
Lopez et al. (2001) Chile	A random sample of 9162 high school students, 12–21 years old; probing assessments of AL at six sites per tooth at all incisors and molars	The prevalence of AL of ≥ 1 mm was 69.2%, of ≥ 2 mm was 16% and of ≥ 3 mm was 4.5%. Al was associated with higher age, female gender, poor oral hygiene, and lower socioeconomic status
Levin et al. (2006) Israel	642 army recruits (87.5% men), 18–30 years old (mean 19.6); radiographic and clinical examination of first molars and incisors	AP prevalence was 5.9% (4.3% LAP, 1.6% GAP); current smoking and north African origin were significantly related to AP

Terms used in all but Levin *et al.* (2006): "localized juvenile periodontitis" instead of "localized aggressive periodontitis" (LAP), and "generalized juvenile periodontitis" instead of "generalized aggressive periodontitis" (GAP).
PD = probing depth; AL = attachment level; CEJ = cemento-enamel junction; AP = aggressive periodontitis.

from IAL, 28% developed localized or generalized aggressive periodontitis, while 30% were reclassified in the no attachment loss group. Molars and incisors were the teeth most often affected in all three affected groups. Thus, the study indicated that these three forms of periodontitis may progress in a similar fashion, and that certain cases of localized, aggressive disease may develop into generalized aggressive periodontitis.

The possibility that *localized aggressive periodontitis* and *prepubertal periodontitis* are associated conditions, i.e. that the former is a development of the latter, has also attracted attention. In a pilot study, Sjödin *et al.* (1989) retrospectively examined radiographs of the primary dentition of 17 subjects with LAP and reported that 16 of the subjects showed a CEJ–bone crest distance of ≥3 mm in at least one tooth site of their deciduous dentition. The same research group (Sjödin & Matsson 1992) examined the CEJ–bone crest distance in radiographs from 128 periodontally healthy children aged 7–9 years, in order to define a threshold value that, if exceeded, would entail periodontal pathology around the deciduous teeth with high probability. Having set this threshold value to 2 mm, Sjödin *et al.* (1993) examined radiographs of

the deciduous dentition retrospectively from 118 patients with aggressive periodontitis and 168 age- and gender-matched periodontally healthy controls. The patients were divided in two groups, one comprising subjects with only one affected site (45 subjects) and another (73 subjects) including subjects with 2–15 sites with bone loss in their permanent dentition. It was found that 52% of the subjects in the latter group, 20% of the subjects in the former group and only 5% of the controls exhibited at least one site with bone loss in their primary dentition. The authors concluded that, at least in some young subjects with aggressive periodontitis, the onset of the disease may be manifested in the primary dentition. Similar results were reported by Cogen *et al.* (1992), from a study in the US. Among systemically healthy young black people with aggressive periodontitis and available radiographs of the primary dentition, 71% showed alveolar bone loss adjacent to one or several primary teeth. Finally, an interesting recent radiographic study of the mixed dentition in Australian children aged 5–12 years was carried out by Darby *et al.* (2005). These authors investigated the prevalence of alveolar bone loss around first permanent molars, and first and second deciduous molars. Based on radiographs of 542 children, 13.0% were found to display definite bone loss, i.e. bone levels >3.0 mm from the CEJ. Half of all lesions with definite bone loss occurred at the second deciduous molars and, in the vast majority, at distal tooth surfaces. In other words, this study showed that the tooth surface of the deciduous dentition most frequently affected by bone loss was the one in close proximity with the most frequent localization of aggressive periodontitis in young age groups, i.e. the mesial surface of the first permanent molar.

Periodontitis and tooth loss

Tooth loss may be the ultimate consequence of destructive periodontal disease. Teeth lost due to the sequels of the disease are obviously not amenable to registration in epidemiological surveys and may, hence, lead to an underestimation of the prevalence and the severity of the disease. The well established epidemiologic concept of *selection bias* (also referred to as the *healthy survivor effect*, indicating that the comparatively healthier subjects will present for an examination while the more severely affected may refuse participation or fail to present because of the morbidity itself) is in this context applicable on the individual tooth level, since the severely affected teeth may have already been extracted/lost. Aspects related to tooth loss on a population basis have been addressed in numerous publications. Important questions that were analyzed included: (1) the relative contribution of periodontitis as a reason underlying tooth extractions in subjects retaining a natural dentition (Cahen *et al.* 1985; Bailit *et al.* 1987; Brown *et al.* 1989; Corbet & Davies 1991; Heft & Gilbert 1991; Klock & Haugejorden 1991; MacDonald Jankowski 1991; Stephens *et al.* 1991; Reich & Hiller 1993; McCaul *et al.* 2001); (2) its role in cases of full-mouth extractions, the so-called *total tooth clearance* (Eklund & Burt 1994; Takala *et al.* 1994), and (3) risk factors for tooth loss (Burt *et al.* 1990; Phipps *et al.* 1991; Krall *et al.* 1994; Drake *et al.* 1995; Hunt *et al.* 1995; Warren *et al.* 2002; Copeland *et al.* 2004; Neely *et al.* 2005; Susin *et al.* 2005b).

Typically, surveys addressing the first topic have utilized questionnaire data obtained from general practitioners instructed to document the reasons for which teeth were extracted over a certain time period. The results indicate that the reason underlying the vast majority of extractions in ages up to 40–45 years is dental caries. However, in older age cohorts, periodontal disease becomes about equally responsible for tooth loss. Overall, periodontitis is thought to account for 30–35% of all tooth extractions while caries and its sequelae for up to 50%. In addition, caries appears to be the principal reason for extractions in cases of total tooth clearance. Finally, identified risk factors for tooth loss include smoking, perceived poor dental health, sociobehavioral traits, and poor periodontal status.

Obviously, it is not feasible to "translate" tooth loss data into prevalence figures of periodontal disease. An evaluation, however, of the periodontal status on a population level, and in particular in older age cohorts, must weigh in information provided by tooth loss data, otherwise underestimation of the occurrence and the sequels of the disease is inevitable (Gilbert *et al.* 2005).

Risk factors for periodontitis

Introduction – definitions

There is an abundance of both empirical evidence and substantial theoretical justification for accepting the widespread belief that many diseases have more than one cause, i.e. that they are of *multi-factorial etiology* (Kleinbaum *et al.* 1982). Consequently, in any particular instance when a *causal relationship* is investigated, the specificity of the relation between exposure to an etiologic agent and effect, i.e. the *necessity* or the *sufficiency* of the condition, may be challenged. In the case of most infectious diseases for example, it is known that the presence of the microbial agent (which we define as the necessary condition) is not always accompanied by signs or symptoms characteristic of that disorder. Thus, the agent itself is not sufficient to cause any pathologic occurrence; rather, the disease development may be dependent on multiple, diverse additional factors, including specific host responses, toxic exposures, nutritional deficiencies, emotional stress, and the complex impact of social influences. In non-infectious diseases (except for genetic abnormalities), there is usually no factor known to be present in every single case of the disease. For example, smoking is not necessary for the development of lung cancer, and no degree of coronary atherosclerosis is a necessary condition for myocardial infarction.

The *causal inference*, i.e. the procedure of drawing conclusions related to the cause(s) of a disease, is a particularly complex issue in epidemiological research. In the 1970s, Hill (1971) formalized the criteria that have to be fulfilled in order to accept a causal relation. These included:

1. *Strength of the association.* The stronger the association is between the potential (*putative*) risk factor and disease presence, the more likely it is that the anticipated causal relation is valid.
2. *Dose–response effect.* An observation that the frequency of the disease increases with the dose or level of exposure to a certain factor supports a causal interpretation.
3. *Temporal consistency.* It is important to establish that the exposure to the anticipated causative factor occurred prior to the onset of the disease. This may be difficult in case of diseases with long latent periods or factors that change over time.

4. *Consistency of the findings.* If several studies investigating a given relationship generate similar results, the causal interpretation is strengthened.
5. *Biological plausibility.* It is advantageous if the anticipated relationship makes sense in the context of current biological knowledge. However, it must be realized that the less that is known about the etiology of a given disease, the more difficult it becomes to satisfy this particular criterion.
6. *Specificity of the association.* If the factor under investigation is found to be associated with only one disease, or if the disease is found to be associated with only one factor among a multitude of factors tested, the causal relation is strengthened. However, this criterion can by no means be used to reject a causal relation, since many factors have multiple effects and most diseases have multiple causes.

It is important to realize that the criteria described above are meant as guidelines when a causal inference is established. None of them, however, is either necessary or sufficient for a causal interpretation. Strict adherence to any of them without concomitant consideration of the other may result in incorrect conclusions.

A distinction has to be drawn between a *causal* factor, assessed as above, and a *risk* factor. In a broad sense, the term risk factor may indicate an aspect of personal behavior or life-style, an environmental exposure, or an inborn or inherited characteristic which, on the basis of epidemiologic evidence, is known to be associated with disease-related conditions. Such an attribute or exposure may be associated with an increased probability of occurrence of a particular disease without necessarily being a causal factor. A risk factor may be modified by intervention, thereby reducing the likelihood that the particular disease will occur.

The principles of the *risk assessment process* were discussed by Beck (1994) and should consist of the following four steps:

1. The *identification* of one or several individual factors that appear to be associated with the disease.
2. In case of multiple factors, a *multi-variate risk assessment model* must be developed that discloses which combination of factors does most effectively discriminate between health and disease.
3. The *assessment* step, in which new populations are screened for this particular combination of factors, with a subsequent comparison of the level of the disease assessed with the one predicted by the model.
4. The *targeting* step, in which exposure to the identified factors is modified by prevention or intervention and the effectiveness of the approach in suppressing the *incidence* of the disease is evaluated.

Thus, according to this process, *potential* or *putative risk factors* (often also referred to as *risk indicators*) are first identified and thereafter tested until their significance as *true risk factors* is proven.

Finally, distinction must be made between *prognostic* factors (or *disease predictors*), i.e. characteristics related to the progression of *pre-existing* disease and *true risk factors*, i.e. exposures related to the *onset* of the disease. For example, it is established in longitudinal studies of periodontal disease (Papapanou *et al.* 1989), that the amount of alveolar bone loss or the number of teeth present at baseline may be used to predict further progression of the disease. These variables are, in fact, alternative measures of the disease itself and express the level of susceptibility of a given subject to periodontal disease. Although they may be excellent predictors for further disease progression, they clearly cannot be considered as risk factors.

There are several ways to study the relation between exposure to a certain factor and the occurrence of a particular disease, as required under point 1. One of these is described in Fig. 7-3 which illustrates a hypothetical situation where exposure to the potential risk factor Z is studied in a cross-sectional

	Exposed	Non-exposed	
Diseased	155	25	180
Healthy	340	480	820
	495	505	1000

Fig. 7-3 Contingency table describing the distribution of a group of 1000 subjects according to exposure to a particular factor and disease status.

study including a sample of 1000 subjects, 180 of whom are found to suffer from the disease D ("diseased") while 820 are disease-free ("healthy"). In this particular setting, it was observed that 155 out of the 180 diseased subjects had been exposed to factor Z but this was also the case for 340 non-diseased subjects. The association between exposure and disease may, in this example, be expressed by the *odds ratio* (OR), which is the ratio of exposure among the diseased and the healthy. For the data in Fig. 7-3, the odds ratio is calculated as (155/25) over (340/480) = (155×480) / (340×25) = 8.75. This indicates that the diseased were 8.75 times more likely to have been exposed to factor Z than the healthy. Note that the OR is frequently misinterpreted to describe the risk of an exposed subject to develop disease, something that is correctly assessed in a prospective cohort rather than a cross-sectional study and is described by the *relative risk*. In the example of Fig. 7-3, if a sample of 495 subjects exposed to factor Z and 505 subjects not exposed to factor Z are prospectively followed over a given time period, and 155 among the exposed and 25 among the non-exposed develop disease D over this period, then the relative risk is calculated as (155/495) over (25/505) = 6.4. In other words, an individual exposed to factor Z is 6.4 times more likely to develop disease D than a non-exposed subject.

In a study of the association between exposure to a risk factor and the occurrence of disease, *confounding* can occur when an additional factor associated with the disease is unevenly distributed among the groups under investigation. For instance, in a study between radon exposure and a form of cancer, smoking may act as a confounder, if the smoking habits of the subjects exposed to radon are different from those of the subjects not exposed.

There are various ways to assess simultaneously the effect of several putative risk factors identified in step 1 and generate the multi-variate model required for step 2. For example, the association between exposure and disease may, for reasons of simplicity, have the form of the following linear equation:

$$y = a + b_1x_1 + b_2x_2 + b_3x_3 + \ldots b_nx_n$$

where y represents occurrence or severity of the disease, a is the intercept (a constant value), x_1, x_2, ... x_n describe the different exposures (putative risk factors), and b_1, b_2, ... b_n are *estimates* defining the relative importance of each individual exposure as determinant of disease, after taking all other factors into account. Such an approach may identify factors with statistically and biologically significant effect and may eliminate the effect of confounders.

In the third step (assessment step), a new population sample that it is independent of the one used in the construction of the multi-variate model is screened for occurrence of disease and presence of the relevant factors included in the multi-variate model of step 2. Alternatively, in the case of a prospective cohort study, exposure to the relevant factors is assessed among the subjects of the new sample, and disease incidence, i.e. the number of new cases of disease, is determined over a time period after a longitudinal follow-up of the subjects. Subsequently, disease predicted by means of the model is compared to the actually observed disease, and the *external validity* of the model (i.e., the "behavior" or "fitness" of the model in the new population) is evaluated.

Lastly, during the targeting step, aspects of causality or risk are verified if disease occurrence is suppressed when exposure is impeded. Ideally, such studies should be designed as randomized clinical trials, in which treatment is randomly assigned in one of two groups and the effectiveness of the intervention is assessed in direct comparison to outcomes in an untreated, control group. Additionally, an evaluation of the particular preventive/therapeutic strategy from a "cost–benefit" point of view is also facilitated in such studies.

In the context of periodontitis, it should be realized that few of the putative risk factors for disease development have been subjected to the scrutiny of all four steps. In fact, risk assessment studies in dental research in general have been frequently confined to the first two steps. Numerous cross-sectional studies identifying potential factors are available, but a relatively limited number of longitudinal studies has involved a multi-variate approach in the identification of exposures of interest while simultaneously controlling for the effect of possible confounders. Intervention studies in the form of randomized clinical trials are sparse. In the following text, the issue of risk factors is addressed according to the principles described above. Results from cross-sectional studies are considered to provide evidence for putative risk factors that may be further enhanced if corroborated by longitudinal studies involving multi-variate techniques, or prospective intervention studies. As reviewed by Borrell and Papapanou (2005), distinction is also made between putative factors that are not amenable to intervention (non-modifiable background factors) and modifiable factors (environmental, acquired, and behavioral).

Non-modifiable background factors

Age

The relationship between age and periodontitis is complex. Early evidence demonstrates that both the prevalence and severity of periodontitis increase with older age, suggesting that age may be a marker for periodontal tissue support loss (van der Velden 1984, 1991; Johnson 1989; Johnson *et al.* 1989; Burt 1994). However, the concept of periodontitis as an inevitable consequence of ageing has been challenged over the years and the alleged 'age effect' likely represents the cumulative effect of prolonged exposure to true risk factors (Papapanou *et al.* 1991). Notably, the association between age and periodontitis appears to be different for pocket depth and clinical attachment loss. While there is a pronounced effect of increasing attachment loss with age, the effect on pocket depth appears to be minimal (Albandar 2002a,b). Interestingly, the effect of age on attachment loss is reduced after adjustment for covariates, such as oral hygiene levels or access to dental care services (Albandar 2002a). However, studies have often failed to adjust for important covariates such as presence of systemic diseases, consumption of multiple medications, and co-morbidities related to nutritional disturbances in the older population. It is therefore difficult to rule out the possibility of an age-related, as opposed to an age-dependent, increased susceptibility to periodontitis in older people.

Gender

There is no established, inherent difference between men and women in their susceptibility to periodontitis, although men have been shown to exhibit worse periodontal health than women in multiple studies from different populations (Okamoto *et al.* 1988; Brown *et al.* 1989; Hugoson *et al.* 1992; Albandar 2002a; Susin *et al.* 2004a). This difference has been traditionally considered to be a reflection of better oral hygiene practices (Hugoson *et al.* 1998b; Christensen *et al.* 2003) and/or increased utilization of oral health care services among women (Yu *et al.* 2001; Dunlop *et al.* 2002; Roberts-Thomson & Stewart 2003). On the other hand, periodontitis is a bacterial infection determined to a large extent by the host immuno-inflammatory response to the bacterial challenge. Although gender-specific differences in these responses have not been unequivocally demonstrated, it is biologically plausible that such differences may in fact exist.

Race/ethnicity

Differences in the prevalence of periodontitis between countries and across continents have been demonstrated (Baelum *et al.* 1996; Albandar 2002a), but no consistent patterns across racial/ethnic groups have been documented when covariates such as age and oral hygiene are accounted for (Burt & Eklund 1999). National surveys in the USA consistently show a racial/ethnic differential pattern in the prevalence of periodontitis, with African Americans exhibiting the highest prevalence of periodontitis followed by Mexican Americans and non-Hispanic white people, and these findings are fairly consistent regardless of the case-definition used (Albandar *et al.* 1999; Arbes *et al.* 2001; Borrell *et al.* 2002; Hyman & Reid 2003). However, race/ethnicity is usually a social construct that determines an array of opportunities related to access, status and resources (Williams 1997, 1999). As a result, race/ethnicity and socioeconomic status (SES) are strongly intertwined, suggesting that the observed racial/ethnic effect may be partially attrib-

uted to confounding by SES due to the unequal meaning of SES indicators across racial/ethnic groups (Williams 1996; Kaufman *et al.* 1997; Krieger *et al.* 1997; Lynch & Kaplan 2000). Corroborating this point, a recent study found that African Americans demonstrated a lower benefit from education and income on periodontal health status than their Mexican American and white peers (Borrell *et al.* 2004). Such findings confirm that socioeconomic indicators across racial/ethnic groups are not commensurable but, probably, reflect the broad implications of historic unequal opportunities among certain racial groups.

Gene polymorphisms

Evidence from classical twin studies (Michalowicz *et al.* 1991) suggests that genetic determinants are significant modifiers of the periodontitis phenotype (Michalowicz 1994; Hart & Kornman 1997; Schenkein 2002) but the role of single nucleotide polymorphisms remains unclear. After the seminal work by Kornman *et al.* (1997) reporting an association of a composite genotype based on specific polymorphisms in the interleukin-1 gene cluster with severe periodontitis in non-smokers, there has been an exponential increase in publications that examined a plethora of gene polymorphisms as severity markers of periodontitis. These include additional investigations of the particular IL-1 gene polymorphism in cross-sectional and case–control settings (Gore *et al.* 1998; Diehl *et al.* 1999; Armitage *et al.* 2000; Mark *et al.* 2000; McDevitt *et al.* 2000; Parkhill *et al.* 2000; Socransky *et al.* 2000; Walker *et al.* 2000; Hodge *et al.* 2001; Laine *et al.* 2001; Papapanou *et al.* 2001; Caffesse *et al.* 2002; Meisel *et al.* 2002, 2003, 2004; Anusaksathien *et al.* 2003; Gonzales *et al.* 2003; Guzman *et al.* 2003; Sakellari *et al.* 2003; Li *et al.* 2004; Quappe *et al.* 2004; Scapoli *et al.* 2005), as well as longitudinal studies (Ehmke *et al.* 1999; De Sanctis & Zucchelli 2000; Lang *et al.* 2000; Cullinan *et al.* 2001; Christgau *et al.* 2003; Jepsen *et al.* 2003). Similar work was quickly expanded to include the study of other gene polymorphisms such as the interleukin-1 receptor antagonist (Tai *et al.* 2002); interleukin-6 (Anusaksathien *et al.* 2003; Trevilatto *et al.* 2003); interleukin-10 (Kinane *et al.* 1999; Yamazaki *et al.* 2001; Gonzales *et al.* 2002; Berglundh *et al.* 2003; Scarel-Caminaga *et al.* 2004); interleukin-4 (Michel *et al.* 2001; Scarel-Caminaga *et al.* 2003; Gonzales *et al.* 2004; Pontes *et al.* 2004); interleukin-2 (Scarel-Caminaga *et al.* 2002); tumor necrosis factor (Galbraith *et al.* 1998; Endo *et al.* 2001; Shapira *et al.* 2001; Craandijk *et al.* 2002; Fassmann *et al.* 2003; Soga *et al.* 2003; Perez *et al.* 2004; Shimada *et al.* 2004); transforming growth factor-beta 1 (TGF-beta 1) (Holla *et al.* 2002b); Fc receptor of immunoglobulin G (Kobayashi *et al.* 1997, 2000a,b, 2001; Sugita *et al.* 1999, 2001; Meisel *et al.* 2001; Chung *et al.* 2003; Loos *et al.* 2003; Yasuda *et al.* 2003; Yamamoto *et al.* 2004; Wolf *et al.* 2006); CD14 receptor (Holla *et al.* 2002a); vitamin D receptor (Hennig *et al.* 1999; Tachi *et al.* 2003; de Brito Junior *et al.* 2004; Park *et al.* 2006); N-acetyltransferase 2 (Meisel *et al.* 2000; Kocher *et al.* 2002); and matrix metalloproteinase 1 and 3 (Holla *et al.* 2004; Itagaki *et al.* 2004).

Typically, the majority of the cross-sectional studies above report positive associations between the investigated polymorphisms and the extent or the severity of periodontitis. The results, however, are not unequivocal, as the strength of the reported associations is not uniformly consistent across populations, the frequency of occurrence of these polymorphisms appears to vary extensively between ethnic groups, the subject samples involved are generally of limited size, the definitions of the outcome variable (periodontitis) vary considerably, and adequate adjustments for other important covariates and risk factors have frequently not been carried out. Importantly, there appear to be differences in the impact of these polymorphisms on early-onset versus adult forms of periodontitis. For example, in the case of IL-1 polymorphisms, while it is the rare allele (allele 2) that has been linked with severe disease in adults, it is allele 1 that has been found to be more prevalent in subjects with early-onset periodontitis (Diehl *et al.* 1999; Parkhill *et al.* 2000).

The relatively few longitudinal studies that have studied specific gene polymorphisms as exposures are similarly conflicting. Ehmke *et al.* (1999) reported no bearing of the IL-1 gene polymorphism on the prognosis of periodontal disease progression following non-surgical periodontal therapy. Jepsen *et al.* (2003) failed to provide evidence that the IL-1 risk genotype was associated with higher gingival crevicular fluid (GCF) volume and percentage bleeding on probing (BoP) during the development of experimental gingivitis. In contrast, Lang *et al.* (2000) concluded that IL-1 genotype-positive subjects have a genetically determined hyper-inflammatory response that is expressed clinically in the periodontal tissues as increased prevalence and incidence of bleeding on probing during maintenance. Three treatment studies examined the impact of this particular polymorphism in regenerative therapy: De Sanctis and Zucchelli (2000) reported that the IL-1 positive genotype was associated with inferior long-term outcome of regenerative therapy of intrabony defects. In contrast, Christgau *et al.* (2003) and Weiss *et al.* (2004) failed to document such an association in similar studies of the regenerative potential of such defects. Finally, in a 5-year prospective study of 295 subjects, Cullinan *et al.* (2001) reported an interaction between the positive genotype, age, smoking and colonization by *Porphyromonas gingivalis* and concluded that the positive genotype is a contributory but non-essential factor for the progression of periodontal disease.

In conclusion, there is insufficient epidemiologic evidence that convincingly establishes any of the above polymorphisms as true risk factors for periodontitis.

Environmental, acquired, and behavioral factors

Specific microbiota

The microbial etiology of gingivitis (Löe *et al.* 1965; Theilade *et al.* 1966) and periodontitis (Lindhe *et al.* 1973) has been established for several decades. Yet, epidemiologic studies that systematically investigated the role of specific microbiota as risk factors for periodontitis were undertaken fairly recently. In a classic paper, Haffajee and Socransky (1994) adapted Koch's postulates to be used in the identification of periodontal pathogens and proposed the following criteria: (1) association, i.e. elevated odds ratios in disease; (2) elimination, i.e. conversion of disease to health when bacteria are suppressed; (3) development of a host response; (4) presence of virulence factors; (5) evidence from animal studies corroborating the observations in humans; and (6) support from risk assessment studies. Based on the above criteria, the consensus report of the 1996 World Workshop in Periodontics identified three species, *Actinobacillus actinomycetemcomitans*, *Porphyromonas gingivalis*, and *Bacteroides forsythus*, as causative factors for periodontitis (since then, two of the three causative species have been renamed: *A. actinomytemcomitans* to *Aggregatibacter actinomycetemcomitans* (Norskov-Lauritsen & Kilian 2006) and *B. forsythus* to *Tanerella forsythia* (Sakamoto *et al.* 2002; Maiden *et al.* 2003)). However, given that only approximately 50% of the bacteria of the oral cavity are currently recognized (Paster *et al.* 2001), it is clear that these three species cannot be considered to be the only causative pathogens, but are rather the ones for which sufficient data have accumulated.

Over the last decade, interesting data have emerged on the prevalence of these causative bacteria in different populations, in states of both periodontal health and disease. Studies performed in children (Tanner *et al.* 2002; Yang *et al.* 2002) that analyzed plaque from the gingival crevice, tooth surface and the dorsum of the tongue revealed that sizeable proportions of subjects harbored *P. gingivalis*, *T. forsythia*, and *A. actinomycetemcomitans* despite absence of overt gingival inflammation. A comparably high carrier state was documented in studies that sampled infants, children, adolescents and adults with good clinical periodontal status (McClellan *et al.* 1996; Könönen 1993; Kamma *et al.* 2000; Lamell *et al.* 2000). Thus, contrary to the conclusions of earlier, culture-based studies that these bacteria occur infrequently in periodontally healthy oral cavities and behave as exogenous pathogens, the above studies that have employed molecular techniques for bacterial identification demonstrate the contrary. However, both the prevalence of and the level of colonization by these pathogens have been shown to vary significantly between populations of different racial or geographic origin (Sanz *et al.* 2000; Ali *et al.* 1994; Haffajee *et al.* 2004; Lopez *et al.* 2004).

Several epidemiologic studies have examined the prevalence of the established periodontal pathogens and its relation to clinical periodontal status in population samples from both developed and developing countries. Griffen *et al.* (1998) examined a convenience sample recruited from a university clinic, and reported that 79% of the diseased and 25% of the healthy subjects were positive for *P. gingivalis*. Interestingly, the prevalence of *P. gingivalis* in the periodontally healthy group varied substantially with race/ethnicity, as it occurred in 22% of white people, 53% of African Americans, and 60% of Asian Americans. In a case–control study of periodontitis patients and age- and gender-matched controls with no or only minimal attachment loss in Sweden, Papapanou *et al.* (2000) reported a high prevalence of *P. gingivalis*, *A. actinomycetemcomitans*, *T. forsythia*, and *Treponema denticola* in periodontitis patients (95%, 83%, 97%, and 93%, respectively), but also similarly high prevalence rates among control subjects (82%, 90%, 82%, and 94%). However, in a quantitative analysis of bacterial load, substantial differences in colonization at high levels (i.e. at an average count $\geq 10^5$ bacterial cells/plaque sample) were observed between patients and controls for three of the four bacteria: 19% versus 3% for *P. gingivalis*, 54% vs. 12% for *T. forsythia*, and 46% vs. 19% for *Tr. denticola*. In contrast, corresponding percentages were similar for *A. actinomycetemcomitans* (1% in both cases and controls). Substantially different prevalence data were reported in a study of blue- and white-collar University employees in Australia (Hamlet *et al.* 2001). These authors detected *A. actinomycetemcomitans* in 23% and *P. gingivalis* in 15% of the subjects.

A number of studies investigated the epidemiology of periodontal pathogens in Asian populations. Timmerman *et al.* (1998) examined a sample of adolescents in rural Indonesia, and detected *P. gingivalis* in 87% and *A. actinomycetemcomitans* in 57% of the subjects. Mombelli *et al.* (1998) examined young factory workers in China and detected *A. actinomycetemcomitans* in 62% and *P. gingivalis* in 55% of the subjects. In contrast, an almost ubiquitous presence of *P. gingivalis* and *T. forsythia* was reported in rural subject samples in China (Papapanou *et al.* 1997) and Thailand (Papapanou *et al.* 2002), while *A. actinomycetemcomitans* was detected in 83% and 93% of the subjects in the Chinese and Thai samples, respectively. Despite this high prevalence, a quantitative analysis of bacterial load correlated well with periodontal status in both studies. For example, a discriminant analysis performed on the data from the Thai study (Papapanou *et al.* 2002) identified threshold levels of average bacterial load which, when exceeded, conferred increased odds for presence of three or more sites with pocket depth ≥ 5 mm. For three species (*P. gingivalis*, *T. forsythia*, and *Tr. denticola*), colonization above these calculated thresholds resulted in statistically significant, elevated odds for periodontitis. In addition, an analysis of the association between colonization at high levels by the "red

complex" bacteria (Socransky *et al.* 1998) and specific periodontal conditions, defined in this particular study by the presence of three or more sites with pocket depth ≥ 5 mm and by two different levels of extent of periodontal tissue loss (≥ 10 and ≥ 30 sites with ≥ 5 mm attachment loss, respectively), revealed statistically significant odds ratios ranging between 3.7 and 4.3 for the "red complex" bacteria and all three disease definitions. Similar cross-sectional associations of statistically significant odd ratios for severe periodontitis conferred by specific bacteria have been also observed in several other studies involving subject samples from the western world (Grossi *et al.* 1994, 1995; Alpagot *et al.* 1996, Craig *et al.* 2001).

Importantly, the association between high levels of colonization by specific periodontal pathogens and the progression of periodontal disease has been corroborated by longitudinal data in untreated populations. For example, in the study by Papapanou *et al.* (1997), a discriminant analysis based on quantitative assessments of subgingival bacterial load classified correctly the substantial majority of the subjects with progression of periodontitis over a preceding 10-year period. Indeed, bacterial profiles classified correctly 75% of the subjects with ten or more sites with longitudinal attachment loss of ≥ 3 mm, and 85% of those that remained stable over the observation period. In a 7-year follow-up study of Indonesian adolescents (Timmerman *et al.* 2000, 2001), and in a subsequent 15-year follow-up of the same cohort (Van der Velden *et al.* 2006), it was shown that subgingival presence of *A. actinomycetemcomitans* was associated with disease progression, defined as presence of longitudinal attachment loss of ≥ 2 mm. In a follow-up of 2–5 years' duration, Machtei *et al.* (1999) reported that subjects colonized by *T. forsythia* at baseline exhibited greater alveolar bone loss, a larger proportion of "loser" sites, and twice as high longitudinal tooth loss than non-colonized subjects. In a 3-year study, Hamlet *et al.* (2004) reported odds ratios of 8.2 for attachment loss in adolescents with persistent colonization with *T. forsythensis*.

Collectively, data generated in the past 15 years have enhanced our knowledge on the role of specific periodontal bacteria as risk factors for periodontitis (Table 7-4), but have also clarified the significance of bacterial load rather than that of mere positive colonization in conferring risk for disease progression. Obviously, the "targeting" criterion of the risk assessment process has been abundantly fulfilled in the case of microbial risk factors. Indeed, a wide body of literature data, recently compiled in systematic reviews, has demonstrated that an antimicrobial approach, including removal of subgingival plaque with or without adjunctive antiseptics or antibiotics followed by adequate maintenance care, is the single most successful and consistent strategy in the treatment of periodontitis (Heitz-Mayfield *et al.* 2002, Herrera *et al.* 2002; Hallmon & Rees 2003).

Table 7-4 Selected studies using bacteria as exposures of significance for periodontitis. (L) indicates a longitudinal study

Authors/country	Sample/methodology	Findings
Beck *et al.* (1990) USA	690 community-dwelling adults, age 65+; probing assessments at mesio- and mid-buccal surfaces, all teeth; logistic regression for advanced AL and deep pocketing; "advanced disease": four or more sites with AL of ≥ 5 mm and one or more of these sites with PD of ≥ 4 mm	Black people: 78% of their sites with attachment loss, mean AL on these sites 4 mm; white people: 65%, 3.1 mm; Odds ratios in black people: tobacco use 2.9; *Porphyromonas gingivalis* > 2% 2.4; *Pr. intermedia* > 2% 1.9; last dental visit > 3 years 2.3; bleeding gums 3.9; in white people: tobacco use 6.2; presence of *P. gingivalis* (+) 2.4; no dental visits for > 3 years plus BANA (+) 16.8
Haffajee *et al.* (1991b) USA	38 subjects, 14–71 years old, with prior evidence of attachment loss; 2-month follow-up; probing assessments at six sites/tooth, all teeth; 28 subgingival samples per subject at baseline, DNA-probe analysis with respect to 14 bacterial species; progression threshold: ≥ 3 mm of LAL; the mean percentage of the total cultivable microbiota was averaged across active and inactive sites; odds ratios computed at different thresholds for each species	Significant odds ratios for new disease: *P. gingivalis* 5.6, *Campylobacter rectus* 3.8, *Veillonella parvula* 0.16, and *Capnocytophaga ochracea* 0.08; discriminant analysis using the significantly related species was useful in predicting subjects at risk for new attachment loss
Grossi *et al.* (1994) USA	Random sample of 1426 subjects, aged 25–74 years, in a metropolitan community; full-mouth probing assessments; multi-variate analysis of risk indicators for attachment loss. Exposures: (1) clinical: supragingival plaque, gingival bleeding, subgingival calculus, PD, CAL; (2) microbial: *Aggregatibacter actinomycetemcomitans*, *Tanerella forsythia*, *C. rectus*, *Eubacterium saburreum*, *Fusobacterium nucleatum*, *P. gingivalis*, *Capnocytophaga spp* and *Pr. intermedia*; (3) co-variates: age, gender, race, education, income, smoking and numbers of packs/year, exposure to occupational hazards, systemic diseases	In a multivariable logistic regression model, *P. gingivalis* (OR 1.59, 95% CI 1.11–2.25) and *T. forsythia* (OR 2.45, 95% CI 1.87–3.24) were positively associated with severity of AL, while *Capnocytophaga* spp. (OR 0.60, 95% CI 0.43–0.84) were protective against AL
Grossi *et al.* (1995) USA	Same sample as in Grossi *et al.* (1994); 1361 subjects, aged 25–74 years; assessments of interproximal bone loss from full-mouth radiographs; the degree of association between bone loss and explanatory variables was analyzed by stepwise logistic regression	In a multivariable logistic regression model, *P. gingivalis* (OR 1.73, 95% CI 1.27–2.37) and *T. forsythia* (OR 2.52, 95% CI 1.98–3.17), were significantly associated with increasing severity of BL
Beck *et al.* (1997) USA (L)	540 dentate adults, aged 65+ years, examined at baseline, 18, 36, and 60 months; incidence of AL was defined as additional AL ≥ 3 mm; microbial variables included presence of *A. actinomycetemcomitans*, *Pr. intermedia*, and *P. gingivalis* and the BANA test; covariates included age, gender, missing teeth, education, smoking, dental visit	BANA (+), and presence of *P. gingivalis* were significantly associated with incident disease
Papapanou *et al.* (1997) China (L)	148 subjects, 30–39 and 50–59 years old in a rural area examined 10 years apart; full-mouth assessments of PD and AL at six sites per tooth; 14 subgingival plaque samples were obtained from each subject at the follow-up examination (1864 in total) and analyzed with respect to 18 bacterial species	Ubiquitous prevalence for the majority of the investigated species on the subject level. Bacterial colonization at high levels by *P. gingivalis*, *Prevotella intermedia*, *Pr. nigrescens*, *T. forsythia*, *F. nucleatum*, *Tr. denticola*, *Micromonas micros*, and *C. rectus* conferred statistically significant odds ratios for being classified as "downhill" (ten or more sites with longitudinal AL loss of ≥ 3 mm)
Machtei *et al.* (1999) USA (L)	A sample of 415 subjects, aged 25–75 years, followed for a period of 2–4 years; full-mouth examination at six sites per tooth at all teeth present; full-mouth intraoral radiographs; bacterial samples obtained from 12 index teeth analyzed with respect to: *A. actinomycetemcomitans*, *T. forsythia*, *C. rectus*, *P. intermedia*, *Capnocytophaga* species, *P. gingivalis*, *E. saburreum*, *F. nucleatum*; covariates included age, gender, smoking (current smokers 15.4%), education, income	Subjects harboring *T. forsythia* at baseline showed significantly higher longitudinal bone loss, greater proportion of "loser" sites (sites with additional AL of ≥ 2 mm) and twice as high tooth mortality

(Continued)

Table 7-4 *Continued*

Authors/country	Sample/methodology	Findings
Timmerman *et al.* (2000) Indonesia (L)	A sample 255 subjects, 15–25 year old, in a rural area, examined 7 years apart; assessments of PD and AL at vestibular surfaces of all teeth; bacterial samples harvested from a variety of intraoral sites and analyzed with respect to *A. actinomycetemcomitans*, *P. gingivalis*, *P. intermedia*, spirochetes, and motile microorganisms	Progressive disease (PDS) was defined as one or more site with longitudinal AL ≥ 2 mm; subgingival presence of *A. actinomycetemcomitans* (OR 4.2, 95% CI 1.4–12.7), *P. gingivalis* (OR 2.3, 95% CI 1.0–5.2) and motile microorganisms (OR 2.2, 95% CI 1.0–5.0) were associated with PDS; in a multivariable logistic model, including age and subgingival calculus, subgingival presence of *A. actinomycetemcomitans* (OR 4.61, p = 0.01) was associated with PDS
Papapanou *et al.* (2002) Thailand	Random sample of 356 subjects 30–39 and 50–59 years old, in a rural area; PD and CAL were assessed at six sites/tooth, at all teeth apart from third molars; subjects were grouped according to different levels of pocketing/attachment loss: subjects with three or more sites with PD ≥ 5 mm (59%, G1); ≥ 10 sites with CAL ≥ 5 mm (50%, G2); and ≥ 30 sites with CAL ≥ 5 mm (24%, G3). Subgingival plaque samples were obtained at maximally 14 sites/subject; checkerboard hybridizations were used to analyze a total of 4343 samples with respect to 27 bacterial species	Odds ratios for heavy colonization by "red complex" species (*P. gingivalis*, *T. forsythia*, *Tr. denticola*) were 3.7 (95% CI 2.3–5.9) for G1; 4.0 (95% CI 2.5–6.6) for G2; and 4.3 (95% CI 2.6–7.1) for G3. Odds ratios for heavy colonization by selected "orange complex" species (*F. nucleatum*, *Pr. intermedia*, *Pr. nigrescens*, *Pe. micros*, *E. nodatum*, *Campylobacter rectus*, and *C. showae*) were 1.5 (95% CI 0.8–2.9) for G1; 1.5 (95% CI 0.8–2.9) for G2; and 1.5 (95% CI 0.8–3.1) for G3
Van der Velden *et al.* (2006) (L)	15-year follow-up of 128 subjects from the above cohort (Timmerman *et al.* 2000)	In a multi-variable logistic model, subgingival presence of *A. actinomycetemcomitans* (OR 4.3, 95% CI 1.2–15.7) was confirmed as a risk factor for the onset of the disease, i.e. longitudinal AL during the first 7-year period, but not for progression of disease during the subsequent 8-year period

PD = probing depth; AL= attachment level; CEJ = cemento-enamel junction; CPITN = Community Periodontal Index of Treatment Needs; BANA = N-benzoyl-DL-arginine-2-naphthylamide; a substrate hydrolyzed in the presence of *Treponema denticola*, *Porphyromonas gingivalis*, and *Tannerella forsythia*.

Cigarette smoking

The biological plausibility of an association between tobacco smoking and periodontitis was founded on the broad effects of multiple tobacco-related substances on cellular structure and function. Smoking has been shown to affect the vasculature, the humoral and cellular immune responses, cell signaling processes, and tissue homeostasis (for recent reviews see Kinane & Chestnutt 2000; Palmer *et al.* 2005). A substantial number of studies, a selection of which is summarized in Table 7-5, established the association of smoking to poor periodontal status (Axelsson *et al.* 1998; Bergström 1989; Goultschin *et al.* 1990; Haber & Kent 1992; Locker 1992; Ragnarsson *et al.* 1992; Haber *et al.* 1993; Jette *et al.* 1993; Stoltenberg *et al.* 1993b; Wouters *et al.* 1993; Martinez Canut *et al.* 1995; Albandar *et al.* 2000; Bergström *et al.* 2000b; Tomar & Asma 2000; Paulander *et al.* 2004b; Susin *et al.* 2004b; Kocher *et al.* 2005). Importantly, the inferior periodontal status of smokers cannot be attributed to poorer plaque control or more severe gingivitis (Bergström 1989). While earlier reports suggested a rather similar composition of the subgingival microflora in smokers and non-smokers (Stoltenberg *et al.* 1993b), recent studies demonstrated that shallow sites in smokers are colonized at higher levels by periodontal pathogens, such as *T. forsythia*, *Treponema denticola*, and *P. gingivalis*, and that these differences are obscured in deep, diseased pockets. In an attempt to quantitate the effects of smoking on the periodontal conditions, Haber *et al.* (1993) suggested that the excess prevalence of periodontal disease in the population attributed solely to smoking is much greater than the that owed to other systemic predispositions, such as diabetes mellitus. Data derived from the NHANES III study (Tomar & Asma 2000) suggested that as many as 42% of periodontitis cases in the US can be attributed to current smoking, and another 11% to former smoking. Similarly, in a study from Brazil, Susin *et al.* (2004b) reported that the attributable fraction of clinical attachment loss due to cigarette smoking was 37.7% and 15.6% among heavy and moderate smokers, respectively. In longitudinal studies, smoking has been found to confer a statistically significant increased risk for periodontitis progression after adjustment for other covariates (Beck *et al.* 1995, 1997; Machtei *et al.* 1999; Norderyd *et al.* 1999; Chen *et al.* 2001; Ogawa *et al.* 2002; Paulander *et al.* 2004b).

Figure 7-4 describes a *meta-analysis* of data from studies studying the association between smoking and periodontal conditions. In essence, meta-analysis is a statistical method which combines results from

Table 7-5 Selected studies using smoking as exposure of significance for periodontitis. **(L)** indicates a longitudinal study

Authors/country	Sample/methodology	Findings
Bergström (1989) Sweden	Patients referred for periodontal therapy (155 subjects, 30, 40 and 50 years old); a random sample of the Stockholm population served as controls; full-mouth probing assessments; sites with PD ≥ 4 mm considered diseased; recording of plaque and gingivitis scores	56% of the patients and 34% of the controls were smokers (odds ratio 2.5); significantly higher frequency of periodontally involved teeth in smokers; no notable difference between smokers and non-smokers with respect to plaque and gingivitis
Haber & Kent (1992) USA	196 patients with PD in a periodontal practice and 209 patients from five general practices; probing assessments at six sites/tooth and full-mouth radiographs; questionnaire on smoking habits; patients with negative history of periodontal therapy from the general practices included as controls; comparison of (1) the prevalence of smoking among the two patient groups, and (2) PD disease severity among current and never smokers	Overall smoking history in the periodontal practice 75%; in the general practice 54%; summary odds ratio for positive smoking history in perio versus general practice patients was 2.6; in the perio group, frequency of current smoking increased with increasing severity of PD
Locker (1992) Canada	907 adults, ≥ 50 years old, living independently in four Ontario communities; partial, probing assessments; half of the participants reported a positive history of smoking and 20% were current smokers	Current smokers had fewer teeth, were more likely to have lost all their natural teeth and had higher extent and severity of PD than those who had never smoked
Haber et al. (1993) USA	132 diabetics and 95 non-diabetics, 19–40 years old; probing assessments at six sites/tooth, all teeth; questionnaire on smoking habits; calculation of the population attributable risk percent (PAR%), as an estimate of the excess prevalence of periodontitis in the study population that is associated with smoking	The prevalence of periodontitis was markedly higher among smokers than non smokers within both the diabetic and non-diabetic groups; PAR% among non diabetics was 51% in ages 19–30 years and 32% in ages 31–40 years
Stoltenberg et al. (1993b) USA	Out of 615 medically healthy adults, 28–73 years old, attending a health maintenance organization, selection of 63 smokers and 126 non-smokers of similar age, sex, plaque, and calculus scores; probing assessments at the proximal surfaces of premolars and molars in a randomly selected posterior sextant; detection of P. gingivalis, Pr. intermedia, A. actinomycetemcomitans, Eikenella corrodens, and F. nucleatum by a semi-quantitative fluorescence immunoassay, in one buccal and one lingual sample per tooth examined; logistic regression to determine if any of the bacteria or smoking were indicators of mean posterior probing depth of ≥ 3.5 mm	Odds ratio for a smoker having a mean PD of ≥ 3.5 mm was 5.3 (95% CI 2.0–13.8); no statistically significant difference between smokers and non-smokers with respect to prevalence of the bacteria examined; the logistic model revealed that a mean PD of ≥ 3.5 mm was significantly associated with the presence of A. actinomycetemcomitans, Pr. intermedia, E. corrodens and smoking; smoking was a stronger indicator than any of the bacteria examined
Jette et al. (1993) USA	1156 community dwellers, age 70+ years; probing assessments at four sites/tooth, all teeth; evaluation if lifelong tobacco use is a modifiable risk factor for poor dental health; multiple regression analysis	18.1% of men and 7.9% of women were tobacco users (overall 12.3%; including 1% smokeless tobacco users); years of exposure to tobacco products was a statistically significant factor for tooth loss, coronal root caries, and periodontal disease, regardless of other social and behavioral factors; periodontal disease (no. of affected teeth) was predicted by longer duration of tobacco use, male sex, and more infrequent practice of oral hygiene
Martinez Canut et al. (1995) Spain	889 periodontitis patients, aged 21–76 years; probing assessments at six sites/tooth, all teeth; analysis of variance to examine the role of smoking on the severity of periodontitis	Smoking was statistically related to increased severity of periodontitis in multi-variate analysis; a dose–response effect was demonstrated, with subjects smoking > 20 cigarettes/day showing significantly higher attachment loss
Kaldahl et al. (1996) USA **(L)**	74 patients with moderate to advanced periodontitis including 31 heavy smokers (≥ 20 cigarettes/day); the effects of cigarette consumption and smoking history on the response to active periodontal treatment and to up to 7 years of supportive periodontal treatment was evaluated. Full-mouth examinations performed at baseline, 4 weeks after mechanical plaque control, 10 weeks following periodontal surgery, and yearly during 7 years of supportive periodontal treatment	Past and never smokers consistently exhibited a significantly greater reduction in PD and greater gains in AL than heavy and light smokers; all groups experienced a similar decrease in the prevalence of BoP following active therapy

(Continued)

Table 7-5 *Continued*

Authors/country	Sample/methodology	Findings
Grossi *et al.* (1997b) USA **(L)**	143 subjects aged 35–65 years with established periodontitis, including 60 current, 55 former, and 28 non-smokers, examined at baseline and 3 months after non-surgical periodontal therapy	Current smokers showed less reduction in PD and less AL gain than former- and non smokers; fewer smokers harbored no *P. gingivalis* or *T. forsythia* after treatment, compared to former and non-smokers
Axelsson *et al.* (1998) Sweden	A random sample of 1093 subjects, aged 35, 50, 65, and 75 years; prevalence of smoking in the four age groups was 35%, 35%, 24%, and 12%, respectively; recordings included AL, CPITN scores, DMF surfaces, plaque, and stimulated salivary secretion rate (SSSR)	In the oldest age group, 41% of the smokers and 35% of the non-smokers were edentulous; in every age group, mean attachment loss was statistically significantly increased in smokers by 0.37, 0.88, 0.85, and 1.33 mm, respectively; smokers had higher CPITN and DMF scores, increased SSSR, but similar plaque levels
Tomar & Asma (2000) USA	12 329 subjects, aged ≥ 18 years, participants in the NHANES III study; probing assessments at mesial and buccal sites in one upper and one lower quadrant; mesial assessments performed from the buccal aspect of the teeth; assessments of gingivitis, PD, and location of the gingival margin in relation to the CEJ; "periodontitis" was defined as one or more site with AL ≥ 4 mm and PD ≥ 4 mm	27.9% of the participants were current smokers and 9.2% met the definition for periodontitis; current smokers were four times as likely to suffer from periodontitis than never smokers, after adjustments for age, gender, race/ethnicity, education, and income: poverty ratio; among current smokers, there was a dose–response relationship between cigarettes/day and periodontitis; 41.9% of periodontitis cases were attributable to current smoking and 10.9% to former smoking
Bergström *et al.* (2000b) Sweden	257 subjects, aged 20–69 years, including 50 current smokers, 61 former smokers, and 133 non-smokers; full mouth clinical and radiographic assessments of the periodontal tissues; smoking exposure defined in terms of consumption (number of cig/day), duration (number of years of smoking) and life-time exposure (product of daily consumption and years of duration-cig/years); threshold levels used: heavy versus light consumption: ≥ 10 cigarettes/day versus < 10 cigarettes/day; duration: ≥ 15 years versus < 15 years; life-time exposure: ≥ 200 cig/years versus < 200 cig/years	Compared to former and non-smokers, current smokers had the highest prevalence of diseased sites (AL ≥ 4 mm); 40–69-year-old current smokers showed a significantly higher prevalence than 20–39-year-old current smokers (27% vs. 4%); the same pattern emerged when comparing heavy versus light smokers according to consumption, duration and life-time exposure; in multiple regression, life-time exposure was highly associated with the frequency of diseased sites and periodontal bone height after adjusting for age, gingival bleeding and plaque index
Albandar *et al.* (2000) USA	705 subjects, aged 21–92 years, 52% males and 87% white; full-mouth examination of PD and AL at six sites; periodontitis was classified as advanced, or mild; cigar, pipe, and cigarette smoking were classified as current, former and never	In multiple linear regression, current and former smoking, regardless of type, was associated with increased percentage of subjects with moderate/advanced periodontitis after adjusting for age, gender, race and numbers of years of being smoking cigarette, cigar and pipe; current smoking was also associated with higher number of missing teeth
Bergström *et al.* (2000a) Sweden **(L)**	10-year follow-up of a sample of 84 dentally aware musicians, including 16 current, 28 former, and 40 non-smokers; full-mouth clinical and radiographic assessments of periodontal status	The prevalence of PD ≥ 4 mm (diseased sites) was 18.7% for current, 11.1% for former, and 8.7% for non-smokers at baseline. At 10 years, these figures were 41.6%, 7.8% and 6.6%; a similar pattern was observed for alveolar bone levels; after adjusting for age, gingival bleeding, plaque index, and frequency of diseased sites at baseline, current smoking was a significant predictor of the increase in diseased sites at 10 years
Susin *et al.* (2004b) Brazil	974 subjects, aged 30–103 years; full mouth examination of PD and AL; severe attachment loss was defined as AL ≥ 5 mm in ≥ 30% of the teeth; exposure to smoking classified as current/former, heavy/moderate/light/none, and quantified as lifetime consumption	Heavy and moderate smokers had significantly higher prevalence of AL ≥ 5 mm than non-smokers; in multivariate analysis heavy (OR 3.6, 95% CI 2.2–6.0) and moderate smoking (OR 2.0, 95% CI 1.4–2.9) conferred higher odds for AL; the attributable fraction of AL due to smoking was 37.7% and 15.6% among heavy and moderate smokers, respectively

PD = probing depth; AL = attachment level; BoP = bleeding on probing; CEJ = cemento-enamel junction; CPITN = Community Periodontal Index of Treatment Needs; DMF = decayed, missing, filled.

Odds ratio

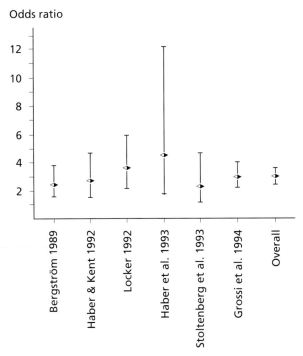

Fig. 7-4 Meta-analysis of smoking as a risk factor for periodontal disease. The studies included are: Bergström (1989), Haber & Kent (1992), Locker (1992), Haber *et al.* (1993), Stoltenberg *et al.* (1993), and Grossi *et al.* (1994). Bars indicate the 95% confidence limits for the depicted odds ratios. From Papapanou (1996), reproduced with permission.

different studies of similar design, in order to gain an overall increased *power*, i.e. an enhanced potential to reveal biological associations which may exist but are difficult to detect (Chalmers 1993; Oakes 1993; Proskin & Volpe 1994). This analysis, initially published as part of the 1996 World Workshop in Periodontics (Papapanou 1996), incorporated data from six studies, including a total of 2361 subjects, with known smoking habits and periodontal status (Bergström & Eliasson 1989; Haber & Kent 1992; Locker 1992; Haber *et al.* 1993; Stoltenberg *et al.* 1993b; Grossi *et al.* 1994). It can be observed that smoking entailed an overall increased, statistically and clinically significant risk for severe disease (estimated overall odds ratio of 2.82; 95% confidence limits 2.36–3.39).

Studies examining the effects of smoking on the outcome of periodontal treatment have demonstrated that treatment responses are modified by cigarette consumption, with current smokers exhibiting poorer responses than former or never smokers (Ah *et al.* 1994; Kaldahl *et al.* 1996; Renvert *et al.* 1996; Grossi *et al.* 1997b; Kinane & Radvar 1997; Boström *et al.* 1998; Machtei *et al.* 1998; Tonetti *et al.* 1998; Scabbia *et al.* 2001; Trombelli *et al.* 2003; Van der Velden *et al.* 2003; Papantonopoulos 2004; Paulander *et al.* 2004a; Rieder *et al.* 2004; Stavropoulos *et al.* 2004; Sculean *et al.* 2005). Notably, these studies have confirmed the negative effect of smoking on the outcome of several periodontal treatment modalities including non-surgical, surgical, and regenerative periodontal therapy. Two recent meta-analyses of the effects of

smoking on the outcome of periodontal therapy (Garcia 2005; Labriola *et al.* 2005) support the above conclusions.

In contrast, smoking cessation was shown to be beneficial to the periodontal tissues. In a longitudinal study (Bolin *et al.* 1993), 349 subjects with ≥20 remaining teeth were examined on two occasions 10 years apart (1970 and 1980). Progression of periodontal disease was assessed on radiographs at all approximal tooth surfaces and was shown to be almost twice as rapid in smokers than in non-smokers. It was also observed that subjects who quit smoking at some time point within the observation period had a significantly retarded progression of bone loss than the one occurring in smokers. Similar observations were made by Krall *et al.* (1997) who reported that, over a mean follow-up period of 6 years, subjects who continued to smoke had a 2.4–3.5-fold risk of tooth loss when compared to non-smokers. Finally, in a 10-year follow-up study, Bergström *et al.* (2000a) observed an increase of periodontally diseased sites concomitant with loss of periodontal bone height in current smokers, as compared to non-smokers whose periodontal health condition remained unaltered throughout the period of investigation. The periodontal health condition in former smokers was similarly stable to that of non-smokers, underscoring the beneficial effects of smoking cessation.

In conclusion, cigarette smoking appears to fulfill the majority of the required steps of the risk assessment process stipulated by Beck (1994) and is considered one of the major risk factors for periodontitis.

Diabetes mellitus

Diabetes as a risk factor for periodontitis has been debated for decades (Genco & Löe 1993), but several biologically plausible mechanisms by which the disease may contribute to impaired periodontal conditions have been identified over the past decade (for reviews see Lalla *et al.* 2000; Mealey & Oates 2006). Table 7-6 summarizes epidemiological evidence based on a number of case–control and prospective cohort studies that examine the periodontal status of patients with diabetes (Hugoson *et al.* 1989; Shlossman *et al.* 1990; Emrich *et al.* 1991; de Pommereau *et al.* 1992; Oliver & Tervonen 1993; Thorstensson & Hugoson 1993; Pinson *et al.* 1995). This association is especially pronounced in subjects with poor metabolic control and a long duration of the disease (Taylor *et al.* 1996; Grossi & Genco 1998; Taylor *et al.* 1998a; Lalla *et al.* 2004). The age of onset of diabetes-related manifestations in the periodontal tissues has also been addressed in studies examining children and adolescents with type 1 diabetes (de Pommereau *et al.* 1992; Pinson *et al.* 1995) and both type 1 and type 2 diabetes (Lalla *et al.* 2006). All three studies documented more pronounced gingival inflammation in subjects with diabetes in ages between 6 and 18 years. The case–control study by Lalla *et al.* (2006) further

Table 7-6 Selected studies using diabetes mellitus as exposure of significance for periodontitis. **(L)** indicates a longitudinal study

Authors/country	Sample/methodology	Findings
Hugoson et al. (1989) Sweden	82 subjects with long- and 72 with short-duration IDDM; 77 non-diabetics (age 20–70 years); full-mouth, probing assessments at four sites/tooth; radiographs of lower molar–premolar regions; subjects assigned into five groups according to increasing severity of periodontal disease; no multi-variate analysis	No notable difference in plaque, calculus, and no. of teeth between diabetics and non-diabetics; long-duration diabetics were more frequently classified in groups 4 and 5 and had significantly more tooth surfaces with PD of ≥ 6 mm than non-diabetics; significantly more extensive ABL in long-duration diabetics 40–49 years old
Shlossman et al. (1990) Arizona, USA	3219 Pima Indians, ≥ 5 years; prevalence of NIDDM 23% (20% in men, 25% in women); probing assessments at six sites/tooth, at six index teeth; alveolar bone loss from panoramic radiographs; 2878 subjects with available radiographic data, probing assessments or both; comparison between diabetics and non-diabetics with respect to AL and ABL	Median attachment loss and alveolar bone loss higher in diabetics for all age groups and in both sexes
Emrich et al. (1991) USA	Sample and methodology same as above (Shlossman et al. 1990); 1342 Pima Indians, 15 years and older, with natural teeth; 19% (254) with diabetes and 12% (158) with impaired glucose tolerance; linear logistic models to predict prevalence and severity of periodontal disease; prevalence: one or more sites with AL of ≥ 5 mm or ABL ≥ 25% of the root length; severity: square root of average AL or ABL	Diabetes, age, and calculus were significant risk markers for periodontitis; odds ratios for a diabetic to have PD was 2.8 (clinically assessed) and 3.4 (radiographically)
de Pommereau et al. (1992) France	85 adolescents with IDDM aged 12–18 years and 38 healthy age-matched controls; probing assessments at six sites/tooth, all teeth; bite-wing radiographs at molars and sites with AL > 2 mm; patients divided according to disease duration (more or less than 6 years); sexual maturation according to Tanner's classification; metabolic control expressed through glycosylated hemoglobin (HbA1c); non-parametric pair-wise analysis	None of the subjects had sites with AL ≥ 3 mm or radiographic signs of periodontitis; despite similar plaque scores, diabetic children had significantly more gingival inflammation; no significant relation between gingival condition and age, Tanner's index, HbA1c level or disease duration
Oliver & Tervonen (1993) USA	114 diabetic patients, 20–64 years old (60% with IDDM and 40% with NIDDM); half-mouth, probing assessments at four sites/tooth; data from the 1985–86 National Survey served as controls	Tooth loss was similar among diabetics and US employed adults; 60% of the diabetics and 16% of the controls had one or more site with PD ≥ 4 mm; attachment level data were comparable in both groups
Thorstensson & Hugoson (1993) Sweden	83 IDDM patients and 99 age- and sex-matched non-diabetics (age 40–70 years); full-mouth, probing assessments at four sites/tooth; radiographs of lower molar-premolar regions; subjects assigned into five groups according to increasing severity of periodontal disease; uni-variate analysis	Diabetics 40–49 years old (mean disease duration 25.6 years) had more periodontal pockets ≥ 6 mm and more extensive alveolar bone loss than non-diabetics, but this was not the case for subjects aged 50–59 or 60–69 years (mean disease duration 20.5 and 18.6 years, respectively). Disease duration appeared to be a significant determinant of periodontitis development
Pinson et al. (1995) USA	26 IDDM children, 7–18 years old and 24 controls, 20 of whom were siblings of the diabetic patients; full-mouth, probing assessments at six sites/tooth; metabolic control assessed through glycosylated hemoglobin (GHb); analysis of covariance	Overall, no statistically significant differences between cases and controls; no association between GHb and clinical variables; after correcting for plaque, diabetics showed more severe gingival inflammation in specific tooth regions
Bridges et al. (1996) USA	A sample of 233 men, aged 24–78 years, including 118 diabetic (46 type 1 and 72 type 2) and 115 non-diabetic subjects, matched for age and BMI	Plaque and gingivitis, bleeding scores, PD, AL, and missing teeth were significantly higher in diabetic than non-diabetic men
Tervonen & Karjalainen (1997) Finland **(L)**	36 patients with type 1 diabetes and 10 controls, aged 24–36 years, received non-surgical periodontal therapy and were followed at 4 weeks, 6 and 12 months; patient with diabetes were further grouped according to diabetic status as: D1 (n = 13) with no diabetic complications and good long-term metabolic control; D2 (n = 15) moderate metabolic control with/without retinopathy; D3 (n = 8) severe diabetes with poor metabolic control and/or multiple complications; periodontal status was monitored radiographically	The periodontal status of the diabetic patients with good control and no complications (D1) and those with moderate control (D2) was similar to non-diabetic controls. Diabetic subjects with poor metabolic control and/or multiple complications (D3) exhibited higher extent of AL ≥ 2 mm at baseline and higher recurrence of PD ≥ 4 mm during follow-up

(Continued)

Table 7-6 *Continued*

Authors/country	Sample/methodology	Findings
Taylor *et al.* (1998a) USA **(L)**	2-year study of 21 patients with type 2 diabetes, including 14 with poor and 7 with better metabolic control, and 338 controls, aged 15–57 years, Native Americans; progression of bone loss was assessed on radiographs; covariates included age, calculus, gingival and plaque indices, time to follow up, alcohol consumption, smoking, obesity (BMI > 27), coronary heart disease, and gender	In multiple logistic regression, poorly controlled diabetic subjects were 11 times more likely (95% CI 2.5–53.3) to have more pronounced bone loss progression than non-diabetic subjects; no such differences were found between better controlled and non-diabetic controls; age, time to follow-up, pronounced bone loss at baseline and calculus index were significant predictors of bone loss progression
Taylor *et al.* (1998b) USA **(L)**	2-year study of 24 subjects with NIDDM and 362 subjects without diabetes, aged 15–57 years; degree of bone loss on panoramic radiographs was assessed in a scale of 0–4	A regression model having progression of bone loss as the dependent variable revealed a cumulative odds ratio for NIDDM of 4.23 (95% CI 1.8–9.9); the association was modified by age, with younger adults exhibiting higher risk for alveolar bone loss progression
Lalla *et al.* (2006) USA	Case–control study of 182 children and adolescents (6–18 years of age) with diabetes (predominantly type 1) and 160 non-diabetic control subjects; half-mouth examination at four sites/tooth in all fully erupted teeth with respect to PD and AL	Children with diabetes had significantly more plaque and gingival inflammation than controls and higher number of teeth with AL; when controlling for age, gender, ethnicity, gingival bleeding, and frequency of dental visits, diabetes remained significantly correlated with attachment loss; body mass index was significantly correlated with AL in children with diabetes

PD = probing depth; AL = attachment level; CEJ = cemento-enamel junction.

IDDM and NIDDM = insulin-dependent and non-insulin-dependent diabetes mellitus, respectively; both terms have been abolished and replaced by type 1 and type 2 diabetes.

reported that attachment loss was more pronounced in young patients with diabetes after adjustment for age, gender, ethnicity, gingival bleeding, and frequency of dental visits. In a subsequent publication, Lalla *et al.* (2007b) reported data on 350 children with either type 1 or type 2 diabetes and found a strong positive association between mean HbA1c levels over the 2 years preceding the dental examination and periodontitis. Finally, in a report including a total of 700 children, 350 with diabetes and 350 non-diabetic controls, Lalla *et al.* (2007a) documented a statistically increased periodontal destruction in children with diabetes across all disease definitions tested and in both age subgroups of 6–11 and 12–18 years.

Several studies suggest a two-way relationship between diabetes and periodontitis, with more severe periodontal tissue destruction in people with diabetes but also a poorer metabolic control of diabetes in subjects with periodontitis (Lalla *et al.* 2000; Soskolne & Klinger 2001; Taylor 2001). Irrespective of the variability in the case definition employed in these studies, subjects with diabetes have higher prevalence, extent, and severity of periodontal disease (Grossi *et al.* 1994; Bridges *et al.* 1996; Firatli 1997; Tervonen & Karjalainen 1997; Taylor *et al.* 1998a,b; Lalla *et al.* 2004). These observations are consistent for both type 1 and type 2 diabetes. In addition, these studies provide evidence of a dose–response relationship between poor metabolic control and the severity as well as the progression of periodontitis

(Seppälä *et al.* 1993; Tervonen & Oliver 1993; Tervonen & Karjalainen 1997; Taylor *et al.* 1998a; Guzman *et al.* 2003). Further expanding this observed dose–response relationship into the pre-diabetic state, a recent study also indicated that the level of glucose intolerance in non-diabetic individuals also correlated with the severity of periodontal disease (Saito *et al.* 2004). In line with the above observations, the outcome of periodontal treatment in well controlled diabetic patients is similar to that of non-diabetic subjects, while poorly controlled diabetics display an inferior outcome (Tervonen & Karjalainen 1997).

Collectively, the above data strongly indicate that diabetes mellitus is a major risk factor for periodontitis.

Obesity

The biologic plausibility of a potential link between obesity and periodontitis has been suggested to involve a hyper-inflammatory state and an aberrant lipid metabolism prevalent in obesity, as well as the pathway of insulin resistance (Saito *et al.* 1998; Nishimura & Murayama 2001) all of which may collectively result in an enhanced breakdown of the periodontal tissue support. Indeed, a number of recent studies point to a positive association between obesity, defined as body mass index (BMI) ≥30, and periodontitis (Anon 2000; Saito *et al.* 2001; Al-Zahrani *et al.* 2003; Wood *et al.* 2003).

Three separate publications have documented such an association in the NHANES III database. In the first publication Al-Zahrani *et al.* (2003) reported a significant association between both BMI and waist-to-hip ratio and periodontitis in younger adults, but no association in middle-aged or older adults (Table 7-1). Wood *et al.* (2003), using a subset of the NHANES III sample including Caucasian subjects aged 18 years and above, reported that BMI, waist-to-hip ratio, visceral fat, and fat-free mass were associated with periodontitis after adjusting for age, gender, history of diabetes, current smoking, and socioeconomic status. Finally, Genco *et al.* (2005), reported that overweight subjects in the upper quartile of insulin resistance index were 1.5 times more likely to have periodontitis compared to their counterparts with high BMI but low insulin resistance index.

In an independent subject sample including 643 apparently healthy Japanese adults, Saito *et al.* (2001) reported that waist-to-hip ratio, BMI, and body fat were significant risk indicators for periodontitis after adjustments for known risk factors. In addition, in a separate analysis of the subsample of subjects with high waist-to-hip ratio, higher BMI and increased body fat significantly increased the adjusted risk of periodontitis, when compared to subjects with low waist-to-hip ratios, BMI or body fat.

Given that the above publications are based on only two population samples, and that inferences on temporality or mechanisms are not possible based on cross-sectional studies, additional research on the role of obesity in periodontitis is warranted.

Osteopenia/osteoporosis

Several cross-sectional studies, of limited sample size and largely confined to postmenopausal women, have suggested that women with low bone mineral density are more likely to have CAL, gingival recession and/or pronounced gingival inflammation (von Wowern *et al.* 1994; Mohammad *et al.* 1996, 1997; Tezal *et al.* 2000). In a radiographic study of 1084 subjects aged 60–75 years, Persson *et al.* (2002) reported a positive association between osteoporosis and periodontitis with an odds ratio of 1.8 (95% CI 1.2–2.5) However, studies that failed to report such an association have been published as well (Weyant *et al.* 1999; Lundström *et al.* 2001).

Based on these studies it has been hypothesized that the systemic loss of bone density in osteoporosis may, in combination with hormone action, heredity, and other host factors, provide a host system that is increasingly susceptible to the infectious destruction of periodontal tissue (Wactawski-Wende 2001). However, the data from longitudinal studies are similarly conflicting. Contrary to Payne *et al.* (1999, 2000) who reported an enhanced longitudinal alveolar bone loss in osteoporotic women versus women with normal mineral bone density, Reinhardt and colleagues (1999) reported no significant impact of

serum estradiol levels on longitudinal attachment loss over a 2-year period. In contrast, Yoshihara *et al.* (2004) found, after adjustments, a significant association between bone mineral density and 3-year longitudinal attachment loss in Japanese subjects ≥70 years old. It appears therefore that additional research is needed to unequivocally establish or refute the role of osteoporosis as a risk factor for periodontitis.

Human immunodeficiency (HIV) infection

After the early studies published in the late 1980s which seemed to indicate that both the prevalence and the severity of periodontitis were exceptionally high in patients with acquired immunodeficiency syndrome (AIDS) (Winkler & Murray 1987), a more tempered picture emerged in subsequent publications. While it cannot be ruled out that the initial reports actually included biased samples, it is also possible that the successful control of immunosuppression in HIV-positive subjects by means of high activity anti-retroviral therapy (HAART) and other continuously evolving drugs has influenced the incidence of periodontal disease progression in HIV-seropositive subjects and has resulted in less severe periodontal manifestations of HIV infection (Chapple & Hamburger 2000). For example, a cross-sectional study of 326 HIV-infected adults (McKaig *et al.* 1998) revealed that, after adjustments for CD4 counts, persons taking HIV-antiretroviral medication were five times less likely to suffer from periodontitis than those not taking such medication, underscoring the importance of the host's immunologic competency in this context.

Nevertheless, publications of the last decade continue to generate conflicting results. Thus, although studies (Smith *et al.* 1995a; Robinson *et al.* 1996; Ndiaye *et al.* 1997; McKaig *et al.* 1998) indicated higher prevalence and severity of periodontitis in HIV-positive subjects when compared to controls, other studies are either not supportive of this notion or indicate that the differences in periodontal status between HIV-seropositive and -seronegative subjects are limited (Cross & Smith 1995; Lamster *et al.* 1997; Scheutz *et al.* 1997; Lamster *et al.* 1998; Vastardis *et al.* 2003). Studies investigating the pathobiology of periodontitis in HIV infected subjects suggested that specific IgG subclass responses to periodontopathic bacteria were similar in HIV-positive and HIV-negative subjects (Yeung *et al.* 2002), while CD4 count levels were not found to correlate with the severity of periodontitis (Martinez Canut *et al.* 1996; Vastardis *et al.* 2003).

The few available longitudinal studies are equally conflicting. Two companion publications reporting from a short-term follow-up study (Cross & Smith 1995; Smith *et al.* 1995b) involved a group of 29 HIV-seropositive subjects who were examined at baseline and 3 months and reported a low prevalence and incidence of attachment loss. The subgingival microbial profiles of the seropositive subjects resembled those obtained from non-systemically affected subjects, and were not correlated to their CD4 and CD8 lymphocyte counts. Similarly, in a small follow-up study of 12 months duration, Robinson *et al.* (2000) found no difference in the progression of periodontitis between HIV-positive and HIV-negative subjects. Hofer *et al.* (2002) demonstrated that compliant HIV-positive subjects can be successfully maintained in a manner similar to non-infected controls. However, a 20-month follow-up study of 114 homosexual or bisexual men by Barr *et al.* (1992) revealed a clear relationship between incidence of attachment loss and immunosupression, expressed through CD4 cell counts. The authors suggested that seropositivity in combination with older age confers an increased risk for attachment loss. Similar observations were reported by Lamster *et al.* (1997) who concluded that periodontitis in the presence of HIV infection is dependent upon the immunologic competency of the host as well as the local inflammatory response to both typical and atypical subgingival microbiota.

It appears therefore that there is no consensus in the literature on the association of HIV/AIDS and periodontitis. Variance due to ongoing advancements in therapy will likely further contribute to the diversity of the findings.

Psychosocial factors

The mechanisms by which psychosocial stress may affect the periodontal status are complex. It has been suggested that one of the plausible pathways may involve behavioral changes leading to smoking and poor oral hygiene that, in turn, may affect periodontal health (Genco *et al.* 1998). In the absence of a biological measure of stress, a limited number of studies have used proxy measures of stress to study its association with periodontitis. In a study of 1426 subjects in Erie County, NY, USA, Genco *et al.* (1999) reported that adult subjects who were under financial strain and exhibited poor coping behaviors were at increased risk of severe periodontitis when compared with subjects who demonstrated good coping behavior patterns under similar financial strain, or with controls under no financial strain. In a limited size study that included 23 employed adults, Linden *et al.* (1996) evaluated the association between occupational stress and the progression of periodontitis and reported that longitudinal attachment loss was significantly predicted by increasing age, lower socioeconomic status, lower job satisfaction, and type A personality, characterized by aggressive, impatient, and irritable behavior. In contrast, a study of 681 subjects carried out in Lithuania (Aleksejuniene *et al.* 2002) could not document an association between psychosocial stress and periodontitis, although they reported that the disease did correlate with lifestyle factors.

Clearly, the study of the role of stress in periodontitis is in its infancy and multiple gaps in our knowledge exist. Nevertheless, given the established role of the sympathetic, parasympathetic, and the peptidergic/sensory nervous systems, as well as that of the hypothalamic–pituitary–adrenal axis on brain-to-immune regulatory pathways, such a role is clearly biologically plausible. Recent experimental animal studies have begun to shed light on basic mechanisms that may explain the link between psychosocial factors and periodontitis. For example, a recent study by Breivik *et al.* (2006) demonstrated that experimentally induced depression in rats accelerated tissue breakdown in a ligature periodontitis model and that pharmacologic treatment of depression attenuated this breakdown. Additional basic and epidemiologic research is needed to fully elucidate this relationship.

Remarks

The analytical epidemiologic studies described above are obviously diverse with respect to important elements of design and methodology, such as definitions of disease, sample size, use of full-mouth or partial-mouth recording protocols, length of follow-up in longitudinal studies, comprehensive or not adjustment for potential confounders, etc. Nevertheless, despite these apparent shortcomings, a number of conclusions can be made with reasonable certainty:

1. Specific bacteria, cigarette smoking, and diabetes mellitus are the major established risk factors for periodontitis. A number of biologically plausible, potentially important additional factors are in need of further investigation in future studies.
2. There is a need to introduce a uniform definition of periodontitis to be used in analytical epidemiologic studies, to facilitate valid comparisons and establish whether seemingly conflicting data reflect true biological variation or are exclusively owed to methodological inconsistencies. To address this point, the Consensus Report of 5th European Workshop in Periodontology (Tonetti & Claffey 2005) suggested a two-level definition of periodontitis as follows: (i) presence of proximal attachment loss of ≥3 mm in two or more non-adjacent teeth, and (ii) presence of proximal attachment loss of ≥5 mm in ≥30% of teeth present. Likewise, the following case definition for the progression of periodontitis was proposed: presence of two or more teeth demonstrating a longitudinal loss of proximal attachment of ≥3 mm, or in cases where attachment level measurements are not available, longitudinal radiographic bone loss of ≥2 mm at two or more teeth may be used as a substitute. Obviously, no definition is devoid of shortcomings and the above proposals are no exception. Nevertheless, a consistent "common denominator" definition across studies will greatly facilitate valid comparisons.

3. Studies need to distinguish clearly between risk factors and disease predictors. Although the use of the latter as explanatory variables in multi-variate models may increase the coefficient of determination (i.e. the proportion of the variance explained by means of the models), it may obscure the significance of true etiologic factors. For example, as shown by Ismail et al. (1990), factors with biologically plausible etiologic potential (such as dental plaque) may not retain their significance in multi-variate models that include alternative expressions of disease such as tooth mobility. It has been demonstrated that baseline levels of disease and morphologic features such as angular bony defects are powerful predictors of future disease progression (Papapanou et al. 1989; Papapanou & Wennström 1991). Haffajee et al. (1991a) showed that age, plaque, and bleeding on probing are related to both baseline disease levels as well as to incident disease. In the search of true exposures of significance for disease onset or progression, inclusion of a factor in a model may thus erroneously discredit a co-varying, biologically significant other factor.

4. The progression pattern of periodontitis over time appears to follow a skewed distribution similar to the skewed distribution of the prevalence of severe periodontitis in the population. In other words, although a majority of subjects may harbor sites which progress over time, it is a small subfraction of subjects that suffer substantial longitudinal attachment loss or bone loss at multiple sites.

Finally, an interesting observation was brought up in a report by Beck et al. (1995). In a longitudinal study, the authors compared characteristics of patients experiencing attachment loss at previously non-diseased sites with those of patients suffering progression of already established disease. While low income and medication with drugs associated with soft tissue reactions were features in common for both groups of patients, new lesions were more frequent in patients who used smokeless tobacco and had a history of oral pain. Risk for progression of established disease was higher in cigarette smokers, subjects with high levels of subgingival P. gingivalis, and individuals with worsening financial problems. These data suggest that periodontitis may be like other diseases for which the factors associated with the initiation of the disease may be different from the ones involved in its progression. If this observation is verified in other studies, such a distinction may have implications for future assessment strategies and may improve the accuracy of the risk/prediction models.

Periodontal infections and risk for systemic disease

During the past decade and a half, an entirely new area of periodontal research has emerged, commonly referred to as "periodontal medicine". Following some initial reports suggesting a link between periodontal infections and a number of systemic conditions, researchers are increasingly dwelling into the exploration of additional epidemiological and experimental evidence as well as possible underlying pathogenic mechanisms. The biological plausibility of the proposed associations between periodontitis and atherosclerosis, cardiovascular and cerebrovascular disease, pregnancy complications, and diabetes mellitus, and the relevant epidemiological evidence available today are summarized in the following text.

Atherosclerosis – cardiovascular/cerebrovascular disease

A wealth of data originating from diverse areas of investigation have implicated chronic, low-level inflammation as an important factor in atherosclerotic cardiovascular disease (CVD) (Ross 1999). Supporting studies stemming from a variety of disciplines, such as cell biology, epidemiology, clinical trials, and experimental animal research, have consistently revealed that atherosclerotic lesions involve an inflammatory component. The cellular interactions in atherogenesis are fundamentally similar to those in chronic inflammatory–fibroproliferative diseases, and atherosclerotic lesions represent a series of highly specific cellular and molecular responses that can best be described, in aggregate, as an inflammatory disease (Ross 1993, 1999).

It is well established that the periodontal diseases represent mixed infections of the periodontal tissues caused by primarily anaerobic, Gram-negative bacteria (Haffajee & Socransky 1994). As discussed above, the prevalence of these infections, especially of mild or moderate severity, may be substantial in certain populations. The deepening of the periodontal sulcus which occurs during the course of these infections is concurrent with a marked bacterial proliferation, resulting in bacterial cell levels reaching 10^9 or 10^{10} bacteria within a single pathological periodontal pocket. The ulcerated epithelial lining of the periodontal pocket may constitute a substantial surface area in cases of generalized periodontitis (Hujoel et al. 2001) and provides a gate through which lipopolysaccharide (LPS) and other antigenic structures of bacterial origin challenge the immune system and elicit a local and systemic host response (Ebersole & Taubman 1994). Importantly, a number of pathogenic species involved in the periodontal infections display tissue invasion properties (Meyer et al. 1991; Sandros et al. 1994; Lamont et al. 1995). Frequent transient bacteremias occurring as a result of daily activities such as tooth brushing or chewing (Silver et al. 1977; Kinane et al. 2005; Forner et al. 2006) may confer a significant systemic bacterial challenge to the host. Circulating levels of several cytokines (IL-1 beta, IL-2, IL-6, and IL-8) induced during the course of several infections (Endo et al. 1992; Humar et al. 1999; Otto *et al.* 1999), but also locally in the periodontal tissues in conjunction with periodontitis (Salvi *et al.* 1998), have been identified as biomarkers of cardiovascular disease (Hackam & Anand 2003; Hansson 2005). Interestingly, these pro-inflammatory cytokines have also been detected within atheromatous lesions (Barath *et al.* 1990a,b; Galea *et al.* 1996). In line with the observation that chronic infection may contribute to a pro-coagulant state, elevated von Willebrand factor antigen, a measure of endothelial cell damage, has been demonstrated in individuals with multiple dental infections (Mattila *et al.* 1989; Torgano *et al.* 1999).

A number of studies have examined the presence of oral bacteria in atheromatic plaque lesions. Chiu (1999) investigated the relationship between the presence of multiple infectious agents in human carotid endarterectomy specimens and pathoanatomic features of the corresponding carotid plaques, and reported positive immunostainings for *P. gingivalis* and *Streptococcus sanguis* in several carotid plaque specimens. The bacteria were immunolocalized in plaque shoulders and within a lymphohistiocytic infiltrate, associated with ulcer and thrombus formation, and adjacent to areas of strong labeling for apoptotic bodies. A similar study using the polymerase chain reaction (Haraszthy *et al.* 2000) reported that 30% of the carotid endarderectomy specimens examined were positive for *T. forsythia*, 26% for *P. gingivalis*, 18% for *A. actinomycetemcomitans*, and 14% positive for *Pr. intermedia*. The validity of these data has been recently confirmed in similar studies (Stelzel *et al.* 2002; Fiehn *et al.* 2005). Corroborating the above observations, in an experimental animal study, oral infection of with *P. gingivalis* promoted atherogenesis and *P. gingivalis* DNA was localized within the aortic tissue of infected mice (Lalla *et al.* 2003).

Emerging evidence from epidemiologic studies indicates that periodontal infections have an impact on a host of peripheral blood markers that have been linked to CVD. For example, periodontitis patients have been shown to display higher white blood cell counts (Kweider *et al.* 1993; Loos *et al.* 2000) and C-reactive protein (CRP) levels (Ebersole *et al.* 1997; Loos *et al.* 2000; Slade *et al.* 2000) than periodontally healthy controls. Wu *et al.* (2000) examined the relation between periodontal health status and serum total and high-density lipoprotein cholesterol, CRP, and plasma fibrinogen. Based on an analysis of a total of 10 146 subjects from NHANES III with available cholesterol and CRP and 4461 subjects with available fibrinogen, poor periodontal status was significantly associated with increased CRP and fibrinogen levels. Slade *et al.* (2000) explored the same database and reported that (1) people with extensive periodontal disease had an increase of approximately one third in mean CRP and a doubling in prevalence of elevated CRP compared with periodontally healthy people, and (2) similarly raised CRP levels in edentulous subjects. Based on data of 2973 participants ≥40 years old from the second phase of NHANES III,

Dye *et al.* (2005) showed that high serum IgG antibody level to *P. gingivalis* was significantly related to elevated serum CRP. In a sample comprising 5552 subjects aged 52–75 years from the Atherosclerosis Risk in Communities study (ARIC) (Slade *et al.* 2003), participants with extensive periodontal disease (≥30% of sites with pocket depth ≥4 mm) had 30% higher CRP levels than participants with extent of periodontal disease between 0 and 30%. In a multi-variate analysis stratified for BMI, extensive periodontal pocketing remained associated with CRP levels when adjusted for age, sex, diabetes mellitus, cigarette use, and use of non-steroidal anti-inflammatory medications. Finally, Schwahn *et al.* (2004) reported on associations between periodontitis, edentulism, and high plasma fibrinogen levels (>3.25 g/l), in 2738 persons aged 20–59 years, participants in the Study of Health in Pomerania (SHIP). In a two-way interaction model adjusted for multiple co-variates (age, gender, BMI, education, alcohol, gastritis, bronchitis, diabetes, use of medications, use of aspirin, LDL, and smoking), presence of ≥15 pockets with probing depth ≥4 mm was significantly associated with high plasma fibrinogen levels with an OR of 1.9 (95% CI 1.2–2.8). Less extensive pocketing or edentulism were not associated with high plasma fibrinogen levels.

Several studies have investigated the association between periodontitis and subclinical atherosclerosis, commonly measured by means of carotid artery intima media thickness (IMT) assessments. Increased IMT has been documented to be directly associated with increased risk or myocardial infarction and stroke (O'Leary *et al.* 1999). Beck *et al.* (2001) provided the first evidence that periodontitis may be linked to subclinical atherosclerosis. These authors analyzed cross-sectional data on 6017 persons, participants in the ARIC study, and demonstrated that severe periodontitis conferred increased odds for higher carotid artery intima media wall thickness (OR 2.09, 95% CI 1.73–2.53 for IMT of ≥1 mm). A couple of years later, the Oral Infection and Vascular Disease Epidemiology Study (INVEST; a prospective population-based cohort study of randomly selected subjects in a tri-ethnic population, comprising a total of 1056 subjects aged ≥55 years, with no baseline history of stroke, myocardial infarction, or chronic inflammatory conditions) investigated the relationship between carotid artery plaque and IMT with tooth loss and measures of periodontitis. In a first report based on data from 711 subjects (Desvarieux *et al.* 2003), tooth loss of 10–19 teeth was associated with increase in prevalence of atherosclerotic plaques in a model adjusted for age, sex, smoking, diabetes, systolic blood pressure, LDL, HDL, ethnicity, education, tooth brushing, social isolation, physical activity, and years of residence (OR 1.9, CI 1.2–3.0). Since in this cohort a higher number of lost teeth paralleled an increased severity of periodontal disease at the remaining teeth, it was assumed that tooth loss reflected, in part, current or cumulative periodontal disease. In a subsequent publication, Engebretson *et al.* (2005) reported on a sub-sample of 203 subjects from the INVEST cohort with available panoramic radiographs. In a logistic regression model, severe bone loss was defined as a whole mouth average bone loss of ≥50% of the root length and was associated with presence of carotid atherosclerotic plaque after adjustment for age, sex, hypertension, coronary artery disease, diabetes, smoking, HDL, and LDL. In addition, log-transformed mean carotid plaque thickness increased over tertiles of periodontal bone loss, suggesting a dose-dependent association. A third INVEST report (Desvarieux *et al.* 2005) included 657 patients with available dental and medical variables as described above, as well as data on the prevalence and level of ten bacterial species, assessed by checkerboard DNA–DNA hybridization (Socransky *et al.* 1994) in up to eight subgingival plaque samples per subject. In this study, "etiological bacterial burden" was defined as the aggregate colonization per subject by *A. actinomycetemcomitans*, *P. gingivalis*, *T. forsythia*, and *Tr. denticola*. The data revealed that IMT and while blood cell counts increased significantly over tertiles of etiologic periodontal bacterial burden in a fully adjusted model including age, BMI, gender, race/ethnicity, smoking, systolic blood pressure, education, diabetes, HDL, and LDL as co-variates. Importantly, the association was exclusively observed for "etiologic bacteria", as increased colonization by putative pathogens of the "orange complex" or a number of health-associated bacteria was not associated with increased IMT.

In an ARIC-based study including a sample of 4585 participants (Beck *et al.* 2005b), serum IgG titers for periodontal pathogens were associated with carotid IMT of ≥1 mm. The strongest association emerged when the combined titer against *Campylobacter rectus* and *Micromonas micros* was used. Similarly, a research group from Finland reported on the association between serum titers to periodontal pathogens and IMT in a sub-sample of 1023 men aged 46–64 from the Kuopio Ischemic Heart Disease Risk Factor study (Pussinen *et al.* 2005). Incident IMT assessed 10 years post baseline in participants with no prior coronary heart disease increased significantly across tertiles of IgA titer levels to *A. actinomycetemcomitans* and *P. gingivalis*.

Another group of epidemiologic studies has focused on the association of periodontal infections with clinical events, primarily coronary heart disease (CHD), myocardial infacrtion (MI) or stroke. An early study by DeStefano *et al.* (1993) used a prospective cohort of 9760 subjects and found a nearly two-fold higher risk of CHD for individuals with periodontal disease. Beck *et al.* (1996) used data from a cohort of 1147 subjects who were medically healthy at baseline, 207 of which developed CHD over an average follow-up of 18 years. Radiographic evidence of alveolar bone loss was used to stratify the subjects according to minimal and severe periodontitis. The results, presented as incidence odds ratios adjusted for age

and race, showed a significant association between severe bone loss and total CHD, fatal CHD, and stroke.

Another ARIC-stemming report based on a sample of 5002 people (Beck *et al.* 2005a) reported no significant association between incipient or severe periodontitis defined by clinical measurements and CHD. However, in regression models adjusted for age, sex, race, diabetes, hypertension, waist-to-hip ratio, HDL and LDL cholesterol, and education, detectable antibody levels to specific periodontal pathogens were associated with prevalent CHD. When stratified for smoking, titers *to Tr. denticola, Prevotella intermedia, Capnocytophaga ochracea*, and *Veillonella parvula* conferred significant odds for CHD in ever smokers, while titers to *Prevotella nigrescens* and *A. actinomycetemcomitans* conferred significant odds for CHD in never smokers. In a retrospective follow-up study of a Finnish cohort of 63 men who were free of CHD at entry, but who developed fatal or non-fatal MI during a subsequent 10-year period, and of 63 age-matched controls, Pussinen *et al.* (2004) analyzed serum samples with respect to IgG and IgA antibodies to different strains of *A. actinomycetemcomitans* and *P. gingivalis*. In logistic regression models adjusted for traditional CHD risk factors such as smoking, serum cholesterol, blood pressure, BMI, and diabetes, increasing serum IgA titers to *P. gingivalis* resulted in significantly increasing odds for MI.

Among the group of studies focusing on the potential association of periodontitis and stroke, an early case–control study by Syrjanen *et al.* (1989) compared the level of dental disease in 40 patients who had suffered a cerebrovascular accident with 40 randomly selected community controls, matched for gender and age, and reported that severe chronic dental infection was associated with cerebral infarction in males under 50 years of age. In another case–control study (Grau *et al.* 1997), multiple logistic regression adjusted for age, social status, and a number of established vascular risk factors revealed that poor dental status was independently associated with cerebrovascular ischemia (OR 2.6, 95% CI 1.18–5.7).

Obviously, critical information on the role of periodontal infection as risk factor for atherosclerotic vascular disease and its sequels should be derived from intervention trials, ideally from randomized, placebo-controlled clinical trials. Unfortunately the design and conduct of such studies is particularly challenging, primarily due to the long time between exposure and manifestation of CVD, the relatively low incidence of CVD-related clinical events necessitating the inclusion of large subject samples, and ethical considerations related to the follow-up of untreated periodontal disease over prolonged time periods. Therefore, intervention trials conducted to date have been limited to the study of the effects of periodontal therapy on surrogate markers of risk for CVD or on pathways related to the pathobiology of the disease. For example, D'Aiuto *et al.* (2004) reported on 94 systemically healthy patients with generalized severe periodontitis who received non-surgical therapy and extractions. In logistic regression analysis, the reduction of CRP-levels 6 months after periodontal therapy was significantly associated with the number of extracted teeth (OR 1.4, CI 1.1–1.8) and a greater than the median probing depth reduction in pockets initially ≥5 mm (OR 4.7, CI 1.4–15.8). In subsequent publications (D'Aiuto *et al.* 2005; D'Aiuto & Tonetti 2005), non-surgical periodontal therapy with and without adjunctive local antibiotics, resulted in a reduction of median CRP-levels at 2 months, with a more pronounced effect in non-smokers than in smokers. Circulating IL-6 levels were significantly reduced only in the group that received adjunctive local antibiotics (intensive treatment), but no significant changes were observed in LDL and HDL cholesterol and triglyceride levels. The same group (D'Aiuto *et al.* 2006) recently reported 6-month data on the effect of standard vs. intensive therapy. In comparison to baseline levels, a significant reduction in white blood cell counts, CRP levels, IL-6 levels, total cholesterol, LDL, and systolic blood pressure was observed in the intensive treatment group, whereas an increase in HDL levels was observed in the standard treatment group. Similarly, Taylor *et al.* (2006) reported that patients undergoing full-mouth extractions who had at least 2 teeth with probing depths ≥6 mm, attachment loss and bleeding on probing showed a significant reduction in CRP levels from 2.5 mg/L to 1.8 mg/L, and this effect was more pronounced in non-smokers.

Finally, another set of studies has focused on the effects of periodontal therapy on endothelial dysfunction, a biomarker of vascular disease (Verma *et al.* 2003). Endothelial dysfunction is defined as the reduced vasodilator capability of peripheral blood vessels and is assessed by measuring the difference in the diameter of a peripheral artery prior to and after reactive hyperemia induced through occlusion of blood flow (Celermajer *et al.* 1992). Endothelial dysfunction was more pronounced in periodontitis subjects than periodontally healthy controls in two studies (Amar *et al.* 2003; Mercanoglu *et al.* 2004). Three intervention studies reporting positive effects of periodontal therapy on endothelial dysfunction are available so far: one using non-surgical periodontal therapy (Mercanoglu *et al.* 2004), one using adjunctive systemic antibiotics (Seinost *et al.* 2005), and a third using a comprehensive "full-mouth disinfection" protocol (Elter *et al.* 2006).

Taken together, the studies above strongly suggest a biologically plausible association between periodontal infections and the pathogenesis of atherosclerotic cardiovascular disease. Obviously studies that have failed to document such an association or that point to a possibility of a more complex, conditional relationship exist as well (Hujoel *et al.* 2000, 2002b; Mattila *et al.* 2000). In particular, it has been suggested that the positive associations in epidemio-logic studies between periodontal infections and atherosclerotic cardiovascular disease may be attributed to residual confounding due to insufficient accounting for the effects of smoking (Hujoel *et al.* 2002a; Spiekerman *et al.* 2003) or may be entirely spurious (Hujoel *et al.* 2003, 2006). While such a possibility is hard to rule out, it appears unreasonable to dismiss as an artifact the entire body of supportive data stemming from diverse investigational approaches (epidemiological, experimental, mechanistic, and intervention studies).

Pregnancy complications

Preterm infants are born prior to completion of 37 weeks of gestation. An estimated 11% (Goldenberg & Rouse 1998) of pregnancies end in preterm birth (PTB), and this rate appears to be on the rise in several developed countries, despite significant advances in obstetric medicine and improvements in prenatal care utilization. Of particular interest are the very preterm infants, born prior to 32 gestational weeks, the majority of which require neonatal intensive care due to their increased perinatal mortality, primarily due to impaired lung development and function. Still, the overall contribution of PTB to infant mortality and morbidity is substantial and includes a number of acute and chronic disorders including respiratory distress syndrome, cerebral palsy, pathologic heart conditions, epilepsy, blindness, and severe learning disabilities (McCormick 1985; Veen *et al.* 1991).

Preterm infants often weigh lower at birth (<2500 g), and low birth weight has been used as a surrogate for prematurity in cases where the exact gestational age at birth is difficult to assess. Birth weight is further classified as very low (<1500 g) or moderately low (between 1500 g and 2500 g). An additional term used is small for gestational age, defined as birth weight within the 10th percentile of normal weight at a particular gestational age. The condition may, thus, affect even full term infants due to intra-uterine growth retardation (Ashworth 1998).

A number of risk factors for preterm birth has been identified (Goldenberg *et al.* 2000). These include young maternal age (Wessel *et al.* 1996; Lao & Ho 1997; Scholl *et al.* 1988), multiple gestation (Lee *et al.* 2006), small weight gain during pregnancy (Honest *et al.* 2005), cervical incompetence (Althuisius & Dekker 2005), smoking, alcohol and drugs of abuse (Myles *et al.* 1998), black race (Kleinman & Kessel 1987; David & Collins 1997), and a number of maternal infections (uterine track infections, bacterial vaginosis, chorioamnionitis) (Romero *et al.* 2001). Obstetric history of PTB is a robust marker of future PTB (Mutale *et al.* 1991). Importantly, approximately 50% of the variance in the incidence of preterm birth remains unexplained (Holbrook *et al.* 1989).

Despite the established role of genito-urinary tract infections in the pathobiology of preterm birth, women with preterm labor do not invariably present with positive amniotic fluid cultures (Romero *et al.* 1988), leading to the hypothesis that PTB may be indirectly mediated through *distant* infections resulting in translocation of bacteria, bacterial vesicles or LPS in the systemic circulation. The possibility that periodontal infections may constitute such maternal infections that adversely influence birth outcome was raised for the first time in the late 1980s (McGregor *et al.* 1988). Transient bacteremias occur commonly in subjects with inflamed gingiva (Ness & Perkins 1980; Kinane *et al.* 2005; Forner *et al.* 2006) and may conceivably reach the placental tissues, providing the inflammatory impetus for labor induction (Offenbacher *et al.* 1998). An interesting publication in this context by Hill (1998) reported that amniotic fluid cultures from women with vaginosis rarely contained bacteria common to the vaginal tract but frequently harbored fusobacteria of oral origin, i.e. common constituents of the periodontal microbiota. Thus, these authors proposed that oral bacteria may reach amniotic fluids and influence maternal fetal tissues via hematogenous spread, resulting in a chorioamniotic challenge. In line with these observations, experimental evidence on the role of oral infections on pregnancy outcomes was first provided is a series of pioneering studies by Collins *et al.* (1994a,b), who demonstrated that injection of *P. gingivalis* in the pregnant hamster resulted in intrauterine growth retardation, smaller fetuses, and an increase in pro-inflammatory mediators such as IL-1beta and PGE_2 in the amniotic fluid. Subsequent studies in pregnant mice (Lin *et al.* 2003a,b) and rabbits (Boggess *et al.* 2005) confirmed and expanded these observations to include experimental infections by *Campylobacter rectus*.

The accumulating body of evidence available from human studies investigating a potential link between oral infections and adverse pregnancy outcomes were recently reviewed (Bobetsis *et al.* 2006; Xiong *et al.* 2006). In an early case–control study, Offenbacher *et al.* (1996) examined 124 mothers, of whom 93 ("cases") gave birth to children with birth weight of less than 2500 g, prior to 37 weeks of gestation. "Controls" were 46 mothers who delivered at term infants of normal birth weight. Assessments included a broad range of known obstetric risk factors, such as tobacco use, drug use, alcohol consumption, level of prenatal care, parity, genitourinary infections, and nutrition. The data showed a small, albeit statistically significant difference, in attachment loss between cases and controls (3.1 vs 2.8 mm). Multivariate logistic regression models, controlling for other risk factors and covariates, demonstrated that periodontitis, defined as ≥60% of all sites with attachment loss of ≥3 mm, conferred adjusted ORs of 7.9 for preterm, low birthweight babies. Following this report, several additional case–control studies were published, most of which reported a positive association between periodontitis and adverse pregnancy outcomes

(Offenbacher *et al.* 1996; Dasanayake *et al.* 2001; Canakci *et al.* 2004; Goepfert *et al.* 2004; Mokeem *et al.* 2004; Radnai *et al.* 2004), although a number of studies that failed to document an association were published as well (Davenport *et al.* 2002; Buduneli *et al.* 2005; Moore *et al.* 2005).

Non-uniform data were also generated by cohort studies, i.e. studies that evaluated the periodontal status of pregnant women prior to completion of the second trimester and compared prospectively the incidence of adverse pregnancy outcomes in women with and without periodontitis. In the first prospective cohort study reporting a positive relationship between periodontitis and prematurity, Jeffcoat *et al.* (2001) assessed the periodontal conditions of 1313 primarily African American pregnant women at 21–24 weeks of gestation and reported that for women with generalized periodontitis, defined as ≥90% of all sites with attachment loss of 3 mm or more, adjusted odds ratios were 4.45 for delivery prior to 37 weeks' gestational age, 5.28 for delivery before 35 weeks' gestational age, and 7.07 for delivery before 32 weeks' gestational age. Corroborating positive data were reported by additional cohorts in the US (Offenbacher *et al.* 2001), Chile (Lopez *et al.* 2002a), and Switzerland (Dortbudak *et al.* 2005). Similar positive associations were reported for very preterm delivery (Offenbacher *et al.* 2006), small-for gestational-age infant (Boggess *et al.* 2006a), pre-eclampsia (Boggess *et al.* 2003), fetal exposure to oral pathogens, assessed by the presence of IgM antibodies in the fetal cord blood (Madianos *et al.* 2001), and with ante-partum vaginal bleeding and risk for premature delivery prior to 35 gestational weeks (Boggess *et al.* 2006b). In contrast, four cohort studies (Romero *et al.* 2002; Holbrook *et al.* 2004; Moore *et al.* 2004; Rajapakse *et al.* 2005) failed to document such an association. Of particular interest is the study by Moore *et al.* (2004) who reported data on 3738 women recruited on attending an ultrasound scan at approximately 12 weeks of pregnancy. Regression analysis indicated no significant relationships between the severity of periodontal disease and either preterm birth or low birth weight, although a positive correlation was reported between poorer periodontal health and late miscarriage.

Five intervention studies on the effects of periodontal treatment on pregnancy outcomes have been published to date. The first (Mitchell-Lewis *et al.* 2001) examined a cohort of 213 young, minority, pregnant, and post-partum women with respect to clinical periodontal status and analyzed the available birth outcome data for 164 women, 74 of whom received oral prophylaxis during pregnancy, and 90 who received no prenatal periodontal treatment. In this cohort with particularly high incidence of preterm low birth weight (PLMW of 16.5%), no differences in clinical periodontal status were observed between PLBW cases and women with normal birth outcomes. However, PLBW mothers harbored statistically significantly higher levels of *T. forsythia* and *C. rectus*, and consistently elevated counts for a number of species examined. Interestingly, PLBW occurred in 18.9% of the women who did not receive periodontal intervention, and in 13.5% (ten cases) of those who received such therapy, reflecting a substantial, although statistically non-significant, incidence reduction of approximately 30%. However, the small sample size in combination with the fact that the participants were not randomly assigned into the two treatment groups were important shortcomings of the study design.

In a pilot intervention study, Jeffcoat *et al.* (2003) recruited 366 women with periodontitis between 21 and 25 weeks' gestation and randomized them to one of three treatment groups with stratification on previous spontaneous preterm birth prior to 35 weeks, BMI <19.8, or bacterial vaginosis assessed by Gram stain of vaginal smear samples. The treatment arms included a group that received supragingival dental prophylaxis and a placebo capsule; a group that received scaling and root planing (SRP) plus a placebo capsule; and a group that received SRP and systemic metronidazole 250 mg t.i.d. for 1 week. An additional group of 723 pregnant women who enrolled in a prospective study served as an untreated reference group. The results revealed that the rate of PTB before 35 gestational weeks was 4.9% in the prophylaxis group, 3.3% in the SRP plus metronidazole group, and 0.8% in the SRP plus placebo group. The corresponding PTB rate in the reference group was 6.3%. Although the difference between the prophylaxis and the SRP plus placebo group approached, but did not reach, statistical significance, the study suggested that periodontal therapy has the potential to reduce PTB, but that adjunctive systemic metronidazole did not enhance the pregnancy outcome. The latter observation is in line with the findings of a multicenter trial that suggested that systemic metronidazole used in the treatment of asymptomatic bacterial vaginosis does not reduce the occurrence of preterm delivery (Carey *et al.* 2000).

In contrast, impressive positive findings were reported from two randomized clinical trials conducted in Chile (Lopez *et al.* 2002b, 2005). In the first trial (Lopez *et al.* 2002b), 400 pregnant women with periodontal disease were enrolled and randomly assigned to either a treatment group which received periodontal therapy before 28 weeks of gestation or to a control group which received treatment after delivery. The incidence of PLBW (i.e. gestational age at birth <37 weeks or birth weight <2500 g) among the 351 women who completed the trial was 1.8% in the treatment group and 10.1% in the control group, resulting in an OR of 5.5 (95% CI 1.6–18.2, p = 0.001). In a multi-variate logistic regression model accounting for previous PLBW, frequency of prenatal visits, and maternal low weight gain, periodontitis remained the strongest factor with OR of 4.7 (95% CI 1.3–17.1). Of note in this trial is the relatively high drop-out rate (12.2%), as well as the fact that approximately one

fifth of the women in the treatment group received adjunctive systemic antibiotics (amoxicillin and metronidazole) for the control of aggressive periodontitis. The second trial from the same group (Lopez *et al.* 2005) examined the effect of treatment of gingivitis on adverse pregnancy outcomes. Out of 870 pregnant women with gingivitis enrolled, two thirds received plaque control, scaling, and daily rinsing with 0.12% clorhexidine prior to 28 weeks of gestation, followed by maintenance every 2–3 weeks until delivery (treatment group) while a control group received therapy after delivery. With 834 women completing the trial, the incidence of PTLBW was 2.1% in the treatment group and 6.7% in the control group (OR 3.3, 95% CI 1.6–6.8; p = 0.0009).

Finally, a multicentre randomized, blinded, controlled trial examined the effect of non-surgical periodontal treatment on preterm birth (Michalowicz *et al.* 2006). After screening a total of 3504 women for a minimum extent and severity of periodontitis to satisfy the study's enrollment criteria, 823 women were randomly assigned to either receive scaling and root planing before 21 weeks (413 women) or after delivery (410 women). Participants in the treatment group underwent additional recall visits. The findings (Fig. 7-5) showed that preterm birth before 37 gestational weeks occurred in 49 of 407 women (12.0%) in the treatment group and in 52 of 405 women (12.8%) in the control group (hazard ratio for treatment group vs. control group, 0.93; p = 0.70; 95% CI 0.63–1.37). There were no significant differences between the treatment and control groups in birth weight or in the rate of delivery of infants that were small for gestational age. However, almost three times as many spontaneous abortions or stillbirths occurred in the control group than in the treatment group (14 vs 5, p = 0.04). Thus, this study failed to document a positive effect of periodontal treatment on rates of preterm birth, low birth weight, or fetal growth restriction, although it demonstrated that periodontal treatment of pregnant women is safe.

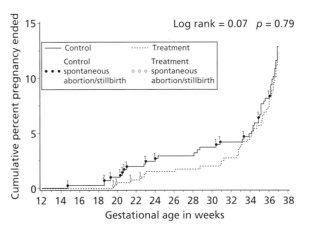

Fig. 7-5 Kaplan–Meier curve for the cumulative incidence of pregnancies ending before 37 weeks in the Obstetrics and Periodontal Therapy study. Adapted from Michalowicz *et al.* 2006, reproduced with permission. Copyright © 2006 Massachusetts Medical Society.

The observed discrepancy in spontaneous abortions and stillbirths between the two groups observed in the above study is clearly intriguing. An effect of periodontal treatment on early adverse outcomes is plausible in light of observational studies that suggest that periodontitis is more strongly associated with late miscarriage (Moore *et al.* 2004), stillbirth, and early spontaneous preterm birth rather than with preterm birth in general. It was suggested therefore (Goldenberg & Culhane 2006) that future studies may preferentially focus on late miscarriage, early stillbirth, and preterm birth prior to 32 weeks, rather than on all preterm births prior to 37 weeks. Additional issues to be addressed in future studies relate to the timing and the intensity of the periodontal intervention, as well as the possibility that such effects may vary with race/ethnicity. Currently, there are at least three randomized controlled trials underway, all of which involve larger subject samples that the study by Michalowicz *et al.* (2006), that will contribute with more definitive answers on whether periodontal treatment has a role in reducing the rate of adverse pregnancy outcomes.

Diabetes mellitus

The role of diabetes as a risk factor for periodontitis has been discussed above; however, limited data seem to suggest that an inverse relationship may also be present. In line with the concept that infections may contribute to impaired metabolic control of diabetes (Rayfield *et al.* 1982; Lang 1992; Ling *et al.* 1994), studies of both type 1 (Thorstensson *et al.* 1996) and type 2 (Taylor *et al.* 1996) diabetic subjects have indicated that periodontal infections may also be detrimental in this context. The former study involved 39 diabetic subjects with severe periodontitis and an equal number of diabetic subjects with gingivitis or mild periodontitis. Both groups had a median duration of diabetes of 25 years. Over a median follow-up period of 6 years, significantly higher prevalence of proteinuria and cardiovascular complications was observed in the severe periodontitis group. A 2-year follow-up study of 90 subjects with type 2 diabetes with good to moderate metabolic control revealed that severe periodontitis at baseline was associated with increased risk for poor glycemic control.

A limited number of studies has examined the effect of treatment of periodontitis on diabetic metabolic control, as reflected by levels of glycated hemoglobin A1c (HbA1c) or plasma glucose. Interestingly, all studies that solely included mechanical periodontal therapy (Seppälä *et al.* 1993; Aldridge *et al.* 1995; Smith *et al.* 1996; Grossi *et al.* 1997a; Christgau *et al.* 1998) but one (Stewart *et al.* 2001) reveal no effect on diabetes metabolic control, regardless of periodontal disease severity, baseline level of metabolic control, type and duration of diabetes. Interestingly, Stewart *et al.* (2001) followed 72 patients with type 2 diabetes for 18 months, half of whom received mechanical

periodontal therapy, but reported that both the periodontally treated and the untreated group showed statistically significant decreases in HbA1c levels (17.1% vs. 6.7%, respectively). In contrast, studies including antibiotics as an adjunct to mechanical therapy (Williams & Mahan 1960; Grossi *et al.* 1997a; Miller *et al.* 1992) reported a limited, short-term improvement in metabolic control. For example, Grossi *et al.* (1997a) reported a 10% improvement in glycated hemoglobin (HbA1c) at 3 months after the completion of non-surgical periodontal therapy combined with adjunctive systemic doxycycline, although this effect was not sustainable at later time points. Interestingly, no such effect on HbA1c was observed in subjects that did not receive adjunctive antibiotic therapy. Rodrigues *et al.* (2003) randomly assigned 30 type 2 patients to two treatment groups, one group receiving non-surgical periodontal therapy with amoxicillin/clavulanic acid and the other receiving only mechanical therapy. At 3 months, HbA1c levels were reduced in both groups, but the reduction was statistically significant only in the group that received scaling and root planing alone. Nevertheless, a recent meta-analysis of ten intervention studies aiming at the quantification of the effects of periodontal treatment on HbA1c level among diabetic patients, including a total of 456 patients, revealed a non-statistically significant decrease in actual HbA1c levels (Janket *et al.* 2005). Indeed, the weighted average decrease in actual HbA1c level was found to be 0.38% for all studies, 0.66% when restricted to type 2 diabetic patients, and 0.71% if adjunctive antibiotics were administered. Clearly, further studies are needed to clarify the conditions under which periodontal treatment can contribute to improved metabolic control, especially in type 1 diabetes.

Concluding remarks

One of the issues related to the descriptive epidemiology of periodontal infections that is still under debate is whether their worldwide prevalence has been decreasing over the last decades. Unfortunately, the data do not allow a clear answer for a number of reasons. First, no universal conclusion is possible, since the prevalence of periodontal disease appears to vary with race and geographic region. Second, the quality of the data available from the developing and the developed countries is clearly not comparable. While some well conducted epidemiologic surveys that provide detailed information have been carried out in a number of countries, the majority of the studies in the developing world have used the CPITN system, which produced data of inadequate detail. Moreover, studies using the exact same methodology to evaluate random samples drawn from the same population over time are sparse. Among the few exceptions is a series of studies from Sweden (Hugoson *et al.* 1998b, 1992, 2005) that documented, by clinical and radiographic means, the frequency

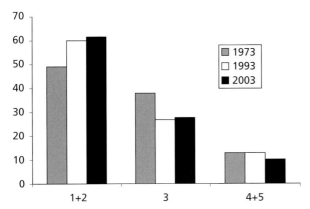

Fig. 7-6 Frequency distribution of subjects with healthy periodontal conditions or gingivitis (groups 1 + 2), moderate periodontitis (group 3), and advanced and severe periodontal disease (groups 4 + 5), in a Swedish cohort in 1973, 1993, and 2003. For definitions see text. Adapted after personal communication with Dr. Anders Hugoson, based on data by Hugoson *et al.* (1992, 1998, 2006).

distribution of various levels of severity of periodontitis in four cross-sectional studies over a 30-year period (in 1973, 1983, 1993, and 2003). In these studies, subjects were grouped according to the severity of their periodontal conditions in five groups: groups 1 and 2 included subjects who were periodontally healthy or only had gingivitis, group 3 included subjects with moderate periodontitis, i.e. whose loss of periodontal tissues support did not extend beyond one third of the root length, while groups 4 and 5 included subjects with more severe destructive disease. As shown in Fig. 7-6, a clear increase in the frequency of subjects in groups 1 and 2 was noted over the 30-year period, from 49% in 1973 to 60% in 1993 to almost 62% in 2003. This increase occurred primarily at the expense of group 3 which declined from 38% in 1973 to 27% in 1993 and apparently reached a plateau at 28% in 2003. Nevertheless, the frequency of subjects in groups 4 and 5 was virtually stable over the 30-year period: 13% in 1973, 13% in 1993 and 10.5% in 2003. Based on these data derived from a population with arguably the best access to and utilization of oral health care in the world, we may conclude that the fraction of the population which is apparently most susceptible to severe periodontitis is apparently not declining in frequency. Instead, the main beneficiaries of the improved oral health awareness, access to care and increased utilization of therapeutic resources that occurred over the last decades appear to be the individuals with moderate levels of periodontitis whose prevalence is clearly lower.

What was also well documented in these and other studies is that the rate of edentulism has decreased substantially over the past 30 years, with elderly groups retaining their natural dentition and higher mean numbers of teeth than their counterparts a generation ago. As a consequence, this fact *per se* should contribute to an increased prevalence of periodontal

disease in older age cohorts, since retained teeth in the elderly are more likely to experience substantial cumulative attachment loss which forms the basis of the assessment of prevalence (Douglass & Fox 1993). It has been argued, however, that such a potential increase, may not necessarily result in increased need for periodontal therapy (Oliver *et al.* 1989). Additional research is clearly required to further elucidate these issues, and an adequate and consistent epidemiological methodology is essential for generating valid comparative data. On the other hand, the need for description of prevalence and incidence of periodontal diseases in every conceivable population has been questioned (Baelum & Papapanou 1996), although such information may be of value for local oral health planners. Instead, the principle task of future epidemiological research is arguably the identification of risk factors for disease development, laying the ground for an enhanced understanding of the pathobiology of periodontitis. Although several risk factors have already been established and a wide array of disease markers has been recognized, the impact of the intervention with such factors on the state of periodontal health on a population level has yet to be documented. To assess the magnitude of the clinical benefit achieved by such modulation, prospective, long-term epidemiological surveys have to be conducted.

Somewhat provocatively, it has been stated that modern science has a tendency to re-discover issues brought up a long time back and (then) rejected. One cannot help bringing the "focal infection" theory in mind, when encountering the emerging plethora of publications dealing with the role of periodontal infections as risk factors for systemic disease. Although the proposed associations appear to be biologically plausible, at this stage, we cannot draw any definitive conclusions on whether these associations are in fact causal, and if so, on the magnitude of their biological effects. Nevertheless, these studies underscore that the oral cavity is an integral part of the human body, and that systemic health must encompass oral, and periodontal, health as well. Last but certainly not least, these studies have provided a unique opportunity for us oral health researchers to expand our investigative sphere, interact fruitfully with our colleagues in medicine, and acquire more knowledge. Irrespective of the definitive conclusions of these research efforts, its by-products may prove to be just as important as the elucidation of the research task *per se*.

Acknowledgments

Some of the tables included in this chapter are partly based on the publication of Papapanou (1986), by permission of the American Academy of Periodontology. Parts of the text on "Risk factors for periodontitis" have been adapted from the review by Borrell and Papapanou (2005).

References

Ah, M.K., Johnson, G.K., Kaldahl, W.B., Patil, K.D. & Kalkwarf, K.L. (1994). The effect of smoking on the response to peri-odontal therapy. *Journal of Clinical Periodontology* **21**, 91–97.

Ainamo, J. (1989). Epidemiology of periodontal disease. In: *Textbook of Clinical Periodontology*. ed. Lindhe, J., 2nd edn, pp. 70–91. Copenhagen: Munksgaard.

Ainamo, J., Barmes, D., Beagrie, G., Cutress, T., Martin, J. & Sardo-Infirri, J. (1982). Development of the World Health Organization (WHO) community periodontal index of treatment needs (CPITN). *International Dental Journal* **32**, 281–291.

Ainamo, J. & Bay, I. (1975). Problems and proposals for record-ing gingivitis and plaque. *International Dental Journal* **25**, 229–235.

Ajwani, S., Mattila, K.J., Tilvis, R.S. & Ainamo, A. (2003). Peri-odontal disease and mortality in an aged population. *Special Care in Dentistry* **23**, 125–130.

Al-Zahrani, M.S., Bissada, N.F. & Borawskit, E.A. (2003). Obesity and periodontal disease in young, middle-aged, and older adults. *Journal of Periodontology* **74**, 610–615.

Albandar, J.M. (2002a). Global risk factors and risk indicators for periodontal diseases. *Periodontology 2000* **29**, 177–206.

Albandar, J.M. (2002b). Periodontal diseases in North America. *Periodontology 2000* **29**, 31–69.

Albandar, J.M., Brunelle, J.A. & Kingman, A. (1999). Destruc-tive periodontal disease in adults 30 years of age and older in the United States, 1988–1994. *Journal of Periodontology* **70**, 13–29.

Albandar, J.M. & Kingman, A. (1999). Gingival recession, gin-gival bleeding, and dental calculus in adults 30 years of age and older in the United States, 1988–1994. *Journal of Peri-odontology* **70**, 30–43.

Albandar, J.M., Streckfus, C.F., Adesanya, M.R. & Winn, D.M. (2000). Cigar, pipe, and cigarette smoking as risk factors for periodontal disease and tooth loss. *Journal of Periodontology* **71**, 1874–1881.

Aldridge, J.P., Lester, V., Watts, T.L., Collins, A., Viberti, G. & Wilson, R.F. (1995). Single-blind studies of the effects of improved periodontal health on metabolic control in type 1 diabetes mellitus. *Journal of Clinical Periodontology* **22**, 271–275.

Aleksejuniene, J., Holst, D., Eriksen, H.M. & Gjermo, P. (2002). Psychosocial stress, lifestyle and periodontal health. *Journal of Clinical Periodontology* **29**, 326–335.

Ali, R.W., Bakken, V., Nilsen, R. & Skaug, N. (1994). Compara-tive detection frequency of 6 putative periodontal patho-gens in Sudanese and Norwegian adult periodontitis patients. *Journal of Periodontology* **65**, 1046–1052.

Alpagot, T., Wolff, L.F., Smith, Q.T. & Tran, S.D. (1996). Risk indicators for periodontal disease in a racially diverse urban population. *Journal of Clinical Periodontology* **23**, 982–988.

Althuisius, S.M. & Dekker, G.A. (2005). A five century evolu-tion of cervical incompetence as a clinical entity. *Current Pharmaceutical Design* **11**, 687–697.

Amar, S., Gokce, N., Morgan, S., Loukideli, M., Van Dyke, T.E. & Vita, J.A. (2003). Periodontal disease is associated with brachial artery endothelial dysfunction and systemic inflam-mation. *Arteriosclerosis, Thrombosis, and Vascular Biology* **23**, 1245–1249.

Anagnou Vareltzides, A., Diamanti Kipioti, A., Afentoulidis, N., Moraitaki Tsami, A., Lindhe, J., Mitsis, F. & Papapanou, P.N. (1996). A clinical survey of periodontal conditions in Greece. *Journal of Clinical Periodontology* **23**, 758–763.

Anon (1999) 1999 International Workshop for a Classification of Periodontal Diseases and Conditions. eds. Caton, J.G. & Armitage, G.C. (Vol. 4), pp. 1–112. Oak Brook, Illinois: Annals of Periodontology.

Anon (2000) Obesity related to periodontal disease. *Journal of the American Dental Association* **131**, 729.

Anusaksathien, O., Sukboon, A., Sitthiphong, P. & Teanpaisan, R. (2003). Distribution of interleukin-1beta(+3954) and IL-1alpha(-889) genetic variations in a Thai population group. *Journal of Periodontology* **74**, 1796–1802.

Arbes, S.J., Jr., Agustsdottir, H. & Slade, G.D. (2001). Environ-mental tobacco smoke and periodontal disease in the United States. *American Journal of Public Health* **91**, 253–257.

Armitage, G.C., Wu, Y., Wang, H.Y., Sorrell, J., di Giovine, F.S. & Duff, G.W. (2000). Low prevalence of a periodontitis-associated interleukin-1 composite genotype in individuals of Chinese heritage. *Journal of Periodontology* **71**, 164–171.

Ashworth, A. (1998). Effects of intrauterine growth retardation on mortality and morbidity in infants and young children. *European Journal of Clinical Nutrition* **52** Suppl 1, S34–41; discussion S41–32.

Axelsson, P., Paulander, J. & Lindhe, J. (1998). Relationship between smoking and dental status in 35-, 50-, 65-, and 75-year-old individuals. *Journal of Clinical Periodontology* **25**, 297–305.

Baelum, V., Chen, X., Manji, F., Luan, W.M. & Fejerskov, O. (1996). Profiles of destructive periodontal disease in differ-ent populations. *Journal of Periodontal Research* **31**, 17–26.

Baelum, V., Fejerskov, O. & Karring, T. (1986). Oral hygiene, gingivitis and periodontal breakdown in adult Tanzanians. *Journal of Periodontal Research* **21**, 221–232.

Baelum, V., Fejerskov, O. & Manji, F. (1988a). Periodontal dis-eases in adult Kenyans. *Journal of Clinical Periodontology* **15**, 445–452.

Baelum, V., Fejerskov, O., Manji, F. & Wanzala, P. (1993a). Influence of CPITN partial recordings on estimates of prev-alence and severity of various periodontal conditions in adults. *Community Dentistry and Oral Epidemiology* **21**, 354–359.

Baelum, V., Luan, W.-M., Fejerskov, O. & Xia, C. (1988b). Tooth mortality and periodontal conditions in 60–80-year-old Chinese. *Scandinavian Journal of Dental Research* **96**, 99–107.

Baelum, V., Manji, F., Fejerskov, O. & Wanzala, P. (1993b). Validity of CPITN's assumptions of hierarchical occurrence of periodontal conditions in a Kenyan population aged 15–65 years. *Community Dentistry and Oral Epidemiology* **21**, 347–353.

Baelum, V., Manji, F., Wanzala, P. & Fejerskov, O. (1995). Rela-tionship between CPITN and periodontal attachment loss findings in an adult population. *Journal of Clinical Periodon-tology* **22**, 146–152.

Baelum, V. & Papapanou, P.N. (1996). CPITN and the epide-miology of periodontal disease. *Community Dentistry and Oral Epidemiology* **24**, 367–368.

Bagramian, R.A., Farghaly, M.M., Lopatin, D., Sowers, M., Syed, S.A. & Pomerville, J.L. (1993). Periodontal disease in an Amish population. *Journal of Clinical Periodontology* **20**, 269–272.

Bailit, H.L., Braun, R., Maryniuk, G.A. & Camp, P. (1987). Is periodontal disease the primary cause of tooth extraction in adults? *Journal of the American Dental Association* **114**, 40–45.

Barath, P., Fishbein, M.C., Cao, J., Berenson, J., Helfant, R.H. & Forrester, J.S. (1990a). Detection and localization of tumor necrosis factor in human atheroma. *American Journal of Car-diology* **65**, 297–302.

Barath, P., Fishbein, M.C., Cao, J., Berenson, J., Helfant, R.H. & Forrester, J.S. (1990b). Tumor necrosis factor gene expres-sion in human vascular intimal smooth muscle cells detected by in situ hybridization. *American Journal of Pathology* **137**, 503–509.

Barr, C., Lopez, M.R. & Rua Dobles, A. (1992). Periodontal changes by HIV serostatus in a cohort of homosexual and bisexual men. *Journal of Clinical Periodontology* **19**, 794–801.

Beck, J., Garcia, R., Heiss, G., Vokonas, P.S. & Offenbacher, S. (1996). Periodontal disease and cardiovascular disease. *Journal of Periodontology* **67**, 1123–1137.

Beck, J.D. (1994). Methods of assessing risk for periodontitis and developing multifactorial models. *Journal of Periodontology* **65**, 468–478.

Beck, J.D., Cusmano, L., Green Helms, W., Koch, G.G. & Offenbacher, S. (1997). A 5-year study of attachment loss in community-dwelling older adults: incidence density. *Journal of Periodontal Research* **32**, 506–515.

Beck, J.D., Eke, P., Heiss, G., Madianos, P., Couper, D., Lin, D., Moss, K., Elter, J. & Offenbacher, S. (2005a). Periodontal disease and coronary heart disease: a reappraisal of the exposure. *Circulation* **112**, 19–24.

Beck, J.D., Eke, P., Lin, D., Madianos, P., Couper, D., Moss, K., Elter, J., Heiss, G. & Offenbacher, S. (2005b). Associations between IgG antibody to oral organisms and carotid intima-medial thickness in community-dwelling adults. *Atherosclerosis* **183**, 342–348.

Beck, J.D., Elter, J.R., Heiss, G., Couper, D., Mauriello, S.M. & Offenbacher, S. (2001). Relationship of Periodontal Disease to Carotid Artery Intima-Media Wall Thickness: The Atherosclerosis Risk in Communities (ARIC) Study. *Arteriosclerosis, Thrombosis, and Vascular Biology* **21**, 1816–1822.

Beck, J.D., Koch, G.G. & Offenbacher, S. (1995). Incidence of attachment loss over 3 years in older adults – new and progressiong lesions. *Community Dentistry and Oral Epidemiology* **23**, 291–296.

Beck, J.D., Koch, G.G., Rozier, R.G. & Tudor, G.E. (1990). Prevalence and risk indicators for periodontal attachment loss in a population of older community-dwelling blacks and whites. *Journal of Periodontology* **61**, 521–528.

Ben Yehouda, A., Shifer, A., Katz, J., Kusner, W., Machtei, E. & Shmerling, M. (1991). Prevalence of juvenile periodontitis in Israeli military recruits as determined by panoramic radiographs. *Community Dentistry and Oral Epidemiology* **19**, 359–360.

Benigeri, M., Brodeur, J.M., Payette, M., Charbonneau, A. & Ismail, A.I. (2000). Community periodontal index of treatment needs and prevalence of periodontal conditions. *Journal of Clinical Periodontology* **27**, 308–312.

Benn, D.K. (1990). A review of the reliability of radiographic measurements in estimating alveolar bone changes. *Journal of Clinical Periodontology* **17**, 14–21.

Berglundh, T., Donati, M., Hahn-Zoric, M., Hanson, L.A. & Padyukov, L. (2003). Association of the -1087 IL 10 gene polymorphism with severe chronic periodontitis in Swedish Caucasians. *Journal of Clinical Periodontology* **30**, 249–254.

Bergström, J. (1989). Cigarette smoking as risk factor in chronic periodontal disease. *Community Dentistry and Oral Epidemiology* **17**, 245–247.

Bergström, J. & Eliasson, S. (1989). Prevalence of chronic periodontal disease using probing depth as a diagnostic test. *Journal of Clinical Periodontology* **16**, 588–592.

Bergström, J., Eliasson, S. & Dock, J. (2000a). A 10-year prospective study of tobacco smoking and periodontal health. *Journal of Periodontology* **71**, 1338–1347.

Bergström, J., Eliasson, S. & Dock, J. (2000b). Exposure to tobacco smoking and periodontal health. *Journal of Clinical Periodontology* **27**, 61–68.

Bhat, M. (1991). Periodontal health of 14–17-year-old US schoolchildren. *Journal of Public Health Dentistry* **51**, 5–11.

Bobetsis, Y.A., Barros, S.P. & Offenbacher, S. (2006). Exploring the relationship between periodontal disease and pregnancy complications. *Journal of the American Dental Association* **137** (Suppl 2), 7S–13S.

Boggess, K.A., Beck, J.D., Murtha, A.P., Moss, K. & Offenbacher, S. (2006a). Maternal periodontal disease in early pregnancy and risk for a small-for-gestational-age infant. *American Journal of Obstetrics and Gynecology* **194**, 1316–1322.

Boggess, K.A., Lieff, S., Murtha, A.P., Moss, K., Beck, J. & Offenbacher, S. (2003). Maternal periodontal disease is associated with an increased risk for preeclampsia. *Obstetrics and Gynecology* **101**, 227–231.

Boggess, K.A., Madianos, P.N., Preisser, J.S., Moise, K.J., Jr. & Offenbacher, S. (2005). Chronic maternal and fetal Porphyromonas gingivalis exposure during pregnancy in rabbits. *American Journal of Obstetrics and Gynecology* **192**, 554–557.

Boggess, K.A., Moss, K., Murtha, A., Offenbacher, S. & Beck, J.D. (2006b). Antepartum vaginal bleeding, fetal exposure to oral pathogens, and risk for preterm birth at <35 weeks of gestation. *American Journal of Obstetrics and Gynecology* **194**, 954–960.

Bolin, A., Eklund, G., Frithiof, L. & Lavstedt, S. (1993). The effect of changed smoking habits on marginal alveolar bone loss. A longitudinal study. *Swedish Dental Journal* **17**, 211–216.

Borrell, L.N., Burt, B.A., Neighbors, H.W. & Taylor, G.W. (2004). Social factors and periodontitis in an older population. *American Journal of Public Health* **94**, 748–754.

Borrell, L.N., Lynch, J., Neighbors, H., Burt, B.A. & Gillespie, B.W. (2002). Is there homogeneity in periodontal health between African Americans and Mexican Americans? *Ethnicity and Disease* **12**, 97–110.

Borrell, L.N. & Papapanou, P.N. (2005). Analytical epidemiology of periodontitis. *Journal of Clinical Periodontology* **32** Suppl 6, 132–158.

Boström, L., Lindér, L.E. & Bergström, J. (1998). Influence of smoking on the outcome of periodontal surgery. A 5-year follow-up. *Journal of Clinical Periodontology* **25**, 194–201.

Bourgeois, D.M., Doury, J. & Hescot, P. (1999). Periodontal conditions in 65–74 year old adults in France, 1995. *International Dental Journal* **49**, 182–186.

Breivik, T., Gundersen, Y., Myhrer, T., Fonnum, F., Osmundsen, H., Murison, R., Gjermo, P., von Horsten, S. & Opstad, P.K. (2006). Enhanced susceptibility to periodontitis in an animal model of depression: reversed by chronic treatment with the anti-depressant tianeptine. *Journal of Clinical Periodontology* **33**, 469–477.

Bridges, R.B., Anderson, J.W., Saxe, S.R., Gregory, K. & Bridges, S.R. (1996). Periodontal status of diabetic and non-diabetic men: effects of smoking, glycemic control, and socioeconomic factors. *Journal of Periodontology* **67**, 1185–1192.

Brown, L.J., Albandar, J.M., Brunelle, J.A. & Löe, H. (1996). Early-onset periodontitis: progression of attachment loss during 6 years. *Journal of Periodontology* **67**, 968–975.

Brown, L.J., Oliver, R.C. & Löe, H. (1989). Periodontal diseases in the U.S. in 1981: Prevalence, severity, extent, and role in tooth mortality. *Journal of Periodontology* **60**, 363–370.

Brown, L.J., Oliver, R.C. & Löe, H. (1990) Evaluating periodontal status of US employed adults. *Journal of the American Dental Association* **121**, 226–232.

Buduneli, N., Baylas, H., Buduneli, E., Turkoglu, O., Kose, T. & Dahlen, G. (2005). Periodontal infections and pre-term low birth weight: a case-control study. *Journal of Clinical Periodontology* **32**, 174–181.

Burt, B.A. (1994) Periodontitis and aging: reviewing recent evidence. *Journal of the American Dental Association* **125**, 273–279.

Burt, B.A. & Eklund, S.A. (1999). *Dentistry, Dental Practice, and the Community*. Philadelphia, PA: W.B. Saunders Company.

Burt, B.A., Ismail, A.I., Morrison, E.C. & Beltran, E.D. (1990). Risk factors for tooth loss over a 28-year period. *Journal of Dental Research* **69**, 1126–1130.

Butterworth, M. & Sheiham, A. (1991). Changes in the Community Periodontal Index of Treatment Needs (CPITN) after periodontal treatment in a general dental practice. *British Dental Journal* **171**, 363–366.

Caffesse, R.G., De LaRosa, M.R., De LaRosa, M.G. & Mota, L.F. (2002). Prevalence of interleukin 1 periodontal genotype in a Hispanic dental population. *Quintessence International* **33**, 190–194.

Cahen, P.M., Frank, R.M. & Turlot, J.C. (1985). A survey of the reasons for dental extractions in France. *Journal of Dental Research* **64**, 1087–1093.

Canakci, V., Canakci, C.F., Canakci, H., Canakci, E., Cicek, Y., Ingec, M., Ozgoz, M., Demir, T., Dilsiz, A. & Yagiz, H. (2004). Periodontal disease as a risk factor for pre-eclampsia: a case control study. *Australian and New Zealand Journal of Obstetrics and Gynaecology* **44**, 568–573.

Carey, J.C., Klebanoff, M.A., Hauth, J.C., Hillier, S.L., Thom, E.A., Ernest, J.M., Heine, R.P., Nugent, R.P., Fischer, M.L., Leveno, K.J., Wapner, R. & Varner, M. (2000). Metronidazole to prevent preterm delivery in pregnant women with asymptomatic bacterial vaginosis. National Institute of Child Health and Human Development Network of Maternal-Fetal Medicine Units. *New England Journal of Medicine* **342**, 534–540.

Carlos, J.P., Wolfe, M.D. & Kingman, A. (1986). The extent and severity index: a simple method for use in epidemiologic studies of periodontal disease. *Journal of Clinical Periodontology* **13**, 500–505.

Celermajer, D.S., Sorensen, K.E., Gooch, V.M., Spiegelhalter, D.J., Miller, O.I., Sullivan, I.D., Lloyd, J.K. & Deanfield, J.E. (1992). Non-invasive detection of endothelial dysfunction in children and adults at risk of atherosclerosis. *Lancet* **340**, 1111–1115.

Chalmers, T.C. (1993). Meta-analytic stimulus for changes in clinical trials. *Statistical Methods in Medical Research* **2**, 161–172.

Chapple, I.L. & Hamburger, J. (2000). The significance of oral health in HIV disease. *Sexually Transmitted Infections* **76**, 236–243.

Chen, X., Wolff, L., Aeppli, D., Guo, Z., Luan, W., Baelum, V. & Fejeskov, O. (2001). Cigarette smoking, salivary/gingival crevicular fluid cotinine and periodontal status. A 10-year longitudinal study. *Journal of Clinical Periodontology* **28**, 331–339.

Chiu, B. (1999). Multiple infections in carotid atherosclerotic plaques. *American Heart Journal* **138**, S534–536.

Christensen, L.B., Petersen, P.E., Krustrup, U. & Kjoller, M. (2003). Self-reported oral hygiene practices among adults in Denmark. *Community Dental Health* **20**, 229–235.

Christgau, M., Aslanidis, C., Felden, A., Hiller, K.A., Schmitz, G. & Schmalz, G. (2003). Influence of interleukin-1 gene polymorphism on periodontal regeneration in intrabony defects. *Journal of Periodontal Research* **38**, 20–27.

Christgau, M., Palitzsch, K.-D., Schmalz, G., Kreiner, U. & Frenzel, S. (1998). Healing response to non-surgical periodontal therapy in patients with diabetes mellitus: clinical, microbiological, and immunological results. *Journal of Clinical Periodontology* **25**, 112–124.

Chung, H.Y., Lu, H.C., Chen, W.L., Lu, C.T., Yang, Y.H. & Tsai, C.C. (2003). Gm (23) allotypes and Fcgamma receptor genotypes as risk factors for various forms of periodontitis. *Journal of Clinical Periodontology* **30**, 954–960.

Clerehugh, V., Lennon, M.A. & Worthington, H.V. (1990). 5-year results of a longitudinal study of early periodontitis in 14- to 19-year-old adolescents. *Journal of Clinical Periodontology* **17**, 702–708.

Cogen, R.B., Wright, J.T. & Tate, A.L. (1992). Destructive periodontal disease in healthy children. *Journal of Periodontology* **63**, 761–765.

Collins, J.G., Smith, M.A., Arnold, R.R. & Offenbacher, S. (1994a). Effects of *Escherichia coli* and *Porphyromonas gingivalis* lipopolysaccharide on pregnancy outcome in the golden hamster. *Infection and Immunity* **62**, 4652–4655.

Collins, J.G., Windley, H.W. 3rd, Arnold, R.R. & Offenbacher, S. (1994b). Effects of a *Porphyromonas gingivalis* infection on inflammatory mediator response and pregnancy outcome in hamsters. *Infection and Immunity* **62**, 4356–4361.

Copeland, L.B., Krall, E.A., Brown, L.J., Garcia, R.I. & Streckfus, C.F. (2004). Predictors of tooth loss in two US adult populations. *Journal of Public Health Dentistry* **64**, 31–37.

Corbet, E.F. & Davies, W.I. (1991). Reasons given for tooth extraction in Hong Kong. *Community Dental Health* **8**, 121–130.

Craandijk, J., van Krugten, M.V., Verweij, C.L., van der Velden, U. & Loos, B.G. (2002). Tumor necrosis factor-alpha gene polymorphisms in relation to periodontitis. *Journal of Clinical Periodontology* **29**, 28–34.

Craig, R.G., Boylan, R., Yip, J., Bamgboye, P., Koutsoukos, J., Mijares, D., Ferrer, J., Imam, M., Socransky, S.S. & Haffajee, A.D. (2001). Prevalence and risk indicators for destructive periodontal diseases in 3 urban American minority populations. *Journal of Clinical Periodontology* **28**, 524–535.

Cross, D.L. & Smith, G.L.F. (1995). Comparison of periodontal disease in HIV seropositive subjects and controls (II). Microbiology, Immunology and prediction of disease progression. *Journal of Clinical Periodontology* **22**, 569–577.

Cullinan, M.P., Westerman, B., Hamlet, S.M., Palmer, J.E., Faddy, M.J., Lang, N.P. & Seymour, G.J. (2001). A longitudinal study of interleukin-1 gene polymorphisms and periodontal disease in a general adult population. *Journal of Clinical Periodontology* **28**, 1137–1144.

Cutress, T.W., Powell, R.N. & Ball, M.E. (1982). Differing profiles of periodontal disease in two similar South Pacific island populations. *Community Dentistry and Oral Epidemiology* **10**, 193–203.

D'Aiuto, F., Nibali, L., Parkar, M., Suvan, J. & Tonetti, M.S. (2005). Short-term effects of intensive periodontal therapy on serum inflammatory markers and cholesterol. *Journal of Dental Research* **84**, 269–273.

D'Aiuto, F., Parkar, M., Nibali, L., Suvan, J., Lessem, J. & Tonetti, M.S. (2006). Periodontal infections cause changes in traditional and novel cardiovascular risk factors: results from a randomized controlled clinical trial. *American Heart Journal* **151**, 977–984.

D'Aiuto, F., Ready, D. & Tonetti, M.S. (2004). Periodontal disease and C-reactive protein-associated cardiovascular risk. *Journal of Periodontal Research* **39**, 236–241.

D'Aiuto, F. & Tonetti, M.S. (2005). Contribution of periodontal therapy on individual cardiovascular risk assessment. *Archives of Internal Medicine* **165**, 1920–1921.

Darby, I.B., Lu, J. & Calache, H. (2005). Radiographic study of the prevalence of periodontal bone loss in Australian school-aged children attending the Royal Dental Hospital of Melbourne. *Journal of Clinical Periodontology* **32**, 959–965.

Dasanayake, A.P., Boyd, D., Madianos, P.N., Offenbacher, S. & Hills, E. (2001). The association between Porphyromonas gingivalis-specific maternal serum IgG and low birth weight. *Journal of Periodontology* **72**, 1491–1497.

Davenport, E.S., Williams, C.E., Sterne, J.A., Murad, S., Sivapathasundram, V. & Curtis, M.A. (2002). Maternal periodontal disease and preterm low birthweight: case-control study. *Journal of Dental Research* **81**, 313–318.

David, R.J. & Collins, J.W., Jr. (1997). Differing birth weight among infants of U.S.-born blacks, African-born blacks, and U.S.-born whites. *New England Journal of Medicine* **337**, 1209–1214.

de Brito Junior, R.B., Scarel-Caminaga, R.M., Trevilatto, P.C., de Souza, A.P. & Barros, S.P. (2004). Polymorphisms in the vitamin D receptor gene are associated with periodontal disease. *Journal of Periodontology* **75**, 1090–1095.

de Pommereau, V., Dargent-Paré, C., Robert, J.J. & Brion, M. (1992). Periodontal status in insulin-dependent diabetic adolescents. *Journal of Clinical Periodontology* **19**, 628–632.

De Sanctis, M. & Zucchelli, G. (2000). Interleukin-1 gene polymorphisms and long-term stability following guided tissue regeneration therapy. *Journal of Periodontology* **71**, 606–613.

DeStefano, F., Anda, R.F., Kahn, H.S., Williamson, D.F. & Russell, C.M. (1993). Dental disease and risk of coronary heart disease and mortality. *British Medical Journal* **306**, 688–691.

Desvarieux, M., Demmer, R.T., Rundek, T., Boden-Albala, B., Jacobs, D.R., Jr., Papapanou, P.N. & Sacco, R.L. (2003). Relationship between periodontal disease, tooth loss, and carotid artery plaque: the Oral Infections and Vascular Disease Epidemiology Study (INVEST). *Stroke* **34**, 2120–2125.

Desvarieux, M., Demmer, R.T., Rundek, T., Boden-Albala, B., Jacobs, D.R., Jr., Sacco, R.L. & Papapanou, P.N. (2005). Periodontal microbiota and carotid intima-media thickness: the Oral Infections and Vascular Disease Epidemiology Study (INVEST). *Circulation* **111**, 576–582.

Diamanti Kipioti, A., Papapanou, P.N., Moraitaki Tsami, A., Lindhe, J. & Mitsis, F. (1993). Comparative estimation of periodontal conditions by means of different index systems. *Journal of Clinical Periodontology* **20**, 656–661.

Diamanti-Kipioti, A., Afentoulidis, N., Moraitaki-Tsami, A., Lindhe, J., Mitsis, F. & Papapanou, P.N. (1995). A radiographic survey of periodontal conditions in Greece. *Journal of Clinical Periodontology* **22**, 385–390.

Diehl, S.R., Wang, Y., Brooks, C.N., Burmeister, J.A., Califano, J.V., Wang, S. & Schenkein, H.A. (1999). Linkage disequilibrium of interleukin-1 genetic polymorphisms with early-onset periodontitis. *Journal of Periodontology* **70**, 418–430.

Dortbudak, O., Eberhardt, R., Ulm, M. & Persson, G.R. (2005). Periodontitis, a marker of risk in pregnancy for preterm birth. *Journal of Clinical Periodontology* **32**, 45–52.

Douglass, C.W. & Fox, C.H. (1993). Cross-sectional studies in periodontal disease: current status and implications for dental practice. *Advances in Dental Research* **7**, 25–31.

Douglass, C.W., Jette, A.M., Fox, C.H., Tennstedt, S.L., Joshi, A., Feldman, H.A., McGuire, S.M. & McKinlay, J.B. (1993). Oral health status of the elderly in New England. *Journal of Gerontology* **48**, M39–M46.

Drake, C.W., Hunt, R.J. & Koch, G.G. (1995). Three-year tooth loss among black and white older adults in North Carolina. *Journal of Dental Research* **74**, 675–680.

Dunlop, D.D., Manheim, L.M., Song, J. & Chang, R.W. (2002). Gender and ethnic/racial disparities in health care utilization among older adults. *The Journals of Gerontology. Series B, Psychological Sciences and Social Sciences* **57**, S221–233.

Dye, B.A., Choudhary, K., Shea, S. & Papapanou, P.N. (2005). Serum antibodies to periodontal pathogens and markers of systemic inflammation. *Journal of Clinical Periodontology* **32**, 1189–1199.

Eaton, K.A., Duffy, S., Griffiths, G.S., Gilthorpe, M.S. & Johnson, N.W. (2001). The influence of partial and full-mouth recordings on estimates of prevalence and extent of lifetime cumulative attachment loss: a study in a population of young male military recruits. *Journal of Periodontology* **72**, 140–145.

Ebersole, J.L., Machen, R.L., Steffen, M.J. & Willmann, D.E. (1997). Systemic acute-phase reactants, C-reactive protein and haptoglobin, in adult periodontitis. *Clinical and Experimental Immunology* **107**, 347–352.

Ebersole, J.L. & Taubman, M.A. (1994). The protective nature of host responses in periodontal diseases. *Periodontology 2000* **5**, 112–141.

Ehmke, B., Kress, W., Karch, H., Grimm, T., Klaiber, B. & Flemmig, T.F. (1999). Interleukin-1 haplotype and periodontal disease progression following therapy. *Journal of Clinical Periodontology* **26**, 810–813.

Eklund, S.A. & Burt, B.A. (1994). Risk factors for total tooth loss in the United States; longitudinal analysis of national data. *Journal of Public Health Dentistry* **54**, 5–14.

Elter, J.R., Hinderliter, A.L., Offenbacher, S., Beck, J.D., Caughey, M., Brodala, N. & Madianos, P.N. (2006). The effects of periodontal therapy on vascular endothelial function: a pilot trial. *American Heart Journal* **151**, 47.

Emrich, L.J., Shlossman, M. & Genco, R.J. (1991). Periodontal disease in non-insulin-dependent diabetes mellitus. *Journal of Periodontology* **62**, 123–131.

Endo, M., Tai, H., Tabeta, K., Kobayashi, T., Yamazaki, K. & Yoshie, H. (2001). Analysis of single nucleotide polymorphisms in the 5′-flanking region of tumor necrosis factor-alpha gene in Japanese patients with early-onset periodontitis. *Journal of Periodontology* **72**, 1554–1559.

Endo, S., Inada, K., Inoue, Y., Kuwata, Y., Suzuki, M., Yamashita, H., Hoshi, S. & Yoshida, M. (1992). Two types of septic shock classified by the plasma levels of cytokines and endotoxin. *Circulatory Shock* **38**, 264–274.

Engebretson, S.P., Lamster, I.B., Elkind, M.S., Rundek, T., Serman, N.J., Demmer, R.T., Sacco, R.L., Papapanou, P.N. & Desvarieux, M. (2005). Radiographic measures of chronic periodontitis and carotid artery plaque. *Stroke* **36**, 561–566.

Fassmann, A., Holla, L.I., Buckova, D., Vasku, A., Znojil, V. & Vanek, J. (2003). Polymorphisms in the +252(A/G) lymphotoxin-alpha and the -308(A/G) tumor necrosis factor-alpha genes and susceptibility to chronic periodontitis in a Czech population. *Journal of Periodontal Research* **38**, 394–399.

Fiehn, N.E., Larsen, T., Christiansen, N., Holmstrup, P. & Schroeder, T.V. (2005). Identification of periodontal pathogens in atherosclerotic vessels. *Journal of Periodontology* **76**, 731–736.

Firatli, E. (1997) The relationship between clinical periodontal status and insulin-dependent diabetes mellitus. Results after 5 years. *Journal of Periodontology* **68**, 136–140.

Forner, L., Larsen, T., Kilian, M. & Holmstrup, P. (2006). Incidence of bacteremia after chewing, tooth brushing and scaling in individuals with periodontal inflammation. *Journal of Clinical Periodontology* **33**, 401–407.

Frost, W.H. (1941). Epidemiology. In: *Papers of Wade Hampton Frost, M.D.* ed. Maxcy, K.E., pp. 493–542. New York: The Commonwealth Fund.

Galbraith, G.M., Steed, R.B., Sanders, J.J. & Pandey, J.P. (1998). Tumor necrosis factor alpha production by oral leukocytes: influence of tumor necrosis factor genotype. *Journal of Periodontology* **69**, 428–433.

Galea, J., Armstrong, J., Gadsdon, P., Holden, H., Francis, S.E. & Holt, C.M. (1996). Interleukin-1 beta in coronary arteries of patients with ischemic heart disease. *Arteriosclerosis, Thrombosis, and Vascular Biology* **16**, 1000–1006.

Garcia, R.I. (2005). Smokers have less reductions in probing depth than non-smokers following nonsurgical periodontal therapy. *Evidence Based Dentistry* **6**, 37–38.

Genco, R.J., Grossi, S.G., Ho, A., Nishimura, F. & Murayama, Y. (2005) A proposed model linking inflammation to obesity, diabetes, and periodontal infections. *Journal of Periodontology* **76**, 2075–2084.

Genco, R.J., Ho, A.W., Grossi, S.G., Dunford, R.G. & Tedesco, L.A. (1999). Relationship of stress, distress and inadequate coping behaviors to periodontal disease. *Journal of Periodontology* **70**, 711–723.

Genco, R.J., Ho, A.W., Kopman, J., Grossi, S.G., Dunford, R.G. & Tedesco, L.A. (1998). Models to evaluate the role of stress in periodontal disease. *Annals of Periodontology* **3**, 288–302.

Genco, R.J. & Löe, H. (1993). The role of systemic conditions and disorders in periodontal disease. *Periodontology 2000* **2**, 98–116.

Gilbert, G.H. & Heft, M.W. (1992). Periodontal status of older Floridians attending senior activity centers. *Journal of Clinical Periodontology* **19**, 249–255.

Gilbert, G.H., Shelton, B.J. & Fisher, M.A. (2005). Forty-eight-month periodontal attachment loss incidence in a population-based cohort study: role of baseline status, incident tooth loss, and specific behavioral factors. *Journal of Periodontology* **76**, 1161–1170.

Goepfert, A.R., Jeffcoat, M.K., Andrews, W.W., Faye-Petersen, O., Cliver, S.P., Goldenberg, R.L. & Hauth, J.C. (2004). Periodontal disease and upper genital tract inflammation in early spontaneous preterm birth. *Obstetrics and Gynecology* **104**, 777–783.

Goldenberg, R.L. & Culhane, J.F. (2006). Preterm birth and periodontal disease. *New England Journal of Medicine* **355**, 1925–1927.

Goldenberg, R.L., Hauth, J.C. & Andrews, W.W. (2000). Intrauterine infection and preterm delivery. *New England Journal of Medicine* **342**, 1500–1507.

Goldenberg, R.L. & Rouse, D.J. (1998). Prevention of premature birth. *New England Journal of Medicine* **339**, 313–320.

Gonzales, J.R., Kobayashi, T., Michel, J., Mann, M., Yoshie, H. & Meyle, J. (2004). Interleukin-4 gene polymorphisms in Japanese and Caucasian patients with aggressive periodontitis. *Journal of Clinical Periodontology* **31**, 384–389.

Gonzales, J.R., Michel, J., Diete, A., Herrmann, J.M., Bodeker, R.H. & Meyle, J. (2002). Analysis of genetic polymorphisms at the interleukin-10 loci in aggressive and chronic periodontitis. *Journal of Clinical Periodontology* **29**, 816–822.

Gonzales, J.R., Michel, J., Rodriguez, E.L., Herrmann, J.M., Bodeker, R.H. & Meyle, J. (2003). Comparison of interleukin-1 genotypes in two populations with aggressive periodontitis. *European Journal of Oral Science* **111**, 395–399.

Gore, E.A., Sanders, J.J., Pandey, J.P., Palesch, Y. & Galbraith, G.M. (1998). Interleukin-1beta+3953 allele 2: association with disease status in adult periodontitis. *Journal of Clinical Periodontology* **25**, 781–785.

Goultschin, J., Cohen, H.D., Donchin, M., Brayer, L. & Soskolne, W.A. (1990). Association of smoking with periodontal treatment needs. *Journal of Periodontology* **61**, 364–367.

Grau, A.J., Buggle, F., Ziegler, C., Schwarz, W., Meuser, J., Tasman, A.J., Buhler, A., Benesch, C., Becher, H. & Hacke, W. (1997). Association between acute cerebrovascular ischemia and chronic and recurrent infection. *Stroke* **28**, 1724–1729.

Griffen, A.L., Becker, M.R., Lyons, S.R., Moeschberger, M.L. & Leys, E.J. (1998). Prevalence of Porphyromonas gingivalis and periodontal health status. *Journal of Clinical Microbiology* **36**, 3239–3242.

Grossi, S.G. & Genco, R.J. (1998). Periodontal disease and diabetes mellitus: a two-way relationship. *Annals of Periodontology* **3**, 51–61.

Grossi, S.G., Genco, R.J., Machtei, E.E., Ho, A.W., Koch, G., Dunford, R., Zambon, J.J. & Hausmann, E. (1995). Assessment of risk for periodontal disease. II. Risk indicators for alveolar bone loss. *Journal of Periodontology* **66**, 23–29.

Grossi, S.G., Skrepcinski, F.B., DeCaro, T., Robertson, D.C., Ho, A.W., Dunford, R.G. & Genco, R.J. (1997a). Treatment of periodontal disease in diabetics reduces glycated hemoglobin. *Journal of Periodontology* **68**, 713–719.

Grossi, S.G., Zambon, J., Machtei, E.E., Schifferle, R., Andreana, S., Genco, R.J., Cummins, D. & Harrap, G. (1997b). Effects of smoking and smoking cessation on healing after mechanical periodontal therapy. *Journal of the American Dental Association* **128**, 599–607.

Grossi, S.G., Zambon, J.J., Ho, A.W., Koch, G., Dunford, R.G., Machtei, E.E., Norderyd, O.M. & Genco, R.J. (1994). Assessment of risk for periodontal disease. I. Risk indicators for attachment loss. *Journal of Periodontology* **65**, 260–267.

Grytten, J. & Mubarak, A. (1989). CPITN (Community Periodontal Index of Treatment Needs) – what is its use and what does it mean? *Norske Tannlaegeforenings Tidende* **99**, 338–343.

Guzman, S., Karima, M., Wang, H.Y. & Van Dyke, T.E. (2003). Association between interleukin-1 genotype and periodontal disease in a diabetic population. *Journal of Periodontology* **74**, 1183–1190.

Haber, J. & Kent, R.L. (1992). Cigarette smoking in a periodontal practice. *Journal of Periodontology* **63**, 100–106.

Haber, J., Wattles, J., Crowley, M., Mandell, R., Joshipura, K. & Kent, R.L. (1993). Evidence for cigarette smoking as a major risk factor for periodontitis. *Journal of Periodontology* **64**, 16–23.

Hackam, D.G. & Anand, S.S. (2003). Emerging risk factors for atherosclerotic vascular disease: a critical review of the evidence. *Journal of the American Medical Association* **290**, 932–940.

Haffajee, A.D., Bogren, A., Hasturk, H., Feres, M., Lopez, N.J. & Socransky, S.S. (2004). Subgingival microbiota of chronic periodontitis subjects from different geographic locations. *Journal of Clinical Periodontology* **31**, 996–1002.

Haffajee, A.D. & Socransky, S.S. (1994). Microbial etiological agents of destructive periodontal diseases. *Periodontology 2000* **5**, 78–111.

Haffajee, A.D., Socransky, S.S., Lindhe, J., Kent, R.L., Okamoto, H. & Yoneyama, T. (1991a). Clinical risk indicators for periodontal attachment loss. *Journal of Clinical Periodontology* **18**, 117–125.

Haffajee, A.D., Socransky, S.S., Smith, C. & Dibart, S. (1991b). Relation of baseline microbial parameters to future periodontal attachment loss. *Journal of Clinical Periodontology* **18**, 744–750.

Hallmon, W.W. & Rees, T.D. (2003). Local anti-infective therapy: mechanical and physical approaches. A systematic review. *Annals of Periodontology* **8**, 99–114.

Hamlet, S., Ellwood, R., Cullinan, M., Worthington, H., Palmer, J., Bird, P., Narayanan, D., Davies, R. & Seymour, G. (2004). Persistent colonization with *Tannerella forsythensis* and loss of attachment in adolescents. *Journal of Dental Research* **83**, 232–235.

Hamlet, S.M., Cullinan, M.P., Westerman, B., Lindeman, M., Bird, P.S., Palmer, J. & Seymour, G.J. (2001). Distribution of *Actinobacillus actinomycetemcomitans*, *Porphyromonas gingivalis* and *Prevotella intermedia* in an Australian population. *Journal of Clinical Periodontology* **28**, 1163–1171.

Hansson, G.K. (2005). Inflammation, atherosclerosis, and coronary artery disease. *New England Journal of Medicine* **352**, 1685–1695.

Haraszthy, V.I., Zambon, J.J., Trevisan, M., Zeid, M. & Genco, R.J. (2000). Identification of periodontal pathogens in atheromatous plaques. *Journal of Periodontology* **71**, 1554–1560.

Hart, T.C. & Kornman, K.S. (1997). Genetic factors in the pathogenesis of periodontitis. *Periodontology 2000* **14**, 202–215.

Heft, M.W. & Gilbert, G.H. (1991). Tooth loss and caries prevalence in older Floridians attending senior activity centers. *Community Dentistry and Oral Epidemiology* **19**, 228–232.

Heitz-Mayfield, L.J., Trombelli, L., Heitz, F., Needleman, I. & Moles, D. (2002). A systematic review of the effect of surgical debridement vs non-surgical debridement for the treatment of chronic periodontitis. *Journal of Clinical Periodontology* **29** (Suppl 3), 92–102; discussion 160–102.

Hennig, B.J., Parkhill, J.M., Chapple, I.L., Heasman, P.A. & Taylor, J.J. (1999). Association of a vitamin D receptor gene polymorphism with localized early-onset periodontal diseases. *Journal of Periodontology* **70**, 1032–1038.

Herrera, D., Sanz, M., Jepsen, S., Needleman, I. & Roldan, S. (2002). A systematic review on the effect of systemic antimicrobials as an adjunct to scaling and root planing in periodontitis patients. *Journal of Clinical Periodontology* **29** (Suppl 3), 136–159; discussion 160–132.

Hill, A.B. (1971). *Principles of Medical Statistics*, 9th edn. New York: Oxford University Press.

Hill, G.B. (1998). Preterm birth: associations with genital and possibly oral microflora. *Annals of Periodontology* **3**, 222–232.

Hirotomi, T., Yoshihara, A., Yano, M., Ando, Y. & Miyazaki, H. (2002). Longitudinal study on periodontal conditions in healthy elderly people in Japan. *Community Dentistry and Oral Epidemiology* **30**, 409–417.

Hobdell, M.H. (2001). Economic globalization and oral health. *Oral Disease* **7**, 137–143.

Hodge, P.J., Riggio, M.P. & Kinane, D.F. (2001). Failure to detect an association with IL1 genotypes in European

Caucasians with generalised early onset periodontitis. *Journal of Clinical Periodontology* **28**, 430–436.

Hofer, D., Hammerle, C.H., Grassi, M. & Lang, N.P. (2002). Long-term results of supportive periodontal therapy (SPT) in HIV-seropositive and HIV-seronegative patients. *Journal of Clinical Periodontology* **29**, 630–637.

Holbrook, R.H., Jr., Laros, R.K., Jr. & Creasy, R.K. (1989). Evaluation of a risk-scoring system for prediction of preterm labor. *American Journal of Perinatology* **6**, 62–68.

Holbrook, W.P., Oskarsdottir, A., Fridjonsson, T., Einarsson, H., Hauksson, A. & Geirsson, R.T. (2004). No link between low-grade periodontal disease and preterm birth: a pilot study in a healthy Caucasian population. *Acta Odontologica Scandinavica* **62**, 177–179.

Holla, L.I., Buckova, D., Fassmann, A., Halabala, T., Vasku, A. & Vacha, J. (2002a). Promoter polymorphisms in the CD14 receptor gene and their potential association with the severity of chronic periodontitis. *Journal of Medical Genetics* **39**, 844–848.

Holla, L.I., Fassmann, A., Benes, P., Halabala, T. & Znojil, V. (2002b). 5 polymorphisms in the transforming growth factor-beta 1 gene (TGF-beta 1) in adult periodontitis. *Journal of Clinical Periodontology* **29**, 336–341.

Holla, L.I., Jurajda, M., Fassmann, A., Dvorakova, N., Znojil, V. & Vacha, J. (2004). Genetic variations in the matrix metalloproteinase-1 promoter and risk of susceptibility and/or severity of chronic periodontitis in the Czech population. *Journal of Clinical Periodontology* **31**, 685–690.

Holm-Pedersen, P., Russell, S.L., Avlund, K., Viitanen, M., Winblad, B. & Katz, R.V. (2006). Periodontal disease in the oldest-old living in Kungsholmen, Sweden: findings from the KEOHS project. *Journal of Clinical Periodontology* **33**, 376–384.

Holmgren, C.J. & Corbet, E.F. (1990). Relationship between periodontal parameters and CPITN scores. *Community Dentistry and Oral Epidemiology* **18**, 322–323.

Honest, H., Bachmann, L.M., Ngai, C., Gupta, J.K., Kleijnen, J. & Khan, K.S. (2005). The accuracy of maternal anthropometry measurements as predictor for spontaneous preterm birth – a systematic review. *European Journal of Obstetrics Gynecology and Reproductive Biology* **119**, 11–20.

Horning, G.M., Hatch, C.L. & Lutskus, J. (1990). The prevalence of periodontitis in a military treatment population. *Journal of the American Dental Association* **121**, 616–622.

Hugoson, A., Koch, G., Gothberg, C., Helkimo, A.N., Lundin, S.A., Norderyd, O., Sjodin, B. & Sondell, K. (2005). Oral health of individuals aged 3–80 years in Jonkoping, Sweden during 30 years (1973–2003). II. Review of clinical and radiographic findings. *Swedish Dental Journal* **29**, 139–155.

Hugoson, A., Laurell, L. & Lundgren, D. (1992). Frequency distribution of individuals aged 20–70 years according to severity of periodontal disease experience in 1973 and 1983. *Journal of Clinical Periodontology* **19**, 227–232.

Hugoson, A., Norderyd, O., Slotte, C. & Thorstensson, H. (1998a). Distribution of periodontal disease in a Swedish adult population 1973, 1983 and 1993. *Journal of Clinical Periodontology* **25**, 542–548.

Hugoson, A., Norderyd, O., Slotte, C. & Thorstensson, H. (1998b). Oral hygiene and gingivitis in a Swedish adult population 1973, 1983 and 1993. *Journal of Clinical Periodontology* **25**, 807–812.

Hugoson, A., Thorstensson, H., Falk, H. & Kuylenstierna, J. (1989). Periodontal conditions in insulin-dependent diabetics. *Journal of Clinical Periodontology* **16**, 215–223.

Hujoel, P.P., Cunha-Cruz, J. & Kressin, N.R. (2006). Spurious associations in oral epidemiological research: the case of dental flossing and obesity. *Journal of Clinical Periodontology* **33**, 520–523.

Hujoel, P.P., Drangsholt, M., Spiekerman, C. & DeRouen, T.A. (2000). Periodontal disease and coronary heart disease risk. *Journal of the American Medical Association* **284**, 1406–1410.

Hujoel, P.P., Drangsholt, M., Spiekerman, C. & DeRouen, T.A. (2002a). Periodontitis-systemic disease associations in the presence of smoking – causal or coincidental? *Periodontology 2000* **30**, 51–60.

Hujoel, P.P., Drangsholt, M., Spiekerman, C. & DeRouen, T.A. (2002b). Pre-existing cardiovascular disease and periodontitis: a follow-up study. *Journal of Dental Research* **81**, 186–191.

Hujoel, P.P., Drangsholt, M., Spiekerman, C. & Weiss, N.S. (2003). An exploration of the periodontitis-cancer association. *Annals of Epidemiology* **13**, 312–316.

Hujoel, P.P., White, B.A., Garcia, R.I. & Listgarten, M.A. (2001). The dentogingival epithelial surface area revisited. *Journal of Periodontal Research* **36**, 48–55.

Humar, A., St Louis, P., Mazzulli, T., McGeer, A., Lipton, J., Messner, H. & MacDonald, K.S. (1999). Elevated serum cytokines are associated with cytomegalovirus infection and disease in bone marrow transplant recipients. *Journal of Infectious Diseases* **179**, 484–488.

Hunt, R.J. (1987). The efficiency of half-mouth examinations in estimating the prevalence of periodontal disease. *Journal of Dental Research*, 1044–1048.

Hunt, R.J., Drake, C.W. & Beck, J.D. (1995). Eighteen-month incidence of tooth loss among older adults in North Carolina. *American Journal of Public Health* **85**, 561–563.

Hunt, R.J. & Fann, S.J. (1991). Effect of examining half the teeth in a partial periodontal recording of older adults. *Journal of Dental Research* **70**, 1380–1385.

Hunt, R.J., Levy, S.M. & Beck, J.D. (1990). The prevalence of periodontal attachment loss in an Iowa population aged 70 and older. *Journal of Public Health Dentistry* **50**, 251–256.

Hyman, J.J. & Reid, B.C. (2003). Epidemiologic risk factors for periodontal attachment loss among adults in the United States. *Journal of Clinical Periodontology* **30**, 230–237.

Ismail, A.I., Eklund, S.A., Striffler, D.F. & Szpunar, S.M. (1987). The prevalence of advanced loss of periodontal attachment in two New Mexico populations. *Journal of Periodontal Research* **22**, 119–124.

Ismail, A.I., Morrison, E.C., Burt, B.A., Caffesse, R.G. & Kavanagh, M.T. (1990). Natural history of periodontal disease in adults: Findings from the Tecumseh Periodontal Disease Study, 1959–87. *Journal of Dental Research* **69**, 430–435.

Itagaki, M., Kubota, T., Tai, H., Shimada, Y., Morozumi, T. & Yamazaki, K. (2004). Matrix metalloproteinase-1 and -3 gene promoter polymorphisms in Japanese patients with periodontitis. *Journal of Clinical Periodontology* **31**, 764–769.

Jamison, H.C. (1963). Prevalence of periodontal disease in the deciduous teeth. *Journal of the American Dental Association* **66**, 208–215.

Janket, S.J., Wightman, A., Baird, A.E., Van Dyke, T.E. & Jones, J.A. (2005). Does periodontal treatment improve glycemic control in diabetic patients? A meta-analysis of intervention studies. *Journal of Dental Research* **84**, 1154–1159.

Jeffcoat, M.K., Geurs, N.C., Reddy, M.S., Cliver, S.P., Goldenerg, R.L. & Hauth, J.C. (2001). Periodontal infection and preterm birth: results of a prospective study. *Journal of the American Dental Association* **132**, 875–880.

Jeffcoat, M.K., Hauth, J.C., Geurs, N.C., Reddy, M.S., Cliver, S.P., Hodgkins, P.M. & Goldenberg, R.L. (2003). Periodontal disease and preterm birth: results of a pilot intervention study. *Journal of Periodontology* **74**, 1214–1218.

Jenkins, W.M. & Kinane, D.F. (1989). The "high risk" group in periodontitis. *British Dental Journal* **167**, 168–171.

Jepsen, S., Eberhard, J., Fricke, D., Hedderich, J., Siebert, R. & Acil, Y. (2003). Interleukin-1 gene polymorphisms and experimental gingivitis. *Journal of Clinical Periodontology* **30**, 102–106.

Jette, A.M., Feldman, H.A. & Tennstedt, S.L. (1993). Tobacco use: A modifiable risk factor for dental disease among the elderly. *American Journal of Public Health* **83**, 1271–1276.

Johnson, B.D., Mulligan, K., Kiyak, H.A. & Marder, M. (1989). Aging or disease? Periodontal changes and treatment considerations in the older dental patient. *Gerodontology* **8**, 109–118.

Johnson, N.W. (1989) Detection of high-risk groups and individuals for periodontal diseases. *International Dental Journal* **39**, 33–47.

Kaldahl, W.B., Johnson, G.K., Patil, K.D. & Kalkwarf, K.L. (1996). Levels of cigarette consumption and response to periodontal therapy. *Journal of Periodontology* **67**, 675–681.

Kamma, J.J., Diamanti-Kipioti, A., Nakou, M. & Mitsis, F.J. (2000). Profile of subgingival microbiota in children with mixed dentition. *Oral Microbiology and Immunology* **15**, 103–111.

Kaufman, J.S., Cooper, R.S. & McGee, D.L. (1997). Socioeconomic status and health in blacks and whites: the problem of residual confounding and the resiliency of race. *Epidemiology* **8**, 621–628.

Kinane, D.F. & Chestnutt, I.G. (2000). Smoking and periodontal disease. *Critical Reviews in Oral Biology and Medicine* **11**, 356–365.

Kinane, D.F., Hodge, P., Eskdale, J., Ellis, R. & Gallagher, G. (1999). Analysis of genetic polymorphisms at the interleukin-10 and tumour necrosis factor loci in early-onset periodontitis. *Journal of Periodontal Research* **34**, 379–386.

Kinane, D.F. & Radvar, M. (1997). The effect of smoking on mechanical and antimicrobial periodontal therapy. *Journal of Periodontology* **68**, 467–472.

Kinane, D.F., Riggio, M.P., Walker, K.F., MacKenzie, D. & Shearer, B. (2005). Bacteraemia following periodontal procedures. *Journal of Clinical Periodontology* **32**, 708–713.

Kingman, A. & Albandar, J.M. (2002). Methodological aspects of epidemiological studies of periodontal diseases. *Periodontology 2000* **29**, 11–30.

Kingman, A., Morrison, E., Löe, H. & Smith, J. (1988). Systematic errors in estimating prevalence and severity of periodontal disease. *Journal of Periodontology* **59**, 707–713.

Kiyak, H.A., Grayston, M.N. & Crinean, C.L. (1993). Oral health problems and needs of nursing home residents. *Community Dentistry and Oral Epidemiology* **21**, 49–52.

Kleinbaum, D.G., Kupper, L.L. & Morgenstern, H. (1982). *Epidemiologic Research. Principles and quantitative methods*, 1st edn. New York, NY: Van Nostrand Reinhold.

Kleinman, J.C. & Kessel, S.S. (1987). Racial differences in low birth weight. Trends and risk factors. *New England Journal of Medicine* **317**, 749–753.

Klock, K.S. & Haugejorden, O. (1991). Primary reasons for extraction of permanent teeth in Norway: changes from 1968 to 1988. *Community Dentistry and Oral Epidemiology* **19**, 336–341.

Kobayashi, T., Sugita, N., van der Pol, W.L., Nunokawa, Y., Westerdaal, N.A., Yamamoto, K., van de Winkel, J.G. & Yoshie, H. (2000a). The Fc gamma receptor genotype as a risk factor for generalized early-onset periodontitis in Japanese patients. *Journal of Periodontology* **71**, 1425–1432.

Kobayashi, T., van der Pol, W.L., van de Winkel, J.G., Hara, K., Sugita, N., Westerdaal, N.A., Yoshie, H. & Horigome, T. (2000b). Relevance of IgG receptor IIIb (CD16) polymorphism to handling of *Porphyromonas gingivalis*: implications for the pathogenesis of adult periodontitis. *Journal of Periodontal Research* **35**, 65–73.

Kobayashi, T., Westerdaal, N.A., Miyazaki, A., van der Pol, W.L., Suzuki, T., Yoshie, H., van de Winkel, J.G. & Hara, K. (1997). Relevance of immunoglobulin G Fc receptor polymorphism to recurrence of adult periodontitis in Japanese patients. *Infection and Immunity* **65**, 3556–3560.

Kobayashi, T., Yamamoto, K., Sugita, N., van der Pol, W.L., Yasuda, K., Kaneko, S., van de Winkel, J.G. & Yoshie, H. (2001). The Fc gamma receptor genotype as a severity factor for chronic periodontitis in Japanese patients. *Journal of Periodontology* **72**, 1324–1331.

Kocher, T., Sawaf, H., Fanghanel, J., Timm, R. & Meisel, P. (2002). Association between bone loss in periodontal disease and polymorphism of N-acetyltransferase (NAT2). *Journal of Clinical Periodontology* **29**, 21–27.

Kocher, T., Schwahn, C., Gesch, D., Bernhardt, O., John, U., Meisel, P. & Baelum, V. (2005). Risk determinants of periodontal disease – an analysis of the Study of Health in Pomerania (SHIP 0). *Journal of Clinical Periodontology* **32**, 59–67.

Könönen, E. (1993). Pigmented Prevotella species in the periodontally healthy oral cavity. *FEMS Immunology and Medical Microbiology* **6**, 201–205.

Kornman, K.S., Crane, A., Wang, H.Y., di Giovine, F.S., Newman, M.G., Pirk, F.W., Wilson, T.G., Jr., Higginbottom, F.L. & Duff, G.W. (1997). The interleukin-1 genotype as a severity factor in adult periodontal disease. *Journal of Clinical Periodontology* **24**, 72–77.

Krall, E.A., Dawson Hughes, B., Papas, A. & Garcia, R.I. (1994). Tooth loss and skeletal bone density in healthy postmenopausal women. *Osteoporosis International* **4**, 104–109.

Krall, E.A., Dawson-Hughes, B., Garvey, A.J. & Garcia, R.I. (1997). Smoking, smoking cessation, and tooth loss. *Journal of Dental Research* **76**, 1653–1659.

Krieger, N., Williams, D.R. & Moss, N.E. (1997). Measuring social class in US public health research: concepts, methodologies, and guidelines. *Annual Review of Public Health* **18**, 341–378.

Kronauer, E., Borsa, G. & Lang, N.P. (1986). Prevalence of incipient juvenile periodontitis at age 16 years in Switzerland. *Journal of Clinical Periodontology* **13**, 103–108.

Krustrup, U. & Erik Petersen, P. (2006). Periodontal conditions in 35–44 and 65–74-year-old adults in Denmark. *Acta Odontologica Scandinavica* **64**, 65–73.

Kweider, M., Lowe, G.D., Murray, G.D., Kinane, D.F. & McGowan, D.A. (1993). Dental disease, fibrinogen and white cell count; links with myocardial infarction? *Scottish Medical Journal* **38**, 73–74.

Labriola, A., Needleman, I. & Moles, D.R. (2005). Systematic review of the effect of smoking on nonsurgical periodontal therapy. *Periodontology 2000* **37**, 124–137.

Laine, M.L., Farre, M.A., Gonzalez, G., van Dijk, L.J., Ham, A.J., Winkel, E.G., Crusius, J.B., Vandenbroucke, J.P., van Winkelhoff, A.J. & Pena, A.S. (2001). Polymorphisms of the interleukin-1 gene family, oral microbial pathogens, and smoking in adult periodontitis. *Journal of Dental Research* **80**, 1695–1699.

Lalla, E., Cheng, B., Lal, S., Kaplan, S., Softness, B., Greenberg, E., Goland, R.S. & Lamster, I.B. (2007a). Diabetes mellitus promotes periodontal destruction in children. *Journal of Clinical Periodontology* **34**, In press.

Lalla, E., Cheng, B., Lal, S., Kaplan, S., Softness, B., Greenberg, E., Goland, R.S. & Lamster, I.B. (2007b). Diabetes-related parameters and periodontal conditions in children. *Journal of Periodontal Research* **42**, 345–349.

Lalla, E., Cheng, B., Lal, S., Tucker, S., Greenberg, E., Goland, R. & Lamster, I.B. (2006). Periodontal changes in children and adolescents with diabetes: a case-control study. *Diabetes Care* **29**, 295–299.

Lalla, E., Lamster, I.B., Drury, S., Fu, C. & Schmidt, A.M. (2000). Hyperglycemia, glycoxidation and receptor for advanced glycation endproducts: potential mechanisms underlying diabetic complications, including diabetes-associated periodontitis. *Periodontology 2000* **23**, 50–62.

Lalla, E., Lamster, I.B., Hofmann, M.A., Bucciarelli, L., Jerud, A.P., Tucker, S., Lu, Y., Papapanou, P.N. & Schmidt, A.M. (2003). Oral infection with a periodontal pathogen accelerates early atherosclerosis in apolipoprotein E-null mice. *Arteriosclerosis, Thrombosis, and Vascular Biology* **23**, 1405–1411.

Lalla, E., Park, D.B., Papapanou, P.N. & Lamster, I.B. (2004). Oral disease burden in Northern Manhattan patients with diabetes mellitus. *American Journal of Public Health* **94**, 755–758.

Lamell, C.W., Griffen, A.L., McClellan, D.L. & Leys, E.J. (2000). Acquisition and colonization stability of Actinobacillus actinomycetemcomitans and Porphyromonas gingivalis in children. *Journal of Clinical Microbiology* **38**, 1196–1199.

Lamont, R.J., Chan, A., Belton, C.M., Izutsu, K.T., Vasel, D. & Weinberg, A. (1995). Porphyromonas gingivalis invasion of gingival epithelial cells. *Infection and Immunity* **63**, 3878–3885.

Lamster, I.B., Grbic, J.T., Bucklan, R.S., Mitchell-Lewis, D., Reynolds, H.S. & Zambon, J.J. (1997). Epidemiology and diagnosis of HIV-associated periodontal diseases. *Oral Disease* **3** (Suppl 1), S141–148.

Lamster, I.B., Grbic, J.T., Mitchell-Lewis, D.A., Begg, M.D. & Mitchell, A. (1998). New concepts regarding the pathogenesis of periodontal disease in HIV infection. *Annals of Periodontology* **3**, 62–75.

Lang, C.H. (1992). Sepsis-induced insulin resistance in rats is mediated by a beta-adrenergic mechanism. *American Journal of Physiology* **263**, E703–711.

Lang, N.P. & Hill, R.G. (1977). Radiographs in periodontics. *Journal of Clinical Periodontology* **4**, 16–28.

Lang, N.P., Tonetti, M.S., Suter, J., Sorrell, J., Duff, G.W. & Kornman, K.S. (2000). Effect of interleukin-1 gene polymorphisms on gingival inflammation assessed by bleeding on probing in a periodontal maintenance population. *Journal of Periodontal Research* **35**, 102–107.

Lao, T.T. & Ho, L.F. (1997). The obstetric implications of teenage pregnancy. *Human Reproduction* **12**, 2303–2305.

Lavstedt, S., Eklund, G. & Henrikson, C.-O. (1975). Partial recording in conjunction with roentgenologic assessment of proximal marginal bone loss. *Acta Odontologica Scandinavica* **33**, 90–113.

Lee, Y.M., Cleary-Goldman, J. & D'Alton, M.E. (2006). Multiple gestations and late preterm (near-term) deliveries. *Seminars in Perinatology* **30**, 103–112.

Levin, L., Baev, V., Lev, R., Stabholz, A. & Ashkenazi, M. (2006). Aggressive periodontitis among young Israeli army personnel. *Journal of Periodontology* **77**, 1392–1396.

Levy, S.M., Warren, J.J., Chowdhury, J., DeBus, B., Watkins, C.A., Cowen, H.J., Kirchner, H.L. & Hand, J.S. (2003). The prevalence of periodontal disease measures in elderly adults, aged 79 and older. *Special Care in Dentistry* **23**, 50–57.

Li, Q.Y., Zhao, H.S., Meng, H.X., Zhang, L., Xu, L., Chen, Z.B., Shi, D., Feng, X.H. & Zhu, X.L. (2004). Association analysis between interleukin-1 family polymorphisms and generalized aggressive periodontitis in a Chinese population. *Journal of Periodontology* **75**, 1627–1635.

Lilienfeld, D.E. (1978). Definitions of epidemiology. *American Journal of Epidemiology* **107**, 87–90.

Lin, D., Smith, M.A., Champagne, C., Elter, J., Beck, J. & Offenbacher, S. (2003a). Porphyromonas gingivalis infection during pregnancy increases maternal tumor necrosis factor alpha, suppresses maternal interleukin-10, and enhances fetal growth restriction and resorption in mice. *Infection and Immunity* **71**, 5156–5162.

Lin, D., Smith, M.A., Elter, J., Champagne, C., Downey, C.L., Beck, J. & Offenbacher, S. (2003b). *Porphyromonas gingivalis* infection in pregnant mice is associated with placental dissemination, an increase in the placental Th1/Th2 cytokine ratio, and fetal growth restriction. *Infection and Immunity* **71**, 5163–5168.

Linden, G.J., Mullally, B.H. & Freeman, R. (1996). Stress and the progression of periodontal disease. *Journal of Clinical Periodontology* **23**, 675–680.

Lindhe, J., Hamp, S.E. & Löe, H. (1973). Experimental periodontitis in the beagle dog. *International Dental Journal* **23**, 432–437.

Ling, P.R., Bistrian, B.R., Mendez, B. & Istfan, N.W. (1994). Effects of systemic infusions of endotoxin, tumor necrosis factor, and interleukin-1 on glucose metabolism in the rat: relationship to endogenous glucose production and peripheral tissue glucose uptake. *Metabolism* **43**, 279–284.

Locker, D. (1992). Smoking and oral health in older adults. *Canadian Journal of Public Health* **83**, 429–432.

Locker, D. & Leake, J.L. (1993). Periodontal attachment loss in independently living older adults in Ontario, Canada. *Journal of Public Health Dentistry* **53**, 6–11.

Löe, H. (1967). The Gingival Index, the Plaque Index and the Retention Index system. *Journal of Periodontology* **38**, 610–616.

Löe, H., Ånerud, Å. & Boysen, H. (1992). The natural history of periodontal disease in man: prevalence, severity, and extent of gingival recession. *Journal of Periodontology* **63**, 489–495.

Löe, H., Ånerud, Å., Boysen, H. & Morrison, E. (1986). Natural history of periodontal disease in man. Rapid, moderate and no loss of attachment in Sri Lankan laborers 14 to 46 years of age. *Journal of Clinical Periodontology* **13**, 431–445.

Löe, H., Ånerud, Å., Boysen, H. & Smith, M. (1978). The natural history of periodontal disease in man. Study design and baseline data. *Journal of Periodontal Research* **13**, 550–562.

Löe, H. & Brown, L.J. (1991). Early onset periodontitis in the United States of America. *Journal of Periodontology* **62**, 608–616.

Löe, H., Theilade, E. & Jensen, S.B. (1965). Experimental gingivitis in man. *Journal of Periodontology* **36**, 177–187.

Loos, B.G., Craandijk, J., Hoek, F.J., Wertheim-van Dillen, P.M. & van der Velden, U. (2000). Elevation of systemic markers related to cardiovascular diseases in the peripheral blood of periodontitis patients. *Journal of Periodontology* **71**, 1528–1534.

Loos, B.G., Leppers-Van de Straat, F.G., Van de Winkel, J.G. & Van der Velden, U. (2003). Fcgamma receptor polymorphisms in relation to periodontitis. *Journal of Clinical Periodontology* **30**, 595–602.

Lopez, N.J., Da Silva, I., Ipinza, J. & Gutierrez, J. (2005). Periodontal therapy reduces the rate of preterm low birth weight in women with pregnancy-associated gingivitis. *Journal of Periodontology* **76**, 2144–2153.

Lopez, N.J., Rios, V., Pareja, M.A. & Fernandez, O. (1991). Prevalence of juvenile periodontitis in Chile. *Journal of Clinical Periodontology* **18**, 529–533.

Lopez, N.J., Smith, P.C. & Gutierrez, J. (2002a). Higher risk of preterm birth and low birth weight in women with periodontal disease. *Journal of Dental Research* **81**, 58–63.

Lopez, N.J., Smith, P.C. & Gutierrez, J. (2002b). Periodontal therapy may reduce the risk of preterm low birth weight in women with periodontal disease: a randomized controlled trial. *Journal of Periodontology* **73**, 911–924.

Lopez, N.J., Socransky, S.S., Da Silva, I., Japlit, M.R. & Haffajee, A.D. (2004). Subgingival microbiota of chilean patients with chronic periodontitis. *Journal of Periodontology* **75**, 717–725.

Lopez, R., Fernandez, O., Jara, G. & Baelum, V. (2001). Epidemiology of clinical attachment loss in adolescents. *Journal of Periodontology* **72**, 1666–1674.

Lundström, A., Jendle, J., Stenström, B., Toss, G. & Ravald, N. (2001). Periodontal conditions in 70-year-old women with osteoporosis. *Swedish Dental Journal* **25**, 89–96.

Lynch, J. & Kaplan, G. (2000). Socioeconomic position. In: Berkman, L. & Kawachi, I. eds. *Social Epidemiology*. New York, NY: Oxford University Press, Inc.

MacDonald Jankowski, D.S. (1991). The detection of abnormalities in the jaws: a radiological survey. *British Dental Journal* **170**, 215–218.

Machtei, E.E., Hausmann, E., Dunford, R., Grossi, S., Ho, A., Davis, G., Chandler, J., Zambon, J. & Genco, R.J. (1999). Longitudinal study of predictive factors for periodontal disease and tooth loss. *Journal of Clinical Periodontology* **26**, 374–380.

Machtei, E.E., Hausmann, E., Schmidt, M., Grossi, S.G., Dunford, R., Schifferle, R., Munoz, K., Davies, G., Chandler, J. & Genco, R.J. (1998). Radiographic and clinical responses to periodontal therapy. *Journal of Periodontology* **69**, 590–595.

Mack, F., Mojon, P., Budtz-Jorgensen, E., Kocher, T., Splieth, C., Schwahn, C., Bernhardt, O., Gesch, D., Kordass, B., John, U. & Biffar, R. (2004). Caries and periodontal disease of the elderly in Pomerania, Germany: results of the Study of Health in Pomerania. *Gerodontology* **21**, 27–36.

Madianos, P.N., Lieff, S., Murtha, A.P., Boggess, K.A., Auten, R.L., Jr., Beck, J.D. & Offenbacher, S. (2001). Maternal periodontitis and prematurity. Part II: Maternal infection and fetal exposure. *Annals of Periodontology* **6**, 175–182.

Maiden, M.F., Cohee, P. & Tanner, A.C. (2003). Proposal to conserve the adjectival form of the specific epithet in the reclassification of Bacteroides forsythus Tanner et al. 1986 to the genus Tannerella Sakamoto et al. 2002 as Tannerella forsythia corrig., gen. nov., comb. nov. Request for an Opinion. *International Journal of Systematic and Evolutionary Microbiology* **53**, 2111–2112.

Mark, L.L., Haffajee, A.D., Socransky, S.S., Kent, R.L., Jr., Guerrero, D., Kornman, K., Newman, M. & Stashenko, P. (2000). Effect of the interleukin-1 genotype on monocyte IL-1beta expression in subjects with adult periodontitis. *Journal of Periodontal Research* **35**, 172–177.

Marshall-Day, C.D., Stephens, R.G. & Quigley, L.F., Jr. (1955). Periodontal disease: prevalence and incidence. *Journal of Periodontology* **26**, 185–203.

Martinez Canut, P., Guarinos, J. & Bagan, J.V. (1996). Periodontal disease in HIV seropositive patients and its relation to lymphocyte subsets. *Journal of Periodontology* **67**, 33–36.

Martinez Canut, P., Lorca, A. & Magan, R. (1995). Smoking and periodontal disease severity. *Journal of Clinical Periodontology* **22**, 743–749.

Matthesen, M., Baelum, V., Aarslev, I. & Fejerskov, O. (1990). Dental health of children and adults in Guinea-Bissau, West Africa, in 1986. *Community Dental Health* **7**, 123–133.

Mattila, K., Rasi, V., Nieminen, M., Valtonen, V., Kesaniemi, A., Syrjala, S., Jungell, P. & Huttunen, J.K. (1989). von Willebrand factor antigen and dental infections. *Thrombosis Research* **56**, 325–329.

Mattila, K.J., Asikainen, S., Wolf, J., Jousimies-Somer, H., Valtonen, V. & Nieminen, M. (2000). Age, dental infections, and coronary heart disease. *Journal of Dental Research* **79**, 756–760.

Maupome, G., Gullion, C.M., White, B.A., Wyatt, C.C. & Williams, P.M. (2003). Oral disorders and chronic systemic diseases in very old adults living in institutions. *Special Care in Dentistry* **23**, 199–208.

McCaul, L.K., Jenkins, W.M. & Kay, E.J. (2001). The reasons for the extraction of various tooth types in Scotland: a 15-year follow up. *Journal of Dentistry* **29**, 401–407.

McClellan, D.L., Griffen, A.L. & Leys, E.J. (1996). Age and prevalence of Porphyromonas gingivalis in children. *Journal of Clinical Microbiology* **34**, 2017–2019.

McCormick, M.C. (1985). The contribution of low birth weight to infant mortality and childhood morbidity. *New England Journal of Medicine* **312**, 82–90.

McDevitt, M.J., Wang, H.Y., Knobelman, C., Newman, M.G., di Giovine, F.S., Timms, J., Duff, G.W. & Kornman, K.S. (2000). Interleukin-1 genetic association with periodontitis in clinical practice. *Journal of Periodontology* **71**, 156–163.

McFall, W.T.J., Bader, J.D., Rozier, R.G., Ramsey, D., Graves, R., Sams, D. & Sloame, B. (1989). Clinical periodontal status of regularly attending patients in general dental practices. *Journal of Periodontology* **60**, 145–150.

McGregor, J.A., French, J.I., Lawellin, D. & Todd, J.K. (1988). Preterm birth and infection: pathogenic possibilities. *American Journal of Reproductive Immunology and Microbiology* **16**, 123–132.

McKaig, R.G., Thomas, J.C., Patton, L.L., Strauss, R.P., Slade, G.D. & Beck, J.D. (1998). Prevalence of HIV-associated periodontitis and chronic periodontitis in a southeastern US study group. *Journal of Public Health Dentistry* **58**, 294–300.

Mealey, B.L. & Oates, T.W. (2006). Diabetes mellitus and periodontal diseases. *Journal of Periodontology* **77**, 1289–1303.

Meisel, P., Carlsson, L.E., Sawaf, H., Fanghaenel, J., Greinacher, A. & Kocher, T. (2001). Polymorphisms of Fc gamma-receptors RIIa, RIIIa, and RIIIb in patients with adult periodontal diseases. *Genes and Immunity* **2**, 258–262.

Meisel, P., Schwahn, C., Gesch, D., Bernhardt, O., John, U. & Kocher, T. (2004). Dose-effect relation of smoking and the interleukin-1 gene polymorphism in periodontal disease. *Journal of Periodontology* **75**, 236–242.

Meisel, P., Siegemund, A., Dombrowa, S., Sawaf, H., Fanghaenel, J. & Kocher, T. (2002). Smoking and polymorphisms of the interleukin-1 gene cluster (IL-1alpha, IL-1beta, and IL-1RN) in patients with periodontal disease. *Journal of Periodontology* **73**, 27–32.

Meisel, P., Siegemund, A., Grimm, R., Herrmann, F.H., John, U., Schwahn, C. & Kocher, T. (2003). The interleukin-1 polymorphism, smoking, and the risk of periodontal disease in the population-based SHIP study. *Journal of Dental Research* **82**, 189–193.

Meisel, P., Timm, R., Sawaf, H., Fanghanel, J., Siegmund, W. & Kocher, T. (2000). Polymorphism of the N-acetyltransferase (NAT2), smoking and the potential risk of periodontal disease. *Archives of Toxicology* **74**, 343–348.

Melvin, W.L., Sandifer, J.B. & Gray, J.L. (1991). The prevalence and sex ratio of juvenile periodontitis in a young racially mixed population. *Journal of Periodontology* **62**, 330–334.

Mercanoglu, F., Oflaz, H., Oz, O., Gokbuget, A.Y., Genchellac, H., Sezer, M., Nisanci, Y. & Umman, S. (2004). Endothelial dysfunction in patients with chronic periodontitis and its improvement after initial periodontal therapy. *Journal of Periodontology* **75**, 1694–1700.

Meyer, D.H., Sreenivasan, P.K. & Fives-Taylor, P.M. (1991). Evidence for invasion of a human oral cell line by Actinobacillus actinomycetemcomitans. *Infection and Immunity* **59**, 2719–2726.

Michalowicz, B.S. (1994). Genetic and heritable risk factors in periodontal disease. *Journal of Periodontology* **65**, 479–488.

Michalowicz, B.S., Aeppli, D., Virag, J.G., Klump, D.G., Hinrichs, J.E., Segal, N.L., Bouchard, T.J., Jr. & Pihlstrom, B.L. (1991). Periodontal findings in adult twins. *Journal of Periodontology* **62**, 293–299.

Michalowicz, B.S., Hodges, J.S., DiAngelis, A.J., Lupo, V.R., Novak, M.J., Ferguson, J.E., Buchanan, W., Bofill, J., Papapanou, P.N., Mitchell, D.A., Matseoane, S. & Tschida, P.A. (2006). Treatment of periodontal disease and the risk of preterm birth. *New England Journal of Medicine* **355**, 1885–1894.

Michel, J., Gonzales, J.R., Wunderlich, D., Diete, A., Herrmann, J.M. & Meyle, J. (2001). Interleukin-4 polymorphisms in early onset periodontitis. *Journal of Clinical Periodontology* **28**, 483–488.

Miller, L.S., Manwell, M.A., Newbold, D., Reding, M.E., Rasheed, A., Blodgett, J. & Kornman, K.S. (1992). The relationship between reduction in periodontal inflammation and diabetes control: a report of 9 cases. *Journal of Periodontology* **63**, 843–848.

Mitchell-Lewis, D., Engebretson, S.P., Chen, J., Lamster, I.B. & Papapanou, P.N. (2001). Periodontal infections and preterm birth: early findings from a cohort of young minority women in New York. *European Journal of Oral Science* **109**, 34–39.

Miyazaki, H., Pilot, T. & Leclercq, M.-H. (1992). Periodontal profiles. An overview of CPITN data in the WHO Global Oral Data Bank for the age group 15–19 years, 35–44 years and 65–75 years. Geneva: World Health Organization.

Miyazaki, H., Pilot, T., Leclercq, M.H. & Barmes, D.E. (1991a). Profiles of periodontal conditions in adolescents measured by CPITN. *International Dental Journal* **41**, 67–73.

Miyazaki, H., Pilot, T., Leclercq, M.H. & Barmes, D.E. (1991b). Profiles of periodontal conditions in adults measured by CPITN. *International Dental Journal* **41**, 74–80.

Mohammad, A.R., Bauer, R.L. & Yeh, C.K. (1997). Spinal bone density and tooth loss in a cohort of postmenopausal women. *International Journal of Prosthodontics* **10**, 381–385.

Mohammad, A.R., Brunsvold, M. & Bauer, R. (1996). The strength of association between systemic postmenopausal osteoporosis and periodontal disease. *International Journal of Prosthodontics* **9**, 479–483.

Mokeem, S.A., Molla, G.N. & Al-Jewair, T.S. (2004). The prevalence and relationship between periodontal disease and pre-term low birth weight infants at King Khalid University Hospital in Riyadh, Saudi Arabia. *Journal of Contemporary Dental Practice* **5**, 40–56.

Mombelli, A., Gmür, R., Frey, J., Meyer, J., Zee, K.Y., Tam, J.O., Lo, E.C., Di Rienzo, J., Lang, N.P. & Corbet, E.F. (1998). *Actinobacillus actinomycetemcomitans* and *Porphyromonas gingivalis* in young Chinese adults. *Oral Microbiology and Immunology* **13**, 231–237.

Moore, S., Ide, M., Coward, P.Y., Randhawa, M., Borkowska, E., Baylis, R. & Wilson, R.F. (2004). A prospective study to investigate the relationship between periodontal disease and adverse pregnancy outcome. *British Dental Journal* **197**, 251–258; discussion 247.

Moore, S., Randhawa, M. & Ide, M. (2005). A case-control study to investigate an association between adverse pregnancy outcome and periodontal disease. *Journal of Clinical Periodontology* **32**, 1–5.

Mühlemann, H.R. & Son, S. (1971). Gingival sulcus bleeding-aleading symptom in initial gingivitis. *Helvetica Odontologica Acta* **15**, 107–113.

Mutale, T., Creed, F., Maresh, M. & Hunt, L. (1991). Life events and low birthweight – analysis by infants preterm and small for gestational age. *British Journal of Obstetrics and Gynaecology* **98**, 166–172.

Myles, T.D., Espinoza, R., Meyer, W., Bieniarz, A. & Nguyen, T. (1998). Effects of smoking, alcohol, and drugs of abuse on the outcome of "expectantly" managed cases of preterm premature rupture of membranes. *Journal of Maternal-Fetal Medicine* **7**, 157–161.

Ndiaye, C.F., Critchlow, C.W., Leggott, P.J., Kiviat, N.B., Ndoye, I., Robertson, P.B. & Georgas, K.N. (1997). Periodontal status of HIV-1 and HIV-2 seropositive and HIV seronegative female commercial sex workers in Senegal. *Journal of Periodontology* **68**, 827–831.

Neely, A.L. (1992). Prevalence of juvenile periodontitis in a circumpubertal population. *Journal of Clinical Periodontology* **19**, 367–372.

Neely, A.L., Holford, T.R., Loe, H., Anerud, A. & Boysen, H. (2005). The natural history of periodontal disease in humans: risk factors for tooth loss in caries-free subjects receiving no oral health care. *Journal of Clinical Periodontology* **32**, 984–993.

Ness, P.M. & Perkins, H.A. (1980). Transient bacteremia after dental procedures and other minor manipulations. *Transfusion* **20**, 82–85.

Nishimura, F. & Murayama, Y. (2001). Periodontal inflammation and insulin resistance–lessons from obesity. *Journal of Dental Research* **80**, 1690–1694.

Norderyd, O., Hugoson, A. & Grusovin, G. (1999). Risk of severe periodontal disease in a Swedish adult population. A longitudinal study. *Journal of Clinical Periodontology* **26**, 608–615.

Norskov-Lauritsen, N. & Kilian, M. (2006). Reclassification of *Actinobacillus actinomycetemcomitans*, *Haemophilus aphrophilus*, *Haemophilus paraphrophilus* and *Haemophilus segnis* as *Aggregatibacter actinomycetemcomitans* gen. nov., comb. nov., *Aggregatibacter aphrophilus* comb. nov. and *Aggregatibacter segnis* comb. nov., and emended description of *Aggregatibacter aphrophilus* to include V factor-dependent and V factor-independent isolates. *International Journal of Systematic and Evolutionary Microbiology* **56**, 2135–2146.

O'Leary, D.H., Polak, J.F., Kronmal, R.A., Manolio, T.A., Burke, G.L. & Wolfson, S.K., Jr. (1999). Carotid-artery intima and media thickness as a risk factor for myocardial infarction and stroke in older adults. Cardiovascular Health Study Collaborative Research Group. *New England Journal of Medicine* **340**, 14–22.

Oakes, M. (1993). The logic and role of meta-analysis in clinical research. *Statistical Methods in Medical Research* **2**, 147–160.

Offenbacher, S., Boggess, K.A., Murtha, A.P., Jared, H.L., Lieff, S., McKaig, R.G., Mauriello, S.M., Moss, K.L. & Beck, J.D. (2006). Progressive periodontal disease and risk of very preterm delivery. *Obstetrics and Gynecology* **107**, 29–36.

Offenbacher, S., Jared, H.L., O'Reilly, P.G., Wells, S.R., Salvi, G.E., Lawrence, H.P., Socransky, S.S. & Beck, J.D. (1998). Potential pathogenic mechanisms of periodontitis associated pregnancy complications. *Annals of Periodontology* **3**, 233–250.

Offenbacher, S., Katz, V., Fertik, G., Collins, J., Boyd, D., Maynor, G., McKaig, R. & Beck, J. (1996). Periodontal infection as a possible risk factor for preterm low birth weight. *Journal of Periodontology* **67**, 1103–1113.

Offenbacher, S., Lieff, S., Boggess, K.A., Murtha, A.P., Madianos, P.N., Champagne, C.M., McKaig, R.G., Jared, H.L., Mauriello, S.M., Auten, R.L., Jr., Herbert, W.N. & Beck, J.D. (2001). Maternal periodontitis and prematurity. Part I: Obstetric outcome of prematurity and growth restriction. *Annals of Periodontology* **6**, 164–174.

Ogawa, H., Yoshihara, A., Hirotomi, T., Ando, Y. & Miyazaki, H. (2002). Risk factors for periodontal disease progression among elderly people. *Journal of Clinical Periodontology* **29**, 592–597.

Okamoto, H., Yoneyama, T., Lindhe, J., Haffajee, A. & Socransky, S. (1988). Methods of evaluating periodontal disease data in epidemiological research. *Journal of Clinical Periodontology* **15**, 430–439.

Oliver, R.C., Brown, L.J. & Loe, H. (1998). Periodontal diseases in the United States population. *Journal of Periodontology* **69**, 269–278.

Oliver, R.C., Brown, L.J. & Löe, H. (1989). An estimate of periodontal treatment needs in the U.S. based on epidemiologic data. *Journal of Periodontology* **60**, 371–380.

Oliver, R.C. & Tervonen, T. (1993). Periodontitis and tooth loss: comparing diabetics with the general population. *Journal of the American Dental Association* **124**, 71–76.

Otto, G., Braconier, J., Andreasson, A. & Svanborg, C. (1999). Interleukin-6 and disease severity in patients with bacteremic and nonbacteremic febrile urinary tract infection. *Journal of Infectious Diseases* **179**, 172–179.

Page, R.C., Bowen, T., Altman, L., Vandesteen, E., Ochs, H., Mackenzie, P., Osterberg, S., Engel, L.D. & Williams, B.L. (1983). Prepubertal periodontitis. I. Definition of a clinical disease entity. *Journal of Periodontology* **54**, 257–271.

Pajukoski, H., Meurman, J.H., Snellman-Grohn, S. & Sulkava, R. (1999). Oral health in hospitalized and nonhospitalized community-dwelling elderly patients. *Oral Surgery, Oral Medicine, Oral Pathology, Oral Radiology, and Endodontics* **88**, 437–443.

Palmer, R.M., Wilson, R.F., Hasan, A.S. & Scott, D.A. (2005). Mechanisms of action of environmental factors–tobacco smoking. *Journal of Clinical Periodontology* **32** Suppl 6, 180–195.

Papantonopoulos, G.H. (2004). Effect of periodontal therapy in smokers and non-smokers with advanced periodontal disease: results after maintenance therapy for a minimum of 5 years. *Journal of Periodontology* **75**, 839–843.

Papapanou, P.N. (1996). Periodontal diseases: epidemiology. *Annals of Periodontology* **1**, 1–36.

Papapanou, P.N., Baelum, V., Luan, W.-M., Madianos, P.N., Chen, X., Fejerskov, O. & Dahlén, G. (1997). Subgingival microbiota in adult Chinese: Prevalence and relation to periodontal disease progression. *Journal of Periodontology* **68**, 651–666.

Papapanou, P.N., Lindhe, J., Sterrett, J.D. & Eneroth, L. (1991). Considerations on the contribution of ageing to loss of periodontal tissue support. *Journal of Clinical Periodontology* **18**, 611–615.

Papapanou, P.N., Neiderud, A.-M., Papadimitriou, A., Sandros, J. & Dahlén, G. (2000). "Checkerboard" assessments of periodontal microbiota and serum antibody responses: a case-control study. *Journal of Periodontology* **71**, 885–897.

Papapanou, P.N., Neiderud, A.-M., Sandros, J. & Dahlén, G. (2001). Interleukin-1 gene polymorphism and periodontal status: a case-control study. *Journal of Clinical Periodontology* **28**, 389–396.

Papapanou, P.N., Teanpaisan, R., Obiechina, N.S., Pithpomchaiyakul, W., Pongpaisal, S., Pisuithanakan, S., Baelum, V., Fejerskov, O. & Dahlén, G. (2002). Periodontal microbiota and clinical periodontal status in a rural sample in Southern Thailand. *European Journal of Oral Science* **110**, 345–352.

Papapanou, P.N. & Wennström, J.L. (1991). The angular bony defect as indicator of further alveolar bone loss. *Journal of Clinical Periodontology* **18**, 317–322.

Papapanou, P.N., Wennström, J.L. & Gröndahl, K. (1988). Periodontal status in relation to age and tooth type. A cross-sectional radiographic study. *Journal of Clinical Periodontology* **15**, 469–478.

Papapanou, P.N., Wennström, J.L. & Gröndahl, K. (1989). A 10-year retrospective study of periodontal disease progression. *Journal of Clinical Periodontology* **16**, 403–411.

Papapanou, P.N., Wennström, J.L. & Johnsson, T. (1993). Extent and severity of periodontal destruction based on partial clinical assessments. *Community Dentistry and Oral Epidemiology* **21**, 181–184.

Papapanou, P.N., Wennström, J.L., Sellén, A., Hirooka, H., Gröndahl, K. & Johnsson, T. (1990). Periodontal treatment needs assessed by the use of clinical and radiographic criteria. *Community Dentistry and Oral Epidemiology* **18**, 113–119.

Park, K.S., Nam, J.H. & Choi, J. (2006). The short vitamin D receptor is associated with increased risk for generalized aggressive periodontitis. *Journal of Clinical Periodontology* **33**, 524–528.

Parkhill, J.M., Hennig, B.J., Chapple, I.L., Heasman, P.A. & Taylor, J.J. (2000). Association of interleukin-1 gene polymorphisms with early-onset periodontitis. *Journal of Clinical Periodontology* **27**, 682–689.

Paster, B.J., Boches, S.K., Galvin, J.L., Ericson, R.E., Lau, C.N., Levanos, V.A., Sahasrabudhe, A. & Dewhirst, F.E. (2001). Bacterial diversity in human subgingival plaque. *Journal of Bacteriology* **183**, 3770–3783.

Paulander, J., Axelsson, P., Lindhe, J. & Wennstrom, J. (2004a). Intra-oral pattern of tooth and periodontal bone loss between the age of 50 and 60 years. A longitudinal prospective study. *Acta Odontologica Scandinavica* **62**, 214–222.

Paulander, J., Wennstrom, J.L., Axelsson, P. & Lindhe, J. (2004b). Some risk factors for periodontal bone loss in 50-year-old individuals. A 10-year cohort study. *Journal of Clinical Periodontology* **31**, 489–496.

Payne, J.B., Reinhardt, R.A., Nummikoski, P.V., Dunning, D.G. & Patil, K.D. (2000). The association of cigarette smoking with alveolar bone loss in postmenopausal females. *Journal of Clinical Periodontology* **27**, 658–664.

Payne, J.B., Reinhardt, R.A., Nummikoski, P.V. & Patil, K.D. (1999). Longitudinal alveolar bone loss in postmenopausal osteoporotic/osteopenic women. *Osteoporosis International* **10**, 34–40.

Perez, C., Gonzalez, F.E., Pavez, V., Araya, A.V., Aguirre, A., Cruzat, A., Contreras-Levicoy, J., Dotte, A., Aravena, O., Salazar, L., Catalan, D., Cuenca, J., Ferreira, A., Schiattino, I. & Aguillon, J.C. (2004). The -308 polymorphism in the promoter region of the tumor necrosis factor-alpha (TNF-alpha) gene and ex vivo lipopolysaccharide-induced TNF-alpha expression in patients with aggressive periodontitis and/or type 1 diabetes mellitus. *European Cytokine Network* **15**, 364–370.

Persson, R.E., Hollender, L.G., Powell, L.V., MacEntee, M.I., Wyatt, C.C., Kiyak, H.A. & Persson, G.R. (2002). Assessment of periodontal conditions and systemic disease in older subjects. I. Focus on osteoporosis. *Journal of Clinical Periodontology* **29**, 796–802.

Petersen, P.E., Bourgeois, D., Bratthall, D. & Ogawa, H. (2005). Oral health information systems–towards measuring progress in oral health promotion and disease prevention. *Bulletin of the World Health Organization* **83**, 686–693.

Petersen, P.E. & Ogawa, H. (2005). Strengthening the prevention of periodontal disease: the WHO approach. *Journal of Periodontology* **76**, 2187–2193.

Phipps, K.R., Reifel, N. & Bothwell, E. (1991). The oral health status, treatment needs, and dental utilization patterns of Native American elders. *Journal of Public Health Dentistry* **51**, 228–233.

Pilot, T. & Miyazaki, H. (1994). Global results: 15 years of CPITN epidemiology. *International Dental Journal* **44**, 553–560.

Pinson, M., Hoffman, W.H., Garnick, J.J. & Litaker, M.S. (1995). Periodontal disease and type I diabetes mellitus in children and adolescents. *Journal of Clinical Periodontology* **22**, 118–123.

Pitiphat, W., Crohin, C., Williams, P., Merchant, A.T., Douglass, C.W., Colditz, G.A. & Joshipura, K.J. (2004). Use of preexisting radiographs for assessing periodontal disease in epidemiologic studies. *Journal of Public Health Dentistry* **64**, 223–230.

Pontes, C.C., Gonzales, J.R., Novaes, A.B., Jr., Junior, M.T., Grisi, M.F., Michel, J., Meyle, J. & de Souza, S.L. (2004). 'Interleukin-4 gene polymorphism and its relation to periodontal disease in a Brazilian population of African heritage'. *Journal of Dentistry* **32**, 241–246.

Proskin, H.M. & Volpe, A.R. (1994). Meta-analysis in dental research: A paradigm for performance and interpretation. *Journal of Clinical Dentistry* **5**, 19–26.

Pussinen, P.J., Alfthan, G., Tuomilehto, J., Asikainen, S. & Jousilahti, P. (2004). High serum antibody levels to Porphyromonas gingivalis predict myocardial infarction. *European Journal of Cardiovascular Prevention and Rehabilitation* **11**, 408–411.

Pussinen, P.J., Nyyssonen, K., Alfthan, G., Salonen, R., Laukkanen, J.A. & Salonen, J.T. (2005). Serum antibody levels to *Actinobacillus actinomycetemcomitans* predict the risk for coronary heart disease. *Arteriosclerosis, Thrombosis, and Vascular Biology* **25**, 833–838.

Quappe, L., Jara, L. & Lopez, N.J. (2004). Association of interleukin-1 polymorphisms with aggressive periodontitis. *Journal of Periodontology* **75**, 1509–1515.

Querna, J.C., Rossmann, J.A. & Kerns, D.G. (1994). Prevalence of periodontal disease in an active duty military population as indicated by an experimental periodontal index. *Military Medicine* **159**, 233–236.

Radnai, M., Gorzo, I., Nagy, E., Urban, E., Novak, T. & Pal, A. (2004). A possible association between preterm birth and early periodontitis. A pilot study. *Journal of Clinical Periodontology* **31**, 736–741.

Ragnarsson, E., Eliasson, S.T. & Olafsson, S.H. (1992). Tobacco smoking, a factor in tooth loss in Reykjavik, Iceland. *Scandinavian Journal of Dental Research* **100**, 322–326.

Rajapakse, P.S., Nagarathne, M., Chandrasekra, K.B. & Dasanayake, A.P. (2005). Periodontal disease and prematurity among non-smoking Sri Lankan women. *Journal of Dental Research* **84**, 274–277.

Ramfjord, S.P. (1959). Indices for prevalence and incidence of periodontal disease. *Journal of Periodontology* **30**, 51–59.

Rayfield, E.J., Ault, M.J., Keusch, G.T., Brothers, M.J., Nechemias, C. & Smith, H. (1982). Infection and diabetes: the case for glucose control. *American Journal of Medicine* **72**, 439–450.

Reich, E. & Hiller, K.A. (1993). Reasons for tooth extraction in the western states of Germany. *Community Dentistry and Oral Epidemiology* **21**, 379–383.

Reinhardt, R.A., Payne, J.B., Maze, C.A., Patil, K.D., Gallagher, S.J. & Mattson, J.S. (1999). Influence of estrogen and osteopenia/osteoporosis on clinical periodontitis in postmenopausal women. *Journal of Periodontology* **70**, 823–828.

Renvert, S., Dahlén, G. & Wikström, M. (1996). Treatment of periodontal disease based on microbiological diagnosis. Relation between microbiological and clinical parameters during 5 years. *Journal of Periodontology* **67**, 562–571.

Rieder, C., Joss, A. & Lang, N.P. (2004). Influence of compliance and smoking habits on the outcomes of supportive periodontal therapy (SPT) in a private practice. *Oral Health and Preventive Dentistry* **2**, 89–94.

Roberts-Thomson, K.F. & Stewart, J.F. (2003). Access to dental care by young South Australian adults. *Australian Dental Journal* **48**, 169–174.

Robinson, P.G., Boulter, A., Birnbaum, W. & Johnson, N.W. (2000). A controlled study of relative periodontal attachment loss in people with HIV infection. *Journal of Clinical Periodontology* **27**, 273–276.

Robinson, P.G., Sheiham, A., Challacombe, S.J. & Zakrzewska, J.M. (1996). The periodontal health of homosexual men with HIV infection: a controlled study. *Oral Disease* **2**, 45–52.

Rodrigues, D.C., Taba, M.J., Novaes, A.B., Souza, S.L. & Grisi, M.F. (2003). Effect of non-surgical periodontal therapy on glycemic control in patients with type 2 diabetes mellitus. *Journal of Periodontology* **74**, 1361–1367.

Romero, B.C., Chiquito, C.S., Elejalde, L.E. & Bernardoni, C.B. (2002). Relationship between periodontal disease in pregnant women and the nutritional condition of their newborns. *Journal of Periodontology* **73**, 1177–1183.

Romero, R., Gomez, R., Chaiworapongsa, T., Conoscenti, G., Kim, J.C. & Kim, Y.M. (2001). The role of infection in preterm labour and delivery. *Paediatric and Perinatal Epidemiology* **15** Suppl 2, 41–56.

Romero, R., Quintero, R., Oyarzun, E., Wu, Y.K., Sabo, V., Mazor, M. & Hobbins, J.C. (1988). Intraamniotic infection and the onset of labor in preterm premature rupture of the membranes. *American Journal of Obstetrics and Gynecology* **159**, 661–666.

Ross, R. (1993). The pathogenesis of atherosclerosis: a perspective for the 1990s. *Nature* **362**, 801–809.

Ross, R. (1999). Atherosclerosis – an inflammatory disease. *New England Journal of Medicine* **340**, 115–126.

Russell, A.L. (1956). A system for classification and scoring for prevalence surveys of periodontal disease. *Journal of Dental Research* **35**, 350–359.

Saito, T., Shimazaki, Y., Kiyohara, Y., Kato, I., Kubo, M., Iida, M. & Koga, T. (2004). The severity of periodontal disease is associated with the development of glucose intolerance in non-diabetics: the Hisayama study. *Journal of Dental Research* **83**, 485–490.

Saito, T., Shimazaki, Y., Koga, T., Tsuzuki, M. & Ohshima, A. (2001). Relationship between upper body obesity and periodontitis. *Journal of Dental Research* **80**, 1631–1636.

Saito, T., Shimazaki, Y. & Sakamoto, M. (1998). Obesity and periodontitis. *New England Journal of Medicine* **339**, 482–483.

Sakamoto, M., Suzuki, M., Umeda, M., Ishikawa, I. & Benno, Y. (2002). Reclassification of *Bacteroides forsythus* (Tanner *et al.* 1986) as *Tannerella forsythensis* corrig., gen. nov., comb. nov. *International Journal of Systematic and Evolutionary Microbiology* **52**, 841–849.

Sakellari, D., Koukoudetsos, S., Arsenakis, M. & Konstantinidis, A. (2003). Prevalence of IL-1A and IL-1B polymorphisms in a Greek population. *Journal of Clinical Periodontology* **30**, 35–41.

Salonen, L.W., Frithiof, L., Wouters, F.R. & Helldén, L.B. (1991). Marginal alveolar bone height in an adult Swedish population. A radiographic cross-sectional epidemiologic study. *Journal of Clinical Periodontology* **18**, 223–232.

Salvi, G.E., Brown, C.E., Fujihashi, K., Kiyono, H., Smith, F.W., Beck, J.D. & Offenbacher, S. (1998). Inflammatory mediators of the terminal dentition in adult and early onset periodontitis. *Journal of Periodontal Research* **33**, 212–225.

Sandros, J., Papapanou, P.N., Nannmark, U. & Dahlén, G. (1994). Porphyromonas gingivalis invades human pocket epithelium in vitro. *Journal of Periodontal Research* **29**, 62–69.

Sanz, M., van Winkelhoff, A.J., Herrera, D., Dellemijn-Kippuw, N., Simon, R. & Winkel, E. (2000). Differences in the composition of the subgingival microbiota of two periodontitis populations of different geographical origin. A comparison between Spain and The Netherlands. *European Journal of Oral Science* **108**, 383–392.

Saxby, M.S. (1987). Juvenile periodontitis: an epidemiological study in the west Midlands of the United Kingdom. *Journal of Clinical Periodontology* **14**, 594–598.

Saxén, L. (1980). Prevalence of juvenile periodontitis in Finland. *Journal of Clinical Periodontology* **7**, 177–186.

Scabbia, A., Cho, K.S., Sigurdsson, T.J., Kim, C.K. & Trombelli, L. (2001). Cigarette smoking negatively affects healing response following flap debridement surgery. *Journal of Periodontology* **72**, 43–49.

Scapoli, C., Trombelli, L., Mamolini, E. & Collins, A. (2005). Linkage disequilibrium analysis of case-control data: an application to generalized aggressive periodontitis. *Genes and Immunity* **6**, 44–52.

Scarel-Caminaga, R.M., Trevilatto, P.C., Souza, A.P., Brito, R.B., Camargo, L.E. & Line, S.R. (2004). Interleukin 10 gene promoter polymorphisms are associated with chronic periodontitis. *Journal of Clinical Periodontology* **31**, 443–448.

Scarel-Caminaga, R.M., Trevilatto, P.C., Souza, A.P., Brito, R.B., Jr. & Line, S.R. (2003). Investigation of IL4 gene polymorphism in individuals with different levels of chronic periodontitis in a Brazilian population. *Journal of Clinical Periodontology* **30**, 341–345.

Scarel-Caminaga, R.M., Trevilatto, P.C., Souza, A.P., Brito, R.B. & Line, S.R. (2002). Investigation of an IL-2 polymorphism in patients with different levels of chronic periodontitis. *Journal of Clinical Periodontology* **29**, 587–591.

Schei, O., Waerhaug, J., Lövdal, A. & Arno, A. (1959). Alveolar bone loss related to oral hygiene and age. *Journal of Periodontology* **30**, 7–16.

Schenkein, H.A. (2002). Finding genetic risk factors for periodontal diseases: is the climb worth the view? *Periodontology 2000* **30**, 79–90.

Scherp, H.W. (1964). Current concepts in periodontal disease research: Epidemiological contributions. *Journal of the American Dental Association* **68**, 667–675.

Scheutz, F., Matee, M.I., Andsager, L., Holm, A.M., Moshi, J., Kagoma, C. & Mpemba, N. (1997). Is there an association between periodontal condition and HIV infection? *Journal of Clinical Periodontology* **24**, 580–587.

Scholl, T.O., Miller, L.K., Shearer, J., Cofsky, M.C., Salmon, R.W., Vasilenko, P. 3rd & Ances, I. (1988). Influence of young maternal age and parity on term and preterm low birthweight. *American Journal of Perinatology* **5**, 101–104.

Schürch, E., Jr. & Lang, N.P. (2004). Periodontal conditions in Switzerland at the end of the 20th century. *Oral Health and Preventive Dentistry* **2**, 359–368.

Schürch, E., Jr., Minder, C.E., Lang, N.P. & Geering, A.H. (1990). Comparison of clinical periodontal parameters with the Community Periodontal Index for Treatment Needs (CPITN) data. *Schweizer Monatsschrift für Zahnmedizin* **100**, 408–411.

Schwahn, C., Volzke, H., Robinson, D.M., Luedemann, J., Bernhardt, O., Gesch, D., John, U. & Kocher, T. (2004). Periodontal disease, but not edentulism, is independently associated with increased plasma fibrinogen levels. Results from a population-based study. *Thrombosis and Haemostasis* **92**, 244–252.

Sculean, A., Stavropoulos, A., Berakdar, M., Windisch, P., Karring, T. & Brecx, M. (2005). Formation of human cementum following different modalities of regenerative therapy. *Clinical Oral Investigations* **9**, 58–64.

Seinost, G., Wimmer, G., Skerget, M., Thaller, E., Brodmann, M., Gasser, R., Bratschko, R.O. & Pilger, E. (2005). Periodontal treatment improves endothelial dysfunction in patients with severe periodontitis. *American Heart Journal* **149**, 1050–1054.

Seppälä, B., Seppälä, M. & Ainamo, J. (1993). A longitudinal study on insulin-dependent diabetes mellitus and periodontal disease. *Journal of Clinical Periodontology* **20**, 161–165.

Shapira, L., Stabholz, A., Rieckmann, P. & Kruse, N. (2001). Genetic polymorphism of the tumor necrosis factor (TNF)-alpha promoter region in families with localized early-onset periodontitis. *Journal of Periodontal Research* **36**, 183–186.

Shimada, Y., Tai, H., Endo, M., Kobayashi, T., Akazawa, K. & Yamazaki, K. (2004). Association of tumor necrosis factor receptor type 2 +587 gene polymorphism with severe chronic periodontitis. *Journal of Clinical Periodontology* **31**, 463–469.

Shlossman, M., Knowler, W.C., Pettitt, D.J. & Genco, R.J. (1990). Type 2 diabetes mellitus and periodontal disease. *Journal of the American Dental Association* **121**, 532–536.

Shlossman, M., Pettitt, D., Arevalo, A. & Genco, R.J. (1986). Periodontal disease in children and young adults on the Gila River Indian Reservation. *Journal of Dental Research* **65**, special issue, abst. # 1127.

Silness, J. & Löe, H. (1964). Periodontal disease in pregnancy. II Corelation between oral hygiene and periodontal condition. *Acta Odontologica Scandinavica* **22**, 112–135.

Silver, J.G., Martin, A.W. & McBride, B.C. (1977). Experimental transient bacteraemias in human subjects with varying degrees of plaque accumulation and gingival inflammation. *Journal of Clinical Periodontology* **4**, 92–99.

Sjödin, B., Crossner, C.G., Unell, L. & Ostlund, P. (1989). A retrospective radiographic study of alveolar bone loss in the primary dentition in patients with localized juvenile periodontitis. *Journal of Clinical Periodontology* **16**, 124–127.

Sjödin, B. & Matsson, L. (1992). Marginal bone level in the normal primary dentition. *Journal of Clinical Periodontology* **19**, 672–678.

Sjödin, B., Matsson, L., Unell, L. & Egelberg, J. (1993). Marginal bone loss in the primary dentition of patients with juvenile periodontitis. *Journal of Clinical Periodontology* **20**, 32–36.

Slade, G.D., Ghezzi, E.M., Heiss, G., Beck, J.D., Riche, E. & Offenbacher, S. (2003). Relationship between periodontal disease and C-reactive protein among adults in the Atherosclerosis Risk in Communities study. *Archives of Internal Medicine* **163**, 1172–1179.

Slade, G.D., Offenbacher, S., Beck, J.D., Heiss, G. & Pankow, J.S. (2000). Acute-phase inflammatory response to periodontal disease in the US population. *Journal of Dental Research* **79**, 49–57.

Slade, G.D., Spencer, A.J., Gorkic, E. & Andrews, G. (1993). Oral health status and treatment needs of non-institutionalized persons aged 60+ in Adelaide, South Australia. *Australian Dental Journal* **38**, 373–380.

Smith, G.L., Cross, D.L. & Wray, D. (1995a). Comparison of periodontal disease in HIV seropositive subjects and controls (I). Clinical features. *Journal of Clinical Periodontology* **22**, 558–568.

Smith, G.L.F., Cross, D.L. & Wray, D. (1995b). Comparison of periodontal disease in HIV seropositive subjects and controls (I). Clinical features. *Journal of Clinical Periodontology* **22**, 558–568.

Smith, G.T., Greenbaum, C.J., Johnson, B.D. & Persson, G.R. (1996). Short-term responses to periodontal therapy in insulin-dependent diabetic patients. *Journal of Periodontology* **67**, 794–802.

Socransky, S.S., Haffajee, A.D., Cugini, M.A., Smith, C. & Kent, R.L., Jr. (1998). Microbial complexes in subgingival plaque. *Journal of Clinical Periodontology* **25**, 134–144.

Socransky, S.S., Haffajee, A.D. & Smith, C. (2000). Microbiological parameters associated with IL-1 gene polymorphisms in periodontitis patients. *Journal of Clinical Periodontology* **27**, 810–818.

Socransky, S.S., Smith, C., Martin, L., Paster, B.J., Dewhirst, F. E. & Levin, A.E. (1994). "Checkerboard" DNA-DNA hybridization. *Biotechniques* **17**, 788–792.

Söder, P.O., Jin, L.J., Söder, B. & Wikner, S. (1994). Periodontal status in an urban adult population in Sweden. *Community Dentistry and Oral Epidemiology* **22**, 106–111.

Soga, Y., Nishimura, F., Ohyama, H., Maeda, H., Takashiba, S. & Murayama, Y. (2003). Tumor necrosis factor-alpha gene (TNF-alpha) -1031/-863, -857 single-nucleotide polymorphisms (SNPs) are associated with severe adult periodontitis in Japanese. *Journal of Clinical Periodontology* **30**, 524–531.

Soskolne, W.A. & Klinger, A. (2001). The relationship between periodontal diseases and diabetes: an overview. *Annals of Periodontology* **6**, 91–98.

Spiekerman, C.F., Hujoel, P.P. & DeRouen, T.A. (2003). Bias induced by self-reported smoking on periodontitis-systemic disease associations. *Journal of Dental Research* **82**, 345–349.

Stavropoulos, A., Mardas, N., Herrero, F. & Karring, T. (2004). Smoking affects the outcome of guided tissue regeneration with bioresorbable membranes: a retrospective analysis of intrabony defects. *Journal of Clinical Periodontology* **31**, 945–950.

Stelzel, M., Conrads, G., Pankuweit, S., Maisch, B., Vogt, S., Moosdorf, R. & Flores-de-Jacoby, L. (2002). Detection of Porphyromonas gingivalis DNA in aortic tissue by PCR. *Journal of Periodontology* **73**, 868–870.

Stephens, R.G., Kogon, S.L. & Jarvis, A.M. (1991). A study of the reasons for tooth extraction in a Canadian population sample [published erratum appears in J Can Dent Assoc 1991 Aug;57(8):611]. *Journal of the Canadian Dental Association* **57**, 501–504.

Stewart, J.E., Wager, K.A., Friedlander, A.H. & Zadeh, H.H. (2001). The effect of periodontal treatment on glycemic control in patients with type 2 diabetes mellitus. *Journal of Clinical Periodontology* **28**, 306–310.

Stoltenberg, J.L., Osborn, J.B., Pihlstrom, B.L., Hardie, N.A., Aeppli, D.M., Huso, B.A., Bakdash, M.B. & Fischer, G.E. (1993a). Prevalence of periodontal disease in a health maintenance organization and comparisons to the national survey of oral health. *Journal of Periodontology* **64**, 853–858.

Stoltenberg, J.L., Osborn, J.B., Pihlstrom, B.L., Herzberg, M.C., Aeppli, D.M., Wolff, L.F. & Fischer, G.E. (1993b). Association between cigarette smoking, bacterial pathogens, and periodontal status. *Journal of Periodontology* **64**, 1225–1230.

Stuck, A.E., Chappuis, C., Flury, H. & Lang, N.P. (1989). Dental treatment needs in an elderly population referred to a geriatric hospital in Switzerland. *Community Dentistry and Oral Epidemiology* **17**, 267–272.

Sugita, N., Kobayashi, T., Ando, Y., Yoshihara, A., Yamamoto, K., van de Winkel, J.G., Miyazaki, H. & Yoshie, H. (2001). Increased frequency of FcgammaRIIIb-NA1 allele in periodontitis-resistant subjects in an elderly Japanese population. *Journal of Dental Research* **80**, 914–918.

Sugita, N., Yamamoto, K., Kobayashi, T., Van Der Pol, W., Horigome, T., Yoshie, H., Van De Winkel, J.G. & Hara, K. (1999). Relevance of Fc gamma RIIIa-158V-F polymorphism to recurrence of adult periodontitis in Japanese patients. *Clinical and Experimental Immunology* **117**, 350–354.

Susin, C. & Albandar, J.M. (2005). Aggressive periodontitis in an urban population in southern Brazil. *Journal of Periodontology* **76**, 468–475.

Susin, C., Dalla Vecchia, C.F., Oppermann, R.V., Haugejorden, O. & Albandar, J.M. (2004a). Periodontal attachment loss in an urban population of Brazilian adults: effect of demographic, behavioral, and environmental risk indicators. *Journal of Periodontology* **75**, 1033–1041.

Susin, C., Kingman, A. & Albandar, J.M. (2005a). Effect of partial recording protocols on estimates of prevalence of periodontal disease. *Journal of Periodontology* **76**, 262–267.

Susin, C., Oppermann, R.V., Haugejorden, O. & Albandar, J.M. (2004b). Periodontal attachment loss attributable to cigarette smoking in an urban Brazilian population. *Journal of Clinical Periodontology* **31**, 951–958.

Susin, C., Oppermann, R.V., Haugejorden, O. & Albandar, J.M. (2005b). Tooth loss and associated risk indicators in an adult urban population from south Brazil. *Acta Odontologica Scandinavica* **63**, 85–93.

Sweeney, E.A., Alcoforado, G.A.P., Nyman, S. & Slots, J. (1987). Prevalence and microbiology of localized prepubertal periodontitis. *Oral Microbiology and Immunology* **2**, 65–70.

Syrjanen, J., Peltola, J., Valtonen, V., Iivanainen, M., Kaste, M. & Huttunen, J.K. (1989). Dental infections in association with cerebral infarction in young and middle-aged men. *Journal of Internal Medicine* **225**, 179–184.

Tachi, Y., Shimpuku, H., Nosaka, Y., Kawamura, T., Shinohara, M., Ueda, M., Imai, H. & Ohura, K. (2003). Vitamin D receptor gene polymorphism is associated with chronic periodontitis. *Life Science* **73**, 3313–3321.

Tai, H., Endo, M., Shimada, Y., Gou, E., Orima, K., Kobayashi, T., Yamazaki, K. & Yoshie, H. (2002). Association of interleukin-1 receptor antagonist gene polymorphisms with early onset periodontitis in Japanese. *Journal of Clinical Periodontology* **29**, 882–888.

Takala, L., Utriainen, P. & Alanen, P. (1994). Incidence of edentulousness, reasons for full clearance, and health status of teeth before extractions in rural Finland. *Community Dentistry and Oral Epidemiology* **22**, 254–257.

Tanner, A.C., Milgrom, P.M., Kent, R.J., Mokeem, S.A., Page, R.C., Riedy, C.A., Weinstein, P. & Bruss, J. (2002). The microbiota of young children from tooth and tongue samples. *Journal of Dental Research* **81**, 53–57.

Taylor, B.A., Tofler, G.H., Carey, H.M., Morel-Kopp, M.C., Philcox, S., Carter, T.R., Elliott, M.J., Kull, A.D., Ward, C. & Schenck, K. (2006). Full-mouth tooth extraction lowers systemic inflammatory and thrombotic markers of cardiovascular risk. *Journal of Dental Research* **85**, 74–78.

Taylor, G.W. (2001). Bidirectional interrelationships between diabetes and periodontal diseases: an epidemiologic perspective. *Annals of Periodontology* **6**, 99–112.

Taylor, G.W., Burt, B.A., Becker, M.P., Genco, R.J. & Shlossman, M. (1998a). Glycemic control and alveolar bone loss progression in type 2 diabetes. *Annals of Periodontology* **3**, 30–39.

Taylor, G.W., Burt, B.A., Becker, M.P., Genco, R.J., Shlossman, M., Knowler, W.C. & Pettitt, D.J. (1996). Severe periodontitis and risk for poor glycemic control in patients with non-insulin-dependent diabetes mellitus. *Journal of Periodontology* **67**, 1085–1093.

Taylor, G.W., Burt, B.A., Becker, M.P., Genco, R.J., Shlossman, M., Knowler, W.C. & Pettitt, D.J. (1998b). Non-insulin dependent diabetes mellitus and alveolar bone loss progression over 2 years. *Journal of Periodontology* **69**, 76–83.

Tervonen, T. & Karjalainen, K. (1997). Periodontal disease related to diabetic status. A pilot study of the response to periodontal therapy in type 1 diabetes. *Journal of Clinical Periodontology* **24**, 505–510.

Tervonen, T. & Oliver, R.C. (1993). Long-term control of diabetes mellitus and periodontitis. *Journal of Clinical Periodontology* **20**, 431–435.

Tezal, M., Wactawski-Wende, J., Grossi, S.G., Ho, A.W., Dunford, R. & Genco, R.J. (2000). The relationship between bone mineral density and periodontitis in postmenopausal women. *Journal of Periodontology* **71**, 1492–1498.

Theilade, E., Wright, W.H., Jensen, S.B. & Loe, H. (1966). Experimental gingivitis in man. II. A longitudinal clinical and bacteriological investigation. *Journal of Periodontal Research* **1**, 1–13.

Thomson, W.M., Broadbent, J.M., Poulton, R. & Beck, J.D. (2006). Changes in periodontal disease experience from 26 to 32 years of age in a birth cohort. *Journal of Periodontology* **77**, 947–954.

Thorstensson, H. & Hugoson, A. (1993). Periodontal disease experience in adult long-duration insulin-dependent diabetics. *Journal of Clinical Periodontology* **20**, 352–358.

Thorstensson, H., Kuylenstierna, J. & Hugoson, A. (1996). Medical status and complications in relation to periodontal disease experience in insulin-dependent diabetics. *Journal of Clinical Periodontology* **23**, 194–202.

Timmerman, M.F., Van der Weijden, G.A., Abbas, F., Arief, E.M., Armand, S., Winkel, E.G., Van Winkelhoff, A.J. & Van der Velden, U. (2000). Untreated periodontal disease in Indonesian adolescents. Longitudinal clinical data and prospective clinical and microbiological risk assessment. *Journal of Clinical Periodontology* **27**, 932–942.

Timmerman, M.F., Van der Weijden, G.A., Arief, E.M., Armand, S., Abbas, F., Winkel, E.G., Van Winkelhoff, A.J. & Van der Velden, U. (2001). Untreated periodontal disease in Indonesian adolescents. Subgingival microbiota in relation to experienced progression of periodontitis. *Journal of Clinical Periodontology* **28**, 617–627.

Timmerman, M.F., Van der Weijden, G.A., Armand, S., Abbas, F., Winkel, E.G., Van Winkelhoff, A.J. & Van der Velden, U. (1998). Untreated periodontal disease in Indonesian adolescents. Clinical and microbiological baseline data. *Journal of Clinical Periodontology* **25**, 215–224.

Tinoco, E.M., Beldi, M.I., Loureiro, C.A., Lana, M., Campedelli, F., Tinoco, N.M., Gjermo, P. & Preus, H.R. (1997). Localized juvenile periodontitis and *Actinobacillus actinomycetemcomitans* in a Brazilian population. *European Journal of Oral Science* **105**, 9–14.

Tomar, S.L. & Asma, S. (2000). Smoking-attributable periodontitis in the United States: findings from NHANES III. National Health and Nutrition Examination Survey. *Journal of Periodontology* **71**, 743–751.

Tonetti, M.S. & Claffey, N. (2005). Advances in the progression of periodontitis and proposal of definitions of a periodontitis case and disease progression for use in risk factor research. *Journal of Clinical Periodontology* **32** Suppl 6, 210–213.

Tonetti, M.S., Muller-Campanile, V. & Lang, N.P. (1998). Changes in the prevalence of residual pockets and tooth loss in treated periodontal patients during a supportive maintenance care program. *Journal of Clinical Periodontology* **25**, 1008–1016.

Torgano, G., Cosentini, R., Mandelli, C., Perondi, R., Blasi, F., Bertinieri, G., Tien, T.V., Ceriani, G., Tarsia, P., Arosio, C. & Ranzi, M.L. (1999). Treatment of *Helicobacter pylori* and *Chlamydia pneumoniae* infections decreases fibrinogen plasma level in patients with ischemic heart disease. *Circulation* **99**, 1555–1559.

Trevilatto, P.C., Scarel-Caminaga, R.M., de Brito, R.B., Jr., de Souza, A.P. & Line, S.R. (2003). Polymorphism at position -174 of IL-6 gene is associated with susceptibility to chronic periodontitis in a Caucasian Brazilian population. *Journal of Clinical Periodontology* **30**, 438–442.

Trombelli, L., Cho, K.S., Kim, C.K., Scapoli, C. & Scabbia, A. (2003). Impaired healing response of periodontal furcation defects following flap debridement surgery in smokers. A controlled clinical trial. *Journal of Clinical Periodontology* **30**, 81–87.

Van der Velden, U. (1984). Effect of age on the periodontium. *Journal of Clinical Periodontology* **11**, 281–294.

van der Velden, U. (1991). The onset age of periodontal destruction. *Journal of Clinical Periodontology* **18**, 380–383.

Van der Velden, U., Abbas, F., Armand, S., Loos, B.G., Timmerman, M.F., Van der Weijden, G.A., Van Winkelhoff, A.J. & Winkel, E.G. (2006). Java project on periodontal diseases. The natural development of periodontitis: risk factors, risk predictors and risk determinants. *Journal of Clinical Periodontology* **33**, 540–548.

van der Velden, U., Abbas, F., Van Steenbergen, T.J., De Zoete, O.J., Hesse, M., De Ruyter, C., De Laat, V.H. & De Graaff, J. (1989). Prevalence of periodontal breakdown in adolescents and presence of *Actinobacillus actinomycetemcomitans* in subjects with attachment loss. *Journal of Periodontology* **60**, 604–610.

Van der Velden, U., Varoufaki, A., Hutter, J.W., Xu, L., Timmerman, M.F., Van Winkelhoff, A.J. & Loos, B.G. (2003). Effect of smoking and periodontal treatment on the subgingival microflora. *Journal of Clinical Periodontology* **30**, 603–610.

Vastardis, S.A., Yukna, R.A., Fidel, P.L., Jr., Leigh, J.E. & Mercante, D.E. (2003). Periodontal disease in HIV-positive individuals: association of periodontal indices with stages of HIV disease. *Journal of Periodontology* **74**, 1336–1341.

Veen, S., Ens-Dokkum, M.H., Schreuder, A.M., Verloove-Vanhorick, S.P., Brand, R. & Ruys, J.H. (1991). Impairments, disabilities, and handicaps of very preterm and very-low-birthweight infants at five years of age. The Collaborative Project on Preterm and Small for Gestational Age Infants (POPS) in The Netherlands. *Lancet* **338**, 33–36.

Verma, S., Buchanan, M.R. & Anderson, T.J. (2003). Endothelial function testing as a biomarker of vascular disease. *Circulation* **108**, 2054–2059.

von Wowern, N., Klausen, B. & Kollerup, G. (1994). Osteoporosis: a risk factor in periodontal disease. *Journal of Periodontology* **65**, 1134–1138.

Wactawski-Wende, J. (2001). Periodontal diseases and osteoporosis: association and mechanisms. *Annals of Periodontology* **6**, 197–208.

Walker, S.J., Van Dyke, T.E., Rich, S., Kornman, K.S., di Giovine, F.S. & Hart, T.C. (2000). Genetic polymorphisms of the IL-1alpha and IL-1beta genes in African-American LJP patients and an African-American control population. *Journal of Periodontology* **71**, 723–728.

Warren, J.J., Watkins, C.A., Cowen, H.J., Hand, J.S., Levy, S.M. & Kuthy, R.A. (2002). Tooth loss in the very old: 13–15-year incidence among elderly Iowans. *Community Dentistry and Oral Epidemiology* **30**, 29–37.

Weiss, O.I., Caton, J., Blieden, T., Fisher, S.G., Trafton, S. & Hart, T.C. (2004). Effect of the interleukin-1 genotype on outcomes of regenerative periodontal therapy with bone replacement grafts. *Journal of Periodontology* **75**, 1335–1342.

Wessel, H., Cnattingius, S., Bergstrom, S., Dupret, A. & Reitmaier, P. (1996). Maternal risk factors for preterm birth and low birthweight in Cape Verde. *Acta Obstetrics and Gynecology Scand* **75**, 360–366.

Weyant, R.J., Jones, J.A., Hobbins, M., Niessen, L.C., Adelson, R. & Rhyne, R.R. (1993). Oral health status of a long-term-care, veteran population. *Community Dentistry and Oral Epidemiology* **21**, 227–233.

Weyant, R.J., Pearlstein, M.E., Churak, A.P., Forrest, K., Famili, P. & Cauley, J.A. (1999). The association between osteopenia and periodontal attachment loss in older women. *Journal of Periodontology* **70**, 982–991.

WHO (1997) *Oral Health Surveys: Basic Methods*: World Health Organization.

WHO Collaborating Centre, M.U., Sweden WHO Oral Health Country/Area Profile Programme. URL http://www.whocollab.odont.lu.se/index.html (accessed on 6/12 2006).

WHO Collaborating Centre, N.U., Japan. WHO Oral Health Country/Area Profile Programme. URL http://www.dent.niigata-u.ac.jp/prevent/perio/contents.html (accessed on 6/12 2006).

Williams, D.R. (1996). Race/ethnicity and socioeconomic status: Measurement and methodological issues. *International Journal of Health Services* **26**, 484–505.

Williams, D.R. (1997). Race and health: basic questions, emerging directions. *Annals of Epidemiology* **7**, 322–333.

Williams, D.R. (1999). Race, socioeconomic status, and health. The added effects of racism and discrimination. *Annals of the New York Academy of Sciences* **896**, 173–188.

Williams, R. & Mahan, C. (1960). Periodontal disease and diabetes in young adults. *Journal of the American Medical Association* **172**, 776–778.

Winkler, J.R. & Murray, P.A. (1987). Periodontal disease. A potential intraoral expression of AIDS may be rapidly progressive periodontitis. *Journal of the California Dental Association* **15**, 20–24.

Wolf, D.L., Neiderud, A.M., Hinckley, K., Dahlen, G., van de Winkel, J.G. & Papapanou, P.N. (2006). Fcgamma receptor polymorphisms and periodontal status: a prospective follow-up study. *Journal of Clinical Periodontology* **33**, 691–698.

Wood, N., Johnson, R.B. & Streckfus, C.F. (2003). Comparison of body composition and periodontal disease using nutritional assessment techniques: Third National Health and Nutrition Examination Survey (NHANES III). *Journal of Clinical Periodontology* **30**, 321–327.

Wouters, F.R., Salonen, L.E., Helldén, L.B. & Frithiof, L. (1989). Prevalence of interproximal periodontal intrabony defects in an adult population in Sweden. A radiographic study. *Journal of Clinical Periodontology* **16**, 144–149.

Wouters, F.R., Salonen, L.W., Frithiof, L. & Helldén, L.B. (1993). Significance of some variables on interproximal alveolar bone height based on cross-sectional epidemiologic data. *Journal of Clinical Periodontology* **20**, 199–206.

Wu, T., Trevisan, M., Genco, R.J., Falkner, K.L., Dorn, J.P. & Sempos, C.T. (2000). Examination of the relation between periodontal health status and cardiovascular risk factors: serum total and high density lipoprotein cholesterol, C-reactive protein, and plasma fibrinogen. *American Journal of Epidemiology* **151**, 273–282.

Xiong, X., Buekens, P., Fraser, W.D., Beck, J. & Offenbacher, S. (2006). Periodontal disease and adverse pregnancy outcomes: a systematic review. *BJOG* **113**, 135–143.

Yamamoto, K., Kobayashi, T., Grossi, S., Ho, A.W., Genco, R.J., Yoshie, H. & De Nardin, E. (2004). Association of Fcgamma receptor IIa genotype with chronic periodontitis in Caucasians. *Journal of Periodontology* **75**, 517–522.

Yamazaki, K., Tabeta, K., Nakajima, T., Ohsawa, Y., Ueki, K., Itoh, H. & Yoshie, H. (2001). Interleukin-10 gene promoter polymorphism in Japanese patients with adult and early-onset periodontitis. *Journal of Clinical Periodontology* **28**, 828–832.

Yang, E.Y., Tanner, A.C., Milgrom, P., Mokeem, S.A., Riedy, C.A., Spadafora, A.T., Page, R.C. & Bruss, J. (2002). Periodontal pathogen detection in gingiva/tooth and tongue flora samples from 18- to 48-month-old children and periodontal status of their mothers. *Oral Microbiology and Immunology* **17**, 55–59.

Yasuda, K., Sugita, N., Kobayashi, T., Yamamoto, K. & Yoshie, H. (2003). FcgammaRIIB gene polymorphisms in Japanese periodontitis patients. *Genes and Immunity* **4**, 541–546.

Yeung, S.C., Taylor, B.A., Sherson, W., Lazarus, R., Zhao, Z.Z., Bird, P.S., Hamlet, S.M., Bannon, M., Daly, C. & Seymour, G.J. (2002). IgG subclass specific antibody response to periodontopathic organisms in HIV-positive patients. *Journal of Periodontology* **73**, 1444–1450.

Yoneyama, T., Okamoto, H., Lindhe, J., Socransky, S.S. & Haffajee, A.D. (1988). Probing depth, attachment loss and gingival recession. Findings from a clinical examination in Ushiku, Japan. *Journal of Clinical Periodontology* **15**, 581–591.

Yoshihara, A., Seida, Y., Hanada, N. & Miyazaki, H. (2004). A longitudinal study of the relationship between periodontal disease and bone mineral density in community-dwelling older adults. *Journal of Clinical Periodontology* **31**, 680–684.

Yu, S.M., Bellamy, H.A., Schwalberg, R.H. & Drum, M.A. (2001). Factors associated with use of preventive dental and health services among U.S. adolescents. *Journal of Adolescent Health* **29**, 395–405.

Part 3: Microbiology

Chapter 8

Oral Biofilms and Calculus

Niklaus P. Lang, Andrea Mombelli, and Rolf Attström

Microbial considerations

Throughout life, all the interface surfaces of the body are exposed to colonization by a wide range of microorganisms. In general, the establishing microbiota live in harmony with the host. Constant renewal of the surfaces by shedding prevents the accumulation of large masses of microorganisms. In the mouth, however, teeth provide hard, non-shedding surfaces for the development of extensive bacterial deposits. The accumulation and metabolism of bacteria on hard oral surfaces is considered the primary cause of dental caries, gingivitis, periodontitis, peri-implant infections, and stomatitis. Massive deposits are regularly associated with localized disease of the subjacent hard or soft tissues. In 1 mm^3 of dental plaque weighing approximately 1 mg, more than 10^8 bacteria are present. Although over 300 species have been isolated and characterized in these deposits, it is still not possible to identify all the species present. In the context of the oral cavity, the bacterial deposits have been termed *dental plaque* or *bacterial plaque*. Classical experiments have demonstrated that accumulation of bacteria on teeth reproducibly induces an inflammatory response in associated gingival tissues (Fig. 8-1a,b). Removal of plaque leads to the disappearance of the clinical signs of this inflammation (Löe *et al.* 1965; Theilade *et al.* 1966). Similar cause and effect relationships have been demonstrated for plaque and peri-implant mucositis (Pontoriero *et al.* 1994).

Germ-free animals provide an experimental model which has demonstrated that the absence of bacteria is associated with optimal dental and gingival health. Clinical studies have convincingly demonstrated that regular daily removal of dental plaque in most patients prevents further dental disease. Dental professionals and patients, therefore, consider regular mechanical removal of all bacterial deposits from non-shedding oral surfaces the primary prerequisite to prevent disease.

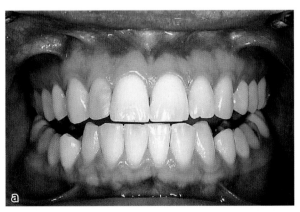
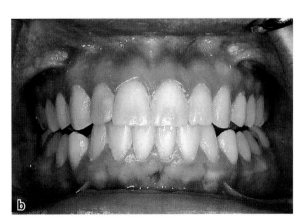

Fig. 8-1 Experimental gingivitis model (Löe *et al.* 1965). (a) Human volunteer with clean teeth and clinically healthy gingival tissues at the start of the period of experimental plaque accumulation. (b) Same human volunteer after 21 days of abolished oral hygiene practices leading to plaque deposits covering almost all tooth surfaces and consequently developing a generalized marginal gingival inflammation.

At first, a direct relationship was often assumed to exist between the total number of accumulated bacteria and the amplitude of the pathogenic effect; biologically relevant differences in the composition of plaque were not usually considered. This bacterial mass, termed *plaque*, was shown to produce a variety of irritants, such as acids, endotoxins, and antigens, which, over time, invariably dissolved teeth and destroyed the supporting tissues. Consequently, the need to discriminate among bacterial deposits from different patients or at healthy or diseased sites was not yet recognized in detail. Individuals with extensive periodontal disease were either suspected of having a weak resistance to bacterial plaque as a whole or were blamed for inadequate home care. Such a view of dental plaque as a biomass is referred to as the *non-specific plaque hypothesis* (Theilade 1986).

The propensity of inflamed sites to undergo permanent tissue destruction was recognized later to be more specific in nature, because not all gingivitis lesions seemed invariably to progress to periodontitis. Most periodontal sites in most subjects do not always show clinical signs of active tissue destruction with loss of connective tissue fiber attachment to the root surface, even though they may constantly be colonized by varying numbers and species of bacteria. Possible pathogens have been suggested among the organisms regularly found at elevated levels in periodontal lesions in relation to those observed under clinically healthy conditions. Longitudinal studies have indicated an increased risk for periodontal breakdown in sites colonized by some potentially pathogenic organisms. Treatment outcomes were better if these organisms could no longer be detected at follow-up examinations (see Chapter 9). If periodontal disease is indeed due to a limited number of bacterial species, the continuous and maximal suppression of plaque as a whole may not be the only possibility to prevent or treat periodontitis. Hence, specific elimination or reduction of presumptive pathogenic bacteria from plaque may become a valid alternative. Treatment may only be necessary in those patients diagnosed as having the specific infection and may be terminated once the pathogenic agents are eliminated. Such a view of periodontitis being caused by specific pathogens is referred to as the *specific plaque hypothesis* (Loesche 1979).

The term *infection* refers to the presence and multiplication of a microorganism in body tissues. The uniqueness of bacterial plaque-associated dental diseases as infections relates to the lack of massive bacterial invasion of tissues. Infections caused by the normal microbiota are sometimes called endogenous infections. Endogenous infections result when indigenous microbes move from their normal habitats into unusual anatomic regions. *Staphylococcus epidermidis*, for instance, is a non-pathogenic, commensal saprophyte on the skin. If this organism reaches the surface of a vascular prosthesis or an orthopedic implant, a serious infection may emerge. Infections caused by endogenous microbes are called *opportunistic infections* if they occur at the usual habitat of the microorganisms. Such infections may be the result of changing ecologic conditions or may be due to a decrease of host resistance. In the prevention of opportunistic infections due to overgrowth of indigenous organisms, continuous control of ecologic conditions regulating bacterial growth has high priority. The majority of microorganisms in periodontitis plaque can also be found occasionally in low proportions in health. These organisms may, therefore, be viewed as putative opportunistic pathogens. A small number of suspected pathogens, e.g. the Gram-negative anaerobe *Porphyromonas gingivalis*, are rare organisms in the mouth of healthy individuals. Some researchers have suggested that such bacteria may be considered exogenous pathogens. If some periodontal microorganisms were indeed exogenous pathogens, avoidance of exposure would become an important goal of prevention, and therapy should be aimed at the elimination of the microorganisms. Their mere presence would be an indication for intervention.

Dental plaque may accumulate supragingivally, i.e. on the clinical crown of the tooth, but also below the gingival margin, i.e. in the subgingival area of the sulcus or pocket. Differences in the composition of the subgingival microbiota have been attributed in part to the local availability of blood products, pocket depth, redox potential, and pO_2. Therefore, the question of whether the presence of specific microorganisms in patients or distinct sites may be the cause or the consequence of disease continues to be a matter of dispute (Socransky *et al.* 1987). Many microorganisms considered to be periodontopathogens are fastidious, strict anaerobes and, as such, may contribute little to the initiation of disease in shallow gingival pockets. If their preferred habitat were the deep periodontal pocket, they would be linked to the progression in sites with pre-existing disease, rather than to the initiation of disease in shallow sites. These microbiologic aspects are to be put in perspective with the host response. Further discussions are presented in Chapter 9.

General introduction to plaque formation

Growth and maturation patterns of bacterial plaque have been studied on natural hard oral surfaces, such as enamel and dentin, or artificial surfaces, such as metal or acrylic, using light and electron microscopy and bacterial culture (Theilade & Theilade 1985). Despite differences in surface roughness, free energy, and charge, the most important features of initial plaque development are similar on all these materials (Siegrist *et al.* 1991).

The ability to adhere to surfaces is a general property of almost all bacteria. It depends on an intricate,

Flow

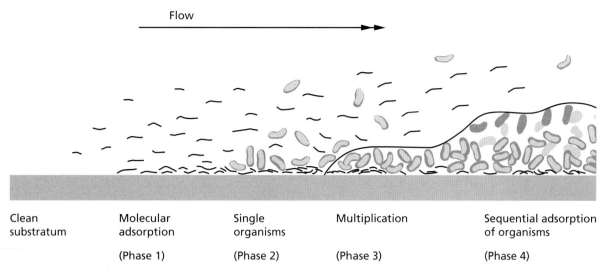

Clean substratum	Molecular adsorption	Single organisms	Multiplication	Sequential adsorption of organisms
	(Phase 1)	(Phase 2)	(Phase 3)	(Phase 4)

Fig. 8-2 Stages in the formation of a biofilm on a clean, hard and non-shedding surface following immersion into a fluid environment. Phase 1: Molecular adsorption to condition the biofilm formation. Phase 2: Bacterial adhesion by single organisms. Phase 3: Growth of extracellular matrix production and multiplication of the adhering bacteria. Phase 4: Sequential adsorption of further bacteria to form a more complex and mature biofilm. Adapted from Marshall (1992).

sometimes exquisitely specific, series of interactions between the surface to be colonized, the microbe, and an ambient fluid milieu (Mergenhagen & Rosan 1985).

Immediately upon immersion of a solid substratum into the fluid media of the oral cavity, or upon cleaning of a solid surface in the mouth, hydrophobic and macromolecules begin to adsorb to the surface to form a conditioning film (Fig. 8-2, Phase 1), termed the acquired pellicle. This film is composed of a variety of salivary glycoproteins (mucins) and antibodies. The conditioning film alters the charge and free energy of the surface, which in turn increases the efficiency of bacterial adhesion. Bacteria adhere variably to these coated surfaces. Some possess specific attachment structures such as extracellular polymeric substances and fimbriae, which enable them to attach rapidly upon contact (Fig. 8-2, Phase 2). Other bacteria require prolonged exposure to bind firmly. Behaviors of bacteria change once they become attached to surfaces. This includes active cellular growth of previously starving bacteria and synthesis of new outer membrane components. The bacterial mass increases due to continued growth of the adhering organisms, adhesion of new bacteria (Fig. 8-2, Phase 4), and synthesis of extracellular polymers. With increasing thickness, diffusion into and out of the biofilm becomes more and more difficult. An oxygen gradient develops as a result of rapid utilization by the superficial bacterial layers and poor diffusion of oxygen through the biofilm matrix. Completely anaerobic conditions eventually emerge in the deeper layers of the deposits. Oxygen is an important ecologic determinant because bacteria vary in their ability to grow and multiply at different levels of oxygen. Diminishing gradients of nutrients supplied by the aqueous phase, i.e. the saliva, are also created.

Reverse gradients of fermentation products develop as a result of bacterial metabolism.

Dietary products dissolved in saliva are an important source of nutrients for bacteria in the supragingival plaque. Once a deepened periodontal pocket is formed, however, the nutritional conditions for bacteria change because the penetration of substances dissolved in saliva into the pocket is very limited. Within the deepened pocket, the major nutritional source for bacterial metabolism comes from the periodontal tissues and blood. Many bacteria found in periodontal pockets produce hydrolytic enzymes with which they can break down complex macromolecules from the host into simple peptides and amino acids. These enzymes may be a major factor in destructive processes of periodontal tissues.

Primary colonization is dominated by facultatively anaerobic Gram-positive cocci. They adsorb onto the pellicle-coated surfaces within a short time after mechanical cleaning. Plaque collected after 24 hours consists mainly of streptococci; *S. sanguis* is the most prominent of these organisms. In the next phase, Gram-positive rods, which are present in very low numbers initially, gradually increase and eventually outnumber the streptococci (Fig. 8-3). Gram-positive filaments, particularly *Actinomyces* spp., are the predominating species in this stage of plaque development (Fig. 8-4). Surface receptors on the deposited Gram-positive cocci and rods allow subsequent adherence of Gram-negative organisms with poor ability to attach directly to pellicle. *Veillonella*, fusobacteria, and other anaerobic Gram-negative bacteria can attach in this way (Fig. 8-5). The heterogeneity of plaque thus gradually increases and, with time, includes large numbers of Gram-negative organisms. A complex array of interrelated bacterial species is the result of this development. Exchange of nutrients

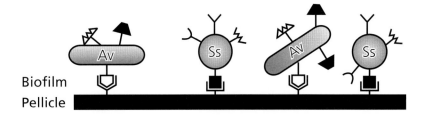

Fig. 8-3 Primary colonization by predominantly Gram-positive facultative bacteria. Ss: *Streptococcus sanguis* is most dominant. Av: *Actinomyces* spp. are also found in 24-hour plaque.

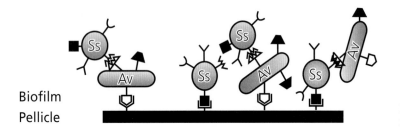

Fig. 8-4 Gram-positive facultative cocci and rods coaggregate and multiply.

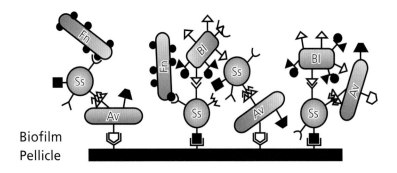

Fig. 8-5 Surface receptors on the Gram-positive facultative cocci and rods allow the subsequent adherence of Gram-negative organisms, which have a poor ability to adhere directly to the pellicle. Fn: *Fusobacterium nucleatum*; BI: *Prevotella intermedia*.

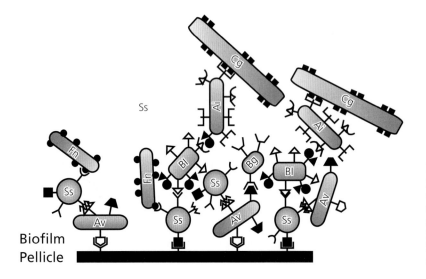

Fig. 8-6 The heterogeneity increases as plaque ages and matures. As a result of ecologic changes, more Gram-negative strictly anaerobic bacteria colonize secondarily and contribute to an increased pathogenicity of the biofilm. Bg: *Porphyromonas gingivalis*; Cg: *Capnocytophaga* sp.

between different species, but also negative interactions, e.g. the production of bacteriocins, play a role in the establishment of a stable bacterial community (Fig. 8-6). Due to the influences of local environmental factors, structurally different types of plaque evolve at different locations. Protection of the growing plaque from shear forces and local availability of certain nutrients are most important. A distinct composition of mature bacterial deposits can eventually be recognized at specific sites and under specific clinical conditions. Examples are the plaque on a smooth enamel surface versus fissure plaque, or the plaque in shallow and less shallow gingival crevices.

Accumulation of plaque along the gingival margin leads to an inflammatory reaction of the soft tissues. The presence of this inflammation has a profound influence on the local ecology. The availability of blood and gingival fluid components promotes growth of Gram-negative bacterial species with an increased periodontopathic potential. Bacterial samples from established gingivitis lesions have increased numbers of these bacteria. Because of the capability enzymatically to digest proteins, many of these organisms do not depend upon a direct availability of dietary carbohydrates. Such bacteria do not produce extracellular polymers and develop only loosely adherent plaque in the developing periodontal pocket. Cultivation of samples from advanced periodontal lesions reveals a predominance of Gram-negative anaerobic rods. Under the microscope, particularly high numbers of anaerobic uncultivable spirochetes can be demonstrated. Further details on the microbial ecology of subgingival plaque are discussed in Chapter 9.

In summary, immediately following immersion of hard, non-shedding surfaces into the fluid environment of the oral cavity, adsorption of macromolecules will lead to the formation of a *biofilm*. Bacterial adhesion to this glycoprotein layer will first involve primary plaque formers, such as Gram-positive facultative cocci and rods. Subsequent colonization on to receptors of these organisms will involve Gram-negative, strictly anaerobic bacteria, while the primary plaque formers also multiply to form colonies. The heterogeneity of the complex biofilm increases with time, as the ecologic conditions gradually change.

Dental plaque as a biofilm

The term *biofilm* describes the relatively undefinable microbial community associated with a tooth surface or any other hard, non-shedding material (Wilderer & Charaklis 1989). In the lower levels of most biofilms a dense layer of microbes is bound together in a polysaccharide matrix with other organic and inorganic materials. On top of this layer is a looser layer, which is often highly irregular in appearance and may extend into the surrounding medium. The fluid layer bordering the biofilm may have a rather "stationary" sublayer and a fluid layer in motion. Nutrient components may penetrate this fluid medium by molecular diffusion. Steep diffusion gradients, especially for oxygen, exist in the more compact lower regions of biofilms. The ubiquity with which anaerobic species are detected from these areas of biofilms provides evidence for these gradients (Ritz 1969).

Accumulation of bacteria on solid surfaces is not an exclusive dental phenomenon. Biofilms are ubiquitous; they form on virtually all surfaces immersed in natural aqueous environments. Biofilms form particularly fast in flow systems where a regular nutrient supply is provided to the bacteria. Rapid formation of visible layers of microorganisms due to extensive bacterial growth accompanied by excretion of copious amounts of extracellular polymers is typical for biofilms. Biofilms effectively protect bacteria from antimicrobial agents. Treatment with antimicrobial substances is often unsuccessful unless the deposits are mechanically removed. Adhesion-mediated infections that develop on permanently or temporarily implanted materials, such as intravascular catheters, vascular prostheses or heart valves, are notoriously resistant to antibiotics and tend to persist until the device is removed. Similar problems are encountered in water conduits, wherein potentially pathogenic bacteria may be protected from chlorination, or on ship hulls, where biofilms increase frictional resistance and turbulence (Gristina 1987; Marshall 1992).

In summary, *dental plaque* as a naturally occurring microbial deposit *represents a true biofilm* which consists of bacteria in a matrix composed mainly of extracellular bacterial polymers and salivary and/or gingival exudate products.

Structure of dental plaque

Supragingival plaque

Supragingival plaque has been examined in a number of studies by light and electron microscopy to gain information on its internal structure (Mühlemann & Schneider 1959; Turesky *et al.* 1961; Theilade 1964; Frank & Brendel 1966; Leach & Saxton 1966; Frank & Houver 1970; Schroeder & De Boever 1970; Theilade & Theilade 1970; Eastcott & Stallard 1973; Saxton 1973; Rönström *et al.* 1975; Tinanoff & Gross 1976; Lie 1978). The introduction of the electron microscope in dental research was a significant development for studies of dental plaque, both because the size of many bacteria approaches the ultimate resolving power of the light microscope, and because the resins used for embedding allowed for sections thinner than the smallest bacterial dimension. The substructure of plaque could therefore be identified.

In studies of the internal details of plaque, samples are required in which the deposits are kept in their original relation to the surface on which they have formed. This may be accomplished by removing the deposits with the tooth. If plaque of known age is the object of study, the tooth surfaces are cleaned at a predetermined time before removal (McDougall 1963; Frank & Houver 1970; Schroeder & De Boever 1970). Pieces of natural teeth or artificial surfaces may also be attached to solid structures in the mouth and removed after a given interval. This method of plaque collection was already used at the beginning of the last century by Black (1911). The systematic use of artificial surfaces for collection of plaque was reintroduced during the 1950s. Thin plastic foils of Mylar® were attached to mandibular incisor teeth for known periods, after which they were removed for histologic, histochemical, and electron microscopic examination of the deposited material (Mandel *et al.* 1957; Mühlemann & Schneider 1959; Zander *et al.* 1960; Schroeder 1963; Theilade 1964). Other types of plastic materials such as Westopal®, Epon®, Araldite®, and *spray plast* have since been employed for this purpose (Berthold *et al.* 1971; Kandarkar 1973; Lie 1975; Listgarten *et al.* 1975; Rönström *et al.* 1975). Results from several such studies indicate that plaque formed

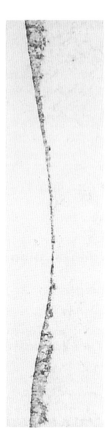

Fig. 8-7 Electron micrographic illustration of a 4-hour dental pellicle. The pellicle has formed on an artificial surface of plastic, which was painted on to the surface of the tooth. The plastic surface was exposed to the environment for a 4-hour period. A thin condensed layer of organic material is covering the film. The material has a relatively homogeneous appearance but varies in thickness over the surface. From Brecx *et al.* (1981).

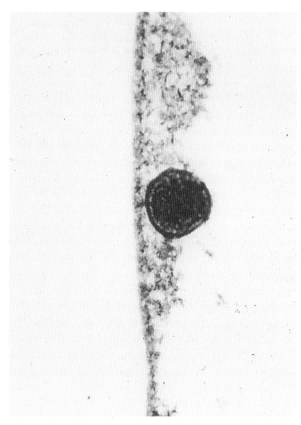

Fig. 8-8 Electron micrographic illustration of a 4-hour dental pellicle with a single bacterium included in the film. The microbe appears attached to the surface. The dental pellicle varies in thickness but has a homogeneous morphology. From Brecx *et al.* (1981).

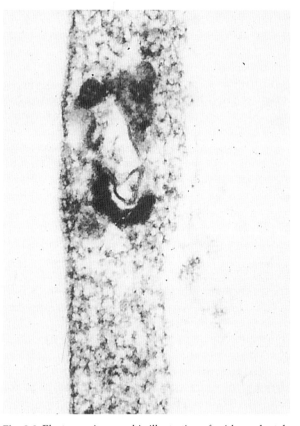

Fig. 8-9 Electron micrographic illustration of a 4-hour dental pellicle, formed on a plastic surface attached to the buccal surface of a tooth. A condensed layer of organic material is observed on the surface and cell remnants are embedded in the film. From Brecx *et al.* (1981).

on natural or artificial surfaces does not differ significantly in structure or microbiology (Hazen 1960; Berthold *et al.* 1971; Nyvad *et al.* 1982; Theilade *et al.* 1982a,b), indicating that at least some of the principal mechanisms involved in plaque formation are unrelated to the nature of the solid surface colonized. However, there are small, but important, differences in the chemical composition of the first layer of organic material formed on these artificial surfaces compared with that formed on natural tooth surfaces (Sönju & Rölla 1973; Sönju & Glantz 1975; Öste *et al.* 1981). Tooth surfaces, enamel as well as exposed cementum, are normally covered by a thin acquired pellicle of glycoproteins (Fig. 8-7). If removed, e.g. by mechanical instrumentation, it reforms within minutes. The pellicle is believed to play an active part in the selective adherence of bacteria to the tooth surface (Fig. 8-8). For details of the proposed mechanisms, see Chapter 9.

The first cellular material adhering to the pellicle on the tooth surface or other solid surfaces consists of coccoid bacteria with numbers of epithelial cells and polymorphonuclear leukocytes (Fig. 8-9). The bacteria are encountered either on (Fig. 8-10) or within the pellicle as single organisms (Fig. 8-11) or as aggregates of microorganisms (Fig. 8-12). Larger

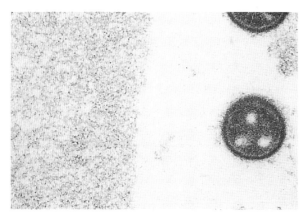

Fig. 8-10 High power electron micrographic illustration of a 4-hour pellicle with bacteria residing in the pellicle at a distance of around one micron from the condensed organic material. The pellicle is rather even in composition and, at the oral side, an irregular condensed organic material is seen close to the bacteria. From Brecx *et al.* (1981).

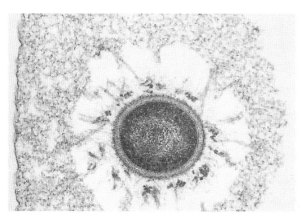

Fig. 8-11 High power electron micrographic illustration of a 4-hour pellicle with an embedded bacterium. The bacterium is deposited on the film surface together with the dental pellicle. Around the bacterium empty spaces are observed representing the radius of extrusions of filaments radiating from the microorganisms. From Brecx *et al.* (1981).

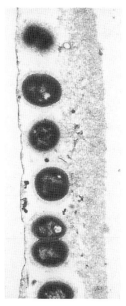

Fig. 8-12 Electron micrographic illustration of a 4-hour dental pellicle with bacteria attached to a plastic surface, which had been adhering to a buccal tooth surface and was exposed to the oral environment. A single row of bacteria attached to the surface is seen to the left. On top of the bacteria, a layer of condensed organic material representing the oral lateral portion of the dental pellicle is noted. From Brecx *et al.* (1981).

numbers of microorganisms may be carried to the tooth surface by epithelial cells.

The number of bacteria found on the surface a few hours after cleaning depends on the procedures applied to the sample before examination, the reason being that adherence to the solid surface is initially very weak. If no special precautions are taken during the preparatory processing, the early deposits are easily lost (Brecx *et al.* 1980). Apparently the adherence of microorganisms to solid surfaces takes place in two steps: (1) a reversible state in which the bacteria adhere loosely, and later (2) an irreversible state, during which their adherence becomes consolidated (Gibbons & van Houte 1980).

Another factor which may modify the number of bacteria in early plaque deposits is the presence of gingivitis, which increases the plaque formation rate so that the more complex bacterial composition is attained earlier (Saxton 1973; Hillam & Hull 1977; Brecx *et al.* 1980). Plaque growth may also be initiated

by microorganisms harbored in minute irregularities in which they are protected from the natural cleaning of the tooth surface.

During the first few hours, bacteria that resist detachment from the pellicle may start to proliferate and form small colonies of morphologically similar organisms (Fig. 8-13). However, since other types of organisms may also proliferate in an adjacent region, the pellicle becomes easily populated by a mixture of different microorganisms (Fig. 8-14). In addition, some organisms seem able to grow between already established colonies (Fig. 8-15). Finally, it is likely that clumps of organisms of different species will become attached to the tooth surface or to the already attached microorganism, contributing to the complexity of the plaque composition after a few days. At this time, different types of organisms may benefit from each other. One example is the corncob configurations resulting from the growth of cocci on the surface of a filamentous microorganism (Listgarten *et al.* 1973). Another feature of older plaque is the presence of dead and lysed bacteria which may provide additional nutrients to the still viable bacteria in the neighborhood (Theilade & Theilade 1970).

The material present between the bacteria in dental plaque is called the intermicrobial matrix and accounts for approximately 25% of the plaque volume. Three sources may contribute to the intermicrobial matrix: the plaque microorganisms, the saliva, and the gingival exudate.

The bacteria may release various metabolic products. Some bacteria may produce various extracellular carbohydrate polymers, serving as energy storage

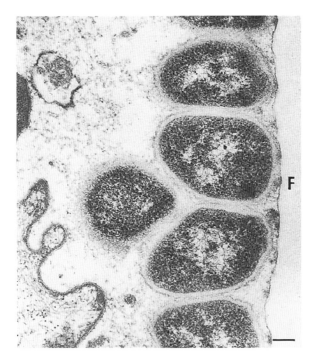

Fig. 8-13 Thin section of plaque colony consisting of morphologically similar bacteria deposited on plastic film (F) applied to the buccal surface of a premolar during an 8-hour period. Magnification ×35 000. Bar: 0.2 μm. From Brecx *et al.* (1980).

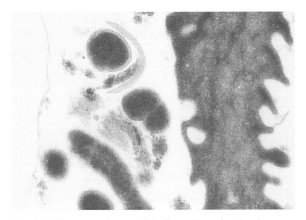

Fig. 8-14 Electron micrographic illustration of early plaque formation. The film surface on which the pellicle and bacteria adhere is located to the left. Bacteria of varying morphology are attached to the film. They are surrounded by organic pellicle material. An epithelial cell remnant is seen in close vicinity to the microbes. From Brecx *et al.* (1981).

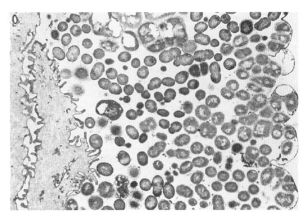

Fig. 8-15 Electron micrographic illustration of 24-hour dental plaque formed on a plastic film surface attached to the buccal surface of the tooth. A multilayer bacterial plaque is noted. A remnant of an epithelial cell has been trapped in the microbial mass. From Brecx *et al.* (1981).

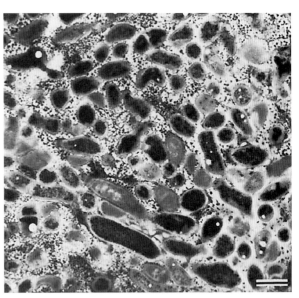

Fig. 8-16 Thin section of old plaque stained for the demonstration of polysaccharides by reacting them with electron-dense material appearing dark in the illustration. Many bacteria contain large amounts of intracellular polysaccharide, and the intermicrobial matrix contains extracellular polysaccharides. Magnification ×7000. Bar: 1 μm. From Theilade & Theilade (1970).

or as anchoring material to secure their retention in plaque (Fig. 8-16). Degenerating or dead bacteria may also contribute to the intermicrobial matrix. Different bacterial species often have distinctly different metabolic pathways and capacity to synthesize extracellular material. The intermicrobial matrix in plaque, therefore, varies considerably from region to region. A fibrillar component is often seen in the matrix between Gram-positive cocci (Fig. 8-17) and is in accordance with the fact that several oral streptococci synthesize levans and glucans from dietary sucrose. In other regions, the matrix appears granular or homogeneous (Fig. 8-18). In parts of the plaque with the presence of Gram-negative organisms, the intermicrobial matrix is regularly characterized by the presence of small vesicles surrounded by a trilaminar membrane, which is similar in structure to that of the outer envelope of the cell wall of the Gram-negative microorganisms (Fig. 8-19). Such vesicles probably contain endotoxins and proteolytic enzymes, and may also be involved in adherence between bacteria (Hofstad *et al.* 1972; Grenier & Mayrand 1987).

It must be remembered, however, that the transmission electron microscope does not reveal all organic components of the intermicrobial matrix. The more soluble constituents may be lost during the

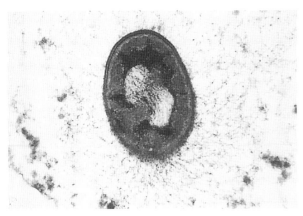

Fig. 8-17 High power electron micrographic illustration of a single bacterium attached to the pellicle by filaments which extend from the bacterial surface to the tooth surface. The surface had been exposed to the oral environment for an 8-hour period. From Brecx *et al.* (1981).

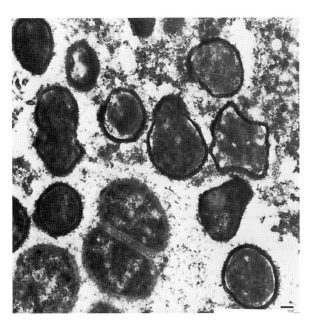

Fig. 8-18 Thin section of plaque with granular or homogeneous intermicrobial matrix. Magnification ×20 000. Bar: 0.1 μm. From Theilade & Theilade (1970).

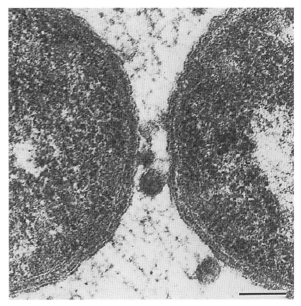

Fig. 8-19 Thin section of plaque with a region predominated by Gram-negative bacteria. Between them, vesicles are surrounded by a trilaminar membrane (two thin electron-dense layers with an electron-lucent layer in between). This substructure is also seen in the outermost endotoxin containing cell wall layer of the adjacent Gram-negative bacteria. Magnification ×110 000. Bar: 0.1 μm. From Theilade & Theilade (1970).

procedures required prior to sectioning and examination of the plaque sample. Biochemical techniques may be used to identify such compounds (Silverman & Klein-berg 1967; Krebel *et al.* 1969; Kleinberg 1970; Hotz *et al.* 1972; Rölla *et al.* 1975; Bowen 1976). Such studies indicate that proteins and carbohydrates constitute the bulk of the organic material while lipids appear in much lower amounts.

The carbohydrates of the matrix have received a great deal of attention, and at least some of the polysaccharides in the plaque matrix are well characterized: fructans (levans) and glucans. Fructans are synthesized in plaque from dietary sucrose and provide a storage of energy which may be utilized by microorganisms in times of low sugar supply. The glucans are also synthesized from sucrose. One type of glucan is dextran, which may also serve as energy storage. Another glucan is mutan, which is not readily degraded, but acts primarily as a skeleton in the matrix in much the same way as collagen stabilizes the intercellular substance of connective tissue. It has been suggested that such carbohydrate polymers may be responsible for the change from a reversible to an irreversible adherence of plaque bacteria.

The small amount of lipids in the plaque matrix are as yet largely uncharacterized. Part of the lipid content is found in the small extracellular vesicles, which may contain lipopolysaccharide endotoxins of Gram-negative bacteria.

Subgingival plaque

Owing to the difficulty of obtaining samples with subgingival plaque preserved in its original position between the soft tissues of the gingiva and the hard tissues of the tooth, there is only a limited number of studies on the detailed internal structure of human subgingival plaque (Schroeder 1970; Listgarten *et al.* 1975; Listgarten 1976; Westergaard *et al.* 1978). From these it is evident that in many respects subgingival plaque resembles the supragingival variety, although the predominant types of microorganisms found vary considerably from those residing coronal to the gingival margin.

Between subgingival plaque and the tooth an electron-dense organic material is interposed, termed a *cuticle* (Fig. 8-20). This cuticle probably contains the remains of the epithelial attachment lamina originally connecting the junctional epithelium to the

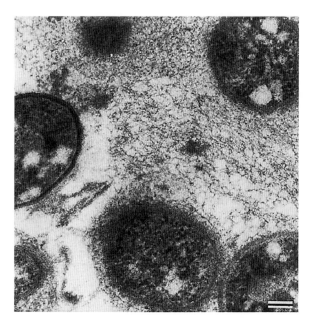

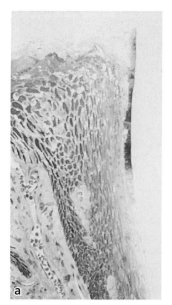

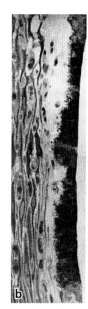

Fig. 8-20 Semithin section of subgingival plaque. An electron-dense cuticle bordering the enamel space is visible to the left. Filamentous bacteria are less than in supragingival plaque. The surface toward the gingival tissue contains many spirochetes (between arrows). Various host tissue cells can be seen on the right side. Magnification ×775. Bar: 10 μm. From Listgarten (1976).

Fig. 8-21 (a) Light microscopic image of the dento-gingival region of a dog with experimental gingivitis. A thin layer of dento-gingival plaque can be seen, extending from the supragingival region approximately 0.5 mm into the gingival sulcus. (b) Higher magnification of a region of the plaque shown in (a). The subgingival plaque has a varying thickness and the epithelial cells are separated from the surface by a layer of leukocytes. There are also numerous leukocytes in the superficial portion of the sulcus epithelium. The apical termination of the plaque is bordered by leukocytes separating the epithelium from direct contact with the plaque bacteria.

tooth, with the addition of material deposited from the gingival exudate (Frank & Cimasoni 1970; Lie & Selvig 1975; Eide *et al.* 1983). It has also been suggested that the cuticle represents a secretory product of the adjacent epithelial cells (Schroeder & Listgarten 1977). Information is lacking concerning its chemical composition, but its location in the subgingival area makes it unlikely that salivary constituents contribute to its formation.

The subgingival plaque structurally resembles supragingival plaque, particularly with respect to plaque associated with gingivitis without the formation of deep pockets (Fig. 8-21). A densely packed accumulation of microorganisms is seen adjacent to the cuticular material covering the tooth surface (Fig. 8-22). The bacteria comprise Gram-positive and Gram-negative cocci, rods, and filamentous organisms. Spirochetes and various flagellated bacteria may also be encountered, especially at the apical extension of the plaque. The surface layer is often less densely packed and leukocytes are regularly interposed between the plaque and the epithelial lining of the gingival sulcus (Fig. 8-23).

When a periodontal pocket has formed, the appearance of the subgingival bacterial deposit becomes much more complex. In this case the tooth surface may either represent enamel or cementum from which the periodontal fibers are detached. Plaque accumulation on the portion of the tooth previously covered by periodontal tissues does not differ markedly from that observed in gingivitis (Fig. 8-24). In this layer, filamentous microorganisms dominate (Figs. 8-25, 8-26, 8-27), but cocci and rods also occur.

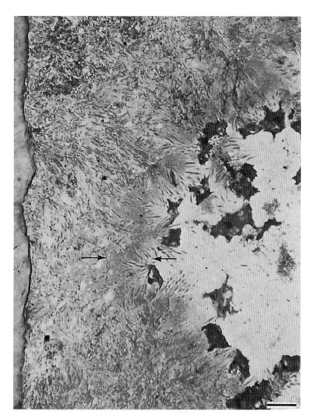

Fig. 8-22 Semithin section of supragingival plaque with layer of predominantly filamentous bacteria adhering to the enamel (to the left). Lighter staining indicates calcification of part of the plaque close to the tooth. Magnification ×750. Bar: 10 μm. From Listgarten (1976).

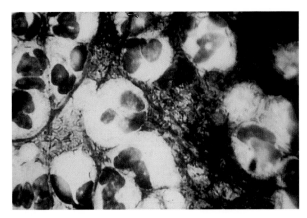

Fig. 8-23 Light microscopic image of a smear sample taken from the dento-gingival region in a subject who had abstained from mechanical oral hygiene during 3 weeks. Numerous leukocytes can be observed embedded in a dense accumulation of bacteria.

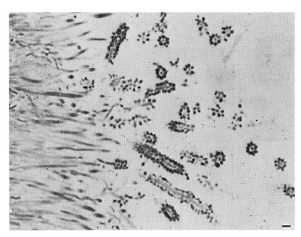

Fig. 8-26 The corncob formations seen at the plaque surface in Fig. 8-24 and 8-25. Magnification ×1300. Bar: 1 μm. From Listgarten (1976).

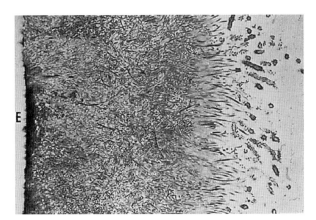

Fig. 8-24 Semithin section of supragingival plaque on enamel (E), which has been dissolved prior to sectioning. Magnification ×750. Bar: 10 μm. From Listgarten (1976).

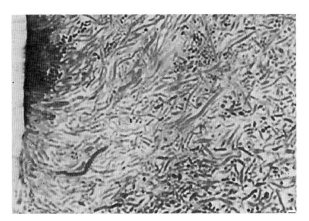

Fig. 8-25 See Fig. 8.24. Filamentous organisms predominate. At the surface some of these organisms are surrounded by cocci. This configuration resembles a corncob. Magnification ×1400. Bar: 1 μm. From Listgarten (1976).

However, in the deeper parts of the periodontal pocket, the filamentous organisms become fewer in number, and in the apical portion they seem to be virtually absent. Instead, the dense, tooth-facing part of the bacterial deposit is dominated by smaller

organisms without particular orientation (Listgarten 1976) (Fig. 8-28).

The surface layers of microorganisms in the periodontal pocket facing the soft tissue are distinctly different from the adherent layer along the tooth surface, and no definite intermicrobial matrix is apparent (Figs. 8-28, 8-29). The microorganisms comprise a larger number of spirochetes and flagellated bacteria. Gram-negative cocci and rods are also present. The multitude of spirochetes and flagellated organisms are motile bacteria and there is no intermicrobial matrix between them. This outer part of the microbial accumulation in the periodontal pocket adheres loosely to the soft-tissue pocket wall (Listgarten 1976).

In cases of juvenile periodontitis (Listgarten 1976; Westergaard *et al*. 1978) the bacterial deposits in deep pockets are much thinner than those found in adult forms of periodontal disease. Areas of the tooth surface in the periodontal pocket may sometimes even be devoid of adherent microbial deposits. The cuticular material has an uneven thickness (Figs. 8-30, 8-31). The adherent layer of microorganisms varies considerably in thickness and shows considerable variation in arrangement. It may exhibit a palisaded organization of the bacteria (Fig. 8-32). The microorganisms in this layer are mainly cocci, rods or filamentous bacteria, primarily of the Gram-negative type (Fig. 8-33). A surface layer with some Gram-positive cocci, frequently associated with filamentous organisms in the typical corncob configuration, may also be found.

Subgingivally located bacteria appear to have the capacity to invade dentinal tubules, the openings of which have become exposed as a consequence of inflammatory driven resorptions of the cementum (Adriaens *et al*. 1988). Such a habitat might serve as the source for bacterial recolonization of the subgingival space following treatment of periodontal disease. The mechanisms involved in such reversed invasion of the subgingival space are unknown.

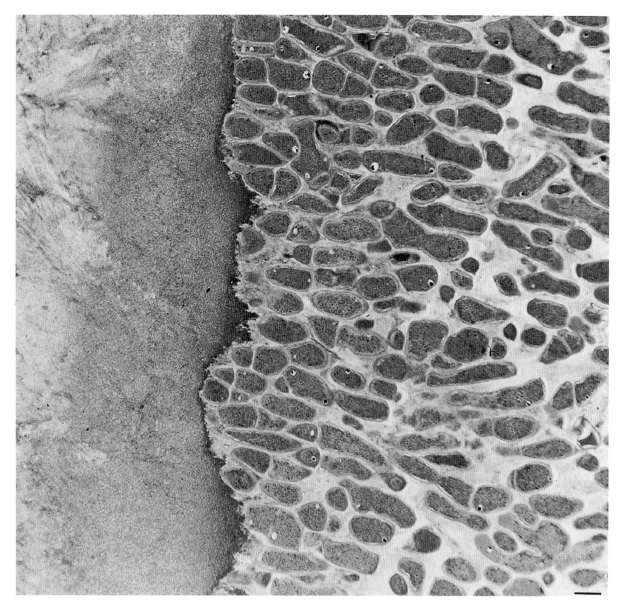

Fig. 8-27 Thin section of supragingival plaque on a root surface (to the left). The Gram-positive bacteria are oriented in a palisading arrangement. Magnification ×6400. Bar: 1 μm. From Listgarten (1976).

The sequential events taking place during the development of subgingival plaque have not been studied in man. However, in dogs, subgingival plaque may develop in the gingival sulcus within a few days, if oral hygiene is discontinued (Matsson & Attström 1979; Ten Napel *et al.* 1983). From these studies it has been established that early dental plaque in the dog has many structural similarities with that occurring in man. This applies to the supragingival plaque (Fig. 8-21a) as well as to the subgingival accumulation (Fig. 8-21b). The deposits may either appear as an apical continuation of the supragingival plaque, or as discrete aggregates at some distance from the supragingival deposit. Old established subgingival plaque shows considerable variation in bacterial composition between dogs: in some, a subgingival microbiota dominated by spirochetes is seen; in others, colonies of Gram-negative cocci

and rods are found in the gingival crevice, whereas spirochetes are virtually absent (Soames & Davies 1975; Theilade & Attström 1985). A characteristic feature of subgingival plaque is the presence of leukocytes interposed between the surfaces of the bacterial deposit and the gingival sulcular epithelium (Fig. 8-34). Some bacteria may be found between the epithelial cells. Evidence of phagocytosis (by polymorphonuclear leukocytes) is frequently encountered (Fig. 8-35).

Although subgingival plaque formation in the dog may not develop identically to that in man, the dog may still serve as a convenient model for investigating the basic phenomena governing the formation of subgingival plaque (Schroeder & Attström 1979).

In summary, there are four distinct subgingival ecologic niches which are probably different in their composition:

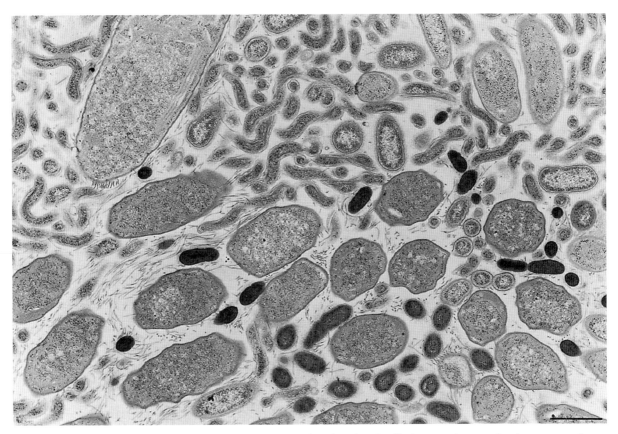

Fig. 8-28 Thin section of subgingival plaque from a deep periodontal pocket. Small microorganisms predominate, many of which are spirochetes. Magnification ×13 000. Bar: 1 µm. From Listgarten (1976).

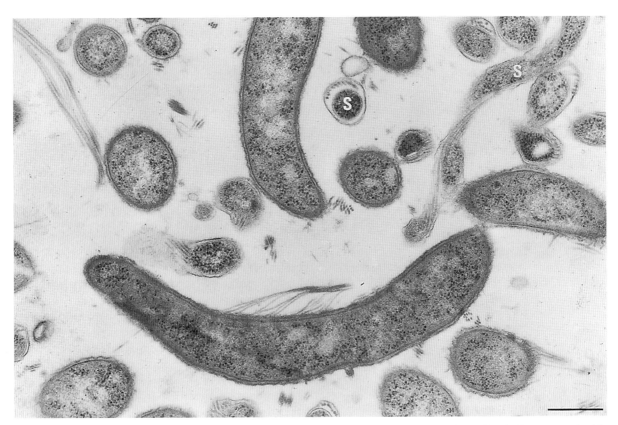

Fig. 8-29 Thin section of subgingival plaque from a deep periodontal pocket with many spirochetes (S), which are recognized by their axial filaments. In the lower part of the figure is a curved organism with flagella at its concave surface. Magnification ×25 000. Bar: 0.5 µm. From Listgarten (1976).

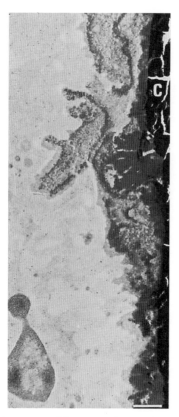

Fig. 8-30 Thin section of deposit in deep pocket of patient with juvenile periodontitis. The cementum (C) is covered with cuticular material and cellular remnants. Magnification ×5500. Bar: 1 μm. From Westergaard *et al.* (1978).

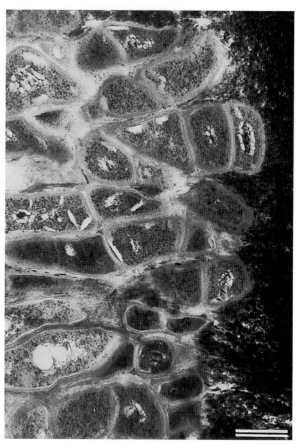

Fig. 8-32 Thin section of plaque in deep pocket of patient with juvenile periodontitis. Densely packed Gram-positive rods grow perpendicular to the cementum to the right in the illustration. Magnification ×23 000. Bar: 0.5 μm. From Westergaard *et al.* (1978).

1. The tooth (or implant) surface
2. The gingival exudate fluid medium
3. The surface of epithelial cells
4. The superficial portion of the pocket epithelium.

The composition of the bacteria in these niches has still not been completely investigated. The influence of the different bacterial compartments on the pathogenesis of the disease process is generally unknown.

Peri-implant plaque

Biofilms form not only on natural teeth, but also on artificial surfaces exposed to the oral environment. As a consequence, the formation of bacterial plaque on oral implants deserves some attention. Although a number of studies have characterized the plaque deposits of the human peri-implant sulcus or pocket using either dark field microscopy (Mombelli *et al.* 1988; Quirynen & Listgarten 1990) or microbiologic culturing techniques (Rams *et al.* 1984; Mombelli *et al.* 1987, 1988; Apse *et al.* 1989; Leonhardt *et al.* 1992), no studies have attempted to document the structure of the supramucosal or the peri-implant (submucosal) microbiota. However, the similarities between peri-implant and subgingival microbial deposits have

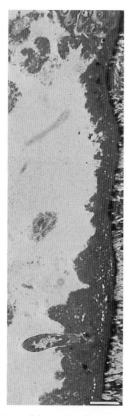

Fig. 8-31 Thin section of deposit in deep pocket of patient with juvenile periodontitis. A cuticle of uneven thickness is seen to the right on the cementum. A small colony of degenerating bacteria adheres to the cuticle in the upper part of the illustration, and below a single rod-shaped microorganism is partly embedded in the cuticle. Magnification ×5500. Bar: 1 μm. From Westergaard *et al.* (1978).

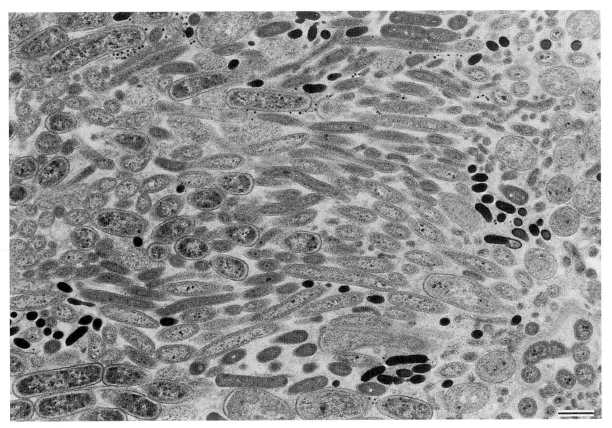

Fig. 8-33 Thin section of plaque in deep pocket of patient with juvenile periodontitis. The bacterial flora is characterized by cocci, rods or filamentous organisms, primarily of the Gram-negative type. Magnification ×9200. Bar: 1 μm. From Westergaard *et al.* (1978).

clearly been demonstrated in cross-sectional (Mombelli *et al.* 1987, 1995) and longitudinal studies (Mombelli *et al.* 1988; Pontoriero *et al.* 1994), and it may be anticipated that the structure of peri-implant plaque deposits may resemble that encountered in the subgingival environment. Micrographs from an implant retrieved because of a peri-implant infection may provide some evidence for the similarity between the structural image of the submucosal peri-implant microbiota (Fig. 8-36).

Dental calculus

Although calculus formation has been reported to occur in germ-free animals as a result of calcification of salivary proteins, dental calculus or tartar usually represents mineralized bacterial plaque.

Clinical appearance, distribution, and clinical diagnosis

Supragingivally, calculus can be recognized as a creamy-whitish to dark yellow or even brownish mass of moderate hardness (Fig. 8-37). The degree of calculus formation is not only dependent on the amount of bacterial plaque present but also on the secretion of the salivary glands. Hence, supragingival calculus is predominantly found adjacent to the excretion ducts of the major salivary glands, such as the lingual aspect of the mandibular anterior teeth and the buccal aspect of the maxillary first molars, where the parotid gland ducts open into the oral vestibule. The duct openings of the submandibular glands are located in the former region. It should be noted that calculus continually harbors a viable bacterial plaque (Zander *et al.* 1960; Theilade 1964; Schroeder 1969).

Subgingivally, calculus may be found by tactile exploration only, since its formation occurs apical to the gingival margin and, hence, is usually not visible to the naked eye. Occasionally, subgingival calculus may be visible in dental radiographs provided that the deposits present an adequate mass (Fig. 8-38). Small deposits or residual deposits following root instrumentation may barely be visualized radiographically. If the gingival margin is pushed open by a blast of air or retracted by a dental instrument, a brownish to black calcified hard mass with a rough surface may become visible (Fig. 8-39). Again, this mineralized mass reflects predominantly bacterial accumulations mixed with products from gingival crevicular fluid and blood. Consequently, subgingival calculus is found in most periodontal pockets, usually extending from the cemento-enamel junction and reaching close to the bottom of the pocket. However, a band of approximately 0.5 mm is usually found coronal to the apical extension of the periodontal pocket (Fig. 8-40). This zone appears to be free of mineralized deposits owing to the fact that gingival crevicular fluid is exuding from the periodontal soft

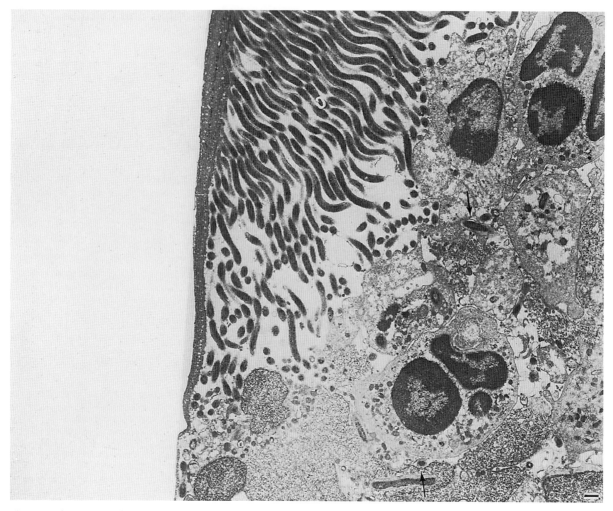

Fig. 8-34 Thin section of old subgingival plaque in a dog with long-standing gingivitis. The most apical colony consists primarily of spirochetes attached to a dense cuticle and surrounded by migrated leukocytes. Single microorganisms are seen between them (arrows). Magnification ×2800. Bar: 1 μm. From Theilade & Attström (1985).

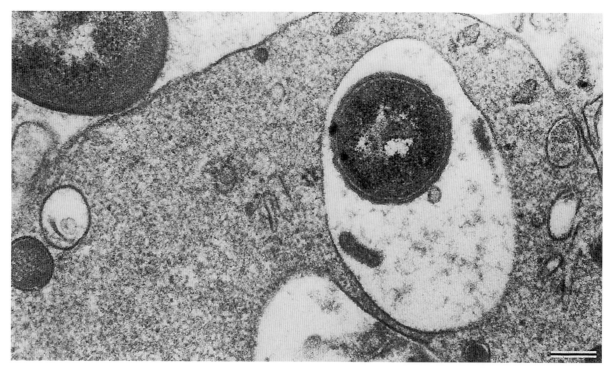

Fig. 8-35 Thin section of part of a leukocyte situated between subgingival plaque and the junctional epithelium of the dog. The large membrane-bound compartment of the leukocyte cytoplasm contains a phagocytized Gram-negative microorganism. Another bacterium is in close apposition to the cytoplasmic membrane of the leukocyte. Magnification ×21 500. Bar: 0.5 μm. From Theilade & Attström (1985).

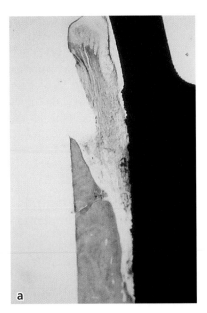
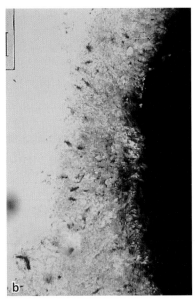

Fig. 8-36 Peri-implant infection. (a) Human explant of an ITI® dental implant affected by a peri-implantitis with an infrabony lesion. Adhering plaque closely resembles the structure of subgingival microbiota encountered in advanced periodontitis. (b) Higher magnification of plaque adhering to the implant surface.

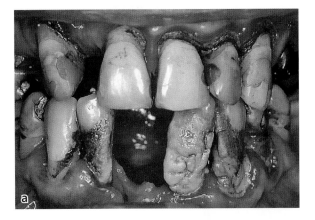
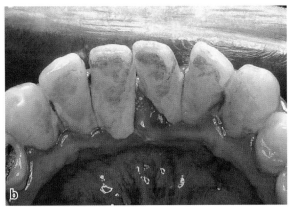
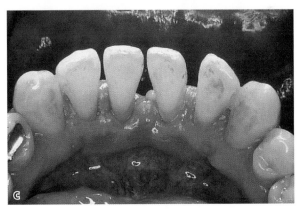

Fig. 8-37 Abundance of supragingival calculus deposits. (a) Gross deposits as a result of long-term neglect of oral hygiene. Two mandibular incisors have been exfoliated. (b) Supragingival plaque usually covering the lingual aspect of mandibular incisors. Note the intense inflammatory reaction adjacent to the deposits. (c) Same patient and region as in Fig. 8-37b following removal of the calculus. The gingival tissues demonstrate healing.

tissues and acting as a gradient against the microbial accumulation. Like supragingival calculus, subgingival calculus also provides an ideal environment for bacterial adhesion (Zander *et al.* 1960; Schroeder 1969).

Plaque mineralization varies greatly between and within individuals and, as indicated above, also within the different regions of the oral cavity.

Not only the formation rate for bacterial plaque (amount of bacterial plaque per time and tooth surface), but also the formation rate for dental calculus (time period during which newly deposited supragingival plaque with an ash weight of 5–10% becomes calcified and yields an ash weight of approximately 80%) is subject to great variability. In some subjects, the time required for the formation of supragingival calculus is 2 weeks, at which time the deposit may already contain approximately 80% of the inorganic material found in mature calculus (Fig. 8-41) (Mühlemann & Schneider 1959; Mandel 1963; Müh-lemann & Schroeder 1964). In fact, evidence of mineralization may already be present after a few days (Theilade 1964). Nevertheless, the formation of dental calculus with the mature crystalline composition of old calculus may require months to years (Schroeder & Baumbauer 1966). Supragingival plaque becomes mineralized saliva and subgingival plaque in the presence of the inflammatory exudate in the pocket. It is, therefore, evident that subgingival calculus represents a secondary product of infection and not a primary cause of periodontitis.

Attachment to tooth surfaces and implants

Dental calculus generally adheres tenaciously to tooth surfaces. Hence, the removal of subgingival calculus may be expected to be rather difficult. The reason for this firm attachment to the tooth surface is the fact that the pellicle beneath the bacterial plaque also calcifies. This, in turn, results in an intimate contact with enamel (Fig. 8-42), cementum (Fig. 8-43) or dentin crystals (Fig. 8-44) (Kopczyk & Conroy 1968; Selvig 1970). In addition, the surface irregularities are also penetrated by calculus crystals and, hence, calculus is virtually locked to the tooth. This is particularly the case on exposed root cementum, where small pits and irregularities occur at the sites

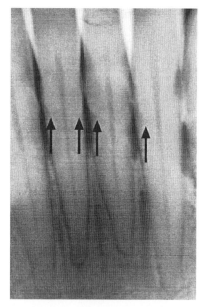

Fig. 8-38 Subgingival calculus may be visible (arrows) on radiographs if abundant deposits are present.

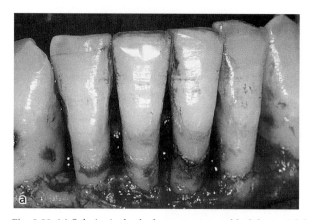 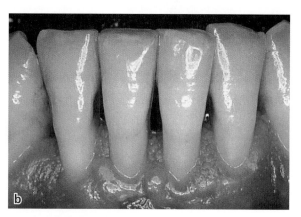

Fig. 8-39 (a) Subgingival calculus presents as a black-brownish hard mass if the gingival margin is retracted or reflected during a surgical procedure. (b) Healing of the site following removal of all hard deposits.

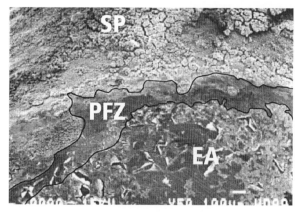

Fig. 8-40 Plaque- and calculus-free zone coronal to the epithelial attachment. SP: subgingival plaque bacteria; PFZ: plaque-free zone; EA: remnants of junctional epithelium.

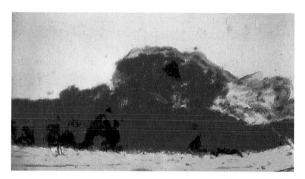

Fig. 8-41 Seven-day-old calcified plaque. Observe the isolated calcification centers indicated by the black areas (van Kossa stain).

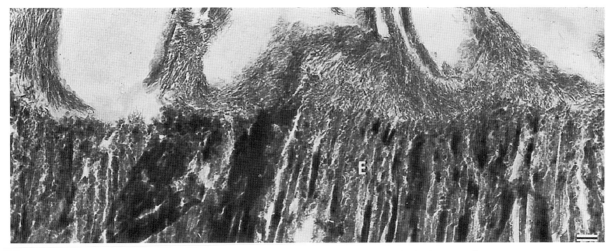

Fig. 8-42 Thin section of enamel surface (E) with overlying calculus. The enamel and calculus crystals are in intimate contact, and the latter extends into the minute irregularities of the enamel. Magnification ×37 500. Bar: 0.1 µm. From Selvig (1970).

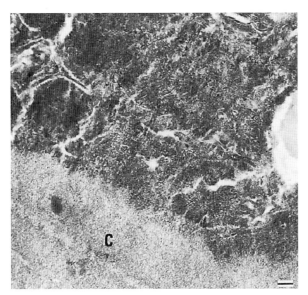

Fig. 8-43 Thin section of cementum surface (C) with overlying calculus. The calculus is closely adapted to the irregular cementum and is more electron-dense and therefore harder than the adjacent cementum. To the right in the illustration, part of an uncalcified microorganism. Magnification ×32 000. Bar: 0.1 µm. From Selvig (1970).

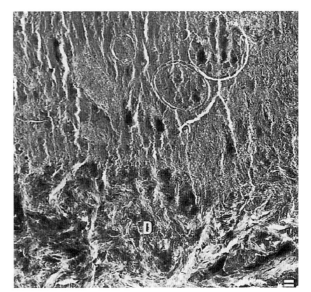

Fig. 8-44 Thin section of dentin (D) surface with overlying calculus. The interface between the calculus and dentin cannot be precisely determined because the calculus crystals fill the irregularities of the dentin surface, which is devoid of cementum as a result of a previous scaling of the root surface. The circular profiles in the calculus completely surround calcified bacteria. Magnification ×19 000. Bar: 1 µm. From Selvig (1970).

of the previous insertion of Sharpey's fibers (Bercy & Frank 1980). Uneven root surfaces may be the result of carious lesions and small areas of cementum may have been lost due to resorption, when the periodontal ligament was still invested into the root surface (Moskow 1969). Under such conditions it may become extremely difficult to remove all calculus deposits without sacrificing some hard tissues of the root.

Although some irregularities may also be encountered on oral implant surfaces, the attachment to commercially pure titanium generally is less intimate than to root surface structures. This in turn, would mean that calculus may be chipped off from oral implants (Fig. 8-45) without detriment to the implant surface (Matarasso *et al.* 1996).

Mineralization, composition, and structure

The mineralization starts in centers which arise intracellularly in bacterial colonies (Fig. 8-46) or extracellularly from matrix with crystallization nuclei (Fig. 8-47). Recent and old calculus consists of four different crystals of calcium phosphate (for review see Schroeder 1969):

1. $CaH (PO_4) \times 2H2O$ = brushite (**B**)
2. $Ca_4H (PO_4)_3 \times 2H2O$ = octa calcium phosphate (**OCP**)
3. $Ca_5(PO_4)_3 \times OH$ = hydroxyapatite (**HA**)
4. $\beta\text{-}Ca_3(PO_4)_2$ = whitlockite (**W**).

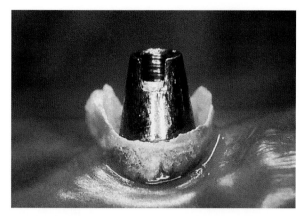

Fig. 8-45 Calculus deposit on an oral implant in a patient without regular maintenance care.

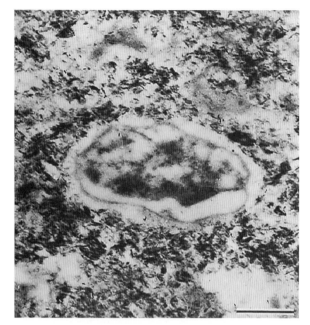

Fig. 8-46 Thin section of old plaque. A degenerating organism is surrounded by intermicrobial matrix in which initial mineralization has started by the deposition of small needle-shaped electron-dense apatite crystals. Magnification ×26 500. Bar: 0.5 μm. From Zander et al. (1960).

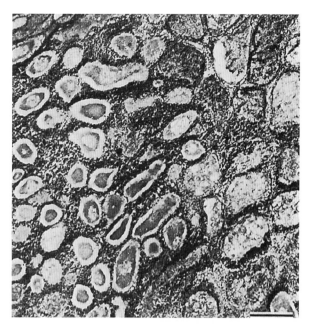

Fig. 8-47 Thin section of old mineralizing plaque. The intermicrobial matrix is totally calcified, and many microorganisms show intracellular crystal deposition. Magnification ×9500. Bar: 1 μm. From Theilade (1964).

Supragingival calculus is clearly built up in layers and yields a great heterogeneity from one layer to another with regard to mineral content. On average, the mineral content is 37%, but ranges from 16% to 51%, with some layers yielding a maximal density of minerals of up to 80% exceptionally (Kani et al. 1983; Friskopp & Isacsson 1984). The predominant mineral in exterior layers is **OCP**, while **HA** is dominant in inner layers of old calculus. **W** is only found in small proportions (Sundberg & Friskopp 1985). **B** is identified in recent calculus, not older than 2 weeks, and appears to form the basis for supragingival calculus formation. The appearance of the crystals is characteristic for **OCP** as forming platelet-like crystals, for **HA** as forming sandgrain or rod-like crystals, while **W** presents with hexagonal (cuboidal, rhomboidal) crystals (Kodaka et al. 1988).

Subgingival calculus appears somewhat more homogeneous since it is built up in layers with an equally high density of minerals. On average the density is 58% and ranges from 32% to 78%. Maximal values of 60–80% have been found (Kani et al. 1983; Friskopp & Isacsson 1984). The predominant mineral is always **W**, although **HA** has been found (Sundberg & Friskopp 1985). **W** contains small proportions (3%) of magnesia (McDougall 1985).

In the presence of a relatively low plaque pH and a concomitant high Ca/P ratio in saliva, **B** is formed which may later on develop into **HA** and **W**. When supragingival plaque mineralizes, **OCP** forms and is gradually changed into **HA**. In the presence of alkaline and anaerobic conditions and concomitant presence of magnesia (or Zn and CO_3), large amounts of **W** are formed, which are a stable form of mineralization.

Clinical implications

Although strong associations between calculus deposits and periodontitis have been demonstrated in experimental (Wærhaug 1952, 1955) and epidemiologic studies (Lövdal et al. 1958), it has to be realized that calculus is always covered by an unmineralized layer of viable bacterial plaque. It has been debated whether or not calculus may exert a detrimental effect on the soft tissues owing to its rough surface. However, it has clearly been established that surface roughness alone does not initiate gingivitis (Wærhaug 1956). On the contrary, in monkeys a normal epithelial attachment with the junctional epithelial cells forming hemidesmosomes and a basement membrane on calculus could be established (Listgarten &

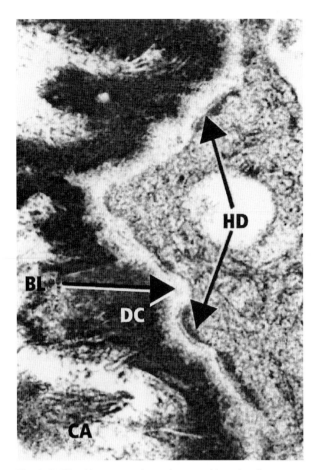

Fig. 8-48 Hemidesmosomal attachment of junctional epithelium on dental calculus in the absence of bacteria following application of chlorhexidine. CA: calculus; HD: hemidesmosomes; BL: basement lamina; DC: dental cuticle. ×32 000. Data from Listgarten & Ellegaard (1973).

by providing an ideal surface configuration conducive to further plaque accumulation and subsequent mineralization.

Nevertheless, calculus deposits may have developed in areas with difficult access for oral hygiene or may – by the size of the deposits – jeopardize proper oral hygiene practices. Calculus may also amplify the effects of bacterial plaque by keeping the bacterial deposits in close contact with the tissue surface, thereby influencing both bacterial ecology and tissue response (Friskopp & Hammarström 1980).

Well controlled animal (Nyman et al. 1986) and clinical (Nyman et al. 1988; Mombelli et al. 1995) studies have shown that the removal of subgingival plaque on top of subgingival calculus will result in healing of periodontal lesions and the maintenance of healthy gingival and periodontal tissues, provided that the supragingival deposits are meticulously removed on a regular basis. One of these studies (Mombelli et al. 1995) clearly demonstrated that the diligent and complete removal of subgingival plaque on top of mineralized deposits after chipping off gross amounts of calculus showed almost identical results in the composition of the microbiota and the clinical parameters to those obtained with routine removal of subgingival calculus by root surface instrumentation. Again, it has to be realized that meticulous supragingival plaque control guarantees the depletion of the supragingival bacterial reservoir for subgingival recolonization. These studies have clearly elucidated the role of subgingival calculus as a plaque-retaining factor.

In summary, dental calculus represents mineralized bacterial plaque. It is always covered by unmineralized viable bacterial plaque, and hence, does not directly come into contact with the gingival tissues. Calculus, therefore, is a secondary etiologic factor for periodontitis. Its presence, however, makes adequate plaque removal impossible and prevents patients from performing proper plaque control. It is the most prominent plaque-retentive factor which has to be removed as a basis for adequate periodontal therapy and prophylactic activities.

Ellegaard 1973) if the calculus surface had been disinfected using chlorhexidine (Fig. 8-48). Furthermore, it has been demonstrated that autoclaved calculus may be encapsulated in connective tissue without inducing marked inflammation or abscess formation (Allen & Kerr 1965).

These studies clearly exclude the possibility of dental calculus being a primary cause of periodontal diseases. The effect of calculus seems to be secondary

References

Adriaens, P.A., De Boever, J.A. & Loesche, W.J. (1988). Bacterial invasion in root cementum and radicular dentin of periodontally diseased teeth in humans. A reservoir of periodontopathic bacteria. *Journal of Periodontology* 59, 222–230.

Allen, D.L. & Kerr, D.A. (1965). Tissue response in the guinea pig to sterile and non-sterile calculus. *Journal of Periodontology* 36, 121–126.

Apse, P., Ellen, R.P., Overall, C.M. & Zarb, G.A. (1989). Microbiota and crevicular fluid collagenase activity in the osseointegrated dental implant sulcus: a comparison of sites in edentulous and partially edentulous patients. *Journal of Periodontal Research* 24, 96–105.

Bercy, P. & Frank, R.M. (1980). Microscopie electronique à balayage de la surface du cément humain normal et carié. *Journal de Biologie Buccale* 8, 331–352.

Berthold, C.H., Berthold, P. & Söder, P.O. (1971). The growth of dental plaque on different materials. *Svensk Tandläkare Tidsskrift* 64, 863–877.

Black, G.V. (1911). Beginnings of pyorrhea alveolaris – treatment for prevention. *Dental Items of Interest* 33, 420–455.

Bowen, W.H. (1976). Nature of plaque. *Oral Sciences Reviews* 9, 3–21.

Brecx, M., Theilade, J. & Attström, R. (1980). Influence of optimal and excluded oral hygiene on early formation of dental plaque on plastic films. A quantitative and descriptive light and electron microscopic study. *Journal of Clinical Periodontology* 7, 361–373.

Brecx, M., Theilade, J. & Attström, R. (1981). Ultrastructural estimation of the effect of sucrose and glucose rinses on dental plaque formed on plastic films. *Scandinavian Journal of Dental Research* 89, 157–164.

Eastcott, A.D. & Stallard, R.E. (1973). Sequential changes in developing human dental plaque as visualized by scanning electron microscopy. *Journal of Periodontology* **44**, 218–244.

Eide, B., Lie, T. & Selvig, K.A. (1983). Surface coatings on dental cementum incident to periodontal disease. I. A scanning electron microscopic study. *Journal of Clinical Periodontology* **10**, 157–171.

Frank, R.M. & Brendel, A. (1966). Ultrastructure of the approximal dental plaque and the underlying normal and carious enamel. *Archives of Oral Biology* **11**, 883–912.

Frank, R.M. & Cimasoni, G. (1970). Ultrastructure de l'epithelium cliniquement normal du sillon et de jonction gingivodentaires. *Zeitschrift für Zellforschung und Mikroskopische Anatomie* **109**, 356–379.

Frank, R.M. & Houver, G. (1970). An ultrastructural study of human supragingival dental plaque formation. In: McHugh, W.D., ed. *Dental Plaque*. Edinburgh: Livingstone, pp. 85–108.

Friskopp, J. & Hammarström, L. (1980). A comparative scanning electron microscopic study of supragingival and subgingival calculus. *Journal of Periodontology* **51**, 553–562.

Friskopp, J. & Isacsson, G. (1984). Mineral content of supragingival and subgingival dental calculus. A quantitative microradiographic study. *Scandinavian Journal of Dental Research* **92**, 417–423.

Gibbons, R.J. & van Houte, J. (1980). Bacterial adherence and the formation of dental plaques. In: Beachey, E.H., ed. *Bacterial adherence*. Receptors and recognition, series B, Vol. 6. London: Chapman, pp. 60–104.

Grenier, D. & Mayrand, D. (1987). Functional characterization of vesicular vesicles produced by *Bacteroides gingivalis*. *Infection and Immunity* **55**, 111–117.

Gristina, A.G. (1987). Biomaterial-centered infection: Microbial adhesion versus tissue integration. *Science* **237**, 1588–1595.

Hazen, S.P. (1960). A study of four week old *in vivo* calculus formation. Thesis. Rochester, NY: University of Rochester.

Hillam, D.G. & Hull, P.S. (1977). The influence of experimental gingivitis on plaque formation. *Journal of Clinical Periodontology* **4**, 56–61.

Hofstad, T., Kristoffersen. T. & Selvig, K.A. (1972). Electron microscopy of endotoxic lipopolysaccharide from *Bacteroides*, *Fusobacterium* and *Sphaerophorus*. *Acta Pathologica and Microbiologica Scandinavia*, Sec B **80**, 413–419.

Hotz, P., Guggenheim, B. & Schmid, R. (1972). Carbohydrates in pooled dental plaque. *Caries Research* **6**, 103–121.

Kandarkar, S.V. (1973). Ultrastructure of dental plaque and acquired pellicle formed on the artificial tooth surface (araldite plate). *Journal of the Indian Dental Association* **45**, 122–129.

Kani, T., Kani, M., Moriwaki, Y. & Doi, Y. (1983). Microbeam x-ray diffraction analysis of dental calculus. *Journal of Dental Research* **62**, 92–95.

Kleinberg, I. (1970). Biochemistry of the dental plaque. *Archives of Oral Biology* **4**, 43–90.

Kodaka, T., Debari, K. & Higashi, S. (1988). Magnesium-containing crystals in human dental calculus. *Journal of Electronic Microscopy* **37**, 73–80.

Kopczyk, R.A. & Conroy, C.W. (1968). The attachment of calculus to root-planed surfaces. *Periodontics* **6**, 78–83.

Krebel, J., Frank, R.M. & Deluzarche, A. (1969). Fractionation of human dental plaque. *Archives of Oral Biology* **14**, 563–565.

Leach, S.A. & Saxton, C.A. (1966). An electron microscopic study of the acquired pellicle and plaque formed on the enamel of human incisors. *Archives of Oral Biology* **11**, 1081–1094.

Leonhardt, Å., Bergenlundh, T., Ericsson, I. & Dahlén, G. (1992). Putative periodontal pathogens on titanium implants and teeth in experimental gingivitis and periodontitis in beagle dogs. *Clinical Oral Implants Research* **3**, 112–119.

Lie, T. (1975). Growth of dental plaque on hydroxy-apatite splints. A method of studying early plaque morphology. *Journal of Periodontal Research* **9**, 137–145.

Lie, T. (1978). Ultrastructural study of early dental plaque formation. *Journal of Periodontal Research* **13**, 391–409.

Lie, T. & Selvig, K.A. (1975). Formation of an experimental dental cuticle. *Scandinavian Journal of Dental Research* **83**, 145–152.

Listgarten, M.A. (1976). Structure of the microbial flora associated with periodontal health and disease in man. A light and electron microscopic study. *Journal of Periodontology* **47**, 1–18.

Listgarten, M.A. & Ellegaard, B. (1973). Electron microscopic evidence of a cellular attachment between junctional epithelium and dental calculus. *Journal of Periodontal Research* **8**, 143–150.

Listgarten, M.A., Mayo, H. & Amsterdam, M. (1973). Ultrastructure of the attachment device between coccal and filamentous microorganisms in "corn cob" formations in dental plaque. *Archives of Oral Biology* **8**, 651–656.

Listgarten, M.A., Mayo, H. & Tremblay, R. (1975). Development of dental plaque in epoxy resin crowns in man. A light and electron microscopic study. *Journal of Periodontology* **46**, 10–26.

Löe, H., Theilade, E. & Jensen, S.B. (1965). Experimental gingivitis in man. *Journal of Periodontology* **36**, 177–187.

Loesche, W.J. (1979). Clinical and microbiological aspects of chemotherapeutic agents used according to the specific plaque hypothesis. *Journal of Dental Research* **58**, 2404–2414.

Lövdal, A., Arnö, A. & Wærhaug, J. (1958). Incidence of clinical manifestations of periodontal disease in light of oral hygiene and calculus formation. *Journal of the American Dental Association* **56**, 21–33.

Mandel, I.D. (1963). Histochemical and biochemical aspects of calculus formation. *Periodontics* **1**, 43–52.

Mandel, I.D., Levy, B.M. & Wasserman, B.H. (1957). Histochemistry of calculus formation. *Journal of Periodontology* **28**, 132137.

Marshall, K.C. (1992). Biofilms: An overview of bacterial adhesion, activity, and control at surfaces. *American Society of Microbiology News* **58**, 202–207.

Matarasso, S., Quaremba, G., Coraggio, F., Vaia, E., Cafiero, C. & Lang, N.P. (1996). Maintenance of implants: an *in vitro* study of titanium implant surface modifications subsequent to the application of different prophylaxis procedures. *Clinical Oral Implants Research* **7**, 64–72.

Matsson, L. & Attström, R. (1979). Histologic characteristics of experimental gingivitis in the juvenile and adult beagle dog. *Journal of Clinical Periodontology* **6**, 334–350.

McDougall, W.A. (1963). Studies on dental plaque. II. The histology of the developing interproximal plaque. *Australian Dental Journal* **8**, 398–407.

McDougall, W.A. (1985). Analytical transmission electron microscopy of the distribution of elements in human supragingival dental calculus. *Archives of Oral Biology* **30**, 603–608.

Mergenhagen, S.E. & Rosan, B. (1985). *Molecular Basis of Oral Microbial Adhesion*. Washington: American Society of Microbiology.

Mombelli, A., Buser, D. & Lang, N.P. (1988). Colonization of osseointegrated titanium implants in edentulous patients: early results. *Oral Microbiology and Immunology* **3**, 113–120.

Mombelli, A., Marxer, M., Gaberthüel, T., Grunder, U. & Lang, N.P. (1995). The microbiota of osseointegrated implants in patients with a history of periodontal disease. *Journal of Clinical Periodontology* **22**, 124–130.

Mombelli, A., Nyman, S., Brägger, N., Wennström, J. & Lang, N.P. (1995). Clinical and microbiological changes associated with an altered subgingival environment induced by periodontal pocket reduction. *Journal of Clinical Periodontology* **22**, 780–787.

Mombelli, A., van Oosten, M.A.C., Schürch, E. & Lang, N.P. (1987). The microbiota associated with successful or failing osseointegrated titanium implants. *Oral Microbiology and Immunology* **2**, 145–151.

Moskow, B.S. (1969). Calculus attachment in cemental separations. *Journal of Periodontology* **40**, 125–130.

Mühlemann, H.R. & Schneider, U.K. (1959). Early calculus formation. *Helvetica Odontologica Acta* **3**, 22–26.

Mühlemann, H.R. & Schroeder, H.E. (1964) Dynamics of supragingival calculus. In: Staple, P.H., ed. *Advances in Oral Biology*. New York: Academic Press, pp. 175–203.

Nyman, S., Sarhed, G., Ericsson, I., Gottlow, J. & Karring, T. (1986). Role of "diseased" root cementum in healing following treatment of periodontal disease. An experimental study in the dog. *Journal of Periodontal Research* **21**, 496–503.

Nyman, S., Westfelt, E., Sarhed, G., & Karring, T. (1988). Role of "diseased" root cementum in healing following treatment of periodontal disease. A clinical study. *Journal of Clinical Periodontology* **15**, 464–468.

Nyvad, B., Fejerskov, O., Theilade, J., Melsen, B., Rölla, G. & Karring, T. (1982). The effect of sucrose or casein on early microbial colonization on Mylar and tooth surfaces in monkeys. *Journal of Dental Research* **61**, 570.

Öste, R., Rönström, A., Birkhed, D., Edwardsson, S. & Stenberg, M. (1981). Gas-liquid chromatographic analysis of amino acids in pellicle formed on tooth surface and plastic film *in vitro*. *Archives of Oral Biology* **26**, 635–641.

Pontoriero, R., Tonelli, M.P., Carnevale, G., Mombelli, A., Nyman, S.R. & Lang, N.P. (1994). Experimentally induced peri-implant mucositis. A clinical study in humans. *Clinical Oral Implants Research* **5**, 254–259.

Quirynen, M. & Listgarten, M.A. (1990). The distribution of bacterial morphotypes around natural teeth and titanium implants *ad modum* Brånemark. *Clinical Oral Implants Research* **1**, 8–12.

Rams, T.E., Roberts, T.W., Taum, H.Jr., Keyes, P.H. (1984). The subgingival microbial flora associated with human dental implants. *Clinical Oral Implants Research* **51**, 529–534.

Ritz, H.L. (1969). Fluorescent antibody staining of Neisseria, Streptococcus and Veillonella in frozen sections of human dental plaque. *Archives of Oral Biology* **14**, 1073–1083.

Rölla, G., Melsen, B. & Sönju, T. (1975). Sulphated macromolecules in dental plaque in the monkeys *Macaca irus*. *Archives of Oral Biology* **20**, 341–343.

Rönström, A., Attström, R. & Egelberg, J. (1975). Early formation of dental plaque on plastic films. 1. Light microscopic observations. *Journal of Periodontal Research* **10**, 28–35.

Saxton, C.A. (1973). Scanning electron microscope study of the formation of dental plaque. *Caries Research* **7**, 102–119.

Schroeder, H.E. (1963). Inorganic content and histology of early calculus in man. *Helvetica Odontologica Acta* **7**, 17–30.

Schroeder, H.E. (1969). *Formation and Inhibition of Dental Calculus*. Berne: Hans Huber Publishers.

Schroeder, H.E. (1970). The structure and relationship of plaque to the hard and soft tissues: electron microscopic interpretation. *International Dental Journal* **20**, 353–381.

Schroeder, H.E. & Attström, R. (1979). Effects of mechanical plaque control on development of subgingival plaque and initial gingivitis in neutropenic dogs. *Scandinavian Journal of Dental Research* **87**, 279–287.

Schroeder, H.E. & Baumbauer, H.U. (1966). Stages of calcium phosphate crystallization during calculus formation. *Archives of Oral Biology* **11**, 1–14.

Schroeder, H.E. & De Boever, J. (1970). The structure of microbial dental plaque. In: McHugh, W.D., ed. *Dental Plaque*. Edinburgh: Livingstone, pp. 49–74.

Schroeder, H.E. & Listgarten, M.A. (1977). *Fine Structure of the Developing Epithelial Attachment of Human Teeth*. Basel: S. Karger.

Selvig, K.A. (1970). Attachment of plaque and calculus to tooth surfaces. *Journal of Periodontal Research* **5**, 8–18.

Siegrist, B.E., Brecx, M.C., Gusberti, F.A., Joss, A. & Lang, N.P. (1991). *In vivo* early human dental plaque formation on different supporting substances. A scanning electron microscopic and bacteriological study. *Clinical Oral Implants Research* **2**, 38–46.

Silverman, G. & Kleinberg, T. (1967). Fractionation of human dental plaque and the characterization of its cellular and acellular components. *Archives of Oral Biology* **12**, 1387–1405.

Soames, J.V. & Davies, R.M. (1975). The structure of subgingival plaque in a beagle dog. *Journal of Periodontal Research* **9**, 333–341.

Socransky, S.S., Haffajee, A.D., Smith, G.L.F. & Dzink, J.L. (1987). Difficulties encountered in the search for the etiologic agents of destructive periodontal disease. *Journal of Clinical Periodontology* **14**, 588–593.

Sönju, T. & Glantz, P.-O. (1975). Chemical composition of salivary integuments formed *in vivo* on solids with some established surface characteristics. *Archives of Oral Biology* **20**, 687–691.

Sönju, T. & Rölla, G. (1973). Chemical analysis of the acquired pellicle formed in two hours on cleaned human teeth. *Caries Research* **7**, 30–38.

Sundberg, J.R. & Friskopp, J. (1985). Crystallography of supragingival and subgingival human dental calculus. *Scandinavian Journal of Dental Research* **93**, 30–38.

Ten Napel, J., Theilade, J., Matsson, L. & Attström, R. (1983). Ultrastructure of developing subgingival plaque in beagle dogs. *Journal of Clinical Periodontology* **12**, 507–524.

Theilade, E. (1986). The non-specific theory in microbial etiology of inflammatory periodontal diseases. *Journal of Clinical Periodontology* **13**, 905–911.

Theilade, E. & Theilade, J. (1970). Bacteriological and ultrastructural studies of developing dental plaque. In: McHugh, W.D., ed. *Dental Plaque*. Edinburgh: Livingstone, pp. 27–40.

Theilade, E. & Theilade, J. (1985). Formation and ecology of plaque at different locations in the mouth. *Scandinavian Journal of Dental Research* **93**, 90–95.

Theilade, E., Theilade, J. & Mikkelsen, L. (1982a). Microbiological studies on early dentogingival plaque on teeth and Mylar strips in humans. *Journal of Periodontal Research* **17**, 12–25.

Theilade, E., Wright, W.H., Jensen, B.S. & Löe, H. (1966). Experimental gingivitis in man. II. A longitudinal clinical and bacteriological investigation. *Journal of Periodontal Research* **1**, 1–13.

Theilade, J. (1964). Electron microscopic study of calculus attachment to smooth surfaces. *Acta Odontologica Scandinavia* **22**, 379–387.

Theilade, J. & Attström, R. (1985). Distribution and ultrastructure of subgingival plaque in beagle dogs with gingival inflammation. *Journal of Periodontal Research* **20**, 131–145.

Theilade, J., Fejerskov, O., Karring, T., Rölla, G. & Melsen, B. (1982b). TEM of the effect of sucrose on plaque formation on Mylar and tooth surfaces in monkeys. *Journal of Dental Research* **61**, 570.

Tinanoff, N. & Gross, A. (1976). Epithelial cells associated with the development of dental plaque. *Journal of Dental Research* **55**, 580–583.

Turesky, S., Renstrup, G. & Glickman, I. (1961). Histologic and histochemical observations regarding early calculus formation in children and adults. *Journal of Periodontology* **32**, 7–14.

Wærhaug, J. (1952). The gingival pocket. *Odontologisk Tidskrift* **60**, Suppl 1.

Wærhaug, J. (1955). Microscopic demonstration of tissue reaction incident to removal of dental calculus. *Journal of Periodontology* **26**, 26–29.

Wærhaug, J. (1956). Effect of rough surfaces upon gingival tissues. *Journal of Dental Research* **35**, 323–325.

Westergaard, J., Frandsen, A. & Slots, J. (1978). Ultrastructure of the subgingival flora in juvenile periodontitis. *Scandinavian Journal of Dental Research* **86**, 421–429.

Wilderer, P.A. & Charaklis, W.G. (1989). Structure and function of biofilms. In: Charaklis, W.G., Wilderer, P.A., eds. *Structure and Function of Biofilms.* Chichester, UK: John Wiley, pp. 5–17.

Zander, H.A., Hazen, S.P. & Scott, D.B. (1960). Mineralization of dental calculus. *Proceedings of the Society of Experimental Biology and Medicine* **103**, 257–260.

Chapter 9

Periodontal Infections

Sigmund S. Socransky and Anne D. Haffajee

Introduction

Periodontal diseases are infections that are caused by microorganisms that colonize the tooth surface at or below the gingival margin. It is estimated that about 700 different species are capable of colonizing the mouth and any individual may typically harbor 150 or more different species. Counts in subgingival sites range from about 10^3 in healthy, shallow sulci to $>10^8$ in deep periodontal pockets. Numbers in supragingival plaque can exceed 10^9 on a single tooth surface. Thus, while hundreds of millions or even billions of bacteria continually colonize the tooth at or below the gingival margin throughout life, most periodontal sites in most individuals do not exhibit new loss of the supporting structures of the teeth at any given time. This recognition is critical. The ecologic relationships between the periodontal microbiota and its host are, by and large, benign, in that damage to the supporting structures of the tooth is infrequent. Occasionally, a subset of bacterial species either is introduced, overgrows or exhibits new properties that lead to the destruction of the periodontium. The resulting stressed equilibrium is usually spontaneously corrected, or corrected by therapy. In either instance, microbial species continue to colonize above and below the gingival margin; hopefully, in a new and "peaceful" equilibrium.

Similarities of periodontal diseases to other infectious diseases

Our concepts of infectious diseases often appear to be influenced by our experiences with acute infections, particularly upper respiratory infections. In acute infections, an agent is acquired by exposure to an individual harboring that agent or from the environment. The agent establishes within tissues or on mucous membranes or skin. Within a short period of time, signs or symptoms of a disease appear at the site of introduction or elsewhere in the individual. A "battle" occurs between the parasite and the host resulting in increasingly obvious clinical signs and symptoms. This host–pathogen interaction often is resolved within a short period of time, usually, but not always, in favor of the host. Thus, daily experience suggests that colonization by a pathogen is rapidly followed by expression of disease. While certain infections follow this pattern, more commonly, colonization by a pathogenic species does not lead to overt disease, at least immediately. For example, 15% of the American population is colonized by *Neisseria meningitidis* (Caugant *et al.* 1988), but only 0.5–1.1 cases of meningitis occur per 100 000 of the population (Summary of Notifiable Diseases – United States 2004, 2006). *Mycobacterium tuberculosis* colonizes about 5% of Americans (Sudre *et al.* 1992), but only 2.6 new cases of tuberculosis per 100 000 of US-born individuals are reported each year (Summary of notifiable diseases – United States 2004, 2006). Finally, about one third of the adult population is colonized by *Haemophilus influenzae* (Kilian & Frederiksen 1981) but only a tiny fraction exhibit disease. Even the highly virulent HIV virus may be detected in individuals for years prior to the development of clinical symptoms.

In a similar fashion, individuals may be colonized continuously by periodontal pathogens at or below the gingival margin and yet not show evidence of ongoing or previous periodontal destruction. Many of the organisms that colonize such sites are members of species thought to be periodontal pathogens. In spite of their presence, periodontal tissue damage does not take place. This is not an anomaly. This phenomenon is consistent with other infectious diseases in which it may be observed that a pathogen is necessary but not sufficient for a disease to occur.

Infectious diseases in a given organ system are caused by one or more of a relatively finite set of pathogens. Further, different species have different tissue specificities and cause diseases in different sites in the body. Lung infections may be caused by a wide range of species that includes *Streptococcus pneumoniae*, *M. tuberculosis*, *Klebsiella pneumoniae*, *Legionella pneumophilia*, and others. Infections of the intestine are caused by *Salmonella typhi*, *Shigella dysenteriae*, *Vibrio cholerae*, *Escherichia coli*, and *Campylobacter* species. In a similar fashion periodontal diseases appear to be caused by a relatively finite group of periodontal pathogens acting alone or in combination. Such species include *Aggregatibacter* (formerly *Actinobacillus*) *actinomycetemcomitans*, *Tannerella forsythia*, *Campylobacter rectus*, *Eubacterium nodatum*, *Fusobacterium nucleatum*, *Peptostreptococcus micros*, *Porphyromonas gingivalis*, *Prevotella intermedia*, *Prevotella nigrescens*, *Streptococcus intermedius*, and *Treponema* sp. (Haffajee & Socransky 1994).

There is a number of other common themes observed in different infectious diseases, particularly those that affect mucous membranes, such as the need to attach to one or more surfaces, the need to "sense" the environment and turn on or off various virulence factors, and the need to overcome or evade host defense mechanisms. Infectious agents have evolved a set of common strategies to perform these tasks and the host has developed a series of responses to combat these infections. Thus, periodontal diseases are infectious diseases that have many properties that are similar to bacterial infections in other parts of the body and to a large extent can be combatted in similar fashions.

Unique features of periodontal infections

Although periodontal diseases have certain features in common with other infectious diseases, there are several features of these diseases that are quite different. In certain ways, periodontal diseases may be among the most unusual infections of the human. The major reason for this uniqueness is *the unusual anatomic feature that a mineralized structure, the tooth, passes through the integument, so that part of it is exposed to the external environment while part is within the connective tissues.* The tooth provides a surface for the colonization of a diverse array of bacterial species. Bacteria may attach to the tooth itself, to the epithelial surfaces of the gingiva or periodontal pocket, to underlying connective tissues, if exposed, and to other bacteria which are attached to these surfaces. In contrast to the outer surface of most parts of the body, the outer layers of the tooth do not "shed" and thus microbial colonization (accumulation) is facilitated. Thus, a situation is set up in which microorganisms colonize a relatively stable surface, the tooth, and are continually held in immediate proximity to the soft tissues of the periodontium. This poses a potential threat to those tissues and indeed to the host itself.

The organisms that cause periodontal diseases reside in biofilms that exist on tooth or epithelial surfaces. The biofilm provides a protective environment for the colonizing organisms and fosters metabolic properties that would not be possible if the species existed in a free-living (planktonic) state. Periodontal infections and another biofilm-induced disease, dental caries, are arguably the most common infectious diseases affecting the human. The onset of these diseases is usually delayed for prolonged periods of time after initial colonization by the pathogen(s). The course of these diseases typically runs for years. The etiologic agents in most instances appear to be members of the indigenous microbiota and, thus, the infections might be thought of as endogenous. The source of the infecting agents for any given individual is usually unknown, although transfer from parents or significant others is thought to play a primary role (Petit *et al.* 1993a,b; Saarela *et al.* 1993; van Steenbergen *et al.* 1993; Preus *et al.* 1994). The major characteristics of these diseases are that they are caused by organisms that reside in biofilms outside the body. Their treatment is complex in that physical, antimicrobial, and ecologic approaches are required.

The presence of a tooth increases the complexity of the host–parasite relationship in a number of ways. The bacteria colonizing the tooth are, by and large, outside the body where they are less able to be controlled by the potent mechanisms which operate within the tissues. The environment within plaque may be conducive for microbial survival, but it is unlikely to be a particularly effective environment for the host to seek out and destroy microorganisms. Factors, such as *hydrogen ion concentration* (pH), *oxidation reduction potential* (Eh), and *proteolytic enzymes*, can affect the performance of host defense mechanisms. In addition, the tooth provides "sanctuaries" in which microorganisms can hide, persist at low levels during treatment and then re-emerge to cause further problems. Bacteria in dentinal tubules, flaws in the tooth, or areas that were demineralized by bacteria are not easily approached by the much larger host cells. In a similar fashion, non-cellular host factors must face diffusion barriers, lytic enzymes, and absorption by the mineral structure of the tooth. Mechanical debridement other than vigorous removal of tooth material cannot reach organisms within the tooth. Chemotherapeutic agents will also have difficulty in reaching the organisms.

Taken together, the infections that affect the tooth and its supporting structures present a formidable problem for both the host and the therapist. The unique anatomic features of this "organ system" must be borne in mind as we attempt to unravel the etiology and pathogenesis of periodontal diseases and plan treatment or prevention strategies for their control.

Historical perspective

The search for the etiologic agents of periodontal diseases has been in progress for over a century. The search started in the "golden age of microbiology" (approx. 1880–1920), when the etiologic agents of many medically important infections were determined. It is not surprising that parallel investigations of the etiology of periodontal diseases were initiated in this era. However, these investigations were not as successful as some of the investigations of extraoral infectious diseases. It seems worthwhile to review briefly the findings of the early era and to understand the effect that the inconclusive nature of many of the studies had on the concepts of etiology and treatment of disease. The references for this section may be found in Socransky and Haffajee (1994).

The early search

Investigators in the period from 1880–1930 suggested four distinct groups of microorganisms as possible etiologic agents; amoeba, spirochetes, fusiforms, and streptococci. The basis of this determination was primarily the seeming association of these organisms with periodontal lesions. The identification of a suspected pathogen was heavily influenced by the nature of the techniques available. The major techniques at that time were wet mount or stained smear microscopy and limited cultural techniques. The different techniques suggested different etiologic agents. A situation not unlike that found today. While a greater variety of improved techniques is available, different techniques can and do emphasize the importance of different organisms.

Amoeba

Certain groups of investigators used stained smears to seek amoeba in bacterial plaque. They found higher proportions of amoeba in lesions of destructive periodontal diseases than in samples taken from sites in healthy mouths or mouths with gingivitis. Local therapies for this organism included the use of dyes or other antiseptic agents to decrease the numbers of amoebae in the oral cavity. Other approaches employed agents such as the emitic, emitin, administered systemically or locally. The role of amoeba in periodontal disease was questioned by some authors because amoeba were found in sites with minimal or no disease and could not be detected in many sites with destructive disease and because of the failure of emitin to ameliorate the symptoms of the disease.

Spirochetes

Other investigators used wet mount preparations or specific stains for spirochetes when they examined dental plaque. They reported higher proportions of spirochetes and other motile forms in lesions of destructive disease when compared with control sites in the same or other individuals. This finding led to the suggestion that spirochetes may be etiologic agents of destructive periodontal disease. Therapies were proposed that sought to control disease by the elimination or suppression of these microorganisms including the systemic administration of Neosalvarsan (compound 606), the anti-spirochetal agent used to treat syphilis, coupled with the use of subgingival scaling to control destructive periodontal disease. Other investigators employed bismuth compounds to treat oral spirochetal infections. Many investigators claimed success in controlling advanced destructive periodontal disease by combining local and systemic therapy. Others questioned the relationship of spirochetes to periodontal diseases.

Fusiforms

The third group of organisms that were frequently suggested to be etiologic agents of destructive periodontal diseases, including Vincent's infection, were the spindle-shaped fusiforms. These organisms were originally recognized on the basis of their frequent appearance in microscopic examination of subgingival plaque samples. The organisms were first related to periodontal disease by Plaut (1894). Vincent (1899) distinguished certain pseudomembranous lesions of the oral cavity and throat from diphtheria and recognized the important role of fusiforms and spirochetes in this disease. In honor of this investigator the infection became known as Vincent's infection. The important role of spirochetes and fusiforms in Vincent's infection was widely recognized in the succeeding 2 decades.

As a footnote to this section, it is worth noting that acute necrotizing ulcerative gingivitis (ANUG) appears to have been declining in many "first world countries" for many decades. Many older practitioners can remember periods when they would see several cases of ANUG a month or even a week. Detection of this disease is much less common today. In reviewing the earlier literature, we were struck with how common the disease appeared to be from about 1915–1930. Most of us are aware of the devastation this disease caused in the combat troops of World War I, when the disease was commonly called trench mouth (due to its frequent occurrence in troops stationed in the trenches of the battlegrounds). What we are less aware of is how common the disease became in countries out of the war zone (e.g. the US) after World War I. For example, Daley (1927a,b) examined over 1000 patients who came to Tufts Dental College in Boston for operative dentistry (not periodontal problems). He found Vincent's infection in one of three people using clinical criteria and stained smears seeking the presence of fusiforms and spirochetes. Daley carefully described the lesions in terms acceptable today; i.e. as ulcerated lesions that bled easily on probing and had a distinctive fetid odor. He further pointed out that the disease was rare in Boston prior to 1917; at which time the troops began to return home. He described an outbreak stemming from a local barracks which led to 75 cases being treated at Tufts within 48 hours. Daley and others in the era felt that the severe outbreak after the war was due to the transmission of more virulent bacteria among an unprotected (not immune) population. Assuming that the disease described in this era was ANUG, it is interesting to note that there was a virtual epidemic. This is particularly intriguing in that it supports the notion that periodontal pathogens can be readily transmitted from one person to another as modern molecular techniques are documenting today.

Streptococci

The fourth group of microorganisms that were proposed as etiologic agents of periodontal diseases in this era were the streptococci. These microorganisms were proposed on the basis of cultural examination of samples of plaque from subgingival sites of periodontal disease. The selection of the streptococci may have been predicated upon the fact these were the only species that could be consistently isolated from periodontitis lesions using the cultural techniques of that era. Since there were no methods available at that time for the specific control of streptococci, workers turned to non-specific agents such as the intramuscular injection of mercury or to the use of vaccines for the control of periodontal diseases.

Vaccines

For the first 3 decades of the twentieth century, vaccines were commonly employed by physicians and dentists in attempts to control bacterial infections. Three types of vaccines were employed for the control of periodontal diseases. These included vaccines prepared from pure cultures of streptococci, and other oral organisms, autogenous vaccines, and stock vaccines such as Van Cott's vaccine, Goldenberg's vaccine or Inava Endocorps vaccine. These vaccines were administered systemically or locally in the periodontal tissues.

Autogenous vaccines were prepared from the dental plaque of patients with destructive periodontal diseases. Plaque samples were removed from the diseased site, "sterilized" by heat, and/or by immersion in iodine or formalin solutions, then re-injected into the same patient, either in the local periodontal lesion or systemically. Proponents of all three techniques claimed great efficacy for the vaccination methods employed, while others using the same techniques were more skeptical.

Other forms of therapy directed against oral microorganisms

The difficulty in controlling microorganisms in the absence of specific antimicrobial agents gave rise to a series of rather remarkable treatment procedures. For example, ultraviolet light was widely used to attempt to control the oral microbiota and to improve the well-being of the local tissue (for review see Rasmussen 1929). Other measures were somewhat more dramatic and in some instances rather frightening. Dental practitioners used electrochemical techniques, caustic agents such as phenol, sulfuric, trichloracetic or chromic acids, nascent copper, castor oil soap (sodium ricolineate), and even radium was used to combat root canal infections. In the last instance radium at levels of up to 0.135 millicuries was placed in canals to "sterilize" them. As might be expected, the reports were glowing. The recent interest in controlling the epithelium in order to maximize re-attachment had antecedents in this era. One technique which appears to have been commonly employed was the use of sodium sulfide to "dissolve" the epithelial lining of the pocket and permit reattachment.

Invasion – the early years

One of the more interesting phenomena of research is the fact that research workers keep rediscovering the same phenomena in a cyclical fashion. Invasion of the periodontal tissues by bacteria was thought to be important in the pathogenesis of periodontal diseases in the early 1900s, forgotten and then rediscovered.

Beckwith *et al.* (1925) used stains specific for bacteria to study biopsy specimens from prisoners at San Quentin who had periodontitis. They regularly observed bacteria both within the epithelium and in the underlying tissues. Bacteria in the epithelium were usually streptococci or "diphtheroids". Gram-negative rods were observed in the connective tissue. They noted the rare occurrence of spiral forms in the tissues, although they were routinely detected in the plaque overlying the tissues. Other investigators also showed invasion into periodontal tissues. Invasion of spirochetes deep into the lesions of Vincent's infection was clearly documented. It was thought that the spirochetes moved into the connective tissues first and were followed by fusiform-shaped species.

Comment

In this early period, literally hundreds of papers were published which suggested certain specific etiologic agents of periodontal diseases or advocated specific therapies directed at microbial control. In spite of this enthusiasm, the concept of the infectious nature of periodontal diseases and the recognition that treatment should be directed at the causative agents, disappeared. Reasons for the demise of this promising area of research could have included the possibility of incorrect etiologic agents, inadequate therapies and multiplicity of diseases. A more likely scenario was the failure of early researchers (and this is still true today) to recognize that periodontal diseases represent an array of infections, each requiring different specific therapies. Indeed, a similar situation exists today where a given adjunctive antibiotic therapy is effective in some individuals and not others. Finally, competing theories explaining the etiology of periodontal diseases in this era appeared to, temporarily at least, gain popularity, due primarily to their nebulous and untestable nature. Such hypotheses as "diffuse alveolar atrophy", "continuing eruption", "lack of function", and "constitutional defects" became acceptable alternatives (to some) to the recognition of the infectious nature of periodontal diseases.

The decline of interest in microorganisms

The initial enthusiasm for the hunt for the etiologic agents of destructive periodontal diseases slowly subsided and by the mid 1930s there were virtually no workers involved in this quest. This state was eloquently described by Belding and Belding (1936) in the aptly titled "Bacteria – Dental Orphans". During the period from the mid 1920s to the early 1960s, the attitude toward the etiology of periodontal diseases changed. In the first 2 decades of this period it was thought that periodontal disease was due to some constitutional defect on the part of the patient,

to trauma from occlusion, to disuse atrophy or to some combination of these factors. Bacteria were thought to be merely secondary invaders in this process or, at most, contributors to the inflammation observed in periodontal destruction.

Non-specific plaque hypothesis

Treatment of patients based on the notion of constitutional defects or trauma from occlusion was not effective in controlling periodontal diseases. Clinicians recognized that plaque control was essential in the satisfactory treatment of periodontal patients. During the late 1950s, a group of clinicians, sometimes referred to as "plaque evangelists", heavily emphasized the need for plaque control in the prevention and treatment of periodontal diseases. Thus, once again bacteria were thought to play a role in the etiology of destructive periodontal disease, but as non-specific causative agents. According to this "non-specific plaque" hypothesis, any accumulations of microorganisms at or below the gingival margin would produce irritants leading to inflammation. The inflammation in turn was responsible for the periodontal tissue destruction. The specific species of microorganisms that accumulated on the teeth was not considered to be particularly significant, providing that their numbers were sufficiently large to trigger a destructive process.

Mixed anaerobic infections

Beginning in the late 1920s, a series of oral and medical microbiologists believed that periodontal disease was the result of "mixed infections". This hypothesis had been considered since the late 1800s when microscopic observations by Vincent in France suggested that certain forms of periodontal disease, particularly ANUG, were due to a combination of microorganisms dominated by fusiforms and spirochetes. These infections were known as fuso-spirochetal infections. In the early 1930s, investigators found that mixtures of microorganisms isolated from lung infections or subgingival plaque would induce lesions when injected subcutaneously into various experimental animals. A combination of a fusiform, a spirochete, an anaerobic vibrio and an alpha hemolytic streptococcus could cause transmissible infections in the guinea pig. Later investigators failed to reproduce their results either with the above combination of microorganisms or with many other combinations they tested. They did demonstrate, however, that mixed infections were due to bacteria (rather than a virus).

Macdonald and co-workers (1956) were later able to produce transmissible mixed infections in the guinea pig groin using combinations of pure cultures. The critical mixture of four organisms included a *Bacteroides melaninogenicus* strain, a Gram-positive anaerobic rod and two other Gram-negative anaerobic rods. This combination of organisms was completely different from those used by earlier investigators to cause transmissible infections. These results led to the concept that mixed infections might be "bacteriologically non-specific but biochemically specific". In other words, any combination of microorganisms capable of producing an array of destructive metabolites could lead to transmissible infections in animals and, by extension, to destructive periodontal infections in humans. Later experiments suggested that members of the *B. melaninogenicus* group were the key species in these infections.

Return to specificity in microbial etiology of periodontal diseases

In the 1960s, interest in the specific microbial etiology of periodontal disease was rekindled by two groups of experiments. The first demonstrated that periodontal disease could be transmitted in the hamster from animals with periodontal disease to animals without periodontal disease by caging them together. Swabs of plaque or feces from diseased animals were effective in transmitting the disease to animals free of disease. It was demonstrated that a pure culture of a Gram-positive pleomorphic rod that later became known as *Actinomyces viscosus* was capable of causing destructive periodontal disease in animals free of disease. Other species isolated from the plaque of hamsters with periodontal disease did not have this capability.

At about the same time, it was demonstrated that spirochetes with a unique ultrastructural morphology could be detected in practically pure culture in the connective tissue underlying lesions of ANUG and within the adjacent epithelium. Control tissue taken from healthy individuals and individuals with other forms of disease did not exhibit a similar tissue invasion. To date, the spirochete associated with ANUG has not been cultivated.

Such findings suggested that there might be more specificity to the microbial etiology of periodontal disease than had been accepted for the previous 4 decades. However, the emphasis of clinicians in the 1960s was on the mechanical control of plaque accumulation. This approach was consistent with the prevailing concept that periodontal disease was due to a non-specific accumulation of bacteria on tooth surfaces. This concept is very much in evidence today and still serves as the basis of preventive techniques in most dental practices. It is also clear that non-specific plaque control is not able to effectively prevent all forms of periodontal disease.

The transmissibility studies stimulated a new concept of periodontal diseases. The organisms which were responsible for the periodontal destruction observed in the hamster clearly differed from other organisms by their ability to form large amounts of bacterial plaque both in the hamster and in *in vitro* test systems. A concept emerged that microorganisms that were capable of forming large amounts of plaque *in vivo* and *in vitro* should be considered as prime suspects in the etiology of periodontal diseases. Human isolates of *Actinomyces* species were shown to have this ability *in vitro* and led to plaque formation and periodontal destruction in animal model systems. These findings reinforced the notion that organisms that formed abundant plaque were responsible for destructive periodontal disease. Unfortunately, later research findings revealed major discrepancies in this hypothesis.

Changing concepts of the microbial etiology of periodontal diseases

By the end of the 1960s it was generally accepted that dental plaque was in some way associated with human periodontal disease. It was believed that the presence of bacterial plaque initiated a series of as yet undefined events that led to the destruction of the periodontium. The composition of plaque was thought to be relatively similar from patient to patient and from site to site within patients. Variability was recognized, but the true extent of differences in bacterial composition was not appreciated. It was thought that the major event triggering destructive periodontal disease was an increase in mass of bacterial plaque, possibly accompanied by a diminution of host resistance. Indeed, in the mid 1960s the classic studies of Loe *et al.* (1965, 1967) and Theilade *et al.* (1966) convincingly demonstrated that plaque accumulation directly preceded and initiated gingivitis. Many investigators believed that gingivitis was harmful, and led to the eventual destruction of the periodontal tissues, probably by host-mediated events.

Yet, certain discrepancies continued to baffle clinicians and research workers alike. If all plaques were more or less alike and induced a particular tissue response in the host, why was periodontal destruction localized, taking place adjacent to one tooth but not another? If plaque mass was a prime trigger for periodontal destruction, why did certain subjects accumulate much plaque, frequently accompanied by gingivitis, but fail, even after many years to develop destruction of the supporting structures? On the other hand, why did some individuals with little detectable plaque or clinical inflammation develop rapid periodontal destruction? If inflammation was the main mediator of tissue destruction, why were so many teeth retained in the presence of continual gingivitis? One explanation may have been that there were inconsistencies in the host response, or disease required the superimposition of local factors such as trauma from occlusion, overhanging fillings etc. Other explanations can be derived from extensive studies of the microbiota adjacent to periodontal tissues.

The recognition of differences in the composition of bacterial plaque from subject to subject and site to site within subjects led to a series of investigations.

Some studies attempted to determine whether specific microorganisms were found in lesion sites as compared to healthy sites. Others studies sought differences in the microorganisms in subgingival plaque samples taken from subjects with clinically different forms of periodontal disease or periodontal health. Newman *et al.* (1976, 1977) and Slots (1976) demonstrated that the microbial composition of subgingival plaque taken from diseased sites differed substantially from the samples taken from healthy sites in subjects with localized aggressive periodontitis (LAP). Tanner *et al.* (1979) and Slots (1977) demonstrated that the microbiota recovered from lesion sites from subjects with chronic periodontitis differed from the microbiota from healthy sites in the same subjects and also from lesion sites in LAP subjects. These studies, along with the demonstration that subjects with LAP could be treated successfully with local debridement and systemic antibiotics, provided the initial impetus to perform larger-scale studies attempting to relate specific microorganisms to the etiology of different periodontal diseases.

Current suspected pathogens of destructive periodontal diseases

Criteria for defining periodontal pathogens

For more than a century, the classical "Koch's postulates" have been used to define a causal relationship between an infectious agent and a disease. These postulates were: (1) the agent must be isolated from every case of the disease, (2) it must not be recovered from cases of other forms of disease or non-pathogenically, and (3) after isolation and repeated growth in pure culture, the pathogen must induce disease in experimental animals (Carter 1987). The criteria for defining pathogens of destructive periodontal diseases initially were based on Koch's postulates but have been amended and extended in recent years. These criteria include association, elimination, host response, virulence factors, animal studies, and risk assessment. The discrimination of a pathogen from a non-pathogenic species is not based on a single criterion but rather on a "weight of evidence" evaluation.

The criterion of association is really the same as Koch's first two postulates; i.e. the species should be found more frequently and in higher numbers in cases of the infection than in individuals without overt disease or with different forms of disease. However, periodontal microbiologists do not expect to find the pathogen in "all cases of the disease" because they currently cannot distinguish "all cases of a given disease". The criterion of elimination is based on the concept that elimination of a species should be accompanied by a parallel remission of disease. If a species is eliminated by treatment and the disease progresses, or if the level of a species remains high or increases in a site and the disease

stops, doubt would be cast on that species' role in pathogenesis. This criterion (like all of the others) has certain problems in that therapy rarely (if ever) eliminates or suppresses only one species at a time. The criterion of host response, particularly the immunological response, appears to be of value in defining periodontal pathogens. If a species (or its antigens) gains access to underlying periodontal tissues and causes damage, it seems likely that the host will produce antibodies or a cellular immune response that is directed specifically to that species. Thus, the host response could act as a pointer to the pathogen(s). Biochemical determinants (virulence factors) may also provide valuable clues to pathogenicity. Potentially damaging metabolites produced, or properties possessed, by certain species may be suggestive that those species could play a role in the disease process.

Animal model systems provide suggestive evidence that a microbial species may play a role in human disease. Particularly noteworthy are studies of experimentally induced disease in dogs or monkeys, which can be manipulated to favor selection of single or subsets of species that may or may not induce pathology. These models usually suggest a possible etiologic role of a species indigenous to the test animal that may have analogues in the human subgingival microbiota. Finally, technological developments, such as checkerboard DNA–DNA hybridization (Fig. 9-1) and polymerase chain reaction (PCR), now permit assessment of specific microorganisms in large numbers of subgingival plaque samples. This allows prospective studies to be performed in which the risk of periodontal disease progression conferred by the presence of an organism at given levels may be assessed.

Periodontal pathogens

The World Workshop in Periodontology (Consensus Report, 1996) designated *A. actinomycetemcomitans*, *P. gingivalis*, and *T. forsythia* as periodontal pathogens. Tables 9-1, 9-2, and 9-3 summarize some of the data that indicate an etiologic role of these species in periodontal diseases, categorized according to the criteria defined above. The summary is by no means exhaustive but does indicate that a growing literature suggests some reasonable candidates as etiologic agents of destructive periodontal diseases.

Aggregatibacter (formerly *Actinobacillus*) *actinomycetemcomitans*

One of the clearest associations between a suspected pathogen and destructive periodontal disease is provided by *A. actinomycetemcomitans*. This species has recently been renamed *Aggregatibacter actinomycetemcomitans* from its former name of *Actinobacillus actinomycetemcomitans* (Norskov-Lauritsen & Kilian 2006). *A. actinomycetemcomitans* is a small, non-motile,

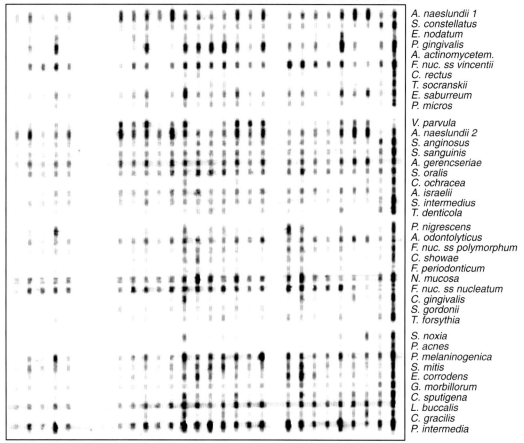

Fig. 9-1 Example of checkerboard DNA–DNA hybridization being used to detect 40 bacterial species in 28 subgingival plaque samples from a single patient. The vertical lanes are the plaque samples numbered from 11 (upper right central incisor) to 47 (lower right second molar). In this subject, teeth 16, 17, 21, and 37 were missing. The two vertical lanes on the right are standards containing either 10^5 or 10^6 cells of each test species. The horizontal lanes contained the indicated DNA probes in hybridization buffer. A signal at the intersection of the vertical and horizontal lanes indicates the presence of a species. The intensity of the signal is related to the number of organisms of that species in the sample. In brief, samples of plaque were placed into individual Eppendorf tubes and the DNA released from the microorganisms by boiling in NaOH. After neutralization, the released DNA was transferred to the surface of a nylon membrane using the 30 channels of a Minislot device (Immunetics, Cambridge, MA). The DNA was fixed to the membrane by UV light and baking and placed in a Miniblotter 45 (Immunetics) with the lanes of DNA at right angles to the 45 channels of the Miniblotter device. Whole genomic DNA probes labelled with digoxigenin were placed in hybridization buffer into 40 of the lanes and hybridized overnight. After stringency washing, the signals were detected using phosphatase-conjugated antibody to digoxigenin and chemifluorescence substrates. Signals were compared to the standards using a Storm Fluorimager and converted to counts.

Table 9-1 Summary of some of the types of data that suggest that *Aggregatibacter actinomycetemcomitans* may be an etiologic agent of destructive periodontal diseases (for literature citations see text and Haffajee & Socransky 1994)

Factor	Data
Association	Elevated in lesions of localized juvenile periodontitis (LJP), prepubertal or adolescent periodontal disease
	Lower in health, gingivitis and edentulous subjects or sites
	Elevated in some adult periodontitis lesions
	Elevated in active lesions of juvenile periodontitis
	Detected in prospective studies
	Detected in apical ares of pocket or in tissues from LJP lesions
Elimination	Elimination or suppression resulted in successful therapy
	Recurrent lesions harbored the species
Host response	Elevated antibody in serum or saliva of LJP patients
	Elevated antibody in serum or saliva of chronic periodontitis patients
	Elevated local antibody in LJP sites
Virulence factors	Leukotoxin; collagenase; endotoxin; epitheliotoxin; fibroblast inhibitory factor; bone resorption inducing factor; induction of cytokine production from macrophages; modification of neutrophil function; degradation of immunoglobulins; cytolethal distending toxin (Cdt); induces apoptotic cell death
	Invades epithelial and vascular endothelial cells *in vitro* and buccal epithelial cells *in vivo*
Animal studies	Induced disease in gnotobiotic rats
	Subcutaneous abscesses in mice

Table 9-2 Summary of some of the types of data that suggest that *Porphyromonas gingivalis* may be an etiologic agent of destructive periodontal diseases (for literature citations see text and Haffajee & Socransky 1994)

Factor	Data
Association	Elevated in lesions of periodontitis
	Lower in sites of health, gingivitis and edentulous subjects
	Elevated in actively progressing lesions
	Elevated in subjects exhibiting periodontal disease progression
	Detected in cells or tissues of periodontal lesions
	Presence indicates increased risk for alveolar bone loss and attachment level loss
Elimination	Elimination resulted in successful therapy
	Recurrent lesions harbored the species
	Successful treatment lowered level and/or avidity of antibody
Host response	Elevated antibody in serum or saliva in subjects with various forms of periodontitis
	Altered local antibody in periodontitis
Virulence factors	Collagenase; endotoxin; proteolytic trypsin-like activity; fibrinolysin; hemolysin; other proteases including gingipain; phospholipase A; degrades immunoglobulin; fibroblast inhibitory factor; H_2S; NH_3; fatty acids; factors that adversely affect PMNs; capsular polysaccharide; bone resorption inducing factor; induction of cytokine production from various host cells; generates chemotactic activities; inhibits migration of PMNs across epithelial barriers; Invades epithelial cells *in vitro*
Animal studies	Important in experimental pure or mixed subcutaneous infections
	Induced disease in gnotobiotic rats
	Studies in sheep, monkeys and dogs
	Immunization diminished disease in experimental animals

Table 9-3 Summary of some of the types of data that suggest that *Tannerella forsythia* may be an etiologic agent of destructive periodontal diseases (for literature citations see text and Haffajee & Socransky 1994)

Factor	Data
Association	Elevated in lesions of periodontitis
	Lower in sites of health or gingivitis
	Elevated in actively progressing lesions
	Elevated in periodontal abscesses
	Increased in subjects with refractory periodontitis
	Detected in epithelial cells of periodontal pockets
	Presence indicates increased risk for alveolar bone loss, tooth and attachment level loss
Elimination	Elimination resulted in successful therapy
	Recurrent lesions harbored the species
	Reduced in successfully treated peri-implantitis
Host response	Elevated antibody in serum of periodontitis subjects and very high in a subset of subjects with refractory periodontitis
Virulence factors	Endotoxin; fatty acid and methylglyoxal production; induces apoptotic cell death; cytokine production from various host cells; invades epithelial cells *in vitro* and *in vivo*
Animal studies	Increased levels in ligature-induced periodontitis and peri-implantitis in dogs
	Induced disease in gnotobiotic rats

Gram-negative, saccharolytic, capnophilic, round-ended rod that forms small, convex colonies with a "star-shaped" center when grown on blood agar plates (Fig. 9-2). This species was first recognized as a possible periodontal pathogen by its increased frequency of detection and higher numbers in lesions of localized aggressive periodontitis (Newman *et al.* 1976; Slots 1976; Newman & Socransky 1977; Slots *et al.* 1980; Mandell & Socransky 1981; Zambon *et al.* 1983a; Chung *et al.* 1989) when compared with numbers in plaque samples from other clinical conditions including periodontitis, gingivitis, and health. Soon thereafter, it was demonstrated that the major-

ity of subjects with localized aggressive periodontitis (LAP) had an enormously elevated serum antibody response to this species (Genco *et al.* 1980; Listgarten *et al.* 1981; Tsai *et al.* 1981; Altman *et al.* 1982; Ebersole *et al.* 1982, 1987) and that there was local synthesis of antibody to this species (Schonfeld & Kagan 1982; Ebersole *et al.* 1985; Smith *et al.* 1985; Tew *et al.* 1985a). When subjects with this form of disease were treated successfully, the species was eliminated or lowered in level; treatment failures were associated with failure to lower the numbers of the species in treated sites (Slots & Rosling 1983; Haffajee *et al.* 1984; Christersson *et al.* 1985; Kornman & Robertson 1985;

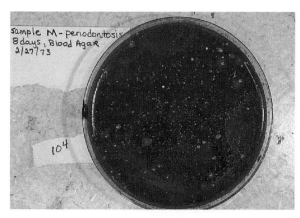

Fig. 9-2 Photograph of a primary isolation plate of a subgingival plaque sample from a diseased site in a subject with LAP. A dilution of the plaque sample was grown for 7 days at 35°C on an enriched blood agar plate in an atmosphere of 80% N_2, 10% H_2, and 10% CO_2. The majority of the small, round, convex colonies on this plate were isolates of *Aggregatibacter actinomycetemcomitans*.

Mandell *et al.* 1986; Preus 1988; Shiloah *et al.* 1998; Tinoco *et al.* 1998). The species produced a number of potentially damaging metabolites, including a leukotoxin (Baehni *et al.* 1979) and a cytolethal distending toxin (Saiki *et al.* 2001; Shenker *et al.* 2001), and induced disease in experimental animals (Irving *et al.* 1978). *A. actinomycetemcomitans* has been shown, *in vitro*, to have the ability to invade cultured human gingival epithelial cells (Blix *et al.* 1992; Sreenivasan *et al.* 1993), human vascular endothelial cells (Schenkein *et al.* 2000) and buccal epithelial cells *in vivo* (Rudney *et al.* 2001). Further, studies have shown that *A. actinomycetemcomitans* induced apoptotic cell death (Arakawa *et al.* 2000; Kato *et al.* 2000).

Perhaps the strongest association data came from studies of "active lesions" in which the species was elevated in actively progressing periodontal lesions when compared with non-progressing sites (Haffajee *et al.* 1984; Mandell 1984; Mandell *et al.* 1987; Haubek *et al.* 2004) and in prospective studies of as yet undiseased siblings of LAP subjects (DiRienzo *et al.* 1994). *A. actinomycetemcomitans* was also elevated in studies of disease progression in young Indonesian subjects (Timmerman *et al.* 2001). Collectively, the data suggest that *A. actinomycetemcomitans* is a probable pathogen of LAP. However, this should not be interpreted as meaning that it is the sole cause of this clinical condition, since a subset of subjects with LAP did not exhibit this species in samples of their subgingival plaque and had no elevated antibody response to the species (Loesche *et al.* 1985; Moore 1987).

The possibility that a subset of *A. actinomycetemcomitans* clonal types was primarily responsible for LAP was raised in studies at the University of Pennsylvania. Strains of *A. actinomycetemcomitans* were isolated from members of 18 families with at least one member with active LAP as well as from from 32 control subjects. Restriction fragment length poly-

morphisms (RFLP) indicated 13 distinct RFLP groups of *A. actinomycetemcomitans* (DiRienzo & McKay 1994). Isolates from LAP subjects fell into predominantly RFLP pattern II, while RFLP patterns XIII and XIV were seen exclusively in isolates from periodontally healthy subjects. Further, disease progression was related strongly to the presence of RFLP group II (DiRienzo *et al.* 1994).

Haubek *et al.* (1996) demonstrated that strains of *A. actinomycetemcomitans* isolated from families, initially of African origin living in geographically different areas, were characterized by a 530 base pair deletion in the leukotoxin gene operon leading to a significantly increased production of leukotoxin. They speculated that this virulent clonal type may account for an increased prevalence of LAP in African Americans and other individuals of African descent. A key isolate of this clonal type, strain JP2, was first isolated from an 8-year-old African American child with prepubertal periodontitis (Tsai *et al.* 1979; Kilian *et al.* 2006). There was a strong association between the presence of the JP2 clonal type of *A. actinomycetemcomitans* and early onset periodontitis in Moroccan school children, but no association between the presence of *A. actinomycetemcomitans* without the 530 bp deletion and early onset periodontitis (Haubek *et al.* 2001). Further, the odds ratio for disease progression in a subject in this population infected with the JP2 clone was 14.5 (Haubek *et al.* 2004). These observations were corroborated in a Brazilian population, where highly leukotoxic strains of *A. actinomycetemcomitans* were more prevalent in aggressive periodontitis than in chronic periodontitis (Cortelli *et al.* 2005). This deletion in the leukotoxin operon was not detected in any strains of *A. actinomycetemcomitans* isolated from adult Chinese subjects (Mombelli *et al.* 1999; Tan *et al.* 2001) or Asian subjects in the United States (Contreras *et al.* 2000). Subjects harboring *A. actinomycetemcomitans* with the 530 bp deletion were 22.5 times more likely to convert to LAP than subjects who had *A. actinomycetemcomitans* variants containing the full-length leukotoxin promoter region (Bueno *et al.* 1998). Interestingly, strains of *A. actinomycetemcomitans* with the RFLP type II pattern described by DiRienzo & McKay (1994) that were found frequently in LAP subjects included strains of the JP2 clonal type (Kilian *et al.* 2006). The above data suggest that *A. actinomycetemcomitans* is a major pathogen of LAP and that the JP2 clonal type is a key pathogen in certain human populations.

A. actinomycetemcomitans has also been implicated in adult forms of destructive periodontal disease, but its role is less clear. The species has been isolated from chronic periodontitis lesions, but less frequently and in lower numbers than from lesions in LAP subjects (Rodenburg *et al.* 1990; Slots *et al.* 1990a). In addition, its numbers in plaque samples from lesions in adults were often not as high as those observed for other suspected pathogens in the same plaque samples. There appear to be at least six serotypes of

A. actinomycetemcomitans (a, b, c, d, e, and f) and these serotypes appear to be clonal in nature (Kilian *et al.* 2006). The most frequently isolated serotype of *A. actinomycetemcomitans* from lesions of LAP in American subjects was serotype b (Zambon *et al.* 1983b), whereas serotype a was more commonly detected in samples from chronic periodontitis subjects (Zambon *et al.* 1983a). This finding was corroborated indirectly by examination of serum antibody levels to the two serotypes. Most elevated responses to *A. actinomycetemcomitans* in LAP subjects were to serotype b while elevated responses to serotype a were more common in adult subjects with chronic periodontitis (Listgarten *et al.* 1981). Some subjects in each group exhibited elevated serum antibody responses to both serotypes. In Finnish subjects, serotypes a and b were more frequently isolated from subjects with periodontal disease and serotype c from periodontally healthy subjects (Asikainen *et al.* 1991). However, this pattern of serotype distribution was not observed in Korea (Chung *et al.* 1989) or Japan (Saito *et al.* 1993; Yoshida *et al.* 2003), where *A. actinomycetemcomitans* serotype c was frequently observed in plaque samples from sites of periodontal pathology. Serotypes d, e, and f, have been recognized more recently (Dogan *et al.* 1999; Mombelli *et al.* 1999) and are found less frequently than serotypes a, b and c. For example, serotypes d, e or f were not detected in a Brazilian population (Teixeira *et al.* 2006) and serotypes d or e were not found in Taiwanese subjects <35 years of age with different forms of periodontitis (Yang *et al.* 2004a).

Antibody data and data from the treatment of *A. actinomycetemcomitans* infected patients with adult or refractory periodontitis provide the most convincing evidence of a possible etiologic role of *A. actinomycetemcomitans* in adult forms of periodontal disease. Thirty-six of 56 adults with destructive periodontal disease examined at multiple time periods at the Forsyth Institute exhibited an elevated serum antibody response to *A. actinomycetemcomitans* serotypes a and/or b. Elevated responses to other suspected periodontal pathogens were far less common. Van Winkelhoff *et al.* (1992) treated 50 adult subjects with "severe generalized periodontitis" and 40 subjects with refractory periodontitis who were culture positive for *A. actinomycetemcomitans* using mechanical debridement and systemically administered amoxicillin and metronidazole. Only one of 90 subjects was culture positive for *A. actinomycetemcomitans* 3–9 months post-therapy (van Winkelhoff *et al.* 1992) and one of 48 subjects was culture positive 2 years post-therapy (Pavicic *et al.* 1994). There was a significant gain in attachment level and decrease in probing pocket depth in virtually all patients after therapy.

It is suspected that *A. actinomycetemcomitans* initially colonizes the oral cavity by attachment to the surfaces of the oral epithelium (Fine *et al.* 2006). There is a specific protein adhesin, Aae, that binds to a carbohydrate receptor on buccal epithelial cells of humans and Old World monkeys. It is thought that *A. actinomycetemcomitans* moves from the buccal epithelial cells to the supragingival plaque, possibly binding to the tooth by fimbriae comprised of repeating subunits of a 6.5 kDa protein, Flp 1. The fimbriae, along with an extracellular carbohydrate polymer, PGA, mediate attachment to hard surfaces (Fine *et al.* 2006). Alternatively, *A. actinomycetemcomitans* may attach to other colonizing bacterial species by coaggregation (Kolenbrander 2000). At some point these organisms may move from the supragingival to the subgingival environment. From this vantage point, they may then attach to and invade the epithelial lining of the periodontal pocket and possibly penetrate the underlying connective tissues (Rudney *et al.* 2001). *A. actinomycetemcomitans* has been shown to be present in the intima of vessel walls (Marques de Silva *et al.* 2005) and has been cultured from atheromatous plaques (Kozarov *et al.* 2005). Finally, *A. actinomycetemcomitans* may leave the oral cavity and cause or contribute to endocarditis, since it has been frequently found in lesions of this condition (Paturel *et al.* 2004).

Porphyromonas gingivalis

P. gingivalis is a second consensus periodontal pathogen that continues to be intensely investigated. Isolates of this species are Gram-negative, anaerobic, non-motile, asaccharolytic rods that usually exhibit coccal to short rod morphologies. *P. gingivalis* is a member of the much investigated "black-pigmented *Bacteroides*" group (Fig. 9-3). Organisms of this group form brown to black colonies (Oliver & Wherry 1921) on blood agar plates and were initially grouped into a single species, *B. melaninogenicus* (*Bacterium melaninogenicum*; Burdon 1928). The black-pigmented *Bacteroides* have a long history of association with periodontal diseases since the early efforts of Burdon (1928) through the mixed infection studies of Macdonald *et al.* (1960) to the current intense interest.

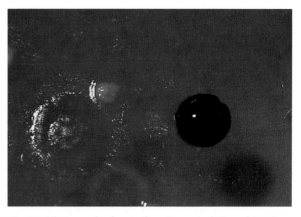

Fig. 9-3 Photograph of part of a primary isolation plate of a subgingival plaque sample from a subject with chronic periodontitis. The medium and growth conditions were as described in Fig. 9-2. The black-pigmented colony was an isolate of *Porphyromonas gingivalis*.

In the late 1970s, it was recognized that the black-pigmented *Bacteroides* contained species that were asaccharolytic (eventually *P. gingivalis*), and either had an intermediate level of carbohydrate fermentation (which eventually led to a group of species including *Prevotella intermedia*) or were highly saccharolytic (leading to the group that includes *Prevotella melaninogenica*).

Early interest in *Porphyromonas gingivalis* and other black-pigmented *Bacteroides* arose primarily because of their essential role in certain experimental mixed infections (Macdonald *et al.* 1956, 1963; Socransky & Gibbons 1965) and their production of an unusually large array of virulence factors (Table 9-2) (Haffajee & Socransky 1994; Deshpande & Khan 1999; Holt & Ebersole 2005). Members of these species produce collagenase, gingipain, an array of proteases (including those that destroy immunoglobulins), hemolysins, endotoxin, fatty acids, ammonia, hydrogen sulfide, indole etc. *P. gingivalis* can inhibit migration of PMNs across an epithelial barrier (Madianos *et al.* 1997), has been shown to affect the production or degradation of cytokines by mammalian cells (Darveau *et al.* 1998; Fletcher *et al.* 1998; Sandros *et al.* 2000). and produces extracellular vesicles that contribute to the loss of membrane-bound CD14 receptors on human macrophage-like cells (Duncan *et al.* 2004).

Studies initiated in the late 1970s and extending to the present have strengthened the association of *P. gingivalis* with disease and demonstrated that the species is uncommon and in low numbers in health or gingivitis but more frequently detected in destructive forms of disease (Table 9-2) (Haffajee & Socransky 1994; O'Brien-Simpson *et al.* 2000; Takeuchi *et al.* 2001; van Winkelhoff *et al.* 2002; Lau *et al.* 2004; Yang *et al.* 2004b). In diseased subjects, there was a strong positive relationship with pocket depth (Kawada *et al.* 2004; Socransky & Haffajee 2005). This species has also been shown to be increased in numbers and or frequency of detection in deteriorating periodontal sites (Dzink *et al.* 1988; Lopez 2000; Kamma *et al.* 2001) or in subjects exhibiting periodontal disease progression (Albandar *et al.* 1997). The species has been shown to be reduced in successfully treated sites but was commonly encountered in sites that exhibited recurrence of disease or persistence of deep periodontal pockets post-therapy (Bragd *et al.* 1987; Haffajee *et al.* 1988a; van Winkelhoff *et al.* 1988; Berglundh *et al.* 1998; Shiloah *et al.* 1998; Winkel *et al.* 1998; Takamatsu *et al.* 1999; Chaves *et al.* 2000; Mombelli *et al.* 2000; Fujise *et al.* 2002; Kawada *et al.* 2004). *P. gingivalis* has been associated with an increased risk of periodontal disease severity and progression (Beck *et al.* 1990, 1992, 1997; Grossi *et al.* 1994, 1995).

P. gingivalis has been shown to induce elevated systemic and local immune responses in subjects with various forms of periodontitis (Table 9-2) (Haffajee & Socransky 1994; Mahanonda *et al.* 1991; O'Brien-Simpson *et al.* 2000). Indeed, there has been an effort in many laboratories, not only to compare the level of antibody response in subjects with and without disease, but to examine relative avidities of antibody (Lopatin & Blackburn 1992; Whitney *et al.* 1992; Mooney *et al.* 1993), subclass of antibody (Lopatin & Blackburn 1992; Wilton *et al.* 1992), the effect of treatment (Chen *et al.* 1991; Johnson *et al.* 1993), and the nature of the antigens which elicit the elevated responses (Ogawa *et al.* 1989; Yoshimura *et al.* 1989; Curtis *et al.* 1991; Papaioannou *et al.* 1991; Duncan *et al.* 1992; Schifferle *et al.* 1993). Noteworthy in this regard were the observations of Ogawa *et al.* (1989), which indicated that an average of approximately 5% of plasma cells in lesions of advanced periodontitis formed antibody to the fimbriae of *P. gingivalis*. The consensus of the antibody studies is that many, but not all, subjects who had experienced periodontal attachment loss exhibited elevated levels of antibody to antigens of *P. gingivalis*, suggesting that this species gained access to the underlying tissues and may have initiated or contributed to the observed pathology.

P. gingivalis-like organisms were also strongly related to destructive periodontal disease in naturally occurring or ligature-induced disease in dogs, sheep or monkeys (Table 9-2). The species or closely related organisms were higher in number in lesion sites than in non-lesion sites in naturally occurring disease. When disease was induced by ligature in dogs or monkeys, the level of the species rose at the diseased sites concomitant with the detection of disease. Of great interest were the observations of Holt *et al.* (1988) who demonstrated that a microbiota suppressed by systemic administration of rifampin (and without detectable *P. gingivalis*) would not cause ligature-induced disease, but the re-introduction of *P. gingivalis* to the microbiota resulted in initiation and progress of the lesions. Ligature-induced periodontitis and peri-implantitis in dogs was also accompanied by a significant increase in the detection of *P. gingivalis* (Nociti *et al.* 2001). Like *A. actinomycetemcomitans*, *P. gingivalis* has been shown to be able to invade human gingival epithelial cells *in vitro* (Lamont *et al.* 1992; Duncan *et al.* 1993; Sandros *et al.* 1993), buccal epithelial cells *in vivo* (Rudney *et al.* 2001), endothelial cells (Takahashi *et al.* 2006) and has been found in higher numbers on or in epithelial cells recovered from the periodontal pocket than in associated plaque (Dzink *et al.* 1989) or healthy sites (Colombo *et al.* 2006). Attachment to and invasion of epithelial cells appears to be mediated by the *P. gingivalis* fimbriae (Njoroge *et al.* 1997; Weinberg *et al.* 1997; Nakajawa *et al.* 2006).

There have been several studies that have attempted to immunize experimental animals against periodontal disease induced by *P. gingivalis*. Studies in monkeys and gnotobiotic rats have indicated that immunization with whole organisms or specific antigens affected the progress of the periodontal lesions. In most instances, periodontal breakdown was decreased (Evans *et al.* 1992; Persson *et al.* 1994a). However, in one study, the disease severity was increased after immunization (Ebersole *et al.* 1991). In the monkey model, the percentage of *P. gingivalis* cells in subgingival plaque was inversely related to the serum antibody titer to this species (Persson *et al.* 1994b). Reductions in alveolar bone loss in the monkey model could also be achieved by immunization with the cysteine protease porphypain-2 from *P. gingivalis* (Moritz *et al.* 1998; Page 2000). In more recent years, investigators have used a mouse "oral challenge" (by cells of *P. gingivalis*) model to study the effects of immunization by various fractions of *P. gingivalis* on alveolar bone loss induced by this species. Immunization by hemagglutinin B (Katz *et al.* 1999), capsular polysaccharide (Gonzalez *et al.* 2003), heat shock protein (Lee *et al.* 2006), gingipain R (Gibson & Genco 2001), and the active sites of RgpA and Kgp proteinases (O'Brien-Simpson *et al.* 2005) protected against alveolar bone loss in the mouse model. Thus, altering the host–*P. gingivalis* equilibrium by raising the level of specific antibodies to *P. gingivalis* antigens markedly affected disease outcome. Such data reinforce the importance of this bacterial species in periodontal disease, at least in the animal model systems employed.

Tannerella forsythia

The third consensus periodontal pathogen, *T. forsythia*, was first described in 1979 (Tanner *et al.* 1979) as a "fusiform" *Bacteroides*. This species was difficult to grow, often requiring 7–14 days for minute colonies to develop. The organism is a Gram-negative, anaerobic, spindle-shaped, highly pleomorphic rod. The growth of the organism was shown to be enhanced by co-cultivation with *F. nucleatum* and indeed it commonly occurred with this species in subgingival sites (Socransky *et al.* 1988). The need for co-cultivation could be overcome by providing N-acetylmuramic acid in the medium (Wyss 1989). Inclusion of this factor markedly enhanced growth and the resulting cells were regularly shaped, short, Gram-negative rods rather than the pleomorphic cells observed in the absence of this factor (Tanner & Izard 2006). A feature that *T. forsythia* cells shares with certain other Gram-negative species is the presence of a serrated S-layer that is easily visible by electron microscopy (Tanner *et al.* 1986) that may contribute to the pathogenicity of the species in periodontal diseases (Sabet *et al.* 2003). The S-layer has been isolated and shown to mediate hemagglutination, adhesion/invasion of epithelial cells, and murine subcutaneous abscess formation. The S-layer is composed of two glycoproteins of molecular mass 200 and 210 kDa (Lee *et al.* 2006). This species has been shown to produce trypsin-like proteolytic activity (BANA test positive) (Loesche *et al.* 1992) and methylglyoxal (Kashket *et al.* 2002), and induce apoptotic cell death (Arakawa *et al.* 2000). In addition, *T.*

forsythia in co-cultures of macrophage and epithelial cells leads to the expression of pro-inflammatory cytokines, chemokines, PGE$_2$, and MMP9 (Bodet *et al.* 2006).

Initially, *T. forsythia* was thought to be a relatively uncommon subgingival species. However, the studies of Gmur *et al.* (1989) using monoclonal antibodies to enumerate the species directly in plaque samples, suggested that the species was more common than previously found in cultural studies and its levels were strongly related to increasing pocket depth. Lai *et al.* (1987) reported similar findings using fluorescent-labeled polyclonal antisera and demonstrated that *T. forsythia* was much higher in subgingival than supragingival plaque samples. Data of Tanner *et al.* (1998) suggested that *T. forsythia* was a major species found at sites that converted from periodontal health to disease. There was a greater risk of periodontal attachment loss in adolescents who were colonized by *T. forsythia* than adolescents in whom the species was not detected (Hamlet *et al.* 2004). *T. forsythia* was in much higher counts, proportions, and prevalence in subjects with various forms of periodontitis than in periodontally healthy subjects (van Winkelhoff *et al.* 2002; Yang *et al.* 2004b; Haffajee *et al.* 2006a). *T. forsythia* was found in higher numbers in sites of destructive periodontal disease or periodontal abscesses than in gingivitis or healthy sites (Lai *et al.* 1987; Herrera *et al.* 2000; Papapanou *et al.* 2000; Lau *et al.* 2004). In addition, *T. forsythia* was detected more frequently and in higher numbers in actively progressing periodontal lesions than inactive lesions (Dzink *et al.* 1988) (Table 9-3). Further, subjects who harbored *T. forsythia* were at greater risk for alveolar bone loss, attachment loss and tooth loss compared with subjects in whom this species was not detected (Machtei *et al.* 1999).

Since these early studies, a large number of additional studies have demonstrated the association of *T. forsythia* with periodontal disease using techniques such as PCR and DNA hybridization (Tanner & Izard 2006). *T. forsythia* has also been shown to be present in the oral cavities of monkeys, cats, and dogs, and species related to *T. forsythia* have been found in insects such as termites (Tanner & Izard 2006). An as yet uncultivated clone similar to *T. forsythia* has been found more frequently in subjects who were periodontally healthy than subjects with periodontitis (Leys *et al.* 2002).

T. forsythia has been shown to be decreased in frequency of detection and counts after successful periodontal therapy, including scaling and root planing (SRP) (Haffajee *et al.* 1997; Takamatsu *et al.* 1999; Cugini *et al.* 2000; Darby *et al.* 2001, 2005; van der Velden *et al.* 2003; Teles *et al.* 2006), periodontal surgery (Levy *et al.* 2002), or systemically administered antibiotics (Feres *et al.* 2000; Winkel *et al.* 1998, 2001; Haffajee *et al.* 2006b; Teles *et al.* 2006). *T. forsythia* was found at higher levels at sites which showed breakdown after periodontal therapy than sites which remained stable or gained attachment (Shiloah *et al.* 1998; Fujise *et al.* 2002). Ligature-induced periodontitis and peri-implantitis in dogs were accompanied by a significant increase in the frequency of detection of *T. forsythia* (Nociti *et al.* 2001). Finally, subjects with a low severity of chronic periodontitis who exhibited a persistent presence of *T. forsythia* at periodontal sites had a 5.3 times greater chance of having at least one site in their mouths losing attachment compared with subjects with occasional or no presence of this species (Tran *et al.* 2001).

Studies using checkerboard DNA–DNA hybridization techniques to examine subgingival plaque samples not only confirmed the high levels of *T. forsythia* detected using fluorescent-labeled antisera but demonstrated that *T. forsythia* was the most common species detected on or in epithelial cells recovered from periodontal pockets (Dibart *et al.* 1998). It was infrequently detected in epithelial cell samples from healthy subjects. Double-labeling experiments demonstrated that *T. forsythia* was both on and in periodontal pocket epithelial cells and indicated the species' ability to invade. Listgarten *et al.* (1993) found that the species most frequently detected in "refractory" subjects was *T. forsythia*. Serum antibody to *T. forsythia* has been found to be elevated in a number of periodontitis patients (Taubman *et al.* 1992) and was often extremely elevated in a subset of refractory periodontal disease subjects. The observation that *T. forsythia* shares antigens with *P. gingivalis* suggests that protective antibody formed to one species may provide protection against both species (Vasel *et al.* 1996).

The role of *T. forsythia* in periodontal diseases has been clarified and strengthened by studies in numerous laboratories involving non-cultural methods of enumeration, such as DNA probes, PCR or immunologic methods. For example, Grossi *et al.* (1994, 1995) considered *T. forsythia* to be the most significant microbial risk factor that distinguished subjects with periodontitis from those who were periodontally healthy.

Spirochetes

Spirochetes are Gram-negative, anaerobic, helical-shaped, highly motile microorganisms that are common in many periodontal pockets (Fig. 9-4). The role of spirochetes in the pathogenesis of destructive periodontal diseases deserves extended comment. Clearly, a spirochete has been implicated as the likely etiologic agent of acute necrotizing ulcerative gingivitis by its presence in large numbers in tissue biopsy specimens from affected sites (Listgarten & Socransky 1964; Listgarten 1965). The role of spirochetes in other forms of periodontal disease is less clear. The organisms have been considered as possible periodontal pathogens since the late 1800s and in the 1980s enjoyed a resurgence of interest for use as pos-

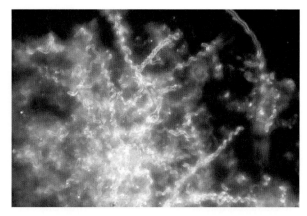

Fig. 9-4 Photomicrograph of a sample of subgingival plaque from a subject with advanced chronic periodontitis viewed by darkfield microscopy. The sample was dominated by large spirochetes with the typical corkscrew appearance.

sible diagnostic indicators of disease activity and/or therapeutic efficacy (Keyes & Rams 1983; Rams & Keyes 1983). The major reason for the interest in this group of organisms has been their increased numbers in sites with increased pocket depth. Healthy sites exhibit few, if any, spirochetes, sites of gingivitis but no attachment loss exhibit low to moderate levels, while many deep pockets harbor large numbers of these organisms. Further, spirochetes such as *Treponema denticola*, have been shown to be at the forefront of periodontal lesions as demonstrated in sections of undisturbed subgingival plaque using immunohistochemical localization (Kigure *et al.* 1995; Noiri *et al.* 2001). The localization of spirochetes next to the epithelial lining of the periodontal pocket may facilitate both attachment of these species to epithelial cells and invasion into the adjacent tissues.

The major difficulty encountered in defining the role of spirochetes has been the difficulty in distinguishing individual species. This is due in large part to difficulty in cultivating spirochetes in general and, in particular, species of spirochetes that are currently uncultivable. There are currently 10 cultivable species of spirochetes (Ellen & Galimanas 2005). At least 50 taxa of subgingival spirochetes can be recognized using 16S rRNA analysis (Dewhirst *et al.* 2000). The cultivable spirochetes require very complex media for their cultivation. These contain infusions of animal organs, trypsin digests of casein, various fatty acids and accessory growth factors, and serum (Ellen & Galimanas 2005). Wyss *et al.* (1999) have developed more defined media for the cultivation of some of the species of oral spirochetes. In spite of the ability to cultivate certain species of oral spirochetes, it has been difficult to use these media to enumerate the spirochetes in subgingival plaque samples. Therefore, in many of the earlier studies of plaque samples, spirochetes were combined either in a single group or groups based on cell size; i.e. small, medium or large. Thus, while there may be pathogens among the spirochetes, their role may have been obscured by unintentionally pooling their numbers with non-pathogenic spirochetes. This would be similar to combining in a single count, organisms with coccal morphologies, such as *P. gingivalis, Veillonella parvula*, and *Streptococcus sanguinis*.

In spite of the limitations of combining spirochetes into a single morphogroup, spirochetes as a group or as individual species have been related to periodontal disease (Ellen & Galimanas 2005). Spirochetes have been associated with an increased risk at a site for the development of gingivitis (Riviere & DeRouen 1998) and periodontitis (Riviere *et al.* 1997). The need to evaluate the role of individual species of spirochetes in periodontal diseases is reinforced by studies of serum antibody responses to different species. When antibody responses to individual species were examined in subjects with chronic or aggressive periodontitis or a healthy periodontium, different responses were observed to different species. Certain spirochetal species elicited an elevated response in one or more of the groups with destructive periodontal disease (Mangan *et al.* 1982; Tew *et al.* 1985c; Lai *et al.* 1986), while others were related to depressed antibody responses in certain patient groups (Steinberg & Gershoff 1968; Tew *et al.* 1985c). Such data suggest that pooling spirochete species into a collective group may obscure meaningful host–parasite interactions.

More recently, specific species of spirochetes have been related to periodontal breakdown using antibody-based or molecular techniques. *Treponema denticola* was found to be more common in periodontally diseased than healthy sites, more common in subgingival than supragingival plaque (Simonson *et al.* 1988; Riviere *et al.* 1992; Albandar *et al.* 1997; Haffajee *et al.* 1998; Yuan *et al.* 2001), and more common in healthy sites that progressed to gingivitis (Riviere & DeRouen 1998). *Tr. denticola* was shown to decrease in successfully treated periodontal sites, but not change or increase in non-responding sites (Simonson *et al.* 1992). Cultural studies suggested that *Tr. denticola* and a "large treponeme" were found more frequently in patients with severe periodontitis than in healthy or gingivitis sites (Moore *et al.* 1982).

Riviere *et al.* (1991,a,b,c, 1992) employed a monoclonal antibody directed against *Treponema pallidum*, the etiologic agent of syphilis, to examine supra- and subgingival plaque samples and/or tissues from healthy, periodontitis and ANUG subjects. This antibody cross-reacted with antigens of uncultivated spirochetes in many of the plaque samples. These "pathogen-related oral spirochetes" (PROS) were the most frequently detected spirochetes in supra- and subgingival plaques of periodontitis patients and were the most numerous spirochetes in periodontitis lesion sites. Their presence in periodontally healthy sites was related to an increased risk of development of periodontitis (Riviere *et al.* 1997). The PROS were also detected in plaque samples from ANUG (Riviere *et al.* 1991c) and tissue biopsies from ANUG lesions using immunohistochemical techniques (Riviere *et al.*

1991a). PROS were also shown to have the ability to penetrate a tissue barrier in *in vitro* systems (Riviere *et al.* 1991b). This property was shared with *Tr. pallidum* but not with other cultivated species of oral spirochetes such as *Tr. denticola, Tr. socranskii, Tr. pectinovorum* or *Tr. vincentii*. In later studies, the PROS were shown by molecular techniques to share 16S rRNA gene sequences with *Tr. vincentii* and *Tr. medium* (Choi *et al.* 1996; Riviere *et al.* 1999). These studies and others suggested that certain specific species of spirochetes were important in the pathogenesis of ANUG and certain forms of periodontitis. Precise evaluation of the role of individual spirochete species appears to be realistic based on their detection in plaque samples by immunologic, PCR or DNA probe techniques. Indeed, enumeration of even uncultivable spirochete taxa is possible using oligonucleotide probes (Tanner *et al.* 1994) or specific antibody as described above. Studies performed using such techniques permit better distinction of species of spirochetes and a clearer understanding of their possible role in disease.

The mechanisms of pathogenicity of the spirochetes have been under active investigation in recent years. Spirochetes demonstrate pathogenicity in animal abscess model systems (Kesavalu *et al.* 1999; Kimizuka *et al.* 2003), and produce a wide range of potential virulence factors (Ellen 2005). Among the virulence factors that may play a major role is a subtilisin family protease, dentilisin, that is encoded by the *prtP* gene. This enzyme affects a wide range of protein substrates including fibronectin, laminin, and fibrinogen (Ishihara *et al.* 1996). It is thought that spirochetes may prolong tissue remodeling and wound healing following periodontal treatment; thus, the chronic periodontal lesion may represent an "ever-healing" wound that is sustained during chronic infection (Ellen & Galimanas, 2005).

Successful treatment of periodontal infections is accompanied by a decrease in the numbers and proportions of oral spirochetes as a group and individual species. Indeed, this reduction is so consistent that it has been used in some studies as a measure of compliance in determining whether subjects used the prescribed antibiotics (Loesche *et al.* 1993).

Prevotella intermedia/Prevotella nigrescens

At present the data for other species as etiologic agents of destructive periodontal diseases are more limited, but certain organisms appear to merit further investigation (Zambon 1996). *Pr. intermedia* is the second black-pigmented *Bacteroides* to receive considerable interest (Fig. 9-5). The levels of this Gram-negative, short, round-ended anaerobic rod have been shown to be particularly elevated in acute necrotizing ulcerative gingivitis (Loesche *et al.* 1982), certain forms of periodontitis (Tanner *et al.* 1979; Dzink *et al.* 1983; Moore *et al.* 1985; Maeda *et al.* 1998; Herrera *et al.* 2000; Papapanou *et al.* 2000; Lee *et al.*

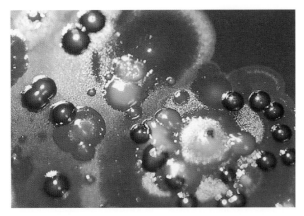

Fig. 9-5 Photograph of part of a primary isolation plate of a subgingival plaque sample from a subject with chronic periodontitis. The medium and growth conditions were as described in Fig. 9-2. The dark-pigmented colonies were isolates of *Prevotella intermedia*.

2003; van Winkelhoff *et al.* 2002; Alves *et al* 2006; Boutaga *et al.* 2006), and progressing sites in chronic periodontitis (Tanner *et al.* 1996; Lopez 2000), and it has been detected by immunohistological methods in the intercellular spaces of periodontal pocket biopsies from rapidly progressive periodontitis subjects (Hillmann *et al.* 1998). Isolates of this species can induce alveolar bone loss in rats (Yoshida-Minami *et al.* 1997). *Pr. intermedia* was reduced more markedly in subgingival plaque samples from subjects who received adjunctive systemically administered amoxicillin plus metronidazole than subjects receiving a placebo (Rooney *et al.* 2002). Persistence of *Pr. intermedia/nigrescens* after standard mechanical therapy has been shown to be associated with a large proportion of sites exhibiting bleeding on probing (Mombelli *et al.* 2000). Berglundh *et al.* (1998) demonstrated that improved clinical parameters after the use of mechanical therapy and systemically administered amoxicillin and metronidazole were associated with a decrease of periodontal pathogens including *Pr. intermedia*.

This species appears to have a number of the virulence properties exhibited by *P. gingivalis* and was shown to induce mixed infections on injection in laboratory animals (Hafstrom & Dahlen 1997). Like *P. gingivalis*, *Pr. intermedia/nigrescens* appears to induce an increased release of MMP-8 and MMP-9 in gingival pockets as well as MMP-9 in plasma (Soder *et al.* 2006). It has also been shown to invade oral epithelial cells *in vitro* (Dorn *et al.* 1998) and induce expression of nitric oxide synthase in tissue culture cells (Kim *et al.* 2004). Elevated seroantibodies to this species have been observed in some but not all subjects with refractory periodontitis (Haffajee *et al.* 1988b). Elevated IgG antibody to *Pr. intermedia* was associated with coronary heart disease (CHD) in past and current smokers, while elevated IgG antibody to *Pr. nigrescens* was associated with CHD in never smokers (Beck *et al.* 2005). Strains of *Pr. intermedia* that show identical phenotypic traits have been sepa-

rated into two species, *Pr. intermedia* and *Pr. nigrescens* (Shah & Gharbia 1992). This distinction makes earlier studies of this "species" difficult to interpret since data from two different species may have been inadvertently pooled. However, new studies which discriminate the species in subgingival plaque samples might strengthen the relationship of one or both species to periodontal disease pathogenesis.

Fusobacterium nucleatum

F. nucleatum is a Gram-negative, anaerobic, spindle-shaped rod that has been recognized as part of the subgingival microbiota for over 100 years (Plaut 1894; Vincent 1899). This species was the most common isolate found in cultural studies of subgingival plaque samples, comprising approximately 7–10% of total isolates from different clinical conditions (Dzink *et al.* 1985, 1988; Moore *et al.* 1985). *F. nucleatum* was prevalent in subjects with periodontitis (Papapanou *et al.* 2000; Colombo *et al.* 2002; Socransky *et al.* 2002; Boutaga *et al.* 2006) and periodontal abscesses (Herrera *et al.* 2000) and was reduced after successful periodontal therapy (van der Velden *et al.* 2003; Haffajee *et al.* 2006b). Although there were differences detected in levels of this species between active and inactive periodontal lesions (Dzink *et al.* 1988), the differences may have been minimized by the inadvertent pooling of subspecies of *F. nucleatum*. Support for this contention may be derived from the antibody responses in subjects with different forms of periodontal disease to different homology groups of *F. nucleatum* (Tew *et al.* 1985b). The role of *F. nucleatum* in periodontal diseases is being clarified by examining the relationship of individual subspecies, such as *F. nucleatum* ss *nucleatum*, *F. nucleatum* ss *polymorphum*, *F. nucleatum* ss *vincentii*, and *F. periodonticum*, to disease status and progression.

IgG and IgM titers in serum against the lipopolysaccharide (LPS) of *F. nucleatum* were higher in subjects with periodontitis than in healthy individuals (Onoue *et al.* 2003). Invasion of this species into human gingival epithelial cells *in vitro* was accompanied by an increased secretion of IL-8 from the epithelial cells (Han *et al.* 2000). The species can induce apoptotic cell death in mononuclear and polymorphonuclear cells (Jewett *et al.* 2001), induces epithelial cells to produce collagenase 3 (Uitto *et al.* 2005), and produces a 65 kDa serine protease (Bachrach *et al.* 2004). In addition, *F. nucleatum* induces cytokine, elastase, and oxygen radical release from leukocytes (Sheikhi *et al.* 2000). Perhaps the most important role of *F. nucleatum* in the subgingival ecosystem is its function as a "bridging" species, facilitating co-aggregation among species as described below.

Campylobacter rectus

C. rectus is a Gram-negative, anaerobic, short, motile vibrio. The organism is unusual in that it utilizes hydrogen or formate as its energy source. It was first described as a member of the "vibrio corroders", a group of short nondescript rods that formed small convex, "dry spreading" or "corroding" (pitting) colonies on blood agar plates. These organisms were eventually shown to include members of a new genus *Wolinella* (most species have been redefined as *Campylobacter*), and *Eikenella corrodens*. *C. rectus* has a 150-kDa protein on its cell surface that forms a paracrystalline lattice or S-layer that surrounds the bacterium (Wang *et al.* 1998, 2000). *C. rectus* may help to initiate periodontitis by increasing the expression of proinflammatory cytokines and the S-layer may help to moderate this response facilitating the survival of the species at the site of infection. *C. rectus* is widely distributed in subgingival sites, even in the primary, mixed and permanent dentitions of children (Umeda *et al.* 2004; Hayashi *et al.* 2006). *C. rectus* has been shown to be present in higher numbers in samples from diseased sites as compared with healthy sites (Moore *et al.* 1983, 1985; Lippke *et al.* 1991; Lai *et al.* 1992; Papapanou *et al.* 1997; Macuch & Tanner 2000; Dogan *et al.* 2003; Ihara *et al.* 2003; Suda *et al.* 2004; Nonnenmacher *et al.* 2005) and it was found in higher numbers and more frequently at sites exhibiting active periodontal destruction (Dzink *et al.* 1985, 1988; Tanner & Bouldin 1989; Rams *et al.* 1993) or converting from periodontal health to disease (Tanner *et al.* 1998). In addition, *C. rectus* was found less frequently and in lower numbers after successful periodontal therapy (Tanner *et al.* 1987; Haffajee *et al.* 1988a; Levy *et al.* 1999; Colombo *et al.* 2005). *C. rectus* was also found in combination with other suspected pathogens in sites of subjects with refractory periodontal diseases (Haffajee *et al.* 1988b) and was in higher levels in subjects with aggressive periodontitis than in subjects with other forms of periodontitis (Gajardo *et al.* 2005). Like *A. actinomycetemcomitans*, *C. rectus* has been shown to produce a leukotoxin. These are the only two oral species known to possess this characteristic (Gillespie *et al.* 1992). The species is also capable of stimulating human gingival fibroblasts to produce IL-6 and IL-8 (Dongari-Bagtzoglou & Ebersole 1996). Higher serum antibody levels to *C. rectus* GroEL was detected in patients with periodontitis when compared with control subjects (Fukui *et al.* 2006).

C. rectus has been associated with a number of systemic conditions. Elevated IgM antibody to *C. rectus* in fetal chord blood has been associated with an increased rate of prematurity (Madianos *et al.* 2001) and increased levels of *C. rectus* along with *Peptostreptococcus micros* in subgingival plaque samples of pregnant females was associated with an increased risk of pre-term low birth weight (Buduneli *et al.* 2005). IgG antibody to these same two species was also associated with increased carotid intima–medial thickness (Beck *et al.* 2005). Finally, *C. rectus*, as well as other oral species, has been detected in atherosclerotic vessels (Fiehn *et al.* 2005) and in occluded arteries in patients with Buerger disease (Iwai *et al.* 2005).

Eikenella corrodens

E. corrodens is a Gram-negative, capnophilic, asaccharolytic, regular, small rod with blunt ends. It has been recognized as a pathogen in other forms of disease, particularly osteomyelitis (Johnson & Pankey 1976), infections of the central nervous system (Emmerson & Mills 1978; Brill *et al.* 1982), and root canal infections (Goodman 1977). This species was found more frequently in sites of periodontal destruction as compared with healthy sites in some (Savitt & Socransky 1984; Muller *et al.* 1997; Yuan *et al.* 2001), but not all studies (Papapanou *et al.* 2000). In addition, *E. corrodens* was found more frequently and in higher levels in actively breaking down periodontal sites (Dzink *et al.* 1985; Tanner *et al.* 1987) and in sites of subjects who responded poorly to periodontal therapy (Haffajee *et al.* 1988b). Successfully treated sites harbored lower proportions of this species (Tanner *et al.* 1987). *E. corrodens* has been found to be elevated in lesions in LAP subjects (Suda *et al.* 2002) as well as in association with *A. actinomycetemcomitans* in such lesions (Mandell 1984; Mandell *et al.* 1987). In tissue culture systems, *E. corrodens* has been shown to stimulate the production of matrix metalloproteinases (Dahan *et al.* 2001) and IL-6 and IL-8 (Yumoto *et al.* 1999, 2001). While there is some association of this species with periodontal disease, to date it has not been particularly strong (Chen *et al.* 1989).

Peptostreptococcus micros

Pe. micros is a Gram-positive, anaerobic, small, asaccharolytic coccus. It has long been associated with mixed anaerobic infections in the oral cavity and other parts of the body (Finegold 1977). Two genotypes can be distinguished, with the smooth genotype being more frequently associated with periodontitis lesions than the rough genotype (Kremer *et al.* 2000). *Pe. micros* has been detected more frequently and in higher numbers at sites of periodontal destruction as compared with gingivitis or healthy sites (Moore *et al.* 1983, 1985; Herrera *et al.* 2000; Papapanou *et al.* 2000; Choi *et al.* 2000; Riggio *et al.* 2001; van Winkelhoff *et al.* 2002; Lee *et al.* 2003; Nonnenmacher *et al.* 2005; Boutaga *et al.* 2006; Gomes *et al.* 2006), was elevated in actively breaking down sites (Dzink *et al.* 1988), and at higher mean levels in current smokers compared with non-smokers (van Winkelhoff *et al.* 2001). The levels and frequency of detection of the species were decreased at successfully treated periodontal sites (Haffajee *et al.* 1988a). Studies of systemic antibody responses to suspected periodontal pathogens indicated that subjects with severe generalized periodontitis had elevated antibody levels to this species when compared with healthy subjects or subjects with LAP (Tew *et al.* 1985a). *Pe. micros* produces proteases (Grenier & Bouclin 2006) and, in a mouse skin model system, it was shown that this species in combination with either *Pr. intermedia* or *Pr. nigrescens* could produce transmissible abscesses (van Dalen *et al.* 1998). In a study of chronic periodontitis subjects with and without acute myocardial infarction, it was found that *Pe. micros* was much higher in the plaque samples of the subjects exhibiting myocardial infarction (Dogan *et al.* 2005).

Selenomonas species

Selenomonas species have been observed in plaque samples using light microscopy for many decades. The organisms may be recognized by their curved shape, tumbling motility, and, in good preparations, by the presence of a tuft of flagella inserted in the concave side. The *Selenomonas* spp. are Gram-negative, curved, saccharolytic rods. The organisms have been somewhat difficult to grow and speciate. However, Moore *et al.* (1987) described six genetically and phenotypically distinct groups isolated from the human oral cavity. *Selenomonas noxia* was found at a higher proportion of shallow sites (pocket depth (PD) <4 mm) in chronic periodontitis subjects compared with similar sites in periodontally healthy subjects (Haffajee *et al.* 1998). Further, *S. noxia* was found to be associated with sites that converted from periodontal health to disease (Tanner *et al.* 1998).

Eubacterium species

Certain *Eubacterium* species have been suggested as possible periodontal pathogens due to their increased levels in diseased sites, particularly those of severe periodontitis (Uematsu & Hoshino 1992). *E. nodatum, Eubacterium brachy,* and *Eubacterium timidum* are Gram-positive strictly anaerobic, small somewhat pleomorphic rods. They are often difficult to cultivate, particularly on primary isolation, and appear to grow better in roll tubes than on blood agar plates. To date, there is greater evidence supporting a possible etiologic role in periodontitis for *E. nodatum* than the other *Eubacterium* species. Moore *et al.* (1982, 1985) used the roll tube cultural technique to examine the proportions of bacterial species in subgingival plaque samples from subjects with various forms of periodontitis, gingivitis, and health. They found that *E. nodatum* was absent or in low proportions in periodontal health and various forms of gingivitis, but was present in higher proportions in moderate periodontitis (2%), generalized early onset periodontitis (8%), LAP (6%), early onset periodontitis (5%), and adult (chronic) periodontitis (2%). *E. nodatum* was in the top 2–14 species enumerated in these different periodontal states. Uematsu and Hoshina (1992) found *Eubacterium* species to be the predominant species in subgingival plaque samples from subjects

with advanced periodontitis using cultural techniques. More recent studies have confirmed an association of *E. nodatum* with periodontitis using molecular techniques. Using species-specific oligonucleotide probes, Booth *et al.* (2004) found that *E. nodatum* was at significantly higher counts in patients than in matched control subjects. The species was also at higher levels in deep compared with shallow pockets. Papapanou *et al.* (2000) found higher counts of *E. nodatum* in 131 periodontitis patients than in 74 periodontally intact controls using checkerboard DNA–DNA hybridization. Colombo *et al.* (2002) also used checkerboard DNA–DNA hybridization to evaluate the microbiota in 25 untreated Brazilian subjects with chronic periodontitis and found a significant positive correlation of *E. nodatum* with mean pocket depth and attachment level. Samples of subgingival plaque were taken from 21 832 periodontal sites in 635 chronic periodontitis and 189 periodontally healthy subjects and examined by checkerboard DNA–DNA hybridization (Haffajee *et al.* 2006a). It was found that *E. nodatum* was strongly associated with chronic periodontitis both in the presence of high levels of *P. gingivalis* and *T. forsythia* and in subjects where these species were in lower proportions. It has also been demonstrated that the percentage of sites colonized by *E. nodatum* was significantly higher in current smokers than non-smokers (Haffajee & Socransky 2001). Some of the *Eubacterium* species elicited elevated antibody responses in subjects with different forms of destructive periodontitis (Tew *et al.* 1985a,b; Vincent *et al.* 1986; Martin *et al.* 1988).

The "milleri" streptococci

Streptococci were frequently implicated as possible etiologic agents of destructive periodontal diseases in the early part of the twentieth century. Cultural studies of the last 2 decades have also suggested the possibility that some of the streptococcal species were associated with, and may contribute to, disease progression. At this time, evidence suggests that the "milleri" streptococci, *Streptococcus anginosus, Streptococcus constellatus,* and *S. intermedius,* might contribute to disease progression in subsets of periodontal patients. The species was found to be elevated at sites which demonstrated recent disease progression (Dzink *et al.* 1988). Walker *et al.* (1993) found *S. intermedius* to be elevated in a subset of patients with refractory disease at periodontal sites which exhibited disease progression. Colombo *et al* (1998a) found that subjects exhibiting a poor response to SRP and then to periodontal surgery with systemically administered tetracycline had higher levels and proportions of *S. constellatus,* than subjects who responded well to periodontal therapy. Refractory subjects also exhibited elevated serum antibody to *S. constellatus* when compared with successfully treated subjects (Colombo *et al.* 1998b). In a study of 161 subjects with acute coronary syndrome (ACS) and 161 control subjects, it was suggested that the oral bacterial load of species including *S. intermedius* and *S. anginosus* may be a risk factor for ACS (Renvert *et al.* 2006). The data on streptococci are somewhat limited, but a continued examination of their role in disease seems warranted.

Other species

It has long been recognized that many taxa in subgingival plaque were not being cultivated based on microscopic observations that revealed cell morphotypes that were never recovered in culture. In addition, there were marked differences between total viable counts (representing cultivable species) and total microscopic counts representing all organisms (Socransky *et al.* 1963; Olsen & Socransky 1981; Moore & Moore 1994). Currently, the best model for exploring microbial diversity is based on isolating DNA from the target environment, amplifying the rDNA using consensus primers and PCR, cloning the amplicons into *Escherichia coli*, and sequencing the cloned 16S rDNA inserts (Pace *et al.* 1986; Hugenholtz & Pace 1996). The resulting sequences are compared with those of known species and phylotypes in sequence databases, such as GenBank and the Ribosomal Database Project (Cole *et al.* 2005). These culture-independent molecular phylogenetic methods have been used to deduce the identity of novel phylotypes from periodontitis subjects (Choi *et al.* 1994; Spratt *et al.* 1999). To date, based on sequence analysis of 16S rRNA clonal libraries from specimens of the oral cavity, over 700 bacterial taxa have been detected, of which over half have not yet been cultivated *in vitro* (Dewhirst *et al.* 2000; Paster *et al.* 2001, 2002; Becker *et al.* 2002; Kazor *et al.* 2003). "New" putative pathogens were tentatively identified in a study in which the presence of 39 bacterial species were determined that were implicated in health or disease based on 16S rRNA clonal analysis. Samples from 66 subjects with chronic periodontitis and 66 age-matched healthy controls were examined for the presence of target species. Associations and relative risks were determined for these species. Several novel taxa, in addition to the classical putative pathogens, were suggested as potential periodontal pathogens or health-related species (Kumar *et al.* 2003).

Interest has grown in groups of cultivable species not commonly found in the subgingival plaque as initiators or possibly contributors to the pathogenesis of periodontal disease, particularly in individuals who have responded poorly to periodontal therapy. Species not commonly thought to be present in subgingival plaque can be found in a proportion of such subjects or even in subjects who have not received periodontal treatment. Studies have examined enteric organisms and staphylococcal species as well as other unusual mouth inhabitants. Slots *et al.* (1990b) used cultural techniques to examine plaque samples from over 3000 chronic periodontitis patients and found that 14% of these patients harbored enteric rods and pseudomonads. *Enterobacter cloacae, Klebsiella pneumoniae, Pseudomonas aeruginosa, Klebsiella oxytoca*, and *Enterobacter agglomerans* comprised more than 50% of the strains isolated. Systemically administered ciprofloxacin improved the treatment response of patients whose periodontal pockets were heavily infected with enteric rods (Slots *et al.* 1990a). This group of investigators also examined 24 subjects with periodontal disease in the Dominican Republic and found that the prevalence of enteric rods in these subjects was higher than levels found in subjects in the US (Slots *et al.* 1991). In the 16 of 24 subjects in whom this group of organisms was detected, they averaged 23% of the cultivable microbiota. Rams *et al.* (1990, 1992) also identified a number of species of staphylococci and enterococci in subjects with various forms of periodontal disease. The presence of unusual species in periodontal lesions suggests the possibility that they may play a role in the etiology of periodontal diseases. However, such roles must be evaluated in the same manner as the species discussed earlier in this section.

In addition to the cultivable and uncultivable bacterial species, a number of studies have suggested that specific viruses, including cytomegalovirus, the Epstein Barr virus, papillomavirus, and herpes simplex virus, may play a role in the etiology or progression of periodontal lesions, possibly by changing the host response to the local subgingival microbiota (for a comprehensive review, see Slots 2005). A suspected role of various viruses was based primarily on association of the viruses with lesion sites when compared with periodontally healthy sites and the effect of successful therapy on reducing the detection frequency of these viruses in treated sites (Klemenc *et al.* 2005; Slots 2005; Slots *et al.* 2006).

Mixed infections

To this point, attention has been paid to the possible role of individual species as risk factors for destructive periodontal diseases. However, the complex mixture of species colonizing the subgingival area can provide a spectrum of relationships with the host, ranging from beneficial (the organisms prevent disease), to harmful (the organisms cause disease). At the pathogenic end of the spectrum, it is conceivable that different relationships exist between pathogens. The presence of two pathogens at a site could have no effect or could diminish the potential pathogenicity of one or the other of the species. Alternatively, pathogenicity could be enhanced either in an additive or synergistic fashion. It seems likely that mixed infections occur in subgingival sites since so many diverse species inhabit this habitat. Evidence to support this concept has been derived mainly from studies in animals in which it was shown that combinations of species were capable of inducing experimental abscesses, even though the components of the mixtures could not (Smith 1930; Proske & Sayers 1934; Cobe 1948; Rosebury *et al.* 1950; Macdonald *et al.* 1956; Socransky & Gibbons 1965). It is not clear whether the combinations suggested in the experimental abscess studies are pertinent to human periodontal diseases. Studies in humans suggest that combinations of *P. gingivalis* and *T. forsythia* may be significant in determining diseased sites and disease progression after treatment (Fujise *et al.* 2002). In addition, it has been observed that species such as *P. gingivalis*, *T. forsythia*, and *A. actinomycetemcomitans* may be components of a polymicrobial intracellular microbiota within human buccal epithelial cells (Rudney *et al.* 2005). At the very least, some species may set the stage for specific pathogens by providing essential nutrients, sites of attachment (co-aggregation), or means to evade or subvert host defenses (e.g. by producing protective capsules or enzymes that destroy host antibody). The relationship of microbial "complexes" to periodontal diseases will be discussed further below.

The nature of dental plaque – the biofilm way of life

Biofilms colonize a widely diverse set of moist surfaces, including the oral cavity, the bottom of boats and docks, the inside of pipes, as well as rocks in streams. Infectious disease investigators are interested in biofilms that colonize a wide array of artificial devices that have been implanted in the human, including catheters, hip and voice prostheses, and contact lenses. Biofilms consist of one or more communities of microorganisms, embedded in a glycocalyx, that are attached to a solid surface. The biofilm allows microorganisms to stick to and multiply on surfaces. Thus, attached bacteria (sessile) growing in a biofilm display a wide range of characteristics that provide a number of advantages over single cell (planktonic) bacteria. The interactions among bacterial species living in biofilms take place at several levels including physical contact, metabolic exchange, small signal molecule mediated communication, and exchange of genetic information (Kolenbrander *et al.* 2006). References to pertinent biofilm literature may be found in the following publications: Newman & Wilson (1999); Socransky & Haffajee (2001); Marsh (2005).

The nature of biofilms

Biofilms are fascinating structures. They are the preferred method of growth for many, perhaps most species of bacteria. This method of growth provides a number of advantages to colonizing species. A major advantage is the protection that the biofilm provides to colonizing species from competing microorganisms, from environmental factors such as host defense mechanisms, and from potentially toxic substances in the environment, such as lethal chemicals or antibiotics. Biofilms also can facilitate processing and uptake of nutrients, cross-feeding (one species providing nutrients for another), removal of potentially harmful metabolic products (often by utilization by other bacteria), as well as the development of an appropriate physicochemical environment (e.g. a properly reduced oxidation reduction potential).

A crude analogy to the development of a biofilm might be the development of a city. Successful human colonization of new environments requires several important factors including a stable nutrient supply, an environment conducive to proliferation, and an environment with limited potential hazards. Cities (like biofilms) develop by an initial "attachment" of humans to a dwelling site followed by multiplication of the existing inhabitants and addition of new inhabitants. Cities and biofilms typically spread laterally and then in a vertical direction often forming columnar habitation sites. Cities and biofilms offer many benefits to their inhabitants. These include shared resources and inter-related activities. Inhabitants of cities or biofilms are capable of "metabolic processes" and synthetic capabilities that could not be performed by individuals in an unattached (planktonic) or nomadic state. An important benefit provided by a city or biofilm is protection both from other potential colonizers of the same species, from exogenous species, and from sudden harmful changes in the environment. Individuals in the "climax community" of a flourishing city/biofilm can facilitate joint activities and live in a far more stable environment than individuals who live in isolation. Cities, like biofilms, require a means to bring in nutrients and raw materials, and to remove waste products. In cities, these are usually roads, water or sewage pipes, in biofilms they may be water channels such as those described below. Cities have maximum practical sizes based on physical constraints and nutrient/waste limits; so do biofilms. Cities that are mildly perturbed, e.g. by a snow storm or a local fire, usually reform a climax community that is similar to that which was present in the first place; as do biofilms. However, major perturbations in the environment such as prolonged drought or a radioactive cloud can lay waste to a city. Major perturbations in the environment such as a toxic chemical can severely affect the composition or existence of a biofilm. Communication between individuals in a city is essential to allow inhabitants to interact optimally. This is usually performed by vocal, written or pictorial means. Communication between bacterial cells within a biofilm is also necessary for optimum community development and is performed by production of signaling molecules such as those found in "quorum sensing" or perhaps by the exchange of genetic information. The long-term survival of the human species as well as a species in a biofilm becomes more likely if that species (or the human) colonizes multiple sites. Thus, detachment of cells from biofilms and establishment in new sites is as important for survival of biofilm dwellers as the migration of individuals and establishment of new cities is for human beings. Thus, we may regard mixed species biofilms as primitive precursors to the more complex organizations observed for eukaryotic species.

Properties of biofilms

Structure

Biofilms are composed of microcolonies of bacterial cells (15–20% by volume) that are non-randomly distributed in a shaped matrix or glycocalyx (75–80% by volume). Earlier studies of thick biofilms (>5 mm) that develop in sewage treatment plants indicated the presence of voids or water channels between the microcolonies that were present in these biofilms. The water channels permit the passage of nutrients and other agents throughout the biofilm acting as a primitive "circulatory" system. Nutrients make contact with the sessile (attached) microcolonies by diffusion from the water channel to the microcolony rather than from the matrix. Microcolonies occur in different shapes in biofilms which are governed by shear forces due to the passage of fluid over the biofilm. At low shear force, the colonies are shaped liked towers or mushrooms, while at high shear force, the colonies are elongated and capable of rapid oscillation. Individual microcolonies can consist of a single species, but more frequently are composed of several different species.

Exopolysaccharides – the backbone of the biofilm

The bulk of the biofilm consists of the matrix or glycocalyx and is composed predominantly of water and aqueous solutes. The "dry" material is a mixture of exopolysaccharides, proteins, salts, and cell material. Exopolysaccharides (EPS), which are produced by the bacteria in the biofilm, are the major components of the biofilm making up 50–95% of the dry weight. They play a major role in maintaining the integrity of the biofilm as well as preventing desiccation and attack by harmful agents. In addition, they may also bind essential nutrients such as cations to create a local nutritionally rich environment favoring specific microorganisms. The EPS matrix could also act as a buffer and assist in the retention of extracellular enzymes (and their substrates) enhancing substrate utilization by bacterial cells. The EPS can be degraded and utilized by bacteria within the biofilm. One distinguishing feature of oral biofilms is that many of the microorganisms can both synthesize and degrade the EPS.

Physiological heterogeneity within biofilms

Cells of the same microbial species can exhibit extremely different physiologic states in a biofilm even though separated by as little as 10 μm. Typically, DNA indicating the presence of bacterial cells is detected throughout the biofilm, but protein synthesis, respiratory activity, and RNA are detected primarily in the outer layers.

The use of micro-electrodes has shown that pH can vary quite remarkably over short distances within a biofilm. Two-photon excitation microscopy of *in vitro* plaque made up of ten intra-oral species showed that, after a sucrose challenge, microcolonies with a pH <3.0 could be detected adjacent to microcolonies with pH values >5.0. The number of metal ions can differ sufficiently in different regions of a biofilm so that difference in ion concentration can produce measurable potential differences. Bacterial cells within biofilms can produce enzymes such as beta-lactamase against antibiotics, catalases, and superoxide dismutases against oxidizing ions released by phagocytes. These enzymes are released into the matrix producing an almost impregnable line of defense. Bacterial cells in biofilms can also produce elastases and cellulases which become concentrated in the local matrix and produce tissue damage. Measurement of oxygen and other gases has demonstrated that certain microcolonies are completely anaerobic even though composed of a single species and grown in ambient air. Carbon dioxide and methane can reach very high concentrations in specific microcolonies in industrial biofilms. Thus, studies to date indicate that sessile cells growing in mixed biofilms can exist in an almost infinite range of chemical and physical microhabitats within microbial communities.

Quorum sensing and exchange of genetic information

Some of the functions of biofilms are dependent on the ability of the bacteria and microcolonies within the biofilm to communicate with one another. Quorum sensing in bacteria "involves the regulation of expression of specific genes through the accumulation of signaling compounds that mediate intercellular communication" (Prosser 1999). Quorum sensing is dependent on cell density. With few cells, signaling compounds may be produced at low levels, however, auto-induction leads to increased concentration as cell density increases. Once the signaling compounds reach a threshold level (quorum cell density), gene expression is activated. Quorum sensing may give biofilms their distinct properties. For example, expression of genes for antibiotic resistance at high cell densities may provide protection. Quorum sensing also has the potential to influence community structure by encouraging the growth of beneficial species (to the biofilm) and discouraging the growth of competitors. It is also possible that physiological properties of bacteria in the community may be altered through quorum sensing. Quoring-sensing signaling molecules produced by putative periodontal pathogens such as *P. gingivalis*, *Pr. intermedia*, and *F. nucleatum* have been detected (Frias *et al.* 2001). Of particular importance may be a recently discovered molecule, autoinducer-2, which is thought to be a universal signal mediating messages among the species in mixed species communities (Kolenbrander *et al.* 2006). This family of molecules has been detected in the cell-free culture supernatants of multiple oral bacterial species. Kolenbrander *et al.* (2006) indicated that commensal bacterial species such as *Streptococcus oralis* and *Actinomyces naeslundii* produce and respond to low levels of autoinducer-2, while pathogens, such as *F. nucleatum*, *Pr. intermedia* and *P. gingivalis*, produce and respond to high levels of these substances. They hypothesized that when the pathogens become established in a mixed species community, their production of high levels of autoinducer-2 may foster the growth of the pathogenic community and minimize the growth of commensal species.

Signaling is not the only way of transferring information in biofilms. The high density of bacterial cells growing in biofilms facilitates exchange of genetic information between cells of the same species and across species or even genera. Conjugation, transformation, plasmid transfer, and transposon transfer have all been shown to occur in naturally occurring or *in vitro* prepared mixed species biofilms (described in greater detail in a later section). Of particular interest, was the demonstration of transfer of a conjugative transposon conferring tetracycline resistance from cells of one genus, *Bacillus subtilis*, to a *Streptococcus* species present in dental plaque grown as a biofilm in a constant depth film fermenter.

Attachment of bacteria

The key characteristic of a biofilm is that the microcolonies within the biofilm attach to a solid surface. Thus, adhesion to a surface is the essential first step in the development of a biofilm. In the mouth, there is a wide variety of surfaces to which bacteria can attach including the oral soft tissues, the pellicle-coated teeth, other bacteria, as well as prosthetic replacements such dentures and implants. Many bacterial species possess surface structures such as fimbriae and fibrils that aid in their attachment to different surfaces. Fimbriae have been detected on a number of oral species including *Actinomyces naeslundii*, *P. gingivalis*, *A. actinomycetemcomitans* and some strains of streptococci such as *Streptococcus salivarius*, *Streptococcus parasanguinis*, and members of the *Streptococcus mitis* group. Fibrils can be found on a number of oral bacterial species. They are morphologically different and shorter than fimbriae and may be densely or sparsely distributed on the cell surface. Oral species that possess fibrils include *S. salivarius*, the *S. mitis* group, *Pr. intermedia*, *Pr. nigrescens*, and *Streptococcus mutans*.

Mechanisms of increased antibiotic resistance of organisms in biofilms

Antibiotics have been and continue to be used effectively in the treatment of periodontal infections. However, the indiscriminate use of antimicrobials and biocides has the potential of leading to the development of resistant bacteria. It has also been suggested that resistance from one type of antimicrobial, such as a biocide, can be transferred to a different type of antimicrobial, such as an antibiotic. Thus, it is important to understand the factors leading to antimicrobial resistance in biofilms such as dental plaque.

It has been recognized for considerable periods of time that organisms growing in biofilms are more resistant to antibiotics than the same species growing in a planktonic (unattached) state. While the mechanisms of resistance to antibiotics of organisms growing in biofilms are not entirely clear, certain general principles have been described. Almost without exception, organisms grown in biofilms are more resistant to antibiotics than the same cells grown in a planktonic state. Estimates of 1000–1500 times greater resistance for biofilm-grown cells than planktonic grown cells have been suggested, although these estimates have been considered to be too high by some investigators. The mechanisms of increased resistance in biofilms differ from species to species, from antibiotic to antibiotic, and for biofilms growing in different habitats. One important mechanism of resistance appears to be the slower rate of growth of bacterial species in biofilms which makes them less susceptible to many but not all antibiotics. It has been shown in many studies that the resistance of bacteria to antibiotics, biocides or preservatives is affected by their nutritional status, growth rate, temperature, pH, and prior exposure to sub-effective concentrations of antimicrobials. Variations in any of these parameters can lead to a varied response to antibiotics within a biofilm. The matrix performs a "homeostatic function", such that cells deep in the biofilm experience different conditions, such as hydrogen ion concentration or redox potentials, than cells at the periphery of the biofilm or cells growing planktonically. Growth rates of these deeper cells will be decreased allowing them to survive better than faster growing cells at the periphery when exposed to antimicrobial agents. In addition, the slower growing bacteria often over-express "non-specific defense mechanisms", including shock proteins and multi-drug efflux pumps, and demonstrate increased exopolymer synthesis.

The exopolymer matrix of a biofilm, although not a significant barrier in itself to the diffusion of antibiotics, does have certain properties that can retard diffusion. For example, strongly charged or chemically highly reactive agents can fail to reach the deeper zones of the biofilm because the biofilm acts as an ion-exchange resin, removing such molecules from solution. In addition, extracellular enzymes, such as beta-lactamases, formaldehyde lyase, and formaldehyde dehydrogenase, may become trapped and concentrated in the extracellular matrix, thus inactivating susceptible, typically positively charged, hydrophilic antibiotics. Some antibiotics such as the macrolides, which are positively charged but hydrophobic, are unaffected by this process. Thus, the ability of the matrix to act as a physical barrier is dependent on the type of antibiotic, the binding of the matrix to that agent, and the levels of the agent employed. Since reaction between the agent and the matrix will reduce the levels of the agent, a biofilm with greater bulk will deplete the agent more readily. Further, hydrodynamics and the turnover rate of the microcolonies will also impact on antibiotic effectiveness.

Alteration of genotype and/or phenotype of the cells growing within a biofilm matrix is receiving increased attention. Cells growing within a biofilm express genes that are not observed in the same cells grown in a planktonic state and they can retain this resistance for some time after being released from the biofilm. For example, it was demonstrated that cells of *Pseudomonas aeruginosa* liberated from biofilms were considerably more resistant to tobramycin than planktonic cells, suggesting that the cells became intrinsically more resistant when growing in a biofilm and retained some of this resistance even outside the biofilm.

The presence of a glycocalyx, a slower growth rate, and development of a biofilm phenotype cannot provide a total explanation for the phenomenon of antibiotic resistance. These features probably delay elimination of the target bacteria, allowing other selection events to take place. Recently, the notion of a subpopulation of cells within a biofilm that are "super-resistant" was proposed. Such cells could explain the remarkably elevated levels of resistance to certain antibiotics that have been suggested in the literature.

Techniques for the detection and enumeration of bacteria in oral biofilm samples

The enumeration of specific bacterial species in oral biofilm samples is a challenging task, in part, because of the large number of bacterial species present in such samples and, in part, because of the fastidious nature of many of the resident species. Ideal methods of enumeration should be able to quantify multiple species, be sensitive, specific, inexpensive, and high throughput. Quantification is essential because the differences in the microbiota between periodontal health and disease, and between pre- and post-periodontal therapy, are quantitative rather than presence or absence of one or more species. The early light microscopy techniques were not satisfactory because they could not distinguish bacterial species

only morphotypes. Cultural techniques are specific in their ability to distinguish species, but are so expensive that the number of samples that can be examined is severely limited. Antibody-based techniques such as immunofluorescence and enzyme-linked immunosorbent assay (ELISA) are very specific and can provide quantitative data. However, antisera to only a limited range of species have been developed and these techniques are somewhat cumbersome, diminishing the number of species and samples that may be conveniently examined. Molecular techniques, including PCR and DNA hybridization, have the advantage of being specific and readily extensible to a wide range of bacterial taxa. PCR is convenient and able to detect low numbers of cells but suffers from the inability to provide quantitative data. Real-time PCR overcomes this limitation, but is expensive and time-consuming, precluding examination of large numbers of species and samples. DNA hybridization using formats such as that described in Fig. 9-1, are sensitive, specific, inexpensive, and high throughput, providing at the moment, perhaps the most useful technique for quantifying a wide range of species in large numbers of biofilm samples.

There has been considerable interest in enumerating the uncultivable or as yet to be cultivated taxa in addition to the cultivable taxa in subgingival biofilms. Recent studies have employed amplification of the 16S rRNA genes directly from plaque samples using PCR and consensus primers. The products were cloned into *Escherichia coli* and the sequences of the inserts determined. These studies provided a remarkably different view of the composition of the subgingival microbiota compared with other techniques such as culture, immunofluorescence, ELISA, PCR, real-time PCR, and DNA hybridization. The results of the cloning–sequencing studies must at present be viewed with considerable caution because these methods failed to detect or detected infrequently known prominent taxa such as *P. gingivalis*, *T. forsythia*, and members of the genera *Fusobacterium* and *Actinomyces*. For more detail on microbiological techniques used to examine biofilm samples see Socransky and Haffajee (2005).

The oral biofilms that lead to periodontal diseases

The section on biofilm biology presented above provided a background to help understand the ecology of the incredibly complex communities of organisms that colonize the tooth surface and lead to periodontal diseases. Figure 9-6 presents a clinical photograph of a subject with less than optimal home care. Evident in this photograph is stain on the tooth surfaces that may have resulted from smoking, coffee or tea drinking. Of greater concern, is the occurrence of a thin film of bacterial plaque on many of the tooth surfaces along with the quite obvious plaque formation in regions such as the mesial buccal surfaces of the

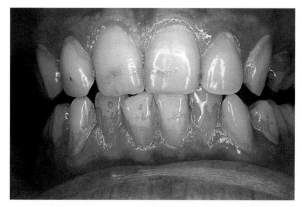

Fig. 9-6 Clinical photograph of a subject exhibiting tooth stain and supragingival dental plaque.

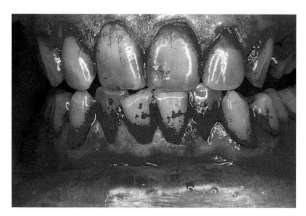

Fig. 9-7 Clinical photograph of the subject in Fig. 9-6 after staining with disclosing solution.

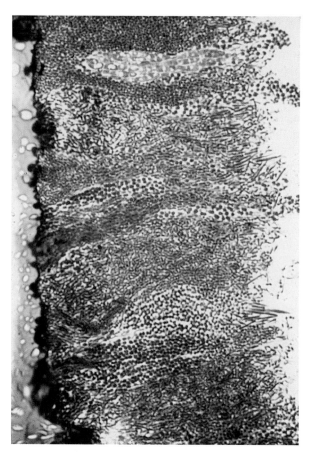

Fig. 9-8 Histological section of human supragingival plaque stained with toluidine blue–methylene blue. The supragingival plaque was allowed to develop for 3 days on an epon crown in a human volunteer. The crown surface is at the left and the saliva interface is towards the right. (Courtesy of Dr. Max Listgarten, University of Pennsylvania.)

upper left and lower right canines. These biofilm (plaque) regions are highlighted in Fig. 9-7, which shows the same dentition after staining with a disclosing solution. The thin films such as those on the lower incisors might consist of biofilm communities that are 50–100 cells thick. Thicker plaques, such as those on the upper left and lower right canines, might consist of biofilms that are 300 or more cell layers in thickness. The number of organisms that reside on the mesial surface of the upper left or lower right canine probably exceeds 300 million. This number is remarkable in that it is similar to the entire human population of the United States. These microbial communities are very complex. Over 700 bacterial species have been detected in the human oral cavity, and over 400 of these can be found in the periodontal pocket (Paster *et al.* 2006). It is thought that about half of these species may be as yet uncultivated. In any given plaque sample, it is not uncommon to detect 30 or more bacterial species. Thus, the biofilms that colonize the tooth surface may be among the most complex biofilms that exist in nature. This complexity is due in large part to the non-shedding surface of the tooth which permits persistent colonization and the opportunity for very complex ecosystems to develop. In addition, the relatively high nutrient abundance as well as the remarkable ability of oral

species to coaggregate with one another may facilitate this complexity.

Figure 9-8 is a section of human supragingival dental plaque grown on an epon crown in a human volunteer (Listgarten *et al.* 1975; Listgarten 1976, 1999). The section demonstrates many of the features of biofilms outlined earlier. Bacterial species adhered to the solid surface, multiplied, and, in this section, formed columnar microcolonies. The heterogeneity of colonizing species is evident even at a morphological level and would be emphasized if the cells within the section had been characterized by cultural or molecular techniques. The surface layers of the biofilm exhibit morphotypes that are not evident in deeper layers and emphasize the role that coaggregation plays in the development of biofilms. Not evident in this section are the water channels in biofilms described earlier. This might be due to preparation or fixation artifacts (Costerton *et al.* 1999) or it might be because the plaque is typical of a "dense" bacterial model. Water channels have been observed in plaque grown in the human oral cavity by confocal microscopy (Wood *et al.* 2000). This dental biofilm has all of the properties of biofilms in other habitats in nature. It has a solid substratum, in this case an epon crown

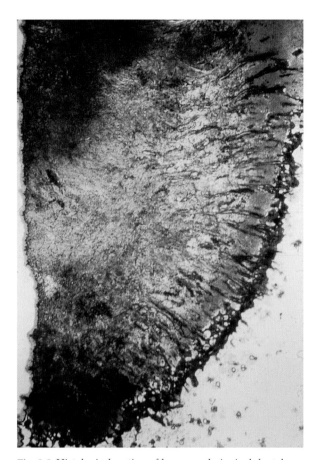

Fig. 9-9 Histological section of human subgingival dental plaque stained with toluidine blue–methylene blue. The tooth surface is to the left and the epithelial lining of the periodontal pocket is to the right. Bacterial plaque attached to the tooth surface is evident towards the upper left of the section, while a second zone of organisms can be observed lining the periodontal pocket wall. (Courtesy of Dr. Max Listgarten, University of Pennsylvania.)

but more typically a tooth, it has the mixed microcolonies growing in a glycocalyx, and it has the bulk fluid interface provided by saliva.

A second biofilm ecosystem is shown in Fig. 9-9. This is a section of human subgingival plaque. The section is at lower magnification than Fig. 9-8 to permit visualization of regions within the biofilm. The plaque attached to the tooth surface is evident in the upper left portion of the section. This tooth-associated biofilm is an extension of the biofilm found above the gingival margin and may be quite similar in microbial composition. A second, possibly epithelial cell-associated biofilm, may be observed lining the epithelial surface of the pocket. This biofilm contains primarily spirochetes and Gram-negative bacterial species (Listgarten *et al.* 1975; Listgarten 1976, 1999). *P. gingivalis* and *Tr. denticola* have been detected in large numbers in the epithelial cell-associated biofilms within the periodontal pocket, by immunocytochemistry (Kigure *et al.* 1995). *T. forsythia* might also be numerous in this zone, since high levels of this species have been detected, using DNA probes, in association with the epithelial cells lining the

periodontal pocket (Dibart *et al.* 1998). Between the tooth-associated and epithelial cell-associated biofilms, a less dense zone of organisms may be observed. These organisms may be "loosely attached" or they might be in a planktonic state. The critical feature of Fig. 9-9 is that there appear to be tooth-associated and epithelial cell-associated regions in subgingival plaque as well as a possible third weakly attached or unattached zone of microorganisms. It is strongly suspected that these regions differ markedly in microbial composition, physiological state, and their response to different therapies.

Microbial complexes

The association of bacteria within mixed biofilms is not random, rather there are specific associations among bacterial species. Socransky *et al.* (1998) examined over 13 000 subgingival plaque samples from 185 adult subjects and used cluster analysis and community ordination techniques to demonstrate the presence of specific microbial groups within dental plaque (Fig. 9-10). Six closely associated groups of bacterial species were recognized. These included specific species of *Actinomyces*, a yellow complex consisting of members of the genus *Streptococcus*, a green complex consisting of *Capnocytophaga* species, *A. actinomycetemcomitans* serotype a, *E. corrodens* and *Campylobacter concisus*, and a purple complex consisting of *V. parvula* and *Actinomyces odontolyticus*. These groups of species are early colonizers of the tooth surface whose growth usually precedes the multiplication of the predominantly Gram-negative orange and red complexes (Fig. 9-10). The orange complex consists of *Campylobacter gracilis*, *C. rectus*, *C. showae*, *E. nodatum*, *F. nucleatum* subspecies, *F. periodonticum*, *Pe. micros*, *Pr. intermedia*, *Pr. nigrescens*, and *S. constellatus*, while the red complex consists of *T. forsythia*, *P. gingivalis*, and *Tr. denticola*. The last two complexes are comprised of the species thought to be the major etiologic agents of periodontal diseases.

Similar relationships have been demonstrated in *in vitro* studies examining interactions between different pairs of oral bacterial species (Kolenbrander *et al.* 2006). These studies of oral bacteria have indicated that cell-to-cell recognition is not random but that each strain has a defined set of partners (Fig. 9-11). Further, functionally similar adhesins found on bacteria of different genera may recognize the same receptors on other bacterial cells. Most human oral bacteria adhere to other oral bacteria. This cell-to-cell adherence is known as coaggregation. It is interesting that the relationships among species determined by pair-wise *in vitro* coaggregation studies depicted in Fig. 9-11 are similar to the microbial complexes (Fig. 9-10) determined by examination of *in vivo* samples suggesting that coaggregation may be a powerful ecological determinant of community development. Figure 9-11 also suggests some of the mechanisms that might control the observed microbial succession

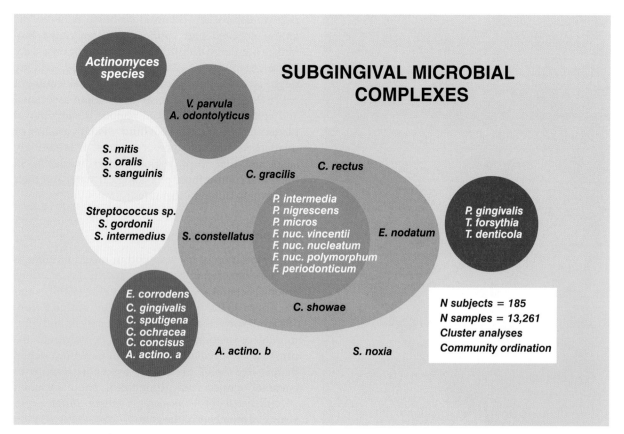

Fig. 9-10 Diagram of the association among subgingival species (adapted from Socransky *et al.* 1998). The data were derived from 13 261 subgingival plaque samples taken from the mesial aspect of each tooth in 185 adult subjects. Each sample was individually analyzed for the presence of 40 subgingival species using checkerboard DNA–DNA hybridization. Associations were sought among species using cluster analysis and community ordination techniques. The complexes to the left are comprised of species thought to colonize the tooth surface and proliferate at an early stage. The orange complex becomes numerically more dominant later and is thought to bridge the early colonizers and the red complex species which become numerically more dominant at late stages in plaque development.

in plaque development that will be discussed below. For example, the ability of many streptococcal species, particularly *S. mitis* and *S. oralis* (Nyvad & Kilian 1987; Li *et al.* 2004), to attach to different receptors found in tooth pellicle as well as to each other may contribute to their critical role as early colonizers of the tooth surface. The streptococci provide receptors for a wide range of species, including other early colonizing species and bridging species, such as *F. nucleatum*, that in turn may coaggregate with late colonizers including many periodontal pathogens.

Factors that affect the composition of subgingival biofilms

Although this chapter emphasizes the effect that microorganisms have on their habitat, the periodontal tissues, it is important to understand that the habitat has a major effect on the composition, metabolic activities, and virulence properties of the colonizing microorganisms. The importance of this axiom, that the microorganisms affect the habitat and the habitat affects the microorganisms, has recently begun to be fully appreciated. Thus, modifications of the supra- and subgingival microbiota certainly affect the outcome, periodontal health or disease; but

changes in the host or local habitat also affect the composition and activities of the microbiota. Understanding this relationship should help to lead us into better approaches to diagnosing the etiology and contributing factors of a patient's disease and to optimizing appropriate therapy. In this section, we will provide examples of some of the factors that are known to modify subgingival microbial composition.

Periodontal disease status

Perhaps the most influential factor on the composition of the subgingival microbiota is the periodontal disease status of the host. Figure 9-12 presents the counts, proportions and percentage of sites colonized at $>10^5$ of 40 subgingival taxa in subjects with chronic periodontitis or periodontal health (Haffajee *et al.* 2006a). Clearly, the major difference between health and disease, *on average*, was the increased counts, proportions, and prevalence of the red complex species, *T. forsythia*, *P. gingivalis*, and *Tr. denticola* in subjects with periodontal disease. In addition, other putative periodontal pathogens of the orange complex were also more prevalent and in higher levels in periodontitis subjects. However, individuals with

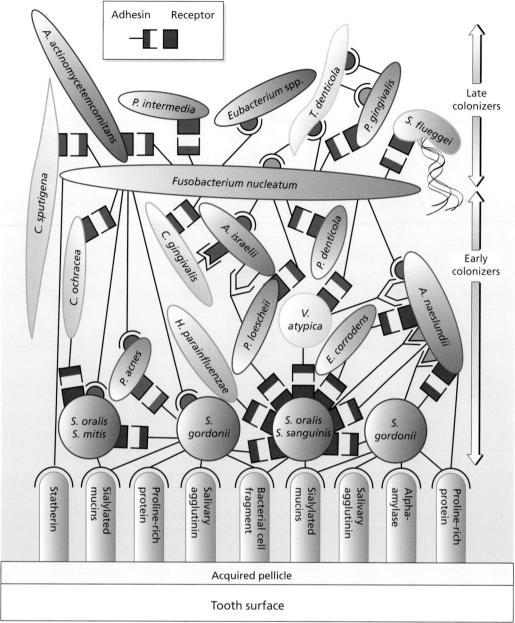

Fig. 9-11 Spatiotemporal model of oral bacterial colonization, showing recognition of salivary pellicle receptors by early colonizing bacteria and coaggregations between early colonizers, fusobacteria and late colonizers of the tooth surface (Kolenbrander *et al*. 2002). Each coaggregation depicted is known to occur in a pairwise test. Collectively, these interactions are proposed to represent development of dental plaque. Starting at the bottom, primary colonizers bind via adhesins (round-tipped black line symbols) to complementary salivary receptors (blue–green vertical round-topped columns) in the acquired pellicle coating the tooth surface. Secondary colonizers bind to previously bound bacteria. Sequential binding results in the appearance of nascent surfaces that bridge with the next coaggregating partner cell. Several kinds of coaggregations are shown as complementary sets of symbols of different shapes. One set is depicted in the box at the top. Proposed adhesins (symbols with a stem) represent cell surface components that are heat inactivated (cell suspension heated to 85°C for 30 minutes) and protease sensitive; their complementary receptors (symbols without a stem) are unaffected by heat or protease. Identical symbols represent components that are functionally similar but may not be structurally identical. Rectangular symbols represent lactose-inhibitable coaggregations. Other symbols represent components that have no known inhibitor. The bacterial species shown are *Aggregatibacter actinomycetemcomitans*, *Actinomyces israelii*, *Actinomyces naeslundii*, *Capnocytophaga gingivalis*, *Capnocytophaga ochracea*, *Capnocytophaga sputigena*, *Eikenella corrodens*, *Eubacterium* spp., *Fusobacterium nucleatum*, *Haemophilus parainfluenzae*, *Porphyromonas gingivalis*, *Prevotella denticola*, *Prevotella intermedia*, *Prevotella loescheii*, *Propionibacterium acnes*, *Selenomonas flueggei*, *Streptococcus gordonii*, *Streptococcus mitis*, *Streptococcus oralis*, *Streptococcus sanguinis*, *Treponema* spp., and *Veillonella atypica*. (Published with permission of Paul Kolenbrander, Kolenbrander *et al*. 2006 and Blackwell Publishing.)

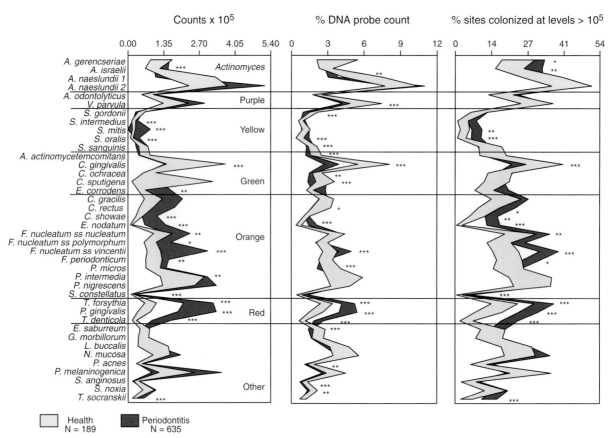

Fig. 9-12 Plots of mean counts (left panel), percents of the total DNA probe count (middle panel) and percentage of sites colonized by 40 bacterial species at counts >10⁵ (right panel) in subgingival plaque samples taken from 189 periodontally healthy and 635 chronic periodontitis subjects. The "bands" represent the mean values ± the 95% confidence intervals after adjusting for 40 comparisons. Mean values for each species were computed by averaging up to 28 samples in each subject, and then averaging across subjects in the two clinical groups. Significance of differences between groups was sought using the non-parametric Mann Whitney test; * $p < 0.05$, ** $p < 0.01$, *** $p < 0.001$ after adjusting for multiple comparisons (Socransky *et al.* 1991). The species were ordered and grouped according to the complexes described by Socransky *et al.* (1998). The yellow profile represents the mean data for the healthy subjects and the red profile represents the data for the periodontitis subjects. Reprinted with permission from Blackwell Publishing (Haffajee *et al.* 2006a, *Oral Microbiology and Immunology*, **21**, 1–14).

different forms of disease have different subgingival microbial profiles. Even subjects with the "same" periodontal disease in terms of both clinical appearance and severity can exhibit quite different subgingival microbiotas (Fig. 9-13).

The local environment

One host factor that markedly influenced the subgingival environment was pocket depth. Figure 9-14 demonstrates that the mean counts of subgingival species differed at sites of different pocket depths. Red complex species, *T. forsythia*, *P. gingivalis*, as well as *Tr. denticola* (data not shown), increased strikingly in numbers with increasing pocket depth. All orange complex species also demonstrated this relationship. *S. sanguinis* and *A. naeslundii* genospecies 2 were typical of the majority of species in the other four complexes that showed little relationship to pocket depth. Thus, red and orange complex species were not only related to periodontal disease status in a subject, but to disease status at the periodontal site. The species of the red and orange complexes were

also elevated at sites exhibiting gingival inflammation, as measured by gingival redness, bleeding on probing, and suppuration (Fig. 9-15). Other species such as *A. naeslundii* genospecies 2 and *S. sanguinis* did not show this relationship.

One remarkable feature of the microbiota of "healthy sites" (defined as sites with pocket depth <4 mm) in subjects with periodontitis was that their microbiota differed markedly from that found in healthy sites in periodontally healthy subjects (Fig. 9-16). The data in Fig. 9-16 once again demonstrate the strong relationship of orange and red complex species with pocket depth in the subjects with periodontitis. However, the figure also demonstrates that subjects who were periodontally healthy had clearly lower levels of periodontal pathogens, such as *E. nodatum*, *P. gingivalis*, *T. forsythia*, and *Tr. denticola*, in their shallow sulci/pockets than were detected in the shallow pockets in periodontitis subjects. This suggests that the "healthy sites" in the subjects with periodontitis would be at more risk for destructive disease initiation and progression than similar sites in periodontally healthy individuals and may

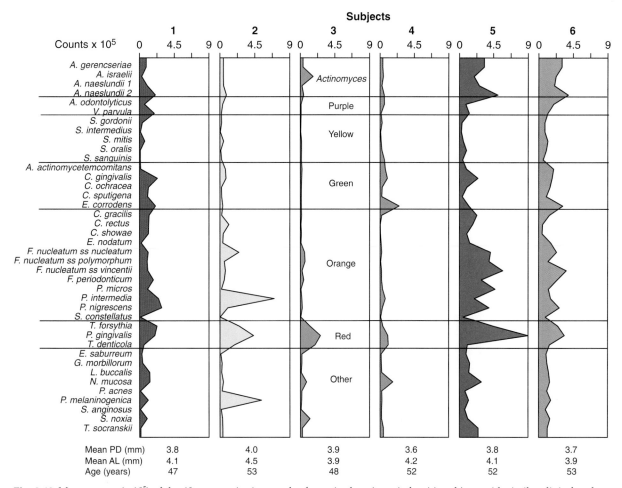

Fig. 9-13 Mean counts ($\times 10^5$) of the 40 test species in samples from six chronic periodontitis subjects with similar clinical and demographic features. Mean values for each species were computed by averaging up to 28 samples in each subject. Each panel represents an individual subject and the mean clinical features of the subjects are presented below each panel. The species were ordered and grouped according to microbial complexes (Socransky *et al.* 1998).

warrant therapy to lower the levels of colonizing pathogens.

Host factors

In addition to the impact of local factors on the composition of subgingival biofilms, host level factors can also affect biofilm composition. Some of these factors include the genetic background of the subject, environmental factors such smoking and diet, systemic conditions such as diabetes and obesity, and even geographic location. For example, subjects who are positive for a specific genotype of the polymorphic IL-1 gene cluster have been found to have increased levels of periodontal disease (Kornman *et al.* 1997) and increased counts of species of the red and orange complexes at sites with pocket depth >6 mm (Socransky & Haffajee 2005). Another condition that has been associated with a heightened inflammatory response, obesity, was associated with increased counts of red complex species in subgingival plaque samples, in particular, increased counts of *T. forsythia* in very obese subjects (Socransky & Haffajee 2005). There are numerous studies in the litera-

ture indicating that subjects who are current smokers have significantly more periodontal disease than past or never smokers and respond less well to mechanical periodontal therapies (Haffajee & Socransky 2000). In addition, it has been shown that current smokers have a larger proportion of their "healthy" sites (pocket depth <4 mm) colonized by red and orange complex species compared to similar sites in subjects who have never smoked (Socransky & Haffajee 2005). Individuals with Sjogren's syndrome, an autoimmune disease, that leads to a variety of host changes including a decrease in salivary flow rates, exhibit decreased levels of supra- and subgingival plaque, but increased proportions of *V. parvula* and *N. mucosa* in supra- and subgingival biofilms (Socransky & Haffajee 2005). Even the geographic location of a subject can influence the composition of subgingival biofilms (Fig. 9-17). Samples of subgingival plaque from the four deepest sites in each subject with chronic periodontitis from five different countries evaluated using checkerboard DNA–DNA hybridization, demonstrated that the proportions of species such as *P. gingivalis*, *Tr. denticola*, and *E. nodatum* differed markedly among subjects. The

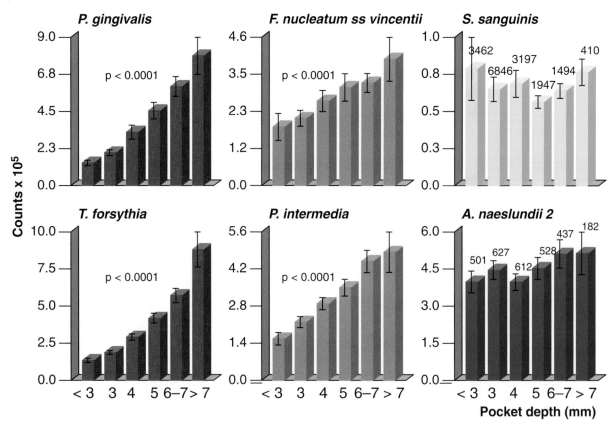

Fig. 9-14 Bar charts of the mean counts ($\times 10^5$, ± SEM) of six subgingival species at selected pocket depths in samples from 635 chronic periodontitis subjects. *T. forsythia* and *P. gingivalis* are representative of the red complex, *F. nucleatum* ss *vincentii* and *Pr. intermedia* are representative of the orange complex species, and *S. sanguinis* and *A. naeslundii* genospecies 2 are typical of other cluster groups. The mean counts of each species at each pocket depth category were computed for each subject and then averaged across subjects. The numbers above the bars in the *S. sanguinis* panel represent the number of sampled sites in each pocket depth category, while the numbers above the bars in the *A. naeslundii* panel represent the number of subjects who provided data for each pocket depth category. Significance of differences among pocket depth categories was tested using the Kruskal-Wallis test and adjusted for 40 comparisons.

differences may have been due to oral hygiene habits, diet, socioeconomic status, genetic background, or transmission among individuals in the community.

Transmission

In planning control of periodontal pathogens, it is essential to clarify their source. If an individual were fortunate enough not to encounter virulent periodontal pathogens, he or she would exhibit minimal periodontal disease even if susceptible. However, most individuals have acquired strains of suspected periodontal pathogens at some time in their lives. For the most part, it appears that subgingival species found in humans are unique to that environment. The subgingival species of the human, by and large, are not commonly encountered in the environment (e.g. soil, air, water) or indeed in the subgingival microbiota of other animal species. Thus, survival of subgingival species in the human requires the transmission of periodontal pathogens from the oral cavity of one individual to the oral cavity of another. Two types of transmission are recognized; "vertical", that is transmission from parent to offspring, and "horizontal",

i.e. passage of an organism between individuals outside the parent–offspring relationship.

Evidence for both forms of transmission has been provided using molecular epidemiology techniques. For many of these techniques, the investigator isolates DNA from strains of a given species recovered from different individuals. The DNA is cut with restriction endonucleases, run on agarose gel electrophoresis and the resulting fingerprint patterns compared, either directly, or with the help of various DNA probes. When these techniques were employed on isolates from subgingival plaque, it was demonstrated that *A. actinomycetemcomitans* and *P. gingivalis* strains isolated from parents and children within the same family exhibited identical restriction endonuclease patterns. Different patterns were found for strains isolated from different families (DiRienzo & Slots 1990; Alaluusua *et al.* 1993; Petit *et al.* 1993a,b). In other studies it was found that *A. actinomycetemcomitans* and *P. gingivalis* strains isolated from husband and wife had the same restriction endonuclease patterns or ribotypes indicating that these species could be transmitted within married couples (Saarela *et al.* 1993; van Steenbergen *et al.* 1993).

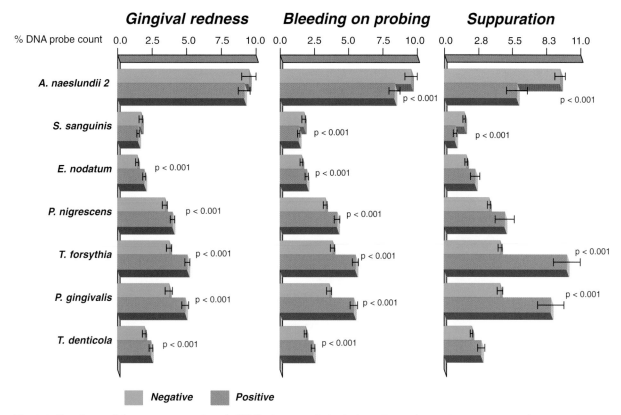

Fig. 9-15 Bar charts of the mean proportions (± SEM) of seven subgingival species at sites positive or negative for gingival redness, BOP and suppuration. *T. forsythia*, *P. gingivalis*, and *T. denticola* are representative of the red complex, *E. nodatum* and *Pr. nigrescens* are representative of the orange complex species, while *A. naeslundii* genospecies 2 and *S. sanguinis* represent other cluster groups. The mean proportions of each species at positive or negative sites for each parameter were computed for each subject and then averaged across subjects. The green bars represent the sites negative for the clinical parameters and the purple bars represent the positive sites. Significance of differences in proportions of species between positive and negative sites was determined using the Wilcoxon signed ranks test and adjusted for 40 comparisons.

The above data should not be surprising in view of the fact that periodontal pathogens have to come from somewhere, and the most likely source would appear to be a family member, whether spouse, sibling or parent. However, while intra-family transmission has been demonstrated, it appears likely that transmission of pathogens also occurs between unrelated individuals. Earlier, the transmission of ANUG was described both within troops in trenches in World War I and in communities outside the war zone after World War I. Another example of transmission between members of different families is provided by the detection of the JP2 clone of *A. actinomycetemcomitans* in individuals of African descent who were located in Africa or had relocated to Europe or the Americas (Kilian *et al.* 2006). Such reports suggest that periodontal pathogens can be transmitted, on occasion, between unrelated individuals. Thus, while there has been an intuitive feeling that the oral microbiota is relatively stable within an individual, it seems likely that new species or different clonal types of the same species can be introduced into an individual at various stages of his or her life. If the newly acquired strain is more virulent than the pre-existing strain of that species, then a change in disease pattern could occur.

Transmission of bacteria is not restricted to passage of strains from one subject to another, but frequently occurs from one type of intraoral biofilm to another. For example, it is thought that a species such as *A. actinomycetemcomitans* may colonize the buccal mucosa long before it can be found in supra- or subgingival biofilms (Fine *et al.* 2006). When a species moves from one oral surface to another, different modes of attachment are employed. For example, for *A. actinomycetemcomitans* a protein adhesin, Aae, may mediate attachment to buccal epithelial cells, while fimbriae and a polysaccharide mediate attachment to tooth surfaces as discussed previously. In a similar fashion streptococcal species, such as *S. mitis*, that are found in high proportions on soft tissue surfaces may be important in dental plaque development on the tooth surfaces from 0–6 hours as described Li *et al.* (2004) and from 1–2 days as described by Socransky and Haffajee (2005). In more mature plaques, these species become a small proportion of the microbiota (Socransky & Haffajee 2005).

There is one more level of intraoral transmission that should be considered and that is the horizontal transfer of genetic material from one bacterial species to another (Roberts & Mullany 2006). This particular mechanism is important not only in providing

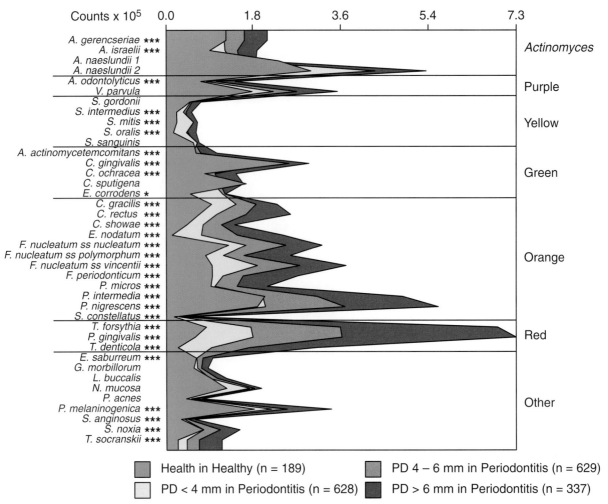

Counts x 10⁵

| | 0.0 | 1.8 | 3.6 | 5.4 | 7.3 |

A. gerencseriae ***
A. israelii ***
A. naeslundii 1
A. naeslundii 2   *Actinomyces*
A. odontolyticus ***
V. parvula   Purple
S. gordonii
S. intermedius ***
S. mitis ***   Yellow
S. oralis ***
S. sanguinis
A. actinomycetemcomitans ***
C. gingivalis ***
C. ochracea ***   Green
C. sputigena
E. corrodens *
C. gracilis ***
C. rectus ***
C. showae ***
E. nodatum ***
F. nucleatum ss nucleatum ***
F. nucleatum ss polymorphum ***
F. nucleatum ss vincentii ***   Orange
F. periodonticum ***
P. micros ***
P. intermedia ***
P. nigrescens ***
S. constellatus ***
T. forsythia ***
P. gingivalis ***   Red
T. denticola ***
E. saburreum ***
G. morbillorum
L. buccalis
N. mucosa
P. acnes   Other
P. melaninogenica ***
S. anginosus ***
S. noxia ***
T. socranskii ***

Health in Healthy (n = 189)   PD 4 – 6 mm in Periodontitis (n = 629)
PD < 4 mm in Periodontitis (n = 628)   PD > 6 mm in Periodontitis (n = 337)

Fig. 9-16 Mean counts (× 10⁵) of 40 species in subgingival plaque samples from periodontal pockets/sulci <4, 4–6 and >6 mm in 635 chronic peridontitis subjects and from periodontally healthy sites in 189 periodontally healthy subjects. Subgingival plaque samples were taken at baseline and analyzed for their content of 40 subgingival species using checkerboard DNA–DNA hybridization. Counts of each species were averaged in each subject for each pocket depth category and then averaged across subjects for each category separately. The species were ordered according to microbial complexes (Socransky *et al*. 1998). Significance of differences among pocket depth categories was sought using the Kruskal Wallis test; * $p < 0.05$, ** $p < 0.01$, *** $p < 0.001$ after adjusting for multiple comparisons (Socransky *et al*. 1991).

potential virulence traits to a pathogenic species, but also in providing information that codes for factors such as adhesins or mechanisms of antibiotic resistance. Mechanisms of horizontal gene transfer include plasmids, conjugative transposons, bacteriophage, and transformation (for review of horizontal gene transfer within the oral cavity see Roberts and Mullany, 2006).

Microbial composition of supra- and subgingival biofilms

The bacteria associated with periodontal diseases reside within biofilms both above and below the gingival margin. The supragingival biofilm is attached to the tooth surface and is predominated by *Actinomyces* species in most plaque samples. Figure 9-18 provides the counts, proportions, and prevalence (percentage of sites colonized) of 40 taxa grouped

according to microbial complexes (Socransky *et al*. 1998) in supragingival plaque samples from periodontally healthy and periodontitis subjects. The *Actinomyces* predominate in both health and disease. Further, all taxa examined could be found (on average) in both health and disease, although counts, proportions, and prevalence (percentage of sites colonized) of periodontal pathogens were significantly higher in the periodontally diseased subjects.

As described above, the nature of subgingival biofilms was more complex with both a tooth-associated and tissue-associated biofilm separated by loosely bound or planktonic cells. Figure 9-12 presented the counts, proportions, and prevalence of 40 taxa in subgingival plaque samples from periodontally diseased and periodontally healthy individuals (Haffajee *et al*. 2006a). Similar to supragingival plaque, the dominant species subgingivally were the *Actinomyces*, but significantly higher counts, proportions, and

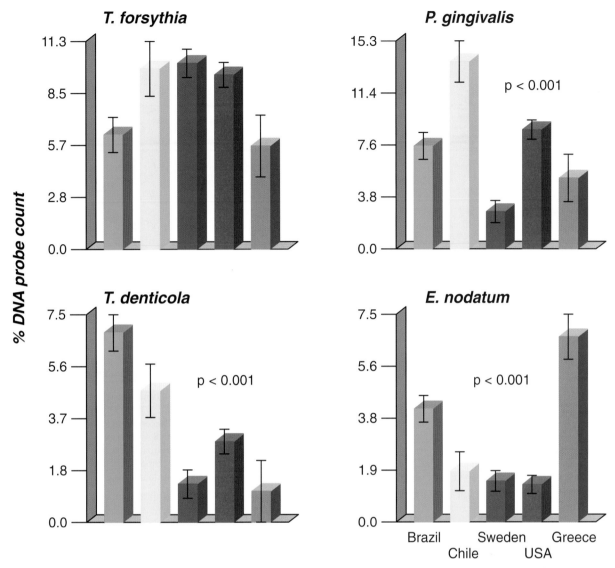

Fig. 9-17 Bar charts of adjusted mean percents (± SEM) of the total DNA probe count of the red complex species, *T. forsythia*, *P. gingivalis*, and *Tr. denticola* and the orange complex species, *E. nodatum*, in baseline subgingival plaque samples taken from the four deepest, sampled periodontal pockets in 58 Brazilian, 26 Chilean, 92 Swedish, 114 American, and 20 Greek chronic periodontitis subjects. The bars represent the mean percents after adjusting for age, mean pocket depth, gender and smoking status. The whiskers indicate the standard error of the mean. Significance of differences among groups for each species was sought using ANCOVA adjusting for age, mean pocket depth, gender and smoking status. The p values were adjusted for 40 comparisons.

prevalence of red and orange complex species were found in the samples from the periodontitis subjects. In particular, there were significantly higher levels, proportions, and prevalence of *P. gingivalis*, *T. forsythia*, and *Tr. denticola* in both supra- and subgingival plaque of periodontitis subjects when compared with similar samples from periodontally healthy individuals. Figure 9-19 summarizes the major differences in microbial complexes between supra- and subgingival plaque in health and periodontitis. As one moves from the supragingival to the subgingival environment and from health to disease, there is a significant decrease in the *Actinomyces* species and an increase in the proportion of members of the red complex.

Development of supra- and subgingival biofilms

Prior to the advent of molecular techniques, few studies had comprehensively examined the microbial shifts that occurred during supra- or subgingival plaque development. Ritz (1967) described the changes that occur in plaque that formed on the labial surfaces of the six upper and six lower anterior teeth from 1–9 days using selective media techniques. The data indicated that streptococci were predominant at 1 day, comprising an average of 46% of the colonies detected. *Neisseria* and *Nocardia* were also high in mean proportions at 1 day but decreased in counts and proportions over time. *Actinomyces* were initially

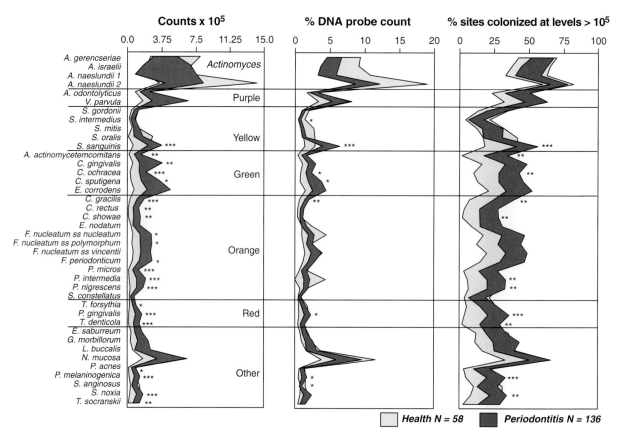

Fig. 9-18 Plots of mean counts (left panel), percents of the total DNA probe count (middle panel) and percentage of sites colonized by 40 bacterial species at counts >10^5 (right panel) in supragingival plaque samples taken from 58 periodontally healthy and 136 chronic periodontitis subjects. The "bands" represent the mean values ± the 95% confidence intervals after adjusting for 40 comparisons. Mean values for each species were computed by averaging up to 28 samples in each subject, and then averaging across subjects in the two clinical groups. Significance of differences between groups was sought using the non-parametric Mann Whitney test; * p < 0.05, ** p < 0.01, *** p < 0.001 after adjusting for multiple comparisons. The species were ordered and grouped according to microbial complexes. The yellow profile represents the mean data for the healthy subjects and the red profile represents the data for the periodontitis subjects.

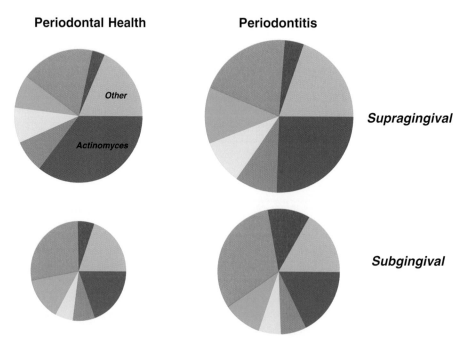

Fig. 9-19 Pie charts of the mean percentage DNA probe count of microbial groups in supragingival plaque samples from 58 periodontally healthy and 136 periodontitis subjects and subgingival plaque samples from 189 periodontally healthy and 635 periodontitis subjects. The species were grouped into seven microbial groups based on the description of Socransky et al. (1998). The areas of the pies were adjusted to reflect the mean total DNA probe counts at each of the sample locations. The significance of differences in mean percentages of the supra- and subgingival complexes in health and disease was tested using the Kruskal Wallis test. All complexes differed significantly among groups at p < 0.001 after adjusting for seven comparisons. The "other" category represents probes to species that did fall into a complex as well as probes to new species whose relationships with other species has not yet been ascertained.

low in proportion (0.18%) but rose to 23% of the microbiota by 9 days. Ritz (1967) felt that there was microbial succession in plaque development with aerobic or facultative species reducing the environment for the subsequent growth of anaerobic species. In a study of five "rapid" and six "slow" plaque formers, a single plaque sample was taken from each subject at days 1, 3, 7, and 14 and evaluated using cultural techniques (Zee *et al.* 1996). Gram-positive bacteria were the predominant cultivable species in both clinical groups, but Gram-negative species increased in proportion more rapidly in the "rapid" plaque formers. At 14 days, the "rapid" plaque formers had a mean of 38% Gram-negative rods compared with 17% in the 14 day samples from the "slow" plaque formers. The majority of cultivable Gram-negative rods were in the genera *Fusobacterium* and *Capnocytophaga*. Striking in their data was the decrease in proportion of Gram-positive cocci from 50–60% at day 1 to <15% at day 14. This decrease was accompanied by an increase in the proportion of *Actinomyces* species and Gram-negative rods.

The introduction of molecular techniques provided a more comprehensive description of biofilm development. Li *et al.* (2004) used checkerboard DNA–DNA hybridization to examine the early development (0–6 hours) of supragingival biofilm on the buccal/labial surfaces of 20 restoration-free tooth surfaces in 15 subjects. Figure 9-20 presents the mean counts of the 40 test species at 0, 2, 4, and 6 hours. Certain species, such as *S. mitis* and *S. oralis*, appeared to be "pioneer" species in supragingival biofilm development since they were the predominant species at 4 and 6 hours. These findings are in accord with *in vivo* cultural studies that demonstrated the early colonization of enamel and root surfaces using cultural techniques (Nyvad & Kilian 1987). The development of the biofilm in the Li *et al.* (2004) study did not appear to be due to simple adsorption of species from saliva, because the microbial profile of saliva samples from the same subjects differed markedly from the biofilm that developed on the teeth (Fig. 9-20).

The development of supragingival and subgingival biofilm, over a 7-day period, in periodontally healthy and diseased subjects has been described (Socransky & Haffajee 2005). Figure 9-21 presents the total DNA probe counts of supra- and subgingival biofilm samples from chronic periodontitis subjects taken pre and post tooth cleaning and at 1, 2, 4, and 7 days in the absence of home care procedures. There was a marked reduction in supra- and subgingival total counts after tooth cleaning, demonstrating that plaque levels could be significantly reduced even in individuals who performed "reasonable" home care procedures. The total numbers of organisms increased

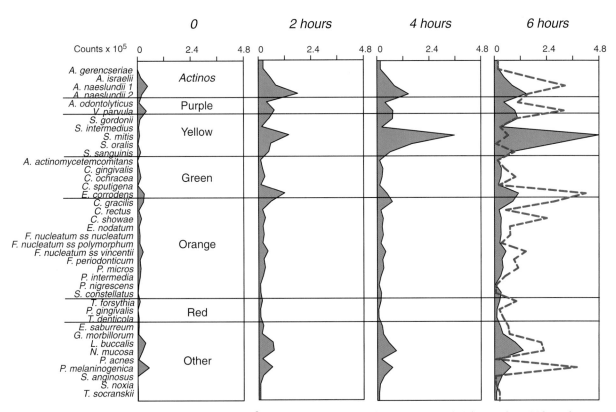

Fig. 9-20 Microbial profiles of the mean counts ($\times 10^5$) of 40 taxa in plaque biofilm samples pooled from at least 20 buccal surfaces immediately post cleaning (0), 2, 4, and 6 hours in 15 subjects. Samples were analyzed for their content of 40 bacterial species using checkerboard DNA–DNA hybridization. Counts of individual species were computed in each subject and then averaged across subjects for each time point. The red dashed profile superimposed on the 6-hour biofilm profile represents the microbial profile of saliva samples from the same subjects taken at baseline. The species are ordered according to the complexes described by Socransky *et al.* (1998). The data were adapted from Li *et al.* (2004).

rapidly, in the absence of oral hygiene, in both the supra- and subgingival areas reaching pre-cleaning levels by 2 days subgingivally and by 4 days supragingivally. These findings were in accord with other studies that demonstrated the rapid return of tooth-associated biofilms after their removal (Sharawy *et al.* 1966; Furuichi *et al.* 1992; Ramberg *et al.* 2003). However, as indicated by the Li *et al.* (2004) study, not all species returned at the same rate.

Figure 9-22 (left panel) presents the mean counts of 4 of 40 tested species in subgingival biofilm samples

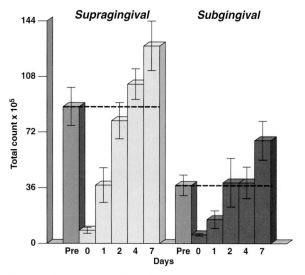

Fig. 9-21 Mean total DNA probe counts ($\times 10^5$, ± SEM) of supra and subgingival plaque samples taken prior to, immediately post-cleaning, and after 1, 2, 4, and 7 days of no oral hygiene in 16 subjects with chronic periodontitis. The dashed horizontal lines are provided to indicate the pre-cleaning levels.

from chronic periodontitis subjects at the six time points described above. All of the species were reduced in counts after tooth cleaning, but *S. oralis* increased rapidly, exceeding baseline (pre-cleaning) levels at 1–2 days. Levels of *F. nucleatum* ss *nucleatum* and *Pr. intermedia* increased more slowly and exceeded baseline levels at between 2 and 4 and 4 and 7 days respectively. The periodontal pathogen, *P. gingivalis*, had not reached baseline values by 7 days. The shifts in the proportions of the same species are presented in Fig. 9-22 (right panel). Proportions of *S. oralis* increased rapidly by 2 days and then declined, while proportions of the two orange complex species, *F. nucleatum* ss *nucleatum* and *Pr. intermedia*, declined initially and slowly increased over the 7-day period. Proportions of *P. gingivalis* decreased over time and were at their lowest levels at 7 days. These findings are instructive in terms of the role that mechanical debridement plays in controlling periodontal infections. While the total number of bacteria returns rapidly after mechanical debridement, reductions in the proportions of certain species, such as *P. gingivalis* and other members of the red and orange complexes, occur and can be maintained for prolonged periods of time. However, it is important to recognize that pathogenic species are not usually eliminated by this form of therapy and can return to pre-treatment levels in periods varying from weeks to years.

Prerequisites for periodontal disease initiation and progression

It is a common feature of many infectious diseases that a pathogenic species may colonize a host and yet

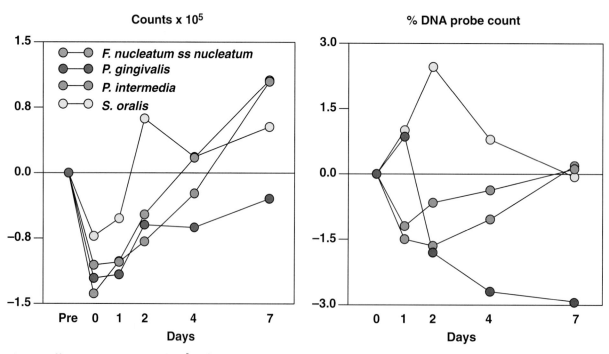

Fig. 9-22 Change in mean counts ($\times 10^5$) (left panel) and percentage of DNA probe count (right panel) of four species in subgingival plaque samples from pre cleaning to immediately post cleaning, and after 1, 2, 4, and 7 days of no oral hygiene in 16 subjects with chronic periodontitis.

the host may not manifest clinical features of that disease for periods of time varying from weeks to decades or ever. Thus, it appears that periodontal disease progression is dependent on the simultaneous occurrence of a number of factors (Socransky & Haffajee 1992, 1993). The host must be susceptible both systemically and locally. The local environment has to contain bacterial species which enhance the infection or at very least do not inhibit the pathogen's activity. The environment also must be conducive to the expression of virulence factors by the pathogen. This might take the form of affecting the regulation of virulence factor expression or stressing the organism so that it manifests properties which lead to tissue damage. The pathogen(s) must achieve sufficient numbers to initiate or cause progression of the infection in that particular individual in the given local environment. Fortunately, the simultaneous occurrence of all these factors does not happen frequently or periodontal disease would be more prevalent and severe in the population.

The virulent periodontal pathogen

Detection of suspected periodontal pathogens in plaque samples from periodontally healthy mouths (Dahlen *et al*. 1989; McNabb *et al*. 1992; Haffajee *et al*. 1998) or healthy sites in periodontally diseased mouths (Socransky *et al*. 1991) raises the question as to whether all strains of a pathogenic species are virulent. A major recognition of the last decade was that all clonal types of a pathogenic species are not equally virulent. For many medically important pathogenic species, a very small proportion of clonal types account for the majority of the disease that is observed (briefly reviewed in Socransky & Haffajee 1991, 1992). The clear association of the virulent JP2 clone of *A. actinomycetemcomitans* in LAP was discusssed above and in greater detail in Fine *et al*. (2006) and Kilian *et al*. (2006). Studies of the pathogenic potential of different strains of *P. gingivalis* in animal model systems support the notion of strain differences in virulence (Grenier & Mayrand 1987a; van Steenbergen *et al*. 1987; Marsh *et al*. 1989; Neiders *et al*. 1989; Sundqvist *et al*. 1991; Baker *et al*. 2000). Certain clonal types of *P. gingivalis* were detected more frequently in samples from periodontitis subjects than control periodontally healthy subjects, suggesting an association of more virulent clonal types with disease (Griffen *et al*. 1999). These studies highlight the fact that there are major differences in virulence of different isolates of *P. gingivalis* and suggest that in some instances when suspected pathogens are found in periodontally healthy sites, the strains may be avirulent. *P. gingivalis fim*A gene encoding fimbrillin, a subunit of fimbriae, has been classified into six genotypes based on their nucleotide sequences. Amano *et al*. (2000) examined the *P. gingivalis fim*A genotypes in dental plaque samples from 380 periodontally healthy adults and 139 periodontitis patients. Type I

and type V genotypes were most common in *P. gingivalis*-positive periodontally healthy adults, while type II and type IV were far more common in subjects with periodontitis. Such data suggest that *fim*A genotype may be an important factor influencing the pathogenicity of *P. gingivalis*.

Another requirement for a pathogen to express virulence is that the organism possess all of the necessary genetic elements. Some of these elements might be missing in a strain inhabiting the gingival crevice area, but could be received from other strains of that species (or possibly other species) via phage, plasmids or transposons (Roberts & Mullany 2006). Thus, periodontally healthy sites might be colonized with periodontal pathogens without a full complement of genes needed to lead to tissue destruction.

Finally, the pathogen must be in the right location in a site (e.g. at the apical area of the pocket or adjacent to the epithelium) in sufficient numbers to initiate disease. There are probably minimum numbers of a pathogen needed to initiate disease.

The local environment

If periodontal disease progression is a comparatively infrequent phenomenon, most of the resident species are likely to be host-compatible and in some instances may be actively beneficial to the host. Thus, microbial interactions play a role in the nature of species that colonize a site and ultimately on the outcome health or disease. Some interactions might be harmful, leading to mixed infections as discussed earlier. Others might be more beneficial to the host. Host-compatible species could colonize sites that otherwise would be colonized by pathogens. They might "dilute" the number of pathogens in a pocket, compete for or alter binding sites for pathogens, or destroy virulence factors produced by pathogens (Socransky & Haffajee 1991).

One carefully studied interbacterial antagonism has implications for our understanding of the ecology of destructive periodontal diseases. Hillman and co-workers (1982, 1985, 1987) became interested in the long-term stability of LAP lesions after treatment with surgery and systemic tetracycline. They surmised that a microbiota was established after treatment that was antagonistic to the return of the presumed pathogen *A. actinomycetemcomitans*. This proved to be the case. It was shown that certain species such as *S. sanguinis*, *Streptococcus uberis* and *A. naeslundii* genospecies 2 produced factors that were inhibitory to the growth of *A. actinomycetemcomitans* (Hillman *et al*. 1985). These species were absent or in low numbers in lesion sites of LAP prior to therapy but in elevated numbers after therapy. The mechanism of inhibition was shown to be hydrogen peroxide formation by the "beneficial" species, (Hillman & Socransky 1987) which either directly, or via a host peroxidase system (Tenovuo & Pruitt 1984), inhibited the pathogen. Stevens *et al*. (1987) and

Hammond *et al.* (1987) demonstrated the reverse antagonism. *A. actinomycetemcomitans* was shown to specifically inhibit the growth of *S. sanguinis*, *S. uberis*, and *A. naeslundii* genospecies 2 (but not other species) by the production of a bacteriocin. This mutual antagonism is highly specific and its outcome may strongly influence whether a subject or a site will exhibit disease due to *A. actinomycetemcomitans*. Such interactions demonstrate the potent role resident microbial species play in permitting or preventing the establishment or spread of pathogenic species. The tremendous controlling pressure of the resident microbiota is reinforced by the difficulty encountered when an investigator attempts to implant a human oral isolate into the microbiota of a conventional animal or purposely attempts to implant strains isolated from one human into the subgingival plaque of another.

The local subgingival environment can affect disease pathogenesis in other ways. One of the more intriguing ways centers around the recognition that virulent strains of pathogenic species do not always express their virulence factors (Socransky & Haffajee 1991). Often, a global "regulon" simultaneously turns on or off the production of multiple virulence factors. The regulon is affected by specific factors in the local environment, such as temperature, osmotic pressure, or the concentration of iron, magnesium or calcium. The effect of environment on protein expression has been shown in subgingival species. For example, the level of iron in the environment will affect the expression of outer membrane proteins of *P. gingivalis* and will also affect virulence of the strain in animal model systems (McKee *et al.* 1986, Barua *et al.* 1990, Bramanti & Holt 1990). Even the presence of specific other species might lead to expression of virulence genes by pathogenic species. For example, the production of a surface protein by *Streptococcus cristatus* caused repression of the *P. gingivalis fim*A gene, possibly influencing the development a pathogenic plaque (Xie *et al.* 2000). The effect of environment on virulence factor expression seems a fertile area for investigation. It may help to explain the long lag phase that occurs prior to disease initiation. Conceivably, a pathogen may reside quietly in an area for years as a compatible member of the microbiota. However, some stress generated by a change in the environment might influence that organism to express long-hidden, rather damaging factors.

Host susceptibility

For a period of time considerably longer than the search for microbial etiologic agents of periodontal diseases, dental practitioners have hypothesized that differences in disease pattern or severity may be due to differences in host susceptibility (in earlier years termed resistance). In spite of these hypotheses, it is remarkable how few "host susceptibly factors" have

been identified. With increased research in this area and better methods for comparing populations, a number of host or environmental factors have been suggested that may impact on the initiation and rate of progression of periodontal diseases. Such factors include defects in polymorphonuclear leukocyte levels or function, a poorly regulated immunological response, smoking, diet, and various systemic diseases (Genco *et al.* 1986; Bergstrom & Eliasson 1987; Greenspan *et al.* 1989; Williams *et al.* 1990; de Pommereau *et al.* 1992; Greenspan & Greenspan 1993; Seppala *et al.* 1993; Thorstensson & Hugoson 1993).

HIV infection

Debilitating systemic illness can alter the host's ability to cope with infections and may exacerbate existing infections. In early studies, it appeared that periodontal diseases were more prevalent and severe in HIV-positive individuals than in patients who were not infected with HIV (Greenspan *et al.* 1989; Williams *et al.* 1990; Greenspan & Greenspan 1993). In some HIV-positive subjects, unusual necrotic, rapidly destructive periodontal lesions were observed. These observations led to speculation that either unusual pathogenic species were involved or that the modification of host resistance was so severe that it led to extreme tissue destruction. Examination of plaque samples taken from periodontitis sites in HIV-positive individuals indicated that the subgingival microbiota was very similar to that seen in non-HIV-infected periodontitis subjects, except that occasionally unusual organisms were encountered (Murray *et al.* 1989, 1991; Zambon *et al.* 1990; Rams *et al.* 1991; Moore *et al.* 1993). Further, suspected periodontal pathogens, including *P. gingivalis*, *Pr. intermedia*, *F. nucleatum*, and *A. actinomycetemcomitans*, were found more frequently in periodontitis sites in HIV-infected subjects than in either gingivitis or, in particular, healthy sites in these subjects (Murray *et al.* 1989). Rams *et al.* (1991) in a study of 14 HIV-infected individuals with periodontitis found that *A. actinomycetemcomitans*, *C. rectus*, *Pe. micros*, and *Pr. intermedia* each averaged 7–16% of the cultivable microbiota in patients positive for the species. In addition, levels of spirochetes were high, while levels of *Candida albicans* and Gram-negative enteric rods were low. Thus, the microbiota of lesions in HIV-positive individuals was quite similar to that in HIV-negative subjects. However, not all HIV-positive subjects exhibit periodontal disease, and certainly not the extremely rapid form of disease. In addition, patients with the mild or rapid forms of disease are successfully treated using conventional periodontal therapies including local debridement, antiseptic mouthwashes, and local and/or systemically administered antimicrobial agents (Williams *et al.* 1990; Winkler & Robertson 1992; Greenspan & Greenspan 1993).

Diabetes

Another systemic illness which has been associated with increased prevalence and incidence of periodontal disease is diabetes. Many studies (de Pommereau *et al.* 1992; Seppala *et al.* 1993; Thorstensson & Hugoson 1993), but not all (Barnett *et al.* 1984; Rylander *et al.* 1987), indicated that periodontitis is more severe in juvenile or adult diabetic subjects than non-diabetic controls. Microbiologic studies of diabetic subjects have indicated that similar periodontal pathogens were found in diseased sites of diabetic subjects as in non-diabetic periodontal patients. *A. actinomycetemcomitans, Capnocytophaga* sp., and "anaerobic vibrios" were found to be elevated in subgingival plaque samples from juvenile diabetic subjects (Mashimo *et al.* 1983), while Sastrowijoto *et al.* (1989) found that *A. actinomycetemcomitans, P. gingivalis,* and *Pr. intermedia* were elevated in diseased sites of adult diabetic subjects. Mandell *et al.* (1992) found that a number of suspected periodontal pathogens were elevated at disease sites in poorly controlled insulin-dependent diabetics, including *Pr. intermedia, Pr. melaninogenica, C. gracilis, E. corrodens, F. nucleatum,* and *C. rectus,* when compared with healthy sites in the same subject. Similar species were found in adult periodontitis patients with non-insulin-dependent diabetes. *Pr. intermedia* was the most frequently detected species, while *C. rectus* and *P. gingivalis* were also very common (Zambon *et al.* 1988).

The intriguing aspect of the studies of HIV-positive and diabetic subjects, is that periodontal lesions, for the most part, appeared to be related to already suspected periodontal pathogens and not to some novel species. Studies such as these suggest that altered host susceptibility may change the rate of disease progression in affected individuals, but by and large the periodontal pathogens are likely to be the same as those found in uncompromised subjects.

Smoking

The deleterious effects of cigarette smoking on the periodontium have been reported in numerous studies (briefly reviewed in Haffajee & Socransky 2000). It has been shown that cigarette smokers have more bone loss, attachment loss, deeper periodontal pockets, and less gingival bleeding than non-smokers. As described in an earlier section, suspected or known periodontal pathogens were more prevalent; i.e. colonized a larger proportion of sites, in current smokers than in past or never smokers. On average, this increased extent of colonization was from 10–25%; i.e. three to seven teeth (of 28) in each subject. The species that differed significantly between smokers and non-smokers were primarily species of the red and orange complexes. The increased extent of colonization appeared to occur primarily at shallow periodontal pockets (<4 mm) rather than deeper pockets. The difference in prevalence of these species helps to explain the greater extent of periodontal destruction in smokers than in non-smokers, since more sites are at risk (colonized by potential pathogens) in subjects who smoke. The reason for this difference in colonization pattern is not clear. Cigarette smoke could directly affect the pathogens or their local habitats. Tobacco usage also could affect the host's ability to control the infection by diminishing the local and systemic immune response. Whatever the reason, the widespread colonization of potential pathogens even at clinically healthy sites is likely to lead to future tissue damage at these sites. Further, the greater extent of colonization by periodontal pathogens could complicate periodontal therapy, since elimination or control of species would be more difficult.

Mechanisms of pathogenicity

Essential factors for colonization of a subgingival species

For a periodontal pathogen to cause disease, it is essential that the pathogen be able to (1) colonize the subgingival area and (2) produce factors that either directly damage the host tissue or lead to the host tissue damaging itself. To colonize subgingival sites, a species must be able to (1) attach to one or more of the available surfaces, (2) multiply, (3) compete successfully against other species desiring that habitat, and (4) defend itself from host defense mechanisms.

Adhesins

To establish in a periodontal site, a species must be able to attach to one or more surfaces, including the tooth (or host-derived substances binding to the tooth), the sulcular or pocket epithelium, or other bacterial species attached to these surfaces. Studies of bacterial adhesion have demonstrated specificity in the involved mechanisms. At the simplest level there are one or more specific receptors on the host cell or other surfaces to which specific "adhesin" molecule(s) on the bacterial surface may attach. It has been demonstrated that there is a multiplicity of receptors on tooth surfaces, epithelial or other mammalian cells, and other bacteria. Some of the adhesins that have been identified on subgingival species include fimbriae (Cisar *et al.* 1984; Clark *et al.* 1986; Sandberg *et al.* 1986, 1988; Isogai *et al.* 1988) and cell-associated proteins (Murray *et al.* 1986, 1988; Mangan *et al.* 1989; Weinberg & Holt 1990). Receptors on tissue surfaces include galactosyl residues (Cisar *et al.* 1984; Murray *et al.* 1988; Sandberg *et al.* 1988; Mangan *et al.* 1989), sialic acid residues (Murray *et al.* 1986), proline-rich proteins or statherin (Clark *et al.* 1986), and type I or

IV collagens (Naito & Gibbons 1988; Winkler *et al.* 1988).

Coaggregation

While many species attach directly to host surfaces, other species attach to bacteria attached to such surfaces. This phenomenon is called coaggregation. It has been shown that there is specificity in the attachment of one species to another in *in vitro* systems and *in vivo* (Kaufman & DiRienzo 1989; Kolenbrander *et al.* 2006). In some instances, coaggregation between non-coaggregating species may be mediated by cellular constituents (e.g. vesicles) of a third species (Ellen & Grove 1989; Grenier & Mayrand 1987b). Further, the mechanism of attachment of cells of a given pair of species appears to be mediated by specific receptor–adhesin interactions. Many of these interactions are lectin-like in that they are based on the attachment of a specific protein on the surface of one species to a specific carbohydrate on the surface of the other (Kinder & Holt 1989; Kolenbrander & Andersen 1989; Kolenbrander *et al.* 1989; Abeygunawardana *et al.* 1990), but other mechanisms exist (Kolenbrander & Andersen 1990; Kolenbrander *et al.* 1989). For example, the *S. sanguinis–A. naeslundii* genospecies 2 interaction was shown to be due to the attachment of a fimbrial-associated lectin on *A. naeslundii* genospecies 2 to a polysaccharide with a repeating heptasaccharide on *S. sanguinis* (Abeygunawardana *et al.* 1990). In certain instances more than one type of adhesin–receptor interaction has been detected between a species pair. It is of interest that the same galactose-binding adhesin of *F. nucleatum* to *P. gingivalis* and *A. actinomycetemcomitans* also binds the cell to human epithelial cells and fibroblasts (Weiss *et al.* 2000).

The initial stages of plaque development involves the adhesion of organisms to the tooth surfaces or pellicle proteins on the tooth surfaces. The early colonizers are dominated by members of the genus *Streptococcus* (Fig. 9-20), followed by the *Actinomyces*, the two genera that commonly exhibit intra-generic coaggregation. This intra-generic coaggregation may help to explain the detection of the yellow complex, which is made up of *Streptococcus* species, and the species forming the *Actinomyces* cluster demonstrated in Fig. 9-10. In addition, there are also frequent coaggregations between species of these two genera. If the *Streptococcus–Actinomyces* coaggregations were random, thousands of potential interactions could result. However, only six specific coaggregation groups of streptococci and six coaggregation groups of *Actinomyces* have been detected (Kolenbrander *et al.* 2006). Sequential colonization of different species during plaque development may be mediated in part by coaggregation. This leads to the concept of bridging species; i.e. one or more species that coaggregate with early colonizers and are in turn attached to by late colonizing species. The colonization would be mediated by specific adhesin–receptor interactions between the early colonizers and the bridging species and a second set of receptor–adhesin interactions between the bridging species and late colonizers. Members of the genus *Fusobacterium* appear to be the major bridging species in dental plaque due to their ability to adhere to a very wide range of dental plaque species.

Multiplication

The gingival crevice and/or periodontal pocket might be considered a lush area for microbial growth, but it is in fact a rather stringent environment for a bacterial species to live in. The mean temperature of the area averages about 35°C and ranges from 30–38°C (Haffajee *et al.* 1992), eliminating whole classes of potential colonizing organisms such as thermophiles and psychrophiles. The pH of 7.0–8.5 is rather restricted (Forscher *et al.* 1954; Kleinberg & Hall 1969; Cimasoni 1983), and numerous microbial species find this range unacceptable. Oxidation reduction potential measurements vary from an Eh of about −300 to +310 mv at pH 7.0 (Onisi *et al.* 1960; Kenney & Ash 1969). The wide range of Eh provides suitable microenvironments for numerous bacterial species, although extremes of Eh in a local environment could be limiting to certain species.

The selective physical environment of the gingival crevice area is accompanied by limited nutritional availability. Three sources of nutrient are available to subgingival organisms (diet, host, and other subgingival species). Certain nutrients essential to some bacterial species must be formed by other species in that area. The vitamin K analogues required by certain *Porphyromonas* and *Prevotella* species (Gibbons & Macdonald 1960) and the hydrogen or formate required by *Campylobacter* species are produced by other species colonizing the subgingival ecosystem. However, the precursors to such substances and certain specific growth factors such as hemin (Evans 1951; Gibbons & Macdonald 1960) must be derived from the host. Gingival crevice fluid (GCF) is not particularly rich in nutrients, creating a major competition for the small amounts available. However, inflammation and damage to the host tissues, as a consequence of the colonizing species, lead to an increase in GCF and breakdown products of tissue, fostering the growth of resident species. Finally, nutrients delivered in relative abundance to the outer layers of plaque may not reach deeper layers.

Interbacterial relationships

Bacterial interactions play important roles in species survival. Some inter-species relationships are favorable, in that one species provides growth factors for, or facilitates attachment of, another. Other relationships are antagonistic due to competition for nutrients and binding sites or to the production of substances which limit or prevent growth of a second species.

A number of types of inter-species interactions have been described. The inter-species agglutinations described above are an important means of bacterial attachment for some species. Bacterial attachment may also be influenced by the production of extracellular enzymes by one set of organisms which uncover binding sites fostering the attachment of a second set of organisms. For example, *S. mitis* and *S. sanguinis* bind in comparable levels to intact epithelial cells, as do strains of *P. gingivalis* and *Pr. intermedia*. However, if epithelial cells are exposed to bacterial neuraminidase the attachment of the streptococci is diminished, but attachment of the *P. gingivalis* and *Pr. intermedia* strains is enhanced (Gibbons 1989). It is suspected that removal of sialic acid reveals galactosyl residues that foster attachment of the suspected pathogens. This mechanism may account for the greater level of such species on cells from periodontal pockets than from healthy sulci (Dzink *et al.* 1989).

Other beneficial interactions are mediated by one species providing growth conditions favorable to another. Such conditions include altered physicochemical parameters such as *Eh* (Socransky *et al.* 1964), *pH* (Kleinberg & Hall 1969), or *temperature* (Haffajee *et al.* 1992). One of the more important environmental parameters is the oxygen level. Subgingival species differ in their ability to grow in the presence or absence of oxygen. Obligate aerobes require oxygen for growth and cannot multiply in its absence. Obligately anaerobic species are killed by even low levels of oxygen, while facultative species can grow in either situation. Dental plaque provides a spectrum of environments with high levels of oxygen available on outer surfaces and adjacent to periodontal tissues, but low levels of oxygen and a low oxidation reduction potential within the plaque. The differences in microenvironments are due in part to location within the periodontal pocket and in part due to the intense reducing abilities of many subgingival species. The survival of some anaerobic species may be due to the presence of facultative or aerobic species that utilize oxygen and/or detoxify its potentially cell damaging activated radicals, such as the hydroxyl radicals. Subgingival species also provide specific growth factors utilized by other species, including branched chain fatty acids and polyamines (Socransky *et al.* 1964), analogues of vitamin K (Gibbons & Macdonald 1960), lactate (Rogosa 1964), formate or hydrogen (Tanner & Socransky 1984).

Colonization of a pathogenic species in the presence of a species that produces substances antagonistic to its survival presents a different challenge to a pathogen. Antagonistic substances vary from those that affect binding (e.g. the enzymes that favored *Pr. intermedia* above probably adversely affected *S. mitis*) to those that kill the species. Factors that kill other species include bacteriocins (Rogers *et al.* 1979; Hammond *et al.* 1987; Stevens *et al.* 1987), hydrogen

peroxide (Holmberg & Hallander 1973; Hillman *et al.* 1985), and organic acids (Mashimo *et al.* 1985). These factors may be considered as virulence factors since they suppress the growth of competing species or different clonal types of the same species (Hillman & Socransky 1989). Defense against such factors varies. The simplest way to avoid such factors is to find sites that are not colonized by antagonistic species. A second method is to produce factors that destroy the antagonistic species. For example, *S. sanguinis* produces hydrogen peroxide which inhibits the growth of *A. actinomycetemcomitans* (Hillman *et al.* 1985), while *A. actinomycetemcomitans* produces a bacteriocin that inhibits *S. sanguinis* (Hammond *et al.* 1987; Stevens *et al.* 1987). Thus, the bacteriocin that protects the suspected pathogen *A. actinomycetemcomitans* from the deleterious effect of the more commonly detected *S. sanguinis* must be considered to be a virulence factor.

Overcoming host defense mechanisms

Subgingival plaque microorganisms appear to overgrow and lead to severe disease in immune-compromised hosts particularly those with neutrophil disorders (Genco *et al.* 1986; Shenker 1987; Winkler *et al.* 1989). Such findings suggest that host defense mechanisms are important in limiting the numbers of bacteria in subgingival plaque and preventing tissue damage.

A bacterial species has a number of host-derived obstacles to overcome when colonizing a subgingival site. These include the flow of saliva and gingival crevice fluid and mechanical displacement by chewing and speaking. Substances in saliva and gingival crevice fluid may aid in the prevention of colonization by blocking the binding of bacterial cells to mammalian surfaces. Such factors include specific antibodies, salivary glycoproteins, mucins, and proline-rich proteins which may act as non-specific blocking agents (Gibbons 1984).

Once a bacterial cell has successfully attached to a surface in the subgingival area, other host mechanisms come into play. Desquamation of epithelial cells presents a new cleansing mechanism, which is overcome by certain species by their ability to bind to underlying epithelial cells (Freter 1985). Other species are able to invade the epithelial cells (Finlay & Falkow 1989; Rudney *et al.* 2001, 2005) and may multiply intracellularly and spread to adjacent cells.

Specific antibody in the subgingival area could act by preventing bacterial attachment or, in some instances, by making the bacterial cell susceptible to various phagocytic or killing mechanisms. A number of subgingival species have evolved mechanisms for evading the effect of specific antibody. Species including *P. gingivalis*, *Pr. intermedia*, *Pr. melaninogenica*, and *Capnocytophaga* species possess IgG and IgA proteases that can destroy antibody (Kilian 1981; Saito *et al.* 1987; Grenier *et al.* 1989). Other species are capable of evading antibody by changing their surface antigens (Gibbons & Qureshi 1980) or possibly by mimicking the host's antigens (Ellen 1985).

Polymorphonuclear leukocytes affect subgingival species in at least two ways: by phagocytosing and ultimately killing bacterial cells or by releasing their lysosomal enzymes into the crevice or pocket. A number of bacterial mechanisms exist that might counteract these effects, including the production of leukotoxin by *A. actinomycetemcomitans* (Baehni *et al.* 1979) and capsules by *P. gingivalis* and other species that inhibit phagocytosis (Okuda & Takazoe 1988). In addition, a number of species have developed strategies to interfere with the killing mechanisms of the polymorphonuclear leukocytes (Boehringer *et al.* 1986; Seow *et al.* 1987, 1989; Sela *et al.* 1988; Yoneda *et al.* 1990).

If a species enters the underlying connective tissue, it has moved into the area where the host's defense mechanisms are the most formidable. Polymorphonuclear leukocytes and antibodies are joined by macrophages and various types of lymphocytes, completing an awesome array of antagonistic cells and their biologically active substances. To be successful in this area a species would have to have evolved sophisticated mechanisms to evade, hide from or destroy opposition. Some of the periodontal pathogens may have devised such mechanisms. For example, it has been shown that *A. actinomycetemcomitans* leukotoxin affects not only polymorphonuclear leukocytes and monocytes (Baehni *et al.* 1979) but also kills mature T and B lymphocyte cell lines (Simpson *et al.* 1988) or facilitates a non-lethal suppression of immune cells (Rabie *et al.* 1988). Other species such as *Pr. intermedia, Porphyromonas endodontalis,* and *Tr. denticola* have been shown to produce substances that suppress immune mechanisms (Shenker *et al.* 1984, Ochiai *et al.* 1989, Shenker & Slots 1989).

Finally, artificial agents, including antiseptics and antibiotics, have been developed that augment the host's natural defense mechanisms against bacterial pathogens. In turn the microorganisms have evolved mechanisms of resistance to these agents and added insult to injury by having the ability to pass these resistance factors to one another, even across species (Guiney & Bouic 1990).

Factors that result in tissue damage

The set of properties that results in a species causing periodontal tissue loss in destructive periodontal diseases is poorly understood. Some or all tissue damage may result from an immunopathologic reaction triggered by a species which is sustained until the species is eliminated or suppressed. However, the fact that disease progression is rare, is associated with specific species, and that inflammation without attachment loss is common, suggest specificity in the properties

of organisms that lead to tissue damage. Two general mechanisms of pathogenesis have been hypothesized. The first involves invasion by subgingival species. The second suggests a "long-range" attack where cells of the pathogenic species remain in the pocket but fragments of cells as well as other "virulence factors" enter the underlying periodontal tissues and either directly damage the tissues or cause "immune pathology" (Allenspach-Petrzilka & Guggenheim 1982; Fillery & Pekovic 1982; Gillette & Johnson 1982; Sanavi *et al.* 1985; Saglie *et al.* 1986, 1988; Christersson *et al.* 1987; Liakoni *et al.* 1987; Listgarten 1988). More details on the mechanisms of pathogenesis may be found in Chapter 11.

Invasion

The possibility of invasion in periodontal infections gained credence with the unequivocal demonstration of invasion by a spirochete with an unique ultrastructural morphology during active episodes of acute necrotizing ulcerative gingivitis (Listgarten & Socransky 1964; Listgarten 1965). Other instances of invasion have been reported in tissues obtained from advanced periodontitis (Frank & Voegel 1978; Vitkov *et al.* 2005), LAP (Gillett & Johnson 1982; Christersson *et al.* 1987), and progressing periodontal lesions (Saglie *et al.* 1988).

As discussed earlier, strains of *A. actinomycetemcomitans* and *P. gingivalis* have been shown to be capable of invading epithelial cells derived from human periodontal pockets or gingival sulci. Other studies demonstrated that *T. forsythia* was present in high numbers in preparations of human periodontal pocket epithelial cells and cells of this species could be detected within the epithelial cells. The property of invasion of epithelial cells is a common property of a wide range of mucosal pathogens including members of the genera *Salmonella, Shigella, Yersinia, Escherichia,* and *Listeria.* The mechanisms of attachment to and subsequent entry differ from species to species. It is thought that fimbriae-mediated adhesion may be a prerequisite for bacterial invasion in periodontitis (Vitkov *et al.* 2005). The ability to enter into and survive within human cells confers an advantage to potential pathogens in that they are protected from many of the host's defense mechanisms.

Adherence to underlying tissues, such as basement membrane and various types of collagen, has been demonstrated (Winkler *et al.* 1987, 1988; Naito & Gibbons 1988). Strains of *F. nucleatum* and *P. gingivalis* adhere well to preparations of basement membrane and type IV collagen. *P. gingivalis* also adheres well to type I collagen, a property that may be useful in invasion of deeper tissues.

Deeper invasion may be important in progression of disease and could be facilitated by the property of motility. The flexible, sinuous spirochete has the physical tools to move through amorphous jelly-like intercellular matrix. If other virulence factors were present, it is likely that spirochetes and other motile forms such as *Selenomonas* and *Campylobacter* would have unique invasive capacities.

Factors that cause tissue damage

The microbial substances that lead to damage of the periodontal tissues are poorly understood, in large part because so many potential "virulence factors" have been described for subgingival species and their roles inadequately evaluated. Virulence factors can be arbitrarily divided into three categories: substances that damage tissue cells (e.g. hydrogen sulphide), substances that cause cells to release biologically active substances (e.g. lipopolysaccharide), and substances that affect the intercellular matrix (e.g. collagenase). There is an unfortunate overlap in this categorization, since some substances elicit more than one response. Further, factors that affect the cells involved in host defense mechanisms may inhibit protective responses and/or lead to the production of substances that can directly damage the tissues.

Some of the suspected virulence factors produced by three periodontal pathogens are summarized in Tables 9-1 to 9-3. Enzymes produced by subgingival species appear to be able to degrade virtually all of the macromolecules found in periodontal tissues. The periodontal pathogen, *P. gingivalis*, produces an unusually wide array of proteases, including those that degrade collagen (Gibbons & Macdonald 1961; Smalley *et al.* 1988; Winkler *et al.* 1988; Jin *et al.* 1989), immunoglobulins (Kilian 1981; Saito *et al.* 1987; Grenier *et al.* 1989), and fibronectin (Wikstrom & Linde 1986; Smalley *et al.* 1988; Lantz *et al.* 1990). Of particular interest are the cysteine proteinases commonly referred to ARG-gingipain and LYS-gingipain which are important to the organism in order to break down proteins to peptides and amino acids necessary for its growth (Abe *et al.* 1998; Genco *et al.* 1999; Kadowaki *et al.* 2000). These proteinases are also important in the processing/maturation of cell surface proteins of *P. gingivalis* such as *fim*A fimbrillin. Other species produce additional or other lytic enzymes. It might be argued that enzymes produced by bacterial species might not be necessary to the pathogenesis of periodontal diseases since similar enzymes can be derived from host tissue. However, if a specific lytic enzyme is essential to disease progression, current data suggest that some subgingival species would form it.

A wide variety of cell preparations or substances have been shown to adversely affect the growth and/ or metabolism of mammalian cells in tissue culture. Some of the substances are low molecular weight end-products of metabolism such as hydrogen sulphide, ammonia, fatty acids or indole (Socransky 1970; Singer & Buckner 1981; van Steenbergen *et al.* 1986). Other factors are less defined and are present in the extracellular milieu of bacterial cultures or extracts of the bacterial cells themselves. The importance of this group of inhibitory factors in the pathogenesis of disease is unclear. However, even minor inhibitions of cell metabolism might adversely affect structural integrity of the periodontal tissues.

It has been known for some time that certain bacterial products can induce organ cultures or tissue cells, including cells involved in host defense, to elaborate biologically active substances. One such factor derived from cultured white blood cells was initially described as osteoclast activating factor, since it accelerated bone resorption in tissue culture systems (Horton *et al.* 1972), but was later recognized as interleukin-1β (Dewhirst *et al.* 1985). Production of this factor was shown to be induced in a number of ways including stimulation by bacterial lipopolysaccharides or whole cells (Uchida *et al.* 2001). Numerous other biologically active mediators including prostaglandins, tumor necrosis factor, thymocyte activating factor, IL-8 (Uchida *et al.* 2001), and chemotactic factors have been shown to be formed in response to the addition of bacterial cells or their products to mammalian cells in tissue culture (Bom-van Noorloos *et al.* 1986; Millar *et al.* 1986; Garrison *et al.* 1988; Hanazawa *et al.* 1988; Lindemann 1988; Lindemann *et al.* 1988; Takada *et al.* 1988; Sismey-Durrant *et al.* 1989; Uitto *et al.* 1989). *P. gingivalis* can perturb the cytokine network not only by stimulating the release of cytokines from host cells, but by removing them from its local environment (Fletcher *et al.* 1997).

Virulence determinants in the genomics era

The study of mechanisms of virulence by oral subgingival species has been ongoing for many years and should exhibit a quantum leap due to the sequencing of the genomes of a number of subgingival species. To date, 308 bacterial genomes have been sequenced, 15 of these represent 13 distinct oral species (Duncan 2005; Kolenbrander *et al.* 2006). The knowledge of the sequences can lead to the development of microarrays to monitor gene expression by suspected periodontal pathogens while colonizing or invading oral tissues. Microarrays are already available for *P. gingivalis*, *S. mutans*, *A. actinomycetemcomitans*, *Tr. denticola*, and *F. nucleatum*. The search of the sequence genomes of periodontal species will undoubtedly reveal a large number of potential virulence factors. Unfortunately, it is an expensive and time-consuming process to evaluate whether the proposed factors actually play a role in human disease.

Effect of therapy on subgingival biofilms

There is an axiom in ecology that perturbations of a complex ecosystem are generally followed by a return

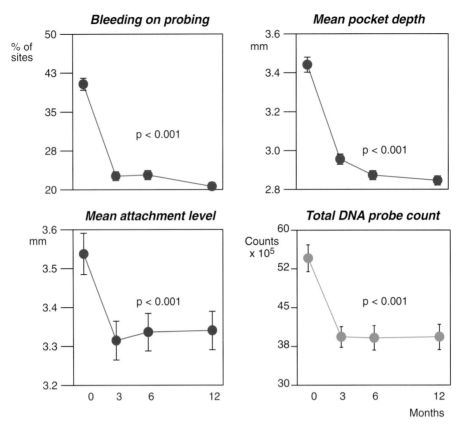

Fig. 9-23 Mean (± SEM) percentage of sites with bleeding on probing, mean pocket depth and attachment level and mean total DNA probe counts at baseline (pre-therapy), and at 3, 6, and 12 months post therapy in 493 chronic periodontitis subjects. The data for each clinical parameter were measured at up to 168 sites in each subject and averaged within a subject and then across subjects at each time point separately. For the microbiological data, mean values were computed by summing the DNA probe counts for each species in up to 28 subgingival plaque samples in each subject, and then averaging across subjects at the four time points separately. The significance of differences over time was determined using the Friedman test.

to an ecosystem of essentially the same composition. Thus, if a clinician alters a complex ecosystem, such as the subgingival biofilm, the expectation of an ecologist would be that, in general, the microbiota would return to a microbiota with a composition similar to that observed pre-therapy. Indeed as discussed earlier, within 4–7 days of biofilm removal by SRP the total numbers of microorganisms at a site had returned to pre-cleaning levels in the absence of home care procedures. Thus, key questions are whether the *composition* of the subgingival biofilm in periodontitis subjects is altered by periodontal therapy to one that is more compatible with health, and if it is, whether the beneficial changes are maintained for prolonged periods of time. Figure 9-23 presents the mean changes in the percentage of sites with bleeding on probing, mean probing pocket depth, and mean clinical attachment level before therapy and at 3, 6, and 12 months post therapy in 493 chronic periodontitis subjects who received different forms of periodontal therapy. All had received SRP and instruction in proper home care and some had received, in addition, periodontal surgery and/ or systemically administered antibiotics. The major

improvement in the clinical parameters occurred between baseline and 3 months post therapy with little change or modest improvement occurring from 3–12 months. Also depicted in this figure are the changes in mean total DNA probe counts at the same time points. The microbiological changes followed the same pattern as the clinical changes and were characterized by marked reductions in total bacterial counts between baseline and 3 months with minimal change thereafter.

Figure 9-24 presents the change in microbial composition of the subgingival biofilm from baseline to 12 months in the subjects presented in Fig. 9-23. There was a major reduction in the counts, proportions, and percentage of sites colonized at levels $>10^5$ for many of the test species. In particular, species of the red and orange complexes, the species associated with the etiology and pathogenesis of periodontal diseases, were significantly reduced by the various forms of therapy and the reductions were still evident 12 months after therapy. Thus, an improvement in mean clinical parameters was accompanied by a mean reduction in total bacterial counts and specifically reductions in the levels of many periodontal patho-

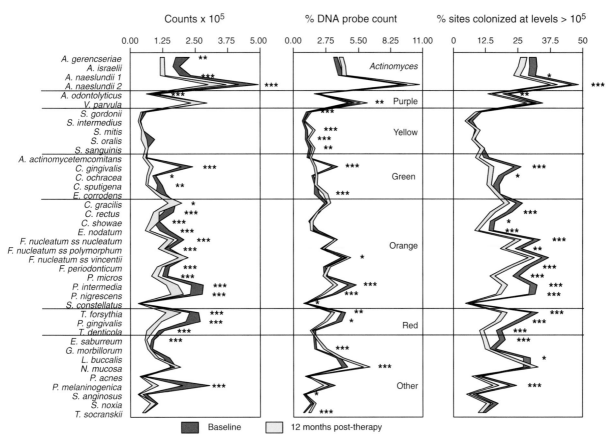

Fig. 9-24 Plots of mean counts (left panel), percents of the total DNA probe count (middle panel) and percentage of sites colonized by 40 bacterial species at counts >10^5 (right panel) in subgingival plaque samples taken from the subjects in Fig. 9-23 at baseline and 12 months post therapy. The "bands" represent the mean values ± SEM. Mean values for each species were computed by averaging up to 28 samples in each subject, and then averaging across subjects at the two time points. Significance of differences between groups was sought using the non-parametric Wilcoxon signed ranks test; * $p < 0.05$, ** $p < 0.01$, *** $p < 0.001$ after adjusting for multiple comparisons (Socransky *et al.* 1991). The species were ordered and grouped according to the complexes described by Socransky *et al.* (1998). The red profiles represent baseline data and the yellow profiles represent data at 12 months. Reprinted with permission from Blackwell Publishing (Haffajee *et al.* 2006b, *Periodontology 2000* **43**, 219–258).

gens. However, not all sites within a subject responded equally well to therapy. Figure 9-25 presents the change in the 40 test species from before therapy to 12 months post therapy at sites that showed improvement in attachment level of >2 mm, sites that showed loss of attachment >2 mm, and sites where the change in attachment level was between these two extremes. There were significant reductions from baseline to 12 months in the mean counts of many of the test species at sites that exhibited change in attachment level ≤2 mm or a "gain" of >2 mm. Not surprisingly the majority of these species were those of the red and orange complexes. In contrast, sites that showed loss of attachment at 12 months post therapy exhibited few changes in the counts of any of the test species, underscoring the association between clinical improvement and reductions in the levels of periodontal pathogens.

As mentioned earlier, not all periodontal therapies work equally well in all subjects, a finding likely related to, among other factors, the nature of the subgingival microbiota prior to therapy. Two systematic

reviews have suggested that adjunctive systemically administered antibiotics can provide better clinical outcomes when compared with scaling and root planing only (Herrera *et al.* 2002; Haffajee *et al.* 2003). Figure 9-26 presents the 12-month microbiological findings in subjects who received SRP only (left panel) and those who received different systemically administered antibiotics as adjuncts to SRP (right panel). While, overall, both therapeutic modalities provided clinical improvements and reductions in bacterial counts, subjects receiving the adjunctive antibiotics exhibited a better clinical response as well as more species, particularly those of the red and orange complexes, with significant reductions which were maintained to 12 months post therapy. The reader may wonder why antibiotics have an effect on the composition of the subgingival microbiota, when these species are living in a protected biofilm environment as described earlier in this chapter. Among the possible explanations would be the disruption of the subgingival biofilm by scaling and root planing during or before antibiotic administration, the

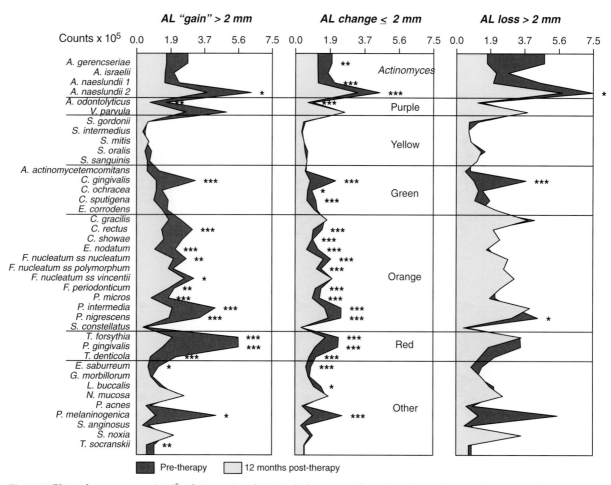

Fig. 9-25 Plots of mean counts ($\times 10^5$) of 40 taxa in subgingival plaque samples at baseline and 12 months at sites that exhibited attachment level "gain" >2 mm, (left panel), change ≤2 mm (middle panel) or loss >2 mm (right panel) from baseline to 12 months. Counts of each species at sites in each of the three attachment level change categories were determined, averaged within a subject, and then averaged across subjects in the three site categories at pre-therapy and 12 months post-therapy separately. Significance of differences between counts at baseline and 12 months was determined using the Wilcoxon signed ranks test and adjusted for multiple comparisons; * p < 0.05; ** p < 0.01; *** p < 0.001. Species were ordered according to microbial complexes. The red panels represent the pre-therapy values and the yellow panels represent the 12 months post-therapy values. Reprinted with permission from Blackwell Publishing (Haffajee *et al.* 2006b, *Periodontology 2000* **43**, 219–258).

location of the red and orange complex species adjacent to the epithelial lining of the periodontal pocket (the site of entry of antibiotics into the periodontal pocket), and the possibility that antibiotics may affect pathogens that are located within mammalian tissue cells. Whatever the reason, it is clear that adjunctive systemic antibiotics lowered the levels of periodontal pathogens and improved clinical parameters significantly more than scaling and root planing alone and may be useful in the treatment of some periodontal infections.

Final comment

Infections of any organ system are caused by a relatively finite set of pathogens sometimes working individually or, occasionally, in small mixtures. For example, lung infections may be caused by any of a variety of organisms, including *M. tuberculosis*, *S.*

pneumoniae, and *K. pneumoniae*. No single therapy is effective against all lung infections. Each of these infections requires the use of a different chemotherapeutic agent and the selection of the agent is based on the findings of diagnostic tests. The analogy to periodontal infections is clear. There is no single cause of these infections, no one treatment can control all the infections, and the choice of treatment should be guided by the nature of the infecting microbiota. Obviously a great deal of additional research is needed to define precisely the contribution of each periodontal pathogen to periodontal disease progression, to devise tests for their presence and to determine the best therapy for each pathogen's suppression. However, when the most appropriate anti-infective therapy is applied to a given subject or site, disease progression should, at least, be stopped and the potential for long-term periodontal stability should be markedly enhanced.

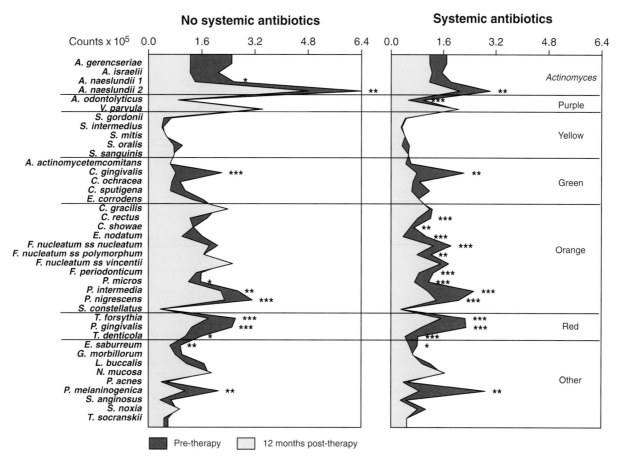

Fig. 9-26 Profiles of mean counts ($\times 10^5$) of 40 taxa in subgingival plaque samples taken pre-therapy and 12 months post-therapy from subjects who did not (left panel) or did receive systemic antibiotics (right panel) as part of their periodontal therapy. Plaque samples were taken from the mesial aspect of each tooth and analyzed separately for their content of 40 species. Data for each species were averaged within in each subject and then across subjects in the two treatment groups for each time point separately. Significance of differences between pre-therapy and 12 months post-therapy was sought using the Wilcoxon test and adjusted for multiple comparisons; * $p < 0.05$; ** $p < 0.01$; *** $p < 0.001$. Species were ordered according to microbial complexes. The red panels represent the pre-therapy values and the yellow panels represent the 12 months post-therapy values. Reprinted with permission from Blackwell Publishing (Haffajee *et al.* 2006b, *Periodontology 2000* **43**, 219–258).

References

Abe, N., Kadowaki, T., Okamoto, K., Nakayama, K., Ohishi, M. & Yamamoto, K. (1998). Biochemical and functional properties of lysine-specific cysteine proteinase (Lys-gingipain) as a virulence factor of *Porphyromonas gingivalis* in periodontal disease. *Journal of Biochemistry (Tokyo)* **123**, 305–312.

Abeygunawardana, C., Bush, C.A. & Cisar, J.O. (1990). Complete structure of the polysaccharide from *Streptococcus sanguis* J22. *Biochemistry* **29**, 234–248.

Alaluusua, S., Saarela, M., Jousimies-Somer, H. & Asikainen, S. (1993). Ribotyping shows intrafamilial similarity in *Actinobacillus actinomycetemcomitans* isolates. *Oral Microbiology & Immunology* **8**, 225–229.

Albandar, J.M., Brown, L.J. & Loe, H. (1997). Putative periodontal pathogens in subgingival plaque of young adults with and without early-onset periodontitis. *Journal of Periodontology* **68**, 973–981.

Allenspach-Petrzilka, G.E. & Guggenheim, B. (1982). *Bacteroides melaninogenicus* subsp. *intermedius* invades rat gingival tissue. *Journal of Dental Research* **61**, 259.

Altman, L.C., Page, R.C., Ebersole, J.L. & Vandesteen, E.G. (1982). Assessment of host defenses and serum antibodies to suspected periodontal pathogens in patients with various types of periodontitis. *Journal of Periodontal Research* **17**, 495–497.

Alves, A.C., Napimoga, M.H., Klein, M.I., Hofling, J.F. & Goncalves, R.B. (2006). Increase in probing depth is correlated with a higher number of *Prevotella intermedia* genotypes. *Journal of Periodontology* **77**, 61–66.

Amano, A. Kuboniwa, M., Nakagawa, I., Akiyama, S., Morisaki, I. & Hamada, S. (2000). Prevalence of specific genotypes of *Porphyromonas gingivalis* fimA and periodontal health status. *Journal of Dental Research* **79**, 1664–1668.

Arakawa, S., Nakajima, T., Ishikura, H., Ichinose, S., Ishikawa, I. & Tsuchida, N. (2000). Novel apoptosis-inducing activity in *Bacteroides forsythus*: a comparative study with three serotypes of *Actinobacillus actinomycetemcomitans*. *Infection and Immunity* **68**, 4611–4615.

Asikainen, S., Lai, CH., Alaluusua, S. & Slots, J. (1991). Distribution of *Actinobacillus actinomycetemcomitans* serotypes in periodontal health and disease. *Oral Microbiology & Immunology* **6**, 115–118.

Bachrach, G., Rosen, G., Bellalou, M., Naor, R. & Sela, M.N. (2004). Identification of a *Fusobacterium nucleatum* 65 kDa serine protease. *Oral Microbiology & Immunology* **19**, 155–159.

Baehni, P., Tsai, C.C., McArthur, W.P., Hammond, B.F. & Taichman, N.S. (1979). Interaction of inflammatory cells and oral microorganisms. VIII. Detection of leukotoxic activity of a plaque-derived gram-negative microorganism. *Infection & Immunity* **24**, 233–243.

Baker, P.J., Dixon, M., Evans, R.T. & Roopenian, D.C. (2000). Heterogeneity of *Porphyromonas gingivalis* strains in the induction of alveolar bone loss in mice. *Oral Microbiology and Immunology* **15**, 27–32.

Barnett, M.L., Baker, R.L., Yancey, J.M., MacMillan, D.R. & Kotoyan, M. (1984). Absence of periodontitis in a population of insulin-dependent diabetes mellitus (IDDM). patients. *Journal of Periodontology* **55**, 402–405.

Barua, P.K., Dyer, D.W. & Neiders, M.E. (1990). Effect of iron limitation on *Bacteroides gingivalis*. *Oral Microbiology & Immunology* **5**, 263–268.

Beck, J.D., Cusmano, L., Green Helms, W., Koch, G.G. & Offenbacher, S. (1997). A 5-year study of attachment loss in community-dwelling older adults: incidence density. *Journal of Periodontal Research* **32**, 506–515.

Beck, J.D., Eke, P., Heiss, G., Madianos, P., Couper, D., Lin, D., Moss, K., Elter, J. & Offenbacher, S. (2005) Periodontal disease and coronary heart disease: a reappraisal of the exposure. *Circulation* **112**, 19–24.

Beck, J.D., Eke, P., Lin, D., Madianos, P., Couper, D., Moss, K., Elter, J., Heiss, G. & Offenbacher, S. (2005). Associations between IgG antibody to oral organisms and carotid intima-medial thickness in community-dwelling adults. *Atherosclerosis* **183**, 342–348.

Beck, J.D., Koch, G.G., Rozier, R.G. & Tudor, G.E. (1990). Prevalence and risk indicators for periodontal attachment loss in a population of older community-dwelling blacks and whites. *Journal of Periodontology* **61**, 521–528.

Beck, J.D., Koch, G.G., Zambon, J.J., Genco, R.J. & Tudor, G.E. (1992). Evaluation of oral bacteria as risk indicators for periodontitis in older adults. *Journal of Periodontology* **63**, 93–99.

Becker, M.R., Paster, B.J., Leys, E.J., Moeschberger, M.L., Kenyon, S.G., Galvin, J.L., Boches, S.K., Dewhirst, F.E. & Griffen, A.L. (2002). Molecular analysis of bacterial species associated with early childhood caries. *Journal of Clinical Microbiology* **40**, 1001–1009.

Beckwith, T.D., Simonton, F.V. & Williams, A. (1925). A histologic study of the gum in pyorrhea. *Journal of the American Dental Association* **12**, 129–153.

Belding, P.H. & Belding, L. J. (1936). Bacteria – dental orphans. *Dental Cosmos* **78**, 506–513.

Berglundh, T., Krok, L., Liljenberg, B., Westfelt, E., Serino, G. & Lindhe, J. (1998). The use of metronidazole and amoxicillin in the treatment of advanced periodontal disease. A prospective, controlled clinical trial. *Journal of Clinical Periodontology* **25**, 354–362.

Bergstrom, J. & Eliasson, S. (1987). Noxious effect of cigarette smoking on periodontal health. *Journal of Periodontal Research* **22**, 513–517.

Blix, I.J., Hars, R., Preus, H.R. & Helgeland, K. (1992). Entrance of *Actinobacillus actinomycetemcomitans* into HEp-2 cells in vitro. *Journal of Periodontology* **63**, 723–728.

Bodet, C., Chandad, F. & Grenier, D. (2006). Inflammatory responses of a macrophage/epitheilial co-culture to mono and mixed infections with *Porphyromonas gingivalis, Treponena denticola* and *Tannerella forsythia*. *Microbes and Infection* **8**, 27–35.

Boehringer, H.R., Berthold, P.H. & Taichman, N.S. (1986). Studies on the interaction of human neutrophils with plaque spirochetes. *Journal of Periodontal Research* **21**, 195–209.

Bom-van Noorloos, A.A., Schipper, C.A., van Steenbergen, T.J.M., de Graaf, J. & Burger, E.H. (1986). *Bacteroides gingivalis* activates mouse spleen cells to produce a factor that stimulates resorptive activity of osteoclasts in vitro. *Journal of Periodontal Research* **21**, 440–444.

Booth, V., Downes, J., Van den Berg, J. & Wade, W.G. (2004). Gram-positive anaerobic bacilli in human periodontal disease. *Journal of Periodontal Research* **39**, 213–220.

Boutaga, K., van Winkelhoff, A.J., Vandenbroucke-Grauls, C.M. & Savelkoul, P.H. (2006). The additional value of real-time PCR in the quantitative detection of periodontal pathogens. *Journal of Clinical Periodontology* **33**, 427–433.

Bragd, L., Dahlen, G., Wikstrom, M. & Slots, J. (1987). The capability of *Actinobacillus actinomycetemcomitans, Bacteroides gingivalis* and *Bacteroides intermedius* to indicate progressive periodontitis; a retrospective study. *Journal of Clinical Periodontology* **14**, 95–99.

Bramanti, T.E. & Holt, S.C. (1990). Iron-regulated outer membrane proteins in the periodontopathic bacterium, *Bacteroides gingivalis*. *Biochemistry & Biophysics Research Communications* **166**, 1146–1154.

Brill, C.B., Pearlstein, L.S., Kaplan, M. & Mancall, E.L. (1982). CNS infections caused by *Eikenella corrodens*. *Achives of Neurology* **39**, 431–432.

Buduneli, N., Baylas, H., Buduneli, E., Turkoglu, O., Kose, T. & Dahlen, G. (2005). Periodontal infections and pre-term low birth weight: a case-control study. *Journal of Clinical Periodontology* **32**, 174–181.

Bueno, L.C., Mayer, M.P. & DiRienzo, J.M. (1998). Relationship between conversion of localized juvenile periodontitis-susceptible children from health to disease and *Actinobacillus actinomycetemcomitans* leukotoxin promter structure. *Journal of Periodontology* **70**, 998–1007.

Burdon K.L. (1928). *Bacterium melaninogenicum* from normal and pathologic tissues. *Journal of Infectious Diseases* **42**, 161–171.

Carter, K.C. (1987). *Essays of Robert Koch*. New York: Greenwood Press, pp. xvii–xix, 161.

Caugant, D.A., Kristiansen, B-E., Froholm, L.O., Bovre, K. & Selander, R.K. (1988). Clonal diversity of *Neisseria meningitidis* from a population of asymptomatic carriers. *Infection & Immunity* **56**, 2060–2068.

Chaves, E.S., Jeffcoat, M.K., Ryerson, C.C. & Snyder, B. (2000). Persistent bacterial colonization of *Porphyromonas gingivalis, Prevotella intermedia* and *Actinobacillus actinomycetemcomitans* in periodontitis and its association with alveolar bone loss after 6 months of therapy. *Journal of Clinical Periodontology* **27**, 897–903.

Chen, C.K., Dunford, P.G., Reynolds, H.S. & Zambon, J.J. (1989). *Eikenella corrodens* in the human oral cavity. *Journal of Periodontology* **60**, 611–616.

Chen, H.A., Johnson, B.D., Sims, T.J., Darveau, R.P., Moncla, B.J., Whitney, C.W., Engel, D. & Page, R.C. (1991). Humoral immune responses to *Porphyromonas gingivalis* before and following therapy in rapidly progressive periodontitis patients. *Journal of Periodontology* **62**, 781–791.

Choi, B.K., Park, S.H., Yoo, Y.J., Choi, S.H., Chai, J.K., Cho, K.S. & Kim, C.K. (2000). Detection of major putative periodontopathogens in Korean advanced adult periodontitis patients using nucleic acid-based approach. *Journal of Periodontology* **71**, 1387–1394.

Choi, B.K., Paster, B.J., Dewhirst, F.E. & Göbel, U. (1994). Diversity of cultivable and uncultivable oral spirochetes from a patient with severe destructive periodontitis. *Infection & Immunity* **62**, 1889–1895.

Choi, B-K., Wyss, C. & Gobel, U.B. (1996). Phylogenetic analysis of pathogen related oral spirochetes. *Journal of Clinical Microbiology* **34**, 1922–1925.

Christersson, L.A., Albini, B., Zambon, J.J., Wikesjo, U.M.E. & Genco, R.J. (1987). Tissue localization of *Actinobacillus actinomycetemcomitans* in human periodontitis. I. Light, immunofluorescence and electron microscopic studies. *Journal of Periodontology* **58**, 529–539.

Christersson, L.A., Slots, J., Rosling, B.G. & Genco, R.J. (1985). Microbiological and clinical effects of surgical treatment of localized juvenile periodontitis. *Journal of Clinical Periodontology* **12**, 465–476.

Chung, H-J., Chung, C-P., Son, S-H. & Nisengard, R.J. (1989). *Actinobacillus actinomycetemcomitans* serotypes and leukotoxicity in Korean localized juvenile periodontitis. *Journal of Periodontology* **60**, 506–511.

Cimasoni, G. (1983). *Crevicular fluid updated*. Monographs in Oral Science 12, Basel: Karger, p. 71.

Cisar, J.O., Sandberg, A.L. & Mergenhagen, S.E. (1984). The function and distribution of different fimbriae on strains of *Actinomyces viscosus* and *Actinomyces naeslundii*. *Journal of Dental Research* **63**, 393–396.

Clark, W.B., Wheeler, T.T., Lane, M.D. & Cisar, J.O. (1986). *Actinomyces* adsorption mediated by Type-1 fimbriae. *Journal of Dental Research* **65**, 1166–1168.

Cobe H.M. (1948). Vincent's infection: experimental reproduction of lesions and the role of streptococci. *Journal of the American Dental Association* **37**, 317–324.

Cole, J.R., Chai, B., Farris, R.J., Wang, Q., Kulam, S.A., McGarrell, D.M., Garrity, G.M. & Tiedje, J.M. (2005). The Ribosomal Database Project (RDP-II): sequences and tools for high-throughput rRNA analysis. *Nucleic Acids Research* **33**, D294–D296.

Colombo, A.P., Haffajee, A.D., Dewhirst, F.E., Paster, B.J., Smith, C.M., Cugini. M.A. & Socransky, S.S. (1998a). Clinical and microbiological features of refractory periodontitis. *Journal of Clinical Periodontology* **25**, 169–180.

Colombo, A.P., Sakellari, D., Haffajee, A.D., Tanner, A., Cugini, M.A. & Socransky, S.S. (1998b). Serum antibodies reacting with subgingival species in refractory periodontitis subjects. *Journal of Clinical Periodontology* **25**, 596–604.

Colombo, A.V., Silva, C.M., Haffajee, A. & Colombo, A.P. (2006). Identification of oral bacteria associated with crevicular epithelial cells from chronic periodontitis lesions. *Journal of Medical Microbiology* **55**, 609–615.

Colombo, A.P., Teles, R.P., Torres, M.C., Rosalem, W., Mendes, M.C., Souto. R.M. & Uzeda, M. (2005). Effects of non-surgical mechanical therapy on the subgingival microbiota of Brazilians with untreated chronic periodontitis: 9 month results. *Journal of Periodontology* **76**, 778–784.

Colombo, A., Teles, R.P., Torres, M.C., Souto, R., Rosalem, W.J., Mendes, M.C. & Uzeda, M. (2002). Subgingival microbiota of Brazilian subjects with untreated chronic periodontitis. *Journal of Periodontology* **73**, 360–369.

Consensus report for periodontal diseases: pathogenesis and microbial factors. (1996). *Annals of Periodontology* **1**, 926–932.

Contreras, A., Rusitanonta, T., Chen, C., Wagner, W.G., Michalowicz, B.S. & Slots, J. (2000). Frequency of 530-bp deletion in *Actinobacillus actinomycetemcomitans* leukotoxin promoter region. *Oral Microbiology and Immunology* **15**, 338–340.

Cortelli, J.R., Cortelli, S.C., Jordan, S., Haraszthy, V.I. & Zambon, J.J. (2005). Prevalence of periodontal pathogens in Brazilians with aggressive or chronic periodontitis. *Journal of Clinical Periodontology* **32**, 860–866.

Costerton, J.W., Cook, G. & Lamont, R. (1999). The community architecture of biofilms: dynamic structures and mechanisms. In: Newman, H.N. & Wilson, M., eds. *Dental Plaque Revisited*. Cardiff: Bioline, pp. 5–14.

Cugini, M.A., Haffajee, A.D., Smith, C., Kent, Jr. R.L. & Socransky, S. (2000). The effect of SRP on the clinical and microbiological parameters of periodontal diseases. 12 month results. *Journal of Clinical Periodontology* **27**, 30–36.

Curtis, M.A., Slaney, J.M., Carman, R.J. & Johnson, N.W. (1991). Identification of the major surface protein antigens of Porphyromonas gingivalis using IgG antibody reactivity of periodontal case-control serum. *Oral Microbiology & Immunology* **6**, 321–326.

Dahan M., Nawrocki, B., Elkaim, R., Soell, M., Bolcato-Bellemin, A.L., Birembaut, P. & Tenenbaum, H. (2001). Expression of matrix metalloproteinases in healthy and diseased human gingiva. *Journal of Clinical Periodontology* **28**, 128–136.

Dahlen, G., Manji, F., Baelum, V. & Fejerskov, O. (1989). Black-pigmented Bacteroides species and *Actinobacillus actinomy-cetemcomitans* in subgingival plaque of adult Kenyans. *Journal of Clinical Periodontology* **16**, 305–310.

Daley, F.H. (1927a). Vincent's gingivitis in Boston in 1926. *Apollonium* **2**, 69–83.

Daley, F.H. (1927b). Vincent's gingivitis in Boston; report no. II. *Apollonium* **2**, 203–206.

Darby, I.B., Hodge, P.J., Riggio, M.P. & Kinane, D.F. (2005). Clinical and microbiological effect of scaling and root planing in smoker and non-smoker chronic and aggressive periodontitis patients. *Journal of Clinical Periodontology* **32**, 200–206.

Darby, I.B., Mooney, J. & Kinane, D.F. (2001). Changes in subgingival microflora and humoral immune response following periodontal therapy. *Journal of Clinical Periodontology* **28**, 796–805.

Darveau, R.P., Belton, C.M., Reife, R.A. & Lamont, R.J. (1998). Local chemokine paralysis, a novel pathogenic mechanism for *Porphyromonas gingivalis*. *Infection and Immunity* **66**, 1660–1665.

de Pommereau, V., Dargent-Pare, C., Robert, J.J. & Brion, M. (1992). Periodontal status in insulin-dependent diabetic adolescents. *Journal of Clinical Periodontology* **19**, 628–632.

Deshpande, R.G. & Khan, M.B. (1999). Purification and characterization of hemolysin from *Porphyromonas gingivalis* A7436. *FEMS Microbiology Letters* **176**, 387–394.

Dewhirst, F.E., Stashenko, P.P., Mole, J.E. & Tsurumachi, T. (1985). Purification and partial sequence of human osteoclast-activating factor: identity with interleukin 1β. *Journal of Immunology* **135**, 2562–2568.

Dewhirst, F.E., Tamer, M.A., Ericson, R.E., Lau, C.N., Levanos, V.A., Boches, S.K., Galvin, J.L. & Paster, B.J. (2000). The diversity of periodontal spirochetes by 16S rRNA analysis. *Oral Microbiology and Immunology* **15**, 196–202.

Dibart, S, Skobe, Z., Snapp, K.R., Socransky, S.S., Smith, C. & Kent, R. (1998). Identification of bacterial species on or in crevicular epithelial cells from healthy and periodontally diseased patients using DNA–DNA hybridization. *Oral Microbiology and Immunology*, **13**, 30–35.

DiRienzo, J.M. & McKay, T.L. (1994). Identification and characterization of genetic cluster groups of *Actinobacillus actinomycetemcomitans* isolated from the human oral cavity. *Journal of Clinical Microbiology* **32**, 75–81.

DiRienzo, J.M. & Slots, J. (1990). Genetic approach to the study of epidemiology and pathogenesis of *Actinobacillus actinomycetemcomitans* in localized juvenile periodontitis. *Archives of Oral Biology* **35** (Suppl), 79S–84S.

DiRienzo, J.M., Slots, J., Sixou, M., Sol, M-A., Harmon, R. & McKay, T.L. (1994). Specific genetic variants of *Actinobacillus actinomycetemcomitans* correlate with disease and health in a regional population of families with localized juvenile periodontitis. *Infection & Immunity* **62**, 3058–3065.

Dogan, B., Antinheimo, J., Cetiner, D., Bodur, A., Emingil, G., Buduneli, E., Uygur, C., Firatli, E., Lakio, L. & Asikainen, S. (2003). Subgingival microflora in Turkish patients with periodontitis. *Journal of Periodontology* **74**, 803–814.

Dogan, B., Buduneli, E., Emingil, G., Atilla, G., Akilli, A., Antinheimo, J., Lakio, L. & Asikainen, S. (2005). Charateristics of periodontal microflora in acute myocardial infarction. *Journal of Periodontology* **76**, 740–748.

Dogan, B., Saarela, M.H., Jousimies-Somer, H., Alaluusua, S. & Asikainen, S. (1999). *Actinobacillus actinomycetemcomitans* serotype e-biotypes, genetic diversity and distribution in relation to periodontal status. *Oral Microbiology and Immunology* **14**, 98–103.

Dongari-Bagtzoglou, A.I. & Ebersole, J.L. (1996). Production of inflammatory mediators and cytokines by human gingival fibroblasts following bacterial challenge. *Journal of Periodontal Research* **31**, 90–98.

Dorn, B.R., Leung, K.L. & Progulske-Fox, A. (1998). Invasion of human oral epithelial cells by *Prevotella intermedia*. *Infection and Immunity* **66**, 6054–6057.

Duncan, A.J., Carman, R.J., Harper, F.H., Griffiths, G.S. & Curtis, M.A. (1992). *Porphyromonas gingivalis*: presence of a species-specific antigen which is discriminatory in chronic inflammatory adult periodontal disease. *Microbial Ecology in Health and Disease* **5**, 15–20.

Duncan, L., Yoshioka, M., Chandad, F. & Grenier, D. (2004). Loss of lipopolysaccharide receptor CD14 from the surface of human macrophage-like cells mediated by *Porphyromonas gingivalis* outer membrane vesicles. *Microbial Pathogenesis* **36**, 319–325.

Duncan, M.J. (2005). Oral microbiology and genomics. *Periodontology 2000* **38**, 63–71.

Duncan, M.J., Nakao, S., Skobe, Z. & Xie, H. (1993). Interactions of *Porphyromonas gingivalis* with epithelial cells. *Infection & Immunity* **61**, 2260–2265.

Dzink, J.L., Gibbons, R.J., Childs, III W.C. & Socransky, S.S. (1989). The predominant cultivable microbiota of crevicular epithelial cells. *Oral Microbiology & Immunology* **4**, 1–5.

Dzink, J.L., Socransky, S.S., Ebersole, J.L. & Frey, D.E. (1983). ELISA and conventional techniques for identification of black-pigmented *Bacteroides* isolated from periodontal pockets. *Journal of Periodontal Research* **18**, 369–374.

Dzink, J.L., Socransky, S.S. & Haffajee, A.D. (1988). The predominant cultivable microbiota of active and inactive lesions of destructive periodontal diseases. *Journal of Clinical Periodontology* **15**, 316–323.

Dzink, J.L., Tanner, A.C.R., Haffajee, A.D. & Socransky, S.S. (1985). Gram negative species associated with active destructive periodontal lesions. *Journal of Clinical Periodontology* **12**, 648–659.

Ebersole, J.L., Brunsvold, M., Steffensen, B., Wood, R. & Holt, S.C. (1991). Effects of immunization with *Porphyromonas gingivalis* and *Prevotella intermedia* on progression of ligature-induced periodontitis in the nonhuman primate Macaca fascicularis. *Infection & Immunity* **59**, 3351–3359.

Ebersole, J.L., Taubman, M.A. & Smith, D.J. (1985). Gingival crevicular fluid antibody to oral microorganisms. II. Distribution and specificity of local antibody responses. *Journal of Periodontal Research* **20**, 349–356.

Ebersole, J.L., Taubman, M.A., Smith, D.J., Frey, D.E., Haffajee, A.D. & Socransky, S.S. (1987). Human serum antibody responses to oral microorganisms IV. Correlation with homologous infection. *Oral Microbiology & Immunology* **2**, 53–59.

Ebersole, J.L., Taubman, M.A., Smith, D.J., Genco, R.J. & Frey D.E. (1982). Human immune responses to oral microorganisms. I. Association of localized juvenile periodontitis (LJP) with serum antibody responses to *Actinobacillus actinomycetemcomitans*. *Clinical Experimental Immunology* **47**, 43–52.

Ellen, R.P. (1985). Specificity of attachment as a tissue-tropic influence on oral bacteria. In: Mergenhagen, S.E. & Rosan, B., eds. *Molecular Basis of Microbial Adhesion*. Washington: American Society for Microbiology, pp. 33–39.

Ellen, R.P. (2005). Virulence determinants of oral treponemes. In: Radolf, J.D. & Lukehart, S.A., eds, *Pathogenic Treponema: Molecular and Cellular Biology*. Wymondham, Norfolk, England: Caister Academic Press, pp. 357–385.

Ellen, R.P. & Galimanas, V.B. (2005). Spirochetes at the forefront of periodontal infections. *Periodontology 2000* **38**, 13–32.

Ellen, R.P. & Grove, D.A. (1989). *Bacteroides gingivalis* vesicles bind to and aggregate *Actinomyces viscosus*. *Infection & Immunity* **57**, 618–620.

Emmerson, A.M. & Mills, F. (1978). Recurrent meningitis and brain abscess caused by *Eikenella corrodens*. *Postgraduate Medical Journal* **54**, 343–345.

Evans, R.J. (1951). Haematin as a growth factor for a strict anaerobe *Fusiformis melaninogenicus*. *Proceedings of the Society for General Microbiology* **5**, XIX.

Evans, R.T., Klausen, B., Sojar, H.T., Bedi, G.S., Sfintescu, C., Ramamurthy, N.S. & Genco, R.J. (1992). Immunization with *Porphyromonas (Bacteroides) gingivalis* fimbriae protects against periodontal destruction. *Infection & Immunity* **60**, 2926–2935.

Feres, M., Haffajee, A.D., Allard, K.A., Som, S. & Socransky, S.S. (2000). Change in subgingival microbial profiles in adult periodontitis subjects receiving either systemically administered amoxicillin or metronidazole. *Journal of Clinical Periodontology* **28**, 597–609.

Fiehn, N.E., Larsen, T., Christiansen, N., Holmstrp, P. & Schroeder, T.V. (2005). Identification of periodontal pathogens in atherosclerotic vessels. *Journal of Periodontology* **76**, 731–736.

Fillery, E.D. & Pekovic, D.D. (1982). Identification of microorganisms in immunological mechanisms on human gingivitis. *Journal of Dental Research* **61**, 253.

Fine, D.H., Kaplan, J.B., Kachlany, S.C. & Scheiner, H.C. (2006). How we got attached to *Actinobacillus actinomycetemcomitans*: a model for infectious diseases. *Periodontology 2000* **42**, 1114–1157.

Finegold, S.M. (1977). *Anaerobic Bacteria and Human Disease*. New York: Academic Press, p. 44.

Finlay, B.B. & Falkow, S. (1989). Common themes in microbial pathogenicity. *Microbiological Reviews* **53**, 210–230.

Fletcher, J., Nair, S., Poole, S., Henderson, B. & Wilson, M. (1998). Cytokine degradation by biofilms of *Porphyromonas gingivalis*. *Current Microbiology* **36**, 216–219.

Fletcher, J., Reddi, K., Poole, S., Nair, S., Henderson, B., Tabona, P. & Wilson, M. (1997). Interactions between periodontopathogenic bacteria and cytokines. *Journal of Periodontal Research* **32**, 200–205.

Forscher, B.K., Paulsen, A.G. & Hess, W.C. (1954). The pH of the periodontal pocket and the glycogen content of the adjacent tissue. *Journal of Dental Research* **33**, 444–453.

Frank, R.M. & Voegel, J.C. (1978). Bacterial bone resorption in advanced cases of human periodontitis. *Journal of Periodontal Research* **13**, 251–261.

Freter, R. (1985). Bacterial adherence, physiological state, and nutrition as interdependent determinants of colonizing ability. In: Mergenhagen, S.E. & Rosan, B., eds. *Molecular Basis of Oral Microbial Adhesion*. Washington: American Society for Microbiology, pp. 61–66.

Frias, J., Olle, E. & Alsina, M. (2001). Periodontal pathogens produce quorum sensing molecules. *Infection and Immunity* **69**, 3431–3434.

Fujise, O., Hamachi, T., Inoue, K., Miura, M. & Maeda, K. (2002). Microbiological markers for prediction and assessment of treatment outcome following non-surgical periodontal therapy. *Journal of Periodontology* **73**, 1253–1259.

Fukui, M., Hinode, D., Yokoyama, M., Tanabe, S. & Yoshioka, M. (2006). Salivary immunoglobulin A directed to oral GroEL in patients with periodontitis and their potential protective role. *Oral Microbiology & Immunology* **21**, 289–295.

Furuichi, Y., Lindhe, J., Ramberg, P. & Volpe, A.R. (1992). Patterens of de novo plaque formation in the human dentition. *Journal of Clinical Periodontology* **19**, 423–433.

Gajardo, M., Silva, N., Gomez, L., Leon, R., Parra, B., Contreras, A. & Gamonal, J. (2005). Prevalence of periodontopathic bacteria in aggressive periodontitis patients in a Chilean population. *Journal of Periodontology* **76**, 289–294.

Garrison, S.W., Holt, S.C. & Nichols, F.C. (1988). Lipopolysaccharide-stimulated PGE2 release from human monocytes. Comparison of lipopolysaccharide prepared from suspected periodontal pathogens. *Journal of Periodontology* **59**, 684–687.

Genco, C.A., Potempa, J., Mikolajczyk-Pawlinska, J. & Travis, J. (1999). Role of gingipains R in the pathogenesis of *Porphyromonas gingivalis*-mediated periodontal disease. *Clinical Infectious Diseases* **28**, 456–465.

Genco, R.J., Slots, J. & Mouton, C. (1980). Systemic immune responses to oral anaerobic organisms. In: Lambe, D.W. Jr,

Genco, R.J. & Mayberry-Carson, K.J., eds. *Anaerobic Bacteria: Selected Topics.* New York: Plenum Press, pp. 277–293.

Genco, R.J., Van Dyke, T.E., Levine, M.J., Nelson, R.D. & Wilson, M.E. (1986). 1985 Kreshover lecture. Molecular factors influencing neutrophil defects in periodontal disease. *Journal of Dental Research* **65**, 1379–1391.

Gibbons, R.J. (1984). Adherent interaction which may affect microbial ecology in the mouth. *Journal of Dental Research* **63**, 378–385.

Gibbons, R.J. (1989). Bacterial adhesion to oral tissues: A model for infectious diseases. *Journal of Dental Research* **68**, 750–760.

Gibbons, R.J. & Macdonald, J.B. (1961). Degradation of collagenous substrates by *Bacteroides melaninogenicus. Journal of Bacteriology* **81**, 614–621.

Gibbons, R.J. & Macdonald, J.B. (1960). Hemin and vitamin K compounds as required factors for the cultivation of certain strains of *Bacteroides melaninogenicus. Journal of Bacteriology* **80**, 164–170.

Gibbons, R.J. & Quereshi, J.V. (1980). Virulence-related physiological changes and antigenic variation of *Streptococcus mutans* colonizing gnotobiotic rats. *Infection & Immunity* **29**, 1082–1091.

Gibson, F.C. 3rd & Genco, C.A. (2001). Prevention of *Porphyromonas gingivalis*-induced oral bone loss following immunization with gingipain R1. *Infection and Immunity* **69**, 7959–7963.

Gillespie, J., De Nardin, E., Radel, S., Kuracina, J., Smutko, J. & Zambon, J.J. (1992). Production of an extracellular toxin by the oral pathogen *Campylobacter rectus. Microbial Pathogenesis* **12**, 69–77.

Gillett, R. & Johnson, N.W. (1982). Bacterial invasion of the periodontium in a case of juvenile periodontis. *Journal of Clinical Periodontology* **9**, 93–100.

Gmur, R., Strub, J.R. & Guggenheim, B. (1989). Prevalence of *Bacteroides forsythus* and *Bacteroides gingivalis* in subgingival plaque of prosthodontically treated patients on short recall. *Journal of Periodontal Research* **24**, 113–120.

Gomes, S.C., Piccinin, F.B., Oppermann, R.V., Susin, C., Nonnenmacher, C.I., Mutters, R. & Marcantonio, R.A. (2006). Periodontal status in smokers and never-smokers: clinical findings and real-time polymerase chain reaction quantification of putative periodontal pathogens. *Journal of Periodontology* **77**, 1483–1490.

Gonzalez, D., Tzianabos, A.O., Genco, C.A. & Gibson, F.C. III (2003). Immunization with *Porphyromonas gingivalis* capsular polysaccharide prevents *P. gingivalis*-elicited oral bone loss in a murine model. *Infection and Immunity* **71**, 2283–2287.

Goodman, A.D. (1977). *Eikenella corrodens* isolated in oral infections of dental origin. *Oral Surgery Oral Medicine Oral Pathology* **44**, 128–134.

Greenspan, D. & Greenspan, J.S. (1993). Oral manifestations of human immunodeficiency virus infection. *Dental Clinics of North America* **37**, 21–32.

Greenspan, J.S., Greenspan, D., Winkler, J.R. & Murray, P.A. (1989). Acquired immunodeficiency syndrome; oral and periodontal changes. In: Genco, R.J., Goldman, H.M. & Cohen, D.W., eds. *Contemporary Periodontics.* Philadelphia: CV Mosby, pp. 298–322.

Grenier, D. & Bouclin, R. (2006). Contribution of proteases and plasmin-acquired activity in migration of *peptostreptococcus micros* through a reconstituted basement membrane. *Oral Microbiology & Immunology* **21**, 319–325.

Grenier, D. & Mayrand, D. (1987a). Selected characteristics of pathogenic and nonpathogenic strains of *Bacteroides gingivalis. Journal of Clinical Microbiology* **25**, 738–740.

Grenier, D. & Mayrand, D. (1987b). Functional characterization of extracellular vesicles produced by *Bacteroides gingivalis. Infection & Immunity* **55**, 111–117.

Grenier, D., Mayrand, D. & McBride, B.C. (1989). Further studies on the degradation of immunoglobulins by black-pigmented *Bacteroides. Oral Microbiology & Immunology* **4**, 12–18.

Griffen, A.L., Lyons, S.R., Becker, M.R., Moeschberger, M.L. & Leys, E.J. (1999). *Porphyromonas gingivalis* strain variability and periodontitis. *Journal of Clinical Microbiology* **37**, 4028–4033.

Grossi, S.G., Genco, R.J., Machtei, E.E., Ho, A.W., Koch, G., Dunford, R.G., Zambon, J.J. & Hausmann, E. (1995). Assessment of risk for periodontal disease. II. Risk indicators for bone loss. *Journal of Periodontology* **66**, 23–29.

Grossi, S.G., Zambon, J.J., Ho, A.W., Koch, G., Dunford, R.G., Machtei, E.E., Norderyd, O.M. & Genco, R.J. (1994). Assessment of risk for periodontal disease. I. Risk indicators for attachment loss. *Journal of Periodontology* **65**, 260–267.

Guiney, D.G. & Bouic, K. (1990). Detection of conjugal transfer systems in oral, black-pigmented *Bacteroides* spp. *Journal of Bacteriology* **172**, 495–497.

Haffajee, A.D., Cugini, M.A., Dibart, S., Smith, C., Kent, R.L. Jr. & Socransky, S.S. (1997). The effect of SRP on the clinical and microbiological parameters of periodontal diseases. *Journal of Clinical Periodontology* **24**, 324–334.

Haffajee, A.D., Cugini, M.A., Tanner, A., Pollack, R.P., Smith, C., Kent, R.L. Jr. & Socransky, S.S. (1998). Subgingival microbiota in healthy, well-maintained elder and periodontitis subjects. *Journal of Clinical Periodontology* **25**, 346–353.

Haffajee, A.D., Dzink, J.L. & Socransky, S.S. (1988a). Effect of modified Widman flap surgery and systemic tetracycline on the subgingival microbiota of periodontal lesions. *Journal of Clinical Periodontology* **15**, 255–262.

Haffajee, A.D. & Socransky, S.S. (1994). Microbial etiological agents of destructive periodontal diseases. In: Socransky, S.S. & Haffajee, A.D., eds. Microbiology and Immunology of Periodontal Diseases. *Periodontology 2000* **5**, 78–111.

Haffajee, A.D. & Socransky, S.S. (2000). Relationship of cigarette smoking to attachment level profiles. *Journal of Clinical Periodontology* **28**, 283–295.

Haffajee, A.D. & Socransky, S.S. (2001). Relationship of cigarette smoking to the subgingival microbiota. *Journal of Clinical Periodontology* **28**, 377–388.

Haffajee, A.D., Socransky, S.S., Dzink, J.L., Taubman, M.A. & Ebersole, J.L. (1988b). Clinical, microbiological and immunological features of subjects with refractory periodontal diseases. *Journal of Clinical Periodontology* **15**, 390–398.

Haffajee, A.D., Socransky, S.S., Ebersole, J.L. & Smith, D.J. (1984). Clinical, microbiological and immunological features associated with the treatment of active periodontosis lesions. *Journal of Clinical Periodontology* **11**, 600–618.

Haffajee, A.D., Socransky, S.S. & Goodson, J.M. (1992). Subgingival temperature. (I). Relation to baseline clinical parameters. *Journal of Clinical Periodontology* **19**, 401–408.

Haffajee, A.D., Socransky, S.S. & Gunsolley, J.C. (2003). Systemic anti-infective periodontal therapy. A systematic review. *Annals of Periodontology*, **8**, 115–181.

Haffajee, A.D., Teles, R.P. & Socransky, S.S. (2006a). Association of *Eubacterium nodatum* and *Treponema denticola* with human periodontitis lesions. *Oral Microbiology & Immunology* **21**, 1–14.

Haffajee, A.D., Teles, R.P. & Socransky, S.S. (2006b). The effect of periodontal therapy on the composition of the subgingival microbiota *Periodontology 2000* **43**, 7–12.

Hafstrom, C. & Dahlen, G. (1997). Pathogenicity of *Prevotella intermedia* and *Prevotella nigrescens* isolates in a wound chamber model in rabbits. *Oral Microbiology and Immunology* **12**, 148–154.

Hamlet, S., Ellwood, R., Cullinan, M., Worthington, H., Palmer, J., Bird, P., Narayanan, D., Davies, R. & Seymour, G. (2004). Persistent colonization with *Tannerella forsythensis* and loss of attachment in adolescents. *Journal of Dental Research* **83**, 232–235.

Hammond, B.F., Lillard, S.E. & Stevens, R.H. (1987). A bacteriocin of *Actinobacillus actinomycetemcomitans. Infection & Immunity* **55**, 686–691.

Han, Y.W., Shi, W., Huang, G.T., Kinder Haake, S., Park, N.H., Kuramitsu, H. & Genco, R.J. (2000). Interactions between periodontal bacteria and human oral epithelial cells: *Fusobacterium nucleatum* adheres to and invades epithelial cells. *Infection and Immunity* **68**, 140–146.

Hanazawa, S., Hirose, K., Ohmori, Y., Amamo, S. & Kitano, S. (1988). *Bacteroides gingivalis* fimbriae stimulate production of thymocyte-activating factor by human gingival fibroblasts. *Infection & Immunity* **56**, 272–274.

Haubek, D., Ennibi, O.K., Poulsen, K., Benzarti, N. & Baelum, V. (2004). The highly leukotoxic JP2 clone of *Actinobacillus actinomycetemcomitans* and progression of periodontal attachment loss. *Journal of Dental Research* **83**, 767–770.

Haubek, D., Ennibi, O.K., Poulsen, K., Poulsen, S., Benzarti, N. & Kilian, M. (2001). Early-onset periodontitis in Morocco is associated with the highly leukotoxic clone of *Actinobacillus actinomycetemcomitans*. *Journal of Dental Research* **80**, 1580–1583.

Haubek, D., Poulsen, K., Westergaard, J., Dahlen, G. & Kilian, M. (1996). Highly toxic clone of *Actinobacillus actinomycetemcomitans* in geographically widespread case of juvenile periodontitis. *Journal of Clinical Microbiology* **32**, 75–81.

Hayashi, F., Okada, M., Soda, Y., Miura, K. & Kozai, K. (2006). Subgingival distribution of *Campylobacter rectus* and *Tannerella forsythensis* in healthy children with primary dentition. *Archives of Oral Biology* **51**, 10–14.

Herrera, D., Roldan, S., Gonzalez, I. & Sanz, M. (2000). The periodontal abscess (I) Clinical and microbiological findings. *Journal of Clinical Periodontology* **27**, 387–394.

Herrera, D., Sanz, M., Jepsen, S., Needleman, I. & Roldan, S. (2002). A systematic review on the effect of systemic antimicrobials as an adjunct to scaling and root planing in periodontitis patients. *Journal of Clinical Periodontology* **29** (Suppl 3), 136–159.

Hillmann, G., Dogan, S. & Geurtsen, W. (1998). Histopathological investigation of gingival tissue from patients with rapidly progressive periodontitis. *Journal of Periodontology* **69**, 195–208.

Hillman, J.D. & Socransky, S.S. (1982). Bacterial interference in the oral ecology of *Actinobacillus actinomycetemcomitans* and its relationship to human periodontosis. *Archives of Oral Biology* **27**, 75–77.

Hillman, J.D. & Socransky, S.S. (1987). Replacement therapy for the prevention of dental disease. *Advances in Dental Research* **1**, 119–125.

Hillman, J.D. & Socransky, S.S. (1989). The theory and application of bacterial interference to oral diseases. In: Myers, H.M., ed. *New Biotechnology in Oral Research*, pp. 1–17. Basel: Karger.

Hillman, J.D., Socransky, S.S. & Shivers, M. (1985). The relationships between streptococcal species and periodontopathic bacteria in human dental plaque. *Archives of Oral Biology* **30**, 791–795.

Holmberg, K. & Hallander, H.O. (1973). Production of bacteriocidal concentrations of hydrogen peroxide by *Streptococcus sanguis*. *Archives of Oral Biology* **18**, 423–434.

Holt, S.C. & Ebersole, J.L. (2005). *Porphyromonas gingivalis*, *Treponema denticola*, and *Tannerella forsythia*: the "red complex", a prototype polybacteria pathogenic consortia in periodontitis. *Periodontology 2000* **38**, 72–122.

Holt, S.C., Ebersole, J., Felton, J., Brunsvold, M. & Kornman, K.S. (1988). Implantation of *Bacteroides gingivalis* in nonhuman primates initiates progression of periodontitis. *Science* **239**, 55–57.

Horton, J.E., Raisz, L.G., Simmons, H.A., Oppenheim, J.J. & Mergenhagen, S.E. (1972). Bone resorbing activity in supernatant fluid from cultures of human peripheral blood leukocytes. *Science* **177**, 793–795.

Hugenholtz, P. & Pace, N.R. (1996). Identifying microbial diversity in the natural environment: a molecular phylogenetic approach. *Trends in Biotechnology* **14**, 190–197.

Ihara, H., Miura, T., Kato, T., Ishihara, K., Nakagawa, T., Yamada, S. & Okuda, K. (2003). Detection of *Campylobacter rectus* in periodontitis sites by monoclonal antibodies. *Journal of Periodontal Research* **38**, 64–72.

Irving, J.T., Socransky, S.S. & Tanner, A.C. (1978). Histological changes in experimental periodontal disease in rats monoinfected with Gram-negative organisms. *Journal of Periodontal Research* **13**, 326–332.

Ishihara, K., Miura, T., Kuramitsu, H.K. & Okuda, K. (1996). Characterization of the treponema deticola prtP gene encoding a prolyl-phenylalanine-specific protease (dentilisin). *Infection & Immunity* **64**, 5178–5186.

Isogai, H., Isogai, E., Yoshimura, F., Suzuki, T., Kagota, W. & Takano, K (1988). Specific inhibition of adherence of an oral strain of *Bacteroides gingivalis* 381 to epithelial cells by monoclonal antibodies against the bacterial fimbriae. *Archives of Oral Biology* **33**, 479–485.

Iwai, T., Inoue, Y., Umeda, M., Huang, Y., Kurihara, N., Koike, M. & Ishikawa, I. (2005). Oral bacteria in the occluded arteries of patients with Buerger disease. *Journal of Vascular Surgery* **42**, 107–115.

Jewett, A., Hume, W.R., Le, H., Huynh, T.N., Han, Y.W., Cheng, G. & Shi, W. (2001). Induction of apoptotic cell death in peripheral blood mononuclear and polymorphonuclear cells by an oral bacterium, *Fusobacterium nucleatum*. *Infection and Immunity* **68**, 1893–1898.

Jin, K.C., Barua, P.k., Zambon, J.J. & Neiders, M.E. (1989). Proteolyic activity in black-pigmented bacteroides species. *Journal of Endodontics* **15**, 463–467.

Johnson, S.M. & Pankey, G.A. (1976). *Eikenella corrodens* osteomyelitis, arthritis, and cellulitis of the hand. *Southern Medical Journal* **69**, 535–539.

Johnson, V., Johnson, B.D., Sims, T.J., Whitney, C.W., Moncla, B.J. & Engel, L.D. (1993). Effects of treatment on antibody titer to *Porphyromonas gingivalis* in gingival crevicular fluid of patients with rapidly progressive periodontitis. *Journal of Periodontology* **64**, 559–565.

Kadowaki T., Nakayama, K., Okamoto, K., Abe, N., Baba, A., Shi, Y. Ratnayake. D.B. & Yamamoto, K. (2000). *Porphyromonas gingivalis* proteinases as virulence factors in progression of periodontal diseases. *Journal of Biochemistry* **128**, 153–159.

Kamma, J.J., Contreras, A. & Slots, J. (2001). Herpes virus and periodontopathic bacteria in early-onset periodontitis. *Journal of Clinical Periodontology* **28**, 879–885.

Kashket, S., Maiden, M., Haffajee, A. & Kasket, E.R. (2003). Accumulation of methylglyoxal in the gingival crevicular fluid of chronic periodontitis patients. *Journal of Clinical Periodontology* **30**, 364–367.

Kato, S., Nakashima, K., Inoue, M., Tomioka, J., Nonaka, K., Nishihar, T. & Kowashi, Y. (2000). Human epithelial cell death caused by *Actinobacillus actinomycetemcomitans* infection. *Journal of Medical Microbiology* **49**, 739–745.

Katz, J., Black, K.P. & Michalek, S.M. (1999). Host responses to recombinant hemagglutinin B of *Porphyromonas gingivalis* in an experimental rat model. *Infection and Immunity* **67**, 4352–4359.

Kaufman, J. & DiRienzo, J.M. (1989). Isolation of a corncob (coaggregation). receptor polypeptide from *Fusobacterium nucleatum*. *Infection & Immunity* **57**, 331–337.

Kawada, M., Yoshida, A., Suzuki, N., Nakano, Y., Saito, T., Oho, T. & Koga, T. (2004). Prevalence of *Porphyromonas gingivalis* in relation to periodontal status assessed by real-time PCR. *Oral Microbiology & Immunology* **19**, 289–292.

Kazor, C.E., Mitchell, P.M., Lee, A.M., Stokes, L.N., Loesche, W.J., Dewhirst, F.E. & Paster, B.J. (2003). Diversity of bacterial populations on the tongue dorsum in halitosis and in health. *Journal of Clinical Microbiology* **41**, 558–563.

Kenney, E.B. & Ash, M.M. (1969). Oxidation-reduction potential of developing plaque, periodontal pockets and gingival sulci. *Journal of Periodontology* **40**, 630–633.

Kesavalu, L., Holt, S.C. & Ebersole, J.L. (1999). Environmental modulation of oral treponeme virulence in a murine model. *Infection & Immunity* **67**, 2783–2789.

Keyes, P.H. & Rams, T.E. (1983). A rationale for management of periodontal diseases: rapid identification of microbial "therapeutic targets" with phase-contrast microscopy. *Journal of the American Dental Association* **106**, 803–812.

Kigure, T., Saito, A., Seida, K., Yamada, S., Ishihara, K. & Okuda, K. (1995). Distribution of *Porphyromonas gingivalis* and *Treponema denticola* in human subgingival plaque at different periodontal pocket depths examined by immunohistochemical methods. *Journal of Periodontal Research* **30**, 332–341.

Kilian, M. (1981). Degradation of immunoglobulins A1, A2 and G by suspected principal periodontal pathogens. *Infection & Immunity* **34**, 757–765.

Kilian, M., Frandsen, E.V.G., Haubek, D. & Poulsen, K. (2006). The etiology of periodontal disease revisited by population genetic analysis. *Periodontology 2000* **42**, 158–179.

Kilian, M. & Frederiksen, W. (1981). Ecology of *Haemophilus*, *Pasteurella* and *Actinobacillus*. In: Kilian, M., Frederiksen, W. & Biberstein, E.L., eds. *Haemophilus, Pasteurella and Actinobacillus*. London: Academic Press Inc., pp. 11–38.

Kim, S.J., Ha, M.S., Choi, E.Y., Choi, J.I. & Choi, I.S. (2004). *Prevotella intermedia* lipopolysaccharide stimulates release of nitric oxide by inducing expression of inducible nitric oxide synthase. *Journal of Periodontal Research* **39**, 424–431.

Kimizuka, R., Kato, T., Ishihara, K. & Okuda, K. (2003). Mixed infections with *Porphyromonas gingivalis* and *Treponema denticola* cause excessive inflammatory responses in a mouse pneumonia model compared with monoinfections. *Microbes & Infection* **5**, 1357–1362.

Kinder, S.A. & Holt, S.C. (1989). Characterization of coaggregation between *Bacteroides gingivalis* T22 and *Fusobacterium nucleatum* T18. *Infection & Immunity* **57**, 3425–3433.

Kleinberg, I. & Hall, G. (1969). pH and depth of gingival crevices in different areas of the mouth of fasting humans. *Journal of Periodontal Research* **4**, 109–117.

Klemenc, P., Skaleric, U., Artnik, B., Nograsek, P. & Marin, J. (2005). Prevalence of some herpesviruses in gingival crevicular fluid. *Journal of Clinical Virology* **34**, 147–152.

Kolenbrander, P.E. (2000). Oral microbial communities: biofilms, interactions, and genetic systems. *Annual Reviews of Microbiology* **54**, 413–437.

Kolenbrander, P.E. & Andersen, R.N. (1989). Inhibition of coaggregation between *Fusobacterium nucleatum* and *Porphyromonas (Bacteroides) gingivalis* by lactose and related sugars. *Infection & Immunity* **57**, 3204–3209.

Kolenbrander, P.E. & Andersen, R.N. (1990). Characterization of *Streptococcus gordonii* (*S. sanguis*) PK488 adhesin-mediated coaggregation with *Actinomyces naeslundii* PK606. *Infection & Immunity* **58**, 3064–3072.

Kolenbrander, P.E., Andersen, R.N., Blehert, D.S., Egland, P.G., Foster, J.S. & Palmer, R.J. Jr. (2002). Communication among oral bacteria. *Microbiology and Molecular Biology Reviews* **66**, 486–505.

Kolenbrander, P.E., Andersen, R.N. & Moore, L.V. (1989). Coaggregation of *Fusobacterium nucleatum*, *Selenomonas flueggei*, *Selenomonas infelix*, *Selenomonas noxia*, and *Selenomonas sputigena* with strains from 11 genera of oral bacteria. *Infection & Immunity* **57**, 3194–3203.

Kolenbrander, P.E., Palmer, R.J. Jr., Rickard, A.H., Jakubobics, N.S., Chalmers, N.I. & Diaz, P.I. (2006). Bacterial interactions and successions during plaque development. *Periodontology 2000* **42**, 47–79.

Kornman, K.S., Crane, A., Wang, H.Y., di Giovine, F.S., Newman, M.G., Pirk, F.W., Wilson, T.G. Jr., Higginbottom, F.L. & Duff, G.W. (1997). The interleukin-1 genotype as a severity factor in adult periodontal disease. *Journal of Clinical Periodontology* **24**, 72–77.

Kornman, K.S. & Robertson, P.B. (1985). Clinical and microbiological evaluation of therapy for juvenile periodontitis. *Journal of Periodontology* **56**, 443–446.

Kozarov, E.V., Dorn, B.R., Shelburne, C.E., Dunn, W.A. Jr. & Progulske-Fox, A. (2005). Human atherosclerotic plaque contains viable invasive *Actinobacillus actinomycetemcomitans* and *Porphyromonas gingivalis*. *Arteriosclerosis, Thrombosis & Vascular Biology* **25**, e17–e18.

Kremer, B.H., Loos, B.G., van der Velden, U., van Winkelhoff, A.J., Craandijk. J., Bulthuis, H.M., Hutter, J., Varoufaki, A.S. & van Steenbergen, T.J. (2000). *Peptostreptococcus micros* smooth and rough genotypes in periodontitis and gingivitis. *Journal of Periodontology* **71**, 209–218.

Kumar, P.S., Griffen, A.L., Barton, J.A., Paster, B.J., Moeschberger, M.L. & Leys, E.J. (2003). New bacterial species associated with chronic periodontitis. *Journal of Dental Research* **82**, 338–344.

Lai, C.-H., Listgarten, M.A., Evian, C.I. & Dougherty, P. (1986). Serum IgA and IgG antibodies to *Treponema vincentii* and *Treponema denticola* in adult periodontitis, juvenile periodontitis and periodontally healthy subjects. *Journal of Clinical Periodontology* **13**, 752–757.

Lai, C.-H., Listgarten, M.A., Shirakawa, M. & Slots, J. (1987). *Bacteroides forsythus* in adult gingivitis and periodontitis. *Oral Microbiology & Immunology* **2**, 152–157.

Lai, C.-H., Oshima, K., Slots, J. & Listgarten, M.A. (1992). *Wolinella recta* in adult gingivitis and periodontitis. *Journal of Periodontal Research* **27**, 8–14.

Lamont, R.J., Oda, D., Persson, R.E. & Persson, G.R. (1992). Interaction of *Porphyromonas gingivalis* with gingival epithelial cells maintained in culture. *Oral Microbiology & Immunology* **7**, 364–367.

Lantz, M.S., Allen, R.D., Bounelis, P., Switalski, L.M. & Hook, M. (1990). *Bacteroides gingivalis* and *Bacteroides intermedius* recognize different sites on human fibrinogen. *Journal of Bacteriology* **172**, 716–726.

Lau, L., Sanz, M., Herrera, D., Morillo, J.M., Martin, C. & Silva, A. (2004). Quantitative real-time polymerase chain reaction versus culture: a comparison between two methods for the detection and quantification of *Actinobacillus actinomycetemcomitans*, *Porphyromonas gingivalis* and *Tannerella forsythensis* in subgingival plaque samples. *Journal of Clinical Periodontology* **31**, 1061–1069.

Lee, J.W., Choi, B.K., Yoo, Y.J., Choi, S.H., Cho, K.S., Chai, J.K. & Kim, C.K. (2003). Distribution of periodontal pathogens in Korean aggressive periodontitis. *Journal of Periodontology* **74**, 1329–1335.

Lee, J.Y., Yi, N.N., Kim, U.S., Choi, J.S., Kim, S.J. & Choi, J.I. (2006). *Porphyromonas gingivalis* heat shock protein vaccine reduces the alveolar bone loss induced by multiple periodontopathogenic bacteria. *Journal of Periodontal Research* **41**, 10–14.

Lee, S.W., Sabet, M., Um, H.S., Yang, J., Kim, H.C. & Zhu, W. (2006). Identification and characterization of the genes encoding a unique surface (S-) layer of *Tannerella forsythia*. *Gene* **371**, 102–111.

Levy, R.M., Giannobile, W.V., Feres, M., Haffajee, A.D., Smith, C. & Socransky, S.S. (1999). The short-term effect of apically repositioned flap surgery on the composition of the subgingival microbiota. *International Journal of Periodontics & Restorative Dentistry* **19**, 555–567.

Levy, R.M., Giannobile, W.V., Feres, M., Haffajee, A.D., Smith, C. & Socransky, S.S. (2002). The effect of apically repositioned flap surgery on clinical parameters and the composition of the subgingival microbiota: 12-month data. *International Journal of Periodontics & Restorative Dentistry* **22**, 209–219.

Leys, E.J., Lyons, S.R., Moeschberger, M.L., Rumpf, R.W. & Griffen, A.L. (2002). Association of *Bacteroides forsythus* and a novel Bacteroides phylotype with periodontitis. *Journal of Clinical Microbiology* **40**, 821–825.

Li, J., Helmerhorst, E.J., Leone, C.W., Troxler, R.F., Yaskell, T., Haffajee, A.D., Socransky, S.S. & Oppenheim, F.G. (2004). Identification of early microbial colonizers in human dental biofilm. *Journal of Applied Microbiology* **97**, 1311–1318.

Liakoni, H., Barber, P. & Newman, H.N. (1987). Bacterial penetration of pocket soft tissues in chronic adult and juvenile periodontitis cases. An ultrastructural study. *Journal of Clinical Periodontology* **14**, 22–28.

Lindemann, R.A. (1988). Bacterial activation of human natural killer cells: role of cell surface lipopolysaccharide. *Infection & Immunity* **56**, 1301–1308.

Lindemann, R.A., Economou, J.S. & Rothermel, H. (1988). Production of interleukin-1 and tumor necrosis factor by human peripheral monocytes activated by periodontal bacteria and extracted lipopolysaccharide. *Journal of Dental Research* **67**, 1131–1135.

Lippke, J.A., Peros, W.J., Keville, M.W., Savitt, E.D. & French, C.K. (1991). DNA probe detection of *Eikenella corrodens*, *Wolinella recta* and *Fusobacterium nucleatum* in subgingival plaque. *Oral Microbiology & Immunology* **6**, 81–87.

Listgarten, M.A. (1965). Electron microscopic observations of the bacterial flora of acute necrotizing ulcerative gingivitis. *Journal of Periodontology* **36**, 328–339.

Listgarten, M.A. (1976). Structure of the microbial flora associated with periodontal health and disease in man. A light and electron microscopic study. *Journal of Periodontology* **47**, 1–18.

Listgarten, M.A. (1988). Bacterial invasion of periodontal tissues (letter). *Journal of Periodontology* **59**, 412.

Listgarten, M.A. (1999). Formation of dental plaque and other oral biofilms. In: Newman, H.N. & Wilson, M., eds. *Dental Plaque Revisited*. Cardiff: Bioline, pp. 187–210.

Listgarten, M.A., Lai, C-H. & Evian, C.I. (1981). Comparative antibody titres to *Actinobacillus actinomycetemcomitans* in juvenile periodontitis, chronic periodontitis and periodontally healthy subjects. *Journal of Clinical Periodontology* **8**, 154–164.

Listgarten, M.A., Lai, C-H. & Young, V. (1993). Microbial composition and pattern of antibiotic resistance in subgingival microbial samples from patients with refractory periodontitis. *Journal of Periodontology* **64**, 155–161.

Listgarten, M.A., Mayo, H.E. & Tremblay, R. (1975). Development of dental plaque on epoxy resin crowns in man. A light and electron microscopic study. *Journal of Periodontology* **46**, 10–26.

Listgarten, M.A. & Socransky, S.S. (1964). Ultrastructural characteristics of a spirochete in the lesion of acute necrotizing ulcerative gingivostomatitis (Vincent's infection). *Archives of Oral Biology* **9**, 95–96.

Loe, H., Theilade, E. & Jensen, S.B. (1965). Experimental gingivitis in man. *Journal of Periodontology* **36**, 177–187.

Loe, H., Theilade, E., Jensen, S.B. & Schiott, C.R. (1967). Experimental gingivitis in man. III. The influence of antibiotics on gingival plaque development. *Journal of Periodontal Research* **2**, 282–289.

Loesche, W.J., Grossman, N. & Giordano, J. (1993). Metronidazole in periodontitis (IV). The effect of patient compliance on treatment parameters. *Journal of Clincial Periodontology* **20**, 96–104.

Loesche, W.J., Lopatin, D.E., Giordano, J., Alcoforado, G. & Hujoel, P.P. (1992). Comparison of the benzoyl-DL-arginine-naphthylamide (BANA). test, DNA probes and immunological reagents for ability to detect anaerobic periodontal infections due to *Porphyromonas gingivalis*, *Treponena denticola* and *Bacteroides forsythus*. *Journal of Clincial Microbiology* **30**, 427–433.

Loesche, W.J., Syed, S.A., Laughon, B.E. & Stoll, J. (1982). The bacteriology of acute necrotizing ulcerative gingivitis. *Journal of Periodontology* **53**, 223–230.

Loesche, W.J., Syed, S.A., Schmidt, E. & Morrison, E.C. (1985). Bacterial profiles of subgingival plaques in periodontitis. *Journal of Periodontology* **56**, 447–456.

Lopatin, D.E. & Blackburn, E. (1992). Avidity and titer of immunoglobulin G subclasses to *Porphyromonas gingivalis* in adult periodontitis patients. *Oral Microbiology & Immunology* **7**, 332–337.

Lopez, N.J. (2000). Occurrence of *Actinobacillus actinomycetemcomitans*, *Porphyromonas gingivalis* and *Prevotella intermedia* in progressing adult periodontitis. *Journal of Periodontology* **71**, 948–954.

Macdonald, J.B., Gibbons, R.J. & Socransky, S.S. (1960). Bacterial mechanisms in periodontal disease. *Annals of the New York Academy of Sciences* **85**, 467–478.

Macdonald, J.B., Socransky, S.S., Gibbons, R.J. (1963). Aspects of the pathogenesis of mixed anaerobic infections of mucous membranes. *Journal of Dental Research* **42**, 529–544.

Macdonald, J.B., Sutton, R.M., Knoll, M.L., Madlener, E.M., Grainger, R.M. (1956). The pathogenic components of an experimental mixed infection. *Journal of Infectious Diseases* **98**, 15–20.

Machtei, E.E., Hausmann, E., Dunford, R., Grossi, S., Ho, A., Chandler, J., Zambon, J. & Genco, R.J. (1999). Longitudinal study of predictive factors for periodontal disease and tooth loss. *Journal of Clinical Periodontology* **26**, 374–380.

Macuch, P.J. & Tanner, A.C. (2000). *Campylobacter* species in health, gingivitis and periodontitis. *Journal of Dental Research* **79**, 785–792.

Madianos, P.N., Lieff, S., Murtha, A.P., Boggess, K.A., Auten, R.L. Jr., Beck, J.D. & Offenbacher, S. (2001). Maternal periodontitis and prematurity. Part II: Maternal infection and fetal exposure. *Annals of Periodontology* **6**, 175–182.

Madianos, P.N., Papapanou, P.N. & Sandros, J. (1997). *Porphyromonas gingivalis* infection of oral epithelium inhibits neutrophil transepithelial migration. *Infection and Immunity* **65**, 3983–3990.

Maeda, N., Okamoto, M., Kondo, K., Ishikawa, H., Osada, R., Tsurumoto, A. & Fujita, H. (1998). Incidence of *Prevotella intermedia* and *Prevotella nigrescens* in periodontal health and disease. *Microbiology and Immunology* **42**, 583–589.

Mahanonda, R., Seymour, G.J., Powell, L.W., Good, M.F. & Halliday, J.W. (1991). Effect of initial treatment of chronic inflammatory periodontal disease on the frequency of peripheral blood T-lymphocytes specific to periodontopathic bacteria. *Oral Microbiology & Immunology* **6**, 221–227.

Mandell, R.L. (1984). A longitudinal microbiological investigation of *Actinobacillus actinomycetemcomitans* and *Eikenella corrodens* in juvenile periodontitis. *Infection & Immunity* **45**, 778–780.

Mandell, R.L., DiRienzo, J., Kent, R., Joshipura, K. & Haber, J. (1992). Microbiology of healthy and diseased periodontal sites in poorly controlled insulin dependent diabetics. *Journal of Periodontology* **63**, 274–279.

Mandell, R.L., Ebersole, J.L. & Socransky, S.S. (1987). Clinical immunologic and microbiologic features of active disease sites in juvenile periodontitis. *Journal of Clinical Periodontology* **14**, 534–540.

Mandell, R.L. & Socransky, S.S. (1981). A selective medium for *Actinobacillus actinomycetemcomitans* and the incidence of the organism in juvenile periodontitis. *Journal of Periodontology* **52**, 593–598.

Mandell, R.L., Tripodi, L.S., Savitt, E., Goodson, J.M. & Socransky, S.S. (1986). The effect of treatment on *Actinobacillus actinomycetemcomitans* in localized juvenile periodontitis. *Journal of Periodontology* **57**, 94–99.

Mangan, D.F., Laughon, B.E., Bower, B. & Lopatin, D.E. (1982). In vitro lymphocyte blastogenic responses and titers of humoral antibodies from periodontitis patients to oral spirochete isolates. *Infection & Immunity* **37**, 445–451.

Mangan, D.F., Novak, M.J., Vora, S.A., Mourad, J. & Kriger, P.S. (1989). Lectinlike interactions of *Fusobacterium nucleatum* with human neutrophiles. *Infection and Immunity* **57**, 3601–3611.

Marques de Silva, R., Caugant, D.A., Lingaas, P.S., Geiran, O., Tronstad, L. & Olsen, I. (2005). Detection of *Actinobacillus actinomycetemcomitans* but not bacteria of the red complex in aortic aneurysms by multiplex polymerase chain reaction. *Journal of Periodontology* **76**, 590–594.

Marsh, P. (2005). Dental plaque: biological significance of a biofilm and community life-style. *Journal of Clinical Periodontology* **32** (Suppl 6), 7–15.

Marsh, P.D., McKee, A.S., McDermid, A.S. & Dowsett, A.B. (1989). Ultrastructure and enzyme activities of a virulent and an avirulent variant of *Bacteroides gingivalis* W50. *FEMS Microbiological Letters* **50**, 181–185.

Martin, S.A. Falkler, W.A., Jr., Vincent, J.W., Mackler, B.F. & Suzuki, J.B. (1988). A comparison of the reactivity of *Eubacterium* species with localized and serum immunoglobulins from rapidly progressive and adult periodontitis patients. *Journal of Periodontology* **59**, 32–39.

Mashimo, P.A., Yamamoto, Y., Nakanura, M., Reynolds, H.S. & Genco, R.J. (1985). Lactic acid production by oral *Streptococcus mitis* inhibits the growth of oral *Capnocytophaga*. *Journal of Periodontology* **56**, 548–552.

Mashimo, P.A., Yamamota, Y., Slots, J., Park, B.H. & Genco, R.J. (1983). The periodontal microflora of juvenile diabetics. Culture, immunofluorescence and serum antibody studies. *Journal of Periodontology* **54**, 420–430.

McKee, A.S., McDermid, A.S., Baskerville, A., Dowsett, A.B. & Ellwood, D.C. (1986). Effect of hemin on the physiology and virulence of *Bacteroides gingivalis* W50. *Infection & Immunity* **52**, 349–355.

McNabb, H., Mombelli, A., Gmur, R., Mathey-Din, S. & Lang, N.P. (1992). Periodontal pathogens in the shallow pockets of immigrants from developing countries. *Oral Microbiology & Immunology* **7**, 267–272.

Millar, S.J., Goldstein, E.G., Levine, M.J. & Hausmann, E. (1986). Modulation of bone metabolism by two chemically distinct lipopolysaccharide fractions from *Bacteroides gingivalis*. *Infection & Immunity* **51**, 302–306.

Mombelli, A., Gmur, R., Lang, N.P., Corbert, E. & Frey, J. (1999). *Actinobacillus actinomycetemcomitans* in Chinese adults. Serotype distribution and analysis of the leukotoxin gene promoter locus. *Journal of Clinical Periodontology* **26**, 505–510.

Mombelli, A., Schmid, B., Rutar, A. & Lang, N.P. (2000). Persistence patterns of *Porphyromonas gingivalis*, *Prevotella intermedia/nigrescens*, and *Actinobacillus actinomycetemcomitans* after mechanical therapy of periodontal disease. *Journal of Periodontology* **71**, 14–21.

Mooney, J., Adonogianaki, E. & Kinane, D.F. (1993). Relative avidity of serum antibodies to putative periodontopathogens in periodontal disease. *Journal of Periodontal Research* **28**, 444–450.

Moore, W.E.C. (1987). Microbiology of periodontal disease. *Journal of Periodontal Research* **22**, 335–341.

Moore, W.E.C., Holdeman, L.V., Cato, E.P., Smibert, R.M., Burmeister, J.A., Palcanis, K.G. & Ranney, R.R. (1985). Comparative bacteriology of juvenile periodontitis. *Infection & Immunity* **48**, 507–519.

Moore, W.E.C., Holdeman, L.V., Cato, E.P., Smibert, R.M., Burmeister, J.A. & Ranney, R.R. (1983). Bacteriology of moderate (chronic) periodontitis in mature adult humans. *Infection & Immunity* **42**, 510–515.

Moore, W.E.C., Holdeman, L.V., Smibert, R.M., Hash, D.E., Burmeister, J.A. & Ranney, R.R. (1982). Bacteriology of severe periodontitis in young adult humans. *Infection & Immunity* **38**, 1137–1148.

Moore, L.V.H., Johnson, J.L. & Moore, W.E.C. (1987). *Selenomonas noxia* sp. nov., *Selenomonas flueggei* sp. nov., *Selenomonas infelix* sp. nov., *Selenomonas dianae* sp. nov. and *Selenomonas artemidis* sp. nov. from the human gingival crevice. *International Journal of Systematic Bacteriology* **36**, 271–280.

Moore, W.E.C. & Moore, L.V.H. (1994). The bacteria of periodontal diseases. *Periodontology 2000* **5**, 66–77.

Moore, L.V.H., Moore, W.E.C., Riley, C., Brooks, C.N., Burmeister, J.A. & Smibert, R.M. (1993). Periodontal microflora of HIV positive subjects with gingivitis or adult periodontitis. *Journal of Periodontology* **64**, 48–56.

Moritz, A.J., Cappelli, D., Lantz, M.S., Holt, S.C. & Ebersole, J.L. (1998). Immunization with *Porphyromonas gingivalis* cysteine protease: effects on experimental gingivitis and ligature-induced periodontitis in *Macaca fascicularis*. *Journal of Periodontology* **69**, 686–697.

Muller, H.P., Heinecke, A., Borneff, M., Knopf, A., Kiencke, C. & Pohl, S. (1997). Microbial ecology of *Actinobacillus actinomycetemcomitans*, *Eikenella corrodens* and *Capnocytophaga* spp. in adult periodontitis. *Journal of Periodontal Research* **32**, 530–542.

Murray, P.A., Grassi, M. & Winkler, J.R. (1989). The microbiology of HIV-associated periodontal lesions. *Journal of Clinical Periodontology* **16**, 635–642.

Murray, P.A., Kern, D.G. & Winkler, J.R. (1988). Identification of a galactose-binding lectin on *Fusobacterium nucleatum* FN-2. *Infection & Immunity* **56**, 1314–1319.

Murray, P.A., Levine, M.J., Reddy, M.S., Tabak, L.A. & Bergey, E.J. (1986). Preparation of a sialic acid-binding protein from *Streptococcus mitis* KS32AR. *Infection & Immunity* **53**, 359–365.

Murray, P.A., Winkler, J.R., Peros, W.J., French, C.K. & Lippke, J.A. (1991). DNA probe detection of periodontal pathogens in HIV-associated periodontal lesions. *Oral Microbiology & Immunology* **6**, 34–40.

Naito, Y. & Gibbons, R.J. (1988). Attachment of *Bacteroides gingivalis* to collagenous substrata. *Journal of Dental Research* **67**, 1075–1080.

Nakajawa, I., Inaba, H., Yamamura, T., Kato, T., Kawai, S., Ooshima, T. & Amano, A. (2006). Invasion of epithelial cells and proteolysis of cellular focal adhesion components by distinct types of *Porphyromonas gingivalis* fimbriae. *Infection & Immunity* **74**, 3773–3782.

Neiders, M.E., Chen, P.B., Suido, H., Reynolds, H.S. & Zambon, J.J. (1989). Heterogeneity of virulence among strains of *Bacteroides gingivalis*. *Journal of Periodontal Research* **24**, 192–198.

Newman, H.N. & Wilson, M. (1999). *Dental Plaque Revisited*. Cardiff: Bioline.

Newman, M.G. & Socransky, S.S. (1977). Predominant cultivable microbiota in periodontosis. *Journal of Periodontal Research* **12**, 120–128.

Newman, M.G., Socransky, S.S., Savitt, E.D., Propas, D.A. & Crawford, A. (1976). Studies of the microbiology of periodontosis. *Journal of Periodontology* **47**, 373–379.

Njoroge, T., Genco, R.J., Sojar, H.T., Hamada, N. & Genco, C.A. (1997). A role for the fimbriae in *Porphyromonas gingivalis* invasion of oral epithelial cells. *Infection and Immunity* **65**, 1980–1984.

Nociti, F.H. Jr., Cesco de Toledo, R., Machado, M.A., Stefani, C.M., Line, S.R. & Goncalves, R.B. (2001). Clinical and microbiological evaluation of ligature-induced peri-implantitis and periodontitis in dogs. *Clincial Oral Implants Research* **12**, 295–300.

Noiri, Y., Li, L. & Ebisu, S. (2001). The localization of periodontal-disease-associated bacteria in human periodontal pockets. *Journal of Dental Research* **80**, 1930–1934.

Nonnenmacher, C., Dalpke, A., Rochon, J., Flores-de-Jacoby, L., Mutters, R. & Heeg, K. (2005). Real-time polymerase chain reaction for detection and quantification of bacteria in periodontal patients. *Journal of Periodontology* **76**, 1542–1549.

Norskov-Lauritsen, N. & Kilian, M. (2006). Reclassification of *Actinobacillus actinomycetemcomitans*, *Haemophilus aphrophilus*, *Haemophilus paraphrophilus* and *Haemophilus segnis* as *Aggregatibacter actinomycetemcomitans* gen. nov., comb. nov., *Aggregatibacter aphrophilus* comb. nov. and *Aggregatibacter segnis* comb. nov., and emended description of *Aggregatibacter aphrophilus* to include V factor-dependent and V factor-independent isolates. *International Journal of Systematic and Evolutionary Microbiology* **56**, 2135–2146.

Nyvad, B. & Kilian, M. (1987). Microbiology of the early colonization of human enamel and root surfaces *in vivo*. *Scandinavian Journal of Dental Research* **95**, 369–380.

O'Brien-Simpson, N.M., Black, C.L., Bhogal, P.S., Cleal, S.M., Slakeski, N., Higgins, T.J. & Reynolds, E.C. (2000). Serum immunoglobulin G (IgG) and IgG subclass responses to the RgpA-Kgp proteinase-adhesin complex of *Porphyromonas gingivalis* in adult periodontitis. *Infection and Immunity* **68**, 2704–2712.

O'Brien-Simpson, N.M., Pathirana, R.D., Paolina, R.A., Chen, Y.Y., Veith, P.D., Tam, V., Ally, N., Pike, R.N. & Reynolds, E.C. (2005). An immune response directed to proteinase and adhesin functional epitopes protects against *Porphyromonas gingivalis*-induced periodontal bone loss. *Journal of Immunology* **175**, 3980–3989.

Ochiai, K., Kurita, T., Nishimura, K. & Ikeda, O.T. (1989). Immunoadjuvant effects of periodontitis-associated bacteria. *Journal of Periodontal Research* **24**, 322–328.

Ogawa, T., McGhee, M.L., Moldoveanu, Z., Hamada, S., Mestecky, J., McGhee, J.R. & Kiyono, H. (1989). *Bacteroides*-specific IgG and IgA subclass antibody-secreting cells isolated from chronically inflamed gingival tissues. *Clinical Experimental Immunology* **76**, 103–110.

Okuda, K. & Takazoe, I. (1988). The role of *Bacteroides gingivalis* in periodontal disease. *Advances in Dental Research* **2**, 260–268.

Oliver, W.W. & Wherry, W.B. (1921). Notes on some bacterial parasites of the human mucous membranes. *Journal of Infectious Diseases* **28**, 341–345.

Olsen, I. & Socransky, S.S. (1981). Comparison of three anaerobic culture techniques and media for viable recovery of subgingival plaque bacteria. *Scandinavian Journal of Dental Research* **89**, 165–174.

Onisi, M., Condo, W., Horiuchi, I. & Uchiyama, Y. (1960). Preliminary report on the oxidation-reduction potentials obtained on surfaces of gingiva and tongue and in intradental space. *Bulletin of the Tokyo Medical Dental University* **7**, 161–164.

Onoue, S., Imai, T., Kumada, H., Umemoto, T., Kaca, W., Isshiki, Y., Kaneko, A. & Kawahara, K. (2003). Serum antibodies of periodontitis patients compared to the lipopolysaccharide of *Porphyromonas gingivalis* and *Fusobacterium nucleatum*. *Microbiology & Immunology* **47**, 51–55.

Pace, N.R., Stahl, D.A., Lane, D.J. & Olsen, G.J. (1986). The analysis of natural microbial populations by ribosomal RNA sequences. *Advances in Microbial Ecology* **9**, 1–55.

Page, R.C. (2000). Vaccination and periodontitis: myth or reality. *Journal of the International Academy of Periodontology* **2**, 31–43.

Papaioannou, S., Marsh, P.D. & Ivanyi, L. (1991). The immunogenicity of outer membrane proteins of haemin-depleted *Porphyromonas (Bacteroides) gingivalis* W50 in periodontal disease. *Oral Microbiology & Immunology* **6**, 327–331.

Papapanou, P.N., Baelum, V., Luan, W.M., Madianos, P.N., Chen, X., Fejerskov, O. & Dahlen, G. (1997). Subgingival microbiota in adult Chinese: prevalence and relation to periodontal disease progression. *Journal of Periodontology* **68**, 651–656.

Papapanou, P.N., Neiderud, A.M., Papadimitriou, A., Sandros, J. & Dahlen, G. (2000). "Checkerboard" assessments of periodontal microbiota and their antibody responses: a case-control study. *Journal of Periodontology* **71**, 885–897.

Paster, B.J., Boches, S.K., Galvin, J.L., Ericson, R.E., Lau, C.N., Levanos, V.A., Sahasrabudhe, A. & Dewhirst, F.E. (2001). Bacterial diversity in human subgingival plaque. *Journal of Bacteriology* **183**, 3770–3783.

Paster, B.J., Falkler, W.A. Jr., Enwonwu, C.O., Idigbe, E.O., Savage, K.O., Levanos, V.A., Tamer, M.A., Ericson, R.L., Lau, C.N. & Dewhirst, F.E. (2002). Predominant bacterial species and novel phylotypes in advanced noma lesions. *Journal of Clinical Microbiology* **40**, 2187–2191.

Paster, B.J., Olsen, I., Aas, J.A & Dewhirst, F.E. (2006). The breadth of bacterial diversity in the human periodontal pocket and other oral sites. *Periodontology 2000* **42**, 80–87.

Paturel, L., Casalta, J.P., Habib, G., Nezri, M. & Raoult, D. (2004). *Actinobacillus actinomycetemcomitans* endocarditis. *Clinical Microbiology & Infection* **10**, 98–118.

Pavicic, M.J.A.M.P., van Winkelhoff, A.J., Douque, N.H., Steures, R.W.R. & de Graaff, J. (1994). Microbiological and clinical effects of metronidazole and amoxicillin in *Actinobacillus actinomycetemcomitans*-associated periodontitis: a 2-year evaluation. *Journal of Clinical Periodontology* **21**, 107–112.

Persson, G.R., Engel, D., Whitney, C., Darveau, R., Weinberg, A., Brunsvold, M., & Page, R.C. (1994a). Immunization against *Porphyromonas gingivalis* inhibits progression of experimental periodontitis in nonhuman primates. *Infection & Immunity* **62**, 1026–1031.

Persson, G.R., Engel, L.D., Whitney, C.W., Weinberg, A., Monla, B.J., Darveau, R.P., Houston, L., Braham, P. & Page, R.C. (1994b). *Macaca fascicularis* as a model in which to assess the safety and efficacy of a vaccine for periodontitis. *Oral Microbiology and Immunology* **9**, 104–111.

Petit, M.D.A., Van Steenbergen, T.J.M., De Graaff, J. & Van der Velden, U. (1993a). Transmission of *Actinobacillus actinomycetemcomitans* in families of adult periodontitis patients. *Journal of Periodontal Research* **28**, 335–345.

Petit, M.D.A., Van Steenbergen, T.J.M., Scholte, L.M.H., Van der Velden, U. & De Graaff, J. (1993b). Epidemiology and transmission of *Porphyromonas gingivalis* and *Actinobacillus actinomycetemcomitans* among children and their family members. *Journal of Clinical Periodontology* **20**, 641–650.

Plaut, H.C. (1894). Studien zur bacteriellen Diagnostik der Diphtherie und der Anginen. *Deutsche Medicinische Wochenschrift* **20**, 920–923.

Preus, H.R. (1988). Treatment of rapidly destructive periodontitis in Papillon-Lefevre syndrome. Laboratory and clinical observations. *Journal of Clinical Periodontology* **15**, 639–643.

Preus, H.R., Zambon, J.J., Dunford, R.G. & Genco, R.J. (1994). The distribution and transmission of *Actinobacillus actinomycetemcomitans* in families with established adult periodontitis. *Journal of Periodontology* **65**, 2–7.

Proske, H.O. & Sayers, R.R. (1934). Pulmonary infections in pneumoconiosis. II. Fuso-spirochetal infection. Experiments in guinea pigs. *Public Health Reports* **29**, 1212–1217.

Prosser, J.I. (1999). Quorum sensing in biofilms. In: Newman, H.N. & Wilson, M., eds. *Dental Plaque Revisited*. Cardiff: Bioline, pp. 79–88.

Rabie, G., Lally, E.T. & Shenker, B.J. (1988). Immunosuppressive properties of *Actinobacillus actinomycetemcomitans* leukotoxin. *Infection & Immunity* **56**, 122–127.

Ramberg, P., Sekino, S., Uzel, N.G., Socransky, S. & Lindhe, J. (2003). Bacterial colonization during de novo plaque formation. *Journal of Clinical Periodontology* **30**, 990–995.

Rams, T.E., Andriola, M. Jr., Feik, D., Abel, S.N., McGiven, T.M. & Slots, J. (1991). Microbiological study of HIV-related periodontitis. *Journal of Periodontology* **62**, 74–81.

Rams, T.E., Feik, D. & Slots, J. (1990). Staphylococci in human periodontal diseases. *Oral Microbiology & Immunology* **5**, 29–32.

Rams, T.E., Feik, D. & Slots, J. (1993). *Campylobacter rectus* in human periodontitis. *Oral Microbiology & Immunology* **8**, 230–235.

Rams, T.E., Feik, D., Young, V., Hammond, B.F. & Slots, J. (1992). Enterococci in human periodontitis. *Oral Microbiology & Immunology* **7**, 249–252.

Rams, T.E. & Keyes, P.H. (1983). A rationale for the management of periodontal diseases: effects of tetracycline on subgingival bacteria. *Journal of the American Dental Association* **107**, 37–41.

Rasmussen, A.T. (1929). Ultraviolet radiation in the treatment of periodontal diseases. *Journal of the American Dental Association* **16**, 3–17.

Renvert, S., Pettersson, T., Ohlsson, O. & Persson, G.R. (2006). Bacterial profile and burden of periodontal infection in subjects with a diagnosis of acute coronary syndrome. *Journal of Periodontology* **77**, 1110–1119.

Riggio, M.P., Lennon, A. & Smith, A. (2001). Detection of peptostreptococcus micros DNA in clinical samples by PCR. *Journal of Medical Microbiology* **50**, 249–254.

Ritz, H.L. (1967). Microbial population shifts in developing human dental plaque. *Archives of Oral Biology* **12**, 15661–1568.

Riviere, G.R. & DeRouen, T.A. (1998). Association of oral spirochetes from periodontally healthy sites with development of gingivitis. *Journal of Periodontology* **69**, 496–501.

Riviere, G.R., DeRouen, T.A., Kay, S.L., Avera, S.P., Stouffer, V.K. & Hawkins, N.R. (1997). Association of oral spirochetes from sites of periodontal health with development of periodontitis. *Journal of Periodontology* **68**, 1210–1214.

Riviere, G.R., Elliot, K.S., Adams, D.F., Simonson, L.G., Forgas, L.B., Nilius, A.M. & Lukehart, S.A. (1992). Relative proportions of pathogen-related oral spirochetes (PROS) and *Treponema denticola* in supragingival and subgingival plaque from patients with periodontitis. *Journal of Periodontology* **63**, 131–136.

Riviere, G.R., Smith, K.S., Willis, S.G. & Riviere, K.H. (1999). Phenotypic and genotypic heterogeneity among comparable pathogen-related oral spirochetes and *Treponema vincentii*. *Journal of Clinical Microbiology* **37**, 3676–3680.

Riviere, G.R., Wagoner, M.A. Baker-Zander, S. Weisz, K.S., Adams, D.F., Simonson, L. & Lukehart, S.A. (1991a). Identification of spirochetes related to *Treponema pallidum* in necrotizing ulcerative gingivitis and chronic periodontitis. *New England Journal of Medicine* **325**, 539–543.

Riviere, G.R., Weisz, K.S., Adams, D.F. & Thomas, D.D. (1991c). Pathogen-related oral spirochetes from dental plaque are invasive. *Infection & Immunity* **59**, 3377–3380.

Riviere, G.R., Weisz, K.S., Simonson, L.G. & Lukehart, S.A. (1991b). Pathogen-related spirochetes identified within gingival tissue from patients with acute necrotizing ulcerative gingivitis. *Infection & Immunity* **59**, 2653–2657.

Roberts, A.P. & Mullany, P. (2006). Genetic basis of horizontal gene transfer among oral bacteria. *Periodontology 2000* **42**, 36–46.

Rodenburg, J.P., van Winkelhoff, A.J., Winkel, E.G., Goene, R.J., Abbas, F. & de Graff, J. (1990). Occurrence of *Bacteroides gingivalis, Bacteroides intermedius* and *Actinobacillus actinomycetemcomitans* in severe periodontitis in relation to age and treatment history. *Journal of Clinical Periodontology* **17**, 392–399.

Rogers, A.H., van der Hoeven, J.S. & Mikx, F.H.M. (1979). Effect of bacteriocin production by *Streptococcus mutans* on the plaque of gnotobiotic rats. *Infection & Immunity* **23**, 571–576.

Rogosa, M. (1964). The genus *Veillonella* I. General, cultural, ecological and biochemical considerations. *Journal of Bacteriology* **87**, 162–170.

Rooney, J., Wade, W.G., Sprague, S.V., Newcombe, R.G. & Addy, M. (2002). Adjunctive effects to non-surgical periodontal therapy of systemic metronidazole and amoxycillin alone and combined. A placebo controlled study. *Journal of Clinical Periodontology* **29**, 342–350.

Rosebury, T., Clarke, A.R., Engel, S.G. & Tergis, F. (1950). Studies of fusospirochetal infection. I. Pathogenicity for guinea pigs of individual and combined cultures of spirochetes and other anaerobic bacteria derived from the human mouth. *Journal of Infectious Diseases* **87**, 217–225.

Rudney, J.D., Chen, R. & Sedgewick, G.J. (2001). Intracellular *Actinobacillus actinomycetemcomitans* and *Porphyromonas gingivalis* in buccal epithelial cells collected from human subjects. *Infection and Immunity* **69**, 2700–2707.

Rudney, J.D., Chen, R. & Sedgewick, G.J. (2005). *Actinobacillus actinomycetemcomitans, Porphyromonas gingivalis* and *Tannerella forsythensis* are components of a polymicrobial intracellular flora within human buccal cells. *Journal of Dental Research* **84**, 59–63.

Rylander, H., Ramberg, P., Blohme, G. & Lindhe, J. (1987). Prevalence of periodontal disease in young diabetics. *Journal of Clinical Periodontology* **14**, 38–43.

Saarela, M., von Troil-Linden, B., Torkko, H., Stucki, A-M., Alaluusua, S., Jousimies-Somer, H. & Asikainen, S. (1993). Transmission of oral bacterial species between spouses. *Oral Microbiology & Immunology* **8**, 349–354.

Sabet, M., Lee, S.W., Nauman, R.K., Sims, T. & Um, H.S. (2003). The surface (S-) layer is a virulence factor of *Bacteroides forsythus*. *Microbiology* **149**, 3617–3627.

Saglie, F.R., Marfany, A. & Camargo, P. (1988). Intragingival occurrence of *Actinobacillus actinomycetemcomitans* and *Bacteroides gingivalis* in active destructive periodonta lesions. *Journal of Periodontology* **59**, 259–265.

Saglie, F.R., Smith, C.T., Newman, M.G., Carranza, F.A. Jr. & Pertuiset, J.J. (1986). The presence of bacteria in the oral epithelium in periodontal disease. II. Immunohistochemical identification of bacteria. *Journal of Periodontology* **57**, 492–500.

Saiki, K., Konishi, K., Gomi, T., Nishihara, T. & Yoshikawa, M. (2001). Reconstitution and purification of cytolethal distending toxin of *Actinobacillus actinomycetemcomitans*. *Microbiology & Immunology* **45**, 497–506.

Saito, A., Hosaka, Y., Nakagawa, T., Seida, K., Yamada, S., Takazoe, I. & Okuda, K. (1993). Significance of serum antibody against surface antigens of *Actinobacillus actinomycetemcomitans* in patients with adult periodontitis. *Oral Microbiology & Immunology* **8**, 146–153.

Saito, M., Otsuka, M., Maehara, R., Endo, J. & Nakamura, R. (1987). Degradation of human secretory immunoglobulin A by protease isolated from the anaerobic periodontopathogenic bacterium, *Bacteroides gingivalis*. *Archives of Oral Biology* **32**, 235–238.

Sanavi, F., Listgarten, M.A., Boyd, F., Sallay, K. & Nowotny, A. (1985). The colonization and establishment of invading bacterium in periodontium of ligature-treated immunosuppressed rats. *Journal of Periodontology* **56**, 273–280.

Sandberg, A.L., Mudrick, L.L., Cisar, J.O., Brennan, M.J., Mergenhagen, S.E. & Vatter, A.E. (1986). Type 2 fimbrial lectin-mediated phagocytosis of oral *Actinomyces* spp. by polymorphonuclear leukocytes. *Infection & Immunity* **54**, 472–476.

Sandberg, A.L., Mudrick, L.L., Cisar, J.O., Metcalf, J.A. & Malech, H.L. (1988). Stimulation superoxide and lactoferrin from polymorphonuclear leukocytes by the Type 2 fimbrial lectin of *Actinomyces viscosus* T14V. *Infection & Immunity* **56**, 267–269.

Sandros, J., Karlsson, C., Lappin, D.F., Madianos, P.N., Kinane, D.F. & Papapanou, P.N. (2000). Cytokine responses of oral epithelial cells to *Porphyromonas gingivalis*. *Journal of Dental Research* **79**, 1808–1814.

Sandros, J., Papapanou, P. & Dahlen, G. (1993). *Porphyromonas gingivalis* invades oral epithelial cells in vitro. *Journal of Periodontal Research* **28**, 219–226.

Sastrowijoto, S.H., Hillemans, P., van Steenbergen, T.J.M., Abraham-Inpijn, L. & de Graaff, J. (1989). Periodontal condition and microbiology of healthy and diseased periodontal pockets in type 1 diabetes mellitus patients. *Journal of Clinical Periodontology* **16**, 316–322.

Savitt, E.D. & Socransky, S.S. (1984). Distribution of certain subgingival microbial species in selected periodontal conditions. *Journal of Periodontal Research* **19**, 111–123.

Schenkein, H.A., Barbour, S.E., Berry, C.R., Kipps, B. & Tew, J.G. (2000). Invasion of human vascular endothelial cells by *Actinobacillus actinomycetemcomitans* via the receptor for platelet-activating factor. *Infection and Immunity* **68**, 5416–5419.

Schifferle, R.E., Wilson, M.E., Levine, M.J. & Genco, R.J. (1993). Activation of serum complement by polysaccharide-containing antigens of *Porphyromonas gingivalis*. *Journal of Periodontal Research* **28**, 248–254.

Schonfeld, S.E. & Kagan, J.M. (1982). Specificity of gingival plasma cells for bacterial somatic antigens. *Journal of Periodontal Research* **17**, 60–69.

Sela, M.N., Weinberg, A., Borinsky, R., Holt, S.C. & Dishon, T. (1988). Inhibition of superoxide production in human polymorphonuclear leukocytes by oral treponemal factors. *Infection & Immunity* **56**, 589–594.

Seppala, B., Seppala, M. & Ainamo, J. (1993). A longitudinal study on insulin-dependent diabetes mellitus and periodontal disease. *Journal of Clinical Periodontology* **20**, 161–165.

Seow, W.K., Bird, P.S., Seymour, G.J. & Thong, Y.H. (1989). Modulation of human neutrophil adherence by periodontopathic bacteria: reversal by specific monoclonal antibodies. *International Achives of Allergy & Applied Immunology* **90**, 24–30.

Seow, W.K., Seymour, G.J. & Thong, Y.H. (1987). Direct modulation of human neutrophil adherence by coaggregating periodontopathic bacteria. *International Achives of Allergy & Applied Immunology* **83**, 121–128.

Shah, H.N. & Gharbia, S.E. (1992). Biochemical and chemical studies on strains designated *Prevotella intermedia* and proposal of a new pigmented species, *Prevotella nigrescens* sp. nov. *International Journal of Systematic Bacteriology* **42**, 542–546.

Sharawy, A.M., Sabharwal, K., Socransky, S.S. & Lobene, R.R. (1966). A quantitative study of plaque and calculus formation in normal and periodontally involved mouths. *Journal of Periodontology* **37**, 495–501.

Sheikhi, M., Gustafsson, A. & Jarstrand, C. (2000). Cytokine, elastase and oxygen radical release by *Fusobacterium nucleatum*-activated leukocytes: a possible pathogenic factor for periodontitis. *Journal of Clinical Periodontology* **27**, 758–762.

Shenker, B.J. (1987). Immunologic dysfunction in the pathogenesis of periodontal diseases. *Journal of Clinical Periodontology* **14**, 489–498.

Shenker, B.J., Hoffmaster, R.H., Zekavat, A., Yamaguchi, N., Lally, E.T. & Demuth, D.R. (2001). Induction of apoptosis in human T cells by *Actinobacillus actinomycetemcomitans* cytolethal distending toxin is a consequence of G(2) arrest of the cell cycle. *Journal of Immunology* **167**, 435–441.

Shenker, B.J., Listgarten, M.A. & Taichman, N.S. (1984). Suppression of human lymphocyte responses by oral spirochetes: a monocyte-dependent phenomenon. *Journal of Immunology* **132**, 2039–2045.

Shenker, B.J. & Slots, J. (1989). Immunomodulatory effects of *Bacteroides* products on in vitro human leukocyte functions. *Oral Microbiology & Immunology* **4**, 24–29.

Shiloah, J., Patters, M.R., Dean, J.W. 3rd., Bland, P. & Toledo, G. (1998). The prevalence of *Actinobacillus actinomycetemcomitans*, *Porphyromonas gingivalis* and *Bacteroides forsythus* in humans 1 year after 4 randomized treatment modalities. *Journal of Periodontology* **69**, 1364–1372.

Simonson, L.G., Goodman, C.H., Bial, J.J. & Morton, H.E. (1988). Quantitative relationship of *Treponema denticola* to severity of periodontal disease. *Infection & Immunity* **56**, 726–728.

Simonson, L.G., Robinson, P.J., Pranger, R.J., Cohen, M.E. & Morton, H.E. (1992). *Treponema denticola* and *Porphyromonas gingivalis* as prognostic markers following periodontal treatment. *Journal of Periodontology* **63**, 270–273.

Simpson, D.L., Berthold, P. & Taichma, N.S. (1988). Killing of human myelomonocytic leukemia and lymphocytic cell lines by *Actinobacillus actinomycetemcomitans* leukotoxin. *Infection & Immunity* **56**, 1162–1166.

Singer, R.E. & Buckner, B.A. (1981). Butyrate and propionate: important components of toxic dental plaque extracts. *Infection & Immunity* **32**, 458–463.

Sismey-Durrant, H.J., Atkinson, S.J., Hopps, R.M. & Heath, J.K. (1989). The effect of lipopolysaccharide from *Bacteroides gingivalis* and muramyl dipeptide on osteoblast collagenase release. *Calcified Tissue International* **44**, 361–363.

Slots, J. (1976). The predominant cultivable organisms in juvenile periodontitis. *Scandinavian Journal of Dental Research* **84**, 1–10.

Slots, J. (1977). The predominant cultivable microflora of advanced periodontitis. *Scandinavian Journal of Dental Research* **85**, 114–121.

Slots, J. (2005). Herpesviruses in periodontal diseases. *Periodontology 2000* **38**, 33–62.

Slots, J., Feik, D. & Rams, T.E. (1990a). *Actinobacillus actinomycetemcomitans* and *Bacteroides intermedius* in human periodontitis: age relationship and mutual association. *Journal of Clinical Periodontology* **17**, 659–662.

Slots, J., Feik, D. & Rams, T.E. (1990b). Prevalence and antimicrobial susceptibility of Enterobacteriaceae, Pseudomonadaceae and Acinetobacter in human periodontitis. *Oral Microbiology & Immunology* **5**, 149–154.

Slots, J., Rams, T.E., Feik, D., Taveras, H.D. & Gillespie, G.M. (1991). Subgingival microflora of advanced periodontitis in the Dominican Republic. *Journal of Periodontology* **62**, 543–547.

Slots, J., Reynolds, H.S. & Genco, R.J. (1980). *Actinobacillus actinomycetemcomitans* in human periodontal disease: a cross-sectional microbiological investigation. *Infection & Immunity* **29**, 1013–1020.

Slots, J. & Rosling, B.G. (1983). Suppression of the periodontopathic microflora in localized juvenile periodontitis by systemic tetracycline. *Journal of Clinical Periodontology* **10**, 465–486.

Slots, J., Saygun, I., Sabeti, M. & Kubar, A. (2006). Epstein-Barr virus in oral diseases. *Journal of Periodontal Research* **41**, 235–244.

Smalley, J.W, Birss, A.J. & Shuttleworth, C.A. (1988). The degradation of type I collagen and human plasma fibronectin by the trypsin-like enzyme and extracellular membrane vesicles of *Bacteroides gingivalis* W50. *Archives of Oral Biology* **33**, 323–329.

Smith, D.T. (1930). Fusospirochetal disease of the lungs produced with cultures from Vincent's angina. *Journal of Infectious Diseases* **46**, 303–310.

Smith, D.J., Gadalla, L.M., Ebersole, J.L. & Taubman, M.A. (1985). Gingival crevicular fluid antibody to oral microorganisms. III. Association of gingival homogenate and gingival crevicular fluid antibody levels. *Journal of Periodontal Research* **20**, 357–367.

Socransky, S.S. (1970). Relationship of bacteria to the etiology of periodontal disease. *Journal of Dental Research* **49**, 203–222.

Socransky, S.S. & Gibbons, R.J. (1965). Required role of Bacteroides melaninogenicus in mixed anaerobic infections. *Journal of Infectious Diseases* **115**, 247–253.

Socransky, S.S., Gibbons, R.J., Dale, A.C., Bortnick, L., Rosenthal, E. & Macdonald, J.B. (1963). The microbiota of the gingival crevice area of man. I. Total microscopic and viable counts and counts of specific organisms. *Archives of Oral Biology* **8**, 275–280.

Socransky, S.S. & Haffajee, A.D. (1991). Microbial mechanisms in the pathogenesis of destructive periodontal diseases: a critical assessment. *Journal of Periodontal Research* **26**, 195–212.

Socransky, S.S. & Haffajee, A.D. (1992). The bacterial etiology of destructive peridontal disease: current concepts. *Journal of Periodontology* **63**, 322–331.

Socransky, S.S. & Haffajee, A.D. (1993). Effect of therapy on periodontal infections. *Journal of Periodontology* **64**, 754–759.

Socransky, S.S. & Haffajee, A.D. (1994). Evidence of bacterial etiology: a historical perspective. In: Socransky, S.S. &

Haffajee, A.D., eds. *Microbiology and Immunology of Periodontal Diseases. Periodontology 2000* **5**, 7–25.

Socransky, S.S. & Haffajee, A.D. (2001). Dental biofilms: difficult therapeutic targets. *Periodontology 2000* **28**, 12–55.

Socransky, S.S. & Haffajee, A.D. (2005). Periodontal microbial ecology. In: Haffajee, A.D. & Socransky, S.S., eds. Microbiology of Periodontal Diseases. *Periodontology 2000* **38**, 135–187.

Socransky, S.S., Haffajee, A.D., Cugini, M.A., Smith, C. & Kent, R.L. Jr. (1998). Microbial complexes in subgingival plaque. *Journal of Clinical Periodontology* **25**, 134–144.

Socransky, S.S., Haffajee, A.D. & Dzink, J.L. (1988). Relationship of subgingival microbial complexes to clinical features at the sampled sites. *Journal of Clinical Periodontology* **15**, 440–444.

Socransky, S.S. Haffajee, A.D., Smith, C. & Dibart, S. (1991). Relation of counts of microbial species to clinical status at the site. *Journal of Clinical Periodontology* **18**, 766–775.

Socransky, S.S., Loesche, W.J., Hubersack, C. & Macdonald, J.B. (1964). Dependency of *Treponema microdentium* on other oral organisms for isobutyrate, polyamines, and a controlled oxidation-reduction potential. *Journal of Bacteriology* **88**, 200–209.

Socransky, S.S., Smith, C. & Haffajee, A.D. (2002). Subgingival microbial profiles in refractory periodontal disease. *Journal of Clinical Periodontology* **29**, 260–268.

Soder, B., Airila Mansson, S., Soder, P.O., Kari, K. & Meurman, J. (2006). Levels of matrix metalloproteinases-8 and -9 with simultaneous presence of periodontal pathogens in gingival crevicular fluid as well as matrix metalloproteinase-9 and cholesterol in blood. *Journal of Periodontal Research* **41**, 411–417.

Spratt, D.A., Weightman, A.J. & Wade, W.G. (1999). Diversity of oral asaccharolytic *Eubacterium* species in periodontitis: identification of novel phylotypes representing uncultivated taxa. *Oral Microbiology & Immunology* **14**, 56–59.

Sreenivasan, P.K., Meyer, D.H. & Fives-Taylor, P.M. (1993). Requirements for invasion of epithelial cells by *Actinobacillus actinomycetemcomitans. Infection & Immunity* **61**, 1239–1245.

Steinberg, A.I. & Gershoff, S.N. (1968). Quantitative differences in spirochetal antibody observed in periodontal disease. *Journal of Periodontology* **39**, 286–289.

Stevens, R.H., Lillard, S.E. & Hammond, B.F. (1987). Purification and biochemical properties of a bacteriocin from *Actinobacillus actinomycetemcomitans. Infection & Immunity* **55**, 686–691.

Suda, R., Kobayashi, M., Nanba, R., Iwamaru, M., Hayashi, Y., Lai, C-H. & Hasegawa, K. (2004). Possible periodontal pathogens associated with clinical symptoms of periodontal disease in Japanese high school students. *Journal of Periodontology* **75**, 1084–1089.

Suda, R., Lai, C-H., Yang, H.W. & Hasegawa, K. (2002). *Eikenella corrodens* in subgingival plaque: relationship to age and periodontal condition. *Journal of Periodontology* **73**, 886–891.

Sudre, P., ten Dam, G. & Kochi, A. (1992). Tuberculosis: a global overview of the situation today. *Bulletin of the World Health Organization* **70**, 149–159.

Summary of notifiable diseases – United States 2004 (2006). *Morbidity and Mortality Weekly Report* **53**, 1–79.

Sundqvist, G., Figdor, D., Hanstrom, L., Sorlin, S. & Sandstrom, G. (1991). Phagocytosis and virulence of different strains of *Porphyromonas gingivalis. Scandinavian Journal of Dental Research* **99**, 117–129.

Takada, H., Ogawa, T., Yoshimura, F., *et al.* (1988). Immunobiological activities of a porin fraction isolated from *Fusobacterium nucleatum* ATCC10953. *Infection & Immunity* **56**, 855–863.

Takahashi, Y., Davey, M., Yumoto, H., Gibson, F.C. 3rd. & Genco C.A. (2006). Fimbria-dependent activation of proinflammatory molecules in *Porphyromonas gingivalis* infected human aortic endothelial cells. *Cellular Microbiology* **8**, 738–757.

Takamatsu, N., Yano, K., He, T., Umeda, M. & Ishikawa, I. (1999). Effect of initial periodontal therapy on the frequency of detecting *Bacteroides forsythus, Porphyromonas gingivalis* and *Actinobacillus actinomycetemcomitans. Journal of Periodontology* **70**, 574–580.

Takeuchi, Y., Umeda, M., Sakamoto, M., Benno, Y., Huang, Y. & Ishikawa, I. (2001). *Treponema socranskii, Treponema denticola,* and *Porphyromonas gingivalis* are associated with severity of periodontal tissue destruction. *Journal of Periodontology* **72**, 1354–1363.

Tan, K.S., Woo, C.H., Ong, G. & Song, K.P. (2001). Prevalence of *Actinobacillus actinomycetemcomitans* in an ethnic adult Chinese population. *Journal of Clinical Periodontology* **28**, 886–890.

Tanner, A. & Bouldin, H. (1989). The microbiology of early periodonitis lesions in adults. *Journal of Clinical Periodontology* **16**, 467–471.

Tanner, A.C.R., Dzink, J.L., Ebersole, J.L. & Socransky, S.S. (1987). *Wolinella recta, Campylobacter concisus, Bacteroides gracilis,* and *Eikenella corrodens* from periodontal lesions. *Journal of Periodontal Research* **22**, 327–330.

Tanner, A.C.R., Haffer, C., Bratthall, G.T., Visconti, R.A. & Socransky, S.S. (1979). A study of the bacteria associated with advancing periodontitis in man. *Journal of Clinical Periodontology* **6**, 278–307.

Tanner, A.C.R. & Izard, J. (2006). *Tannerella forsythia*, a periodontal pathogen entering the genomic era. *Periodontology 2000* **42**, 88–113.

Tanner, A., Kent, R., Maiden, M.F. & Taubman, M.A. (1996). Clinical, microbiological and immunological profile of health, gingivitis, and putative active periodontal subjects. *Journal of Periodontal Research* **31**, 195–204.

Tanner, A.C.R., Listgarten, M.A., Ebersole, J.L. & Strzempko, M.N. (1986). *Bacteroides forsythus* sp. nov., a slow growing fusiform *Bacteroides* sp. from the human oral cavity. *International Journal of Systematic Bacteriology* **36**, 213–221.

Tanner, A., Maiden, M.F., Macuch, P.J., Murray, L.L. & Kent, R.L. Jr. (1998). Microbiota of health, gingivitis and initial periodontitis. *Journal of Clinical Periodontology* **25**, 85–98.

Tanner, A., Maiden, M.F.J., Paster, B.J. & Dewhirst, F.E. (1994). The impact of 16S ribosomal RNA-based phylogeny on the taxonomy of oral bacteria. In: Socransky, S.S. & Haffajee, A.D., eds. Microbiology and Immunology of Periodontal Diseases. *Periodontology 2000* **5**, 26–51.

Tanner, A.C.R. & Socransky, S.S. (1984). Genus *Wolinella*. In: Buchanan, N. & Gibbons, N., eds. *Bergey's Manual of Determinative Bacteriology*, 8th edn. Baltimore: Williams and Wilkins Co, pp. 646–650.

Taubman, M.A., Haffajee, A.D., Socransky, S.S., Smith, D.J. & Ebersole, J.L. (1992). Longitudinal monitoring of humoral antibody in subjects with destructive periodontal diseases. *Journal of Periodontal Research* **27**, 511–521.

Teixeira, R.E., Mendes, E.N., Roque de Carvalho, M.A., Nicoli, J.R., Farias, Lde, M. & Magalhaes, P.P. (2006). *Actinobacillus actinomycetemcomitans* serotype-specific genotypes and periodontal status in Brazilian subjects. *Canadian Journal of Microbiology* **52**, 182–188.

Teles, R.P., Haffajee, A.D. & Socransky, S.S. (2006). Microbiological goals of periodontal therapy. *Periodontology 2000* **43**, 180–218.

Tenovuo, J. & Pruitt, K.M. (1984). Relationship of the human salivary peroxidase system to oral health. *Journal of Oral Pathology* **13**, 573–584.

Tew, J.G., Marshall, D.R., Burmeister, J.A. & Ranney, R.R. (1985a). Relationship between gingival crevicular fluid and serum antibody titers in young adults with generalized and localized periodontitis. *Infection & Immunity* **49**, 487–493.

Tew, J.G., Marshall, D.R., Moore, W.E., Best, A.M., Palcanis, K.G. & Ranney, R.R. (1985b). Serum antibody reactive with predominant organisms in the subgingival flora of young adults with generalized severe periodontitis. *Infection & Immunity* **48**, 303–311.

Tew, J.G., Smibert, R.M., Scott, E.A., Burmeister, J.A. & Ranney, R.R. (1985c). Serum antibodies in young adult humans reactive with periodontitis associated treponemes. *Journal of Periodontal Research* **20**, 580–590.

Theilade, E., Wright, W.H., Jensen, S.B. & Loe, H. (1966). Experimental gingivitis in man. II. A longitudinal clinical and bacteriological investigation. *Journal of Periodontal Research* **1**, 1–13.

Thorstensson, H. & Hugoson, A. (1993). Periodontal disease experience in adult long-duration insulin-dependent diabetics. *Journal of Clinical Periodontology* **20**, 352–358.

Timmerman, M.F., van der Weijden, G.A., Arief, E.M., Armand, S., Abbas, F., Winkel, E.G., van Winkelhoff, A.J. & van der Velden, U. (2001). Untreated periodontal disease in Indonesian adolescents: subgingival microbiota in relation to experienced progression of periododontitis. *Journal of Clinical Periodontology* **28**, 617–627.

Tinoco, E.M., Beldi, M.I., Campedelli, F., Lana, M., Loureiro, C.A., Bellini, H.T., Rams, T.E., Tinoco, N.M., Gjermo, P. & Preus, H.R. (1998). Clinical and microbiological effects of adjunctive antibiotics in the treatment of localized juvenile periodontitis. A controlled clinical trial. *Journal of Periodontology* **69**, 1355–1363.

Tran, S.D., Rudney, J.D., Sparks, B.S. & Hodges, J.S. (2001). Persistent presence of *Bacteroides forsythus* as a risk factor for attachment loss in a population with low prevalence and severity of adult periodontitis. *Journal of Periodontology* **72**, 1–10.

Tsai, C-C., McArthur, W.P., Baehni, P.C., Evian, C., Genco, R.J. & Taichman, N.S. (1981). Serum neutralizing activity against *Actinobacillus actinomycetemcomitans* leukotoxin in juvenile periodontitis. *Journal of Clinical Periodontology* **8**, 338–348.

Tsai, C-C., McArthur, W.P., Baehni, P.C., Hammond, B.F. & Taichman, N.S. (1979). Extraction and partial characterization of leukotoxin from a plaque-derived Gram-negative microorganism. *Infection & Immunity* **25**, 427–439.

Uchida, Y., Shiba, H., Komatsuzawa, H., Takemoto, T., Sakata, M., Fujita, T., Kawaguchi, H., Sugai, M. & Kurihara, H. (2001). Expression of IL-1 beta and IL-8 by human gingival epithelial cells in response to *Actinobacillus actinomycetemcomitans*. *Cytokine* **7**, 152–161.

Uematsu, H. & Hoshino, E. (1992). Predominant obligate anaerobes in human periodontal pockets. *Journal of Periodontal Research* **27**, 15–19.

Uitto, V.J., Baillie, D., Wu, Q., Gendron, R., Grenier, D., Putnins, E.E., Kanervo, A. & Firth, J.D. (2005). *Fusobacterium nucleatum* increases collagenase 3 production and migration of epithelial cells. *Infection & Immunity* **73**, 1171–1179.

Uitto, V.J., Larjava, H., Heino, J. & Sorsa, T. (1989). A protease of *Bacteroides gingivalis* degrades cell surface and matrix glycoproteins of cultured gingival fibroblasts and induces secretion of collagenase and plasminogen activator. *Infection & Immunity* **57**, 213–218.

Umeda, M., Miwa, Z., Takeuchi, Y., Ishizuka, M., Huang, Y., Noguchi, K., Tanaka, M., Takagi, Y. & Ishikawa, I. (2004). The distribution of periodontopathic bacteria among Japanese children and their parents. *Journal of Periodontal Research* **39**, 398–404.

van Dalen, P.J., van Deutekom-Mulder, E.C., de Graaff, J. & van Steenbergen, T.J. (1998). Pathogenicity of *Peptostreptococcus micros* morphotypes and *Prevotella* species in pure and mixed cultures. *Journal of Medical Microbiology* **47**, 135–140.

van der Velden, U., Varoufaki, A., Hutter, J.W., Xo, L., Timmerman, M.F., van Winkelhoff, A.J. & Loos, B.J. (2003). Effect of smoking and periodontal treatment on the subgingival microflora. *Journal of Clinical Periodontology* **30**, 603–610.

van Steenbergen, T.J.M., Delemarre, F.G., Namavar, F. & de Graaff, J. (1987). Differences in virulence within the species *Bacteroides gingivalis*. *Antonie Van Leeuwenhoek* **53**, 233–244.

van Steenbergen, T.J., Petit, M.D., Scholte, L.H., Van der Velden, U. & de Graaff, J. (1993). Transmission of *Porphyromonas gingivalis* between spouses. *Journal of Clinical Periodontology* **20**, 340–345.

van Steenbergen, T.J.M., van der Mispel, L.M.S. & de Graaff, J. (1986). Effects of ammonia and volatile fatty acids produced by oral bacteria on tissue culture cells. *Journal of Dental Research* **65**, 909–912.

van Winkelhoff, A.J., Bosch-Tijhof, C.J., Winkel, E.G. & van der Reijden, W.A. (2001). *Porphyromonas gingivalis, Bacteroides forsythus* and other putative periodontal pathogens in subjects with and without periodontal destruction. *Journal of Periodontology* **72**, 666–671.

van Winkelhoff, A.J., Loos, B.G., van der Reijden, W.A. & van der Velden, U. (2002). *Porphyromonas gingivalis, Bacteroides forsythus* and other putative periodontal pathogens in subjects with and without periodontal destruction. *Journal of Clinical Periodontology* **29**, 1023–1028.

van Winkelhoff, A.J., Tijhof, C.J. & de Graaff, J. (1992). Microbiological and clinical results of metronidazole plus amoxicillin therapy in *Actinobacillus actinomycetemcomitans*-associated periodontitis. *Journal of Periodontology* **63**, 52–57.

van Winkelhoff, A.J., van der Velden, U. & de Graaf, J. (1988). Microbial succession in recolonizing deep periodontal pockets after a single course of supra- and subgingival debridement. *Journal of Clinical Periodontology* **15**, 116–122.

Vasel, D., Sims, T.J., Bainbridge, B., Houston, L., Darveau, R. & Page, R.C. (1996). Shared antigens of *Porphyrominas gingivalis* and *Bacteroides forsythus*. *Oral Microbiology and Immunology* **11**, 226–235.

Vincent, J.W., Falkler, W.A., Jr. & Suzuki, J.B. (1986). Systemic antibody response of clinically characterized patients with antigens of *Eubacterium brachy* initially and following periodontal therapy. *Journal of Periodontology* **57**, 625–631.

Vincent, M.H. (1899). Recherches bacteriologiques sur l'angine a bacilles fusiformes. *Annales de L'Institut Pasteur* **8**, 609–620.

Vitkov, L., Krautgartner, W.D. & Hannig, M. (2005). Bacterial internalization in periodontitis. *Oral Microbiology & Immunology* **20**, 317–321.

Walker, C., Gordon, J., Magnusson, I. & Clark, W.B. (1993). A role for antibiotics in the treatment of refractory periodontitis. *Journal of Periodontology* **64**, 772–781.

Wang, B., Kraig, E. & Kolodrubetz, D. (1998). A new member of the S-layer protein family: charaterization of the *crs* gene from *Campylobacter rectus*. *Infection & Immunity* **66**, 1521–1526.

Wang, B., Kraig, E. & Kolodrubetz, D. (2000). Use of defined mutants to assess the role of the *Campylobacter rectus* S-layer in bacterium-epithelial cell interactions. charaterization of the *crs* gene. *Infection & Immunity* **68**, 1465–1473.

Weinberg, A., Belton, C.M., Park, Y. & Lamont, R.J. (1997). Role of fimbriae in *Porphyromonas gingivalis* invasion of gingival epithelial cells. *Infection and Immunity* **65**, 313–316.

Weinberg, A. & Holt, S.C. (1990). Interaction of *Treponema denticola* TD-4, GM-1, and MS25 with human gingival fibroblasts. *Infection & Immunity* **58**, 1720–1729.

Weiss, E.I., Shaniztki, B., Dotan, M., Ganeshkumar, N., Kolenbrander, P.E. & Metzger, Z. (2000). Attachment of *Fusobacterium nucleatum* PK1594 to mammalian cells and its coaggregation with periodontopathic bacteria are mediated by the same galactose-binding adhesin. *Oral Microbiology and Immunology* **15**, 371–377.

Whitney, C., Ant, J., Moncla, B., Johnson, B., Page, R.C. & Engel, D. (1992). Serum immunoglobulin G antibody to *Porphyromonas gingivalis* in rapidly progressive periodontitis: titer, avidity, and subclass distribution. *Infection & Immunity* **60**, 2194–2200.

Wikstrom, M. & Linde, A. (1986). Ability of oral bacteria to degrade fibonectin. *Infection & Immunity* **51**, 707–711.

Williams, C.A., Winkler, J.R., Grassi, M. & Murray, P.A. (1990). HIV-associated periodontitis complicated by necrotizing stomatitis. *Oral Surgery Oral Medicine Oral Pathology* **69**, 351–355.

Wilton, J.M., Hurst, T.J. & Austin, A.K. (1992). IgG subclass antibodies to *Porphyromonas gingivalis* in patients with destructive periodontal disease. A case: control study. *Journal of Clinical Periodontology* **19**, 646–651.

Winkel, E.G., van Winkelhoff, A.J. & van der Velden, U. (1998). Additional clinical and microbiological effects of amoxicillin and metronidazole after initial periodontal therapy. *Journal of Clinical Periodontology* **25**, 857–864.

Winkler, J.R. & Robertson, P.B. (1992). Periodontal disease associated with HIV infection. *Oral Surgery Oral Medicine Oral Pathology* **73**, 145–150.

Winkler, J.R., John, S.R., Kramer, R.H., Hoover, C.I. & Murray, P.A. (1987). Attachment of oral bacteria to a basement-membrane-like matrix and to purified matrix proteins. *Infection & Immunity* **55**, 2721–2726.

Winkler, J.R., Matarese, V., Hoover, C.I., Kramer, R.H. & Murray, P.A. (1988). An in vitro model to study bacterial invasion of periodontal tissues. *Journal of Periodontology* **59**, 40–45.

Winkler, J.R., Murray, P.A., Grassi, M. & Hammerle, C. (1989). Diagnosis and management of HIV-associated periodontal lesions. *Journal of the American Dental Association* **119**, 25S-34S.

Wood, S.R., Kirkham, J., Marsh, P.D., Shore, R.C., Nattress, B. & Robinson, C. (2000). Architecture of intact natural human plaque biofilms studied by confocal lasers canning microscopy. *Journal of Dental Research* **79**, 21–27.

Wyss, C. (1989). Dependence of proliferation of *Bacteroides forsythus* on exogenous N-acetylmuramic acid. *Infection & Immunity* **57**, 1757–1759.

Wyss, C., Choi, B.K., Schupbach, P., Moter, A., Guggenheim, B. & Gobel, U.B. (1999). *Treponema lecithinolyticum* sp. nov., a small saccharolytic spirochaete with phospholipase A and C activities associated with periodontal diseases. *International Journal of Systematic Bacteriology* **49**, 1329–1339.

Xie, H., Cook, G.S., Costerton, J.W., Bruce, G., Rose, T.M. & Lamont, R.J. (2000). Intergeneric communication in dental plaque biofilms. *Journal of Bacteriology* **182**, 7067–7069.

Yang, H.W., Asikainen, S., Dogan, B., Suda, R. & Lai, C.H. (2004a). Relationship of *Actinobacillus actinomycetemcomitans* serotype b to aggressive periodontitis: frequency in pure cultured isolates. *Journal of Periodontology* **75**, 592–599.

Yang, H.W., Huang, Y.F. & Chou, M.Y. (2004b). Occurrence of *Porphyromonas gingivalis* and *Tannerella forsythensis* in periodontally diseased and healthy subjects. *Journal of Periodontology* **75**, 1077–1083.

Yoneda, M., Maida, K. & Aono, M. (1990). Suppression of bacteriocidal activity of human polymorphonuclear leukocytes by *Bacteroides gingivalis*. *Infection & Immunity* **58**, 406–411.

Yoshida, Y., Suzuki, N., Nakano, Y., Shibuya, K., Ogawa, Y. & Koga T. (2003). Distribution of *Actinobacillus actinomycetemcomitans* serotypes and *Porphyromonas gingivalis* in Japanese adults. *Oral Microbiology and Immunology* **18**, 135–139.

Yoshida-Minami, I., Suzuki, A., Kawabata, K., Okamoto, A., Nishihara, Y., Nagashima, S., Morisaki, I. & Ooshima, T. (1997). Alveolar bone loss in rats infected with a strain of *Prevotella intermedia* and *Fusobacterium nucleatum* isolated from a child with prepubertal periodontitis. *Journal of Periodontology* **68**, 12–17.

Yoshimura, F., Watanabe, K., Takasawa, T., Kawanami, M. & Kato, H. (1989). Purification and properties of a 75-kilodalton major protein, an immunodominant surface antigen, from the oral anaerobe *Bacteroides gingivalis*. *Infection & Immunity* **57**, 3646–3652.

Yuan, K., Chang, C.J., Hsu, P.C., Sun, H.S., Tseng, C.C. & Wang, J.R. (2001). Detection of putative periodontal pathogens in non-insulin-dependent diabetes mellitus and non-diabetes mellitus by polymerase chain reaction. *Journal of Periodontal Research* **36**, 18–24.

Yumoto, H., Nakae, H., Fujinaka, K., Ebisu, S. & Matsuo, T. (1999). Interleukin-6 (IL-6). and IL-8 are induced in human oral epithelial cells in response to exposure to periodontopathic *Eikenella corrodens*. *Infection and Immunity* **67**, 384–394.

Yumoto, H., Nakae, H., Yamada, M., Fujinaka, K., Shinohara, C., Ebisu, S. & Matsuo, T. (2001). Soluble products from *Eikenella corrodens* stimulate oral epithelial cells to induce inflammatory mediators. *Oral Microbiology & Immunology* **16**, 298–305.

Zambon, J.J. (1996). Periodontal diseases: microbial factors. *Annals of Periodontology* **1**, 879–925.

Zambon, J.J., Christersson, L.A. & Slots, J. (1983a). *Actinobacillus actinomycetemcomitans* in human periodontal disease. Prevalence in patient groups and distribution of biotypes and serotypes within families. *Journal of Periodontology* **54**, 707–711.

Zambon, J.J., Reynolds, H., Fisher, J.G., Shlossman, M., Dunford, R. & Genco, R.J. (1988). Microbiological and immunological studies of adult periodontitis in patients with noninsulindependent diabetes mellitus. *Journal of Periodontology* **59**, 23–31.

Zambon, J.J., Reynolds, H.S. & Genco, R.J. (1990). Studies of the subgingival microflora in patients with acquired immunodeficiency syndrome. *Journal of Periodontology* **61**, 699–704.

Zambon, J.J., Slots, J. & Genco, R.J. (1983b). Serology of oral *Actinobacillus actinomycetemcomitans* and serotype distribution in human periodontal disease. *Infection & Immunity* **41**, 19–27.

Zee, K.Y., Samaranayake, L.P. & Attstrom, R. (1996). Predominant cultivable supragingival plaque in Chinese "rapid" and "slow" plaque formers. *Journal of Clinical Periodontology* **23**, 1025–1031.

Chapter 10

Peri-implant Infections

Ricardo P. Teles, Anne D. Haffajee, and Sigmund S. Socransky

Introduction

The introduction of dental implants as a procedure to replace natural teeth lost due to dental caries, trauma or periodontal diseases has been a major advance in the management of edentulous and partially edentulous individuals. The insertion of these "new surfaces" also presents a new opportunity for bacterial colonization. One might surmise that the presence of these implant surfaces with different physical properties from teeth might select for bacterial species that are unique to this habitat, leading to a microbiota that may be substantially different from that found on natural teeth. This chapter will examine the nature of the microbiota on implant surfaces in individuals who have clinically healthy implants in the edentulous or in the partially edentulous dentition. After examining the microbiota associated with healthy implants, the nature of the microbiota associated with peri-implantitis will be described.

Early biofilm development on implant surfaces

When an implant is inserted into the oral cavity, it provides a new and physically different surface for the colonization of microorganisms that might already be resident in the oral cavity or enter the oral cavity during biofilm development. The scanning electron micrographs provided in Fig. 10-1 indicate that implant surfaces are readily colonized by a variety of different bacterial morphotypes. The colonization of osseointegrated implants was studied using an immunoblot technique for the detection of antigens to six different species: *Porphyromonas gingivalis*, *Prevotella intermedia*, *Actinomyces naeslundii* genospecies 2 (formerly *Actinomyces viscosus*), *Fusobacterium nucleatum*, *Treponema socranskii*, and *Treponema denticola* (Koka *et al.* 1993). Supra- and subgingival plaque samples were collected from teeth close to the implants before implant exposure and at

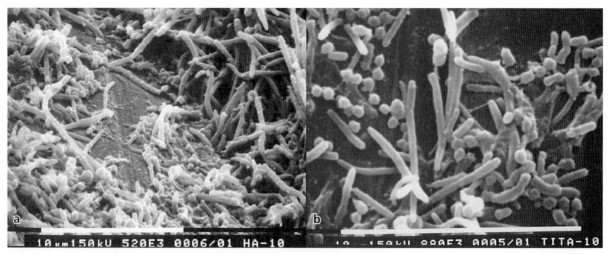

Fig. 10-1 Scanning electron micrographs of the subgingival microbiota on a titanium smooth collar of a hydroxyapatite plasma spray-coated dental implant (a) and on the smooth collar of a titanium dental implant (b). Courtesy of Dr. Charles Cobb.

14 and 28 days after exposure. Samples were taken from the implants 14 and 28 days after the second-stage surgery. The six test species were present in supragingival biofilm samples from the teeth at baseline, but *F. nucleatum* and *Tr. denticola* were not found in subgingival samples at this time point. The frequency of detection on teeth of most of the test species remained constant during the 28 days of observation. *Tr. denticola* was not detected at any time point in subgingival plaque samples from both teeth and implants. All six species were recovered from supragingival plaque samples from implant fixtures after 14 days of exposure, while only *A. naeslundii* genospecies 2 could be detected in the subgingival samples of implants at this time point. After 28 days of implant exposure, all but one species (*Tr. denticola*) could be recovered from subgingival plaque samples of implants. The data suggested that implants in partially edentulous subjects were colonized by periodontal pathogens as early as 14 days after exposure to the oral environment and that establishment of a complex subgingival microbiota occurred as early as 28 days after exposure.

Biofilm development on teeth and implants was also compared during a 3-week study of experimental gingivitis and experimental peri-implant mucosi-tis using phase contrast microscopy (Pontoriero *et al.* 1994). Biofilm samples revealed similar proportions of coccoid cells, motile rods, and spirochetes on both teeth and implants at baseline and after 3 weeks of plaque accumulation. The results were similar to those reported by Löe *et al.* (1965) and Theilade *et al.* (1966) of experimental gingivitis in dentate subjects, in which higher proportions of motile rods and spirochetes and lower proportions of coccoid cells were detected after 3 weeks of plaque accumulation. The authors suggested that plaque accumulated at similar rates on both teeth and implant surfaces.

The development of biofilms on the surface of implants was examined in partially edentulous subjects who required implants (Quirynen *et al.* 2006). Samples were taken from implant and teeth sites using paper points at 2, 4, 12, and 26 weeks after implant exposure and evaluated for their content of 40 bacterial species using checkerboard DNA–DNA hybridization. The mean counts (x 10^5) of the 40 test species evaluated in the samples from the teeth and implant surfaces at the different time points are presented in Fig. 10-2. Higher counts of red and orange complex species (for a description of the microbial complexes, see Chapter 9) were detected on the tooth surfaces at all time points, particularly at 2 weeks. At

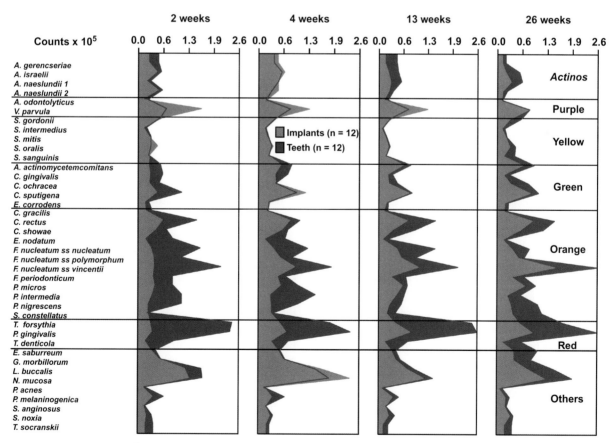

Fig. 10-2 Mean counts (×10^5) of 40 species in samples from 48 implants and 48 teeth in 12 subjects at 2, 4, 13, and 26 weeks after implant exposure. Mean counts of each species were computed by averaging the data for each site category separately in each subject, and then averaging across subjects at each time point separately. Significance of differences between site categories was sought using the Mann Whitney test. No significant differences were found after adjusting for multiple comparisons (Socransky *et al.* 1991). The species were ordered and grouped according to the complexes described by Socransky *et al.* (1998).

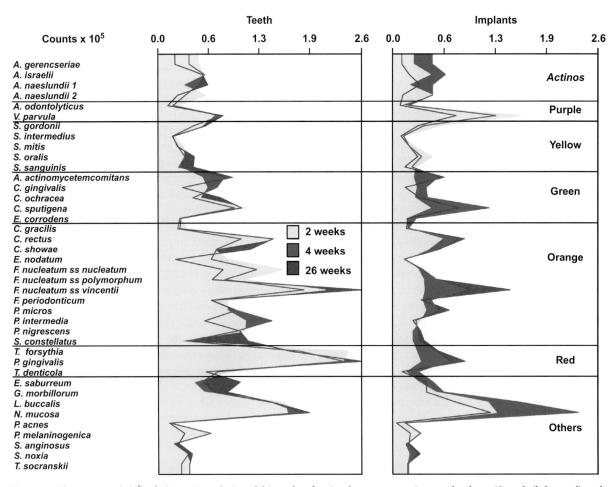

Fig. 10-3 Mean counts ($\times 10^5$) of 40 species at 2, 4, and 26 weeks after implant exposure in samples from 48 teeth (left panel) and 48 implants (right panel) from 12 subjects. Mean counts of each species were computed by averaging the data for each site category separately in each subject, and then averaging across subjects at each time point separately. Significance of differences over time was sought using the Friedman test. No significant differences were detected after adjusting for multiple comparisons (Socransky *et al.* 1991). The species were ordered and grouped according to the complexes described by Socransky *et al.* (1998).

later time points the differences between the different sampled sites were less marked, although red and some orange complex species were still at higher levels in the samples from the teeth. Figure 10-3 presents the mean counts of the 40 test bacteria at tooth (left panel) and implant sites (right panel) at 2, 4, and 26 weeks after implant exposure. There was little change in the mean microbial profiles at the tooth sites over time. However, at the implant sites, there was an increase in counts of certain species including *F. nucleatum* ss *vincentii*, *Peptostreptococcus micros*, *Prevotella nigrescens*, and *P. gingivalis*. Figures 10-2 and 10-3 are interesting because they suggest that species thought to be "early colonizers" on teeth, dentures, and soft tissues (Socransky & Haffajee 2005; Kolenbrander *et al.* 2006), such as *Streptococcus mitis* and *Streptococcus oralis*, appear on implants by 2 weeks and are maintained at their initial levels for periods of 2 to 26 weeks. Other species, such as members of the genus *Fusobacterium*, *Pe. micros*, and *P. gingivalis*, may be detected at early time intervals, but their levels increase more slowly over time. Some species thought to be periodontal pathogens, such as *Eubacterium nodatum* and *Tr. denticola*

(Haffajee *et al.* 2006), were initially present in low numbers on implants with little evidence of an increase by 6 months at these clinically healthy implant sites.

The above studies indicated that the early development of biofilms on implant surfaces was similar to that observed on natural teeth and other restorative materials that were placed in the oral cavity. It is likely that in the first step, proteins of saliva may form a pellicle on the surface of the implant providing receptors for the adhesins that occur on oral bacterial species. In this regard, Edgerton *et al.* (1996) examined *in vitro*, experimental salivary pellicles formed on titanium surfaces. Several salivary components previously described in enamel pellicles were also found on titanium, including high-molecular weight mucins, α-amylase, secretory IgA, and proline-rich proteins. However, cystatins and low-molecular weight mucins, commonly found on enamel, were not detected on titanium surfaces. These differences in pellicle composition could result in qualitative differences in early biofilm formation on implants compared to teeth. Data comparing the initial bacterial colonization on titanium, hydroxyapatite, and amalgam surfaces suggested that this may not be the case (Leonhardt *et al.* 1995). Biofilm accumulation was examined at 10 minutes and 1, 3, 6, 24, and 72 hours in healthy volunteers who wore intraoral removable splints containing small sections of the three different materials. No significant differences were found in the species colonizing the three surfaces at any time point. It was concluded that although the salivary pellicle that formed on titanium surfaces might differ from that on enamel surfaces, these differences did not seem to influence the bacterial composition of the early biofilms formed on these surfaces.

It has been shown in studies of biofilm development on natural teeth that attachment of bacteria occurred within minutes (Socransky *et al.* 1977) and that increases in specific species could be detected in time periods as short as 2–6 hours (Li *et al.* 2004). It is likely that biofilm development on the implant follows a similar course and that "maturation" is well under way by 2 weeks. Data supporting this conjecture were provided by Quirynen *et al.* (2005b) who examined biofilm development on implant surfaces 1 week after their insertion and showed that there were quite marked differences in the microbiotas on the implants with either shallow or deep pockets compared with the microbiota found in shallow and deep pockets adjacent to the natural teeth. The differences had decreased by 2 weeks and were markedly reduced by 6 months, as shown in Figs. 10-2 and 10-3. It must be pointed out that colonization of a pristine implant surface may be different from that of a previously cleaned tooth. The pristine surfaces of the implant are devoid of an indigenous microbiota and may require initial colonization by early colonizers to set the stage for the subsequent complex community (Kolenbrander *et al.* 2006). The cleaned tooth is likely to have remnants of an attached microbiota (Li *et al.* 2004; Socransky & Haffajee 2005) that can immediately multiply and provide surfaces for attachment of later colonizing species. This may also account for the longer time period required for the biofilm developing on implant surfaces to reach a more complex climax community.

Time of implant exposure and climax community complexity

Studies on early plaque development clearly demonstrated development of multi-species supra- and subgingival biofilms on implant fixtures within weeks of their exposure to the oral cavity (Fig. 10-1). However, microbiological data from fully and partially edentulous subjects suggested that the complete maturation of the implant biofilm might take months, if not years to occur. The microbial changes that took place over time on 68 implants inserted in 22 subjects with a history of advanced aggressive periodontitis were examined by De Boever and De Boever (2006). Microbial samples were collected at various time points after installation of transmucosal implants and processed using DNA probes. The frequency of detection of *P. gingivalis* and *Tannerella forsythia* at levels $>10^5$ increased from 0% of implants at 1 month after insertion to 10% and 4% respectively at the end of the 6-month follow-up (Fig. 10-4).

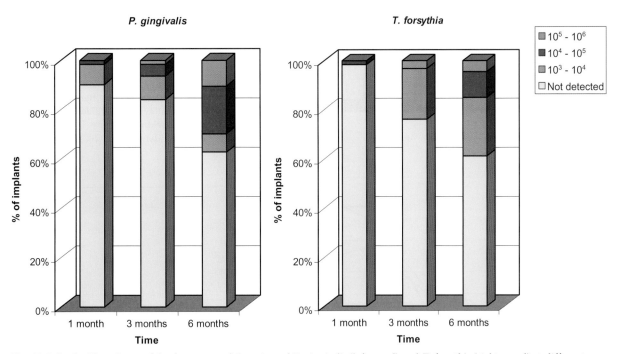

Fig. 10-4 Stacked bar charts of the frequency of detection of *P. gingivalis* (left panel) and *T. forsythia* (right panel) at different levels on 68 implants inserted in 22 advanced aggressive periodontitis subjects at different time points. The bar colors indicate the different levels of detection of *P. gingivalis* and *T. forsythia* using DNA probes. Data adapted from De Boever & De Boever (2006).

The levels of subgingival species over time on implants inserted in subjects with a history of periodontitis were examined using cultural techniques (Leonhardt *et al.* 1993). The mean percentage of total viable counts increased between 2 and 36 months for periodontal pathogens including *P. gingivalis* (0.3% to 1.8%), *Pr. intermedia* (1.1% to 1.9%), and *Aggregatibacter actinomycetemcomitans* (formerly known as *Actinobacillus actinomycetemcomitans*) (0.1% to 1.0%). In a second study, the colonization of implant fixtures over a period of 12 months was examined (van Winkelhoff *et al.* 2000). The percentage of subjects positive for the orange complex species *Pr. intermedia* (60%), *Pe. micros* (90%), and *F. nucleatum* (85%) were already high 1 month after implant exposure, while the red complex species, *T. forsythia*, was detected in 55% of subjects at 6 months.

Microbial colonization on implants that had been in place for up to 5 years was examined using darkfield microscopy in subjects treated for generalized aggressive periodontitis and up to 3 years in subjects treated for chronic periodontitis (Mengel *et al.* 2001; Mengel & Flores-de-Jacoby 2005). A clear increase in the complexity of the subgingival peri-implant microbiota over time was observed, with an increase in the proportions of motile rods, fusiforms, spirochetes, and filaments and a decrease in the proportion of coccoid cells. Interestingly, in the aggressive periodontitis group, there was a marked increase in the proportions of spirochetes, fusiforms, and motile rods between the 4- and 5-year time-points (Fig. 10-5) which was preceded by an increase in mean Gingival Index scores, mean pocket depth, and mean attachment level (Fig. 10-6). This change in the local habitat, in terms of increased inflammation and deeper pockets, may have been responsible for the observed shifts in the peri-implant microbiota.

Indirect evidence of an increase in biofilm complexity over time has been provided by studies comparing the microbiota on implants exposed to the oral environment for different lengths of time. Implants present in the oral cavity for 3–4 years were significantly more frequently colonized by *A. actinomycetemcomitans* and/or *P. gingivalis/Pr. intermedia* (44.4% of sites), compared to implants present for only 1–2 years (2.6%) (George *et al.* 1994). The implant microbiota in partially edentulous subjects harbored increased proportions of spirochetes and motile rods at implant sites with longer intraoral exposure times (Papaioannou *et al.* 1995). A statistically significant

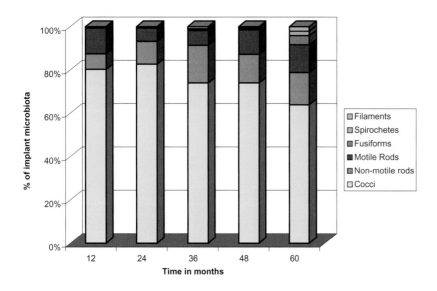

Fig. 10-5 Stacked bar chart of the distribution of bacterial morphotypes on ten implants from five aggressive periodontitis subjects at different time points. The bar colors indicate the percentage of the microbiota comprised by the different morphotypes identified using darkfield microscopy. Data adapted from Mengel *et al.* (2001).

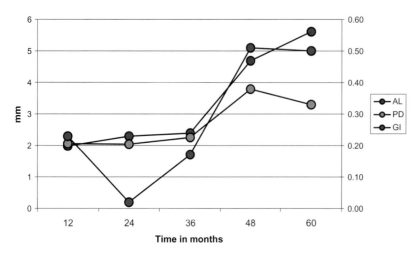

Fig. 10-6 Mean attachment level (AL), pocket depth (PD), and gingival index (GI) values around ten implants from five aggressive periodontitis subjects at different time points. The left Y-axis represents the scale for AL and PD in mm, while the right Y-axis presents the scale for the GI. Data adapted from Mengel *et al.* (2001).

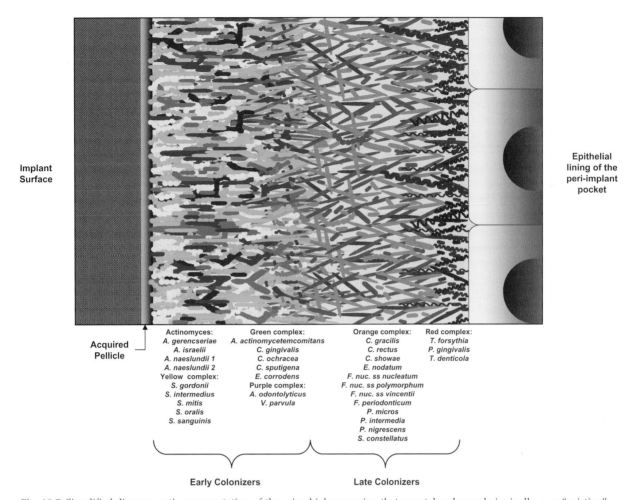

Fig. 10-7 Simplified diagrammatic representation of the microbial succession that may take place subgingivally on a "pristine" implant surface exposed to the oral environment. Microbial species are colored according to the microbial complexes described by Socransky *et al*. (1998).

increase in the proportion of motile rods around implants from 1 year (2.7%) to 2 years (5%) after implant loading has also been reported (Sbordone *et al*. 1999). The sequence of colonization of microbial complexes at implants with different loading times, determined using checkerboard DNA–DNA hybridization, was found to be similar to that described on tooth surfaces (Lee *et al*. 1999a). Levels of yellow and green complex species (early colonizers) were relatively stable at all loading times examined. Orange complex species were detected at lower levels than the streptococci, and their levels appeared to peak 12–24 months after loading. Red complex species were either absent or detected at low levels on implants exposed for only 3 months and only increased at later times. *P. gingivalis* and *T. forsythia* were detected at their highest levels between 7 to 12 months after loading.

Studies on early colonization of "pristine" implant surfaces and on the impact of length of time of implant presence on the composition of the microbiota suggest a pattern and sequence of microbial succession on these surfaces quite similar to the one described for tooth surfaces (Socransky & Haffajee 2005; Kolenbrander *et al*. 2006). A salivary acquired

pellicle forms on implant surfaces, providing the binding sites for adhesins on the surface of early colonizers such as members of the yellow complex (streptococci species) and *Actinomyces* spp. Multiplication and coaggregation of these early colonizers will result in a dense accumulation of bacteria attached to the implant surface and/or to each other. A second wave of early colonizers will adhere to the coaggregates attached to the implant surface. These include members of the green and purple complexes, which will, in turn, form their own coaggregates. Members of the orange complex will form a more "loosely attached" mass of microorganisms interspersed between the implant-associated biofilm and the epithelial-associated biofilm, composed in large part by red complex species. Species that participate in multiple coaggregates, such as the fusobacteria, will act as coaggregation bridges between early and late colonizers (Fig. 10-7).

The microbiota on implants in edentulous subjects

Early reports characterizing the microbiota on successful implants in fully edentulous subjects using darkfield microscopy described coccoid bacteria as the main morphotype, with a low proportion of spirochetes, fusiforms, and motile and curved rods. Results obtained using cultural techniques confirmed these findings and described high levels of Gram-positive facultative cocci, high levels of *Actinomyces* and *Veillonella* spp., low total anaerobic counts, low levels of Gram-negative anaerobic rods, low frequency of *Fusobacterium* spp. and "black-pigmented *Bacteroides*", and no detection of *P. gingivalis* (Mombelli *et al.* 1987, 1988; Mombelli & Mericske-Stern 1990). The levels of *A. actinomycetemcomitans*, *P. gingivalis*, and *Pr. intermedia* were measured on successful implants exposed to the oral environment for 3–38 months (Ong *et al.* 1992). *P. gingivalis* was not cultured from any sample, while *A. actinomycetemcomitans* was present in only one sample and *Pr. intermedia* was detected in 7/37 sampled sites. These data suggested that the microbiota colonizing clinically healthy implant fixtures in fully edentulous subjects was very similar to the microbiota associated with healthy periodontal sites in periodontally healthy subjects (Socransky & Haffajee 2005).

It was suggested that extraction of all of the teeth resulted in elimination of *P. gingivalis* and *A. actinomycetemcomitans* from the oral microbiota (Danser *et al.* 1994, 1995, 1997). *A. actinomycetemcomitans* and *P. gingivalis* could not be detected in samples from the oral mucosa and saliva 1–3 months after full-mouth extraction, even in subjects where these microorganisms were detected prior to tooth extraction (Danser *et al.* 1994). The prevalence of these pathogens in denture-wearing subjects with a history of periodontitis and an average of 9.3 years of edentulism was also investigated. *A. actinomycetemcomitans* was not detected and *P. gingivalis* was found in only 2/26 subjects in samples obtained from saliva, the oral mucous membranes, and biofilm accumulating on the dentures (Danser *et al.* 1995). These observations implied that the subgingival environment was the primary habitat of these periodontal pathogens and that the intraoral surfaces of edentulous subjects did not constitute a reservoir for these species. Indeed, the same group of investigators did not detect these periodontal pathogens in samples from the oral mucosa or from the peri-implant pockets in edentulous subjects with a past history of periodontitis who had received implants as part of the reconstruction of their dentition (Danser *et al.* 1997). The data suggested that even after the reestablishment of a "subgingival" environment by implant insertion, there was no intraoral reservoir of the two test species to re-colonize the peri-implant sulcus. Other investigators also reported a paucity of periodontal pathogens such as *P. gingivalis* and spirochetes around healthy implants inserted in fully edentulous subjects, even after 5 years in function (Mombelli & Mericske-Stern 1990). However, both *P. gingivalis* and *A. actinomycetemcomitans* were detected in peri-implantitis cases

occurring 5 years or more after loading in edentulous subjects (Leonhardt *et al.* 1999).

Later publications using molecular techniques to identify periodontal pathogens in the peri-implant microbiota have indicated a higher prevalence of pathogens around implants in fully edentulous subjects than initially described (Lee *et al.* 1999b; Hultin *et al.* 2002; Quirynen *et al.* 2005a; Devides & Franco 2006). The implant microbiota in fully and partially edentulous subjects was examined using checkerboard DNA–DNA hybridization (Lee *et al.* 1999b). Periodontal pathogens including *P. gingivalis*, *T. forsythia*, and *A. actinomycetemcomitans* could be detected in samples from implants in the edentulous subjects, although less frequently than in samples from implants in partially dentate subjects. In addition, *P. gingivalis*, *Pr. intermedia*, *Pr. nigrescens*, *T. forsythia*, *A. actinomycetemcomitans*, *F. nucleatum*, *Tr. denticola*, *Pe. micros*, and *Streptococcus intermedius* were detected by checkerboard DNA–DNA hybridization in subgingival samples obtained from stable implants in edentulous subjects, although at levels below 10^6 cells (Hultin *et al.* 2002). The microbiota of 37 fully edentulous subjects restored with overdentures or fixed full prostheses for at least 10 years was also examined using checkerboard DNA–DNA hybridization. Pooled subgingival plaque samples were collected from the overdenture subjects and two implants in the canine area in the fixed denture group (Quirynen *et al.* 2005a). The detection frequencies of several periodontal pathogens were higher than previously reported: *A. actinomycetemcomitans* (35/37), *P. gingivalis* (33/37), and *T. forsythia* (10/37). The counts of most species were <10^5 cells. However, some subjects showed levels of key pathogens above 10^5 cells: *A. actinomycetemcomitans* (8/37), *P. gingivalis* (29/37), and *T. forsythia* (3/37). Other pathogens such as *Tr. denticola* and *Tr. socranskii* were rarely detected.

The prevalence of *A. actinomycetemcomitans*, *P. gingivalis*, and *Pr. intermedia* at implant sites in the mandible of fully edentulous subjects was also investigated using polymerase chain reaction (PCR) to detect the species (Devides & Franco 2006). The presence of these pathogens was evaluated before implant insertion, and at 4 and 6 months after restoration of the implants with immediately loaded fixed prostheses. Prior to implant placement, *A. actinomycetemcomitans* and *Pr. intermedia* were detected in 13.3% and 46.7% of subjects respectively, while *P. gingivalis* was not detected. The values for these species at 4 and 6 months after prosthesis insertion were: 60.0% and 73.3%; 46.7% and 53.3%; 46.7% and 53.3%, for *A. actinomycetemcomitans*, *P. gingivalis*, and *Pr. intermedia*, respectively. The data indicated a higher frequency of detection of periodontal pathogens around implants in fully edentulous subjects than had been described based on cultural techniques and latex agglutination assays, and also suggested an increased colonization of the fixtures over time. These data were in accord with a study that compared checkerboard DNA–DNA hybridization and culture methods for the detection of 18 subgingival species in samples from teeth and implants from the same subjects (Leonhardt *et al.* 2003). The frequency of detection of all test species in implant samples was lower when culture rather than checkerboard DNA–DNA hybridization was employed. Molecular techniques have also been shown to be more sensitive than culture for the detection of periodontal pathogens in periodontally healthy subjects (Borrell & Papapanou 2005). The use of molecular techniques has demonstrated a greater prevalence of periodontal pathogens at implant sites in fully edentulous subjects than was previously recognized.

The pre- and post-implantation microbiota on implants and the dorsum of the tongue were examined in fully edentulous subjects using checkerboard DNA–DNA hybridization (Lee *et al.* 1999b). The results demonstrated that species such as *Streptococcus sanguinis*, *A. naeslundii*, *Capnocytophaga ochracea*, and *Campylobacter rectus* were infrequently found in peri-implant samples when not present on the dorsum of the tongue. The authors concluded that the tongue may be the source of bacteria initially colonizing implant fixtures and suggested that other soft tissue surfaces might also be reservoirs. The microbiota in the oral cavity of edentulous subjects without implants has been examined using checkerboard DNA–DNA hybridization (Socransky & Haffajee 2005). Periodontal pathogens were detected in samples of saliva and in samples from different intraoral surfaces, such as: dorsum, lateral and ventral surfaces of the tongue; floor of the mouth; hard palate; attached gingiva; buccal mucosa; vestibule and the surface of the dentures. These data suggested that the soft tissues of edentulous subjects harbor periodontal pathogens and are the likely source for colonization of implants after insertion in fully edentulous subjects.

The microbiota on implants in partially edentulous subjects

The literature comparing the microbiota around implants in edentulous subjects with the microbiota in partially edentulous subjects seemed to reinforce the role of the remaining dentition as a major source for colonization of implants by periodontal pathogens. Reported microbiological differences between samples from implants in partially and fully edentulous subjects included a higher percentage and frequency of detection of "black-pigmented *Bacteroides*" (Nakou *et al.* 1987; Apse *et al.* 1989; Hultin *et al.* 1998), fewer coccoid cells and significantly more motile rods and spirochetes (Quirynen & Listgarten 1990; Papaioannou *et al.* 1995), and a higher frequency of detection of *P. gingivalis* and *Pr. intermedia* on implant surfaces in partially edentulous subjects (George *et al.* 1994; Kalykakis *et al.* 1998).

Investigations comparing the peri-implant microbiota with the microbiota of neighboring teeth described several similarities in the composition of the two. For instance, counts of different morphotypes did not differ significantly between subgingival samples from implants and natural teeth in partially edentulous subjects (Quirynen & Listgarten 1990). Similarities in the subgingival microbiota of implants and natural teeth were also found using darkfield microscopy and the benzoyl-DL-arginine-naphthylamide (BANA) test, which detected the presence of trypsin-like enzymes produced primarily by the red complex species (Palmisano *et al.* 1991). The intraoral transmission of bacteria from teeth to implants was investigated in partially edentulous subjects using phase contrast microscopy (Quirynen *et al.* 1996). The results suggested that implants harbored more spirochetes and motile rods when teeth were present in the same jaw and when the pockets around teeth presented a pathogenic microbiota. The microbiota of implants that had been in function for 10 years in partially edentulous subjects was examined using DNA probes (Hultin *et al.* 2000). It was found that there were no significant differences between the microbiota around the natural teeth and fixtures and that the most common species isolated from both surfaces were *Tr. denticola*, *S. intermedius*, and *Pe. micros*. The microbiota of successfully osseointegrated implants in partially edentulous subjects was investigated using checkerboard DNA–DNA hybridization (Lee *et al.* 1999a). *S. intermedius*, *S. oralis*, *S. sanguinis*, *Streptococcus gordonii*, *Veillonella parvula*, *F. nucleatum*, and *Capnocytophaga gingivalis* were the dominant species in biofilms that formed on the fixtures. It was also demonstrated that the microbiota of healthy implants and clinically comparable crowned teeth present in the same subject were quite similar, suggesting that the major influence on the peri-implant microbiota was the microbiota on the remaining teeth.

The studies reporting similarities in the composition of the microbiota on teeth and implants were suggested but did not prove that teeth were the primary source of colonizing microorganisms for implant fixtures. Using pulsed field gel electrophoresis (PFGE), chromosomal DNA segmentation patterns of isolates of *P. gingivalis* and *Pr. intermedia* obtained from implants and natural teeth in the same subjects were compared (Sumida *et al.* 2002). The PFGE patterns of *P. gingivalis* strains isolated from the implant and tooth samples from the same subject were identical, while PFGE patterns differed among samples from different subjects. Similarly, the PFGE patterns of *Pr. intermedia* strains from teeth and implants were identical in two of three subjects examined. In another study using the same methodology, it was found that 75% of the *P gingivalis* isolates in samples from teeth and implants were the same in a subject, while 100% of the *Pr. intermedia* strains within a subject were a perfect match, clearly demonstrating transmission from the natural teeth to the implant fixtures (Takanashi *et al.* 2004). Unfortunately, PFGE patterns were not examined for the same test species isolated from soft tissues. Although the remaining dentition seems to be the primary source of bacteria for the colonization of implant surfaces in partially edentulous subjects, the potential role of soft tissues surfaces and saliva as reservoirs for implant infection cannot be discarded.

The microbiota on implants in subjects with a history of periodontal disease

Since the remaining dentition has been implicated as a source of microorganisms that colonize implants, it might be surmised that higher levels of periodontal pathogens would colonize implants in subjects with a history of periodontal infection. The early colonization of dental implants in subjects who had been treated for aggressive periodontitis was examined in 22 subjects who were on a maintenance program for periods ranging from 12–240 months (De Boever & De Boever 2006). 68 non-submerged implants were microbiologically sampled at 10 days and 1, 3, and 6 months after implant installation. DNA probes were used to determine the levels of subgingival species such as *A. actinomycetemcomitans*, *P. gingivalis*, *Pr. intermedia*, *T. forsythia*, and *Tr. denticola*. The implants were colonized by all five periodontal pathogens as early as 10 days after implant insertion and an increase in the frequency of detection of most pathogens was observed over time. The number of implants with at least one periodontal pathogen increased from 36 to 66 implants after 6 months in the oral environment. However, some subjects presented with only low levels (10^3–10^4 cells) of these pathogens.

Other studies found that the composition of the microbiota on the implant fixtures in partially edentulous subjects was similar to the subgingival microbiota of the residual teeth, although lower levels of most species were detected on the implants. For example, subgingival plaque samples from teeth and implant fixtures in partially edentulous subjects previously treated for periodontal disease were evaluated for the presence of *A. actinomycetemcomitans*, *P. gingivalis*, and *Pr. intermedia* using cultural techniques, (Leonhardt *et al.* 1993). The prevalence of subjects positive for the test bacterial species at both teeth and fixtures was similar after 6 months of implant exposure. The composition of the subgingival microbiota around implants and teeth 1 and 2 years after implant loading was examined in 25 subjects who had previously been treated for moderate to severe chronic periodontitis (Sbordone *et al.* 1999). There was an increase in the percentage of motile rods on implants over time and also an increase in the frequency of detection of *A. actinomycetemcomitans* and *P. gingivalis*. Although periodontal pathogens were present at low levels on both teeth and implants (<1% of the total cultivable microbiota), *P. gingivalis* and *Capnocytophaga* spp. were the most frequent isolates around implants at both 1 and 2 years after loading.

Mombelli *et al.* (1995) also examined the colonization of implants placed in partially edentulous subjects previously treated for periodontal disease. Subgingival plaque samples were collected from the deepest residual periodontal pocket of each quadrant in 20 subjects prior to installation of single-stage implants or prior to exposure of two-stage implants in the oral cavity. After 3 and 6 months of exposure of the implant fixtures to the oral environment, the implants and the residual deepest pocket in each quadrant were also sampled. Darkfield microscopy demonstrated that, after 3 months, samples from implants presented a distribution of morphotypes similar to samples from the residual deepest pockets. Further, the composition of the implant microbiota did not change between 3 and 6 months. The frequency of detection of subgingival species identified by cultural methods on implants was similar to the frequency of detection in the deepest residual pocket samples. When *P. gingivalis*, *Pr. intermedia*, and *Fusobacterium* spp. were found in high proportions in baseline samples from the residual deep pockets, they were also found in elevated proportions in the 3-month implant samples. The findings supported the notion that the residual pockets acted as reservoirs for colonization of the implant surfaces. They also suggested that compared with implants in fully edentulous and periodontally healthy subjects, the prevalence of periodontal pathogens on implants was higher in partially dentate periodontitis subjects.

A prospective study was designed to follow the clinical and microbiological outcomes at implants placed in subjects with a history of generalized aggressive and chronic periodontitis (Mengel *et al.* 1996, 2001; Mengel & Flores-de-Jacoby 2005). Fifteen generalized aggressive periodontitis (GAP), 12 generalized chronic periodontitis, and 12 periodontally healthy subjects were monitored for 3 years. Microbiological samples were collected yearly from both implants and teeth and examined using darkfield microscopy and DNA probe analysis for the detection of *A. actinomycetemcomitans*, *P. gingivalis*, and *Pr. intermedia*. The subjects with disease were extensively treated over a period for several years. This reduced the numbers and complexity of the colonizing microbiota on the natural dentition. Thus, after implant placement the microbiota colonizing the implants in samples from the two disease categories and periodontal health were similar in composition and dominated by coccoid cells over a period of 3 years. The clinical results indicated a continuous loss of attachment at both teeth and implants in GAP subjects. These subjects also exhibited the greatest amount of bone loss at teeth and implants. A small subset of five subjects with GAP was followed for up to 5 years. In these subjects, the microbiota around implants demonstrated a sharp increase in spirochetes, motile rods, filaments, and fusiforms from year 4 to year 5 (Fig. 10-5). Further, the levels of *P. gingivalis* and *Pr. intermedia* increased during the last 3 years of observation. These microbiological changes were preceded by a clear deterioration in the implant clinical parameters between years 3 and 4 (Fig. 10-6). The implant success rate for this subgroup was only 88.8%, compared to a 3-year success rate of 97.9% for the entire sample of 15 subjects.

The microbiota on implants and teeth from subjects with a previous history of periodontitis enrolled in a supportive maintenance program was also examined (Agerbaek *et al*. 2006). A total of 128 peri-implant samples and 1060 subgingival tooth samples were processed using checkerboard DNA–DNA hybridization. Overall, the proportions of the majority of the 40 test subgingival species were similar in implant and tooth samples; only the proportions of the *Actinomyces* spp. and the purple complex species (*V. parvula* and *Actinomyces odontolyticus*) were higher at tooth sites. Taken together, the data indicated that the microbiota colonizing implants in subjects with periodontitis was similar to that observed in the samples from periodontal pockets in the same individuals and harbored more pathogenic species than observed in fully or partially edentulous subjects with minimal or no periodontal disease.

The microbiota of peri-implantitis sites

Marked differences were found in the distribution of different morphotypes in the biofilms of successful implants (n = 10) in subjects with only healthy implants when compared with successful implants (control sites, n = 6) and peri-implantitis sites (test sites, n = 8) in subjects with peri-implantitis (Mombelli *et al*. 1987). Stable implants in healthy subjects were colonized primarily by coccoid cells, while fusiforms and motile rods were present at very low levels and spirochetes were absent. Spirochetes and fusiforms were detected in low proportions in samples from the healthy implants in peri-implantitis subjects. No significant differences could be found in the microbiotas of samples from healthy implants in subjects with or without peri-implantitis. The microbiota at peri-implantitis sites presented much higher levels of motile rods, spirochetes, and fusiforms, while coccoid cells accounted for only 50% of the microbiota (Fig. 10-8). Checkerboard DNA–DNA hybridization was employed to study the microbiota associated with peri-implantitis in 22 subjects with peri-implantitis sites, and eight control subjects with healthy implants (Salcetti *et al*. 1997). Forty subgingival taxa were examined and only four species were found to be positively associated with peri-implantitis versus healthy implants: *Pr. nigrescens*, *Pe. micros*, *F. nucleatum ss vincentii*, and *F. nucleatum ss nucleatum*. Although not statistically significant, there was a trend for a higher prevalence of *P. gingivalis*, *T. forsythia*, and *Tr. denticola* on implants present in subjects with failing implants compared to healthy implants from the control group. The healthy implants in the control subjects also displayed a tendency towards greater detection frequencies of streptococci, especially *S. gordonii* and *S. mitis*, as well as *Pr. intermedia*.

The presence of microorganisms in 18 samples of granulation tissue surgically removed from peri-implant infrabony pockets (>5 mm) from edentulous subjects was examined using cultural techniques

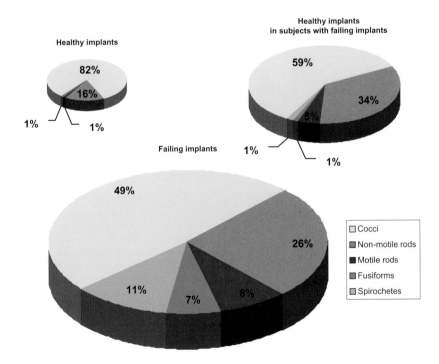

Fig. 10-8 Pie charts of the mean percentage of different morphotypes in the microbiota of samples from ten healthy implant sites in subjects with successful implants only, samples from six healthy implant sites and from eight peri-implantitis sites in subjects with peri-implantitis. The numbers correspond to the mean percentage of each morphotype within the microbiota. The areas of the pies have been adjusted to reflect mean total counts of each site category. Data adapted from Mombelli *et al*. (1987).

(Augthun & Conrads 1997). The species most frequently isolated were: "Bacteroidaceae" (16/18), *A. actinomycetemcomitans* (16/18 samples), *F. nucleatum* (4/18), *Capnocytophaga spp* (5/18), and *Eikenella corrodens* (3/18). The microbiota associated with peri-implantitis in 37 subjects with failing implants was compared with the microbiota in 51 subjects with healthy implants (Leonhardt *et al.* 2003). Microbiological samples were analyzed using cultural methods for the occurrence of *Pr. intermedia/nigrescens*, *A. actinomycetemcomitans*, *P. gingivalis*, enterics, yeast, and *Staphylococcus* spp. There were four groups of subjects. None of the test species were detected in the healthy edentulous subjects. In the healthy dentate patient group *Pr. intermedia/nigrescens* was detected in 26% of subjects but *A. actinomycetemcomitans* and *P. gingivalis* were detected in only one subject each. The edentulous peri-implantitis group exhibited *P. gingivalis*, *A. actinomycetemcomitans* and *Pr. intermedia/nigrescens* in 25%, 13%, and 38% of subjects respectively, while 31%, 3%, and 66% of dentate peri-implantitis subjects exhibited these species. *Staphylococcus epidermidis* was found in 17% of the dentate peri-implantitis subjects, enterics were found in 30% of the peri-implantitis group, but in only 8% of the healthy group (p < 0.001). *Candida albicans* was isolated in samples from 10% of the dentate peri-implantitis subjects.

The distribution of periodontal pathogens recovered from peri-implantitis sites and teeth with chronic or recurrent periodontitis was examined using microbial samples sent to the Microbiological Testing Laboratory at University of Pennsylvania by different dental practitioners (Listgarten & Lai 1999). Forty-one consecutive samples from subjects with failing implants, chronic periodontitis or recurrent periodontitis were examined using darkfield microscopy and cultural methods for the detection of: *A. actinomycetemcomitans*, *C. rectus*, *Pr. intermedia/nigrescens*, *E. corrodens*, *P. micros*, *Capnocytophaga*, *Fusobacterium* spp., *Staphylococcus aureus*, *Staphylococcus* spp., and yeast. *P. gingivalis* and *T. forsythia* were detected by indirect immunofluorescence. *T. forsythia* was the most frequently detected species and was found in 83% of samples from chronic periodontitis, 85% of recurrent periodontitis samples, and 59% of samples of peri-implantitis sites, although at low levels (1–3% of the total cultivable microbiota). Most bacterial species had a higher frequency of detection and were present in higher levels in samples from teeth than in samples from implants. On the other hand, enteric rods were more prevalent (10% of subjects) and present in higher proportions on implants and in recurrent periodontitis compared with the chronic periodontitis. Yeasts were more prevalent in chronic periodontitis samples than on failing implants and *S. aureus* and *Staphylococcus* spp. were detected infrequently.

Checkerboard DNA–DNA hybridization was employed to examine the levels of 12 microorganisms in subgingival samples obtained from five different categories of sites: (1) peri-implantitis sites in partially edentulous subjects (n = 14); (2) healthy implant sites from the same subjects with peri-implantitis (n = 17); (3) teeth from the same group with peri-implantitis (n = 17); (4) healthy implant sites from partially edentulous (n = 13) and fully edentulous subjects (n = 6) with only healthy implant sites; (5) teeth from subjects with healthy implant sites (n = 13) (Hultin *et al.* 2002). Periodontal pathogens, such as *P. gingivalis*, *Pr. intermedia*, *T. forsythia*, *A. actinomycetemcomitans*, and *Tr. denticola*, were present in samples from all categories of sites, however, species were recovered at levels above 10^6 cells only around failing fixtures. When peri-implantitis sites and healthy sites from the same subjects were compared, peri-implantitis sites had higher levels of *A. actinomycetemcomitans*, *F. nucleatum*, and *Tr. denticola* (Fig. 10-9). Further, *C. rectus* and *S. noxia* were only found around implants in subjects with

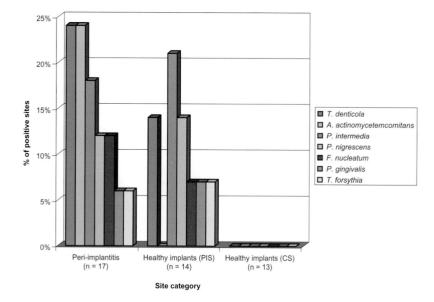

Fig. 10-9 Bar chart of the mean frequency of detection of seven subgingival species in different implant site categories: implants affected by peri-implantitis, healthy implants in subjects with peri-implantitis (PIS) and healthy implants in partially edentulous control subjects (CS). Data adapted from Hultin *et al.* (2002).

peri-implantitis. Using cultural methods, Botero *et al.* (2005) compared the microbiota associated with 16 implants with peri-implantitis in 11 subjects with the microbiota on 15 healthy implants in 8 subjects. All subjects were partially edentulous and the microbiota associated with the remaining teeth in subjects with peri-implantitis was also examined. *P. gingivalis* was detected only in peri-implantitis samples (43.7% of the samples), while peri-implant lesions harbored statistically significantly higher levels of enteric rods and *Pr. intermedia/nigrescens*.

For the most part, the literature on the microbiota of failing implants describes the presence of elevated levels of species previously associated with periodontal infections. Other microorganisms, not commonly implicated as etiological agents of periodontal diseases, have also been recovered from peri-implant lesions, including staphylococci, enteric rods, and yeast, although a causal relationship between these microorganisms and peri-implant infections is premature.

Summary

Although the microbiology of the dental implant in clinically healthy and diseased situations has been studied less intensively than the microbiology of the natural dentition, available data suggest the following:

1. The new "hard tissue" surface presented to the oral environment by the implant provides a surface for the attachment of salivary proteins, peptides, and other substances. These substances rapidly form a pellicle that is probably quite similar to the pellicle formed on natural teeth.

2. The pellicle provides receptors for the adhesins on specific species of oral bacteria that form the early colonizers of the implant. These species appear to be similar to those that colonize the teeth and include members of the genera *Streptococcus, Actinomyces,* and *Veillonella.*

3. The insertion of the implant appears to "set the clock back" for the development of the mature biofilm; i.e. for a number of years the microbial composition of biofilms on healthy implants may be similar to that observed on the surfaces of periodontally healthy teeth in the adolescent.

4. With time, varying from months to years, the implant microbiota becomes more complex. Pockets may develop around the implant, which harbor increased numbers and proportions of orange and red complex species in a fashion analogous to the increase in these species in deep periodontal pockets adjacent to natural teeth.

5. The development of peri-implantitis appears to be accompanied in large part by an increase in bacterial species that have been found to increase in periodontitis. These include periodontal pathogens, such as *P. gingivalis, T. forsythia,* and *A. actinomycetemcomitans,* as well as additional taxa including staphylococci and enteric rods.

6. The microbiota of implants in partially edentulous subjects who have had periodontitis appears to harbor more periodontal pathogens than the microbiota at implants in partially edentulous subjects without periodontitis and implants in fully edentulous subjects. The presence of these species appears to increase the long-term risk for peri-implantitis in subjects with a history of periodontitis.

References

Agerbaek, M.R., Lang, N.P. & Persson, G.R. (2006). Comparisons of bacterial patterns present at implant and tooth sites in subjects on supportive periodontal therapy. I. Impact of clinical variables, gender and smoking. *Clinical Oral Implants Research* 17, 18–24.

Apse, P., Ellen, R.P., Overall, C.M. & Zarb, G.A. (1989). Microbiota and crevicular fluid collagenase activity in the osseointegrated dental implant sulcus: a comparison of sites in edentulous and partially edentulous patients. *Journal of Periodontal Research* 24, 96–105.

Augthun, M. & Conrads, G. (1997). Microbial findings of deep peri-implant bone defects. *International Journal of Oral and Maxillofacial Implants* 12, 106–112.

Borrell, L.N. & Papapanou, P.N. (2005). Analytical epidemiology of periodontitis. *Journal of Clinical Periodontology* 32 Suppl 6, 132–158.

Botero, J.E., Gonzalez, A.M., Mercado, R.A., Olave, G. & Contreras, A. (2005). Subgingival microbiota in peri-implant mucosa lesions and adjacent teeth in partially edentulous patients. *Journal of Periodontology* 76, 1490–1495.

Danser, M.M., van Winkelhoff, A.J., de Graaff, J., Loos, B.G. & van der Velden, U. (1994). Short-term effect of full-mouth extraction on periodontal pathogens colonizing the oral mucous membranes. *Journal of Clinical Periodontology* 21, 484–489.

Danser, M.M., van Winkelhoff, A.J., de Graaff, J. & van der Velden, U. (1995). Putative periodontal pathogens colonizing oral mucous membranes in denture-wearing subjects with a past history of periodontitis. *Journal of Clinical Periodontology* 22, 854–859.

Danser, M.M., van Winkelhoff, A.J. & van der Velden, U. (1997). Periodontal bacteria colonizing oral mucous membranes in edentulous patients wearing dental implants. *Journal of Periodontology* 68, 209–216.

De Boever, A.L. & De Boever, J.A. (2006). Early colonization of non-submerged dental implants in patients with a history of advanced aggressive periodontitis. *Clinical Oral Implants Research* 17, 8–17.

Devides, S.L. & Franco, A.T. (2006). Evaluation of peri-implant microbiota using the polymerase chain reaction in completely edentulous patients before and after placement of implant-supported prostheses submitted to immediate load. *International Journal of Oral and Maxillofacial Implants* 21, 262–269.

Edgerton, M., Lo, S.E. & Scannapieco, F.A. (1996). Experimental salivary pellicles formed on titanium surfaces mediate adhesion of streptococci. *International Journal of Oral and Maxillofacial Implants* 11, 443–449.

George, K., Zafiropoulos, G.G., Murat, Y., Hubertus, S. & Nisengard, R.J. (1994). Clinical and microbiological status of osseointegrated implants. *Journal of Periodontology* **65**, 766–770.

Haffajee, A.D., Teles, R.P. & Socransky, S.S. (2006). Association of *Eubacterium nodatum* and *Treponema denticola* with human periodontitis lesions. *Oral Microbiology and Immunology* **21**, 269–282.

Hultin, M., Bostrom, L. & Gustafsson, A. (1998). Neutrophil response and microbiological findings around teeth and dental implants. *Journal of Periodontology* **69**, 1413–1418.

Hultin, M., Gustafsson, A., Hallstrom, H., Johansson, L.A., Ekfeldt, A. & Klinge, B. (2002). Microbiological findings and host response in patients with peri-implantitis. *Clinical Oral Implants Research* **13**, 349–358.

Hultin, M., Gustafsson, A. & Klinge, B. (2000). Long-term evaluation of osseointegrated dental implants in the treatment of partly edentulous patients. *Journal of Clinical Periodontology* **27**, 128–133.

Kalykakis, G.K., Mojon, P., Nisengard, R., Spiekermann, H. & Zafiropoulos, G.G. (1998). Clinical and microbial findings on osseo-integrated implants; comparisons between partially dentate and edentulous subjects. *European Journal of Prosthodontics and Restorative Dentistry* **6**, 155–159.

Koka, S., Razzoog, M.E., Bloem, T.J. & Syed, S. (1993). Microbial colonization of dental implants in partially edentulous subjects. *Journal of Prosthetic Dentistry* **70**, 141–144.

Kolenbrander, P.E., Palmer, R.J., Jr., Rickard, A.H., Jakubovics, N.S., Chalmers, N.I. & Diaz, P.I. (2006). Bacterial interactions and successions during plaque development. *Periodontology 2000* **42**, 47–79.

Lee, K.H., Maiden, M.F., Tanner, A.C. & Weber, H.P. (1999a). Microbiota of successful osseointegrated dental implants. *Journal of Periodontology* **70**, 131–138.

Lee, K.H., Tanner, A.C., Maiden, M.F. & Weber, H.P. (1999b). Pre- and post-implantation microbiota of the tongue, teeth, and newly placed implants. *Journal of Clinical Periodontology* **26**, 822–832.

Leonhardt, A., Adolfsson, B., Lekholm, U., Wikstrom, M. & Dahlen, G. (1993). A longitudinal microbiological study on osseointegrated titanium implants in partially edentulous patients. *Clinical Oral Implants Research* **4**, 113–120.

Leonhardt, A., Bergstrom, C. & Lekholm, U. (2003). Microbiologic diagnostics at titanium implants. *Clinical Implant Dentistry and Related Research* **5**, 226–232.

Leonhardt, A., Olsson, J. & Dahlen, G. (1995). Bacterial colonization on titanium, hydroxyapatite, and amalgam surfaces in vivo. *Journal of Dental Research* **74**, 1607–1612.

Leonhardt, A., Renvert, S. & Dahlen, G. (1999). Microbial findings at failing implants. *Clinical Oral Implants Research* **10**, 339–345.

Li, J., Helmerhorst, E.J., Leone, C.W., Troxler, R.F., Yaskell, T., Haffajee, A.D., Socransky, S.S. & Oppenheim, F.G. (2004). Identification of early microbial colonizers in human dental biofilm. *Journal of Applied Microbiology* **97**, 1311–1318.

Listgarten, M.A. & Lai, C.H. (1999). Comparative microbiological characteristics of failing implants and periodontally diseased teeth. *Journal of Periodontology* **70**, 431–437.

Löe, H., Theilade, E. & Jensen, S.B. (1965). Experimental gingivitis in man. *Journal of Periodontology* **36**, 177–187.

Mengel, R. & Flores-de-Jacoby, L. (2005). Implants in patients treated for generalized aggressive and chronic periodontitis: a 3-year prospective longitudinal study. *Journal of Periodontology* **76**, 534–543.

Mengel, R., Schroder, T. & Flores-de-Jacoby, L. (2001). Osseointegrated implants in patients treated for generalized chronic periodontitis and generalized aggressive periodontitis: 3- and 5-year results of a prospective long-term study. *Journal of Periodontology* **72**, 977–989.

Mengel, R., Stelzel, M., Hasse, C. & Flores-de-Jacoby, L. (1996). Osseointegrated implants in patients treated for general-

ized severe adult periodontitis. An interim report. *Journal of Periodontology* **67**, 782–787.

Mombelli, A., Buser, D. & Lang, N.P. (1988). Colonization of osseointegrated titanium implants in edentulous patients. Early results. *Oral Microbiology and Immunology* **3**, 113–120.

Mombelli, A., Marxer, M., Gaberthuel, T., Grunder, U. & Lang, N.P. (1995). The microbiota of osseointegrated implants in patients with a history of periodontal disease. *Journal of Clinical Periodontology* **22**, 124–130.

Mombelli, A. & Mericske-Stern, R. (1990). Microbiological features of stable osseointegrated implants used as abutments for overdentures. *Clinical Oral Implants Research* **1**, 1–7.

Mombelli, A., van Oosten, M.A., Schurch, E. Jr & Land, N.P. (1987). The microbiota associated with successful or failing osseointegrated titanium implants. *Oral Microbiology and Immunology* **2**, 145–151.

Nakou, M., Mikx, F.H., Oosterwaal, P.J. & Kruijsen, J.C. (1987). Early microbial colonization of permucosal implants in edentulous patients. *Journal of Dental Research* **66**, 1654–1657.

Ong, E.S., Newman, H.N., Wilson, M. & Bulman, J.S. (1992). The occurrence of periodontitis-related microorganisms in relation to titanium implants. *Journal of Periodontology* **63**, 200–205.

Palmisano, D.A., Mayo, J.A., Block, M.S. & Lancaster, D.M. (1991). Subgingival bacteria associated with hydroxylapatite-coated dental implants: morphotypes and trypsin-like enzyme activity. *International Journal of Oral and Maxillofacial Implants* **6**, 313–318.

Papaioannou, W., Quirynen, M., Nys, M. & van Steenberghe, D. (1995). The effect of periodontal parameters on the subgingival microbiota around implants. *Clinical Oral Implants Research* **6**, 197–204.

Pontoriero, R., Tonelli, M.P., Carnevale, G., Mombelli, A., Nyman, S.R. & Lang, N.P. (1994). Experimentally induced peri-implant mucositis. A clinical study in humans. *Clinical Oral Implants Research* **5**, 254–259.

Quirynen, M., Alsaadi, G., Pauwels, M., Haffajee, A., van Steenberghe, D. & Naert, I. (2005a). Microbiological and clinical outcomes and patient satisfaction for two treatment options in the edentulous lower jaw after 10 years of function. *Clinical Oral Implants Research* **16**, 277–287.

Quirynen, M. & Listgarten, M.A. (1990). Distribution of bacterial morphotypes around natural teeth and titanium implants ad modum Branemark. *Clinical Oral Implants Research* **1**, 8–12.

Quirynen, M., Papaioannou, W. & van Steenberghe, D. (1996). Intraoral transmission and the colonization of oral hard surfaces. *Journal of Periodontology* **67**, 986–993.

Quirynen, M., Vogels, R., Pauwels, M., Haffajee, A.D., Socransky, S.S., Uzel, N.G. & van Steenberghe, D. (2005b). Initial subgingival colonization of "pristine" pockets. *Journal of Dental Research* **84**, 340–344.

Quirynen, M., Vogels, R., Peeters, W., van Steenberghe, D., Naert, I. & Haffajee, A. (2006). Dynamics of initial subgingival colonization of "pristine" peri-implant pockets. *Clinical Oral Implants Research* **17**, 25–37.

Salcetti, J.M., Moriarty, J.D., Cooper, L.F., Smith, F.W., Collins, J.G., Socransky, S.S. & Offenbacher, S. (1997). The clinical, microbial, and host response characteristics of the failing implant. *International Journal of Oral and Maxillofacial Implants* **12**, 32–42.

Sbordone, L., Barone, A., Ciaglia, R.N., Ramaglia, L. & Iacono, V.J. (1999). Longitudinal study of dental implants in a periodontally compromised population. *Journal of Periodontology* **70**, 1322–1329.

Socransky, S.S. & Haffajee, A.D. (2005). Periodontal microbial ecology. *Periodontology 2000* **38**, 135–187.

Socransky, S.S., Haffajee, A.D., Cugini, M.A., Smith, C. & Kent, R.L., Jr. (1998). Microbial complexes in subgingival plaque. *Journal of Clinical Periodontology* **25**, 134–144.

Socransky, S.S., Haffajee, A.D., Smith, C. & Dibart, S. (1991). Relation of counts of microbial species to clinical status at the sampled site. *Journal of Clinical Periodontology* **18**, 766–775.

Socransky, S.S., Manganiello, A.D., Propas, D., Oram, V. & van Houte, J. (1977). Bacteriological studies of developing supragingival dental plaque. *Journal of Periodontal Research* **12**, 90–106.

Sumida, S., Ishihara, K., Kishi, M. & Okuda, K. (2002). Transmission of periodontal disease-associated bacteria from teeth to osseointegrated implant regions. *International Journal of Oral and Maxillofacial Implants* **17**, 696–702.

Takanashi, K., Kishi, M., Okuda, K. & Ishihara, K. (2004). Colonization by Porphyromonas gingivalis and Prevotella intermedia from teeth to osseointegrated implant regions. *Bulletin of Tokyo Dental College* **45**, 77–85.

Theilade, E., Wright, W.H., Jensen, S.B. & Löe, H. (1966). Experimental gingivitis in man. II. A longitudinal clinical and bacteriological investigation. *Journal of Periodontal Research* **1**, 1–13.

van Winkelhoff, A.J., Goene, R.J., Benschop, C. & Folmer, T. (2000). Early colonization of dental implants by putative periodontal pathogens in partially edentulous patients. *Clinical Oral Implants Research* **11**, 511–520.

Part 4: Host–Parasite Interactions

Chapter 11

Pathogenesis of Periodontitis

Denis F. Kinane, Tord Berglundh, and Jan Lindhe

Introduction

Inflammatory and immune reactions to microbial plaque are the predominant features of gingivitis and periodontitis. The inflammatory reaction is visible both clinically and microscopically in the affected periodontium.

Inflammatory and immune processes operate in the gingival tissues to protect against local microbial attack and prevent microorganisms or their damaging products from spreading into or invading the tissues. These host defense reactions are, however, also considered potentially harmful to the host in that inflammation can damage surrounding cells and connective tissue structures. Furthermore, inflammatory and immune reactions that extend deep into the connective tissue beyond the cemento-enamel junction (CEJ) may include loss of connective tissue attachment to the tooth involved as well as loss of alveolar bone. These "defensive" processes could therefore paradoxically contribute to the tissue injury observed in gingivitis and periodontitis.

Whilst inflammatory and immune reactions within the periodontal tissues may appear similar to those seen elsewhere in the body, there are significant differences. To some extent this is a consequence of the anatomy of the periodontium, e.g. the permeable junctional epithelium that has remarkable cell and fluid dynamics, with its prime purpose to preserve epithelial continuity across the hard and soft tissue interface. Another important feature is that the "defensive processes" in the periodontal tissues occur in response to large numbers and varieties of microbes

that reside on the tooth surface in a biofilm community, close to rather than within the gingiva.

Periodontal disease has sometimes been referred to as a "mixed bacterial infection" to denote that multiple microbial species contribute to the development of disease. Microbial species interact, and although some may not be overtly pathogenic they may still influence the disease process by aiding and assisting the pathogenic bacteria also contained within the microbial biofilm. Thus, purportedly 'commmensal' microbes may endorse the virulence potential of other microbes by providing specific growth conditions or defensive factors; this calls into question our definition of commensal and pathogen with respect to biofilm related diseases.

The microorganisms in the biofilm within periodontal pockets are in a continual state of flux; species, which are relevant at one stage of disease, may not be important at other disease phases. In other words, tissue destruction may result from combinations of bacterial factors, which vary over time. This contrasts with most other classical infectious diseases (e.g. tuberculosis, syphilis, gonorrhea) where the host contends with one organism and the diagnosis of the disease is indicated by the presence or absence of this particular pathogen.

The pathogenicity of microorganisms relates as much to the individual host's innate and/or inflammatory and/or immune capability, as to the virulence of the bacteria themselves. For example, periodontal tissue breakdown could result from microbial enzymes that directly digest the tissue but also, and more likely, from host responses to these enzymes. Furthermore, tissue destructive responses might result from the host's inflammatory or immune reaction to normal physiological components of the bacteria such as the lipopolysaccharides found in the outer membrane of Gram-negative bacteria.

Epidemiological studies have shown that even within the same individual, the severity of periodontal tissue injury often varies from tooth to tooth and from one tooth surface to another. Thus, whilst many teeth within an individual mouth may exhibit advanced loss of connective tissue attachment and alveolar bone, other teeth or tooth surfaces (sites) may be almost unaffected and surrounded by a normal periodontium. Hence, a patient who is susceptible to, and is exhibiting, periodontal disease is not afflicted with a "homogeneous" condition (see Chapter 18). Each affected site in his/her mouth represents an "individualized" or "specific" microenvironment. In some sites, the inflammatory lesion may be contained within the gingiva (gingivitis) for prolonged periods of time without any apparent progression of the disease into deeper tissues. In other sites, active periodontal tissue destruction (periodontitis) may occur and may be a consequence of a variety of host and parasite factors.

However, it is not presently understood why in some patients the inflammatory lesions remain confined to the marginal portion of the gingival tissues, whilst in other susceptible subjects they progress to involve more apical portions of the periodontium and cause loss of connective tissue attachment and alveolar bone. The same arguments are true for individual sites within a susceptible individual. Clearly some imbalance of the host–parasite relationship is occurring in the destructive lesions. This imbalance may be unique to that site and to gingivitis- and periodontitis-susceptible individuals generally.

Clinically healthy gingiva

"*Clinically healthy gingiva*" is a term used to describe the level of gingival health that may be attained by patients who clean their teeth in a meticulous manner. The oral surface of clinically healthy gingiva consists of keratinized oral epithelium that is continuous with the junctional epithelium (Fig. 11-1a) that is attached to the tooth surface by hemidesmosomes. Supporting the oral and junctional epithelia is a network of connective tissue that includes prominent collagen fibers, which maintain the shape of the gingival tissues and assist the relatively weak hemidesmosomal attachment of the junctional epithelium to the tooth. Immediately inside the junctional epithelium there is a dentogingival plexus, containing large numbers of venules, which supplies the epithelium with various nutrients as well as defense cells (leukocytes) (Fig. 11-1b,c).

The clinically healthy gingiva consistently features a small infiltrate of inflammatory cells that involves both the junctional epithelium and the subjacent connective tissue (Page & Schroeder 1976). This inflammatory reaction occurs in response to the continuous presence of bacterial products in the crevice region (Fig. 11-2). The small inflammatory lesion also harbors lymphocytes and macrophages. Transudates and exudates of fluid that contains varying amounts of plasma proteins leave the vessels of the dentogingival plexus and arrive in the gingival crevice region as the gingival crevicular fluid (GCF) (Egelberg 1967; Cimasoni 1983). Among the leukocytes, neutrophils (polymorphonuclear (PMN) cells) predominate in the crevice region (sulcus) and appear to migrate continuously through the junctional epithelium into the crevice (Figs. 11-3, 11-4). The recruitment of leukocytes from the gingival tissue to the crevice is due to the chemoattractant actions of products derived from the biofilm as well as from factors release by the host.

Sites with *clinically healthy gingiva* appear to deal with continuous microbial challenges without progressing to clinical gingivitis (redness, swelling, bleeding on probing), probably because of several defensive factors that include:

- The intact barrier provided by the junctional epithelium
- The regular shedding of epithelial cells into the oral cavity
- The positive flow of fluid to the gingival crevice which may wash away unattached microorganisms and noxious products
- The presence in GCF of antibodies to microbial products
- The phagocytic function of neutrophils and macrophages
- The detrimental effect of complement on the microbiota.

The host–microbial interplay or balance, which constitutes the situation in clinically healthy gingiva, must clearly change if *gingivitis* is to follow. Gingivitis will follow if there is sufficient plaque accumulation and retention such that microbial products evoke a more substantive inflammatory response. Lesions characteristic of gingivitis occupy a larger volume than those present in clinically healthy gingiva and are accompanied by more pronounced loss of collagen (Fig. 11-4). The inflammatory reaction will also initiate and perpetuate immune responses to the oral microorganisms. Gingival lesions may persist for many years without concomitant loss of periodontal attachment, destruction of periodontal ligament or evidence of bone loss. Clearly certain individuals (and sites), however, go on to develop periodontitis from gingivitis lesions. It is well known that individuals with obvious defects of the inflammatory system, e.g. neutrophil depletion or dysfunction, may rapidly develop advanced periodontitis.

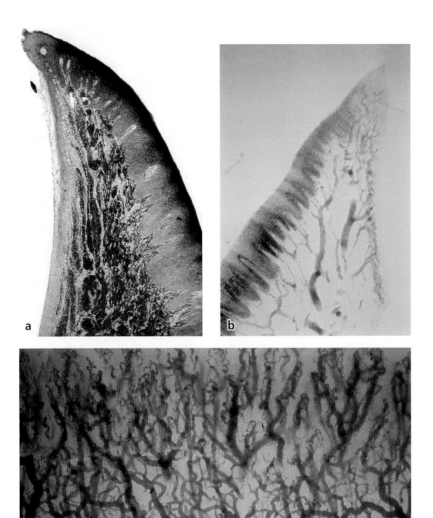

Fig. 11-1 (a) Buccal–lingual section of a normal beagle dog gingiva. The oral epithelium is continuous with a junctional epithelium, which is facing the enamel surface. (b) Micrograph of a buccal–lingual section of a normal (pristine) beagle dog gingiva illustrating the vasculature of the gingival unit. A thin vascular network is present beneath the junctional epithelium. (c) The thin vascular network (plexus) is shown in a mesial-distal section.

There is an accumulating body of evidence, which suggests that the host's immune response to periodontal pathogens may be quite different in subjects that become affected by advanced chronic periodontitis and those who will not progress beyond gingivitis.

Gingival inflammation

The classical phases of "acute" and "chronic" inflammation are not easily applied in periodontal disease, probably because in clinically healthy gingiva a small lesion similar to an acute inflammatory reaction is already present. Subsequently developing chronic inflammatory changes become superimposed so that both acute and chronic elements co-exist in most gingival lesions.

Histopathological features of gingivitis

The clinical symptoms of inflammation may appear subtle in the early stages of gingivitis but the underlying histopathological changes, albeit present in a small compartment of the gingival tissues, are quite marked. Alterations in the vascular network occur with many capillary beds being opened up. Exudation of GCF and proteins from the dentogingival plexus will increase and this will make the tissue edematous and swollen. Inflammatory cells leave the vasculature and accumulate in the connective tissue lateral to the junctional epithelium. The connective tissue infiltrate is at first mainly comprised of macrophages and lymphocytes. As the cellular infiltrate becomes enlarged, plasma cells dominate the lesion and collagen depletion becomes quite substantial.

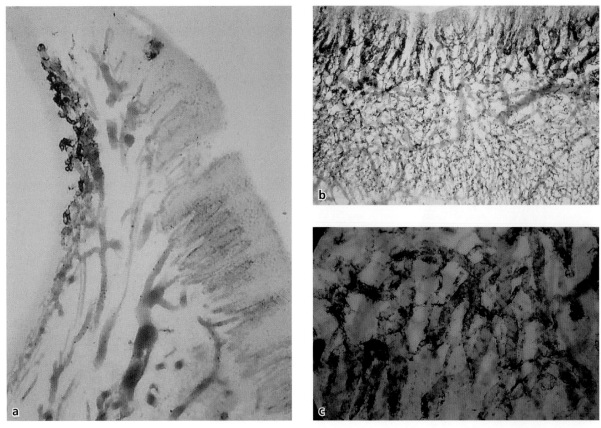

Fig. 11-2 (a) Microphotograph of a buccal–lingual section of a normal beagle dog gingiva. A filter paper strip has been introduced between the junctional epithelium and the tooth. An increased permeability of the gingival vessels has occurred, identified by the presence of carbon particles, which were injected intravenously prior to biopsy. The carbon particles have become trapped in the open endothelial junctions, and so-called vascular labelling has occurred. (b) A mesio-distal section of the same gingival unit as in (a). (c) Higher magnification of (b) (from Egelberg 1967).

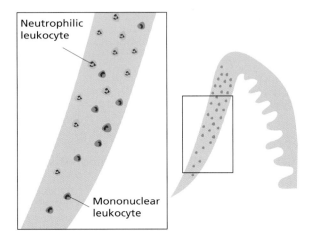

Fig. 11-3 Leukocytes in the junctional epithelium. Observe that the volume of leukocytes decreases in an apical direction and approaches 0 in the most apical portion. Within the junctional epithelium, the mononuclear leukocytes are located in more basal layers, while the neutrophilic granulocytes are present primarily in the superficial portions of the junctional epithelium.

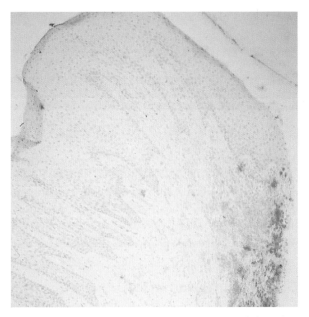

Fig. 11-4 Immunostained section showing neutrophils in the junctional epithelium of healthy gingiva.

In this context it is important to emphasize that the lesion in the gingiva is closely related to the presence and extension of the biofilm on the associated tooth surface. Thus, findings from analyses of human autopsy material (Waerhaug 1952) indicated that the distance between plaque and calculus on the tooth surface and the inflammatory lesion in the gingiva never exceeded 1–2 mm.

Different lesions in gingivitis/periodontitis

In 1976, Page and Schroeder divided the progressing lesion in the gingival/periodontal tissues into four phases: *initial, early, established,* and *advanced* stages or lesions. The descriptions of the initial and early lesion were intended to characterize the histopathology of clinically healthy gingiva and early stages of gingivitis, while the established lesion featured "chronic" gingivitis. The advanced lesion was considered to reflect the phase when gingivitis progressed to periodontitis and was a lesion that was consistently associated with attachment and bone loss. The evidence on which these descriptions were based was the prevailing information generated predominantly from animal biopsy material and some human adolescent samples.

Below we have used the terms initial, early, established, and advanced lesion to describe some features of the developing inflammatory process in the gingival and periodontal tissues. We have, however, not consistently adhered to the definitions and descriptions used in the original publication by Page and Schroeder.

The initial lesion

Inflammation soon develops as plaque is allowed to form on the gingival third of the tooth surface. Within 24 hours marked changes are evident in the dentogingival plexus as more blood is brought to the area. Dilation of the arterioles, capillaries, and venules of the vascular network becomes a prominent feature (Fig. 11-2). Hydrostatic pressure within the microcirculation increases and intercellular gaps form between adjacent endothelial cells in the capillaries. Thus, an increase in the permeability of the microvascular bed results, so that proteins and, subsequently, fluids may exude into the tissues (Fig. 11-5).

The flow of GCF increases. Noxious substances released from the biofilm are diluted both inside the gingival tissue and in the crevice. Furthermore, bacteria and their products may be flushed away from the crevice region and end up in the saliva. Plasma proteins are part of GCF and include defensive proteins such as antibodies, complement and protease inhibitors, and other macromolecules with numerous functions. Already during this initial phase of the host response, PMN cell migration is facilitated by the presence of various adhesion molecules (intercellular adhesion molecule-1 (ICAM-1), endothelial leukocyte adhesion molecule-1 (ELAM-1)), and other adhesions in the dentogingival vasculature. These molecules assist the binding of PMN cells to the venules and subsequently they help the cells to leave the blood vessel (Fig. 11-6). The PMNs migrate up a chemo-attractant gradient to the crevice and are further assisted in their movement (1) by other adhesion molecules uniquely present on the junctional epithelial cells (Moughal *et al.* 1992) and (2) by the presence of microbial chemotactic factors. Lymphocytes are retained in the connective tissues on contact with antigens, cytokines or adhesion molecules and are therefore not so readily lost through the junctional epithelium and into the oral cavity, as are PMNs. Most lymphocytes have the ability to produce CD44 (CD, cluster determinant) receptors on their surfaces, which permit the binding of the cell to the connective tissue framework.

Within 2–4 days of plaque build-up the cellular response described above is probably well established and is maintained by chemotactic substances originating from the plaque microbiota as well as from host cells and secretions (Fig. 11-7).

The early lesion

An ensuing and somewhat different gingival lesion will become present after several days of plaque accumulation (Fig. 11-8). The vessels in the dentogingival plexus remain dilated, but their numbers increase due to the opening up of previously inactive capillary beds. The increased size and enhanced numbers of vascular units are reflected in increased redness of the marginal gingiva that is a characteristic clinical symptom during this phase (Egelberg 1967; Lindhe & Rylander 1975).

Lymphocytes and PMNs are also the predominant leukocytes in the infiltrate at this stage of gingivitis and very few plasma cells are noted within the expanding lesion (Listgarten & Ellegaard 1973; Payne *et al.* 1975; Seymour *et al.* 1983; Brecx *et al.* 1987). Several fibroblasts within the lesion exhibit signs of degeneration. This probably occurs through apoptosis and serves to remove fibroblasts from the area, thus permitting more leukocyte infiltration (Page & Schroeder 1976; Takahashi *et al.* 1995). Similarly breakdown of collagen fibers occurs in the infiltrated area. This net loss of collagen fibers will provide space for the infiltrating cells.

The basal cells of the junctional and sulcular epithelium now proliferate. This represents an attempt by the body to enhance the "mechanical" barrier to plaque bacteria and their products. Epithelial rete pegs can be seen invading the coronal portion of the lesion in the connective tissue (Schroeder 1970; Schroeder *et al.* 1973). Tissue alterations during this phase also involve the loss of the coronal portion of the junctional epithelium. A niche forms between the

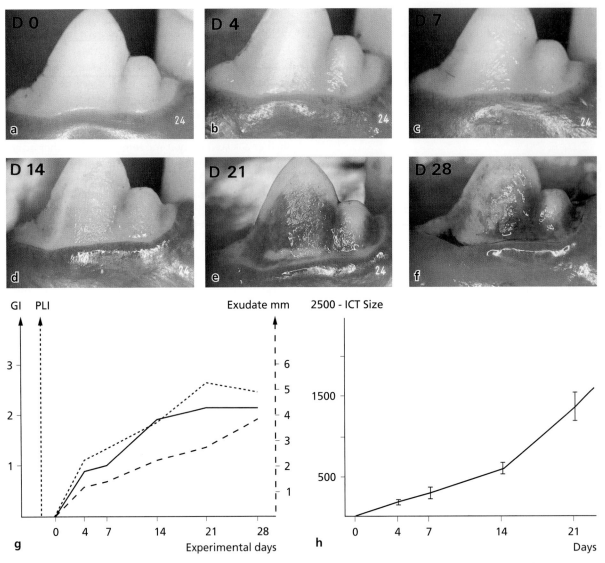

Fig. 11-5 Gingival alterations which occurred during a 28-day period of plaque accumulation and gingivitis development in beagles. (a) Normal gingiva. (b) Day 4. (c) Day 7. (d) Day 14. (e) Day 21. (f) Day 28 of undisturbed plaque accumulation. Note the gradually developing plaque on the tooth surfaces and the inflammatory changes in the gingiva. The vascular reaction is illustrated by a gradually increasing number of vessels in the gingival margin. (g) Gingival index (GI), plaque index (PLI) and gingival exudate alterations (exudate) that occurred during the experimental gingivitis period. (h) In gingival biopsy specimens obtained at various time intervals it can be seen that the inflammatory cell infiltrate (ICT) in the gingiva gradually increased in size.

epithelium and the enamel surface and a subgingival biofilm may now form.

This so-called early lesion may persist for long periods and the variability in time required to produce an established lesion may reflect variance in susceptibility between subjects.

The established lesion

As the exposure of plaque continues there is a further enhancement of the inflammatory response of the gingival tissue. The flow of GCF is increased. The connective tissue as well as the junctional epithelium is transmigrated by an increased number of leukocytes.

The lesion, as defined by Page and Schroeder (1976), is dominated by plasma cells. This conclusion was based mainly on data from animal experiments. Results from examinations of human biopsies, however, revealed that in young individuals lymphocytes occupied a somewhat larger proportion of the infiltrate than plasma cells (Brecx et al. 1988; Fransson et al. 1996). On the other hand, in old subjects, plasma cells were the dominant cell type in established gingivitis lesions (Fransson et al. 1996).

Collagen loss continues as the inflammatory cell infiltrate expands, resulting in collagen-depleted spaces extending deeper into the tissues, which then become available for infiltration and accumulation of leukocytes (Figs. 11-9, 11-10). During this time the dentogingival epithelium continues to proliferate and the rete pegs extend deeper into the connective tissue in an attempt to maintain epithelial integrity and a barrier to microbial entry. The junctional

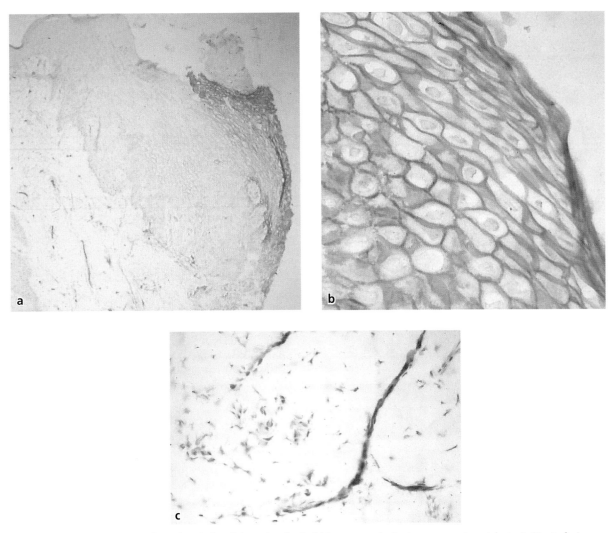

Fig. 11-6 (a) ICAM-1 immunohistochemical staining of a gingival biopsy sample during an experimental gingivitis study in humans after day 7. ICAM-1 positive blood vessels and junctional epithelium can be clearly seen. (b) Higher magnification of (a) showing the extensive junctional epithelium staining. (c) Higher magnification of (a) showing the ICAM-1 positive vessels within the connective tissue.

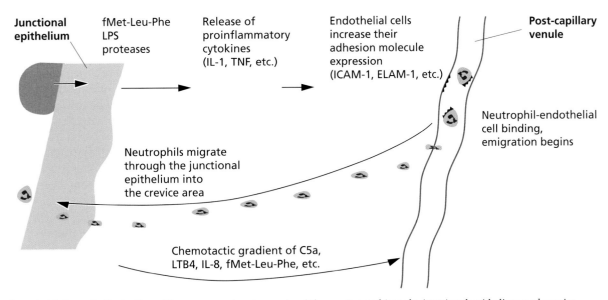

Fig. 11-7 Schematic illustration of the process whereby neutrophils are attracted into the junctional epithelium and crevice region.

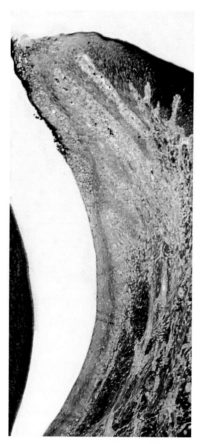

Fig. 11-8 Buccal–lingual section of beagle dog gingiva with an early lesion. Note the epithelial rete pegs in the coronal portion of the lesion.

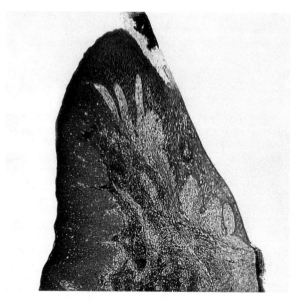

Fig. 11-9 Buccal–lingual section of beagle dog gingiva exhibiting an established lesion. The junctional epithelium is replaced by a pocket epithelium and rete pegs extend deep into the infiltrated connective tissue.

epithelium is substituted by a pocket epithelium that is not attached to the tooth surface. This allows for a further apical migration of the biofilm. The pocket epithelium harbors large numbers of leukocytes, predominantly PMNs. In comparison to the original

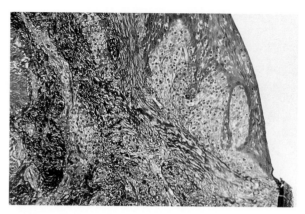

Fig. 11-10 Detail of Fig. 11-9. Note the large number of leukocytes in the inflammatory cell infiltrate and the pocket epithelium.

junctional epithelium, the pocket epithelium is more permeable to the passage of substances into and out of the underlying connective tissue. This pocket epithelium may be ulcerated in places. Figure 11-11 schematically illustrates the alterations which occur during the development of gingivitis and periodontitis.

Two types of established lesion appear to exist: one remains stable and does not progress for months or years (Lindhe *et al.* 1975; Page *et al.* 1975), while the second becomes more active and converts more rapidly to a progressive and destructive advanced lesion.

The advanced lesion

As the pocket deepens, the biofilm continues its apical downgrowth and flourishes in this anaerobic ecological niche. The gingival tissues offer reduced resistance to periodontal probing.

The inflammatory cell infiltrate extends further apically into the connective tissues. The advanced lesion has many of the characteristics of the established lesion but differs importantly in that loss of connective tissue attachment and alveolar bone occurs (Fig. 11-12). The damage to the collagen fibers is extensive. The pocket epithelium migrates apically from the cemento-enamel junction, and there are widespread manifestations of inflammation and immunopathological tissue damage. The lesion is no longer localized to the gingival tissues, but the inflammatory cell infiltrate extends laterally and apically into the connective tissue of the true attachment apparatus. It is generally accepted that plasma cells are the dominant cell type in the advanced lesion (Garant & Mulvihill 1972; Berglundh & Donati 2005).

In summary, in the progression from health to gingivitis and on to periodontitis there are many unknown factors related to timing. In addition, there is extensive subject and site variability in both exacerbating factors and innate susceptibility.

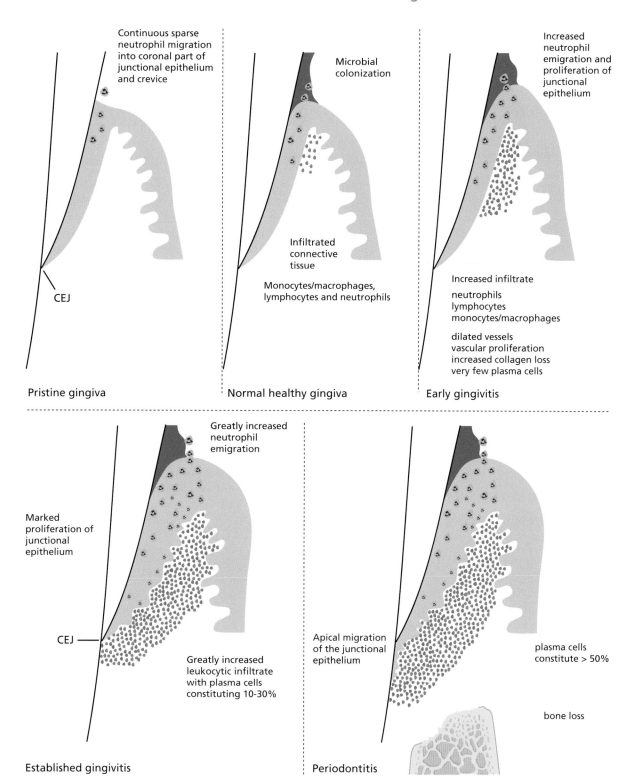

Continuous sparse neutrophil migration into coronal part of junctional epithelium and crevice

CEJ

Pristine gingiva

Microbial colonization

Infiltrated connective tissue

Monocytes/macrophages, lymphocytes and neutrophils

Normal healthy gingiva

Increased neutrophil emigration and proliferation of junctional epithelium

Increased infiltrate

neutrophils
lymphocytes
monocytes/macrophages

dilated vessels
vascular proliferation
increased collagen loss
very few plasma cells

Early gingivitis

Greatly increased neutrophil emigration

Marked proliferation of junctional epithelium

CEJ

Greatly increased leukocytic infiltrate with plasma cells constituting 10-30%

Established gingivitis

Apical migration of the junctional epithelium

plasma cells constitute > 50%

bone loss

Periodontitis

Fig. 11-11 Schematic illustration of the changes in the gingival tissues during the development of gingivitis and periodontitis. The most significant differences are in the extent and composition of the inflammatory infiltrate and the epithelial proliferation in gingivitis, and the apical migration of epithelium and bone loss seen in periodontitis lesions. CEJ: cemento-enamel junction.

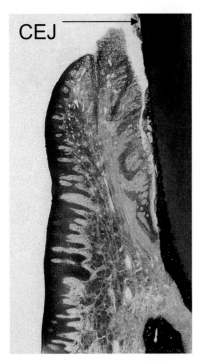

Fig. 11-12 Buccal–lingual section of a periodontitis (advanced) lesion in a beagle dog. Note the apical extension of the inflammatory cell infiltrate and the loss of connective tissue attachment and supporting bone. CEJ: cemento-enamel junction.

Host–parasite interactions

Microbial virulence factors

Periodontal disease is initiated and sustained by factors (substances) produced by the subgingival microbiota (the biofilm). Some of these substances can directly injure host cells and tissues. Other microbial constituents may activate inflammatory or cellular and humoral immune systems that cause damage to the periodontal tissues. It is the latter pathway which accounts for most injury to the periodontal tissues.

Microbial invasion

The invasion of the dentogingival epithelium by spirochetes was conclusively documented by Listgarten (1965) who studied the histopathology of lesions of necrotizing ulcerative gingivitis (ANUG). Although there have been numerous reports of microbial invasion in other forms of gingivitis and periodontitis, the significance of these observations is unclear. Even if bacteria can be found in the tissues, it is not known whether this represents true invasion (i.e. microbial colonization and proliferation within the tissues) or displacement or translocation of bacteria from the biofilm into the soft tissues. In conclusion, it is not known yet whether microbial invasion presents an important challenge to the host or represents an artifact.

Enzymes

Microorganisms produce a variety of soluble enzymes that may digest extracellular host proteins and other molecules and thereby produce nutrients for bacterial growth. In addition to enzymes, bacteria also release numerous, harmful metabolic waste products, such as ammonia, indole, hydrogen sulfide, and butyric acid.

Amongst the enzymes released by bacteria in the biofilm, *proteases* (proteinases) are capable of digesting collagen, elastin, fibronectin, fibrin, and various other components of the intercellular matrix of both epithelial and connective tissues. One protease that has attracted much attention is the Arg1-protease produced by *Porphyromonas gingivalis* for which high potency is claimed. This protease, in addition, has the capability to induce a strong humoral immune response (Aduse-Opoku *et al.* 1995). Another protease, leukotoxin, was a focus of interest for many years, but as yet no *in vivo* evidence exists for its claimed role in periodontal tissue destruction (Haubek *et al.* 1995). This leukotoxin has been studied in both America and Europe but it appears that the strains of *Aggregatibacter actinomycetemcomitans* that produce the protease differed (Haubek *et al.* 1995). It seems that the more virulent form, which produces leukotoxin in excess and thus has great capacity to kill leukocytes, is common in strains from America but virtually absent in strains from Europe, despite identical disease prevalence.

Endotoxin

Lipopolysaccharides (LPSs) of Gram-negative microorganisms are capable of invoking both the inflammatory and immune responses as they interact with host cells. Many of the functions attributed to LPS are associated with their ability to stimulate the production of cytokines. LPS also has profound effects on blood coagulation and on the complement system. The properties of LPS, as well as of *lipoteichoic acids* (LTAs) of Gram-positive bacteria, are numerous and may be influenced by many other molecules that interact with these outer membrane structures. LPS and LTA are produced and released from microorganisms present in the subgingival biofilm and cause release of chemical mediators of inflammation to produce vascular permeability and encourage, through chemotactic actions, inflammatory cells to move into and accumulate in the gingival tissues. Furthermore, leukocytes are stimulated to release pro-inflammatory agents and cytokines.

Summary: Microbes are capable of producing a variety of substances which either directly or indirectly harm the host. The main detrimental effect may be the host's own innate, inflammatory, and immune response to the foreign molecules and antigens of the microbe.

Host defense processes

Host–parasite reactions can be divided into innate (non-specific) and adaptive (specific) responses. Innate reactions include the inflammatory response and do not involve immunological mechanisms. Adaptive reactions that include immunological responses tend to be very effective as the host response is specifically "tailored" to the offending pathogen(s).

Important aspects of host defense processes

Inflammatory processes

The host has an extensive repertoire of defensive responses to ward off invasion by pathogens. Such responses may either result in a rapid resolution of the lesion (e.g. a staphylococcal abscess which heals) or that no lesion at all develops in the affected tissue (e.g. smallpox infection in a successfully vaccinated host). An ineffective response may result in a chronic lesion that does not resolve (e.g. tuberculosis) or if excessively deployed, in a lesion in which the host responses contribute significantly to tissue destruction (e.g. rheumatoid arthritis or asthma).

In the classical description of inflammation, a tissue is presented that appears macroscopically red, swollen, hot, and painful, and with possible loss of function in specific sites. Redness and heat are due to vasodilatation and increased blood flow. Swelling is a result of increased vascular permeability and leakage of plasma proteins that create an osmotic potential that draws fluid into the inflamed tissues. Related to the vascular changes there is an accumulation of inflammatory cells infiltrating the lesion. Pain is rarely experienced in aggressive and chronic periodontal disease, but could theoretically occur due to stimulation of afferent nerves by chemical mediators of inflammation in necrotizing periodontal disease. Impairment of function is classically illustrated in arthritically swollen joints.

Molecules, cells, and processes

Proteinases (proteases)

Periodontal disease results in tissue degradation, and thus proteases, derived both from the host and from bacteria, are central to the disease processes. Proteinases (collagenase, elastase-like and trypsin-like, as well as serine and cysteine proteinases) cleave proteins by hydrolyzing peptide bonds and may be classified into two major classes, *endopeptidases* and *exopeptidases*, depending on the location of activity of the enzyme on its substrate. Efforts have been made to assess endopeptidase activity in gingival tissues and in GCF. A reduction of protease levels following treatment was obtained in several studies.

Proteinase inhibitors

Release of proteinases in the gingiva and the crevicular area promotes inflammatory reactions and contributes to connective tissue damage via several pathways. In contrast, *proteinase inhibitors* would dampen the inflammatory process. Among such inhibitors alpha-2 macroglobulin (A2-M) and alpha1 antitrypsin (A1-AT) must be recognized. In fact, gingival collagenase inhibition by A2-M has been demonstrated to occur in gingival tissues and polymorphonuclear leukocyte (PMN) collagenase is also inhibited by A1-AT.

Many host and microbial enzymes are likely to be present in the crevice at any one time. Realizing the potentially destructive features of such enzymes, consideration should be given to the source of these enzymes, their relative proportions and the inhibitory mechanisms available within the crevice. The main enzyme activity is host derived and specific and non-specific inhibitors are plentiful within the crevice and thus enzyme activity will be localized and short-lived.

Matrix metalloproteinases

The periodontium is structurally comprised of fibrous elements, including collagen, elastin, and glycoproteins (laminin, fibronectin, proteoglycans), minerals, lipids, water, and tissue-bound growth factors. In addition there exists a large variety of extracellular matrix components, including tropocollagen, proteoglycans, and other proteins (elastin, osteocalcin, osteopontin, bone sialoprotein, osteonectin, and tenascin). All of these matrix components are constantly in a state of turnover and thus there is much matrix enzyme activity in health, disease, and tissue repair and remodeling (Kinane 2001). Matrix metalloproteinases (MMPs) are responsible for remodeling and degradation of the matrix components.

One of the MMPs that has received much attention is the *neutrophil (PMN) collagenase* that is found in higher concentrations in inflamed gingival specimens than in clinically healthy gingiva. The increased presence of these MMP enzymes in diseased over healthy sites (Ohlsson *et al.* 1973), their increase during experimental gingivitis (Kowashi *et al.* 1979), and decrease after periodontal treatment (Haerian *et al.* 1995, 1996) suggest that MMPs from PMNs are involved in periodontal tissue breakdown.

The periodontal ligament is one of the most metabolically active tissues in the body, and collagen metabolism represents most of this activity. The biological reason for this activity probably relates to its ability to adapt to occlusal forces generated during function. An important feature of connective tissues in general and the periodontal ligament in particular, is the process of constant renewal of the extracellular matrix components involving MMP.

It is evident that the activity of MMPs and their inhibitors is associated with tissue turnover as well as with gingivitis, destructive periodontitis, and with the healing of the periodontal tissues following therapy.

Cytokines

Cytokines are soluble proteins, secreted by cells involved in both the innate and adaptive host response, and act as messenger molecules that transmit signals to other cells. They have numerous actions that include initiation and maintenance of immune and inflammatory responses and regulation of growth and differentiation of cells. Cytokines are numerous, many have overlapping functions, and they are interlinked to form an active network which controls the host response. Control of cytokine release and action is complex and involves inhibitors and receptors. Many cytokines are capable of acting back on the cell that produced them so as to stimulate (or downgrade) their own production and the production of other cytokines.

Interleukins are important members of the cytokine group and are primarily involved in communication between leukocytes and other cells, such as epithelial cells, endothelial cells, and fibroblasts engaged in the inflammatory process. In addition, *interleukin (IL)-1a, IL-1b*, and *tumor necrosis factor (TNF)-alpha* stimulate bone resorption and inhibit bone formation.

A series of more than 20 molecules has been identified, that act to recruit defense cells (PMNs, macrophages, lymphocytes) to areas where they are required. These chemotactic cytokines play an important role in cell-mediated immune responses.

Prostaglandins

Prostaglandins are derivatives of arachidonic acid and are important mediators of inflammation. Macrophages in particular, but also several other cells produce prostaglandins, particularly PGE_2 which is a potent vasodilator and inducer of cytokine production by various cells. PGE_2 acts on fibroblasts and osteoclasts to induce production of MMPs, which are of importance for tissue turnover and tissue destruction in gingivitis and periodontitis (see above).

Polymorphonuclear leukocytes

The PMN is the predominant leukocyte within the gingival crevice/pocket in both health and disease. PMNs are attracted from the circulation to the affected area via chemotactic stimuli elicited from, for example, microorganisms in the biofilm, and host-derived chemokines. *Elastase*, a serine protease, is contained in the primary granules of the PMN. Elastase may cause tissue breakdown and is present with increased activity at sites of gingival inflammation. *Lactoferrin* is contained in the secondary granules of

the PMN, and is released during PMN migration and is associated with PMN activation. Differences in the relative amounts of elastase and lactoferrin were found in periodontal sites with varying degrees of inflammation. A greater proportion of lactoferrin to elastase was found in advanced periodontitis lesions than in gingivitis sites. This variation in the release of primary and secondary granule enzymes by PMNs may indicate alterations in PMN function in different disease environments (Fig. 11-13).

Bone destruction

Tissue destruction is one of the hallmarks of periodontitis and involves connective tissue structures and alveolar bone. Degradation of collagen and matrix components in the connective tissue is regulated by inflammatory processes in the periodontitis lesion and includes the production of various MMPs (see above).

Bone resorption is mediated by osteoclasts and takes place concomitant with the breakdown of the connective tissue attachment during disease progression. Thus, the mechanisms involved in bone resorption respond to signals from inflammatory cells in the lesion and initiate degradation of bone in order to maintain a "safety" distance to the periphery of the inflammatory cell infiltrate. Analyses of human autopsy material and biopsy specimens from animal experiments have demonstrated that the alveolar bone in periodontitis is separated from the inflammatory cell infiltrate by a 0.5–1 mm wide zone of a non-infiltrated connective tissue. This encapsulation of the lesion is an important feature of host defense mechanisms in periodontitis and bone resorption is thus required to re-establish dimensions of the connective tissue capsule following a phase of attachment loss during disease progression.

Osteoclasts are multinucleated cells that develop from osteoclast progenitor cells/macrophages and exhibit specific abilities to degrade organic and inorganic components of bone. As mentioned above, different mediators such as IL-1 beta, PGE_2 and TNF-alpha but also IL-6, IL-11 and IL-17 may act as activators on osteoclasts. Another and more important system in osteoclast activation includes the receptor activator of nuclear factor-kappa beta (RANK), the RANK ligand (RANKL) and osteoprotegrin (OPG). RANK is a receptor expressed by osteoclast progenitor cells. RANKL and OPG are cytokines that belong to the TNF family and are produced by osteoblasts and bone marrow stromal cells. While RANKL promotes activation of osteoclasts, OPG has the opposite effect. Thus, the binding of RANKL to the RANK will result in the differentiation of osteoclast progenitor cells into active osteoclasts, while OPG that binds to RANKL will inhibit the differentiation process (for review see Lerner 2006). Analyses of human biopsy specimens revealed that levels of RANKL were higher and levels of OPG were lower in sites with

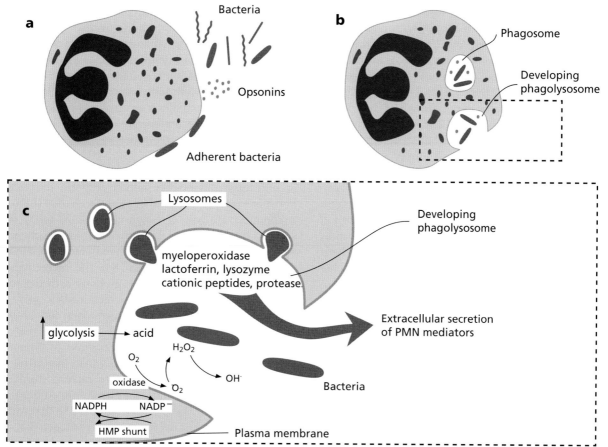

Fig. 11-13 Major events in the encounter between PMNs and invading microorganisms. (a) Once PMNs emigrate from the microcirculation, they migrate toward bacteria under the influence of chemotactic factors. Upon contact PMNs adhere to the organisms (many types of bacteria must be opsonized to facilitate PMN adherence and phagocytosis). (b) Coincident with adhesion, PMNs begin to phagocytose these organisms. This is accomplished as the plasma membrane flows around and then invaginates to internalize attached organisms which are now contained within phagosomes. Several bacteria can be phagocytosed simultaneously by the PMN. (c) As these events occur PMNs demonstrate dramatic metabolic alterations including: an elevation in glycolysis; a marked rise in oxygen consumption; and increased glucose utilization by the hexose monophosphate shunt. Glycolytic metabolism of glucose provides the energy required by phagocytosis and also results in a drop in intracellular pH due to the formation of lactate. The oxidative burst is largely the result of NADPH oxidase activity (an enzyme associated with the cell membrane), which oxidizes NADPH to NADP and results in the reduction of oxygen to various free radicals. These oxidants are released into the phagosome to kill bacteria. The hexose monophosphate shunt provides for the regeneration of NADPH. At the same time, lysosomes are mobilized toward the developing phagosome and fuse with the phagosome membrane, giving rise to a phagolysosome. Lysosomal antimicrobial compounds (myeloperoxidase, lysozyme, lactoferrin, cationic proteins, etc.) are discharged into the vacuole. The combination of oxidative and non-oxidative (acid pH, lysosomal agents) pathways explains how PMNs kill ingested organisms. Lysozyme and neutral proteases (particularly elastase) derived from lysosomes digest and dispose of the dead organisms. Before invagination is completed, biologically active products can be released from the phagosome into the external environment. These agents play a role in extracellular killing of microorganisms but also may adversely affect surrounding host cells and tissue structures.

periodontitis than in sites representing healthy gingiva (Crotti *et al*. 2003; Liu *et al*. 2003).

The RANK/RANKL/OPG system is also involved in bone degradation processes that are induced by pro-inflammatory cytokines such as PGE_2, TNF-alpha, IL-1 beta, IL-6, IL-11, and IL-17. In addition, the production of the RANKL is not confined to osteoblasts and bone marrow stromal cells. Thus, the contribution of RANKL by T cells and other cells in inflammation must be considered. The role of T cells, however, is unclear given that this cell not only produces RANKL but also inhibitors of RANKL, such as interferon (IFN)-gamma and IL-4 (Takayanagi 2005).

In summary, bone resorption is part of the encapsulation process of the inflammatory cell infiltrate in periodontitis. Osteoclasts develop from osteoclast progenitor cells or macrophages and are regulated by the RANK/RANKL/OPG system and/or pro-inflammatory cytokines.

The innate defense systems

Innate immune mechanisms operate without any previous contact with the disease-causing microorganism. These mechanisms include the *barrier function* of the oral epithelia and *vascular* and *cellular* aspects of the *inflammatory responses*.

The gingival crevice is the first region of the periodontium that comes into contact with microorganisms that attempt to attach and colonize the area. Several innate mechanisms serve to prevent such microbial colonization and include (1) the mechanical washing effect of the *saliva* and *GCF*, and (2) the detrimental effect on bacterial growth of *constituents* of these fluids (e.g. antibodies and proteases, complement, salivary lactoferrin, and other proteins).

The oral mucosa itself is not simply a barrier but has a chemical composition that may be harmful to bacteria. Furthermore, the cells of the epithelium can respond to the bacteria by (1) producing antimicrobial peptides, including beta-defensin etc., that kill the microbes, (2) releasing other molecules, such as IL-1 beta, capable of inducing or enhancing the local inflammatory reaction, and (3) releasing IL-8, a chemokine which attracts host defense cells such as neutrophils and macrophages to reduce the microbial insult. The epithelium can also respond by increasing the expression of surface molecules such as cell adhesion molecules that, in turn, may interact with proinflammatory cytokines and chemokines to assist the recruitment of leukocytes to the crevice.

Molecules in saliva, such as *lactoferrin*, may bind iron, change the local environment, and hence prevent microbial proliferation. In addition, lactoferrin is highly bactericidal. Molecules present in the GCF include *complement*, which can kill bacteria directly or together with antibodies, and can bring PMNs to the region (via chemotaxis) and hereby initiate and facilitate the process of phagocytosis.

The concept that epithelial and endothelial cells and fibroblasts are structural cells not involved in specific immune or inflammatory reactions has been disproved. Toll-like receptors are structures evolved to detect bacterial challenge and are present on all human cells, including epithelial and endothelial cells, and may bind microbial cell molecules, such as lipopolysaccharides, microbial fimbriae, and lipoteichoic acid. This suggests that even innate responses of the host may be tailored to particular bacteria. The host and its pathogens have developed together over millions of years and have learned to recognize, mimic, and utilize each other's systems in highly sophisticated ways.

Innate immune processes

The primary etiologic agent in the initiation of the gingivitis is the accumulation of the bacterial plaque biofilm in the gingival crevice. Irritation of the gingival tissues induces an "inflammatory response". The rapid inflammatory process that occurs in gingivitis is an early step in the initiation of the overall immune and inflammatory response, and is part of the *innate immune* system; i.e. it is part of the inherent biologic responses that require no prior experience. Inflammation is an extremely well coordinated process that comprises increased vascular permeability, migration of PMN leukocytes, monocytes, and lymphocytes into the affected tissues, and activation of cells to secrete inflammatory mediators that guide an amplifying cascade of biochemical and cellular events. Although inflammation was once considered a nonspecific arm of the immune response, the inflammatory response is actually a relatively specific event, which is carefully orchestrated through a wide-ranging repertoire of receptors and corresponding ligands.

The specific nature of inflammation allows rapid identification and a better tailored response to infection. For example, bacterial lipopolysaccharide (LPS), a common antigen of Gram-negative bacteria, is specifically recognized by host receptors such as soluble LPS binding protein, membrane-associated CD14 and toll-like receptors (TLRs). The interactions between LPS and these host proteins activate an intracellular cascade of events which leads to secretion of specific inflammatory mediators and antimicrobial proteins. These specific interactions may explain why the inflammatory response to Gram-positive bacteria is less pronounced than the inflammatory response to Gram-negative bacteria during *in vitro* and *in vivo* inflammatory assays. In addition, the discovery that there is a group of TLRs that can recognize a wide but restricted set of pathogen-associated molecular structures may explain how different bacteria induce different responses. In fact, even LPS from different bacteria may activate different TLRs, and induce a different response. These interactions enable the host to sample and sort its current environmental condition, to discriminate between pathogenic bacterial challenges, and to mount a selective and appropriate response. Recent data indicate that TLRs may respond to bacterial and non-bacterial challenges, such as oxidized low-density lipoprotein cholesterol. Thus the host may respond through inflammation to a range of challenges, from bacteria to cholesterol. However, the nature of the response differs and its character depends on the microbial triggering of specific receptors, the signal transduction pathways, and the way cells and tissues respond to these signals in terms of cytokine and defensive protein production.

During experimental gingivitis studies, individual variations in the rate of development of gingival inflammation have been noted (see Chapter 17) and the difference in gingivitis susceptibility is not simply due to plaque differences. Trombelli *et al.* (2004) have also shown that while all individuals will develop some degree of inflammation, there are interindividual differences in response to dental plaque. These differences may be explained by genetics or environment. Using the "twin study approach", Michalowicz *et al.* (2000), could not demonstrate an association between gingival inflammation and genetics, perhaps due to the cross-sectional approach of the study. However, their data support the major role of genetics in the development of periodontitis, in which gingival inflammation is considered as a major part of the pathogenesis. In summary, all of the above studies are consistent with the hypothesis of genetically based host modulation of gingival inflammation.

Variation in microbial modulation of innate responses

Innate immunity represents the inherited resistance to microbial infection, which is detected by pattern-recognition receptors (PRRs). PRRs are strategically located at the interface between the mammalian host and the microbes, and have evolved to recognize conserved microbial motifs, known as microbe-associated molecular patterns (MAMPs). TLRs constitute an evolutionarily ancient PRR family, which plays a central role in the induction of innate immune and inflammatory responses. Not surprisingly, TLRs are expressed predominantly in cells which mediate first-line defense, such as neutrophils, monocytes/macrophages, and dendritic cells, as well as epithelial cells. Distinct members of the TLR family respond to different types of MAMPs, endowing the innate response with a relative specificity. The discovery of TLRs and the identification of their ligand repertoire have prompted the "bar code" hypothesis of innate recognition of microbes. According to this concept, TLRs read a "bar code" on microbes which is then decoded intracellularly to tailor the appropriate type of innate response. For instance, simultaneous activation of TLR5 and TLR4 would be interpreted as infection with a flagellated Gram-negative bacterium, whereas activation of TLR2 together with TLR5 would likely indicate the presence of a flagellated Gram-positive bacterium. However, this "bar code" detection system would not readily distinguish between pathogens and commensals, since they both share similar invariant structures (e.g., LTA, LPS, or flagellae). The immune system, however, generally elicits a vigorous inflammatory response against pathogens aimed at eliminating them, whereas it normally tolerates commensals.

The immune or adaptive defense system

In contrast to the innate host response, the adaptive response utilizes strategies of recognition, memory, and binding to support the effector systems in the elimination of challenging elements. Thus, the host response to factors released by microbial plaque in periodontal diseases involves a series of different effector mechanisms that are activated by the *innate* immune response. The effector mechanisms in this first line of defense may be insufficient to eliminate a given pathogen. The *adaptive* immune response, which is a second line of defense, is then activated. The adaptive response improves the host's ability to recognize the pathogen.

Immune memory and *clonal expansion* of immune cells are the hallmarks of adaptive immunity.

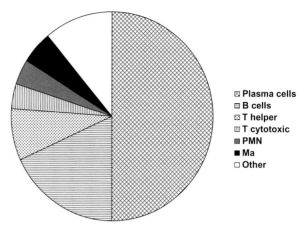

Fig. 11-14 Distribution of cell proportions in periodontitis lesions. Adapted from Berglundh & Donati (2005).

Although the effector mechanisms activated by the adaptive system appear to be similar to those of the innate system, the antimicrobial activities in adaptive immunity are specialized functions regulated by lymphocytes. This means that the defense mechanisms in the gingiva are synchronized by the communication through signals (cytokines) between specific groups of cells.

The cells involved in the adaptive response and which reside in the inflammatory lesion in sites with periodontitis have been described in several studies that included a histopathological analysis of the composition of the cell infiltrate. In a recent review on aspects of adaptive host response in periodontitis a meta-analysis was made with regard to the cell composition in periodontitis lesions (Berglundh & Donati 2005). Plasma cells represent about 50% of cells, while B cells comprise about 18%. The proportion of B cells is larger than that of all T cells. T helper cells occur in larger numbers than T cytotoxic cells. PMN cells and macrophages represent less than 5% of cells (Fig. 11-14). In the review it was further observed that lesions in aggressive and chronic forms of periodontitis exhibit similar features with respect to cellular composition. In both chronic and aggressive forms of periodontitis the proportions of plasma cells and B cells appear to be larger in lesions obtained from sites representing severe periodontitis than in lesions from areas with moderate or mild periodontitis.

The following outline provides an overview of T cell and B cell characteristics and immunoregulatory mechanisms of adaptive host response in periodontitis (Fig. 11-15).

Antigen presentation

The biofilm is consistently challenging the host. The antigens produced include proteins from Gram-positive bacteria and LPSs (endotoxins) from Gram-negative microorganisms. Antigen-presenting cells (APCs) have a unique ability to internalize and process antigens. Langerhans cells, macrophages,

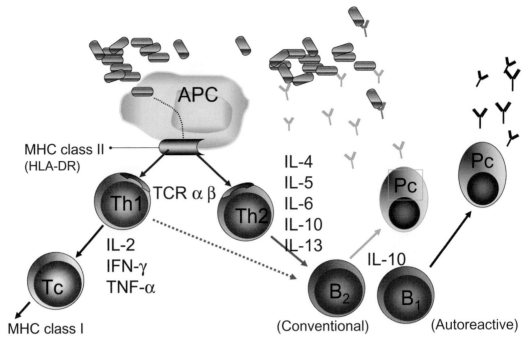

Fig. 11-15 Immune regulation in periodontal disease.

and dendritic cells are professional APCs and contribute to antigen recognition and early response mechanisms in host defense. B cells are considered to be important APCs in periodontitis and use the capacity of their memory systems in antigen presentation within the adaptive host response. The processed antigen (e.g. a peptide) inside the APC binds to an important carrying molecule. This molecule, termed *class-II* molecule of the major histocompatibility complex (MHC), transports the peptide to the cell surface. The peptide will thus, together with the MHC class-II molecule, become identifiable (i.e. presented) to T cells.

T cell receptors

The presentation of the processed antigen involves interactions with receptors on the T cells: T cell receptors (TCRs). It is in this context important to realize that the resulting immune response from this presentation varies with the build up of the TCR. The TCR is comprised of two glycoprotein chains, mainly alpha and beta (Fig. 11-15). The external portion of these alpha and beta chains contains a variable segment, which has many features in common with the antigen-binding site at immunoglobulins. This means that the composition of the variable segment in the alpha or the beta chain determines the type of immune reaction that will occur.

It is well known that the composition, or expression, of the variable chains of TCRs (TCR alpha/beta phenotype or genes) is of importance in several autoimmune diseases (Bröker *et al.* 1993) and also in periodontal disease (Nakajima *et al.* 1996; Yamazaki *et al.* 1997; Geatch *et al.* 1997; Berglundh *et al.* 1998). The results reported on TCRs in periodontitis have con-

sistently revealed that the TCR repertoire of T cells in the local periodontitis lesions differs from that of T cells in peripheral blood. In other words, factors present at the local site, i.e. antigens released from microorganisms in the subgingival biofilm, may influence the expression of TCRs in the periodontitis lesion (Mathur *et al.* 1995). This fact also explains the differences observed in the distribution of TCRs in gingival tissues before and after periodontal therapy (Berglundh *et al.* 1999) as well as between adult subjects with advanced chronic periodontitis and children with aggressive periodontitis (Berglundh *et al.* 2001).

T cell dependent (mediated) processes

Cytokines produced by T helper (Th) cells regulate most functions within the adaptive defense system in the periodontal tissues. Th cells occur as Th-1 and Th-2 cells. Both Th-1 and Th-2 cells express the CD4 marker but are distinguished from each other by their cytokine production (cytokine profiles) (Fig. 11-15). Th-1 cells produce *IL-2*, *IFN-gamma*, and *TNF-alpha*. These cytokines have several functions and may activate other T cells, including the so-called cytotoxic T cells (Tc).

Tc cells express the CD8 marker and serve as guards against microorganisms that are capable of invading host cells, i.e. viruses and invasive bacteria. In the infected host cells, the antigen (e.g. a peptide) produced by the intracellularly located pathogen binds to MHC class-I molecules, which carry the peptide to the surface of the infected host cell. The Tc cell has the ability to recognize this alteration in the MHC class-I molecules and exerts its host defense action by destroying the membrane of the infected cell and by activating its nucleases. This cell-mediated host response orchestrated by the Tc cell also includes activation of macrophages.

It is well established that CD8-positive cells are found in smaller numbers in gingivitis/periodontitis lesions than CD4-positive cells (Yamazaki *et al.* 1995; Berglundh *et al.* 2002a; Berglundh & Donati 2005). It may therefore be anticipated that viruses and other invasive microorganisms do not constitute a major part of the antigens in peridodontitis.

B cell regulation processes

The large amounts of soluble and accessible antigens occurring in the periodontal environment require the involvement of host defense systems different from those involved in cell-mediated immunity. Specific antibodies (immunoglobulins), occurring in fluids such as plasma or GCF, have the ability to bind to antigens. This type of host defense is called *humoral immune response*. In the process through which the antigen becomes bound to the antibody, certain effector systems, e.g. *complement*, are activated. The activation of the complement system, in turn, mediates PMN and macrophage migration to the site and phagocytosis is initiated. The process in which the antibody contributes to the elimination of antigens by enhancing phagocytosis is termed *opsonization.*

Antibodies are produced by plasma cells that represent the final stage in B cell proliferation. The activation and differentiation of B cells require the presence of certain cytokines, IL-4, IL-5, and IL-6, that are mainly produced by Th-2 cells (Gemmell & Seymour 1998). Since plasma cells and B cells constitute a major part of the leukocytes in advanced periodontitis lesions, it is reasonable to assume that Th-2 functions may dominate over those dependent on Th-1. In early studies it was indeed suggested that the immunoregulatory mechanisms in the advanced periodontitis lesions involve Th-2 cells to a larger extent than Th-1 cells (Seymour *et al.* 1993, 1996). Several later studies have, however, failed to confirm this observation (Yamazaki *et al.* 1994, 1997; Fujihashi *et al.* 1996; Prabhu *et al.* 1996; Yamamoto *et al.* 1997). Berglundh *et al.* (2002a) reported that the connective tissue lesions in advanced periodontitis contained similar proportions of cells expressing cytokine profiles characteristic for Th-1 (IFN-gamma and IL-2) and Th-2 (IL-4 and IL-6) cells. Current data thus suggest that chronic periodontitis lesions are regulated by a combined Th-1 and Th-2 function.

The immunoglobulins produced by plasma cells in the gingival lesions are mainly directed towards antigens present in the subgingival biofilm. Data have been presented, however, which indicate that antibodies directed against host tissue components, i.e. *autoantibodies*, may also occur in the gingival lesion (Hirsch *et al.* 1988, 1989; Jonsson *et al.* 1991). *Auto-reactive B cells*, also referred to as *B-1 cells*, are associated with the production of auto-antibodies.

Large amounts of B-1 cells are present in the peripheral blood of patients with autoimmune disease, such as rheumatoid arthritis and Sjögren's syndrome (Youinou *et al.* 1988). The presence of circulating auto-reactive B cells in periodontitis patients has also been described. Thus, Afar *et al.* (1992) and Berglundh *et al.* (1998, 2002b) reported that B-1 cells occur in large numbers in the peripheral blood of patients with advanced chronic periodontitis. The gingival lesion in patients with such advanced periodontitis also contains a substantial number of B cells out of which about 30% exhibit auto-reactive characteristics (Sugawara *et al.* 1992; Berglundh *et al.* 2002b).

In this context it should be recognized that clinically successful, non-surgical periodontal therapy (i.e. resolution of gingivitis and reduction of sites with deep pockets) failed to alter the proportion of B-1 cells in peripheral blood (Berglundh *et al.* 1999). It was suggested that the elevated levels of B-1 cells in peripheral blood may not entirely reflect a response to microorganisms in the subgingival biofilm. Rather, it appears that the effector systems in the humoral immune response in periodontitis may also include production of antibodies directed to the periodontal tissues of the host.

In the humoral immune response the function, i.e. the avidity (binding strength to the antigen) of the antibody most also be considered. Thus, some but not all antibodies have a strong ability to opsonize bacteria and thereby prevent bacterial colonization. Account must also given to issues such as (1) whether antibody levels in the GCF or in serum or both are of importance for the protection of the host, (2) whether local levels of antibodies are merely a reflection of serum levels, or (3) whether significant antibody production by plasma cells present in the gingiva is taking place. In addition, there is evidence that the subclass of immunoglobulin produced has a bearing on aspects of its function such as complement fixation and opsonization. Thus, in aggressive periodontitis there seems to be a preponderance of IgG2 production over IgG1. This means that the functionally less effective IgG2 may play a role in rendering such patients more susceptible to periodontal tissue destruction (Wilson *et al.* 1995). Several studies suggest that assessments of the titer and avidity (the binding strength) of a patient's antibody to various microorganisms in the subgingival biofilm may be useful in the differential diagnosis and classification of periodontal diseases (Mooney *et al.* 1993).

IgG has four subclasses and IgA has two subclasses. Antibodies of different subclasses have different properties. Thus, IgG2 antibodies are effective against carbohydrate antigens (LPS) whereas the other subclasses are mainly directed against proteins. Kinane *et al.* (1997) studied the immunoglobulin subclasses (IgG1–4 and IgA1–2) produced by plasma cells in the gingival lesion of periodontitis patients (Fig. 11-16). The proportions of plasma cells producing IgG and IgA subclasses were similar to the

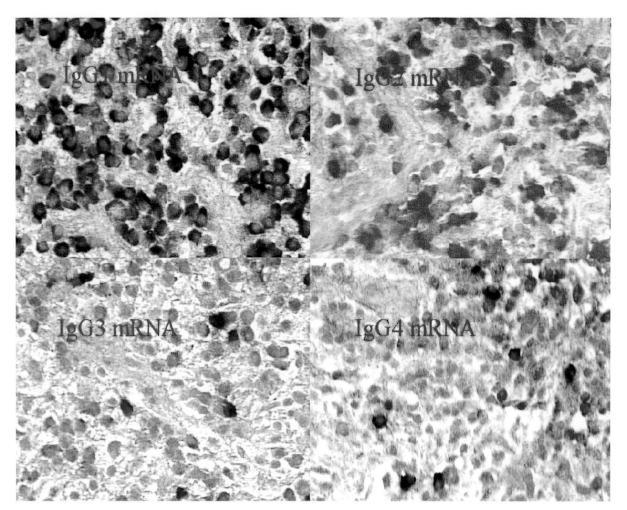

Fig. 11-16 Plasma cells within the periodontal gingiva. The mRNA for immunoglobulin production is noted in abundance within the plasma cell cytoplasms indicating that gingival plasma cells have the ability to produce antibodies locally (Kinane *et al.* 1997).

proportions of these immunoglobulin subclasses in serum. IgG1-producing plasma cells were predominant (mean 63%) in the gingival lesions; 23% of all IgG-producing plasma cells produced IgG2 antibodies, while IgG3- and IgG4-producing cells were present in much smaller numbers (3% and 10% respectively).

The protective role of the immune responses

Recruitment of leukocytes into areas of injury or infection is essential for an effective host defense. The constant migration of T cells and other leukocytes to tissues throughout the body allows the immune system to protect the host from a variety of antigenic challenges.

Leukocyte migration into tissues is particularly prominent during inflammatory responses and results from the cytokine-induced expression of adhesion molecules on the surface of vascular endothelial cells (Kinane *et al.* 1991) (Fig. 11-7). Endothelial leukocyte adhesion molecule-1 (ELAM-1) and intercellular adhesion molecule-1 (ICAM-1) are crucial for

cellular trafficking (Fig. 11-6). The changes in vascular adhesion molecule expression and numbers of infiltrating leukocytes during a 21-day experimental gingivitis episode were investigated by Moughal *et al.* (1992). ELAM-1 and ICAM-1 positive vessels as well as PMNs and T cells were identified within gingival biopsy specimens taken on days 0, 7, 14, and 21. Vascular endothelium expressed ELAM-1 and ICAM-1 both in clinically "healthy" tissue (day 0) and in experimentally inflamed tissue (days 7–21). Positive vessels were found mainly in the connective tissue subjacent to the junctional epithelium where the highest numbers of T cells and neutrophils were also seen. A gradient of ICAM-1 was found to exist in the junctional epithelium, with the strongest staining in the marginal (crevicular) portion. This observation, together with the vascular expression of ELAM-1 and ICAM-1 in both clinically "healthy" and inflamed tissue, suggests that the function of the adhesion molecules is crucial and that these molecules direct leukocyte migration towards the gingival crevice (Fig. 11-7). The importance of these mechanisms is highlighted by the rapid progress of periodontitis that is found in patients with insufficient levels of ELAM-1

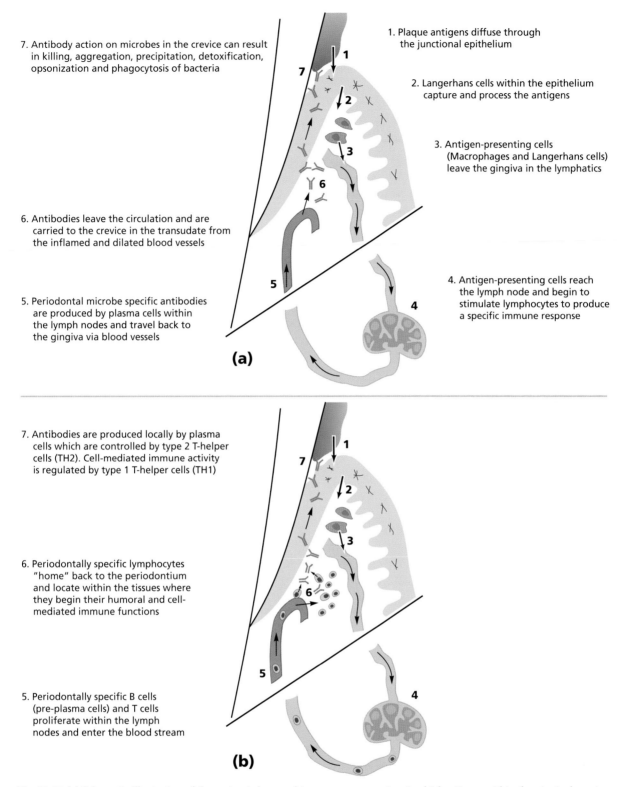

7. Antibody action on microbes in the crevice can result in killing, aggregation, precipitation, detoxification, opsonization and phagocytosis of bacteria

1. Plaque antigens diffuse through the junctional epithelium

2. Langerhans cells within the epithelium capture and process the antigens

3. Antigen-presenting cells (Macrophages and Langerhans cells) leave the gingiva in the lymphatics

6. Antibodies leave the circulation and are carried to the crevice in the transudate from the inflamed and dilated blood vessels

4. Antigen-presenting cells reach the lymph node and begin to stimulate lymphocytes to produce a specific immune response

5. Periodontal microbe specific antibodies are produced by plasma cells within the lymph nodes and travel back to the gingiva via blood vessels

(a)

7. Antibodies are produced locally by plasma cells which are controlled by type 2 T-helper cells (TH2). Cell-mediated immune activity is regulated by type 1 T-helper cells (TH1)

6. Periodontally specific lymphocytes "home" back to the periodontium and locate within the tissues where they begin their humoral and cell-mediated immune functions

5. Periodontally specific B cells (pre-plasma cells) and T cells proliferate within the lymph nodes and enter the blood stream

(b)

Fig. 11-17 (a) Schematic illustration of the systemic humoral immune response to microbial antigens within the gingival crevice region. (b) Schematic illustration of the local cellular immune response within the gingival crevice region and how this is invoked by microbial antigens and the mechanism by which pertinent periodontal immune cells traffic to the periodontium.

and ICAM-1, i.e. subjects suffering from *leukocyte adhesion deficiency syndrome* (LAD).

Specific antibody responses

P. gingivalis and *A. actinomycetemcomitans* are considered to be important pathogens in various forms of periodontal disease. Several studies have demonstrated that the antibody titers to these two organisms are increased in patients with periodontitis compared with subjects without disease (Kinane *et al.* 1993, 1999; Mooney & Kinane 1994).

Furthermore, Naito *et al.* (1987) and Aukhil *et al.* (1988) demonstrated that the serum titer to

P. gingivalis was *reduced* in subjects with advanced periodontitis following successful treatment. In this regard a study by Mooney *et al.* (1995) must be recognized. They reported on specific antibody titer and avidity to *P. gingivalis* and *A. actinomycetemcomitans* in chronic periodontitis patients before and after periodontal therapy. The authors observed that *IgG avidities* (the binding strength of the antibodies) to *P. gingivalis* increased significantly and specific *IgA levels* more than doubled as a result of treatment. Interestingly, only patients who had high levels of antibody before treatment showed a significant increase in antibody avidity. In addition, patients who originally had high levels of IgG and IgA to *P. gingivalis* also had better treatment outcomes, in terms of a reduced number of deep pockets and sites which bled on probing, than patients with initially lower titers.

Antibody levels are probably dependent on a number of factors including previous exposure to the subgingival microbiota and the host's ability to respond to particular antigens. The effect of treatment on antibody level and avidity may be the result of an inoculation (transient bacteremia) effect that occurs during scaling and root planing. The reduction in the amount of bacteria, i.e. the antigen load, which occurs after subgingival scaling and root planing, may allow the activation of B cells (clones) that produce antibodies with high avidity.

The findings described above suggest that periodontal therapy affects the magnitude and quality of the humoral immune response to periodontal pathogens, that this effect is dependent on initial serostatus, and that, thus, initial serostatus may have a bearing on treatment outcome.

In conclusion, the humoral immune response, especially IgG and IgA, is considered to have a protective role in the pathogenesis of periodontal disease but the precise mechanisms are still unknown. Peri-odontal therapy may improve the magnitude and quality of the humoral immune response through a process of immunization.

Homing – recruitment of cells to the periodontium

As explained previously, the recruitment of leukocytes into areas of injury or infection (homing) is essential for an effective host defense and the constant migration of leukocytes into the inflamed periodontal tissues results from the cytokine-induced expression of adhesion molecules on the surface of vascular endothelial cells. It has been suggested that antigen-presenting cells set up humoral immune response functions within peripheral lymph nodes (Fig. 11-17). Evidence exists, however, that homing of cells involved in both humoral and cellular immune responses is pronounced in diseased periodontal tissues. Recently Zitzmann *et al.* (2005a,b) reported on the specific "homing receptor" MadCAM-1 in periodontitis lesions. It is also possible that local proliferation of such leukocytes may occur in periodontitis. In an experimental gingivitis study in subjects who were treated for severe chronic periodontitis, Zitzmann *et al.* (2005b) reported that the presence of a residual inflammatory infiltrate influenced the reactions to *de novo* plaque formation. Thus, the increase of (1) the size of the gingival lesion, (2) the proportions of T and B cells, and (3) the expression of vascular adhesion molecules (including MadCAM-1) that occurred during the 21-day plaque formation period was more pronounced in sites that contained residual inflammatory infiltrates than in sites with no or only small remaining lesions. In other words, the large number of T cells and B cells that occur in the periodontitis lesion may be attracted to the diseased site through selective homing which is enhanced by local T and B cell presence.

References

Aduse-Opoku, J., Muir, J., Slaney, J.M., Rangarajan, M. & Curtis, M.A. (1995). Characterisation, genetic analysis, and expression of a protease antigen (PrpPI) of *Porphyromonas gingivalis* W50. *Infection and Immunity* **63**, 4744–4754.

Afar, B., Engel, D. & Clark, E.A. (1992). Activated lymphocyte subsets in adult periodontitis. *Journal of Periodontal Research* **2**, 126–133.

Aukhil, I., Lopatin, D.E., Syed, S.A., Morrison, E.C., & Kowalski, C.J. (1988). The effects of periodontal therapy on serum antibody (IgG) levels to plaque microorganisms. *Journal of Clinical Periodontology* **15**, 544–550.

Berglundh, T. & Donati, M. (2005). Aspects of adaptive host response in periodontitis. *Proceedings from the 5th European Workshop on Periodontology. Journal of Clinical Periodontology* **32** (Suppl), 87–107.

Berglundh, T., Liljenberg, B., Tarkowski, A. & Lindhe, J. (1998). Local and systemic TCR V gene expression in advanced periodontal disease. *Journal of Clinical Periodontology* **25**, 125–133.

Berglundh, T., Liljenberg, B. & Lindhe, J. (1999). Some effects of periodontal therapy on local and systemic immunological parameters. *Journal of Clinical Periodontology* **26**, 91–98.

Berglundh, T., Liljenberg, B. & Lindhe, J. (2002a). Some cytokine profiles of T-helper cells in lesions of advanced periodontitis. *Journal of Clinical Periodontology* **29**, 705–709.

Berglundh, T., Liljenberg, B., Tarkowski, A. & Lindhe, J. (2002b). The presence of local and circulating autoreactive B cells in patients with advanced periodontitis. *Journal of Clinical Periodontology* **29**, 281–286.

Berglundh, T., Wellfelt, B., Liljenberg, B. & Lindhe, J. (2001). Some local and systemic immunological features of prepubertal periodontitis. *Journal of Clinical Periodontology* **28**, 113–121.

Brecx, M.C., Fröhlicher, I., Gehr, P. & Lang, N.P. (1988). Stereological observations on long-term experimental gingivitis in man. *Journal of Clinical Periodontology* **15**, 621–627.

Brecx, M.C., Gautschi, M., Gehr, P. & Lang, N.P. (1987). Variability of histologic criteria in clinically healthy human gingiva. *Journal of Periodontal Research* **22**, 468–472.

Bröker, B.M., Korthauer, U., Heppt, P., Weseloh, G., de la Camp, R., Kroczek, R.A. & Emmrich, F. (1993). Biased T cell receptor V gene usage in rheumatoid arthritis. Oligoclonal expansion of T cells expressing Va2 genes in synovial fluid but not in peripheral blood. *Arthritis and Rheumatism* **36**, 1234–1243.

Cimasoni, G. (1983). *Crevicular Fluid Updated*. Basel: Karger.

Crotti, T., Smith, M.D., Hirsch, R., Soukoulis, S., Weedon, H., Capone, M., Ahern, M.J. & Haynes, D. (2003). Receptor activator NF kappaB ligand (RANKL) and osteoprotegerin (OPG) protein expression in periodontitis. *Journal of Periodontal Research* **38**, 380–387.

Egelberg, J. (1967). The topography and permeability of vessels at the dentogingival junction in dogs. *Journal of Periodontal Research* **20**, Suppl 1.

Fransson, C., Berglundh, T. & Lindhe, J. (1996). The effect of age on the development on gingivitis. *Journal of Clinical Periodontology*, **23**, 379–385.

Fujihashi, K., Yamamoto, M., Hiroi, T., Bamberg, T.V., McGhee, J.R. & Kiyono, H. (1996). Selected Th1 and Th2 cytokine mRNA expression by CD4(+) T cells isolated from inflamed human gingival tissues. *Clinical and Experimental Immunology* **103**(3), 422–428.

Garant, P.R. & Mulvihill, J.E. (1972). The fine structure of gingivitis in the beagle. III. Plasma cell infiltration of the subepithelial connective tissue. *Journal of Periodontal Research* **7**, 161–172.

Geatch, D.R., Ross, D.A., Heasman, P.A. & Taylor, J.J. (1997). Expression of T-cell receptor Vbeta2, 6 and 8 gene families in chronic adult periodontal disease. *European Journal of Oral Science* **105**, 397–404.

Gemmell, E. & Seymour, G.J. (1998). Cytokine profiles of cells extracted from humans with periodontal diseases. *Journal of Dental Research* **77**, 16–26.

Haerian, A., Adonogianaki, E., Mooney, J., Docherty, J. & Kinane, D.F. (1995). Gingival crevicular stromelysin, collagenase and tissue inhibitor of metalloproteinases levels in healthy and diseased sites. *Journal of Clinical Periodontology* **22**, 505–509.

Haerian, A., Adonogianaki, E., Mooney, J., Manos, A. & Kinane, D.F. (1996). Effects of treatment on gingival crevicular collagenase, stromelysin and tissue inhibitor of metalloproteinases and their ability to predict response to treatment. *Journal of Clinical Periodontology* **23**, 83–91.

Haubek, D., Poulsen, K. & Kilian, M. (1995). Evidence for absence in northern Europe of especially virulent clonal types of *Actinobacillus actinomycetemcomitans*. *Journal of Clinical Microbiology* **33**, 395–401.

Hirsch, H.Z., Tarkowski, A., Koopman, W.J. & Mestecky, J. (1989). Local production of IgA- and IgM-rheumatoid factors in adult periodontal disease. *Journal of Clinical Immunology* **9**, 273–278.

Hirsch, H.Z., Tarkowski, A., Miller, E.J., Gay, S., Koopman, W.J. & Mestecky, J. (1988). Autoimmunity to collagen in adult periodontal disease. *Journal of Oral Pathology* **17**, 456–459.

Jonsson, R., Pitts, A., Lue, C., Gay, S. & Mestecky, J. (1991). Immunoglobulin isotype distribution of locally produced autoantibodies to collagen type I in adult periodontitis. *Journal of Clinical Periodontology* **18**, 703–707.

Kinane, D.F. (2001). Regulators of tissue destruction and homeostasis as diagnostic aids in periodontology. *Periodontology 2000* **24**, 215–225.

Kinane, D.F., Adonogianaki, E., Moughal, N., Mooney, J. & Thornhill, M. (1991). Immunocytochemical characterisation of cellular infiltrate, related endothelial changes and determination of GCF acute phase proteins during human experimental gingivitis. *Journal of Periodontal Research* **26**, 286–288.

Kinane, D.F., Lappin, D.F., Koulouri, O. & Buckley, A. (1999). Humoral immune responses in periodontal disease may have mucosal and systemic immune features. *Clinical and Experimental Immunology* **115**, 534–541.

Kinane, D.F., Mooney, J., MacFarlane, T.W. & McDonald, M. (1993). Local and systemic antibody response to putative periodontopathogens in patients with chronic periodontitis: correlation with clinical indices. *Oral Microbiology and Immunology* **8**, 65–68.

Kinane, D.F., Takahashi, K. & Mooney, J. (1997). Crevicular fluid and serum IgG subclasses and corresponding mRNA expressing plasma cells in periodontal lesions. *Journal of Periodontal Research* **32**, 176–178.

Kowashi, Y., Jaccard, F. & Cimasoni, G. (1979). Increase of free collagenase and neutral protease activities in the gingival crevice during experimental gingivitis in man. *Archives of Oral Biology* **34**, 645–650.

Lerner, U.H. (2006) Inflammation-induced bone remodeling in periodontal disease and the influence of post-menopausal osteoporosis. *Journal of Dental Research* **85**, 596–607.

Lindhe, J., Hamp, S-E. & Löe, H. (1975). Plaque-induced periodontal disease in beagle dogs. A 4-year clinical, roentgenographical and histometric study. *Journal of Periodontal Research* **10**, 243–255.

Lindhe, J. & Rylander, H. (1975). Experimental gingivitis in young dogs. *Scandinavian Journal of Dental Research* **83**, 314–326.

Listgarten, M.A. (1965). Electron microscopic observations on the bacterial flora of acute necrotizing ulcerative gingivitis. *Journal of Periodontology* **36**, 328–339.

Listgarten, M.A. & Ellegaard, B. (1973). Experimental gingivitis in the monkey. Relationship of leucocyte in junctional epithelium, sulcus depth and connective tissue inflammation scores. *Journal of Periodontology* **8**, 199–214.

Liu, D., Xu, J.K., Figliomeni, L., Huang, L., Pavlos, N.J., Rogers, M., Tan, A., Price, P. & Zheng, M.H. (2003). Expression of RANKL and OPG mRNA in periodontal disease: possible involvement in bone destruction. *International Journal of Molecular Medicine* **11**, 17–21.

Mathur, A., Michalowicz, B., Yang, C. & Aeppli, D. (1995). Influence of periodontal bacteria and disease status on Vb expression in T cells. *Journal of Periodontal Research* **30**, 369–373.

Michalowicz, B.S., Diehl, S.R., Gunsolley, J.C., Sparks, B.S., Brooks, C.N., Koertge, T.E., Califano, J.V., Burmeister, J.A. & Schenkein, H.A. (2000). Evidence of a substantial genetic basis for risk of adult periodontitis. *Journal of Periodontology* **71**, 1699–1707.

Mooney, J., Adonogianaki, E. & Kinane, D.F. (1993). Relative avidity of serum antibodies to putative periodontopathogens in periodontal disease. *Journal of Periodontal Research* **28**, 444–450.

Mooney J., Adonogianaki, E., Riggio, M., Takahashi, K., Haerian, A. & Kinane, D.F. (1995). Initial serum antibody titer to *Porphyromonas gingivalis* influences development of antibody avidity and success of therapy for chronic periodontitis. *Infection and Immunity* **63**, 3411–3416.

Mooney, J. & Kinane, D.F. (1994). Humoral immune responses to *Porphyromonas gingivalis* and *Actinobacillus actinomycetemcomitans* in adult periodontitis and rapidly progressive periodontitis. *Oral Microbiology and Immunology* **9**, 321–326.

Moughal, N.A., Adonogianaki, E., Thornhill, M.H. & Kinane, D.F. (1992). Endothelial cell leukocyte adhesion molecule-1 (ELAM-1) and intercellular adhesion molecule-1 (ICAM-1) expression in gingival tissue during health and experimentally induced gingivitis. *Journal of Periodontal Research* **27**, 623–630.

Naito, Y., Okuda, K. & Takazoe, I. (1987). Detection of specific antibody in adult human periodontitis sera to surface antigens of Bacteroides gingivalis. *Infection and Immunity* **55**, 832–834.

Nakajima, T., Yamazaki, K. & Hara, K. (1996). Biased T cell receptor V gene usage in tissues with periodontal disease. *Journal of Periodontal Research* **31**, 2–10.

Ohlsson, K., Olsson, I. & Tynelius-Brathall, G. (1973). Neutrophil leukocyte collagenase, elastase and serum protease inhibitors in human gingival crevices. *Acta Odontologica Scandinavica* **31**, 51–59.

Page, R.C. & Schroeder, H.E. (1976). Pathogenesis of inflammatory periodontal disease. A summary of current work. *Laboratory Investigation* **33**, 235–249.

Page, R.C., Simpson, D.M. & Ammons, W.F. (1975). Host tissue response in chronic inflammatory periodontal disease. IV. The periodontal and dental status of a group of aged great apes. *Journal of Periodontology* **46**, 144–155.

Payne, W.A., Page, R.C., Ogilvie, A.L. & Hall, W.B. (1975). Histopathologic features of the initial and early stages of experimental gingivitis in man. *Journal of Periodontal Research* **10**, 51–64.

Prabhu, A., Michalowicz, B.S. & Mathur, A. (1996). Detection of local and systemic cytokines in adult periodontitis. *Journal of Periodontology* **67**, 515–522.

Schroeder, H.E. (1970). Quantitative parameters of early human gingival inflammation. *Archives of Oral Biology* **15**, 383–400.

Schroeder, H.E., Münzel-Pedrazzoli, S. & Page, R.C. (1973). Correlated morphometric and biochemical analysis of gingival tissue in early chronic gingivitis in man. *Archives of Oral Biology* **18**, 899–923.

Seymour, G.J., Gemmell, E., Kjeldsen, M., Yamazaki, K., Nakajima, T. & Hara, K. (1996). Cellular immunity and hypersensitivity as components of periodontal destruction. *Oral Diseases* **2**, 96–101.

Seymour, G.J., Gemmell, E., Reinhardt, R.A., Eastcotyt, J. & Taubman, M.A. (1993). Immunopathogenesis of chronic inflammatory periodontal disease: cellular and molecular mechanisms. *Journal of Periodontal Research* **28**, 478–486.

Seymour, G.J., Powell, R.N., Cole, K.L., Aitken, J.F., Brooks, D., Beckman, I., Zola, H., Bradley, J. & Burns, G.F. (1983). Experimental gingivitis in humans. A histochemical and immunological characterisation of the lymphoid cell subpopulations. *Journal of Periodontal Research* **18**, 375–385.

Sugawara, M., Yamashita, K., Yoshie, H. & Hara, K. (1992). Detection of, and anti-collagen antibody produced by, CD5 positive B cells in inflamed gingival tissues. *Journal of Periodontal Research* **27**, 489–498.

Takayanagi, H. (2005). Inflammatory bone destruction and osteoimmunology. *Journal of Periodontal Research* **40**, 287–293.

Takahashi, K., Poole, I. & Kinane, D.F. (1995). Detection of IL-1 MRNA-expressing cells in human gingival crevicular fluid by in situ hybridization. *Archives of Oral Biology* **40**, 941–947.

Trombelli, L., Tatakis, D.N., Scapoli, C., Bottega, S., Orlandini, E. & Tosi, M. (2004). Modulation of clinical expression of plaque-induced gingivitis. II. Identification of "high-responder" and "low-responder" subjects. *Journal of Clinical Periodontology* **31**, 239–252.

Waerhaug, J. (1952) The gingival pocket; anatomy, pathology, deepening and elimination. *Odontologisk Tidskrift* **60** (Suppl 1), 1–186.

Wilson, M.E., Bronson, P.M. & Hamilton, R.G. (1995). Immunoglobulin G2 antibodies promote neutrophil killing of Actinobacillus actinocetemcomitans. *Infection and Immunity* **63**, 1070–1075.

Yamamoto, M., Fujihashi, K., Hiroi, T., McGhee, J.R., Van Dyke, T.E. & Kiyono, H. (1997). Molecular and cellular mechanisms for periodontal diseases: role of Th1 and Th2 type cytokines in induction of mucosal inflammation. *Journal of Periodontal Research* **32**, 115–119.

Yamazaki, K., Nakajima, T., Gemmell, E., Polak, B., Seymour, G.J. & Hara, K. (1994). IL-4 and IL-6 producing cells in human periodontal disease tissue. *Journal of Oral Pathology and Medicine* **23**, 347–353.

Yamazaki, K., Nakajima, T. & Hara, K. (1995). Immunohistological analysis of T cell functional subsets in chronic inflammatory periodontal disease. *Clinical and Experimental Immunology* **99**, 384–391.

Yamazaki, K., Nakajima, T., Kubota, Y., Gemmell, E., Seymour, G.J. & Hara, K. (1997). Cytokine messenger RNA expression in chronic inflammatory periodontal disease. *Oral Microbiology and Immunology* **12**, 281–287.

Youinou, P., Mackenzie, L., le Masson, G., Papadopoulos, N. M., Jouguan, J., Pennec, Y.L., Angelidis, P., Katsakis, P., Moutsopoulos, H.M. & Lydyard, P.M. (1988). CD5-expressing B lymphocytes in the blood and salivary glands of patients with primary Sjögren's syndrome. *Journal of Autoimmunology* **1**, 185–194.

Zitzmann, N., Berglundh, T. & Lindhe, J. (2005a). Remaining inflammatory cell infiltrates following periodontal therapy including gingivectomy or open flap debridement. *Journal of Clinical Periodontology* **32**, 139–146.

Zitzmann, N., Lindhe, J. & Berglundh, T. (2005b). Reactions to de novo plaque formation at periodontitis sites treated with either resective or non-resective periodontal therapy *Journal of Clinical Periodontology* **32**, 1175–1180.

Chapter 12

Modifying Factors

Richard Palmer and Mena Soory

Diabetes, pregnancy, and tobacco smoking have profound and far-reaching effects on the host, including effects on the:

1. Physiological response
2. Vascular system
3. Inflammatory response
4. Immune system
5. Tissue repair.

They therefore have the potential to modify the:

1. Susceptibility to disease
2. Plaque microbiota
3. Clinical presentation of periodontal disease
4. Disease progression
5. Response to treatment.

Diabetes and smoking were cited as risk factors for periodontitis in Chapter 7 and the epidemiological evidence for their association with periodontitis was dealt with. Both factors are particularly important because they may affect the individual over a great many years, usually decades, and challenge the host to varying degrees. In contrast, pregnancy is of relatively short duration (although possibly with multiple episodes) but should be considered in relation to other hormonal changes which occur at puberty, menopause, and in women on hormonal contraceptives.

These three modifying factors are extremely important in many other disease processes, for example cardiovascular disease, which also affects

people to varying degrees. Much of this variation in susceptibility is probably due to genetic interactions, and there is increasing evidence of important associations with many genetic polymorphisms. There will undoubtedly be emerging genetic evidence to link periodontal disease susceptibility to modifying factors considered in this chapter.

Diabetes mellitus

Diabetes mellitus (DM) is a complex disease with varying degrees of systemic and oral complications, depending on the extent of metabolic control, presence of infection, and underlying demographic variables. This has led to conflicting results in epidemiologic studies, with regard to periodontal disease presentation in diabetic patients and their response to treatment. This section deals with diabetes and its implications on the host response to bacterial plaque, in the context of clinical and laboratory data pertaining to periodontal disease.

Type 1 and type 2 diabetes mellitus

DM is categorized as type 1 and type 2 DM. Type 1 DM develops due to impaired production of insulin, while type 2 DM is caused by deficient utilization of insulin. Type 1 DM results from destruction of the insulin-producing β cells of the pancreas. This can occur when genetically predisposed individuals succumb to an inducing event such as a viral infection or other factors that trigger a destructive autoimmune response (Szopa *et al.* 1993). Approximately

10–20% of all diabetics are insulin-dependent or type 1. They usually have a rapid onset of symptoms associated with a deficiency or total lack of insulin and the condition may be difficult to control. Nearly 90% are diagnosed before the age of 21 years.

Type 2 DM results from insulin resistance, which also contributes to cardiovascular and other metabolic disturbances (Murphy & Nolan 2000). However, insulin production may decrease later in the disease process and require supplementation (Slavkin 1997), in addition to controlling diet or using oral hypoglycemic agents. The onset of symptoms in type 2 DM is more gradual and less severe, usually presenting after the age of 40 years.

Clinical symptoms

The typical signs and symptoms of diabetes are polyuria, polydipsia, polyphagia, pruritus, weakness, and fatigue. These features are more pronounced in type 1 than in type 2 DM, and are a result of hyperglycemia. The complications of DM include retinopathy, nephropathy, neuropathy, macrovascular disease, and impaired wound healing (Lalla *et al.* 2000; Soory 2000a). The treatment of DM is aimed at reducing blood glucose levels to prevent such complications.

There is conclusive evidence of the importance of glycemic control in the prevention of diabetic complications. Patients regularly use blood glucose monitors to provide effective feedback for adjustment of insulin dosage to meet individual requirements (Mealey 1998). Recent studies have shown significant improvement in reducing complications associated with type 2 DM with controlled blood glucose levels (UKPDS 1998a,b). In these studies of over 5000 type 2 DM patients, the risk of retinopathy and nephropathy was reduced by 25% with effective glycemic control, using sulfonylureas, metformin or insulin. The risk of developing hypoglycemia needs to be monitored in these patients on intensive treatment regimes, particularly those on insulin.

Oral and periodontal effects

Poorly controlled diabetic subjects may complain of diminished salivary flow and burning mouth or tongue. Diabetic subjects on oral hypoglycemic agents may suffer from xerostomia, which could predispose to opportunistic infections with *Candida albicans*. Candidiasis has been reported in patients with poorly controlled DM (Ueta *et al.* 1993), associated with suppressed oxygen free radical release by polymorphonuclear cells (PMNs) and reduced phagocytosis.

There is good evidence to support the concept that there is an association between poorly controlled diabetes mellitus and periodontitis (Fig. 12-1). Any differences in periodontal health between type 1 and type 2 DM patients may relate to differences in management of glycemic control, age, duration of disease, utilization of dental care, periodontal disease susceptibility, and habits such as smoking. Type 1 DM patients have an increased risk of developing periodontal disease with age, and with the severity and duration of their diabetes.

Periodontal attachment loss has been found to occur more frequently in moderate and poorly controlled diabetic patients, of both type 1 and type 2 DM, than in those under good control (Westfelt *et al.* 1996). In addition, diabetics with more advanced systemic complications present with a greater frequency and severity of periodontal disease (Karjalainen *et al.* 1994). Conversely, initial phase periodontal treatment comprising motivation and debridement of periodontal pockets in type 2 diabetic patients resulted in improved metabolic control of diabetes (Stewart *et al.* 2001). A recent study by Kiran *et al.* (2005) confirmed these findings. In a study population of patients with type 2 DM and glycosylated hemoglobin values of 6–8%, initial phase periodontal treatment resulted in a significant improvement in glycaemic control. Total cholesterol, triglyceride, and low density lipoprotein levels also decreased in the test group and increased in the control group. These

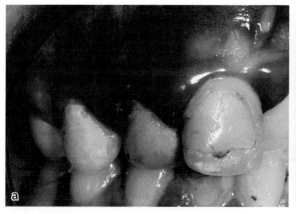 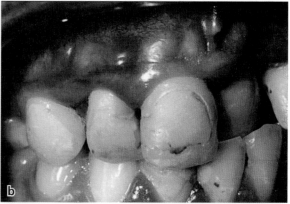

Fig. 12-1 Poorly controlled type 1 diabetes mellitus in a young female aged 19 years. (a) Very inflamed and swollen gingival tissues. Early attachment loss was present. (b) The same patient after responding to a course of non-surgical periodontal treatment and improved oral hygiene.

findings demonstrate that the status of periodontal disease control can contribute to metabolic control of DM (Faria-Almeida *et al.* 2006). The release of cytokines such as tumor necrosis factor (TNF)-α have implications on glucose and lipid metabolism (Cutler & Iacopino 2005) relevant to DM (Iacopino 2001) and cardiovascular disease. There are similar potential interactions between other systemic conditions and oral diseases (Pihlstrom *et al.* 2005; Kinane *et al.* 2006; Meurman & Hamalainen 2006). Insulin resistance can develop in response to chronic bacterial infection seen in periodontal disease, resulting in worse metabolic control in diabetic patients (Grossi *et al.* 1996). There is evidence to support the hypothesis that adequate control of severe inflammatory periodontal disease could alleviate symptoms of co-existing systemic diseases in susceptible individuals. In a population of Pima Indians with type 2 DM and severe periodontal disease, the risk of cardiorenal mortality and diabetic nephropathy was three times greater than amongst those with mild or moderate disease (Saremi *et al.* 2005).

Probably the most classic description of the undiagnosed or poorly controlled diabetic is the patient presenting with multiple periodontal abscesses, leading to rapid destruction of periodontal support (Figs. 12-2, 12-3). Harrison *et al.* (1983) reported a case of deep neck infection of the submental, sublingual, and submandibular spaces, secondary to periodontal abscesses involving the mandibular incisors, in a poorly controlled diabetic patient. In a population study Ueta *et al.* (1993) demonstrated that DM was a predisposing factor for periodontal and periapical abscess formation due to suppression of neutrophil function. The effects on the host response, and in particular neutrophil function, may account for this finding.

Association of periodontal infection and diabetic control

The presence of acute infection can predispose to insulin resistance (Atkinson & Maclaren 1990). This can occur independently of a diabetic state and persist for up to 3 weeks after resolution of the infection (Yki-Jarvinen *et al.* 1989). In a longitudinal study of subjects with type 2 DM, it was demonstrated that subjects with severe periodontal disease demonstrated significantly worse control of their diabetic condition than those with minimal periodontal

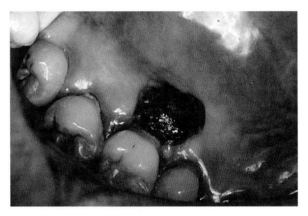

Fig. 12-2 A localized palatal periodontal abscess associated with a periodontal pocket in a 42-year-old poorly controlled diabetic patient.

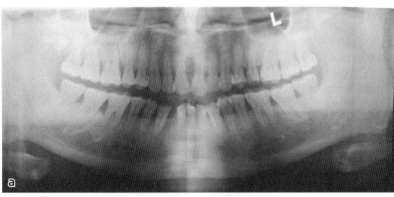

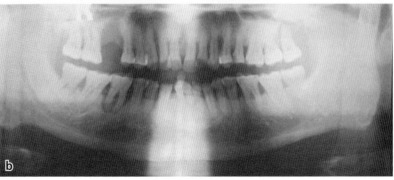

Fig. 12-3 Radiographs of a 50-year-old male who developed type 2 diabetes mellitus in the period between the two radiographs which were taken 3 years apart. There has been rapid bone loss and tooth loss associated with recurrent multiple periodontal abscesses.

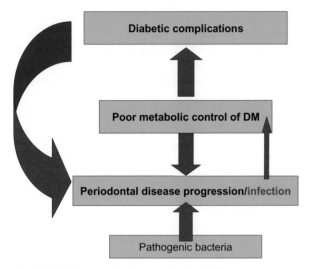

Fig. 12-4 Diabetes control and periodontal disease progression.

involvement (Taylor *et al*. 1996) (Fig. 12-4). The incidence of proteinuria and cardiovascular complications, as a result of uncontrolled diabetes, was found to be significantly greater in diabetics with severe periodontal disease than those with gingivitis or early periodontal disease (Thorstensson *et al*. 1996). Some studies have shown that stabilization of the periodontal condition with mechanical therapy, in combination with systemic tetracycline, improves the diabetic condition in such patients (Grossi *et al*. 1997b). Reduced insulin dosage in type 1 diabetics following periodontal treatment has also been reported (Sastrowijoto *et al*. 1990). However, other studies have not shown improvement in diabetic control following non-surgical periodontal treatment (Aldridge *et al*. 1995). These effects of periodontal therapy may be more pronounced in poorly controlled diabetic patients with severe periodontal disease.

Significant inflammatory lesions in severe periodontal disease could contribute to exacerbation of diabetes. Markers of inflammation common to diabetes and periodontal disease are an indication of disease control (Soory 2002, 2004).

Modification of the host–bacteria relationship in diabetes

Effects on microbiota

Hyperglycemia in uncontrolled diabetics has implications on the host response (Gugliucci 2000) and affects the regional microbiota. This can potentially influence the development of periodontal disease and caries in poorly controlled type 1 and type 2 DM patients. *Capnocytophaga* species have been isolated as the predominant cultivable organisms from periodontal lesions in type 1 diabetics, averaging 24% of the cultivable flora (Mashimo *et al*. 1983). A similar distribution of the predominant putative pathogens, *Prevotella intermedia*, *Campylobacter rectus*, *Porphy-*

romonas gingivalis, and *Aggregatibacter actinomycetemcomitans* (formerly known as *Actinobacillus actinomycetemcomitans*), to those associated with chronic adult periodontal disease was detected in periodontal lesions of type 2 diabetics (Zambon *et al*. 1988), with potential for disease activity during poor metabolic control. In an insulin-dependent diabetic population with a large proportion of poorly controlled diabetics, Seppala and Ainamo (1996) showed significantly increased percentages of spirochetes and motile rods and decreased levels of cocci in periodontal lesions, compared with well controlled patients.

Effects on the host response

Diabetes mellitus has far-reaching effects on the host response (Fig. 12-5).

Polymorphonuclear leukocytes
Reduced PMN function (Marhoffer *et al*. 1992) and defective chemotaxis in uncontrolled diabetics can contribute to impaired host defenses and progression of infection (Ueta *et al*. 1993). Crevicular fluid collagenase activity, originating from PMNs, was found to be increased in diabetic patients and this could be inhibited *in vitro* by tetracycline through its enzyme inhibitory effects (Sorsa *et al*. 1992). The PMN enzymes beta-glucuronidase (Oliver *et al*. 1993) and elastase, in association with diabetic angiopathy (Piwowar *et al*. 2000), have been detected at significantly higher levels in poorly controlled diabetic patients.

Cytokines, monocytes, and macrophages
Diabetic patients with periodontitis have significantly higher levels of interleukin (IL)-1β and prostaglandin E_2 (PGE$_2$) in crevicular fluid compared to non-diabetic controls with a similar degree of periodontal disease (Salvi *et al*. 1997). In addition, the release of these cytokines (IL-1β, PGE$_2$, TNF-α) by monocytes has been shown to be significantly greater in diabetics than in non-diabetic controls. Chronic hyperglycemia results in non-enzymatic glycosylation of numerous proteins, leading to the accumulation of advanced glycation end products (AGE), which play a central role in diabetic complications (Brownlee 1994). Increased binding of AGEs to macrophages and monocytes (Brownlee 1994) can result in a destructive cell phenotype with increased sensitivity to stimuli, resulting in excessive release of cytokines. Altered macrophage phenotype due to cell surface binding with AGE, prevents the development of macrophages associated with repair. This could contribute to delayed wound healing seen in diabetic patients (Iacopino 1995).

Connective tissue
A hyperglycemic environment, due to decreased production or utilization of insulin, can reduce growth,

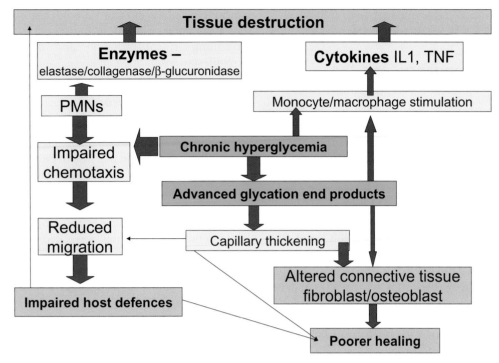

Fig. 12-5 Effects of diabetes mellitus on the host response.

proliferation, and matrix synthesis by gingival and periodontal ligament fibroblasts and osteoblasts. The formation of AGE results in reactive oxygen species, which are damaging to cellular function in gingival tissues, due to oxidative stress (Schmidt *et al*. 1996). The accumulation of AGE in tissues alters the function of several intercellular matrix components, including vascular wall collagen, resulting in deleterious complications (Ulrich & Cerami 2001). This has adverse effects on cell–matrix interactions and vascular integrity, potentially affecting periodontal disease presentation and treatment responses in uncontrolled diabetics. Vascular changes, such as thickening of the capillary basement membrane in a hyperglycemic environment, can impair oxygen diffusion, metabolic waste elimination, PMN migration, and diffusion of antibodies. Binding of AGE to vascular endothelial cells can trigger responses that induce coagulation, leading to vasoconstriction and microthrombus formation (Esposito *et al*. 1992), resulting in impaired perfusion of tissues. Recent work using a cell culture model has demonstrated that glucose, AGE, and nicotine inhibit the synthesis of steroid markers of wound healing (Rahman & Soory 2006). This inhibition was overcome by the antioxidant glutathione and insulin-like growth factor (IGF), which also functions as an antioxidant. These findings can be extrapolated to the 'in vivo' situation, demonstrating the relevance of oxidative stress-induced mechanisms in periodontal disease and DM, with therapeutic implications of medications with antioxidant effects (Soory & Tilakaratne 2003). These findings may be extrapolated to healing responses in the uncontrolled dia-

betic smoker with periodontal disease (Graves *et al*. 2006).

Effects on healing and treatment response

Wound healing is impaired due to the cumulative effects on cellular functions as described above. In summary, these factors include:

1. Decreased synthesis of collagen by fibroblasts
2. Increased degradation by collagenase
3. Glycosylation of existing collagen at wound margins
4. Defective remodeling and rapid degradation of newly synthesized, poorly cross-linked collagen.

Periodontal treatment

The treatment of well controlled DM patients would be similar to that of non-diabetic patients for most routine dental procedures. The short-term non-surgical treatment response of stable diabetics has been found to be similar to that of non-diabetic controls, with similar trends in improved probing depths, attachment gain, and altered subgingival microbiota (Christgau *et al*. 1998). Well controlled diabetics with regular supportive therapy have been shown to maintain treatment results 5 years after a combination of non-surgical and surgical treatment (Westfelt *et al*. 1996). However, a less favorable treatment outcome may occur in long-term maintenance therapy of poorly controlled diabetics, who may succumb to more rapid recurrence of initially deep pockets (Tervonen & Karjalainen 1997).

Puberty, pregnancy, and the menopause

The hormonal variations experienced by women during physiological and non-physiological conditions (such as hormone replacement therapy and use of hormonal contraceptives) result in significant changes in the periodontium, particularly in the presence of pre-existing, plaque-induced gingival inflammation. The implications of these changes on the tissues of the periodontium have been reviewed comprehensively (Mascarenhas et al. 2003; Guncu et al. 2005). Periods of hormonal flux are known to occur during puberty, menstruation, pregnancy, and the menopause. Changes in hormone levels occur when the anterior pituitary secretes follicle-stimulating hormone (FSH) and luteinizing hormone (LH), resulting in the maturation of the ovary and cyclical production of estrogen and progesterone.

The gingiva is a target tissue for the actions of steroid hormones. Clinical changes in the tissues of the periodontium have been identified during periods of hormonal fluctuation. The effects of estrogen and progesterone on the periodontium have received significant research attention. The main potential effects of these hormones on the periodontal tissues can be summarized as:

- Estrogen affects salivary peroxidases, which are active against a variety of microorganisms (Kimura et al. 1983), by changing the redox potential.
- Estrogen has stimulatory effects on the metabolism of collagen and angiogenesis (Sultan et al. 1986).
- Estrogen can trigger autocrine or paracrine polypeptide growth factor signaling pathways, whose effects may be partially mediated by the estrogen receptor itself (Chau et al. 1998).
- Estrogen and progesterone can modulate vascular responses and connective tissue turnover in the periodontium, associated with interaction with inflammatory mediators (Soory 2000b).

The interaction of estrogen and progesterone with inflammatory mediators may help to explain the increased levels of inflammation seen during periods of hormonal fluctuation. For example, when cultured human gingival fibroblasts were incubated with progesterone concentrations common in late pregnancy, there was a 50% reduction in the formation of the inflammatory mediator IL-6, compared with control values (Lapp et al. 1995). IL-6 induces the synthesis of tissue inhibitor of metalloproteinases (TIMP) in fibroblasts (Lotz & Guerne 1991), reduces the levels of TNF and enhances the formation of acute phase proteins (Le & Vilcek 1989). A progesterone-induced reduction in IL-6 levels could result in less TIMP,

more proteolytic enzyme activity, and higher levels of TNF at the affected sites, due to less inhibition, resulting in inflammation and obvious clinical manifestations.

Puberty and menstruation

During puberty, there are raised levels of testosterone in males and estradiol in females. Several studies have demonstrated an increase in gingival inflammation in children of circumpubertal age, with no change in plaque levels (Sutcliffe 1972). In a longitudinal study, Mombelli et al. (1989) reported that the mean papillary bleeding scores and percentage of interdental bleeding sites correlated with the development of secondary sexual characteristics at puberty, while other studies did not find a significant correlation between the onset of puberty and gingival changes in parapubescent women (Tiainen et al. 1992). These discrepancies may be attributed to factors such as the oral hygiene status of the population and study design.

The prevalence of certain periodontal pathogens reported during puberty may have a direct association with the hormones present and their utilization by selected pathogens. For example *Prevotella intermedia* is able to substitute progesterone and estrogen for menadione (vitamin K) as an essential nutrient (Kornman & Loesche 1979). An association between pubertal gingivitis, *P. intermedia* and serum levels of testosterone, estrogen, and progesterone has been reported in a longitudinal study (Nakagawa et al. 1994).

Pre-existing plaque-induced gingivitis may be an important factor in detecting hormone-induced changes during the menstrual cycle. Holm-Pedersen and Loe (1967) demonstrated that women with gingivitis experienced increased inflammation with an associated increase in crevicular fluid exudate during menstruation compared with healthy controls. Most female patients are not aware of any changes in their gingivae during the menstrual cycle (Amar & Chung 1994), while a few experience enlarged hemorrhagic gingivae in the days preceding menstrual flow. This has been associated with more gingivitis, increased crevicular fluid flow, and tooth mobility (Grant et al. 1988). Early studies demonstrated similar findings during the menstrual cycle in a population with pre-existing gingivitis, in response to fluctuations in the levels of estrogen and progesterone (Lindhe & Attstrom 1967).

Pregnancy

During pregnancy, the increased levels of sex steroid hormones are maintained from the luteal phase which results in implantation of the embryo, until parturition. Pregnant women, near or at term, produce large quantities of estradiol (20 mg/day), estriol (80 mg/day), and progesterone (300 mg/day).

Gingival inflammation initiated by plaque, and exacerbated by these hormonal changes in the second and third trimester of pregnancy, is referred to as pregnancy gingivitis. Parameters, such as gingival probing depths (Hugoson 1970; Miyazaki *et al.* 1991), bleeding on probing (Miyazaki *et al.* 1991), and crevicular fluid flow (Hugoson 1970), were found to be increased. These inflammatory features can be minimized by maintaining good plaque control.

According to early reports, the prevalence of pregnancy gingivitis ranges from 35% (Hasson 1966) to 100% (Lundgren *et al.* 1973). In a study of 130 pregnant women, Machuca *et al.* (1999) demonstrated gingivitis in 68% of the population, ranging from 46% in technical executives to 88% in manual workers. Cross-sectional studies examining pregnant and postpartum women have shown that pregnancy is associated with significantly more gingivitis than at postpartum, despite similar plaque scores (Silness & Loe 1963). Further observations were made by Hugoson (1970) in a longitudinal study of 26 women during and following pregnancy, which also demonstrated that the severity of gingival inflammation correlated with the gestational hormone levels during pregnancy (Fig. 12-6). A more recent study of a rural population of Sri Lankan women (Tilakaratne *et al.* 2000a) showed increased gingivitis of varying degrees of significance amongst all the pregnant women investigated, compared with matched non-pregnant controls. There was a progressive increase in inflammation with advancing pregnancy which was more significant in the second and third trimesters of pregnancy, despite the plaque levels remaining unchanged. At the third month after parturition, the level of gingival inflammation was similar to that observed in the first trimester of pregnancy. This suggests a direct correlation between gingivitis and sustained, raised levels of gestational hormones during pregnancy, with regression during the postpartum period. In investigations by Cohen *et al.* (1969) and Tilakaratne *et al.* (2000a), the values for loss of attachment remained unchanged during pregnancy and 3 months postpartum.

Effects on the microbiota

There is an increase in the selective growth of periodontal pathogens such as *P. intermedia* in subgingival plaque during the onset of pregnancy gingivitis at the third to fourth month of pregnancy. The gestational hormones act as growth factors, by satisfying the naphthoquinone requirement for bacteria (Di Placido *et al.* 1998). These findings were also confirmed by Muramatsu and Takaesu (1994) who showed that from the third to fifth month of pregnancy, the number of gingival sites which bled on probing corresponded with the percentage increase in *P. intermedia*. During pregnancy, progesterone is less actively catabolized to its inactive products, resulting in higher levels of the active hormone (Ojanotko-Harri *et al.* 1991). A 55-fold increase in the proportion of *P. intermedia* has been demonstrated in pregnant women compared with non-pregnant controls (Jensen *et al.* 1981), implying a role for gestational hormones in causing a change in microbial ecology in the gingival pocket. Although an overall association has been demonstrated, a cause and effect relationship may be less clear.

Effects on the tissues and host response

The increase in severity of gingivitis during pregnancy has been partly attributed to the increased circulatory levels of progesterone and its effects on the capillary vessels (Lundgren *et al.* 1973). Elevated progesterone levels in pregnancy enhance capillary permeability and dilatation, resulting in increased gingival exudate. The effects of progesterone in stimulating prostaglandin synthesis can account for some of the vascular changes (Miyagi *et al.* 1993).

The elevated levels of estrogen and progesterone in pregnancy affect the degree of keratinization of the

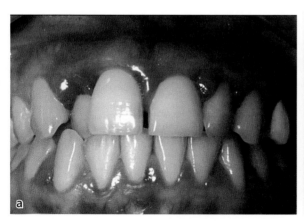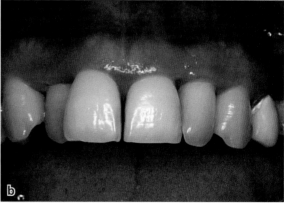

Fig. 12-6 Gingivitis associated with pregnancy. (a) A patient in the last trimester of pregnancy with very inflamed edematous gingival tissue which tended to bleed with the slightest provocation. (b) The improvement in gingival health 6 months after birth of the baby and an intensive course of non-surgical periodontal treatment.

gingival epithelium and alter the connective tissue ground substance. The decreased keratinization of the gingivae, together with an increase in epithelial glycogen, are thought to result in decreased effectiveness of the epithelial barrier in pregnant women (Abraham-Inpijn *et al.* 1996). Hormonal factors that affect the epithelium and increase vascular permeability can contribute to an exaggerated response to bacterial plaque during pregnancy. The influence of gestational hormones on the immune system can contribute further to the initiation and progression of pregnancy gingivitis. High levels of progesterone and estrogen associated with pregnancy (and the use of some oral contraceptives) have been shown to suppress the immune response to plaque (Sooriyamoorthy & Gower 1989). Neutrophil chemotaxis and phagocytosis, along with antibody and T cell responses, have been reported to be depressed in response to high levels of gestational hormones (Raber-Durlacher *et al.* 1993).

Pregnancy granuloma or epulis

A pedunculated, fibrogranulomatous lesion can sometimes develop during pregnancy and is referred to as a pregnancy granuloma or epulis. A combination of the vascular response induced by progesterone and the matrix stimulatory effects of estradiol contributes to the development of pregnancy granulomas, usually at sites with pre-existing gingivitis (Fig. 12-7). The vascular effects result in a bright red, hyperemic, and edematous presentation. The lesions often occur in the anterior papillae of the maxillary teeth and usually do not exceed 2 cm in diameter. They can bleed when traumatized and their removal is best deferred until after parturition, when there is often considerable regression in their size (Wang *et al.* 1997). Surgical removal of the granuloma during pregnancy can result in recurrence due to a combination of poor plaque control and hormone-mediated growth of the lesion. Careful oral hygiene and debridement during pregnancy are important in preventing its occurrence (Wang *et al.* 1997).

Periodontal treatment during pregnancy

Pregnant women need to be educated on the consequences of pregnancy on gingival tissues and thoroughly motivated in plaque control measures, with professional treatment as required. They are likely to be more comfortable to receive dental treatment during the second trimester than in the first or third trimester of pregnancy, although emergency treatment is permissible at any stage during pregnancy (Amar & Chung 1994). Since most medications cross the placental barrier and organogenesis occurs mainly in the first trimester, pregnant women are best treated in the second trimester, to avoid the occurrence of developmental defects. Any form of medication during pregnancy must only be used if the gravity of the condition being treated outweighs the consequences. Amongst the antibiotics, tetracycline, vancomycin, and streptomycin can contribute to staining of teeth and ototoxic and nephrotoxic effects during the fourth to ninth months of pregnancy; erythromycin, penicillins, and cephalosporins are relatively safer, but any medication must only be administered in consultation with the patient's obstetrician (Lynch *et al.* 1991).

Menopause and osteoporosis

During menopause there is a decline in hormonal levels due to decreased ovarian function. This is characterized by tissue changes such as desquamation of gingival epithelium (Fig. 12-8) and osteoporosis (Fig. 12-9) which may be attributed to hormone deficiency. It has been demonstrated that women with early onset of menopause have a higher incidence of osteoporosis and significantly lower bone mineral density (Kritz-Silverstein & Barrett-Connor 1993).

A third of women over age 60 are affected by postmenopausal osteoporosis (Baxter 1987). The changes involved are a reduction in bone density, affecting its mass and strength without significantly affecting its chemical composition. An alteration in the calcium–phosphate equilibrium due to deficient

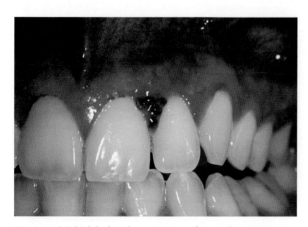

Fig. 12-7 Multi-lobulated appearance of an early pregnancy epulis, demonstrating vascular elements and tissue oedema.

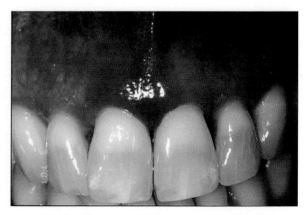

Fig. 12-8 Clinical appearance of anterior maxillary gingiva with pronounced desquamation in a woman during menopause.

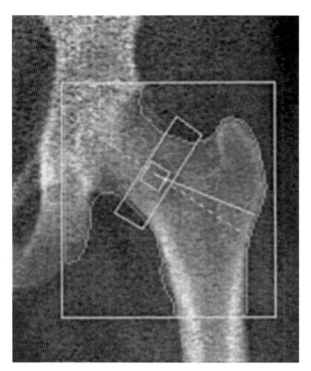

Fig. 12-9 A DEXA scan used to measure mineral bone density in the hip. This technique is not routinely applied to the jaws.

absorption of dietary calcium and increased excretion due to diminished estrogen levels can account for some of the bone changes seen in postmenopausal women (Shapiro *et al.* 1985), usually involving the mandible more than the maxilla.

Estrogen replacement therapy has been shown to prevent osteoporosis and maintain bone mineral content at several sites throughout the skeleton (Moore *et al.* 1990), with a 5% increase in bone mineral content in the region of the head compared to those taking placebo (Gotfredsen *et al.* 1986). The influence of estrogen on bone mineral density has been demonstrated in these studies, but a cause and effect relationship with periodontal disease is less clear.

A 2-year follow-up study of 42 171 postmenopausal women (Grodstein *et al.* 1996) showed that the risk of tooth loss was significantly lower amongst hormone users. These findings reinforce those of Paganini-Hill (1995), who showed a 36% decrease in tooth loss in estrogen users compared with non-users. There is evidence to suggest that use of estrogen is necessary to protect against bone loss (Grady *et al.* 1992). Although osteoporosis in postmenopausal women may not be the cause of periodontal disease, it may affect the severity of pre-existing disease. The circulating levels of estrogen have been shown to have an influence on alveolar bone density in postmenopausal women (Payne *et al.* 1997).

Effect of smoking on osteoporosis

A negative association between smoking and bone density has been demonstrated by Krall and Dawson-Hughes (1991). Smokers can differ from non-smokers in weight, caffeine intake, age at menopause, and alcohol consumption (Lindquist & Bengtsson 1979; Rigotti 1989); all these factors can potentially confound an association between smoking and bone density. A study on female twins by Hopper and Seeman (1994) showed that in the 20 pairs who varied most, by 20 or more pack years, the differences in bone density within pairs were 9.3% at the lumbar spine, 5.8% at the femoral neck, and 6.5% at the femoral shaft. This study also demonstrated increased serum levels of FSH and LH in smokers, implying reduced circulating levels of estrogen, leading to increased bone resorption. Other investigators have demonstrated the effects of smoking on the synthesis and degradation of estrogen (Jensen *et al.* 1985). The study by Jensen *et al.* (1985) investigated 136 postmenopausal women who were treated with three different doses of estrogen–progesterone or placebo. They showed reduced levels of estrogen in smokers (range of 1–30 cigarettes/day in the previous 6 months, mean 12.4), compared with non-smokers (not smoked in the previous 3 months). There was also a significant inverse correlation between the number of cigarettes smoked per day and the serum levels of estrogen, suggestive of increased hepatic metabolism of estrogen in postmenopausal smokers, resulting in lower serum levels of these hormones.

Treatment of osteoporosis

In osteoporotic patients, the rate of bone loss during the early postmenopausal period increases to 3–4% per year. Estrogen replacement therapy, which slows bone turnover, results in increased bone density in the trabecular spaces during remodeling (Frost 1989). The increased skeletal bone mass which occurs in response to estrogen replacement therapy is apparent in the first 2 years of treatment and maintained with continuation of treatment (Kimmel *et al.* 1994). The effects of estrogen in regaining bone mass to premenopausal levels and in preventing/reversing postmenopausal osteoporotic changes in the long bones and spine have been demonstrated in several studies (Armamento-Villareal *et al.* 1992; Takahashi *et al.* 1994).

There is some controversy with regard to the benefits of hormone replacement due to the risk factors involved. Fractures due to osteoporosis and heart disease in postmenopausal women can be reduced by 50% with estrogen replacement therapy. However, hormone replacement with estrogen alone exposes such patients to the risk of endometrial cancer. Long-term hormone replacement therapy has been shown to correlate with an increased risk of breast cancer. Modern formulations utilize combined therapy with a suitable dose of progesterone in combination with estrogen in order to minimize some of these risk factors (Whitehead & Lobo 1988).

Hormonal contraceptives

Contraceptives utilize synthetic gestational hormones (estrogen and progesterone), to reduce the likelihood of ovulation/implantation (Guyton 1987). Less dramatic but similar effects to pregnancy are sometimes observed in the gingivae of hormonal contraceptive users. The most common oral manifestation of elevated levels of ovarian hormones is an increase in gingival inflammation with an accompanying increase in gingival exudate (Mariotti 1994).

There are reported systemic risk factors associated with long-term use of hormonal contraceptives. The correlation between hormonal contraceptive use and significant cardiovascular disease associated with arterial and venous thromboembolic episodes has been reviewed by Westhoff (1996). Estrogen is responsible for both arterial and venous effects, while progesterone effects arterial changes. Women using oral contraceptives show elevated plasma levels of several clotting factors, related to the dose of estrogen. Raised levels of factors VIIc and XIIc are significant, since they increase the likelihood of coagulation and in men these factors have a strong positive correlation with ischemic heart disease. However, the relative risk is dependent on the contraceptive formulation used and there may not be a consistent biological plausibility to explain this association (Davis 2000).

There are several different formulations of hormonal contraceptives (Davis 2000) including:

1. Combined oral contraceptives containing artificial analogues of estrogen and progesterone
2. Progesterone-based mini-pill
3. Slow release progesterone implants placed subdermally that last up to 5 years (e.g. Norplant)
4. Depo Provera, a very effective progestin injection given by a doctor every 3 months.

Current combined oral contraceptives consist of low doses of estrogens (50 µg/day) and/or progestins (1.5 mg/day) (Mariotti 1994). The formulations used in the early periodontal studies contained higher concentrations of gestational hormones, e.g. 50 µg estrogen with 4 mg progestin (El-Ashiry *et al.* 1971), 100 µg estrogen with 5 mg progestin (Lindhe & Bjorn 1967). The results obtained in these studies would partly reflect the contraceptive preparation used. In one early study (Knight & Wade 1974) women who were on hormonal contraceptives for more than 1.5 years exhibited greater periodontal destruction compared to the control group of comparable age and oral hygiene. This could partly reflect higher dose of gestagens used in older contraceptive preparations. However, a recent study on a population of rural Sri Lankan women confirmed these findings (Tilakaratne *et al.* 2000b), showing significantly higher levels of gingivitis in contraceptive users (0.03 mg estradiol and 0.15 mg of a progestin), than non-users, despite similar plaque scores. There was also significant periodontal breakdown in those who used the pro-

gesterone injection (a depot preparation of 150 mg progesterone) 3-monthly for 2–4 years, compared with those who used it for less than 2 years. These findings may be attributed to the duration of use, and the effects of progesterone in promoting tissue catabolism, resulting in increased periodontal attachment loss. However, if low plaque levels are established and maintained for the duration of use, these effects could be minimized.

Effect on tissue response

Both estrogen and progesterone are known to cause increased gingival exudate, associated with inflammatory edema (Lindhe & Bjorn 1967). A 53% increase in crevicular fluid volume has been demonstrated in hormonal contraceptive users compared with controls. El-Ashiry *et al.* (1971) observed that the most pronounced effects on the gingiva occurred in the first 3 months of contraceptive treatment, but the dose of gestational hormones was higher in the older formulations compared with those used currently (Davis 2000), accounting for a more florid response in the tissues.

It has been suggested that the interaction of estrogen with progesterone results in the mediation of the effects characteristic of progesterone. Human gingiva has receptors for progesterone and estrogen (Vittek *et al.* 1982; Staffolani *et al.* 1989), providing evidence that gingiva is a target tissue for both gestational hormones. In *in vitro* studies of cultured gingival fibroblasts, estrogen enhanced the formation of anabolic androgen metabolites, while progesterone caused a diminished response. The combined effect of both gestational hormones on the yield of androgens was less pronounced than with estrogen alone, implying a more catabolic role for progesterone (Tilakaratne & Soory 1999).

Progesterone causes increased vascular permeability, resulting in the infiltration of polymorphonuclear leukocytes and raised levels of PGE_2 in the sulcular fluid (Miyagi *et al.* 1993). Increased capillary permeability may be induced by estrogen by stimulating the release of mediators such as bradykinin, prostaglandins, and histamine. However, the main effects of estrogen are in controlling blood flow. Hence the combination of estrogen and progesterone in the contraceptive pill can contribute to vascular changes in the gingivae. The resultant gingivitis can be minimized by establishing low plaque levels at the beginning of oral contraceptive therapy (Zachariasen 1993).

Tobacco smoking

Tobacco smoking is very common, with cigarettes being the main product smoked. In the European Union, an average of 29% of the adult population smoke, ranging from 17.5% in Sweden to 45% in Greece (http://www.ash.org.uk). The figure is higher for men (35%) than for women (24%). Most smokers start the habit as teenagers, with the highest prevalence in the 20–24-year-old age group. Socioeconomic differences also exist with higher smoking in the lower socioeconomic groups. These data are similar for the US population (Garfinkel 1997; http://www.cdc.gov/tobacco/) where an estimated 44.5 million adults smoke. Reported smoking rates for third world countries are even higher. Smoking is associated with a wide spectrum of disease including stroke, coronary artery disease, peripheral artery disease, gastric ulcer, and cancers of the mouth, larynx, esophagus, pancreas, bladder, and uterine cervix. It is also a major cause of chronic obstructive pulmonary disease and a risk factor for low birth weight babies. Approximately 50% of regular smokers are killed by their habit and smoking causes 30% of cancer deaths.

Cigarette smoke is a very complex mixture of substances with over 4000 known constituents. These include carbon monoxide, hydrogen cyanide, reactive oxidizing radicals, a high number of carcinogens, and the main psychoactive and addictive molecule – nicotine (Benowitz 1996). Many of these components could modify the host response in periodontitis. In most of the *in vitro* studies considered in the latter parts of this chapter the experimenters utilized simple models with nicotine alone. Tobacco smoke has a gaseous phase and solid phase which contains tar droplets. The tar and nicotine yields of cigarettes have been reduced due to physical characteristics of the filters. However, there has been little change in the tar and nicotine content of the actual tobacco and the dose an individual receives is largely dependent upon the way in which they smoke (Benowitz 1989). Inter-subject smoking variation includes: frequency of inhalation; depth of inhalation; length of the cigarette stub left; presence or absence of a filter; and the brand of cigarette (Benowitz 1988).

The patient's exposure to tobacco smoke can be measured in a number of ways, including interviewing the subject using simple questions or more sophisticated questionnaires and biochemical analyses (Scott *et al.* 2001). The latter tests include exhaled carbon monoxide in the breath, which is commonly measured in smoking cessation clinics, and cotinine (a metabolite of nicotine) in saliva, plasma/serum or urine (Wall *et al.* 1988). Cotinine measurements are more reliable in determining a subject's exposure to tobacco smoke because the half-life is 14–20 hours compared with the shorter half-life of nicotine which is 2–3 hours (Jarvis *et al.* 1988). The mean plasma and salivary cotinine concentrations of regular smokers are approximately 300 ng/ml and urine concentrations are about 1500 ng/ml. Non-smokers typically have plasma/saliva concentrations under 2 ng/ml, but this may be raised slightly due to environmental exposure (passive smoking).

Inhalation of tobacco smoke allows very rapid absorption of nicotine into the blood and transport to the brain, which is faster than an intravenous infusion. Nicotine in tobacco smoke from most cigarettes is not well absorbed through the oral mucosa because the nicotine is in an ionized form as a result of the pH (5.5). In contrast cigar and pipe smoke is more alkaline (pH 8.5), which allows good absorption of un-ionized nicotine through the buccal mucosa (Benowitz 1988). Nicotine is absorbed rapidly in the lung where the smoke is well buffered. The administration of nicotine causes a rise in the blood pressure, an increase in heart rate, an increase in respiratory rate, and decreased skin temperature due to peripheral vasoconstriction. However, at other body sites, such as skeletal muscle, nicotine produces vasodilatation.

These differing actions of nicotine have led to some controversy over its action in the periodontal tissues. Clarke and co-workers (1981) showed that the infusion of nicotine resulted in a transient decrease in gingival blood flow in a rabbit model. However, Baab and Öberg (1987) using laser Doppler flowmetry to monitor relative gingival flow in 12 young smokers, observed an immediate but transient increase in relative gingival blood flow during smoking, compared to the presmoking or resting measurements. The authors hypothesized that the steep rise in heart rate and blood pressure due to smoking could lead to an increase in the gingival circulation during smoking. These results were confirmed by Meekin *et al.* (2000) who showed that subjects who smoked only very occasionally experienced an increase in blood flow to the head, whereas regular smokers showed no change in blood flow, demonstrating tolerance in the regular smoker. The increase in blood flow to the gingival and forehead skin following an episode of smoking in 13 casual consumers of tobacco was confirmed by Mavropoulos *et al.* (2003) and Morozumi *et al.* (2004) showed that the gingival blood flow significantly increased at 3 days following quitting, providing important information on the recovery of gingival tissue following quitting smoking.

Periodontal disease in smokers

Pindborg (1947) was one of the first investigators to study the relationship between smoking and periodontal disease. He discovered a higher prevalence of acute necrotizing ulcerative gingivitis, a finding that was confirmed in many subsequent studies of this condition (Fig. 12-10) (Pindborg 1949; Kowolik & Nisbet 1983; Johnson & Engel 1986). Early studies showed that smokers had higher levels of periodontitis but they also had poorer levels of oral hygiene (Brandzaeg & Jamison 1984) and higher levels of calculus (Fig. 12-11) (Alexander 1970; Sheiham 1971). Later studies which took account of oral hygiene status and employed more sophisticated statistical analyses showed that smokers had more disease regardless of oral hygiene (Ismail *et al.* 1983; Bergstrom 1989; Bergstrom & Preber 1994).

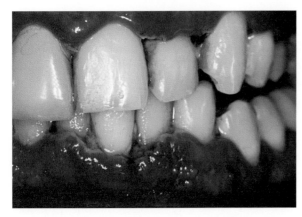

Fig. 12-10 The typical appearance of necrotizing ulcerative gingivitis in a heavy smoker with poor oral hygiene.

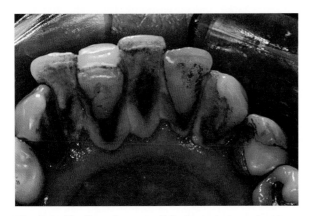

Fig. 12-11 The lingual aspects of the lower incisors showing gross supragingival calculus formation and relatively little gingival inflammation in a female patient who has smoked 20 cigarettes per day for over 20 years.

A large number of studies have established that in comparing smokers and non-smokers with periodontitis, smokers have:

1. Deeper probing depths and a larger number of deep pockets (Feldman *et al.* 1983; Bergstrom & Eliassson 1987a; Bergstrom *et al.* 2000a)
2. More attachment loss including more gingival recession (Grossi *et al.* 1994; Linden & Mullally 1994; Haffajee & Socransky 2001a)
3. More alveolar bone loss (Bergstrom & Floderus Myhred 1983; Bergstrom & Eliasson 1987b; Feldman *et al.* 1987; Bergstrom *et al.* 1991, 2000b; Grossi *et al.* 1995)
4. More tooth loss (Osterberg & Mellstrom 1986; Krall *et al.* 1997)
5. Less gingivitis and less bleeding on probing (Feldman *et al.* 1983; Preber & Bergstrom 1985; Bergstrom & Preber 1986; Haffajee & Socransky 2001a)
6. More teeth with furcation involvement (Mullally & Linden 1996).

The finding of less gingival bleeding on probing is associated with less inflamed marginal tissue and lower bleeding scores when probing the depth of the pockets. The typical clinical appearance of the smoker's gingival tissue is shown in Fig. 12-12, which demonstrates relatively low levels of marginal inflammation and a tendency to a more fibrotic appearance with little edema. Despite the clinical appearance of the gingival tissue, the patient has deep pockets,

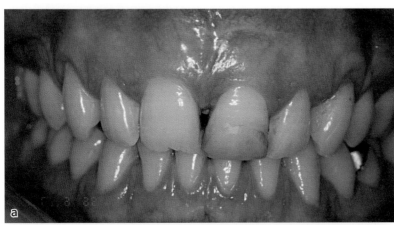

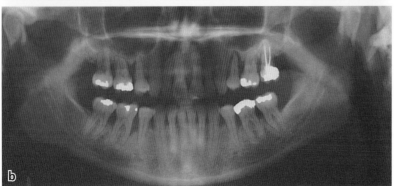

Fig. 12-12 A 30-year-old female smoker with advanced periodontitis. (a) The clinical appearance shows marginal gingiva with little signs of inflammation. Probing depths greater than 6 mm were present at most interproximal sites, but with little bleeding on probing. (b) Generalized advanced bone loss in this patient.

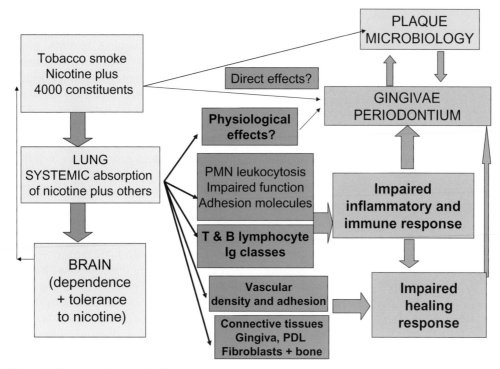

Fig. 12-13 Effects of tobacco smoking on the host response.

advanced attachment loss, and bone loss, as shown in Fig. 12-12b.

Modification of the host–bacteria relationship in smoking

There are several theories as to why smokers have more periodontal disease than non-smokers, involving both bacterial aspects and the host response (Barbour *et al.* 1997; Palmer *et al.* 2005). The potential interactions are illustrated in Fig. 12-13.

Effects on plaque bacteria

Smokers may have higher levels of plaque than non-smokers, which may be accounted for by poorer levels of oral hygiene rather than higher rates of supragingival plaque growth (Bergstrom 1981; Bergstrom & Preber 1986). Several studies have shown that smokers harbor more microbial species which are associated with periodontitis than non-smokers, including *P. gingivalis*, *A. actinomycetemcomitans*, *Tanerella forsythia* (*Bacteroides forsythus*) (Zambon *et al.* 1996), *P. intermedia*, *Peptostreptococcus micros*, *Fusobacterium nucleatum*, *Campylobacter rectus* (van Winkelhoff *et al.* 2001), *Staphylococcus aureus*, *Eschericia coli*, and *Candida albicans* (Kamma *et al.* 1999). Smokers may have a higher proportion of sites harboring these putative periodontal pathogens, in particular the palatal aspects of the maxillary teeth and the upper and lower incisor regions (Haffajee & Socransky 2001a,b). In contrast several studies have failed to show differences in the bacterial species between smokers and non-smokers (Preber *et al.*

1992; Darby *et al.* 2000; Bostrom *et al.* 2001; van der Velden *et al.* 2003). Microbiological studies differ in their methodology, ability to identify and quantify putative pathogens, and the number of subjects included. Changes in the pocket environment secondary to the effect of smoking on the host tissues could result in a different microflora in smokers.

Effects on the host response

The relationship between plaque accumulation and development of inflammation in smokers has been studied in classical experimental gingivitis studies (Bergstrom & Preber 1986). They demonstrated that there is no difference in plaque accumulation when comparing smokers and non-smokers. However, the development of inflammation was very much retarded in the smoking group with less sites exhibiting redness or bleeding on probing. They also showed lower amounts of gingival crevicular fluid (GCF) during the development of gingivitis. Smoking may result in lower resting GCF flow rate (Persson *et al.* 1999) and an episode of smoking may produce a transient increase in GCF flow rate (McLaughlin *et al.* 1993). The reduced bleeding has previously been proposed to be caused by nicotine-induced vasoconstriction, but as previously described in this chapter, more recent evidence has failed to show a reduction in blood flow to the gingiva following smoking a cigarette in regular smokers (Meekin *et al.* 2000). The reduced bleeding on the other hand is probably due to long-term effects on the inflammatory lesion. Histological comparisons of the lesions from smokers and non-smokers have shown fewer blood vessels in the inflammatory lesions of smokers (Rezavandi *et al.* 2001). It is pertinent to note that gingival bleeding on probing has been shown to increase within 4–6 weeks of quitting smoking (Nair *et al.* 2003), and this parallels reported recovery of reduced serum ICAM levels (Palmer *et al.* 2002).

Smoking has a profound effect on the immune and inflammatory system (reviewed by Barbour *et al.* 1997; Palmer *et al.* 2005). Smokers have an increased number of leukocytes in the systemic circulation (Sorenson *et al.* 2004), but fewer cells may migrate into the gingival crevice/pocket (Eichel & Shahrik 1969). Smoking is associated with chronic obstructive pulmonary disease (Barnes 2000) and many of the mechanisms indicated are paralleled in findings related to periodontal disease. It is thought that the main cell type responsible for destruction of lung parenchyma is the neutrophil, which is delayed in its transit through the pulmonary vasculature (McNee *et al.* 1989), where it is stimulated to release proteases including elastase, cathepsins, and matrix metalloproteases (Barnes 2000). These destructive molecules are balanced by inhibitors such as α-1-antitrypsin and tissue inhibitors of matrix metalloproteases.

Studies *in vitro* have shown a direct inhibition of neutrophil and monocyte–macrophage defensive functions by high concentrations of nicotine that may be achieved in patients using smokeless tobacco (Pabst *et al.* 1995). MacFarlane and co-workers (1992) examined patients with refractory periodontitis and found a high proportion of smokers in this diagnostic group. These investigators demonstrated abnormal PMN phagocytosis associated with a high level of cigarette smoking.

The PMN is a fundamental defense cell in the periodontal tissue. There is a constant traffic of PMNs from the gingival vasculature through the connective tissue and junctional epithelium into the gingival sulcus/pocket. This is described in some detail in Chapter 11. The PMN is the first line of defense and is chemotactically attracted to bacterial challenge at the dentogingival junction. The PMN contains a powerful battery of enzymes including elastase and other collagenases that have been implicated in tissue destruction in periodontitis and pulmonary disease. Eichel and Shahrik (1969) suggested decreased PMN migration into the oral cavity of smokers. Subsequently, PMNs harvested from the gingival sulcus of smokers were shown to have reduced phagocytic capacity compared to PMNs from non-smokers (Kenney *et al.* 1977). Neutrophil defects have been associated with an increased susceptibility to periodontitis, including cyclic neutropenia where there is a reduction in the number of neutrophils, and conditions such as leukocyte adhesion deficiency (LAD 1 and LAD 2), which may be responsible for cases of generalized prepubertal periodontitis as described by Page *et al.* (1983). It is proposed that smoking causes alterations to PMN function which could be

considered to be minor variations of these more profound defects.

The normal passage of the PMN from the microvasculature to the periodontal tissues involves a classic series of events including capture, rolling on the endothelium, firm adhesion to the endothelium, and transmigration through the vessel wall into the connective tissue (Ley 1996). This involves a complex interaction between receptors and ligands on the leukocyte surface and endothelium including selectins, ICAM-1 and LFA1 (CD18, CD11b) (Crawford & Watanabe 1994; Gemmel *et al.* 1994). Defects in the functional ligands for the selectins have been implicated in LAD 2 and mutations in the gene encoding CD18 resulting in absence of the β 2 integrins with LAD 1. Subjects with LAD are susceptible to serious and life-threatening infections and have tremendous destruction of the periodontal tissues, often leading to total tooth loss in the deciduous dentition. These serious and rare conditions illustrate the overwhelming importance of the adhesion molecules and suggest that minor defects in them may also give rise to more subtle conditions that could lead to increased susceptibility to periodontal destruction. In this respect, it has been shown that smokers are affected by upregulation of molecules such as ICAM-1 on the endothelium and they have higher levels of circulating soluble ICAM-1 which could interfere with the normal receptor ligand binding and function of the leukocyte in the defense of the periodontal tissue (Koundouros *et al.* 1996; Palmer *et al.* 1999; Scott *et al.* 2000a). A potential destructive mechanism is the release of elastase from neutrophils following binding of ICAM with CD18 (Mac 1 and LFA 1) (Barnett *et al.* 1996). Lower levels of elastase detected in the gingival fluid of smokers compared to non-smokers, may indicate more elastase release within the tissues (Alavi *et al.* 1995), and this is especially important considering the effects of smoking on protease inhibitors.

Tobacco smoking has a chronic effect on the elevated levels of soluble ICAM (sICAM) and there is evidence that the subject may return to more normal levels after quitting smoking (Scott *et al.* 2000b; Palmer *et al.* 2002). These molecules can be detected in the serum and in the GCF. It has also been shown that cotinine is present in the GCF in about the same concentration as it appears in serum, but the levels of sICAM are much lower in smokers despite very much higher serum levels than non-smokers (Fraser *et al.* 2001). Many other molecules have been studied in the GCF of smokers with many reporting reduced levels compared to non-smokers. Alavi *et al.* (1995) showed significantly lower concentrations of elastase and elastase complexed with α1-antitrypsin in smokers GCF. Although Bostrom *et al.* (1999) showed higher levels of TNF-α in GCF in smokers, they reported no differences in levels of IL-6 (Bostrom *et al.* 2000). Rawlinson *et al.* (2003) found levels of IL-1beta and IL-1ra to be significantly lower in GCF from diseased sites in smokers compared to non-smokers, and Petropoulos *et al.* (2004) showed that the concentration of IL-1alpha in GCF of smokers was approximately half that found in non-smokers.

PMN-related periodontal tissue destruction may also be related to suppression or exacerbation of the respiratory burst and generation of reactive oxygen species. For example Gustafsson *et al.* (2000) have shown that the priming capacity of TNF-α, measured as generation of oxygen radicals from stimulated neutrophils, is higher in neutrophils from smokers, compared to neutrophils from non-smokers. Thus, inappropriate activation of periodontal neutrophils is thought to contribute to the degradation of gingival tissues and the progression of inflammatory periodontal disease (Deas *et al.* 2003).

The effects of smoking on lymphocyte function and antibody production are very complex, with the various components having the potential to cause immunosuppression or stimulation. It is likely that the particulate phase of cigarette smoke confers immunosuppressive properties. Acute or chronic exposure to hydrocarbons may stimulate or inhibit the immune response, the net effect being dependent upon the dose and duration of the exposure to components of tobacco smoke. The leukocytosis observed in smokers results in increased numbers of circulating T and B lymphocytes (reviewed in Sopori & Kozak 1998). Studies that have examined T cell subsets report different findings of either reduced, increased or no change in the number of CD4 T cells (Loos *et al.* 2004). Smoking appears to affect both B and T cell function, inducing functional unresponsiveness in T cells.

It has been reported that serum IgG levels in smokers may be reduced (Quinn *et al.* 1998) with depression of IgG2, particularly in some racial groups (Quinn *et al.* 1996; Graswinkel *et al.* 2004). Reported levels of serum IgA and IgM classes are variable and IgE may be elevated (Burrows *et al.* 1981).

The clinical change in the tissues of smokers was described above. It is not surprising that histological evaluation of smokers' tissues has shown that there is a decrease in the vascularity of the tissues (Rezavandi *et al.* 2001). This is a chronic effect due to smoking and may also be associated with alterations in the expression of adhesion molecules within the endothelium. The effect of tobacco smoking on the expression of adhesion molecules on leukocytes, within the inflammatory lesion, in the junctional epithelium and cells of the pocket epithelium could have important implications on the progession of periodontitis in smokers. The effect of smoking on macrovasular disease is well documented (Powell 1998) and its effects on microvascular disease could also be of importance in periodontal disease and in healing.

Effects on healing and treatment response

The healing potential of tissues has important implications in any chronic inflammatory lesion and in repair following treatment. Smoking has been identified as an important cause of impaired healing in orthopedic surgery, plastic surgery, dental implant surgery (Bain & Moy 1993), and in all aspects of periodontal treatment including non-surgical treatment, basic periodontal surgery, regenerative periodontal surgery, and mucogingival plastic periodontal surgery (Preber & Bergstrom 1986; Miller 1987; Tonetti *et al.* 1995; Grossi *et al.* 1996, 1997a; Kaldahl *et al.* 1996; Bostrom *et al.* 1998; Tonetti 1998; Kinane & Chestnutt 2000; Heasman *et al.* 2006).

In non-surgical treatment, smoking is associated with poorer reductions in probing depth and gains in clinical attachment. In most studies smokers have a lower level of bleeding at baseline, and following treatment bleeding scores are reduced in smokers in a similar manner to those in non-smokers. The poorer reductions in probing depths and gains in attachment level amount to a mean of approximately 0.5 mm. Much of this may be due to less recession of the marginal tissues in smokers as there is less edema and more fibrosis in the gingiva. The same may be true for the deeper tissues of the periodontium where there is less of an inflammatory infiltrate and vascularity at the depth of the pocket. These differences in the tissues between smokers and non-smokers in the untreated state may largely account for the differences in response to non-surgical treatment. It has been proposed that these differences may be manifest by differences in probe penetration in smokers and non-smokers, particularly in deep pockets (Biddle *et al.* 2001).

The poor response of smokers to non-surgical treatment may also apply to those treated with adjunctive antibiotics (Kinane & Radvar 1997; Palmer *et al.* 1999). Response to non-surgical treatment may be seen merely as resolution of inflammation and improvement of the epithelial attachment together with some formation of collagen. However, the response following periodontal surgery is more complex and involves an initial inflammatory reaction followed by organization of the clot, and formation of granulation tissue consisting of capillary buds and fibroblasts laying down collagen. The surgical flaps have to revascularize and the epithelial attachment has to reform on the surface. In regenerative surgery there also has to be formation of a connective tissue attachment and cementogenesis. Tobacco smoke and nicotine undoubtedly affect the microvasculature, the fibroblasts and connective tissue matrix, the bone and also the root surface itself. It has been shown in *in vitro* studies that fibroblasts are affected by nicotine in that they demonstrate reduced proliferation, reduced migration and matrix production, and poor attachment to surfaces (Raulin *et al.* 1988; Tipton & Dabbous 1995; James *et al.* 1999; Tanur *et al.* 2000). The root surfaces in smokers are additionally contaminated by products of smoking such as nicotine, cotinine, acrolein, and acetaldehyde, and these molecules may affect the attachment of cells (Raulin *et al.* 1988; Cattaneo *et al.* 2000; Gamal & Bayomy 2002; Poggi *et al.* 2002). Smoking has a direct effect on bone and is an established risk factor in osteoporosis. It has also been proposed that it may have a direct affect on bone loss in periodontitis (Bergstrom *et al.* 1991) and it undoubtedly delays healing of bone in fracture wound repair. It is not surprising therefore that tobacco smoking has been implicated in poorer responses to periodontal surgical treatment.

Smoking cessation

All patients should be assessed for smoking status and given advice to quit the habit. About 70% of people who smoke would like to quit and should be assisted. They should be referred to specialist cessation services if the treating practitioner does not feel confident in this area. They can be advised about nicotine replacement therapy. People's success with quitting is considerably improved using nicotine replacement therapy and drugs such as buproprion hydrochloride. Former smokers more closely resemble non-smokers in their periodontal health status and response to treatment, but the time required to revert to this status has not been defined. In one of the few papers that have attempted to combine a quit smoking and periodontal treatment interventional study, Preshaw *et al.* (2005) showed a more favorable periodontal treatment outcome in those subjects that managed to quit using well established quit smoking strategies including counseling, nicotine replacement therapy and bupropion. From the original group of 49 subjects there were only 11 continuous quitters at 12 months. It would be of great interest to determine what changes in periodontal status would have occurred with just the quit smoking intervention, and more randomized controlled clinical trials are required in this area.

References

Abraham-Inpijn, L., Polsacheva, D.V. & Raber-Durlacher, J.E. (1996). The significance of endocrine factors and microorganisms in the development of gingivitis in pregnant women. *Stomatolgiia* **75**, 15–18.

Alavi, A.L., Palmer, R.M., Odell, E.W., Coward, P.Y. & Wilson, R.F. (1995). Elastase in gingival crevicular fluid from smokers and non-smokers with chronic inflammatory periodontal disease. *Oral Diseases* **1**, 103–105.

Aldridge, J.P., Lester, V., Watts, T.L., Collins, A., Viberti, G. & Wilson, R.F. (1995). Single blind studies on the effects of improved periodontal health on metabolic control in type 1 diabetes mellitus. *Journal of Clinical Periodontology* **22**, 271–275.

Alexander, A.G. (1970). The relationship between tobacco smoking, calculus and plaque accumulation and gingivitis. *Dental Health* **9**, 6–9.

Amar, S. & Chung, K.M. (1994). Influence of hormonal variation on the periodontium in women. *Periodontology 2000* **6**, 79–87.

Armamento-Villareal, R., Villareal, D.T., Avioli, L.V. & Civitelli, R. (1992). Estrogen status and heredity are major determinants of premenopausal bone mass. *Journal of Clinical Investigation* **90**, 2464–2471.

Atkinson, M.A. & Maclaren, N.K. (1990). What causes diabetes? *Scientific American* **263**, 62–63, 66–71.

Baab, D.A. & Öberg, P.A. (1987). The effect of cigarette smoking on gingival blood flow in humans. *Journal of Clinical Periodontology* **14**, 418–424.

Bain, C.A. & Moy, P.K. (1993). The association between the failure of dental implants and cigarette smoking. *International Journal of Oral & Maxillofacial Implants* **8**, 609–615.

Barbour, S.E., Nakashima, K., Zhang, J.B. *et al.* (1997). Tobacco and smoking: environmental factors that modify the host response (immune system) and have an impact on periodontal health. *Critical Reviews in Oral Biology & Medicine* **8**, 437–460.

Barnes, P.J. (2000). Chronic obstructive pulmonary disease. *New England Journal of Medicine* **343**, 269–280.

Barnett, C.C, Moore, E.E, Moore, F.A., Biffl, W.L. & Partrick D.A. (1996). Soluble intercellullar adhesion molecule-1 provokes polymorphonuclear leukocyte elastase release by CD18. *Surgery* **120**, 395–402.

Baxter, J.C. (1987). Osteoporosis: oral manifestations of a systemic disease. *Quintessence International* **18**, 472–479.

Benowitz, N.L. (1988). Pharmacological aspects of cigarette smoking and nicotine addiction. *New England Journal of Medicine* **319**, 1318–1330.

Benowitz, N.L. (1989). Health and public policy implications of the low yield cigarette. *New England Journal of Medicine* **320**, 1619–1621.

Benowitz N.L. (1996). Pharmacology of nicotine: addiction and therapeutics. *Annual Reviews in Pharmacology and Toxicology* **36**, 597–613.

Bergstrom J. (1981). Short-term investigation on the influence of cigarette smoking upon plaque accumulation. *Scandinavian Journal of Dental Research* **89**, 235–238.

Bergstrom, J. (1989). Cigarette smoking as a risk factor in chronic periodontal disease. *Community Dentistry and Oral Epidemiology* **17**, 245–247.

Bergstrom, J. & Eliasson, S. (1987a). Noxious effect of cigarette smoking on periodontal health. *Journal of Periodontal Research* **22**, 513–517.

Bergstrom, J. & Eliasson, S. (1987b). Cigarette smoking and alveolar bone height in subjects with high standard of oral hygiene. *Journal of Clinical Periodontology* **14**, 466–469.

Bergstrom, J., Eliasson, S. & Dock, J. (2000a). A 10-year prospective study of tobacco smoking and periodontal health. *Journal of Periodontology* **71**, 1338–1347.

Bergstrom, J., Eliasson, S. & Dock, J. (2000b). Exposure to smoking and periodontal health. *Journal of Clinical Periodontology* **27**, 61–68.

Bergstrom, J., Eliasson, S. & Preber, H. (1991). Cigarette smoking and periodontal bone loss. *Journal of Periodontology* **62**, 244–246.

Bergstrom, J. & Floderus Myrhed, B. (1983). Co-twin control study of the relationship between smoking and some periodontal disease factors. *Community Dentistry and Oral Epidemiology* **11**, 113–116.

Bergstrom, J., Persson, L. & Preber, H. (1988). Influence of cigarette smoking on vascular reaction during experimental gingivitis. *Scandinavian Journal of Dental Research* **96**, 34–39.

Bergstrom, J. & Preber, H. (1986). The influence of tobacco smoking on the development of experimental gingivitis. *Journal of Periodontal Research* **21**, 668–676.

Bergstrom, J. & Preber, H. (1994). Tobacco use as a risk factor. *Journal of Periodontology* **65**, 545–550.

Biddle, A., Palmer, R.M., Wilson, R.F. & Watts, T.L.P. (2001). Comparison of periodontal probing measurements in smokers and non-smokers. *Journal of Clinical Periodontology* **28**, 806–812.

Bostrom, L., Linder, L.E. & Bergstrom, J. (1998). Influence of smoking on the outcome of periodontal surgery. A 5-year follow-up. *Journal of Clinical Periodontology* **25**, 194–201.

Bostrom L., Linder L.E. & Bergstrom, J. (1999). Smoking and crevicular fluid levels of IL-6 and TNF-alpha in periodontal disease. *Journal of Clinical Periodontology* **26**, 352–357.

Bostrom, L., Linder, L. & Bergstrom, J. (2000). Smoking and GCF levels of IL-1β and IL-1-ra in periodontal disease. *Journal of Clinical Periodontology* **27**, 250–255.

Bostrom, L., Bergstrom, J., Dahlén, G. & Linder, L. (2001). Smoking and subgingival microflora in periodontal disease. *Journal of Clinical Periodontology* **28**, 212–219.

Brandzaeg, P. & Jamison, H.C. (1984). A study on periodontal health and oral hygiene in Norwegian army recruits. *Journal of Periodontology* **35**, 303–307.

Brownlee, M. (1994). Glycation and diabetic complications. *Diabetes* **43**, 836–841.

Burrows, B., Halonen, M., Barbee, R.A. & Lebowitz, M.D. (1981). The relationship of serum immunoglobulin E to cigarette smoking. *American Review of Respiratory Disease* **124**, 523–525.

Cattaneo, V., Getta, G., Rota, C., Vezzoni, F., Rota, M., Gallanti, A., Boratto, R. & Poggi, P. (2000). Volatile components of cigarette smoke: Effect of acroleine and acetaldehyde on human gingival fibroblasts *in vitro*. *Journal of Periodontology* **71**, 425–432.

Chau, D., Mancoll, J.S., Lee, S., Zhao, J., Phillips, L.G., Gittes, G.K. & Longaker, M.T. (1998). Tamoxifen downregulates TGFβ-production in keloid fibroblasts. *Annals of Plastic Surgery* **40**, 490–493.

Christgau, M., Palitzsch, K.D., Schmalz, G., Kreiner, U. & Frenzel, S. (1998). Healing response to non-surgical periodontal therapy in patients with diabetes mellitus: clinical, microbiological and immunological results. *Journal of Clinical Periodontology* **25**, 112–124.

Clarke, N.G., Shepherd, B.C. & Hirsch, R.S. (1981). The effects of intra-arterial epinephrine and nicotine on gingival circulation. *Oral Surgery, Oral Medicine, Oral Pathology* **52**, 577–582.

Cohen, D.W., Friedman, L., Shapiro, J. & Kyle, G.C. (1969). A longitudinal investigation of the periodontal changes during pregnancy. *Journal of Periodontology* **40**, 563–570.

Crawford, J.M. & Watanabe K. (1994). Cell adhesion molecules in inflammation and immunity: relevance to periodontal diseases. *Critical Reviews in Oral Biology & Medicine* **5**, 91–123.

Cutler, C.W. & Iacopino, A.M. (2003). Periodontal disease: links with serum lipid/triglyceride levels? Review and new data. *Journal of the International Academy of Periodontology* **5**, 47–51.

Darby, I., Hodge, P., Riggio, M. & Kinane, D. (2000). Microbial comparison of smoker and non-smoker adult and early onset patients by polymerase chain reaction. *Journal of Clinical Periodontology* **27**, 417–424.

Davis, A.J. (2000). Advances in contraception (review). *Obstetrics and Gynaecology Clinics of North America* **27**, 597–610.

Deas, D.E., Mackey, S.A. & McDonnell, H.T. (2003). Systemic disease and periodontitis: manifestations of neutrophil dysfunction. *Periodontology 2000* **32**, 82–104.

Di Placido, G., Tumini, V., D'Archivio, D. & Peppe, G. (1998). Gingival hyperplasia in pregnancy II. Aetiopathogenic factors and mechanisms. *Minerva Stomatologica* **47**, 223–229.

Eichel, G. & Shahrik, H.A. (1969). Tobacco smoke toxicity: loss of human oral leucocyte function and fluid cell metabolism. *Science* **166**, 1424–1428.

El-Ashiry, G.M., El-Kafrawy, A.H., Nasr, M.F. *et al.* (1971). Effects of oral contraceptives on the gingiva. *Journal of Periodontology* **56**, 18–20.

Esposito, C., Gerlach, H., Brett, J., Stern, D. & Vlassara, H. (1992). Endothelial receptor mediated binding of glucose-modified albumin is associated with increased monolayer permeability and modulation of cell-surface coagulant properties. *Journal of Experimental Medicine* **170**, 1387–1407.

Faria-Almeida, R., Navarro, A. & Bascones, A. (2006). Clinical and metabolic changes after conventional treatment of Type 2 diabetic patients with chronic periodontitis. *Journal of Periodontology* **77**, 591–598.

Feldman, R.S., Alman, J.E. & Chauncey, H.H. (1987). Periodontal disease indexes and tobacco smoking in healthy ageing men. *Gerodontics* **1**, 43–46.

Feldman, R.S., Bravacos, J.S. & Rose, C.L. (1983). Association between smoking different tobacco products and periodontal disease indexes. *Journal of Periodontology* **54**, 481–487.

Fraser, H.S., Palmer, R.M., Wilson, R.F., Coward, P.Y. & Scott, D.A. (2001). Elevated systemic concentrations of soluble ICAM-1 are not reflected in the gingival crevicular fluid of smokers with periodontitis. *Journal of Dental Research* **80**, 1643–1647.

Frost, H.M. (1989). Some effects of basic multicellular unit-based remodelling on photon absorptiometry of trabecular bone. *Bone and Mineral* **7**, 47–65.

Gamal, A.Y. & Bayomy, M.M. (2002). Effect of cigarette smoking on human PDL fibroblasts attachment to periodontally involved root surfaces *in vitro*. *Journal of Clinical Periodontology* **29**, 763–770.

Garfinkel, L. (1997). Trends in cigarette smoking in the United States. *Preventive Medicine* **26**, 447–450.

Gemmell, E., Walsh, L.J., Savage, N.W. & Seymour, G.J. (1994). Adhesion molecule expression in chronic inflammatory periodontal disease tissue. *Journal of Periodontal Research* **29**, 46–53.

Gotfredsen, A., Nilas, L., Riis, B.J., Thomsen, K. & Christiansen, C. (1986). Bone changes occurring spontaneously and caused by oestrogen in early post-menopausal women: a local or generalised phenomenon? *British Medical Journal* **292**, 1098–1100.

Grady, D., Rubin, S.M., Petitti, D.B. *et al.* (1992). Hormone therapy to prevent disease and prolong life in post-menopausal women. *Annals of Internal Medicine* **117**, 1016–1037.

Grant, D., Stern, J. & Listgarten, M. (1988). The epidemiology, etiology and public health aspects of periodontal disease. In: Grant, D., Stern, J. and Listgarten, M., eds. *Periodontics*. St. Louis: CV Mosby Co, pp. 229, 332–335.

Graswinkel, J.E., van der Velden, U., van Winkelhoff, A.J., Hoek, F.J. & Loos, B.G. (2004). Plasma antibody levels in periodontitis patients and controls. *Journal of Clinical Periodontology* **31**, 562–568.

Graves, D.T., Liu, R., Alikhani, M., Al-Mashat, H. & Trackman, P.C. (2006). Diabetes-enhanced inflammation and apoptosis – impact on periodontal pathology. *Journal of Dental Research* **85**, 15–21.

Grodstein, F., Colditz, G.A. & Stampfer, M.J. (1996). Post-menopausal hormone use and tooth loss: a prospective study. *Journal of the American Dental Association* **127**, 370–377.

Grossi, S.G., Genco, R.J., Machtei, E.E. *et al.* (1995). Assessment of risk for periodontal disease. II. Risk indicators for alveolar bone loss. *Journal of Periodontology* **66**, 23–29.

Grossi, S.G., Skrepcinski, F.B., DeCaro, T., Zambon, J.J., Cummin, D. & Genco, R.J. (1996). Response to periodontal therapy in diabetics and smokers. *Journal of Periodontology* **67**, 1094–1102.

Grossi, S.G., Skrepcinski, F.B., DeCaro, T., Zambon, J.J., Cummin, D. & Genco, R.J. (1997). Treatment of periodontal disease in diabetics reduces glycated haemoglobin. *Journal of Periodontology* **68**, 713–719.

Grossi, S.G., Zambon, J.J., Ho, A.W. *et al.* (1994). Assessment of risk for periodontal disease. I. Risk indicators for attachment loss. *Journal of Periodontology* **65**, 260–267.

Grossi, S.G., Zambon, J., Machtei, E.E. *et al.* (1997). Effects of smoking and smoking cessation on healing after mechanical therapy. *Journal of the American Dental Association* **128**, 599–607.

Gugliucci, A. (2000). Glycation as the glucose link to diabetic complications (review). *Journal of the American Osteopathic Association* **100**, 621–634.

Guncu, G.N., Tozum, T.F. & Caglayan, F. (2005). Effects of endogenous sex hormones on the periodontium – review of the literature. *Australian Dental Journal* **50**, 138–145.

Gustafsson, A., Asman, B. & Bergstrom, K. (2000). Cigarette smoking as an aggravating factor in inflammatory tissue-destructive diseases. Increase in tumor necrosis factor-alpha priming of peripheral neutrophils measured as generation of oxygen radicals. *International Journal of Clinical & Laboratory Research* **30**, 187–190.

Guyton, A.C. (1987). *Human Physiology and Mechanisms of Disease*, 4th edn. Philadelphia: W.B. Saunders Co.

Haber, J., Wattles, J., Crowley, M., Mandell, R., Joshipura, K. & Kent, R.L. (1993). Evidence for cigarette smoking as a major risk factor for periodontitis. *Journal of Periodontology* **64**, 16–23.

Haffajee, A.D. & Socransky, S.S. (2001a). Relationship of cigarette smoking to attachment level profiles. *Journal of Clinical Periodontology* **28**, 283–295.

Haffajee, A.D. & Socransky, S.S. (2001b). Relationship of cigarette smoking to the subgingival microbiota. *Journal of Clinical Periodontology* **28**, 377–388.

Harrison, G.A., Schultz, T.A. & Schaberg, S.J. (1983). Deep neck infection complicated by diabetes mellitus. *Oral Surgery* **55**, 133–137.

Hasson, E. (1966). Pregnancy gingivitis. *Harefuah* **58**, 224–230.

Heasman, L., Stacey, F., Preshaw, P.M., McCracken, G.I., Hepburn, S. & Heasman, P.A. (2006). The effect of smoking on periodontal treatment response: a review of clinical evidence. *Journal of Clinical Periodontology* **33**, 241–253.

Holm-Pedersen, P. & Loe, H. (1967). Flow of gingival exudate as related to menstruation and pregnancy. *Journal of Periodontal Research* **2**, 13–20.

Hopper, J.L. & Seeman, E. (1994). The bone density of female twins discordant for tobacco use. *New England Journal of Medicine* **330**, 387–392.

Hugoson, A. (1970). Gingival inflammation and female sex hormones. *Journal of Periodontal Research* **5** (Suppl), 9.

Iacopino, A.M. (1995). Diabetic periodontitis: possible lipid induced defect in tissue repair through alteration of macrophage phenotype function. *Oral Diseases* **1**, 214–229.

Iacopino, A.M. (2001). Periodontitis and diabetes interrelationships: role of inflammation. *Annals of Periodontology* **6**, 125–127.

Ismail, A.I., Burt, B.A. & Eklund, S.A. (1983). Epidemiologic patterns of smoking and periodontal disease in the United States. *Journal of the American Dental Association* **106**, 617–621.

James, J.A., Sayers, N.S., Drucker, D.B. & Hull, P.S. (1999). Effects of tobacco products on the attachment and growth of periodontal ligament fibroblasts. *Journal of Periodontology* **70**, 518–525.

Jarvis, M.J., Russell, M.A.H., Benowitz, N.L. & Feyerabend, C. (1988). Elimination of cotinine from body fluids: implications for non-invasive measurement of tobacco smoke exposure. *American Journal of Public Health* **78**, 696–698.

Jarvis, M.J., Tunstall-Pedoe, H., Feyerabend, C., Vesey, C. & Saloojee, Y. (1987). Comparison of tests used to distinguish smokers from non-smokers. *American Journal of Public Health* **77**, 1435–1438.

Jensen, J., Christiansen, C. & Rodbro, P. (1985). Cigarette smoking, serum oestrogens and bone loss during hormone-replacement therapy early after menopause. *New England Journal of Medicine* **313**, 973–975.

Jensen, J., Liljemark, W. & Bloomquist, C. (1981). The effect of female sex hormones on subgingival plaque. *Journal of Periodontology* **52**, 599–602.

Johnson, B.D. & Engel, D. (1986). Acute necrotizing ulcerative gingivitis. A review of diagnosis, etiology and treatment. *Journal of Periodontology* **57**, 141–150.

Kaldahl, W.B, Johnson, G.K, Patil, K. & Kalkwarf, K.L. (1996). Levels of cigarette consumption and response to periodontal therapy. *Journal of Periodontology* **67**, 675–681.

Kamma, J.J., Nakou, M. & Baehni, P.C. (1999). Clinical and microbiological characteristics of smokers with early onset periodontitis. *Journal of Periodontal Research* **34**, 25–33.

Karjalainen, K.M., Knuuttila, M.L. & von Dickhoff, K.J. (1994). Association of the severity of periodontal disease with organ complications in type 1 diabetic patients. *Journal of Periodontology* **65**, 1067–1072.

Kenney, E.B., Kraal, J.H., Saxe, S.R. & Jones, J. (1977). The effect of cigarette smoke on human oral polymorphonuclear leukocytes. *Journal of Periodontal Research* **12**, 227–234.

Kimmel, D.B., Slovik, D.M. & Lane, N.E. (1994). Current and investigational approaches for reversing established osteoporosis. *Rheumatoid Disease Clinics of North America* **20**, 735–758.

Kimura, S., Elce, J.S. & Jellinek, P.H. (1983). Immunological relationship between peroxidases in eosinophils, uterus and other tissues of the rat. *Biochemical Journal* **213**, 165–169.

Kinane, D.F. & Chestnutt, I.G. (2000). Smoking and periodontal disease. *Critical Reviews in Oral Biology and Medicine* **11**, 356–365.

Kinane, D.F. & Radvar M. (1997). The effect of smoking on mechanical and antimicrobial periodontal therapy. *Journal of Periodontology* **68**, 467–472.

Kinane, D.F., Peterson, M. & Stathopoulou, P.G. (2006). Environmental and other modifying factors of the periodontal diseases. *Periodontology 2000* **40**, 107–119.

Kiran, M., Arpak, N., Unsal, E. & Erdogan, M.F. (2005). The effect of improved periodontal health on metabolic control in type 2 diabetes mellitus. *Journal of Clinical Periodontology* **32**, 266–272.

Knight, G.M. & Wade, A.B. (1974). The effects of hormonal contraceptives on the human periodontium. *Journal of Periodontal Research* **9**, 18–22.

Kornman, K.S. & Loesche, W.J. (1979). Effects of oestradiol and progesterone on *Bacteroides melaninogenicus*. *Journal of Dental Research* **58A**, 107.

Koundouros, E., Odell, E., Coward, P.Y., Wilson, R.F. & Palmer, R.M. (1996). Soluble adhesion molecules in serum of smokers and non-smokers, with and without periodontitis. *Journal of Periodontal Research* **31**, 596–599.

Kowolik, M.J. & Nisbet, T. (1983). Smoking and acute ulcerative gingivitis. *British Dental Journal* **154**, 241–242.

Kraal, J.H. & Kenney, R.B. (1979). The response of polymorphonuclear leucocytes to chemotactic stimulation for smokers and non-smokers. *Journal of Periodontal Research* **14**, 383–389.

Krall, E.A. & Dawson-Hughes, B. (1991). Smoking and bone loss among post-menopausal women. *Journal of Bone and Mineral Research* **6**, 331–338.

Krall, E.A., Dawson-Hughes, B., Garvey, A.J. & Garcia, R.I. (1997). Smoking, smoking cessation and tooth loss. *Journal of Dental Research* **76**, 1653–1659.

Kritz-Silverstein, D. & Barrett-Connor, E. (1993). Early menopause, number of reproductive years and bone mineral density in postmenopausal women. *American Journal of Public Health* **83**, 983–988.

Lalla, E., Lamster, I.B., Drury, S., Fu, C. & Schmidt, A.M. (2000). Hyperglycaemia, glycooxidation and receptor for advanced glycation end products: potential mechanisms underlying diabetic complications, including diabetes-associated periodontitis (review). *Periodontology 2000* **23**, 50–62.

Lapp, C.A., Thomas, M.E. & Lewis, J.B. (1995). Modulation by progesterone of interleukin-6 production by gingival fibroblasts. *Journal of Periodontology* **66**, 279–284.

Le, J. & Vilcek, J. (1989). Interleukin-6: A multifunctional cytokine regulating immune reactions and the acute phase response. *Laboratory Investigation* **61**, 588–602.

Ley, K. (1996). Molecular mechanisms of leukocyte recruitment in the inflammatory process. *Cardiovascular Research* **32**, 733–742.

Linden, G.J. & Mullally, B.H. (1994). Cigarette smoking and periodontal destruction in young adults. *Journal of Periodontology* **65**, 718–723.

Lindhe, J. & Attstrom, R. (1967). Gingival exudation during the menstrual cycle. *Journal of Periodontal Research* **2**, 194–198.

Lindhe, J. & Bjorn, A.L. (1967). Influence of hormonal contraceptives on the gingivae of women. *Journal of Periodontal Research* **2**, 1–6.

Lindquist, O. & Bengtsson, C. (1979). Menopausal age in relation to smoking. *Acta Medica Scandinavica* **205**, 73–77.

Loos, B.G., Roos, M.T., Schellekens, P.T., van der Velden, U. & Miedema, F. (2004). Lymphocyte numbers and function in relation to periodontitis and smoking. *Journal of Periodontology* **75**, 557–564.

Lotz, M. & Guerne, P-A. (1991). Interleukin-6 induces the synthesis of tissue inhibitor of metalloproteinase-1/erythroid potentiating activity (TIMP-1/EPA). *Journal of Biological Chemistry* **266**, 2017–2020.

Lundgren, D., Magnussen, B. & Lindhe, J. (1973). Connective tissue alterations in gingiva of rats treated with oestrogens and progesterone. *Odontologisk Revy* **24**, 49–58.

Lynch, C.M., Sinnott, J.T., Holt, D.A. & Herold, A.H. (1991). Use of antibiotics during pregnancy. *American Family Physician* **43**, 1365–1368.

MacFarlane, G.D., Herzberg, M.C., Wolff, L.F. & Hardie, N.A. (1992). Refractory periodontitis associated with abnormal polymorphonuclear leukocyte phagocytosis and cigarette smoking. *Journal of Periodontology* **63**, 908–913.

Machuca, G., Khoshfeiz, O., Lacalle, J.R., Machuca, C. & Bullon, P. (1999). The influence of general health and socio-cultural variables on the periodontal condition of pregnant women. *Journal of Periodontology* **70**, 779–785.

Marhoffer, W., Stein, M., Maeser, E. & Federlin, K. (1992). Impairment of polymorphonuclear leucocyte function and metabolic control of diabetes. *Diabetes Care* **15**, 156–260.

Mariotti, A. (1994). Sex steroid hormones and cell dynamics in the periodontium. *Critical Reviews in Oral Biology and Medicine* **5**, 27–53.

Mascarenhas P., Gapski R., Al-Shammari K. & Wang, H-L. (2003). Influence of sex hormones on the periodontium. *Journal of Clinical Periodontology* **30**, 671–81.

Mashimo, P.A., Yamamoto, Y., Slots, J., Park, B.H. & Genco, R.J. (1983). The periodontal microflora of juvenile diabetics. Culture, immunofluorescence, and serum antibody studies. *Journal of Periodontology* **54**, 420–430.

Mavropoulos, A., Aars, H. & Brodin, P. (2003). Hyperaemic response to cigarette smoking in healthy gingiva. *Journal of Clinical Periodontology* **30**, 214–221.

McLaughlin, W.S., Lovat, F.M., Macgregor, I.D. & Kelly, P.J. (1993). The immediate effects of smoking on gingival fluid flow. *Journal of Clinical Periodontology* **20**, 448–451.

McNee, W., Wiggs, B., Belzberg, A.S. & Hogg, J.C. (1989). The effect of cigarette smoke on neutrophil kinetics in human lungs. *New England Journal of Medicine* **321**, 924–928.

Mealey, B.L. (1998). Impact of advances in diabetes care on dental treatment of the diabetic patient. *Compendium of Continuing Education in Dentistry* **19**, 41–58.

Meekin, T.N., Wilson, R.F., Scott, D.A., Ide, M. & Palmer, R.M. (2000). Laser Doppler flowmeter measurement of relative gingival and forehead skin blood flow in light and regular smokers during and after smoking. *Journal of Clinical Periodontology* **23**, 236–242.

Meurman, J.H. & Hamalainen, P. (2006). Oral health and morbidity – implications of oral infections on the elderly. *Gerodontology* **23**, 3–16.

Miller, P.D. (1987). Root coverage with free gingival grafts. Factors associated with incomplete coverage. *Journal of Periodontology* **58**, 674–681.

Miyagi, M., Morishita, M. & Iwamoto, Y. (1993). Effects of sex hormones on production of prostaglandin E2 by human peripheral monocytes. *Journal of Periodontology* **64**, 1075–1078.

Miyazaki, H., Yamashita, Y., Shirahama, R., Goto-Kimura, K., Shimada, N., Sogame, A. & Takehara, T. (1991). Periodontal condition of pregnant women assessed by CPITN. *Journal of Clinical Periodontology* **18**, 751–754.

Mombelli, M., Gusberti, F.A., van Oosten, M.A.C. & Lang, N.P. (1989). Gingival health and gingivitis development during puberty. *Journal of Clinical Periodontology* **16**, 451–456.

Moore, M., Bracker, M., Sartoris, D., Saltman, P. & Strause, L. (1990). Long-term oestrogen replacement therapy in postmenopausal women sustains vertebral bone mineral density. *Journal of Bone and Mineral Research* **5**, 659–664.

Morozumi, T., Kubota, T., Sato, T., Okuda, K. & Yoshie, H. (2004). Smoking cessation increases gingival blood flow and gingival crevicular fluid. *Journal of Clinical Periodontology* **31**, 267–272.

Mullally, B.H. & Linden, G.J. (1996). Molar furcation involvement associated with cigarette smoking in periodontal referrals. *Journal of Clinical Periodontology* **23**, 658–661.

Muramatsu, Y. & Takaesu, Y. (1994). Oral health status related to subgingival bacterial flora and sex hormones in saliva during pregnancy. *Bulletin of the Tokyo Dental College* **35**, 139–151.

Murphy, E. & Nolan, J.J. (2000). Insulin sensitiser drugs (review). *Expert Opinion on Investigational Drugs* **9**, 347–361.

Nair, P., Sutherland, G., Palmer, R., Wilson, R. & Scott, D. (2003). Gingival bleeding on probing increases after quitting smoking. *Journal of Clinical Periodontology* **30**, 435–437.

Nakagawa, S., Fujii, H., Machida, Y. & Okuda, K. (1994). A longitudinal study from prepuberty to puberty of gingivitis. Correlation between the occurrence of *Prevotella intermedia* and sex hormones. *Journal of Clinical Periodontology* **21**, 658–665.

Ojanotko-Harri, A.O., Harri, M.P., Hurttia, H.M. & Sewon, L.A. (1991). Altered tissue metabolism of progesterone in pregnancy gingivitis and granuloma. *Journal of Clinical Periodontology* **18**, 262–266.

Oliver, R.C., Tervonen, T., Flynn, D.G. & Keenan, K.M. (1993). Enzyme activity in crevicular fluid in relation to metabolic control of diabetes and other periodontal risk factors. *Journal of Periodontology* **64**, 358–362.

Osterberg, T. & Mellstrom, D. (1986). Tobacco smoking: a major risk factor for loss of teeth in three 70-year-old cohorts. *Community Dentistry and Oral Epidemiology* **14**, 367–370.

Pabst, M.J., Pabst, K.M., Collier, J.A. *et al.* (1995). Inhibition of neutrophil and monocyte defensive functions by nicotine. *Journal of Periodontology* **66**, 1047–1055.

Paganini-Hill, A. (1995). The benefits of oestrogen relacement therapy on oral health. *Archives of Internal Medicine* **155**, 325–329.

Page, R.C., Bowen, T., Altman, L., Vandesteen, E., Ochs, H., Mackenzie, P., Osterberg, S., Engel, L.D. & Williams, B.L. (1983). Prepubertal periodontitis I. Definition of a clinical disease entity. *Journal of Periodontology* **54**, 257–271.

Palmer, R.M., Matthew, J.P. & Wilson, R.F. (1999). Non-surgical periodontal treatment with and without adjunctive metronidazole in smokers and non-smokers. *Journal of Clinical Periodontology* **26**, 158–163.

Palmer, R.M., Scott, D.A., Meekin, T.N., Wilson, R.F., Poston, R.N. & Odell, E.W. (1999). Potential mechanisms of susceptibility to periodontitis in tobacco smokers. *Journal of Periodontal Research* **34**, 363–369.

Palmer, R.M., Stapleton, J.A., Sutherland, G., Coward, P.Y., Wilson, R.F. & Scott, D.A. (2002). Effect of nicotine replacement and quitting smoking on circulating adhesion molecule profiles (sICAM-1, sCD44v5, sCD44v6). *European Journal of Clinical Investigation* **32**, 852–857.

Palmer, R.M., Wilson, R.F., Hasan, A.S. & Scott, D.A. (2005) Mechanisms of action of environmental factors – tobacco smoking. *Journal of Clinical Periodontology* **32** (Suppl 6), 180–195.

Payne, J.B., Zachs, N.R., Reinhardt, R.A., Nummikoski, P.V. & Patil, K. (1997). The association between oestrogen status and alveolar bone density changes in post-menopausal women with a history of periodontitis. *Journal of Periodontology* **68**, 24–31.

Persson, L., Bergstrom, J., Gustafsson, A. & Åsman, B. (1999). Tobacco smoking and gingival neutrophil activity in young adults. *Journal of Clinical Periodontology* **26**, 9–13.

Petropoulos, G., McKay, I. & Hughes, F. (2004). The association between neutrophil numbers and interleukin-1α concentrations in gingival crevicular fluid of smokers and non-smokers with periodontal disease. *Journal of Clinical Periodontology* **31**, 390–395.

Pihlstrom, B.L., Michalowicz, B.S. & Johnson N.W. (2005). Periodontal diseases. *Lancet* **366**, 1809–1820.

Pindborg, J.J. (1947). Tobacco and gingivitis. I. Statistical examination of the significance of tobacco in the development of ulceromembranous gingivitis and in the formation of calculus. *Journal of Dental Research* **26**, 261–264.

Pindborg, J.J. (1949). Tobacco and gingivitis. II Correlation between consumption of tobacco, ulceromembranous gingivitis and calculus. *Journal of Dental Research* **28**, 460–463.

Piwowar, A., Knapik-Kordecka, M. & Warwas, M. (2000). Concentrations of leukocyte elastase in plasma and polymorphonuclear neutrophil extracts in type 2 diabetes. *Clinical Chemistry & Laboratory Medicine* **38**, 1257–1261.

Poggi, P., Rota, M. & Boratto, R. (2002). Volatile fraction of cigarette smoke induces alterations in the human gingival fibroblast skeleton. *Journal of Periodontal Research* **37**, 230–235.

Powell J.T. (1998). Vascular damage from smoking: disease mechanisms at the arterial wall. *Vascular Medicine* **3**, 21–28.

Preber, H. & Bergstrom, J. (1985). Occurrence of gingival bleeding in smoker and non-smoker patients. *Acta Odontologica Scandinavica* **43**, 315–320.

Preber, H. & Bergstrom, J. (1986). The effect of non-surgical treatment on periodontal pockets in smokers and non-smokers. *Journal of Clinical Periodontology* **13**, 319–323.

Preber, H., Bergstrom, J. & Linder, L.E. (1992). Occurrence of periopathogens in smoker and non-smoker patients. *Journal of Clinical Periodontology* **19**, 667–671.

Preshaw, P.M., Heasman, L., Stacey, F., Steen, N., McCracken, G.I. & Heasman, P.A. (2005). The effect of quit smoking on chronic periodontitis. *Journal of Clinical Periodontology* **32**, 869–879.

Quinn, S.M., Zhang, J.B., Gunsolley, J.C., Schenkein, J.G., Schenkein, H.A. & Tew, J.G. (1996). Influence of smoking and race on immunoglobulin G subclass concentrations in early-onset periodontitis patients. *Infection & Immunity* **64**, 2500–2505.

Quinn, S.M., Zhang, J.B., Gunsolley, J.C., Schenkein, H.A. & Tew, J.G. (1998). The influence of smoking and race on adult periodontitis and serum 1gG2 levels. *Journal of Periodontology* **69**, 171–177.

Raber-Durlacher, J.E., Leene, W., Palmer-Bouva, C.C.R., Raber, J. & Abraham-Inpijn, L. (1993). Experimental gingivitis during pregnancy and post-partum: Immunological aspects. *Journal of Periodontology* **64**, 211–218.

Rahman, Z.A. & Soory, M. (2006). Antioxidant effects of glutathione and IGF in a hyperglycaemic cell culture model of fibroblasts: Some actions of advanced glycaemic end products and nicotine. *Endocrine, Metabolic & Immune Disorders – Drug Targets* **6** (3), 279–286.

Rawlinson, A., Grummit, J., Walsh, T. & Douglas, I. (2003). Interleukin-1 and receptor antagonist levels in gingival crevicular fluid in heavy smokers versus non-smokers. *Journal of Clinical Periodontology* **30**, 42–48.

Raulin, L.A., McPherson, J.C., McQuade, M.J. & Hanson, B.S. (1988). The effect of nicotine on the attachment of human fibroblasts to glass and human root surfaces in vitro. *Journal of Periodontology* **59**, 318–325.

Rezavandi, K., Palmer, R.M., Odell, E.W., Scott, D.A. & Wilson, R.F. (2001). Expression of E-Selectin and ICAM-1 in gingival tissues of smokers and non-smokers with periodontitis. *Journal of Oral Pathology and Medicine* **31**, 59–64.

Rigotti, N.A. (1989). Cigarette smoking and body weight. *New England Journal of Medicine* **320**, 931–933.

Salvi, G.E., Yalda, B., Collins, J.G., Jones, B.H., Smith, F.W., Arnold, R.R. & Offenbacher, S. (1997). Inflammatory mediator response as a potential risk marker for periodontal diseases in insulin-dependent diabetes mellitus patients. *Journal of Periodontology* **68**, 127–135.

Saremi, A., Nelson, R.G., Tulloch-Reid, M., Hanson, R.L., Sievers, M.L., Taylor, G.W., Shlossman, M., Bennet, P.H., Genco, R. & Knowler, W.C. (2005). Periodontal disease and mortality in Type 2 Diabetes. *Diabetes Care* **28**, 27–32.

Sastrowijoto, S.H., van der Velden, U., van Steenbergen, T.J.M. et al. (1990). Improved metabolic control, clinical periodontal status and subgingival microbiology in insulin-dependent diabetes mellitus. A prospective study. *Journal of Clinical Periodontology* **17**, 233–242.

Schmidt, A.M., Weidman, E., Lalla, E. et al. (1996). Advanced glycation end products (AGEs) induce oxidant stress in the gingiva: a potential mechanism underlying accelerated periodontal disease associated with diabetes. *Journal of Periodontal Research* **31**, 508–515.

Scott, D.A., Palmer, R.M. & Stapleton, J.A. (2001). Validation of smoking status in clinical research into inflammatory periodontal disease: a review. *Journal of Clinical Periodontology* **28**, 712–722.

Scott, D.A., Stapleton, J.A., Wilson, R.F. et al. (2000b). Dramatic decline in circulating intercellular adhesion molecule-1 concentration on quitting tobacco smoking. *Blood Cells, Molecules and Diseases* **26**, 255–258.

Scott, D.A., Todd, D.H., Wilson, R.F. et al. (2000a). The acute influence of tobacco smoking on adhesion molecule expression on monocytes and neutrophils and on circulating adhesion molecule levels in vivo. *Addiction Biology* **5**, 195–205.

Seppala, B. & Ainamo, J. (1996). Dark field microscopy of the subgingival microflora in insulin-dependent diabetes. *Journal of Clinical Periodontology* **23**, 63–67.

Shapiro, S., Bomberg, J., Benson, B.W. et al. (1985). Postmenopausal osteoporosis: dental patients at risk. *Gerodontics* **1**, 220–225.

Sheiham, A. (1971) Periodontal disease and oral cleanliness in tobacco smokers. *Journal of Periodontology* **42**, 259–263.

Silness, J. & Loe, H. (1963). Periodontal disease in pregnancy. II. Correlation between oral hygiene and periodontal condition. *Acta Odontologica Scandinavica* **22**, 121–135.

Slavkin, H.C. (1997). Diabetes, clinical dentistry and changing paradigms. *Journal of the American Dental Association* **128**, 638–644.

Sooriyamoorthy, M. & Gower, D.B. (1989). Hormonal influences on gingival tissue: relationship to periodontal disease. *Journal of Clinical Periodontology* **16**, 201–208.

Soory, M. (2000a). Hormonal factors in periodontal disease. *Dental Update* **27**, 380–383.

Soory, M. (2000b). Targets for steroid hormone mediated actions of periodontal pathogens, cytokines and therapeutic agents: some implications on tissue turnover in the periodontium. *Current Drug Targets* **1**, 309–325.

Soory, M (2002). Hormone mediation of immune responses in the progression of diabetes, rheumatoid arthritis and periodontal diseases. *Current Drug Targets – Immune Endocrine & Metabolic Disorders* **2**, 13–25.

Soory, M (2004). Biomarkers of diabetes mellitus and rheumatoid arthritis associated with oxidative stress, applicable to periodontal diseases. *Current Topics in Steroid Research* **4**, 1–17.

Soory, M. & Tilakaratne, A. (2003). Anabolic potential of fibroblasts from chronically inflamed gingivae grown in hyperglycaemic culture medium in the presence or absence of insulin and nicotine. *Journal of Periodontology* **74**, 1771–1777.

Sopori, M.L. & Kozak, W. (1998). Immunomodulatory effects of cigarette smoke. *Journal of Neuroimmunology* **83**, 148–156.

Sorensen, L.T., Nielsen, H.B., Kharazmi, A. & Gottrup, F. (2004). Effect of smoking and abstention on oxidative burst and reactivity of neutrophils and monocytes. *Surgery* **136**, 1047–1053.

Sorsa, T., Ingman, T., Suomalainen, K. *et al.* (1992). Cellular source and tetracycline inhibition of gingival crevicular fluid collagenase of patients with labile diabetes mellitus. *Journal of Clinical Periodontology* **19**, 146–149.

Staffolani, N., Guerra, M. & Pugliese, M. (1989). Hormonal receptors in gingival inflammation. *Minerva Stomatologica* **38**, 823–826.

Stewart, J.E., Wager, K.A., Friedlander, A.H. & Zadeh, H.H. (2001). The effect of periodontal treatment on glycaemic control in patients with type 2 diabetes mellitus. *Journal of Clinical Periodontology* **28**, 306–310.

Sultan, C., Loire, C. & Kern, P. (1986). Collagen and hormone steroids. *Annals of Biological Clinics* **44**, 285–288.

Sutcliffe, P. (1972). A longitudinal study of gingivitis and puberty. *Journal of Periodontal Research* **7**, 52–58.

Szopa, T.M., Titchener, P.A., Portwood, N.D. & Taylor, K.W. (1993). Diabetes mellitus due to viruses – some recent developments. *Diabetologia* **36**, 687–695.

Takahashi, K., Tsuboyama, T., Matsushita, M. *et al.* (1994). Effective intervention of low peak bone mass and bone remodelling in the spontaneous murine model of senile osteoporosis, SAM-P/6, by Ca supplement and hormone treatment. *Bone* **15**, 209–215.

Tanur, E., McQuade, M., McPherson, J., Al-Hashami, I. & Rivera-Hidalgo, F. (2000). Effects of nicotine on the strength of gingival fibroblasts to glass and non-diseased human root surfaces. *Journal of Periodontology* **71**, 717–722.

Taylor, G.W., Burt, B.A., Becker, M.P. *et al.* (1996). Severe periodontitis and risk for poor glycemic control in patients with non-insulin-dependent diabetes mellitus. *Journal of Periodontology* **67** (Suppl), 1085–1093.

Tervonen, T. & Karjalainen, K. (1997). Periodontal disease related to diabetic status. A pilot study of the response to periodontal therapy in Type 1 diabetes. *Journal of Clinical Periodontology* **24**, 505–510.

Tervonen, T. & Oliver, R. (1993). Long-term control of diabetes mellitus and periodontitis. *Journal of Clinical Periodontology* **20**, 431–435.

Thorstensson, H., Kuylenstierna, J. & Hugoson, A. (1996). Medical status and complications in relation to periodontal disease experience in insulin-dependent diabetics. *Journal of Clinical Periodontology* **23**, 194–202.

Tiainen, L., Asikainen, S. & Saxen, L. (1992). Puberty-associated gingivitis. *Community Dentistry & Oral Epidemiology* **20**, 87–89.

Tilakaratne, A. & Soory, M. (1999). Modulation of androgen metabolism by oestradiol-17β and progesterone, alone and in combination, in human gingival fibroblasts in culture. *Journal of Periodontology* **70**, 1017–1025.

Tilakaratne, A., Soory, M., Ranasinghe, A.W., Corea, S.M.X., Ekanayake, S.L. & De Silva, M. (2000a). Periodontal disease status during pregnancy and 3 months post-partum in a rural population of Sri-Lankan women. *Journal of Clinical Periodontology* **27**, 787–792.

Tilakaratne, A., Soory, M., Ranasinghe, A.W., Corea, S.M.X., Ekanayake, S.L. & De Silva, M. (2000b). Effects of hormonal contraceptives on the periodontium in a population of rural Sri-Lankan women. *Journal of Clinical Periodontology* **27**, 753–757.

Tipton, D.A. & Dabbous, M.K. (1995). Effects of nicotine on proliferation and extracellular matrix production of human gingival fibroblasts in vitro. *Journal of Periodontology* **66**, 1056–1064.

Tonetti, M.S. (1998). Cigarette smoking and periodontal diseases: etiology and management of disease. *Annals of Periodontology* **3**, 88–101.

Tonetti, M.S., Pini-Prato, G. & Cortellini, P. (1995). Effect of cigarette smoking on periodontal healing following GTR in infrabony defects. A preliminary retrospective study. *Journal of Clinical Periodontology* **22**, 229–234.

Ueta, E., Osaki, T., Yoneda, K. & Yamamoto, T. (1993). Prevalence of diabetes mellitus in odontogenic infections and oral candidiasis: an analysis of neutrophil suppression. *Journal of Oral Pathology and Medicine* **22**, 168–174.

UKPDS (1998a). UK Prospective Diabetes Study Group. Intensive blood-glucose control with sulfonylureas or insulin compared with conventional treatment and risk of complications in patients with Type 2 diabetes. *Lancet* **352**, 837–853.

UKPDS (1998b). UK Prospective Diabetes Study Group. Effect of intensive blood-glucose control with metformin on complications in overweight patients with Type 2 diabetes. *Lancet* **352**, 854–865.

Ulrich, P. & Cerami, A. (2001). Protein glycation, diabetes and aging. *Recent Progress in Hormone Research* **56**, 1–21.

van der Velden, U., Varoufaki, A., Hutter, J., Xu, L., Timmerman, M., van Winkelhoff, A. & Loos, B. (2003). Effect of smoking and periodontal treatment on subgingival microflora. *Journal of Clinical Periodontology* **30**, 603–610.

van Winkelhoff. A.J., Bosch-Tijhof, C.J., Winkel, E.G. & van der Reijden, W.A. (2001). Smoking affects the subgingival microflora in periodontitis. *Journal of Periodontology* **72**, 666–671.

Vittek, J., Munnangi, P.R., Gordon, G.G., Rappaport, S.G. & Southren, A.L. (1982). Progesterone receptors in human gingiva. *IRCS, Medical Science* **10**, 381.

Wall, M.A., Johnson, J., Jacob, P. & Benowitz, NL (1988). Cotinine in the serum, saliva and urine of nonsmokers, passive smokers and active smokers. *American Journal of Public Health* **78**, 699–701.

Wang, P.H., Chao, H.T., Lee, W.L., Yuan, C.C. & Ng, H.T. (1997). Severe bleeding from a pregnancy tumour. A case report. *Journal of Reproductive Medicine* **42**, 359–362.

Westfelt, E., Rylander, H., Blohme, G., Joanasson, P. & Lindhe, J. (1996). The effect of periodontal therapy in diabetes. *Journal of Clinical Periodontology* **23**, 92–100.

Westhoff, C.L. (1996). Oral contraceptives and venous thromboembolism: should epidemiological associations drive clinical decision making? *Contraception* **54**, 1–3.

Whitehead, M.I. & Lobo, R.A. (1988). Progestogen use in postmenopausal women. Consensus conference. *Lancet* **ii**, 1243–1244.

Yki-Jarvinen, H., Sammalkorpi, K., Koivisto, V.A. & Nikkila, E.A. (1989). Severity, duration and mechanisms of insulin resistance during acute infections. *Journal of Clinical Endocrinology and Metabolism* **69**, 317–323.

Zachariasen, R.D. (1993). The effect of elevated ovarian hormones on periodontal health: oral contraceptives and pregnancy. *Women and Health* **20**, 21–30.

Zambon, J.J., Grossi, S.G., Machtei, E.E., Ho, A.W., Dunford, R. & Genco, R.J. (1996). Cigarette smoking increases the risk for subgingival infection with periodontal pathogens. *Journal of Periodontology* **67**, 1050–1054.

Zambon, J.J., Reynolds, H., Fisher, J.G., Shlossman, M., Dunford, R. & Genco, R.J. (1988). Microbiological and immunological studies of adult periodontitis in patients with non-insulin dependent diabetes mellitus. *Journal of Periodontology* **59**, 23–31.

Chapter 13

Susceptibility

Bruno G. Loos, Ubele van der Velden, and Marja L. Laine

Introduction

Periodontitis is a chronic infectious disease of the supporting tissues of the teeth. Due to the bacterial infection, the periodontal tissues become inflamed and are slowly destroyed by the action of the inflammatory process. If left untreated, the teeth lose their ligamentous support to the alveolar bone, become mobile, and are eventually lost.

Periodontitis is considered to be a complex disease. Common features of complex human diseases (for example Alzheimer's disease, Crohn's disease, and cardiovascular diseases) are that these conditions present mostly with a relatively mild phenotype, and are slowly progressive and chronic in nature (Tabor *et al.* 2002). Furthermore, these types of disease are of relatively late onset (mostly adult onset) and relatively common. The pathophysiology of complex diseases is characterized by various biological pathways, leading to similar clinical phenomena. Importantly, complex diseases are associated with variations in multiple genes, each having a small overall contribution and relative risk for the disease process. Complex diseases are typically polygenic, i.e. multiple genes play each a limited role (low penetrance genes); the disease genes in complex diseases are therefore considered disease-modifying genes (Hart *et al.* 2000b). Analogous to other complex diseases, we estimate that for periodontitis, at least 10 and as many as 20 disease-modifying genes may be involved. However, it is important to realize that the number

and type of disease-modifying genes for the same condition may not be equal for different forms of periodontitis and different ethnic populations; they are also influenced by environmental factors (gene–environment interactions).

Disease-modifying genes contrast to major disease genes. Aberrant allelic forms (see Box 13-1) of major genes are responsible for disease expression according to Mendel's laws (Hart *et al.* 2000b). For example, the fatal inherited disease cystic fibrosis is caused by a recessive mutation in the cystic fibrosis transmembrane conductance regulator (*CFTR*) gene (Brennan & Geddes 2002). This gene encodes for a protein that functions as a plasma membrane chloride channel in epithelial tissues, in particular in lung epithelium. If a person is homozygous for the *rare* disease allele (*R*-allele), then he/she will develop cystic fibrosis. On the other hand, individuals will not develop the disease if they are homozygous for the *normal (N)* allele (so called *wild type*) or when they are heterozygous, i.e. they have both the dominant *N*-allele and the recessive *R*-allele.

A genetic component in the etiology of periodontal disease was proposed as early as 1935 (reviewed in Loevy 1976). From the late 1990s a substantial increase in papers on putative genetic risk factors for susceptibility to and severity of periodontitis has appeared in the periodontal literature (Michalowicz *et al.* 1991; Hart 1994; Hart & Kornman 1997; Hart *et al.* 1997, 2000b; Page 1999; Page & Sturdivant 2002). The presence of genetic risk factors directly increases

Box 13-1 Human genes, polymorphisms and other definitions

Each normal human being has 23 pairs of chromosomes (the diploid human genome), 22 pairs of *autosomal* chromosomes and 1 pair of sex chromosomes (XX for females and XY for males) (Fig. 13-1). From each pair, one chromosome is inherited from the father and one from the mother. Chromosomes show differences in size and have characteristic lateral series of bands (G-banding); therefore each chromosome can be identified by its characteristic size and banding pattern.

Each chromosome contains a long duplex of deoxyribonucleic acid (DNA). DNA consists of chemically linked sequences of nucleotides; these are the "building blocks" of the DNA and always contain a nitrogenous base. Four nitrogenous bases exist: adenine (A), guanine (G), cytosine (C), and thymine (T). The bases are linked to a sugar (2-deoxyribose), where a phosphate group is also added. The *haploid* human genome (i.e. one copy of 22 autosomal chromosomes and one sex chromosome) consist of 3.3×10^9 nucleotides (also written as 3.3×10^9 base pairs (bp)). In the chromosomes, DNA is arranged in a double helix model: two polynucleotide chains in the duplex are associated together by hydrogen bonding between the nitrogenous bases. These reactions are described as base pairing and they are complementary: G pairs only with C, and A pairs only with T. Therefore, if one chain of DNA is sequenced, the complementary chain of the duplex can be deduced.

DNA contains the genetic code and a given specific sequence of nucleotides encodes for the sequence of amino acids that constitutes the corresponding protein (Fig. 13-2). The genetic code is read in groups of three nucleotides; each trinucleotide sequence (triplet) is called a codon. Written in the conventional direction from left to right, the nucleotide sequence of the DNA strand, a gene can be deciphered. A gene consists of two parts (Fig. 13-2): (1) a *coding region*, i.e. a reading frame starting at nucleotide position +1, containing a multitude of triplets that codes for a sequence of amino acids to form a protein; and (2) a *promoter region*, i.e. a sequence of nucleotides upstream (left) of the coding region starting with nucleotide position −1 read from right to left, that is not organized in a series of triplets but contains stretches of nucleotides that are essential for the regulation of the transcription of the coding region. Within the coding region intermittent areas of non-coding DNA exist; these regions are called introns. The true coding areas within the coding region are called exons (Fig. 13-2). From the recent results of the human genome project, it is estimated that about 25 000 human genes exist.

Variant forms (polymorphisms) of a gene that can occupy a specific chromosal site *(locus)* are called *alleles*. Two or more alleles for a given locus may exist in nature throughout evolution, but may develop at any time. A *polymorphic* locus is one whose alleles are such that the most common, *normal* variant (*N*-allele) among them occurs with <99% frequency in the population. Thus, if a locus is for example *bi-allelic*, the *rarer* allele (designated *R*-allele) must occur with a frequency >1% in the population. In this way, when different alleles of a given gene co-exist in the human population, we speak about *genetic polymorphisms*.

Polymorphisms arise as a result of gene mutations. All organisms undergo spontaneous mutations as a result of normal cellular function or random interactions with the environment. An alteration that changes only a single base pair is called a point mutation. Not all point mutations are repaired and can therefore be transmitted by inheritance through generations. The most common class of point mutations is the *transition*, comprising the substitution of a G-C (guanine–cytosine) pair with an A-T (adenine–thymine) pair or vice versa. The variation at the site harboring such changes has recently been termed a "single nucleotide polymorphism" (SNP) (Schork *et al.* 2000).

The SNP may have no effects or may have some important biological effects. For example, if a transition has taken place within the coding region of a gene, it may result in an amino acid substitution and therefore an altered protein structure, which may then alter its function. Or, when such mutations have taken place in the promoter region of the gene, it may alter gene regulation, for example resulting in (completely) inhibited or reduced gene expression or, alternatively, result in over-expression of the gene, perhaps with biological consequences. SNPs occur more frequently than any other type of genetic polymorphism; the frequency of SNPs across the human genome is estimated at every 0.3–1 kilobases (Kb).

Other SNPs result from *insertions* or *deletions*. The simple form of this polymorphism is where a single nucleotide pair may be deleted or may be inserted with the same potential effects as described above for the *transition*. Another common type of insertion/deletion polymorphism is the existence of variable numbers of repeated bases or nucleotide patterns in a genetic region. Repeated base patterns can consist of several hundreds of base pairs, known as "variable number of tandem repeats" (VNTRs or *mini-satellites*). Also common are *micro-satellites*, which consist of two, three or four nucleotide repeats, on a variable number of occasions.

(Continued)

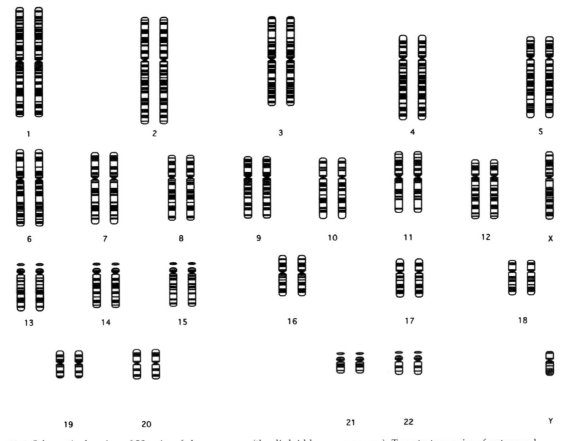

Fig. 13-1 Schematic drawing of 23 pairs of chromosomes (the diploid human genome). Twenty-two pairs of autosomal chromosomes and one pair of sex chromosomes are present. In this case the genome of a male is shown (one X and one Y chromosome). In the case of a female, two X chromosomes would have been present. G-banding generates a characteristic lateral series of bands in each member of the chromosome set. Adapted from Hart *et al.* (2000a).

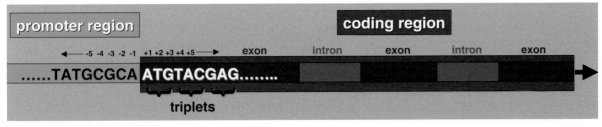

Fig. 13-2 Schematic representation of a gene. The gene consists of a promoter and a coding region. Within the coding region, intermittent areas of non-coding DNA exist (intron). Exons contain triplets of nucleotides (codons) that code for a specific amino acid. The number and length of exons and introns within the coding region is variable per gene. Nucleotides are numbered throughout the whole coding region starting with number 1 for the first nucleotide. The nucleotides in the promoter region are also numbered, starting with −1.

the probability of periodontal disease developing, and, if they are absent, this possibility is reduced. Genetic risk factors are part of the causal chain, or expose the host to the causal chain. Notably, it may be possible that an allele, which is originally defined as *R*-allele, is associated with absence of disease; in such cases, the *R*-allele could be considered protective.

Evidence for the role of genetics in periodontitis

In the past it was thought that periodontitis would eventually develop in subjects with a longstanding history of poor oral hygiene and gingivitis. However, during the last decades the concept of high-risk groups was introduced. This concept arose on the basis of the results from epidemiologic studies as well as from longitudinal clinical studies and has been one of the factors that supported the development of the theory that periodontitis may have a genetic background.

A study from 1966 is one of the earliest studies from which it could be deduced that certain individuals are more at risk for periodontitis than others (Trott & Cross 1966). In this study the principal reasons for tooth extractions in over 1800 subjects were investigated. The figures showed that in each age category the percentage of teeth lost due to periodontal disease is always higher than the percentages of patients who lost teeth due to periodontal disease. This means that relatively many teeth are lost in relatively few patients. This phenomenon could be confirmed in a 28 year longitudinal study of an American population. It was found that in a group of subjects who had a full dentition at a mean age of 28 years, 28 years later 22% of the subjects were responsible for 77% of all teeth lost (Burt *et al.* 1990). The same phenomenon was found in two longitudinal studies evaluating the effect of periodontal therapy in periodontitis patients over more than 15 years (Hirschfeld & Wasserman 1978; McFall 1982). These studies showed that 20% of the patient populations accounted for about 75% of all lost teeth. The concept of high risk for the development of periodontitis was further confirmed in longitudinal studies investigating the natural history of periodontal disease. In a Sri Lankan population without dental care and absence of oral hygiene, investigators (Löe *et al.* 1986) were able to identify three subpopulations: a group with no progression (11%), a group with moderate progression (81%), and a group with rapid progression of periodontal breakdown (8%). In a recent study the initiation and progression of periodontal breakdown was studied in a population deprived from regular dental care in a remote village on Western Java (van der Velden *et al.* 2006). The authors found that 20% of the subjects developed severe breakdown whereas the remaining population developed minor to moderate breakdown.

The phenomenon that a relatively small proportion of the population is at risk for developing severe forms of periodontitis may suggest that not everybody is equally susceptible to periodontitis. The microbial causation of inflammatory periodontal diseases is well established (Löe *et al.* 1965; Socransky & Haffajee 1992). In addition the prevalence and proportions of periodontal pathogens are higher in periodontitis patients compared to healthy controls (Griffen *et al.* 1998; van Winkelhoff *et al.* 2002). However if periodontitis is simply and solely caused by one or more specific periodontal pathogens, the disease should develop in the majority of subjects infected by these organisms. In contrast, periodontal pathogens show a relatively high prevalence in subjects with gingivitis or minor periodontitis. For example, it was found in a large group of subjects with gingivitis or minor periodontitis (mean age 52 years) that there was a prevalence of 38% for *Aggregatibacter actinomycetemcomitans*, 32% for *Porphyromonas gingivalis*, and 42% for *Prevotella intermedia* (Wolff *et al.* 1993). Therefore the existence of high-risk groups cannot be explained by the microbiology alone. There are, however, other factors that may play a major role in the development of periodontitis, i.e. the inflammatory and immune response both locally and systemically. These factors include systemic diseases, such as diabetes, and environmental factors, such as smoking and possible stress (Kinane *et al.* 2006). It is likely that the effectiveness of an individual's immune response influences the extent of periodontal destruction, which can be regarded as the susceptiblity of a subject to periodontitis.

Heritability of aggressive periodontitis (early onset periodontitis)

Some time ago it was recognized that siblings of patients with juvenile periodontitis (JP) frequently also suffer from periodontitis. This was mainly based on case reports of one or a few families ascertained on the basis of one subject (the proband) with JP. In an American study on 77 siblings of 39 probands with localized (L) or generalized (G) JP, it was shown that almost 50% of the siblings also suffered from JP (Boughman *et al.* 1992). In 11 families a co-occurrence of LJP and GJP was present. As an epidemiological survey in the US showed that the prevalence of JP varies between 0.16 and 2.49% (Löe & Brown 1991), the high prevalence of JP in these families suggests a genetic background for the disease.

The largest JP family study included 227 probands with aggressive periodontitis (Marazita *et al.* 1994). There were 26 GJP individuals whose earlier records were consistent with LJP, i.e. demonstrating progression from the localized to a more generalized form. Furthermore, there were 16 families with co-occurrence of LJP and GJP, confirming the findings of Boughman *et al.* (1992). Out of the 227 probands, 104 had at least one first-degree relative clinically examined. Now it was possible to carry out a segregation analysis on 100 families (four families each had two probands). Segregation analysis is a formal method of studying families with a disease to assess the likelihood that the condition is inherited as a genetic trait. The family members included 527 subjects: 60 with LJP, 72 with GJP, 254 unaffected subjects, and 141 subjects with an unknown periodontal condition. The group of unaffected subjects included edentulous subjects, subjects with adult periodontitis, and periodontally healthy subjects. The majority of the families were of African American origin. The authors concluded that the most likely mode of inheritance was autosomal dominant in both African American and Caucasian kindred, with penetrance of 70% in African Americans and 73% in Caucasians.

Heritability of chronic periodontitis (adult periodontitis)

Very few investigations exist with regard to family studies of probands with chronic (adult) periodontitis or younger subjects with minor periodontitis. In an early study of nuclear families, path models were used to investigate the relative influences of genetic and environmental factors in a large Hawaiian population in the age range of 14 to over 60 years (Chung et al. 1977). They concluded that the data failed to detect significant heritability, and common family environment proved to be a major determinant in the variation of periodontal health. In a periodontal study of families in the US published in 1993, 75 families consisting of 178 subjects largely <40 years of age were investigated (Beaty et al. 1993). To determine familiar aggregation, standard familial correlations were computed, i.e. father–mother, parent–offspring, sibling–sibling, etc. The results showed a statistically significant family effect for mean plaque index, but not for mean gingival index and mean attachment loss. Both the gingival index and attachment loss showed a stronger correlation between mothers and offspring compared to fathers and offspring. Yet another study analyzed the periodontal condition in an untreated population in Guatemala consisting of 109 siblings from 40 nuclear families with an age range of 35–60 years (Dowsett et al. 2002). They failed to show a familial clustering for periodontal disease.

The effect of sibling relationship on the periodontal condition was investigated in an epidemiologic study of a group of young Indonesians deprived of regular dental care (van der Velden et al. 1993). The study population included 23 family units consisting of three or more siblings. In all, 78 subjects aged 15–25 years were studied. The results of the analysis showed a significant sibling relationship effect for plaque, calculus, and loss of attachment but not for pocket depth. In order to study familial aspects of chronic (adult) periodontitis in a Dutch population, 24 families were selected at the Academic Center for

Dentistry, Amsterdam (Petit et al. 1994), each consisting of a proband with chronic (adult) periodontitis, a spouse and one to three children. The mean age of the probands was 39 years, with a range from 30–50 years. In total 49 children were investigated with an age range of 3 months to 15 years. The results showed that none of the children under the age of 5 years was affected by periodontitis, whereas in the group of 5–15 years, 21% had at least 1 pocket ≥5 mm in conjunction with loss of attachment. In the group of 10–15 years this was 45%. This contrasts with the results of a cross-sectional epidemiological study carried out in the city of Amsterdam; it was shown that the prevalence of pockets ≥5 mm in conjunction with loss of attachment in 15-year-old adolescents is about 5% (van der Velden et al. 1989). Thus, and on the basis of the Petit et al. (1994) study, it can be suggested that chronic (adult) periodontitis may aggregate in families.

A gene mutation with major effect on human disease and its association with periodontitis

This chapter focuses mainly on putative genetic risk factors that have been identified by the candidate gene approach, i.e. investigators have plausible arguments of a conceptual, biologic, and epidemiologic nature to investigate the association of the selected genetic polymorphism(s) with periodontitis. Nevertheless, by linkage analysis in specific families with several generations available and having among them one or more proband(s) with a strong disease phenotype, new disease genes may still be identified. Before the candidate genes and their respective genetic polymorphisms are explored in their association with periodontitis, we first discuss the discovery of a major disease gene associated with prepubertal periodontitis and Papillon-Lefèvre syndrome (PLS).

Periodontitis is recognized as a component of many single gene syndromes (Kinane & Hart 2003). Many of these disorders are characterized either by immune or structural deficiencies; of these syndromic disorders, PLS is relatively unique, in that periodontitis forms a significant component of the disease along with hyperkeratosis of the palms of the hands and soles of the feet.

The gene mutated in PLS was mapped to a specific band on the long arm of chromosome 11 (Fischer et al. 1997; Laass et al. 1997; Hart et al. 1998). Subsequently, this location was refined and a candidate gene within this region was identified that encoded for the lysosomal protease cathepsin C: the *CTSC* gene (Toomes et al. 1999). Cathepsin C is a proteinase, which is found in neutrophils and lymphocytes as well as in epithelial cells. Toomes et al. (1999) elucidated its genomic organization, demonstrated mutations in the *CTSC* gene in eight families, and showed that these mutations result in an almost complete loss of function of the enzyme. This was immediately con-

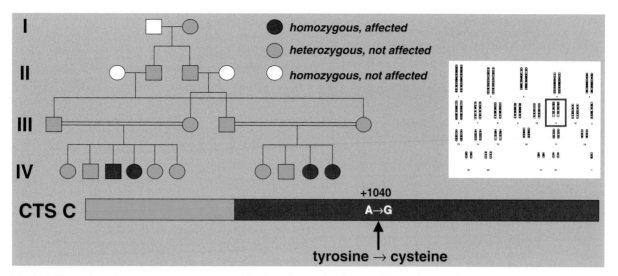

Fig. 13-3 Through an internal marriage event in a family of Jordanian descent, Hart and co-workers have identified and localized a gene on chromosome 11 that is responsible for a severe form of prepubertal periodontitis (Hart *et al.* 2000a). Starting with four affected children from generation IV of two families, a disease causing *R*-allele of the cathepsin C (CTS C) gene was discovered. Cathepsin C is a proteinase which is found in neutrophils and lymphocytes as well as epithelial cells. Affected children, but not their brothers and sisters, were homozygous for an A to G transition polymorphism at gene position +1040. This resulted in a substitution of the amino acid tyrosine by a cysteine. This polymorphism was shown to be functional as there was a decreased cathepsin C activity (Hart *et al.* 2000a). However, the mechanism by which an altered function of cathepsin C plays a role in the pathogenesis of the prepubertal form of periodontitis is unknown.

firmed (Hart *et al.* 1999) and Hart and co-workers demonstrated similar mutations in other families. To date more than 40 mutations have been reported in the *CTSC* gene (Selvaraju *et al.* 2003; de Haar *et al.* 2004; Noack *et al.* 2004). Furthermore, interesting data from analyses in a single family with four different *CTSC* mutations were reported (Hewitt *et al.* 2004) and the investigators proposed that minimal cathepsin C activity (~13%) was necessary to prevent the clinical features of PLS. However, the exact mechanism by which an altered function of cathepsin C plays a role in the pathogenesis of the prepubertal form of periodontitis is unknown.

CTSC mutations have also been identified in families with prepubertal periodontitis suggesting that this condition is allelic to PLS (Hart *et al.* 2000a) (Fig. 13-3). However, these mutations are not different to those observed in classical PLS and, notably, all cases of prepubertal periodontitis do not have mutations in *CTSC*. This suggests that prepubertal periodontitis is a genetically heterogeneous condition with some cases representing a variant of PLS (Hewitt *et al.* 2004). There has also been speculation that polymorphic functional variants of *CTSC* may be involved in the more common type of aggressive periodontitis. However, given that carriers of a mutant copy of the gene are phenotypically unaffected and that very little cathepsin C activity appears to be necessary in order to prevent the disease, this seems an unlikely hypothesis. Indeed, evidence against this hypothesis was provided (Hewitt *et al.* 2004); it was shown that there was no difference in cathepsin C activity between 30 cases of aggressive periodontitis and controls.

Disease-modifying genes in relation to periodontitis

Periodontitis develops in a limited subset of humans. About 10–15% of the population will develop severe forms of destructive periodontal disease. The disease is importantly influenced by the microorganisms in the subgingival biofilm, by acquired systemic diseases that reduce or hamper an "optimal" host response, and by environmental factors. Specific bacteria in the microbial biofilm and smoking are accepted as true rather than putative risk factors. On top of the above risk factors are disease-modifying genes, which contribute to susceptibility and severity of periodontitis. For these disease-modifying genes, Mendelian principles do not apply (Hart 1996; Hart *et al.* 2000b), because both heterozygous and homozygous subjects for a given disease-modifying gene may not necessarily develop the disease; other genetic risk factors (gene–gene interactions) and/or environmental risk factors (gene–environmental interactions) also need to be present simultaneously (definition of complex disease).

Currently, very little is known about which genes may be involved in periodontitis as disease-modifying genes. Table 13-1 summarizes the candidate gene polymorphisms investigated in relation to periodontitis. It is clear from this summary that, as the immune system plays a crucial role in the pathogenesis of periodontitis, researchers have concentrated on the identification of genetic polymorphisms in several aspects of host immunity.

Below we summarize the epidemiological findings in various studies of candidate genes as risk

---

Table 13-1 Summary of candidate genes, and the corresponding encoded proteins, for which gene polymorphisms have been investigated as putative risk factors for periodontitis

Gene	Coded protein
ACE	Angiotensin-converting enzyme
CARD15 (NOD2)	Caspase recruitment domain-15
CCR5	Chemokine receptor-5
CD14	CD-14
ER2	Estrogen receptor-2
ET1	Endothelin-1
FBR	Fibrinogen
FcγRIIa	Fc γ receptor IIa
FcγRIIb	Fc γ receptor IIb
FcγRIIIa	Fc γ receptor IIIa
FcγRIIIb	Fc γ receptor IIIb
FPR1	N-formylpeptide receptor-1
IFNGR1	Interferon γ receptor-1
IL1A	Interleukin-1α
IL1B	Interleukin-1β
IL1RN	Interleukin-1 receptor antagonist
IL2	Interleukin-2
IL4	Interleukin-4
IL6	Interleukin-6
IL10	Interleukin-10
LTA	Lymphotoxin-α
MMP1	Matrix metalloproteinase-1
MMP3	Matrix metalloproteinase-3
MMP9	Matrix metalloproteinase-9
MPO	Myeloperoxidase
NAT2	N-acetyltransferase-2
PAI1	Plasminogen-activator-inhibitor-1
RAGE	Receptor for advanced glycation end products
TGFB	Transforming growth factor-β
TIMP2	Tissue inhibitor of matrix metalloproteinase
TLR2	Toll-like receptor-2
TLR4	Toll-like receptor-4
TNFA	Tumor necrosis factor-α
TNFR2	Tumor necrosis factor receptor-2
VDR	Vitamin D receptor

factors (Loos et al. 2005). We have grouped some candidate genes together and possible mechanisms of action are given in boxes, i.e. which arguments have been used and which hypotheses have been proposed to study the various modifying genes in relation to periodontitis.

IL-1 and TNF-α gene polymorphisms

In Box 13-2, several arguments have been summarized to justify why the genes encoding for interleukin-1 (IL-1) and tumor necrosis factor-α (TNF-α) appear to be good candidates for genetic studies in relation to periodontitis.

Epidemiological findings for gene polymorphisms in the IL1 gene cluster

The genes IL1A, IL1B, and IL1RN encoding for the proteins IL-1α, IL-1β, and IL-RA respectively, are

located in close proximity in the IL1 gene cluster on chromosome 2. Kornman et al. (1997) reported first on polymorphisms for the IL1 genes in relation to periodontitis. This study reports on an IL1 composite genotype (see below), however no data are presented for the carriage rates of the individual IL1 R-alleles (IL1A, IL1B, IL1RN). To date, the following IL1 genetic polymorphisms have been studied in relation to periodontitis: IL1A −889 (in linkage with +4845), IL1B −511 (in linkage with −31), IL1B +3954 (also mentioned in the literature as +3953) and IL1RN VNTR (in linkage with +2018).

It has become clear that among the different studies with exclusively Caucasian subjects, considerable variation is seen for the carriage rates of the IL1 R-alleles. For example for the polymorphic IL1A −889 (+4845), the carriage rate for the R-allele varies from 34–64% for patients and 35–60% for controls. None of the studies involving Caucasians and non-Caucasians have found a significant association between periodontitis and/or disease severity and IL1A −889 (+4845) as single risk factor, except when combined with other IL1 polymorphisms. The carriage rate of the IL1A −889 (+4845) R-allele in Chileans was comparable to that reported by other reports (Quappe et al. 2004), while the carriage rate among Japanese people appears lower (Tai et al. 2002). The latter finding demonstrates an important issue, that is that carriage rate of genetic polymorphisms may vary among different ethnic populations. Therefore, possible positive associations between a genetic polymorphism and disease within one population may not necessarily be extrapolated to other populations.

Three studies have reported carriage rates for the IL1B −511 (−31) R-allele, and to date this genetic polymorphism has not been associated with periodontitis. The carriage of the R-allele was higher among Japanese people (67–78%) than among Caucasians (59%) (Gore et al. 1998; Tai et al. 2002; Soga et al. 2003).

The SNP IL1B +3954 (+3953) initially appeared promising as risk factor for periodontitis among Caucasians. However there are conflicting results. Galbraith et al. (1998) found an association between the R-allele and periodontitis and Gore et al. (1998) observed an association with the severity of periodontal destruction. Quappe et al. (2004) reported that the N-allele might indeed be protective for periodontitis in Chileans. By contrast, Parkhill et al. (2000) observed an over-representation of the N-allele among early onset periodontitis (EOP) patients, and they concluded that the N-allele, and in particular in smokers, is associated with periodontitis, rather than the R-allele. The latter observation was also shown in a family linkage analysis, which included both families of African American and Caucasian heritage, therefore implying a role in the disease process for the N-allele (Diehl et al. 1999). Among Japanese subjects, the carriage rate of the IL1B +3954 (+3953) is

Box 13-2 Why are genes encoding for IL-1 and TNF good candidates as modifying disease genes for periodontitis?

There is evidence to suggest that IL-1 and TNF-α play important roles in the pathogenesis of periodontitis. IL-1α, IL-1β, and TNF-α are potent immunologic mediators with pro-inflammatory properties. Moreover, IL-1 and TNF-α have the capacity to stimulate bone resorption and they can regulate fibroblast cell proliferation, of both gingival and periodontal ligament origin. IL-1 and TNF-α levels are increased in the gingival crevicular fluid of periodontitis subjects and these cytokines are found in higher levels in inflamed periodontal tissues compared to healthy tissues.

Various studies have suggested that polymorphisms in the genes of the *IL1* cluster and in the *TNFA* gene, could predispose subjects to elevated IL-1 (decreased IL-1 receptor antagonist (RA)) and TNF-α protein levels. The majority of these cited studies suggest that the *R*-allele of a given polymorphism in the promoter region results in an upregulation of protein production. These studies have often been performed with isolated cells of healthy individuals or with cultured cell lines or cell constructs (transfected cells).

Inherent (most likely genetically determined) inter-individual differences have also been observed for IL-1 and TNF-α production by peripheral blood mononuclear cells or oral leukocytes, isolated from individuals with and without periodontitis. It is conceivable that these differences in IL-1 and TNF-α production and secretion play a role as risk factors, however insufficient evidence currently exists to conclude that this is a key phenomenon occurring in the pathophysiology of periodontitis. Nevertheless, the concept is attractive and may explain some of the epidemiologic findings of genetic polymorphisms associated with the susceptibility to and severity of periodontitis.

Some *IL1* and *TNFA R*-alleles have been suggested as potential genetic markers for other complex diseases. For example, *IL1* and *TNFA* gene polymorphisms have been associated with several inflammatory and infectious disease processes, including inflammatory bowel disease, Sjögren syndrome, rheumatoid arthritis, meningococcal disease, systemic lupus erythematosus, and psoriasis.

importantly low (<10%), and given this low carriage rate, no association with periodontitis can be expected. Clearly, large-scale studies in homogeneous populations are needed to further investigate the potential of the *IL1* +3954 (+3953) genotypes as risk factors for periodontitis.

Few studies have investigated polymorphisms in the *IL1RN* gene and again conflicting results are reported. In Caucasians the *R*-allele was not associated as single risk factor with periodontitis, however in combination with other *IL1* SNPs it was reported to have a possible relationship with periodontitis prevalence and severity (Laine *et al.* 2001; Meisel *et al.* 2002). In Japanese subjects the *IL1RN R*-allele was significantly associated with periodontitis (Tai *et al.* 2002). In contrast, Parkhill *et al.* (2000) observed the *IL1RN N*-allele in combination with the *IL1B* +3954 *N*-allele and smoking to be associated with early onset periodontitis (EOP).

Kornman *et al.* (1997) reported that the combined presence of the *R*-allele of the *IL1A* gene at nucleotide position −889 and the *R*-allele of the *IL1B* gene at nucleotide position +3954 (+3953) was associated with severity of periodontitis in non-smoking Caucasian patients. This combined carriage rate of the *R*-alleles was designated the *IL1* composite genotype (Kornman *et al.* 1997). Since that time a considerable number of studies investigating the *IL1* composite genotype in Caucasians and non-Caucasians has been published. An association between the *IL1* com-

posite genotype and the severity of periodontal destruction has also been reported by two other cross-sectional studies (McDevitt *et al.* 2000; Papapanou *et al.* 2001). However, other studies have failed to corroborate that *IL1* composite genotype alone may behave as a risk factor for periodontitis severity (Gore *et al.* 1998; Ehmke *et al.* 1999; Cattabriga *et al.* 2001; Laine *et al.* 2001; Meisel *et al.* 2002, 2003, 2004). In contrast to the results of Kornman *et al.* (1997), Meisel *et al.* (2002, 2003, 2004) observed the *IL1* composite genotype to be associated with periodontitis in smokers. These conflicting results cast doubt on the utility of the *IL1* composite genotype as a putative risk factor for severity of periodontitis in Caucasians. Nevertheless, it has also been reported that patients with the *IL1* composite genotype more often harbored putative periodontal pathogens and have increased counts of these pathogens (Socransky *et al.* 2000). Interestingly, Laine *et al.* (2001) reported increased frequency of the *R*-alleles of the *IL1A*, *IL1B*, and *IL1RN* genes in non-smoking patients in whom *P. gingivalis* and *A. actinomycetemcomitans* could not be detected. These latter results suggest that *IL1* gene polymorphisms may play a role in the absence of other (putative) risk factors (Meisel *et al.* 2002, 2003, 2004).

Studies among Chinese Americans and African Americans have not resulted in interpretable findings, because the *IL1* composite genotype was hardly present in these ethnic populations (Armitage *et al.*

2000; Walker *et al*. 2000). In South American subjects the carriage rate of the *IL1* composite genotype (up to 25%) was somewhat lower than that reported for Europeans and North American study subjects (up to 48%) and no associations with periodontitis have been found.

Several longitudinal studies on *IL1* polymorphisms have been performed. From these studies it may be possible to assess whether a given genotype can be considered a true risk factor. For example, it was reported among periodontitis patients in maintenance over 5–14 years, that the *IL1* composite genotype increased the risk of tooth loss by 2.7-fold (McGuire & Nunn 1999). The *IL1* composite genotype in combination with heavy smoking increased the risk of tooth loss by 7.7-fold (McGuire & Nunn 1999). In an Australian study 295 gingivitis and moderate periodontitis subjects were followed for 5 years and the *IL1* composite genotype was determined (Cullinan *et al*. 2001); the investigators reported that among non-smoking subjects >50 years, those that were *IL1* composite genotype positive, had deeper probing depths than *IL1* composite genotype negative subjects. Furthermore, a significant interaction was found between carriage of the *IL1* composite genotype and age, smoking, and the presence of *P. gingivalis*, which suggests that the *IL1* composite genotype is a contributory but non-essential risk factor (Cullinan *et al*. 2001).

In summary, for the global population, polymorphisms in the *IL1* gene cluster cannot be regarded as (putative) risk factors for periodontitis or severity of periodontal destruction. For Caucasian patients with chronic periodontitis the role of the *IL1* composite genotype seems to hold some promise, however to date no clear evidence has emerged and there are currently too many conflicting and negative results. Large cohort studies of homogeneous composition should be initiated, in which all of the currently accepted non-genetic (putative) risk factors are included. Multi-variate analyses should be employed to estimate relative contributions of all factors.

Epidemiological findings for *TNFA* gene polymorphisms

The *TNFA* gene is located on chromosome 6 within the major histocompatibility complex (MHC) gene cluster. Several case–control studies in both Caucasians and non-Caucasians have investigated genetic polymorphisms in the *TNFA* gene as putative risk factors for periodontitis. SNPs in the gene encoding TNF-α are mainly studied in the promoter region at positions −1031, −863, −367, −308, −238 but also in the coding region in the first intron at position +489.

Similar to findings for genes of the *IL1* cluster, differences for the carriage rate of the *R*-alleles between Caucasians and other ethnic populations were apparent; at position −308 the *R*-allele carriage rate for Caucasians varied between 20% and 3%, while this was 2–3% for Japanese subjects. For the *TNFA* −238 the frequencies of *R*-alleles were comparable between both ethnic populations (<10%). The carriage rates of the *R*-alleles at positions −367 and −238 were <10%, making them less likely to be associated with periodontitis; indeed no associations have been found with periodontitis for these SNPs (Galbraith *et al*. 1998; Craandijk *et al*. 2002; Soga *et al*. 2003).

Among Japanese subjects, associations with periodontitis have been observed for the SNPs *TNFA* −1031 and −863 (Soga *et al*. 2003); these polymorphisms have not been tested in Caucasians. Among Caucasians, the only association of a *TNFA* polymorphism was observed at position −308 by Galbraith *et al*. (1998) and this was not corroborated by other studies with Caucasians in the study population. Among families with a high prevalence of EOP, the *TNFA* −308 gene polymorphisms have also been investigated, but were found not to be associated with EOP (Shapira *et al*. 2001). Another marker in the TNF-α gene was investigated in relation to susceptibility for aggressive periodontitis. This marker was based on a variable number of micro-satellite repeats, but was not found to be associated with generalized juvenile periodontitis (GJP) (Kinane *et al*. 1999).

Investigations into the severity of periodontitis in relation to any of the *TNFA R*-alleles did not reveal a positive association. The carriage of the *R*-allele at nucleotide positions −308 and −238 revealed no association between the percentage of teeth with ≥50% bone loss (Craandijk *et al*. 2002). Moreover, the carriage rates of the *R*-alleles at nucleotide positions −376, −308, −238, and +489 were not different between patients with moderate or severe periodontitis. Others reported also a lack of association of *TNFA* genetic polymorphisms with the severity of periodontitis (Kornman *et al*. 1997; Galbraith *et al*. 1998).

Based on the available literature to date, there is very limited data to support associations between any of the reported *TNFA* gene variations and periodontitis. *TNFA* −1031 and −863 may have promise, but they have only been tested in one study among Japanese subjects. More studies are needed to address *TNFA* polymorphisms and these studies should also involve investigations into other genetic polymorphisms in genes like *IL1*, for possible gene–gene interactions that may play a role in the complex pathogenesis of periodontitis.

FcγR gene polymorphisms

In Box 13-3, some background has been summarized to explain why the genes encoding for Fc gamma receptors (FcγR) seem good candidates for genetic studies in relation to periodontitis.

Several studies have investigated the *FcγRIIa* polymorphisms in relation to periodontitis in several populations. In Caucasians and African Americans, the carriage rate of the *R*-allele is relatively high: 63–77% (Colombo *et al*. 1998; Meisel *et al*. 2001; Fu *et al*.

Box 13-3 Why are genes encoding for FcγR good candidates as disease-modifying genes for periodontitis?

Leukocytes from both the myeloid and lymphoid lineages express receptors (FcγR) for the constant (Fc) region of immunoglobulin G molecules. Indeed, FcγR are found on a wide variety of immune cells in the periodontal tissues. FcγRs are likely to play a role in the pathogenesis of periodontitis, as a bridge between the cellular and humoral branches of the immune system. Microorganisms and bacterial antigens, opsonized with antibody, can be phago-cytosed via FcγR on neutrophils or internalized via FcγR by a variety of antigen-presenting cells (APCs), including monocytes, macrophages and B cells. T cells and natural killer (NK) cells may become acti-vated, when IgG-opsonized bacteria are bound to these cells via FcγR; a variety of cytokines and che-mokines may also be released. When one or several of the FcγR-mediated leukocyte functions are com-promised or exaggerated due to genetic polymor-phisms in the FcγR genes, it is conceivable that the susceptibility to and/or severity of periodontitis is affected. This concept was proposed more than a decade ago.

The leukocyte *FcγR* genes are found on chromo-some 1, and encode three main receptor classes: FcγRI (CD64), FcγRII (CD32), and FcγRIII (CD16). These classes are further subdivided into subclasses: FcγRIa and b, FcγRIIa, b, and c, and FcγRIIIa and b.

FcγRIIa is found on all granulocytes, on APCs, platelets, endothelial cells, and a subset of T cells. FcγRIIIa is present on monocytes and macrophages, NK cells and a subset of T cells. The FcγRIIIb is the most abundantly expressed IgG receptor on neutrophils.

Structural and functional differences in FcγRIIa, IIIa and b have been described (Fig. 13-4). G to A transition polymorphisms in the FcγRIIa gene result in the substitution of histidine (H) for arginine (R) at amino acid position 131 of the receptor. FcγRIIa-H131 binds IgG2 immune complexes efficiently, whereas the FcγRIIa-R131 allotype cannot mediate this interaction. The G to T transition polymorphism in the FcγRIIIa gene, results in an amino acid 158-valine (V) substitution for 158-phenylalanine (F). The FcγRIIIa-V158 has a higher affinity for IgG1 and 3 than FcγRIIIa-F158. Moreover, FcγRIIIa-V158 can bind IgG4 while FcγRIIIa-F158 is unable to do so. A bi-allelic polymorphism in the FcγRIIIb gene under-lies the FcγRIIIb-neutrophil antigen (NA) 1 or NA2 allotype. This is caused by four amino acid substitu-tions in the Fc-binding region resulting in differ-ences in glycosylation. The NA2 type binds less efficiently human IgG1 and IgG3 immune com-plexes than FcγRIIIb-NA1.

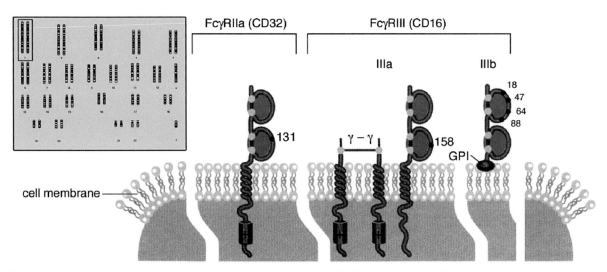

Fig. 13-4 Schematic drawing of three of the human Fc receptors for IgG. They have an extracellular part, a transmembrane region and a cytoplasmic tail (except FcγRIIIb, which is anchored in the outer leaflet of the cell membrane via a glycosyl-phosphatidyl-inositol (GPI) molecule). The extracellular part of leukocyte FcγR class II and III consists of two immunoglobulin-like domains. The + sign in the intracellular signaling motifs (cylinder) indicates the capacity of signaling to the cytoplasmic environment of the cell. The FcγRIIa-mediated effector functions can be established through the intracellular signaling motif (cylinder) within the cytoplasmic tail of the molecule. The FcγRIIIa is associated with a γ-chain homodimer, which serves as signaling subunit. The FcγRIIIb-mediated effector functions are transmitted through the GPI. The functional genetic polymorphisms are depicted as black dots (•) in the extracellular Ig-like domains. For the FcγRIIa at amino acid position 131, arginine (R) or histidine (H) is present. For the FcγRIIIa at amino acid position 158, valine (V) or phenylalanine (F) is present. The FcγRIIIb polymorphism is caused by four amino acid substitutions at positions 18, 47, 64, and 88 and results in glycosylation differences, affecting receptor affinity. The CD indication in parentheses indicates the numbering within the cluster of differentiation system of immunological markers (van der Pol & van de Winkel 1998).

2002; Loos *et al.* 2003; Yamamoto *et al.* 2004). In Japanese people the carriage rate is lower: 39–50%. In Japanese people and African Americans, the *FcγRIIa* polymorphisms are not associated with periodontitis or with the severity of the disease. However, in Caucasians some studies showed an association, with the *N*-allele rather than the expected *R*-allele (Loos *et al.* 2003; Yamamoto *et al.* 2004). A weak relationship with aggressive periodontitis was observed for the *FcγRIIa N*-allele (Loos *et al.* 2003). Moreover, periodontitis patients (aggressive and chronic periodontitis) homozygous for the *N*-allele (H/H131 genotype) have more periodontal bone loss than the other patients carrying one or two *R*-alleles. Homozygosity for the *N*-allele was significantly more prevalent in periodontitis (Yamamoto *et al.* 2004).

For the *FcγRIIIa* gene again a lower *R*-allele carriage rate is seen in Japanese than in Caucasian and African American subjects. The *FcγRIIIa N*-allele (V158) seems as a putative risk factor for periodontitis (Meisel *et al.* 2001; Loos *et al.* 2003). However, in Japan, both the *FcγRIIIa R*-allele (F158), as well as the *FcγRIIIa N*-allele, were proposed as risk factors. It is apparent that there are conflicting results and comparisons between the different studies are difficult as the prevalences of *FcγR* genotypes are different among subjects of different ethnic background.

In Japanese patients, the *FcγRIIIb R*-allele (NA2) was associated with generalized (G)-EOP (Kobayashi *et al.* 2000) and was found more often in adult patients with disease recurrence (Kobayashi *et al.* 1997). The carriage rate of the *FcγRIIIb R*-allele in Caucasians is relatively high (>75%) and to date no associations with periodontitis have been found.

The possibility that genes encoding for Fcγ receptors are associated with periodontitis in different ethnic groups seems promising. However, to date no clear and convincing data are present to definitively designate one or more of the *FcγR* gene polymorphisms as true risk factors for periodontitis. Further research is needed in larger groups of subjects from different global populations to confirm the current observations. Furthermore, functional studies among subjects with different FcγR genotypes need to be undertaken to investigate the corresponding phenotypes and unravel the role of the Fcγ receptors in the pathogenesis of periodontitis.

Gene polymorphisms in the innate immunity receptors

There are some good arguments why the genes encoding for proteins of the innate immune response are good candidate genes in relation to periodontitis (Box 13-4).

Two studies with Caucasian subjects investigated the *CD14* −260 polymorphism in chronic periodontitis, but did not find associations (Holla *et al.* 2002; Folwaczny *et al.* 2004a). However after stratification of the cohort according to gender, it was found that the *CD14* −260 *N*-allele was more prevalent among females with periodontitis (67%) than among healthy control subjects (44%) (Folwaczny *et al.* 2004a). In a Japanese study, again no association was found between the *CD14* −260 polymorphism and periodontitis (Yamazaki *et al.* 2003). Nevertheless, Holla *et al.* (2002) found among Caucasians a tendency for an increased frequency of the *CD14* −260 *R/R* genotype in patients with severe disease (19.2%) compared with the patients with moderate disease (8.3%). The *CD14* −260 *R/R* genotype was also associated with severe periodontitis in Dutch Caucasians; even stronger association was found after adjusting for age, gender, smoking, and presence of *P. gingivalis* and *A. actinomycetemcomitans* (Laine *et al.* 2005). Results for another polymorphism in the *CD14* gene have also been reported (Holla *et al.* 2002); a higher frequency of the *N*-allele and the *N/N* genotype of the *CD14* −1359 polymorphism was found in patients with severe periodontal disease than in patients with moderate periodontitis.

Two studies have attempted to associate *TLR* polymorphisms with periodontitis (Folwaczny *et al.* 2004b; Laine *et al.* 2005). However, despite the perceived importance of these functional *TLR* polymorphisms, no relation with periodontitis has been observed.

Although the polymorphisms of the *CARD15* (*NOD2*) gene are strongly associated with Crohn's disease (Hugot *et al.* 2001), to date they have not been associated with periodontitis (Folwaczny *et al.* 2004c; Laine *et al.* 2004).

Vitamin D receptor gene polymorphisms

Several arguments have been put forward for the vitamin D receptor (*VDR*) gene to be proposed as candidate gene in relation to periodontitis (see Box 13-5).

Several studies have identified a *VDR* polymorphisms in relation to periodontitis at positions *Taq-1*, *Bsm-1*, and *Fok-1* (Hennig *et al.* 1999; Tachi *et al.* 2001, 2003; Yoshihara *et al.* 2001; Sun *et al.* 2002; Taguchi *et al.* 2003; de Brito Junior *et al.* 2004). The studies on the *Taq-1* and *Bsm-1* SNPs of the *VDR* gene have found some associations with periodontitis, however not unconditionally. The carriage rate of the *R*-allele ranges between 12 and 66% across different ethnic populations, among Brazilians it was in the higher range (45–66%) and in Japanese the lower rate (5–12%). In the study by Hennig *et al.* (1999) the carriage rate of the *R*-allele ranged between 32 and 37%. Nevertheless, in five case–control studies an association of the *R*-allele with several forms of periodontitis have been observed (Hennig *et al.* 1999; Tachi *et al.* 2001; Yoshihara *et al.* 2001; Sun *et al.* 2002; de Brito Junior *et al.* 2004), while in one Japanese study an association with the *N*-allele has been found (Tachi *et al.* 2003). The apparent discrepancy cannot be explained, however it may relate to different

Box 13-4 Why are genes encoding for receptors of the innate immune response good candidates as disease-modifying genes for periodontitis?

The innate immune response is the first line of defense in infectious diseases. Without having to wait until an antigen-specific immune response is in full action (3–5 days), the host is challenged to detect the pathogen and to mount a rapid, immediate defensive response. The innate immune system recognizes pathogen-associated molecular patterns (PAMPs) that are expressed on microorganisms, but not on host cells. Extra- and intracellular receptors like CD14, CARD15, and toll-like receptors (TLRs) recognize PAMPs of Gram-positive and Gram-negative bacteria and mediate the production of cytokines necessary for further development of effective immune response (Fig. 13-5). Both TLR2 and TLR4 use CD14 as a co-receptor.

The R-allele in the promoter region of CD14 at position −260 (−159) enhances the transcriptional activity of the gene. Individuals homozygous for the R-allele have increased serum levels of soluble (s) CD14 and an increased density of CD14 in mono-

cytes. The CD14 −260 SNP has previously been associated of increased risk with myocardial infarction and Crohn's disease. Furthermore, increased serum levels of sCD14 have been associated with periodontitis.

Two common co-segregating missense polymorphisms of TLR4, Asp299Gly and Thr399Ile, affect the extracellular domain of the TLR4 protein, leading to an attenuated efficacy of signaling and a reduced capacity to elicit inflammation. The TLR4 Asp299Gly gene polymorphism has been correlated with hypo-responsiveness to inhaled LPS, sepsis, and infections caused by Gram-negative bacteria.

The 3020insC and 2104 C > T polymorphisms of the CARD15 (NOD2) gene lead to impaired activation of nuclear factor-kappa B, resulting in altered transcription of pro-inflammatory cytokine genes and reduced expression of these cytokines. These polymorphisms are strongly associated with Crohn's disease.

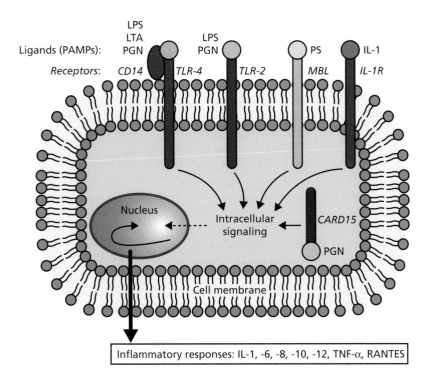

Fig. 13-5 Schematic drawing of a cell and the intracellular activation of the NF-kappa B pathway. The NF-kappa B pathway stimulates the nucleus to increase production of inflammatory mediators. Extra- and intracellular receptors, toll-like receptors 4 and 2 (TLR-4 and TLR-2), MBL, IL-1 receptor (IL-1R) and CARD15, recognize pathogen-associated molecular patterns (PAMPs) of Gram-positive and Gram-negative bacteria and mediate the production of cytokines necessary for further development of effective immune response. Both TLR-2 and TLR-4 use CD14 as a co-receptor. PAMPs are lipopolysaccharide (LPS), lipoteichoic acid (LTA), peptidoglygan (PGN), and polysaccharide (PS).

gene–environment interactions affecting different ethnic populations and/or it is related to differences in the type of periodontitis being investigated. Moreover, we cannot exclude that there is a lack of consistency in "case definition" for each disease type between studies.

The VDR gene is an interesting candidate gene for its association with periodontitis, because it affects both bone metabolism and immune functions. More-

over some encouraging results have been found for different ethnic populations. Further studies should be engaged to confirm the current preliminary data.

IL-10 gene polymorphisms

There are some interesting arguments why the gene encoding for interleukin-10 (IL-10) is a candidate gene for periodontitis (Box 13-6).

Box 13-5 Why is the gene encoding for vitamin D receptor a good candidate as a disease-modifying gene for periodontitis?

Alveolar bone destruction results from the periodontitis disease process. If left untreated, consequences of periodontitis are tooth mobility and eventually tooth exfoliation. Therefore, it is conceivable that mediators of bone metabolism play a role in the pathophysiology of periodontitis. With this is in mind investigators have identified genetic polymorphisms in genes coding for mediators in bone homeostasis, in particular the *VDR* gene. Bone homeostasis mediators are linked to factors affecting bone mineral density and have been related to disorders of bone metabolism, such as osteoporosis and osteoarthritis. Interestingly, genetic polymorphisms in the *VDR* gene have also been associated with infectious diseases, in particular tuberculosis. In addition to mediating bone homeostasis, vitamin D and its receptor play a role in phagocytosis by monocytes and affect monocyte differentiation.

Box 13-6 Why is the gene encoding for IL-10 a good candidate as a disease-modifying gene for periodontitis?

The gene encoding IL-10 is located on chromosome 1, in a cluster with closely related interleukin genes, including *IL19*, *IL20*, and *IL24*. IL-10 is produced by monocytes/macrophages and T cells and plays a role in the regulation of pro-inflammatory cytokines such as IL-1 and TNF-α. In particular, IL-10 is considered an anti-inflammatory cytokine, down-regulating the pro-inflammatory immune response of the monocyte/macrophage and stimulating the production of protective antibodies. However, it has also been suggested that IL-10 can stimulate the generation of auto-antibodies. As a matter of fact, auto-antibodies may play a role in periodontitis. Functional disturbance in the *IL10* gene due to genetic polymorphisms could be detrimental to host tissues and could be linked to periodontal disease susceptibility. The *IL10* SNPs have been associated with altered IL-10 production. *IL10* genetic polymorphisms have been associated with systemic lupus erythematosus and rheumatoid arthritis.

IL10 gene microsatellite markers have been investigated in relation to aggressive periodontitis (Kinane *et al.* 1999). However, no significant differences in frequencies of various *IL10* alleles between patients and periodontally healthy controls were observed. In Japanese patients either with G-EOP or with adult periodontitis (AP), as well as controls, three polymorphisms in the promoter region of the *IL10* gene were analyzed (Yamazaki *et al.* 2001). No significant differences for the carriage rates of the polymorphism in the *IL10* gene were seen between all patients and controls. Also no significant differences were observed for these latter haplotypes between AP and EOP.

The *IL10* −1087 polymorphism may be an interesting polymorphism for future studies among Caucasians. It has been shown in one study that the *N*-allele is more abundant in periodontitis in particular in non-smokers (Berglundh *et al.* 2003). These observations have led the authors to speculate that the *N*-allele prevalence in periodontitis patients may result in higher levels of auto-antibodies, which may lead to increased periodontal destruction (Berglundh *et al.* 2003). These observations were not corroborated by a Brazilian study (Scarel-Caminaga *et al.* 2004); the latter study observed a trend for increased carriage of the *IL10* −1087 *N*-allele among controls.

In summary, a limited number of studies have investigated genetic variations at three positions in the *IL10* promoter region, but to date *IL10* is not a strong candidate gene due to the mixed results in the various studies in the literature.

Miscellaneous gene polymorphisms

Table 13-2 lists various other candidate gene polymorphisms that have been studied in relation to periodontitis. These are not discussed as the other candidates above, since mainly negative results have been obtained and/or too few studies are published for a meaningful analysis. However, the table illustrates the variety of candidates and the difficulty in interpreting results; if some positive results are reported, these are often in subgroups or conditional. Clearly, further studies are needed employing larger patient numbers, which focus on candidate genes that have a proven role in the pathophysiology of periodontitis, where gene polymorphisms result in functional changes or are linked to other gene polymorphisms which in turn are strong markers of inflammatory and/or infectious diseases.

Disease-modifying genes in relation to implant failures and peri-implantitis

The success of implant dentistry is often reported as survival rate (i.e. the implant is functional and present in the mouth after a given observation period). Several longitudinal studies have reported survival rates of around 90–95% over periods of 5–10 years (Esposito *et al.* 1998; Berglundh *et al.* 2002; Roos-Jansaker *et al.* 2006). However, complications do

Table 13-2 Polymorphisms in miscellaneous genes studied in relation to periodontitis and reported association (adapted from Loos *et al.* 2005)

Polymorphism in gene	Number of studies	Associated with periodontitis reported respectively
ACE	1	– (+ [1])
CCR5	1	–
ER2	1	–
ET1	1	–
FBR	1	+ [2]
FcγRIIb	1	+
FPR1	1	– (+ [3])
IL2	1	– (+ [4])
IL4	4 and 1	– and +
IL6	1 and 2	+ and – (+ [5, 6])
INFGR1	1	– (+ [7])
LTA	1 and 1	+ and – (+ [8])
MMP1	2 and 1	– and – (+ [9])
MMP3	1	–
MMP9	1	–
MPO	1	– (+ [10])
NAT2	1 and 1	– (+ [11]) and + (+ [11])
PAI1	1	+
RAGE	1	+
TGFB	1 and 1	– and – (+ [12])
TIMP2	1	–
TNFR2	1	+

Symbols: – = association not found; + = association found.
[1] in combination with LTA.
[2] R-allele associated with higher serum fibrinogen.
[3] associated with LJP in African-Americans.
[4] R-allele associated with severity.
[5] R-allele protective.
[6] R-allele associated with higher serum levels of IL-6.
[7] R-allele in combination with smoking.
[8] N-allele protective in combination with TNFA-308.
[9] R-allele associated in non-smokers.
[10] R-allele protective for females.
[11] NAT2 slow phenotype associated with severity.
[12] R-allele possibly small effect in relation to severity.

Table 13-3 Summary of candidate genes, and corresponding encoded proteins, for which gene polymorphisms have been investigated as markers for early or late implant failure and/or peri-implantitis

Gene	Coded protein
CTR	Calcitonin receptor
BMP4	Bone morphogenetic protein
IL1A	Interleukin-1α
IL1B	Interleukin-1β
IL1RN	Interleukin-1 receptor antagonist
IL2	Interleukin-2
IL6	Interleukin-6
MMP1	Matrix metalloproteinase-1
MMP9	Matrix metalloproteinase-9
TGFB1	Transforming growth factor-β
TNFA	Tumor necrosis factor-α

late implant failures and/or bone loss occurring around dental implants.

Early failures in implant dentistry

The IL-1 gene cluster polymorphisms in association with early failures

To date four studies have reported on the *IL1A* –889, *IL1B* –511, *IL1B* +3954, and *IL1RN* VNTR polymorphisms in early implant failures, either separately or in a combination (composite genotype; carriers of the R-allele in *IL1A* –889 and *IL1B* +3954). Homozygosity of the *IL1B* –511 R-allele has been reported to be associated with marginal bone loss around the dental implants in Japanese patients (Shimpuku *et al.* 2003). However, another study did not observed an association between the *IL1B* –511 R-allele homozygosity and early implant loss in white Brazilians (Campos *et al.* 2005). No other associations have been reported for *IL1* gene cluster polymorphisms and early implant failures/complications.

Miscellaneous gene polymorphisms in association with early failures

Polymorphisms in the *IL2, IL6, TNFA, TGFB1, MMP1*, and *MMP9* genes (Table 13-3) have been studied in white Brazilians, and *CTR* and *BMP4* gene polymorphisms in a Japanese population. One study reported that carriage of the *MMP1* –1607 R-allele is associated with early implant loss (Santos *et al.* 2004). All patients who lost at least one implant during the first year appeared to be carriers of the R-allele of *MMP1*, while 38% of those who did not lose implants were carriers of the R-allele of *MMP1*.

Bone morphogenetic protein (BMP) plays an important role in bone remodeling, and the R-allele of the *AluI* polymorphism of the *BMP4* gene has been associated with marginal bone loss around implants in Japanese patients (Shimpuku *et al.* 2003).

occur; in the latter studies early implant loss has been reported to occur in 1–7% of the implants and late implant loss with a follow-up of 5–14 years can occur in 2–13% of the implants.

Previous studies have indicated that peri-implantitis and implant failures appear to cluster in subsets of individuals and that a patient who has lost one dental implant is at elevated risk of experiencing another implant loss (Weyant & Burt 1993; Hutton *et al.* 1995). These observations have led to the question of whether there is a common denominator for susceptibility to implant failures and/or complications. At this time, little is known about the genetic susceptibility and genetic polymorphisms involved in peri-implant complications; however, several scientific papers have appeared in the literature investigating this aspect. Table 13-3 summarizes the candidate genes studied in association with early or

Late failures in implant dentistry

The follow-up period of late implant failures in the available studies varied from 1–15 years and only genetic variation in the genes of the *IL1* cluster have been investigated. Two studies reported on the *IL1A* −889, *IL1B* −511, *IL1B* +3954, and *IL1RN* VNTR polymorphisms separately in association with late implant failures (Rogers *et al.* 2002; Laine *et al.* 2006). One study found an association between the carriage of the *IL1RN* VNTR *R*-allele and late implant failure, but not for the other *IL1* gene polymorphisms (Laine *et al.* 2006).

As has been studied in relation to periodontitis, the composite *IL1* genotype (carriage of the *R*-allele in *IL1A* −889 and *IL1B* +3954) has also been investigated in relation to late implant failures. Two out of five available studies found only a conditional association between the late implant failures and *IL1* composite genotype; the other studies reported negative findings. In the first positive study, 90 Caucasian patients were investigated for peri-implant bone loss at the time of re-examination (mean 5.6 years after prosthetic rehabilitation) (Feloutzis *et al.* 2003). Twenty-eight patients carrying the *IL1* composite genotype were stratified into non-smokers, former smokers, and heavy smokers. Heavy smokers were found to have more total and annual bone loss, when compared with non-smokers or former smokers. The other study also reported that the *IL1* composite genotype and smoking were significantly associated with peri-implant bone loss after 8 years in function (Gruica *et al.* 2004). However, the results from both studies need to be interpreted with care; the number of subjects in both studies after stratification for genotype carriage and heavy smoking was so low that the power of the studies is severely compromised (see below).

In summary, there are several studies that have shown an association between early or late dental implant failures in relation to genetic polymorphisms. However most of them still need to be confirmed in another study cohort, consisting of larger numbers of study subjects. For Caucasians who smoke, the *IL-1* composite genotype may be a possible marker for late implant failures; this was also a genetic marker possibly associated with periodontitis. It is important to emphasize that is difficult to compare and summarize the available literature due to the fact that there is diversity of definitions for the dental implant failure and peri-implant disease, as well as heterogeneity in study design and implant systems.

Conclusions and future developments

An important problem related to research in the heredity of periodontitis is that, whatever the cause of the disease is, the symptoms are the same; specifically, deepening of the periodontal pocket, loss of attachment, and alveolar bone loss. It is likely that overlapping clinical phenotypes exist between different forms of periodontitis. It is important that globally accepted definitions of "cases" of chronic, and localized and generalized aggressive forms of periodontitis are used in future studies, to allow valid comparisons to be made between gene polymorphism data from different parts of the world. In the majority of cases, it is likely that the development of periodontitis in an individual depends on the collective presence of a number of environmental risk factors in conjunction with a number of genetic risk factors at a given time point during life. The more genetic risk factors an individual has inherited, the greater the genetic predisposition and the higher the chance of early development of periodontitis. Whenever an individual has inherited a major disease gene mutation, we would expect early development of periodontitis. However to date, major disease gene mutations have not been identified, which result in the periodontitis phenotype in otherwise systemically healthy individuals. Since the children of patients with chronic periodontitis show a relatively high prevalence of incipient periodontitis, it is likely that some forms of early periodontitis share a common pathogenic pathway with that of chronic periodontitis in adults.

A multitude of polymorphisms in genes, most of which code aspects of the host immune response, have been explored. There are indications that some polymorphisms in the *IL1* gene cluster, the *FcγR* gene cluster and in the genes encoding the vitamin D receptor and IL-10, may be associated with periodontitis in certain ethnic groups. However, in general, even among studies with subjects of the same ethnic background, no consistent results have been obtained. Often, only by defining small subgroups of individuals or after stratification, researchers have found some significant associations, but the studies appear underpowered for proper interpretation. Moreover, carriage of specific combinations of alleles within a given locus (haplotype analysis) and among various genes (gene-gene interactions) have only been sparsely investigated. Therefore we conclude that until now no specific genetic risk factor for periodontitis has been identified.

In general, the genetic studies in relation to periodontitis are hampered by population heterogeneity and differences in patient selection and diagnostic criteria. At the same time, it is also possible that inconsistent results may reflect the underlying complexity and heterogeneity of genetic influence in periodontitis. The heterogeneity in periodontitis case definitions is still one of the major problems in the interpretation of the various studies available in the literature in relation to genetic risk factors for periodontitis.

Another problem encountered in the literature, is that many studies have investigated putative genetic risk factors without considering other, established risk factors for periodontitis as co-variates. For example, most would agree that in periodontal research, age, gender, and smoking, should always be included in multivariate statistical analyses. Further, the vast majority of studies has not considered the infectious component (gene–environment interaction). We recommend strongly that, where possible, the bacterial microorganisms or appropriate surrogate measures of bacterial infection should be included as co-variates in the analyses.

Future studies applying the candidate gene approach could be guided by results from genome-wide searches or by results from gene expression signatures (Papapanou *et al.* 2004) or family linkage analyses (Diehl *et al.* 1999; Li *et al.* 2004). Furthermore, these types of studies need to be large scale, in consortium-based approaches, because single studies are greatly underpowered. It is estimated that meaningful results for the candidate gene approach may only be obtained with thousands of patients, since most associations refer to small odds ratios (range 1.1–1.50) (Ioannidis *et al.* 2003). Useful reviews and recommendations have been published on the topic of the candidate gene approach for complex diseases (Clayton & McKeigue 2001; Tabor *et al.* 2002; Colhoun *et al.* 2003; Ioannidis 2003).

References

Armitage, G.C., Wu, Y., Wang, H.Y., Sorrell, J., di Giovine, F.S. & Duff, G.W. (2000). Low prevalence of a periodontitis-associated interleukin-1 composite genotype in individuals of Chinese heritage. *Journal of Periodontology* **71**, 164–171.

Beaty, T.H., Colyer, C.R., Chang, Y.C., Liang, K.Y., Graybeal, J.C., Muhammad, N.K. & Levin, L.S. (1993). Familial aggregation of periodontal indices. *Journal of Dental Research* **72**, 544–551.

Berglundh, T., Donati, M., Hahn-Zoric, M., Hanson, L.A. & Padyukov, L. (2003). Association of the −1087 IL 10 gene polymorphism with severe chronic periodontitis in Swedish Caucasians. *Journal of Clinical Periodontology* **30**, 249–254.

Berglundh, T., Persson, L. & Klinge, B. (2002). A systematic review of the incidence of biological and technical complications in implant dentistry reported in prospective longitudinal studies of at least 5 years. *Journal of Clinical Periodontology* **29** (Suppl 3), 197–212; discussion 232–193.

Boughman, J.A., Astemborski, J.A. & Suzuki, J.B. (1992). Phenotypic assessment of early onset periodontitis in sibships. *Journal of Clinical Periodontology* **19**, 233–239.

Brennan, A.L. & Geddes, D.M. (2002). Cystic fibrosis. *Current Opinions in Infectious Diseases* **15**, 175–182.

Burt, B.A., Ismail, A.I., Morrison, E.C. & Beltran, E.D. (1990). Risk factors for tooth loss over a 28-year period. *Journal of Dental Research* **69**, 1126–1130.

Campos, M.I., Santos, M.C., Trevilatto, P.C., Scarel-Caminaga, R.M., Bezerra, F.J. & Line, S.R. (2005). Evaluation of the relationship between interleukin-1 gene cluster polymorphisms and early implant failure in non-smoking patients. *Clinical Oral Implants Research* **16**, 194–201.

Cattabriga, M., Rotundo, R., Muzzi, L., Nieri, M., Verrocchi, G., Cairo, F. & Pini Prato, G. (2001). Retrospective evaluation of the influence of the interleukin-1 genotype on radiographic bone levels in treated periodontal patients over 10 years. *Journal of Periodontology* **72**, 767–773.

Chung, C.S., Kau, M.C., Chung, S.S. & Rao, D.C. (1977). A genetic and epidemiologic study of periodontal disease in Hawaii. II. Genetic and environmental influence. *American Journal of Human Genetics* **29**, 76–82.

Clayton, D. & McKeigue, P.M. (2001). Epidemiological methods for studying genes and environmental factors in complex diseases. *Lancet* **358**, 1356–1360.

Colhoun, H.M., McKeigue, P.M. & Davey Smith, G. (2003). Problems of reporting genetic associations with complex outcomes. *Lancet* **361**, 865–872.

Colombo, A.P., Eftimiadi, C., Haffajee, A.D., Cugini, M.A. & Socransky, S.S. (1998). Serum IgG2 level, Gm(23) allotype and FcgammaRIIa and FcgammaRIIIb receptors in refractory periodontal disease. *Journal of Clinical Periodontology* **25**, 465–474.

Craandijk, J., van Krugten, M.V., Verweij, C.L., van der Velden, U. & Loos, B.G. (2002). Tumor necrosis factor-alpha gene polymorphisms in relation to periodontitis. *Journal of Clinical Periodontology* **29**, 28–34.

Cullinan, M.P., Westerman, B., Hamlet, S.M., Palmer, J.E., Faddy, M.J., Lang, N.P. & Seymour, G.J. (2001). A longitudinal study of interleukin-1 gene polymorphisms and periodontal disease in a general adult population. *Journal of Clinical Periodontology* **28**, 1137–1144.

de Brito Junior, R.B., Scarel-Caminaga, R.M., Trevilatto, P.C., de Souza, A.P. & Barros, S.P. (2004). Polymorphisms in the vitamin D receptor gene are associated with periodontal disease. *Journal of Periodontology* **75**, 1090–1095.

de Haar, S.F., Jansen, D.C., Schoenmaker, T., De Vree, H., Everts, V. & Beertsen, W. (2004). Loss-of-function mutations in cathepsin C in two families with Papillon-Lefevre syndrome are associated with deficiency of serine proteinases in PMNs. *Human Mutation* **23**, 524.

Diehl, S.R., Wang, Y., Brooks, C.N., Burmeister, J.A., Califano, J.V., Wang, S. & Schenkein, H.A. (1999). Linkage disequilibrium of interleukin-1 genetic polymorphisms with early-onset periodontitis. *Journal of Periodontology* **70**, 418–430.

Dowsett, S.A., Archila, L., Foroud, T., Koller, D., Eckert, G.J. & Kowolik, M.J. (2002). The effect of shared genetic and environmental factors on periodontal disease parameters in untreated adult siblings in Guatemala. *Journal of Periodontology* **73**, 1160–1168.

Ehmke, B., Kress, W., Karch, H., Grimm, T., Klaiber, B. & Flemmig, T.F. (1999). Interleukin-1 haplotype and periodontal disease progression following therapy. *Journal of Clinical Periodontology* **26**, 810–813.

Esposito, M., Hirsch, J.M., Lekholm, U. & Thomsen, P. (1998). Biological factors contributing to failures of osseointegrated oral implants. (I). Success criteria and epidemiology. *European Journal of Oral Sciences* **106**, 527–551.

Feloutzis, A., Lang, N., Tonetti, M., Burgin, W., Bragger, U., Buser, D., Duff, G. & Kornman, K. (2003). IL-1 gene polymorphism and smoking as risk factors for peri-implant bone loss in a well-maintained population. *Clinical Oral Implants Research* **14**, 10–17.

Fischer, J., Blanchet-Bardon, C., Prud'homme, J.F., Pavek, S., Steijlen, P.M., Dubertret, L. & Weissenbach, J. (1997). Mapping of Papillon-Lefevre syndrome to the chromosome 11q14 region. *European Journal of Human Genetics* **5**, 156–160.

Folwaczny, M., Glas, J., Torok, H.P., Fricke, K. & Folwaczny, C. (2004a). The CD14 −159C-to-T promoter polymorphism in periodontal disease. *Journal of Clinical Periodontology* **31**, 991–995.

Folwaczny M., Glas, J., Torok, H.P., Limbersky, O. & Folwaczny, C. (2004b). Toll-like receptor (TLR) 2 and 4 mutations in periodontal disease. *Clinical and Experimental Immunology* **135**, 330–335.

Folwaczny, M., Glas, J., Torok, H.P., Mauermann, D. & Folwaczny, C. (2004c). The 3020insC mutation of the NOD2/CARD15 gene in patients with periodontal disease. *European Journal of Oral Sciences* **112**, 316–319.

Fu, Y., Korostoff, J.M., Fine, D.H. & Wilson, M.E. (2002). Fc gamma receptor genes as risk markers for localized aggressive periodontitis in African-Americans. *Journal of Periodontology* **73**, 517–523.

Galbraith, G.M., Steed, R.B., Sanders, J.J. & Pandey, J.P. (1998). Tumor necrosis factor alpha production by oral leukocytes: influence of tumor necrosis factor genotype. *Journal of Periodontology* **69**, 428–433.

Gore, E.A., Sanders, J.J., Pandey, J.P., Palesch, Y. & Galbraith, G.M. (1998). Interleukin-1beta+3953 allele 2: association with disease status in adult periodontitis. *Journal of Clinical Periodontology* **25**, 781–785.

Griffen, A.L., Becker, M.R., Lyons, S.R., Moeschberger, M.L. & Leys, E.J. (1998). Prevalence of *Porphyromonas gingivalis* and periodontal health status. *Journal of Clinical Microbiology* **36**, 3239–3242.

Gruica, B., Wang, H.Y., Lang, N.P. & Buser, D. (2004). Impact of IL-1 genotype and smoking status on the prognosis of osseointegrated implants. *Clinical Oral Implants Research* **15**, 393–400.

Hart, T.C. (1994). Genetic considerations of risk in human periodontal disease. *Current Opinion in Periodontology* 3–11.

Hart, T.C. (1996). Genetic risk factors for early-onset periodontitis. *Journal of Periodontology* **67**, 355–366.

Hart, T.C. & Kornman, K.S. (1997). Genetic factors in the pathogenesis of periodontitis. *Periodontology 2000* **14**, 202–215.

Hart, T.C., Stabholz, A., Meyle, J., Shapira, L., Van Dyke, T.E., Cutler, C.W. & Soskolne, W.A. (1997). Genetic studies of syndromes with severe periodontitis and palmoplantar hyperkeratosis. *Journal of Periodontal Research* **32**, 81–89.

Hart, T.C., Bowden, D.W., Ghaffar, K.A., Wang, W., Cutler, C.W., Cebeci, I., Efeoglu, A. & Firatli, E. (1998). Sublocalization of the Papillon-Lefevre syndrome locus on 11q14-q21. *American Journal of Medical Genetics* **79**, 134–139.

Hart, T.C., Hart, P.S., Bowden, D.W., Michalec, M.D., Callison, S.A., Walker, S.J., Zhang, Y. & Firatli, E. (1999). Mutations of the cathepsin C gene are responsible for Papillon-Lefevre syndrome. *Journal of Medical Genetics* **36**, 881–887.

Hart, T.C., Hart, P.S., Michalec, M.D., Zhang, Y., Marazita, M.L., Cooper, M., Yassin, O.M., Nusier, M. & Walker, S. (2000a). Localisation of a gene for prepubertal periodontitis to chromosome 11q14 and identification of a cathepsin C gene mutation. *Journal of Medical Genetics* **37**, 95–101.

Hart, T.C., Marazita, M.L. & Wright, J.T. (2000b). The impact of molecular genetics on oral health paradigms. *Critical Reviews in Oral Biology and Medicine* **11**, 26–56.

Hennig, B.J., Parkhill, J.M., Chapple, I.L., Heasman, P.A. & Taylor, J.J. (1999). Association of a vitamin D receptor gene polymorphism with localized early-onset periodontal diseases. *Journal of Periodontology* **70**, 1032–1038.

Hewitt, C., McCormick, D., Linden, G., Turk, D., Stern, I., Wallace, I., Southern, L., Zhang, L., Howard, R., Bullon, P., Wong, M., Widmer, R., Gaffar, K.A., Awawdeh, L., Briggs, J., Yaghmai, R., Jabs, E.W., Hoeger, P., Bleck, O., Rudiger, S.G., Petersilka, G., Battino, M., Brett, P., Hattab, F., Al-Hamed, M., Sloan, P., Toomes, C., Dixon, M., James, J., Read, A.P. & Thakker, N. (2004). The role of cathepsin C in Papillon-Lefevre syndrome, prepubertal periodontitis, and aggressive periodontitis. *Human Mutation* **23**, 222–228.

Hirschfeld, L. & Wasserman, B. (1978). A long-term survey of tooth loss in 600 treated periodontal patients. *Journal of Periodontology* **49**, 225–237.

Holla, L.I., Buckova, D., Fassmann, A., Halabala, T., Vasku, A. & Vacha, J. (2002). Promoter polymorphisms in the CD14 receptor gene and their potential association with the severity of chronic periodontitis. *Journal of Medical Genetics* **39**, 844–848.

Hugot, J.P., Chamaillard, M., Zouali, H., Lesage, S., Cezard, J.P., Belaiche, J., Almer, S., Tysk, C., O'Morain, C.A., Gassull, M., Binder, V., Finkel, Y., Cortot, A., Modigliani, R., Laurent-Puig, P., Gower-Rousseau, C., Macry, J., Colombel, J.F., Sahbatou, M. & Thomas, G. (2001). Association of NOD2 leucine-rich repeat variants with susceptibility to Crohn's disease. *Nature* **411**, 599–603.

Hutton, J.E., Heath, M.R., Chai, J.Y., Harnett, J., Jemt, T., Johns, R.B., McKenna, S., McNamara, D.C., van Steenberghe, D., Taylor, R. *et al.* (1995). Factors related to success and failure rates at 3-year follow-up in a multicenter study of overdentures supported by Branemark implants. *International Journal of Oral Maxillofacial Implants* **10**, 33–42.

Ioannidis, J.P. (2003). Genetic associations: false or true? *Trends in Molecular Medicine* **9**, 135–138.

Ioannidis, J.P., Trikalinos, T.A., Ntzani, E.E. & Contopoulos-Ioannidis, D.G. (2003). Genetic associations in large versus small studies: an empirical assessment. *Lancet* **361**, 567–571.

Kinane, D.F. & Hart, T.C. (2003). Genes and gene polymorphisms associated with periodontal disease. *Critical Reviews in Oral Biology and Medicine* **14**, 430–449.

Kinane, D.F., Hodge, P., Eskdale, J., Ellis, R. & Gallagher, G. (1999). Analysis of genetic polymorphisms at the interleukin-10 and tumour necrosis factor loci in early-onset periodontitis. *Journal of Periodontal Research* **34**, 379–386.

Kinane, D.F., Peterson, M. & Stathopoulou, P.G. (2006). Environmental and other modifying factors of the periodontal diseases. *Periodontology 2000* **40**, 107–119.

Kobayashi, T., Westerdaal, N.A., Miyazaki, A., van der Pol, W.L., Suzuki, T., Yoshie, H., van de Winkel, J.G. & Hara, K. (1997). Relevance of immunoglobulin G Fc receptor polymorphism to recurrence of adult periodontitis in Japanese patients. *Infection and Immunity* **65**, 3556–3560.

Kobayashi, T., Sugita, N., van der Pol, W.L., Nunokawa, Y., Westerdaal, N.A., Yamamoto, K., van de Winkel, J.G. & Yoshie, H. (2000). The Fcgamma receptor genotype as a risk factor for generalized early-onset periodontitis in Japanese patients. *Journal of Periodontology* **71**, 1425–1432.

Kornman, K.S., Crane, A., Wang, H.Y., di Giovine, F.S., Newman, M.G., Pirk, F.W., Wilson, T.G., Jr., Higginbottom, F.L. & Duff, G.W. (1997). The interleukin-1 genotype as a severity factor in adult periodontal disease. *Journal of Clinical Periodontology* **24**, 72–77.

Laass, M.W., Hennies, H.C., Preis, S., Stevens, H.P., Jung, M., Leigh, I.M., Wienker, T.F. & Reis, A. (1997). Localisation of a gene for Papillon-Lefevre syndrome to chromosome 11q14-q21 by homozygosity mapping. *Human Genetics* **101**, 376–382.

Laine, M.L., Farre, M.A., Gonzalez, G., van Dijk, L.J., Ham, A.J., Winkel, E.G., Crusius, J.B., Vandenbroucke, J.P., van Winkelhoff, A.J. & Pena, A.S. (2001). Polymorphisms of the interleukin-1 gene family, oral microbial pathogens, and smoking in adult periodontitis. *Journal of Dental Research* **80**, 1695–1699.

Laine, M.L., Leonhardt, A., Roos-Jansaker, A.M., Pena, A.S., van Winkelhoff, A.J., Winkel, E.G. & Renvert, S. (2006). IL-1RN gene polymorphism is associated with peri-implantitis. *Clinical Oral Implants Research* **17**, 380–385.

Laine, M.L., Murillo, L.S., Morre, S.A., Winkel, E.G., Pena, A.S. & van Winkelhoff, A.J. (2004). CARD15 gene mutations in periodontitis. *Journal of Clinical Periodontology* **31**, 890–893.

Laine, M.L., Morre, S.A., Murillo, L.S., van Winkelhoff, A.J. & Pena, A.S. (2005). CD14 and TLR4 gene polymorphisms in adult periodontitis. *Journal of Dental Research* **84**, 1042–1046.

Li, Y., Xu, L., Hasturk, H., Kantarci, A., DePalma, S.R. & Van Dyke, T.E. (2004). Localized aggressive periodontitis is linked to human chromosome 1q25. *Human Genetics* **114**, 291–297.

Löe, H., Theilade, E. & Jensen, S.B. (1965). Experimental gingivitis in man. *Journal of Periodontology* **36**, 177–187.

Löe, H., Anerud, A., Boysen, H. & Morrison, E. (1986). Natural history of periodontal disease in man. Rapid, moderate and no loss of attachment in Sri Lankan laborers 14 to 46 years of age. *Journal of Clinical Periodontology* **13**, 431–445.

Löe, H. & Brown, L.J. (1991). Early onset periodontitis in the United States of America. *Journal of Periodontology* **62**, 608–616.

Loevy, H.T. (1976). Genetic aspects of periodontal disease. *Quintessence International* **5**, 1–4.

Loos, B.G., John, R.P. & Laine, M.L. (2005). Identification of genetic risk factors for periodontitis and possible mechanisms of action. *Journal of Clinical Periodontology* **32** (Suppl 6), 159–179.

Loos, B.G., Leppers-Van de Straat, F.G., van de Winkel, J.G. & van der Velden, U. (2003). Fcgamma receptor polymorphisms in relation to periodontitis. *Journal of Clinical Periodontology* **30**, 595–602.

Marazita, M.L., Burmeister, J.A., Gunsolley, J.C., Koertge, T.E., Lake, K. & Schenkein, H.A. (1994). Evidence for autosomal dominant inheritance and race-specific heterogeneity in early-onset periodontitis. *Journal of Periodontology* **65**, 623–630.

McDevitt, M.J., Wang, H.Y., Knobelman, C., Newman, M.G., di Giovine, F.S., Timms, J., Duff, G.W. & Kornman, K.S. (2000). Interleukin-1 genetic association with periodontitis in clinical practice. *Journal of Periodontology* **71**, 156–163.

McFall, W.T., Jr. (1982). Tooth loss in 100 treated patients with periodontal disease. A long-term study. *Journal of Periodontology* **53**, 539–549.

McGuire, M.K. & Nunn, M.E. (1999). Prognosis versus actual outcome. IV. The effectiveness of clinical parameters and IL-1 genotype in accurately predicting prognoses and tooth survival. *Journal of Periodontology* **70**, 49–56.

Meisel, P., Carlsson, L.E., Sawaf, H., Fanghaenel, J., Greinacher, A. & Kocher, T. (2001). Polymorphisms of Fc gamma-receptors RIIa, RIIIa, and RIIIb in patients with adult periodontal diseases. *Genes and Immunity* **2**, 258–262.

Meisel, P., Schwahn, C., Gesch, D., Bernhardt, O., John, U. & Kocher, T. (2004). Dose-effect relation of smoking and the interleukin-1 gene polymorphism in periodontal disease. *Journal of Periodontology* **75**, 236–242.

Meisel, P., Siegemund, A., Dombrowa, S., Sawaf, H., Fanghaenel, J. & Kocher, T. (2002). Smoking and polymorphisms of the interleukin-1 gene cluster (IL-1alpha, IL-1beta, and IL-1RN) in patients with periodontal disease. *Journal of Periodontology* **73**, 27–32.

Meisel, P., Siegemund, A., Grimm, R., Herrmann, F.H., John, U., Schwahn, C. & Kocher, T. (2003). The interleukin-1 polymorphism, smoking, and the risk of periodontal disease in the population-based SHIP study. *Journal of Dental Research* **82**, 189–193.

Michalowicz, B.S., Aeppli, D., Virag, J.G., Klump, D.G., Hinrichs, J.E., Segal, N.L., Bouchard, T.J., Jr. & Pihlstrom, B.L. (1991). Periodontal findings in adult twins. *Journal of Periodontology* **62**, 293–299.

Noack, B., Gorgens, H., Hoffmann, T., Fanghanel, J., Kocher, T., Eickholz, P. & Schackert, H.K. (2004). Novel mutations in the cathepsin C gene in patients with pre-pubertal aggressive periodontitis and Papillon-Lefevre syndrome. *Journal of Dental Research* **83**, 368–370.

Page, R.C. (1999). Milestones in periodontal research and the remaining critical issues. *Journal of Periodontal Research* **34**, 331–339.

Page, R.C. & Sturdivant, E.C. (2002). Noninflammatory destructive periodontal disease (NDPD). *Periodontology 2000* **30**, 24–39.

Papapanou, P.N., Abron, A., Verbitsky, M., Picolos, D., Yang, J., Qin, J., Fine, J.B. & Pavlidis, P. (2004). Gene expression signatures in chronic and aggressive periodontitis: a pilot study. *European Journal of Oral Sciences* **112**, 216–223.

Papapanou, P.N., Neiderud, A.M., Sandros, J. & Dahlen, G. (2001). Interleukin-1 gene polymorphism and periodontal status. A case-control study. *Journal of Clinical Periodontology* **28**, 389–396.

Parkhill, J.M., Hennig, B.J., Chapple, I.L., Heasman, P.A. & Taylor, J.J. (2000). Association of interleukin-1 gene polymorphisms with early-onset periodontitis. *Journal of Clinical Periodontology* **27**(9):682–689.

Petit, M.D., Van Steenbergen, T.J.M., Timmerman, M.F., De Graaff, J. & van der Velden, U. (1994). Prevalence of periodontitis and suspected periodontal pathogens in families of adult periodontitis patients. *Journal of Clinical Periodontology* **21**, 76–85.

Quappe, L., Jara, L. & Lopez, N.J. (2004). Association of interleukin-1 polymorphisms with aggressive periodontitis. *Journal of Periodontology* **75**, 1509–1515.

Rogers, M.A., Figliomeni, L., Baluchova, K., Tan, A.E., Davies, G., Henry, P.J. & Price, P. (2002). Do interleukin-1 polymorphisms predict the development of periodontitis or the success of dental implants? *Journal of Periodontal Research* **37**, 37–41.

Roos-Jansaker, A.M., Lindahl, C., Renvert, H. & Renvert, S. (2006). Nine- to fourteen-year follow-up of implant treatment. Part I: implant loss and associations to various factors. *Journal of Clinical Periodontology* **33**, 283–289.

Santos, M.C., Campos, M.I., Souza, A.P., Trevilatto, P.C. & Line, S.R. (2004). Analysis of MMP-1 and MMP-9 promoter polymorphisms in early osseointegrated implant failure. *International Journal of Oral Maxillofacial Implants* **19**, 38–43.

Scarel-Caminaga, R.M., Trevilatto, P.C., Souza, A.P., Brito, R.B., Camargo, L.E. & Line, S.R. (2004). Interleukin 10 gene promoter polymorphisms are associated with chronic periodontitis. *Journal of Clinical Periodontology* **31**, 443–448.

Schork, N.J., Fallin, D. & Lanchbury, J.S. (2000). Single nucleotide polymorphisms and the future of genetic epidemiology. *Clinical Genetics* **58**, 250–264.

Selvaraju, V., Markandaya, M., Prasad, P.V., Sathyan, P., Sethuraman, G., Srivastava, S.C., Thakker, N. & Kumar, A. (2003). Mutation analysis of the cathepsin C gene in Indian families with Papillon-Lefevre syndrome. *BMC Medical Genetics* **4**, 5.

Shapira, L., Stabholz, A., Rieckmann, P. & Kruse, N. (2001). Genetic polymorphism of the tumor necrosis factor (TNF)-alpha promoter region in families with localized early-onset periodontitis. *Journal of Periodontal Research* **36**, 183–186.

Shimpuku, H., Nosaka, Y., Kawamura, T., Tachi, Y., Shinohara, M. & Ohura, K. (2003). Genetic polymorphisms of the interleukin-1 gene and early marginal bone loss around endosseous dental implants. *Clinical Oral Implants Research* **14**, 423–429.

Socransky, S.S. & Haffajee, A.D. (1992). The bacterial etiology of destructive periodontal disease: current concepts. *Journal of Periodontology* **63**, 322–331.

Socransky, S.S., Haffajee, A.D., Smith, C. & Duff, G.W. (2000). Microbiological parameters associated with IL-1 gene polymorphisms in periodontitis patients. *Journal of Clinical Periodontology* **27**, 810–818.

Soga, Y., Nishimura, F., Ohyama, H., Maeda, H., Takashiba, S. & Murayama, Y. (2003). Tumor necrosis factor-alpha gene (TNF-alpha) −1031/−863, −857 single-nucleotide polymorphisms (SNPs) are associated with severe adult periodontitis in Japanese. *Journal of Clinical Periodontology* **30**, 524–531.

Sun, J.L., Meng, H.X., Cao, C.F., Tachi,, Y., Shinohara M., Ueda, M., Imai, H. & Ohura, K. (2002). Relationship between vitamin D receptor gene polymorphism and periodontitis. *Journal of Periodontal Research* **37**, 263–267.

Tabor, H.K., Risch, N.J. & Myers, R.M. (2002). Opinion: Candidate-gene approaches for studying complex genetic traits: practical considerations. *Nature Reviews. Genetics* **3**, 391–397.

Tachi, Y., Shimpuku, H., Nosaka, Y., Kawamura, T., Shinohara, M., Ueda, M., Imai, H., Ohura, K., Sun, J., Meng, H. & Cao, C. (2001). Association of vitamin D receptor gene polymorphism with periodontal diseases in Japanese and Chinese. *Nucleic Acids Research* Suppl, 111–112.

Tachi, Y., Shimpuku, H., Nosaka, Y., Kawamura, T., Shinohara, M., Ueda, M., Imai, H. & Ohura, K. (2003). Vitamin D receptor gene polymorphism is associated with chronic periodontitis. *Life Sciences* **73**, 3313–3321.

Taguchi, A., Kobayashi, J., Suei, Y., Ohtsuka, M., Nakamoto, T., Tanimoto, K., Sanada, M., Tsuda, M. & Ohama, K. (2003). Association of estrogen and vitamin D receptor gene polymorphisms with tooth loss and oral bone loss in Japanese postmenopausal women. *Menopause* **10**, 250–257.

Tai, H., Endo, M., Shimada, Y., Gou, E., Orima, K., Kobayashi, T., Yamazaki, K. & Yoshie, H. (2002). Association of interleukin-1 receptor antagonist gene polymorphisms with early onset periodontitis in Japanese. *Journal of Clinical Periodontology* **29**, 882–888.

Toomes, C., James, J., Wood, A.J., Wu, C.L., McCormick, D., Lench, N., Hewitt, C., Moynihan, L., Roberts, E., Woods, C.G., Markham, A., Wong, M., Widmer, R., Ghaffar, K.A., Pemberton, M., Hussein, I.R., Temtamy, S.A., Davies, R., Read, A.P., Sloan, P., Dixon, M.J. & Thakker, N.S. (1999). Loss-of-function mutations in the cathepsin C gene result in periodontal disease and palmoplantar keratosis. *Nature Genetics* **23**, 421–424.

Trott, J.R. & Cross, H.G. (1966). An analysis of the principle reasons for tooth extractions in 1813 patients in Manitoba. *The Dental Practitioner and Dental Record* **17**, 20–27.

van der Pol, W. & van de Winkel, J.G. (1998). IgG receptor polymorphisms: risk factors for disease. *Immunogenetics* **48**, 222–232.

van der Velden, U., Abbas, F., Armand, S., de Graaff, J., Timmerman, M.F., van der Weijden, G.A., van Winkelhoff, A.J. & Winkel, E.G. (1993). The effect of sibling relationship on the periodontal condition. *Journal of Clinical Periodontology* **20**, 683–690.

van der Velden, U., Abbas, F., Armand, S., Loos, B.G., Timmerman, M.F., Van der Weijden, G.A., van Winkelhoff, A.J. & Winkel, E.G. (2006). Java project on periodontal diseases. The natural development of periodontitis: risk factors, risk predictors and risk determinants. *Journal of Clinical Periodontology* **33**, 540–548.

van der Velden, U., Abbas, F., Van Steenbergen, T.J., De Zoete, O.J., Hesse, M., De Ruyter, C., De Laat, V.H. & De Graaff, J. (1989). Prevalence of periodontal breakdown in adolescents and presence of *Actinobacillus actinomycetemcomitans* in subjects with attachment loss. *Journal of Periodontology* **60**, 604–610.

van Winkelhoff, A.J., Loos, B.G., van der Reijden, W.A. & van der Velden, U. (2002). *Porphyromonas gingivalis*, *Bacteroides forsythus* and other putative periodontal pathogens in subjects with and without periodontal destruction. *Journal of Clinical Periodontology* **29**, 1023–1028.

Walker, S.J., Van Dyke, T.E., Rich, S., Kornman, K.S., di Giovine, F.S. & Hart, T.C. (2000). Genetic polymorphisms of the IL-1alpha and IL-1beta genes in African-American LJP patients and an African-American control population. *Journal of Periodontology* **71**, 723–728.

Weyant, R.J. & Burt, B.A. (1993). An assessment of survival rates and within-patient clustering of failures for endosseous oral implants. *Journal of Dental Research* **72**, 2–8.

Wolff, L.F., Aeppli, D.M., Pihlstrom, B., Anderson, L., Stoltenberg, J., Osborn, J., Hardie, N., Shelburne, C. & Fischer, G. (1993). Natural distribution of 5 bacteria associated with periodontal disease. *Journal of Clinical Periodontology* **20**, 699–706.

Yamamoto, K., Kobayashi, T., Grossi, S., Ho, A.W., Genco, R.J., Yoshie, H. & De Nardin, E. (2004). Association of Fcgamma receptor IIa genotype with chronic periodontitis in Caucasians. *Journal of Periodontology* **75**, 517–522.

Yamazaki, K., Tabeta, K., Nakajima, T., Ohsawa, Y., Ueki, K., Itoh, H. & Yoshie, H. (2001). Interleukin-10 gene promoter polymorphism in Japanese patients with adult and early-onset periodontitis. *Journal of Clinical Periodontology* **28**, 828–832.

Yamazaki, K., Ueki-Maruyama, K., Oda, T., Tabeta, K., Shimada, Y., Tai, H., Nakajima, T., Yoshie, H., Herawati, D. & Seymour, G.J. (2003). Single-nucleotide polymorphism in the CD14 promoter and periodontal disease expression in a Japanese population. *Journal of Dental Research* **82**, 612–616.

Yoshihara, A., Sugita, N., Yamamoto, K., Kobayashi, T., Miyazaki, H. & Yoshi, H. (2001). Analysis of vitamin D and Fcgamma receptor polymorphisms in Japanese patients with generalized early-onset periodontitis. *Journal of Dental Research* **80**, 2051–2054.

Part 5: Trauma from Occlusion

Chapter 14

Trauma from Occlusion: Periodontal Tissues

Jan Lindhe, Sture Nyman, and Ingvar Ericsson

Definition and terminology

Trauma from occlusion is a term used to describe pathologic alterations or adaptive changes which develop in the periodontium as a result of undue force produced by the masticatory muscles. *Trauma from occlusion* is only one of many terms that have been used to describe such alterations in the periodontium. Other terms often used are: *traumatizing occlusion, occlusal trauma, traumatogenic occlusion, periodontal traumatism, overload*, etc. In addition to producing damage in the periodontal tissues, excessive occlusal force may also cause injury in, for example, the temporomandibular joint, the masticatory muscles, and the pulp tissue. This chapter deals exclusively with the effects of *trauma from occlusion* on the periodontal tissues.

Trauma from occlusion was defined by Stillman (1917) as "a condition where injury results to the supporting structures of the teeth by the act of bringing the jaws into a closed position". The World Health Organization (WHO) in 1978 defined *trauma from occlusion* as "damage in the periodontium caused by stress on the teeth produced directly or indirectly by teeth of the opposing jaw". In "Glossary of Periodontic Terms" (American Academy of Periodontology 1986), *occlusal trauma* was defined as "an injury to the attachment apparatus as a result of excessive occlusal force".

Traumatizing forces may act on an individual tooth or on groups of teeth in premature contact relationship; they may occur in conjunction with parafunctions such as clenching and bruxism, or in conjunction with loss or migration of premolar and molar teeth with an accompanying, gradually developing spread of the anterior teeth of the maxilla, etc.

In the literature, the tissue injury associated with trauma from occlusion is often divided into *primary* and *secondary*. The *primary* form includes a tissue reaction (damage), which is elicited around a tooth with normal height of the periodontium, while the *secondary* form is related to situations in which occlusal forces cause injury in a periodontium of reduced height. The distinction between a *primary* and a *secondary* form of injury – *primary* and *secondary occlusal trauma* – serves no meaningful purpose, since the alterations which occur in the periodontium as a consequence of trauma from occlusion are similar and independent of the height of the target tissue, i.e. the periodontium. It is, however, important to understand that symptoms of trauma from occlusion may develop only in situations when the magnitude of the load elicited by occlusion is so high that the periodontium around the exposed tooth cannot properly withstand and distribute the resulting force with unaltered position and stability of the tooth involved. This means that in cases of severely reduced height of the periodontium even comparatively small forces may produce traumatic lesions or adaptive changes in the periodontium.

Trauma from occlusion and plaque-associated periodontal disease

Ever since Karolyi (1901) postulated that an interaction may exist between "*trauma from occlusion*" and "*alveolar pyrrohea*", different opinions have been presented in the literature regarding the validity of this claim. In the 1930s, Box (1935) and Stones (1938) reported experiments in sheep and monkeys, the result of which seemed to indicate that "trauma from occlusion is an etiologic factor in the production of that variety of periodontal disease in which there is vertical pocket formation associated with one or a varying number of teeth" (Stones 1938). The experiments by Box and Stones, however, have been criticized because they lacked proper controls and because the experimental design of the studies did not justify the conclusions drawn.

The interaction between trauma from occlusion and plaque-associated periodontal disease in humans was frequently discussed in the period 1955–1970 in connection with "report of a case", "in my opinion" statements, etc. Even if such anecdotal data may have some value in clinical dentistry, it is obvious that conclusions drawn from research findings are much more pertinent. The research-based conclusions are not always indisputable but they invite the reader to a critique which anecdotal data do not. In this chapter, therefore, the presentation will be limited to findings collected from research endeavors involving: (1) human autopsy material, (2) clinical trials, and (3) animal experiments.

Analysis of human autopsy material

Results reported from carefully performed research efforts involving examinations of human autopsy material have been difficult to interpret. In the specimens examined (1) the histopathology of the lesions in the periodontium have been described, as well as (2) the presence and apical extension of microbial deposits at adjacent root surfaces, (3) the mobility of the teeth involved, and (4) "the occlusion" of the sites under scrutiny. It is obvious that assessments made in specimens from cadavers have a limited to questionable value when "cause–effect" relationships between occlusion, plaque, and periodontal lesions are to be described. It is not surprising, therefore, that *conclusions* drawn from this type of research can be controversial. This can best be illustrated if "Glickman's concept" is compared with "Waerhaug's concept" of what autopsy studies have revealed regarding trauma from occlusion and periodontal disease.

Glickman's concept

Glickman (1965, 1967) claimed that the pathway of the spread of a plaque-associated gingival lesion can be changed if forces of an abnormal magnitude are acting on teeth harboring subgingival plaque. This would imply that the character of the progressive tissue destruction of the periodontium at a "traumatized tooth" will be different from that characterizing a "non-traumatized" tooth. Instead of an even destruction of the periodontium and alveolar bone (suprabony pockets and horizontal bone loss), which, according to Glickman, occurs at sites with uncomplicated plaque-associated lesions, sites which are also exposed to abnormal occlusal force will develop angular bony defects and infrabony pockets.

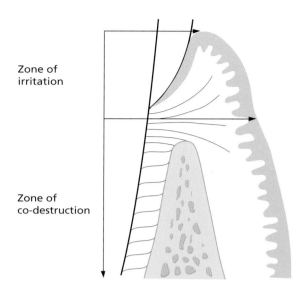

Fig. 14-1 Schematic drawing of the zone of irritation and the zone of co-destruction according to Glickman.

Since Glickman's concept regarding the effect of trauma from occlusion on the spread of the plaque-associated lesion is often cited, a more detailed presentation of his theory seems pertinent. The periodontal structures can be divided into two zones (Fig. 14-1):

1. The zone of irritation
2. The zone of co-destruction.

The *zone of irritation* includes the marginal and interdental gingiva. The soft tissue of this zone is bordered by hard tissue (the tooth) only on one side and is not affected by forces of occlusion. This means that gingival inflammation cannot be induced by trauma from occlusion but is the result of irritation from microbial plaque. The plaque-associated lesion at a "non-traumatized" tooth propagates in the apical direction by first involving the alveolar bone and only later the periodontal ligament area. The progression of this lesion results in an even (horizontal) bone destruction.

The *zone of co-destruction* includes the periodontal ligament, the root cementum, and the alveolar bone, and is coronally demarcated by the trans-septal (interdental) and the dento-alveolar collagen fiber bundles (Fig. 14-1). The tissue in this zone may become the seat of a lesion caused by trauma from occlusion.

The fiber bundles which separate the zone of co-destruction from the zone of irritation can be affected from two different directions:

1. From the inflammatory lesion maintained by plaque in the *zone of irritation*
2. From trauma-induced changes in the *zone of co-destruction*.

Through this exposure from two different directions the fiber bundles may become dissolved and/or orientated in a direction parallel to the root surface. The spread of an inflammatory lesion from the *zone of irritation* directly down into the periodontal ligament (i.e. not via the interdental bone) may hereby be facilitated (Fig. 14-2). This alteration of the "normal" pathway of spread of the plaque-associated inflammatory lesion results in the development of angular bony defects. Glickman (1967) stated in a review paper that *trauma from occlusion* is an etiologic factor (co-destructive factor) of importance in situations where angular bony defects combined with infrabony pockets are found at one or several teeth (Fig. 14-3).

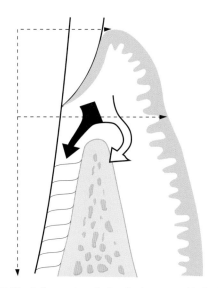

Fig. 14-2 The inflammatory lesion in the zone of irritation can, in teeth not subjected to trauma, propagate into the alveolar bone (open arrow), while in teeth also subjected to trauma from occlusion, the inflammatory infiltrate spreads directly into periodontal ligament (filled arrow).

Waerhaug's concept

Waerhaug (1979) examined autopsy specimens (Fig. 14-4) similar to Glickman's, but in addition measured the distance between the subgingival plaque and (1) the periphery of the associated inflammatory cell infiltrate in the gingiva, and (2) the surface of the adjacent alveolar bone. He concluded from his analysis that angular bony defects and infrabony pockets occur equally often at periodontal sites of teeth which are not affected by trauma from occlusion as in traumatized teeth. In other words, he refuted the hypothesis that trauma from occlusion played a role in the spread of a gingival lesion into the "zone of codestruction". The loss of connective attachment and the resorption of bone around teeth are, according to Waerhaug, exclusively the result of inflammatory lesions associated with subgingival plaque. Waerhaug concluded that angular bony defects and infrabony pockets occur when the subgingival plaque of one tooth has reached a more apical level than the microbiota on the neighboring tooth, and when the volume of the alveolar bone surrounding the roots is comparatively large. Waerhaug's observations support findings presented by Prichard (1965) and Manson (1976) which imply that the pattern of loss of supporting structures is the result of an interplay between the form and volume of the alveolar bone and the apical extension of the microbial plaque on the adjacent root surfaces.

It is obvious, as stated above, that examinations of autopsy material have a limited value when determining "cause–effect" relationships with respect to trauma and progressive periodontitis. As a consequence, the conclusions drawn from this field of research have not been generally accepted. A number of authors tend to accept Glickman's conclusions that trauma from occlusion is an aggravating factor in

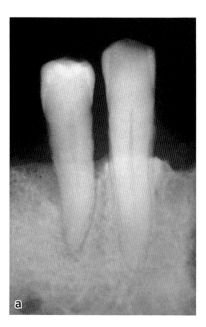
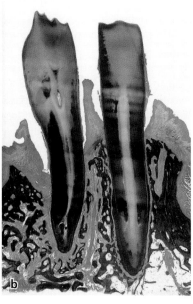

Fig. 14-3 (a) A radiograph of a mandibular premolar–canine region. Note the angular bony defect at the distal aspect of the premolar. (b) Histologic mesiodistal section of the specimen illustrated in (a). Note the infrabony pocket at the distal aspect of the premolar. From Glickman & Smulow (1965).

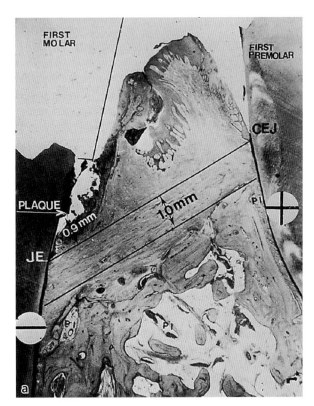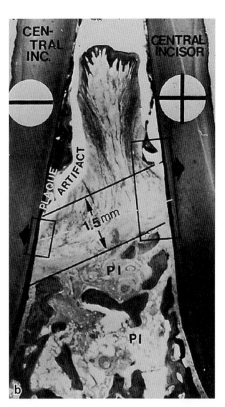

Fig. 14-4 Microphotographs illustrating two interproximal areas with angular bony defects. "–" denotes a tooth not subjected and "+" denotes a tooth subjected to trauma from occlusion. In categories "–" and "+" the distance between the apical cells of the junctional epithelium and the supporting alveolar bone is about 1–1.5 mm, and the distance between the apical extension of plaque and the apical cells of the junctional epithelium about 1 mm. Since the apical cells of the junctional epithelium and the subgingival plaque are located at different levels on the two adjacent teeth, the outline of the bone crest becomes oblique. A radiograph from such a site would disclose the presence of an angular bony defect at a non-traumatized ("–") tooth.

periodontal disease (e.g. Macapanpan & Weinmann 1954; Posselt & Emslie 1959; Glickman & Smulow 1962, 1965) while others accept Waerhaug's concept, i.e. that there is no relationship between occlusal trauma and the degree of periodontal tissue breakdown (e.g. Lovdahl *et al.* 1959; Belting & Gupta 1961; Baer *et al.* 1963; Waerhaug 1979).

Clinical trials

In addition to the presence of angular bony defects and infrabony pockets, *increased tooth mobility* is frequently listed as an important sign of occlusal trauma. For details regarding tooth mobility, see Chapter 51. Conflicting data have also been reported regarding the periodontal conditions of mobile teeth. In one clinical study by Rosling *et al.* (1976) patients with advanced periodontal disease associated with multiple angular bony defects and mobile teeth were exposed to antimicrobial therapy (i.e. subgingival scaling after flap elevation). Healing was evaluated by probing attachment level measurements and radiographic monitoring. The authors reported that "the infrabony pocket located at hypermobile teeth exhibited the same degree of healing as those adjacent to firm teeth". In another study, however, Fleszar *et al.* (1980) reported on the influence of tooth mobility on healing following periodontal therapy includ-

ing both root debridement and occlusal adjustment. They concluded that "pockets of clinically mobile teeth do not respond as well to periodontal treatment as do those of firm teeth exhibiting the same disease severity".

A third study (Pihlstrom *et al.* 1986) studied the association between trauma from occlusion and periodontitis by assessing a series of clinical and radiographic features at maxillary first molars. Parameters included in this study were: probing depth, probing attachment level, tooth mobility, wear facets, plaque and calculus, bone height, widened periodontal space, etc. Pihlstrom and his associates concluded from their measurements and examinations that teeth with increased mobility and widened periodontal ligament space had, in fact, deeper pockets, more attachment loss, and less bone support than teeth without these symptoms.

Burgett *et al.* (1992) studied the effect of occlusal adjustment in the treatment of periodontitis. Fifty subjects with periodontitis were examined at baseline and subsequently treated for their periodontal condition with root debridement ± flap surgery. Twenty-two out of the 50 patients, in addition, received comprehensive occlusal therapy. Re-examinations performed 2 years later disclosed that probing attachment gain was on average about 0.5 mm larger in patients who received the combined treatment, i.e. scaling and occlusal adjustment, than in patients in whom the occlusal adjustment was not included.

Nunn and Harrel (2001) and Harrel and Nunn (2001) examined the relationship between occlusal discrepancies and periodontitis in two studies. Their sample included about 90 subjects that had been referred for treatment of periodontal disease and who had at least two (≥1 year apart) complete periodontal records, including occlusal analysis. The patients were examined with respect to probing pocket depth (PPD), tooth mobility, and furcation involvement (at multirooted teeth). In addition, some occlusal contact relationships were studied such as (1) discrepancies in centric relation and centric occlusion, (2) premature occlusal contacts in protrusive movements (lateral and frontal) of the mandible in working and non-working quadrants. A treatment plan, including both periodontal and occlusal measures, was subsequently designed for each patient. About one third of the subjects decided to abstain from treatment, about 20 subjects accepted only a non-surgical approach of therapy (SRP), while about 50% of the patients accepted and received comprehensive treatment that included surgical pocket elimination (surgery) as well as occlusal adjustment (if indicated). Some teeth in the SRP group received occlusal therapy while other teeth with occlusal discrepancies were left untreated. It was observed that teeth with occlusal discrepancies had significantly deeper PPD values and higher mobility scores than teeth without occlusal "trauma" and also that teeth exposed to occlusal adjustment responded better (reduction in PPD) to non-surgical periodontal therapy than teeth with remaining occlusal discrepancies.

The findings in some of the clinical studies referred to above lend some support to the concept that trauma from occlusion (and increased tooth mobility) may have a detrimental effect on the periodontium. Neiderud et al. (1992), however, in a beagle dog study demonstrated that tissue alterations which occur at mobile teeth with clinically healthy gingivae (and normal height of the tissue attachment) may reduce the resistance offered by the periodontal tissues to probing. In other words, if the probing depth at two otherwise similar teeth – one non-mobile and one hypermobile – is recorded, the tip of the probe will penetrate 0.5 mm deeper at the mobile than at the non-mobile tooth. This finding must be taken into consideration when the above clinical data are interpreted.

Since neither analysis of autopsy material nor data from clinical trials can be used to properly determine the role trauma from occlusion may play in periodontal pathology, it is necessary to describe the contributions made by means of animal research in this particular field. Results from such experiments, describing the reactions of the normal and subsequently the diseased periodontium to occlusal forces, are presented below.

Animal experiments

Orthodontic type trauma

The reaction of the periodontal tissues to traumatic forces initiated by occlusion has been studied principally in animal experiments. In early experiments the reaction of the normal periodontium was studied following the application of forces which were inflicted on teeth in one direction only. Biopsy specimens, including tooth and periodontium, were harvested after varying experimental time intervals and prepared for histologic examinations. Analysis of the tissue sections (Häupl & Psansky 1938; Reitan 1951; Mühlemann & Herzog 1961; Ewen & Stahl 1962; Waerhaug & Hansen 1966; Karring et al. 1982) revealed the following: when a tooth is exposed to unilateral forces of a magnitude, frequency or duration that its periodontal tissues are unable to withstand and distribute while maintaining the stability of the tooth, certain well defined reactions develop in the periodontal ligament, eventually resulting in an adaptation of the periodontal structures to the altered functional demand. If the crown of a tooth is affected by such horizontally directed forces, the tooth tends to tilt (tip) in the direction of the force (Fig. 14-5). This tilting force results in the development of *pressure* and *tension zones* within the marginal and apical parts of the periodontium. The tissue reactions which develop in the *pressure zone* are characterized by increased vascularization, increased vascular permeability, vascular thrombosis, and disorganization of cells and collagen fiber bundles. If the magnitude of forces is within certain limits, allowing the maintenance of the vitality of the periodontal ligament cells,

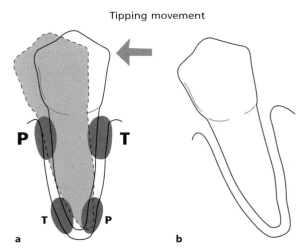

Fig. 14-5 (a) If the crown of a tooth is exposed to excessive, horizontally directed forces (arrow), pressure (P) and tension (T) zones will develop within the marginal and apical parts of the periodontium. The supra-alveolar connective tissue remains unaffected by force application. Within the pressure and tension zones tissue alterations take place which eventually allow the tooth to tilt in the direction of the force. (b) When the tooth is no longer subjected to the trauma, complete regeneration of the periodontal tissues takes place. There is no apical downgrowth of the dentogingival epithelium.

bone-resorbing osteoclasts soon appear on the bone surface of the alveolus in the *pressure zone*. A process of bone resorption is initiated. This phenomenon is called "*direct bone resorption*".

If the force applied is of higher magnitude, the result may be necrosis of the periodontal ligament tissue in the *pressure zone*, i.e. decomposition of cells, vessels, matrix, and fibers (*hyalinization*). "Direct bone resorption" therefore cannot occur. Instead, osteoclasts appear in marrow spaces within the adjacent bone tissue where the stress concentration is lower than in the periodontal ligament and a process of undermining or "*indirect bone resorption*" is initiated. Through this reaction the surrounding bone is resorbed until there is a breakthrough to the hyalinized tissue within the *pressure zone*. This breakthrough results in a reduction of the stress in this area, and cells from the neighboring bone or adjacent areas of the periodontal ligament can proliferate into the *pressure zone* and replace the previously hyalinized tissue, thereby re-establishing prerequisites for "direct bone resorption". Irrespective of whether the bone resorption is of a direct or an indirect nature the tooth moves (tilts) further in the direction of the force.

Concomitant with the tissue alterations in the *pressure zone*, apposition of bone occurs in the *tension zone* in order to maintain the normal width of the periodontal ligament in this area. Because of the tissue reactions in the *pressure* and *tension* zones the tooth becomes, temporarily, hypermobile. When the tooth has moved (tilted) to a position where the effect of the forces is nullified, healing of the periodontal tissues takes place in both the *pressure* and the *tension* zones and the tooth becomes stable in its new position. In orthodontic tilting (tipping) movements, neither gingival inflammation nor loss of connective tissue attachment will occur in a healthy periodontium and, as long as the tooth is not moved through the envelope of the alveolar process, there is no apical migration of the dentogingival epithelium. In other words, since the supraalveolar connective tissue is only bordered by hard tissue (the tooth) on one side (in the direction of the force), this structure remains unaffected by this type of force.

These tissue reactions do not differ fundamentally from those which occur as a consequence of *bodily tooth movement* in orthodontic therapy (Reitan 1951). The main difference is that the *pressure* and *tension* zones, depending on the direction of the force, are more extended in an apical–coronal direction along the root surface than in conjunction with tipping movement (Fig. 14-6). The supra-alveolar connective tissue is not affected by the force, either in conjunction with tipping or in conjunction with bodily movements of the tooth. Unilateral forces directed to the crown of teeth, therefore, will not induce inflammatory reactions in the gingiva or cause loss of connective tissue attachment.

Studies have demonstrated, however, that orthodontic forces producing bodily (or tipping) move-

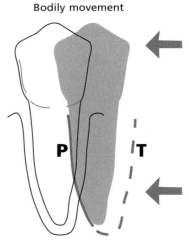

Fig. 14-6 When a tooth is exposed to forces which produce "bodily tooth movement", e.g. in orthodontic therapy, the pressure (P) and tension (T) zones, depending on the direction of the force, are extended over the entire tooth surface. The supra-alveolar connective tissue is not affected in conjunction either with tipping or with bodily movements of teeth. Forces of this kind, therefore, will not induce inflammatory reactions in the gingiva. No apical downgrowth of the dentogingival epithelium occurs.

ment of teeth may result in gingival recession and loss of connective tissue attachment (Steiner *et al.* 1981; Wennström *et al.* 1987). This breakdown of the attachment apparatus occurred at sites with gingivitis when, in addition, the tooth was moved through the envelope of the alveolar process. At such sites bone dehiscence becomes established and, if the covering soft tissue is thin (in the direction of the movement of the tooth), recession (attachment loss) may occur.

Criticism has been directed, however, at experiments in which only unilateral trauma is exerted on teeth (Wentz *et al.* 1958). It has been suggested that in humans, unlike in the animal experiments described above, the occlusal forces act alternately in one and then in the opposite direction. Such forces have been termed *jiggling forces*.

Jiggling-type trauma

Healthy periodontium with normal height
Experiments have been reported in which traumatic forces were exerted on the crowns of the teeth, alternately in buccal and lingual or mesial and distal directions, and in which the teeth were not allowed to move away from the force (e.g. Wentz *et al.* 1958; Glickman & Smulow 1968; Svanberg & Lindhe 1973; Meitner 1975; Ericsson & Lindhe 1982). In conjunction with "*jiggling-type trauma*" no clearcut *pressure* and *tension zones* can be identified but rather there is a combination of pressure and tension on both sides of the jiggled tooth (Fig. 14-7).

The tissue reactions in the periodontal ligament provoked by the combined *pressure* and *tension* forces were found to be similar, however, to those reported

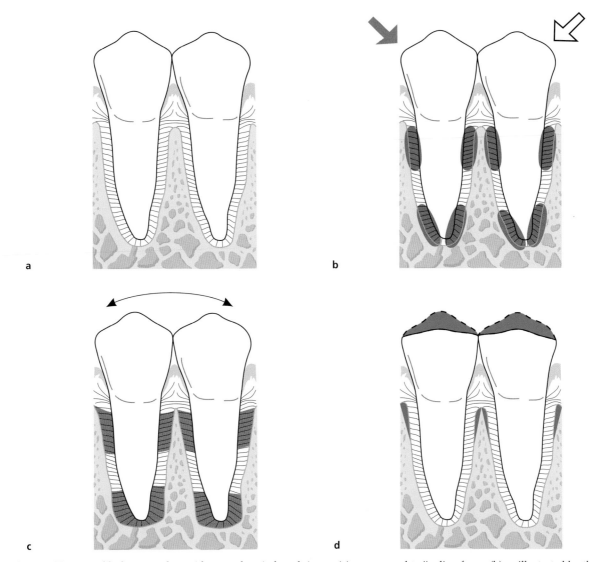

Fig. 14-7 Two mandibular premolars with normal periodontal tissues (a) are exposed to jiggling forces (b) as illustrated by the two arrows. The combined tension and pressure zones (encircled areas) are characterized by signs of acute inflammation including collagen resorption, bone resorption, and cementum resorption. As a result of bone resorption the periodontal ligament space gradually increases in size on both sides of the teeth as well as in the periapical region. (c) When the effect of the force applied has been compensated for by the increased width of the periodontal ligament space, the ligament tissue shows no sign of inflammation. The supra-alveolar connective tissue is not affected by the jiggling forces and there is no apical downgrowth of the dentogingival epithelium. (d) After occlusal adjustment the width of the periodontal ligament becomes normalized and the teeth are stabilized.

for the pressure zone at orthodontically moved teeth, with the one difference that the periodontal ligament space at jiggling gradually increased in width on both sides of the tooth. During the phase when the periodontal space gradually increased in width, (1) inflammatory changes were present in the ligament tissue, (2) active bone resorption occurred, and (3) the tooth displayed signs of gradually increasing (*progressive*) mobility. When the effect of the forces applied had been compensated for by the increased width of the periodontal ligament space, the ligament tissue showed no signs of increased vascularity or exudation. The tooth was hypermobile but the mobility was no longer *progressive* in character. Distinction should thus be made between *progressive* and *increased* tooth mobility.

In *jiggling-type trauma* experiments, performed on animals with a normal periodontium, the supra-alveolar connective tissue was not influenced by the occlusal forces, the reason being that this tissue compartment is bordered by hard tissue on one side only. This means that a gingiva which was uninflamed at the start of the experiment remained uninflamed, but also that an overt inflammatory lesion residing in the supra-alveolar connective tissue was not aggravated by the jiggling forces.

Healthy periodontium with reduced height

Progressive periodontal disease is characterized by gingival inflammation and a gradually developing loss of connective tissue attachment and alveolar bone. Treatment of periodontal disease, i.e. removal

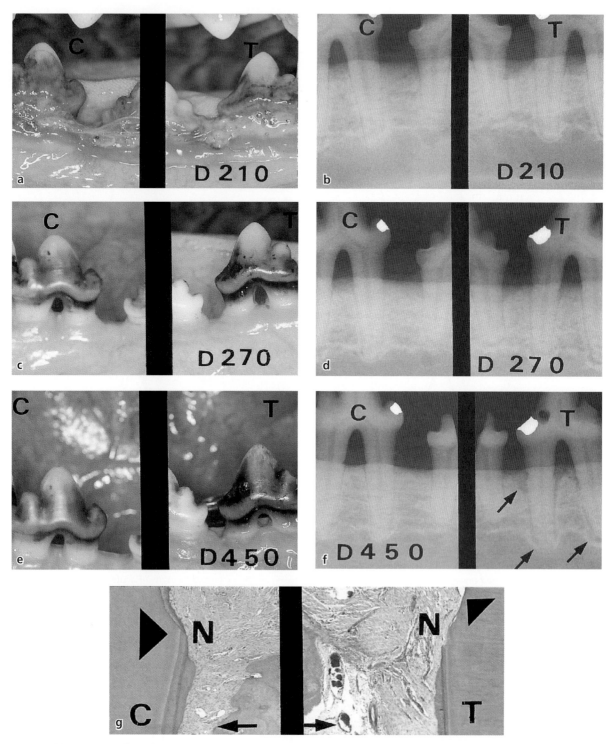

Fig. 14-8 (a) Dogs were allowed to accumulate plaque and calculus in the mandibular premolar regions over a 210-day period. (b) When around 40–50% of the periodontal tissue support had been lost the animals were treated by scaling, root planing, and pocket elimination. During surgery, a notch was prepared in the root at the level of the bone crest. (c, d) The dogs were subsequently placed on a plaque-control program and 2 months later (day 270) all experimental teeth (the lower fourth premolars; 4P and P4) were surrounded by a healthy periodontium with reduced height. (e) The mandibular left fourth premolar (T) was exposed to jiggling forces. (f) As a consequence, a widened periodontal ligament and increased tooth mobility resulted. (g) This increase in tooth mobility and the development of widened periodontal ligament space did not, however, result in apical downgrowth of the dentogingival epithelium. Arrowheads indicate the apical extension of the junctional epithelium which coincides with the apical border of the notch (N), prepared in the root surface prior to jiggling. C = control tooth; T = test tooth.

of plaque and calculus and elimination of pathologically deepened pockets, will result in the re-establishment of a healthy periodontium but with reduced height. The question is whether a healthy periodontium with reduced height has a capacity similar to that of the normal periodontium to adapt to traumatizing occlusal forces (secondary occlusal trauma).

This problem has also been examined in animal experiments (Ericsson & Lindhe 1977). Destructive periodontal disease was initiated in dogs by allowing the animals to accumulate plaque and calculus for a period of 6 months (Fig. 14-8). When around 50% of the periodontal tissue support had been lost (Fig. 14-8a,b), the progressive disease was subjected to treatment by scaling, root planing, and pocket elimination (Fig. 14-8c). During a subsequent 8-month period, the animals were enrolled in a careful plaque-control program. During this period certain premolars were exposed to traumatizing jiggling forces. The periodontal tissues in the combined *pressure* and *tension zones* reacted to the forces by vascular proliferation, exudation, and thrombosis, as well as by bone resorption. In radiographs, widened periodontal ligaments (Fig. 14-8d) could be found around the traumatized teeth, which displayed signs of *progressive* tooth mobility at clinical examination. The gradual increase

in the width of the periodontal ligament and the resulting progressive increase in tooth mobility took place during a period of several weeks but eventually terminated. The active bone resorption ceased and the markedly widened periodontal ligament tissue regained its normal composition; healing had occurred (Fig. 14-8e). The teeth were hypermobile but surrounded by periodontal structures which had adapted to the altered functional demands.

During the entire experimental period the supra-alveolar connective tissue remained unaffected by the jiggling forces. There was no further loss of connective tissue attachment and no further downgrowth of dentogingival epithelium (Fig. 14-8e). The results from this study clearly reveal that within certain limits a healthy periodontium with reduced height has a capacity similar to that of a periodontium with normal height to adapt to altered functional demands (Fig. 14-9).

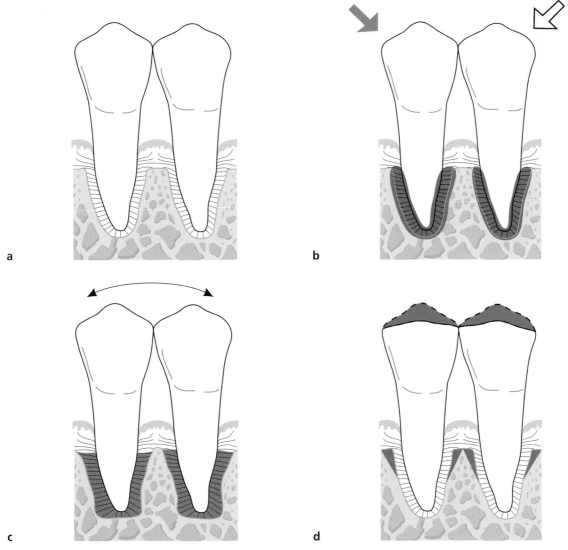

Fig. 14-9 (a) Two mandibular premolars are surrounded by a healthy periodontium with reduced height. (b) If such premolars are subjected to traumatizing forces of the jiggling type a series of alterations occurs in the periodontal ligament tissue. (c) These alterations result in a widened periodontal ligament space and in an increased tooth mobility but do not lead to further loss of connective tissue attachment. (d) After occlusal adjustment the width of the periodontal ligament is normalized and the teeth are stabilized.

Plaque-associated periodontal disease

Experiments carried out on humans and animals have demonstrated that *trauma from occlusion* cannot induce pathologic alterations in the supra-alveolar connective tissue, i.e. cannot produce inflammatory lesions in a normal gingiva or aggravate a gingival lesion associated with plaque and cannot induce loss of connective tissue attachment. The question remains if abnormal occlusal forces can influence the spread of the plaque-associated lesion and enhance the rate of tissue destruction in periodontal disease. This has been studied in animal experiments (Lindhe & Svanberg 1974; Meitner 1975; Nyman *et al.* 1978; Ericsson & Lindhe 1982; Polson & Zander 1983). In these experiments progressive and destructive periodontal disease was first initiated in dogs or monkeys by allowing the animals to accumulate plaque and calculus. Teeth thus involved in a progressive periodontal disease process were also subjected to trauma from occlusion.

"Traumatizing" jiggling forces (Lindhe & Svanberg 1974) were exerted on premolars and were found to induce certain tissue reactions in the combined *pressure/tension zones*. Within a few days of the onset of the jiggling forces, the periodontal ligament tissue in these zones displayed signs of inflamma-tion, had increased numbers of vessels, showed increased vascular permeability and exudation, thrombosis, as well as retention of neutrophils and macrophages. On the adjacent bone surfaces there were a large number of osteoclasts. Since the teeth could not orthodontically move away from the jiggling forces, the periodontal ligament of both sides of the tooth gradually increased in width, the teeth became hypermobile (*progressive* tooth mobility) and angular bony defects could be detected in the radiographs. The forces were eventually nullified by the increased width of the periodontal ligament.

If the forces applied were of a magnitude to which the periodontal structures could adapt, the *progressive* increase of the tooth mobility terminated within a few weeks. The active bone resorption ceased but the angular bone destruction persisted as well as the increased tooth mobility. The periodontal ligament had an increased width but a normal tissue composition. Histologic examination of biopsy specimens revealed that this adaptation had occurred with no greater apical proliferation of the dentogingival epithelium than was caused by the plaque-associated lesion (Fig. 14-10) (Meitner 1975). This means that occlusal forces which allow adaptive alterations to develop in the *pressure/tension* zones of the periodon-

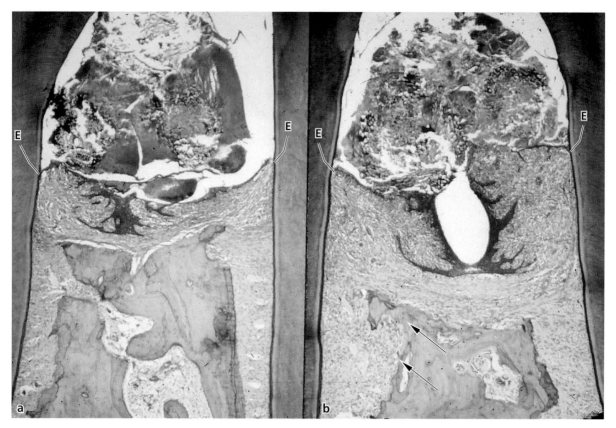

Fig. 14-10 (a) A composite photomicrograph illustrating the interdental space between two pairs of teeth. The teeth have been subjected to experimental, ligature-induced periodontitis and in (b) also to repetitive mechanical injury. In (b), there is considerable loss of alveolar bone and an angular widening of the periodontal ligament space (arrows). However, the apical downgrowth of the dentogingival epithelium in the two areas (a) and (b) is similar. E indicates the apical level of the dentogingival epithelium. Courtesy of Dr. S.W. Meitner.

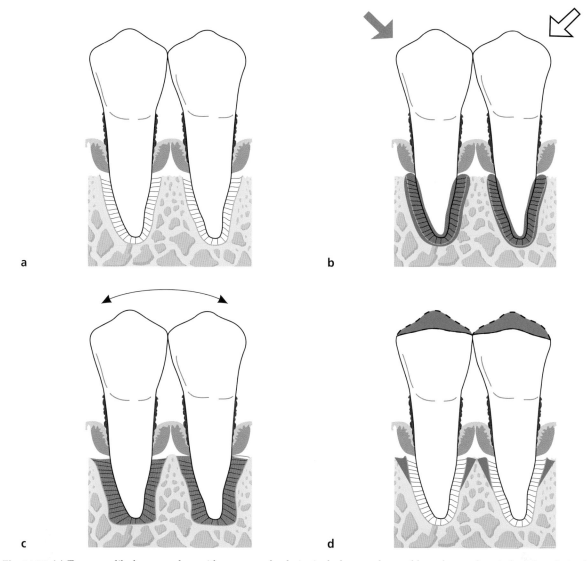

Fig. 14-11 (a) Two mandibular premolars with supra- and subgingival plaque, advanced bone loss and periodontal pockets of a suprabony character. Note the connective tissue infiltrate (shadowed areas) and the uninflamed connective tissue between the alveolar bone and the apical portion of the infiltrate. (b) If these teeth are subjected to traumatizing forces of the jiggling type, pathologic and adaptive alterations occur within the periodontal ligament space. (c) These tissue alterations, which include bone resorption, result in a widened periodontal ligament space and increased tooth mobility but no further loss of connective tissue attachment. (d) Occlusal adjustment results in a reduction of the width of the periodontal ligament and in less mobile teeth.

tal ligament will not aggravate a plaque-associated periodontal disease (Fig. 14-11).

If, however, the magnitude and direction of the jiggling forces were such that, during the course of the study (6 months), the tissues in the pressure/tension zones could not become adapted, the injury in the *zones of co-destruction* had a more permanent character. For several months the periodontal ligament in the pressure/tension zones displayed signs of inflammation (vascular proliferation, exudation, thrombosis, retention of neutrophils and macrophages, collagen destruction). Osteoclasts residing on the walls of the alveolus maintained the bone-resorptive process, which resulted in a gradual widening of the periodontal ligament in the pressure/tension zones (Fig. 14-12). As a consequence, the resulting angular bone destruction was continuous and the mobility of the teeth remained progres-

sive. The plaque-associated lesion in the "zone of irritation" and the inflammatory lesion in the "zone of co-destruction" merged; the dentogingival epithelium proliferated in an apical direction and periodontal disease was aggravated (Figs. 14-13, 14-14) (Lindhe & Svanberg 1974).

Similar findings were reported from another experiment in the dog (Ericsson & Lindhe 1982) in which the effect was assessed of a *prolonged* period of jiggling force application on the rate of progression of plaque-associated, marginal periodontitis. Thus, in dogs with continuing periodontal disease, certain teeth were exposed to jiggling forces during a period of 10 months. Control teeth were not jiggled. Figure 14–15a illustrates the marked periodontal tissue breakdown around a tooth which was exposed to plaque infection combined with jiggling trauma for several months and Fig. 14-15b illustrates a control tooth which was exposed to plaque infection only.

On the other hand, more short-term experiments in the monkey (Polson & Zander 1983), evaluating the effect of *trauma from occlusion* on teeth involved in an ongoing process of periodontitis, failed to support the findings by Lindhe and Svanberg (1974) and Ericsson and Lindhe (1982). Polson and Zander (1983) observed that trauma superimposed on periodontal lesions associated with angular bony defects (1) caused increased loss of alveolar bone but (2) failed to produce additional loss of connective tissue attachment.

Conclusions

Experiments carried out in humans as well as animals, have produced convincing evidence that neither unilateral forces nor jiggling forces, applied to teeth with a healthy periodontium, result in pocket formation or in loss of connective tissue attachment. *Trauma from occlusion cannot induce periodontal tissue breakdown.* Trauma from occlusion does, however, result in resorption of alveolar bone leading to an increased tooth mobility which can be of a transient or permanent character. This bone resorption with resulting increased tooth mobility should be regarded as a physiologic adaptation of the periodontal ligament and surrounding alveolar bone to the traumatizing forces, i.e. to altered functional demands.

In teeth with progressive, plaque-associated periodontal disease, trauma from occlusion may, under certain conditions, enhance the rate of progression of the disease, i.e. act as a co-factor in the destructive process. From a clinical point of view, this knowledge strengthens the demand for proper treatment of plaque associated with periodontal disease. This treatment will arrest the destruction of the periodontal tissues even if the occlusal trauma persists. Treatment directed towards the trauma alone, however, i.e. occlusal adjustment or splinting, may reduce the mobility of the traumatized teeth and result in some regrowth of bone, but it will not arrest the rate of further breakdown of the supporting apparatus caused by plaque. (For a detailed discussion of treatment of teeth exhibiting increased mobility, see Chapter 51.)

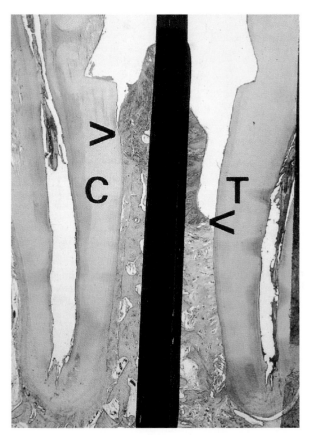

Fig. 14-13 Microphotographs from one control (C) and one test (T) tooth after 240 days of experimental periodontal tissue breakdown and 180 days of trauma from occlusion of the jiggling type (T). The arrowheads denote the apical position of the dentogingival epithelium. The attachment loss is more pronounced in T than in C. From Lindhe & Svanberg (1974).

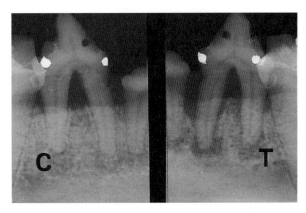

Fig. 14-12 Radiographic appearance of one test tooth (T) and one control tooth (C) at the termination of an experiment in which periodontitis was induced by ligature placement and plaque accumulation and in which trauma of the jiggling type was induced. Note angular bone loss particularly around the mesial root of the mandibular premolar (T) and the absence of such a defect at the mandibular premolar (C). From Lindhe & Svanberg (1974).

Fig. 14-15 (a) Periodontal conditions around a tooth which has been exposed to trauma from occlusion (of the jiggling type) for 300 days in combination with plaque-associated experimental periodontitis. (b) Condition of a control tooth from the same dog in which experimental periodontitis but no jiggling trauma had been in operation. Note the difference between (a) and (b) regarding the degree of bone destruction and loss of connective tissue attachment. Note also in (a) the location of the subgingival plaque at the apex of the root. From Ericsson & Lindhe (1982).

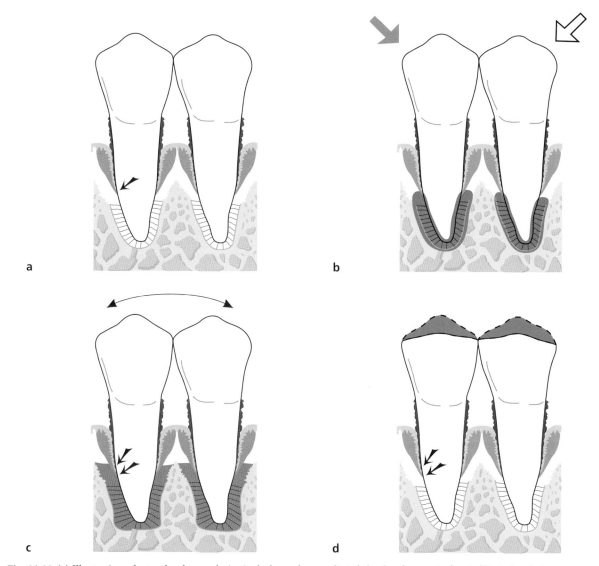

Fig. 14-14 (a) Illustration of a tooth where subgingival plaque has mediated the development of an infiltrated soft tissue (shadowed area) and an infrabony pocket. (b) When trauma from occlusion of the jiggling type is inflicted (arrows) on the crown of this tooth, the associated pathologic alterations occur within a zone of the periodontium which is also occupied by the inflammatory cell infiltrate (shadowed area). In this situation the increasing tooth mobility may also be associated with an enhanced loss of connective tissue attachment and further downgrowth of dentogingival epithelium; compare arrows in (c) and (d). Occlusal adjustment will result in a narrowing of the periodontal ligament, less tooth mobility, but no improvement of the attachment level (d) (Lindhe & Ericsson 1982).

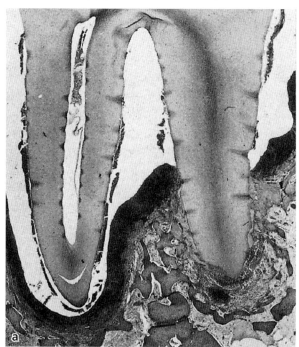

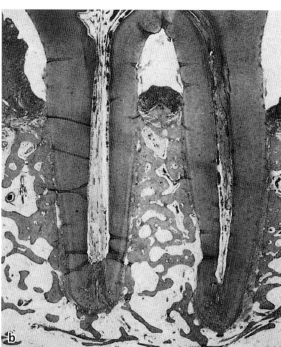

References

Baer, P., Kakehashi, S., Littleton, N.W., White, C.L. & Lieberman, J.E. (1963). Alveolar bone loss and occlusal wear. *Periodontics* **1**, 91.

Belting, C.M. & Gupta, O.P. (1961). The influence of psychiatric disturbances on the severity of periodontal disease. *Journal of Periodontology* **32**, 219–226.

Box, H.K. (1935). Experimental traumatogenic occlusion in sheep. *Oral Health* **25**, 9–25.

Burgett, F., Ramfjord, S., Nissle, R., Morrison, E., Charbeneau, T. & Caffesse, R. (1992). A randomized trial of occlusal adjustment in the treatment of periodontitis patients. *Journal of Clinical Periodontology* **19**, 381–387.

Ericsson, I. & Lindhe, J. (1977). Lack of effect of trauma from occlusion on the recurrence of experimental periodontitis. *Journal of Clinical Periodontology* **4**, 114–127.

Ericsson, I. & Lindhe, J. (1982). The effect of longstanding jiggling on experimental marginal periodontitis in the beagle dog. *Journal of Clinical Periodontology* **9**, 497–503.

Ewen, S.J. & Stahl, S.S. (1962). The response of the periodontium to chronic gingival irritation and long-term tilting forces in adult dogs. *Oral Surgery, Oral Medicine, Oral Pathology* **15**, 1426–1433.

Fleszar, T.J., Knowles, J.W., Morrison, E.C., Burgett, F.G., Nissle, R.R. & Ramfjord, S.P. (1980). Tooth mobility and periodontal therapy. *Journal of Clinical Periodontology* **7**, 495–505.

Glickman, I. (1965). Clinical significance of trauma from occlusion. *Journal of the American Dental Association* **70**, 607–618.

Glickman, I. (1967). Occlusion and periodontium. *Journal of Dental Research* **46** (Suppl 1), 53.

Glickman, I. & Smulow, J.B. (1962). Alterations in the pathway of gingival inflammation into the underlying tissues induced by excessive occlusal forces. *Journal of Periodontology* **33**, 7–13.

Glickman, I. & Smulow, J.B. (1965). Effect of excessive occlusal forces upon the pathway of gingival inflammation in humans. *Journal of Periodontology* **36**, 141–147.

Glickman, I. & Smulow, J.B. (1968). Adaptive alteration in the periodontium of the Rhesus monkey in chronic trauma from occlusion. *Journal of Periodontology* **39**, 101–105.

Harrel, S. & Nunn, M. (2001). Longitudinal comparison of the periodontal status of patients with moderate to severe periodontal disease receiving no treatment, non-surgical treatment and surgical treatment utilizing individual sites for analysis. *Journal of Periodontology* **72**, 1509–1519.

Häupl, K. & Psansky, R. (1938). Histologische Untersuchungen der Wirdungsweise der in der Funktions-Kiefer-Orthopedie verwendeten Apparate. *Deutsche Zahn-, Mund- und Kieferheilkunde* **5**, 214.

Karolyi, M. (1901). Beobachtungen über Pyorrhea alveolaris. *Osterreichisch-Ungarische Viertel Jahresschrift für Zahnheilkunde* **17**, 279.

Karring, T., Nyman, S., Thilander, B. & Magnusson, I. (1982). Bone regeneration in orthodontically produced alveolar bone dehiscences. *Journal of Periodontal Research* **17**, 309–315.

Lindhe, J. & Ericsson, I. (1982). The effect of elimination of jiggling forces on periodontally exposed teeth in the dog. *Journal of Periodontology* **53**, 562–567.

Lindhe, J. & Svanberg, G. (1974). Influences of trauma from occlusion on progression of experimental periodontitis in the Beagle dog. *Journal of Clinical Periodontology* **1**, 3–14.

Lovdahl, A., Schei, O., Waerhaug, J. & Arno, A. (1959). Tooth mobility and alveolar bone resorption as a function of occlusal stress and oral hygiene. *Acta Odontologica Scandinavica* **17**, 61–77.

Macapanpan, L.C. & Weinmann, J.P. (1954). The influence of injury to the periodontal membrane on the spread of gingival inflammation. *Journal of Dental Research* **33**, 263–272.

Manson, J.D. (1976). Bone morphology and bone loss in periodontal disease. *Journal of Clinical Periodontology* **3**, 14–22.

Meitner, S.W. (1975). *Co-destructive factors of marginal periodontitis and repetitive mechanical injury.* Thesis. Rochester, USA: Eastman Dental Center and The University of Rochester, USA.

Mühlemann, H.R. & Herzog, H. (1961). Tooth mobility and microscopic tissue changes reproduced by experimental occlusal trauma. *Helvetica Odontologia Acta* **5**, 33–39.

Neiderud, A-M., Ericsson, I. & Lindhe, J. (1992). Probing pocket depth at mobile/nonmobile teeth. *Journal of Clinical Periodontology* **19**, 754–759.

Nunn, M. & Harrel, S. (2001). The effect of occlusal discrepancies on periodontitis. I. Relationship of initial occlusal discrepancies to initial clinical parameters. *Journal of Periodontology* **72**, 485–494.

Nyman, S., Lindhe, J. & Ericsson, I. (1978). The effect of progressive tooth mobility on destructive periodontitis in the dog. *Journal of Clinical Periodontology* **7**, 351–360.

Pihlstrom, B.L., Anderson, K.A., Aeppli, D. & Schaffer, E.M. (1986). Association between signs of trauma from occlusion and periodontitis. *Journal of Periodontology* **57**, 1–6.

Polson, A. & Zander, H. (1983). Effect of periodontal trauma upon infrabony pockets. *Journal of Periodontology* **54**, 586–591.

Posselt, U. & Emslie, R.D. (1959). Occlusal disharmonies and their effect on periodontal diseases. *International Dental Journal* **9**, 367–381.

Prichard, J.F. (1965). *Advanced Periodontal Disease.* Philadelphia: W.B. Saunders.

Reitan, K. (1951). The initial tissue reaction incident to orthodontic tooth movement as related to the influence of function. *Acta Odontologica Scandinavica* **10**, Suppl 6.

Rosling, B., Nyman, S. & Lindhe, J. (1976). The effect of systematic plaque control on bone regeneration in infrabony pockets. *Journal of Clinical Periodontology* **3**, 38–53.

Steiner, G.G., Pearson, J.K. & Ainamo, J. (1981). Changes of the marginal periodontium as a result of labial tooth movement in monkeys. *Journal of Periodontology* **56**, 314–320.

Stillman, P.R. (1917). The management of pyorrhea. *Dental Cosmos* **59**, 405.

Stones, H.H. (1938). An experimental investigation into the association of traumatic occlusion with periodontal disease. *Proceedings of the Royal Society of Medicine* **31**, 479–495.

Svanberg, G. & Lindhe, J. (1973). Experimental tooth hypermobility in the dog. A methodological study. *Odontologisk Revy* **24**, 269–282.

Waerhaug, J. (1979). The infrabony pocket and its relationship to trauma from occlusion and subgingival plaque. *Journal of Periodontology* **50**, 355–365.

Waerhaug, J. & Hansen, E.R. (1966). Periodontal changes incident to prolonged occlusal overload in monkeys. *Acta Odontologica Scandinavica* **24**, 91–105.

Wennström, J., Lindhe, J., Sinclair, F. & Thilander, B. (1987). Some periodontal tissue resections to orthodontic tooth movement in monkeys. *Journal of Clinical Periodontology* **14**, 121–129.

Wentz, F.M., Jarabak, J. & Orban, B. (1958). Experimental occlusal trauma imitating cuspal interferences. *Journal of Periodontology* **29**, 117–127.

Chapter 15

Trauma from Occlusion: Peri-implant Tissues

Niklaus P. Lang and Tord Berglundh

Introduction

Enosseous osseointegrated oral implants have been suggested to serve as anchorage for orthodontic appliances where the existing dentition does not provide sufficient anchorage (see Chapter 58). Both clinical (Turley *et al.* 1988; Ödman *et al.* 1988, 1994; Haanaes *et al.* 1991) and experimental (Wehrbein & Diedrich 1993; Wehrbein *et al.* 1996) studies have demonstrated that osseointegrated implants were able to provide sufficient and stable anchorage for tooth movement during the period of orthodontic therapy, hereby eliminating the need of observing Newton's third law (1687) according to which an applied force can be divided into an *action* component and an equal and opposite *reaction* moment.

In long-term clinical studies of various two-stage submerged implant systems, however, implant loss has been attributed to *overloading or excessive loading*. In patients with edentulous (Adell *et al.* 1981; Lindquist *et al.* 1988) and partially edentulous jaws (Jemt *et al.* 1989; Quirynen *et al.* 1992) most of the losses of implants were considered to be the result of excessive occlusal loading. While it has been shown that early loading of oral implants may impede successful osseointegration (Sagara *et al.* 1993), the effect of excessive occlusal functional forces following successful osseointegration has not been documented so far. However, studies by Isidor (1996, 1997) have demonstrated that loading of implants through the creation of a massive supra-occlusion, leading to excessive, and most likely unphysiologic, laterally directed occlusal forces, established a high risk for the loss of osseointegration. Nevertheless, in one out of four experimental animals, even such excessive loading forces were unable to jeopardize the interfacial union of the alveolar bone with the implant surface.

The forces applied in the studies mentioned were characterized as being very high and of short dura-

tion. However, they could not be quantified. None of the experimental studies performed up to date allowed for the analysis of a direct relationship between changes in the stress and strain applied to oral implants which are encountered during functional loading and of the tissue reactions of the surrounding alveolar bone. Such information would appear to be of crucial importance for the evaluation of the etiology and pathogenesis of implant loss due to overload.

Orthodontic loading and alveolar bone

In order to evaluate the tissue reactions adjacent to oral implants following loading with well defined forces and to relate the strain values applied on the trabecular surface of the alveolar bone, an animal study was performed using finite element analysis (FEA) to determine the cellular activity (Melsen & Lang 2001).

In six adult monkeys, the lower first and the second premolars as well as the second molars were removed. After 6 months, two specially designed screw implants were inserted in the region of the lower left second premolar and second molar. After further 3 months, a square rod with three notches at different levels was inserted and tightened to the top of the implants. The notches served as reference for the measurements of the implant displacement. A flat disk was placed between the implant and the rod. To this disk two extensions were welded buccally and lingually in a way that a coil spring could be placed as close as possible to the estimated level of the center of resistance (Fig. 15-1). Immediately before buccal and lingual springs were inserted, the extensions were placed on the occlusal surface of the implants. Impressions of each segment were taken.

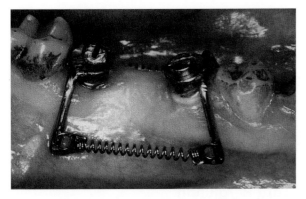

Fig. 15-1 Clinical picture demonstrating the Ni-Ti coil springs applied for a continuous loading through the centre of resistance. From Melsen & Lang (2001).

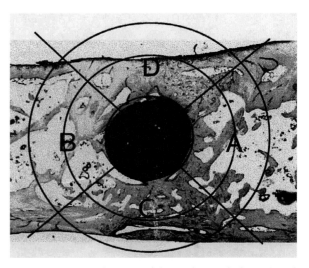

Fig. 15-2 Horizontal section of the implant with the projected grid used for the histomorphometrical evaluation of different regions surrounding the implant. Region A is submitted to compression, region B to tension, and regions C and D to shearing forces. From Melsen & Lang (2001).

Subsequently, two measurements were performed with an electronic strain gauge-based measuring device. For anchorage of the device, a cast splint was fitted to the anterior segment of the dentition and each of the implant screws. One measurement was made between the notches close to the implant connection, and another between the notches close to the top of the square rod extensions. These were repeated after 11 weeks, i.e. at the termination of orthodontic loading period. The direction and magnitude of the displacement of the implant as a result of loading could thus be calculated in the sagittal plane.

Following the baseline recordings, springs extending from the anterior to the posterior implant were attached to the power arms buccally and lingually (Fig. 15-1). Forces applied to the implants varied from 100 cN to each implant to a total load of 300 cN per implant. One monkey served as control, i.e. the implants in this animal were not subjected to any loading.

At the end of the experiment, the monkeys were sacrificed. Subsequently, parallel horizontal tissue sections from the coronal to the apical end of the implants were cut and stained with fast green. A grid consisting of three concentric circular gridlines was projected on to the sections (Fig. 15-2). The circular grid lines were intersected by four equidistant radial lines starting at the center of the grid and coinciding with the central axis of the implants. The four radial lines divided the regions between the circles and into eight areas, two in the direction of the force (A: compression zone), two in the opposite direction (B: tension zone), and four lateral to the implants (C and D: shear zone) (Fig. 15-2).

At a magnification of ×160, the extent of resorption lacunae and the extent of osteoid covered surfaces as a fraction of the total surface of trabecular bone were assessed. Also, using morphometry, bone density was evaluated within each quadrant. Furthermore, to measure the amount of osseointegration, the proportion of direct bone-to-implant contact was calculated by projecting a grid consisting of 32 radial lines extending from the center of the implants on to the section to be analyzed (Fig. 15-3).

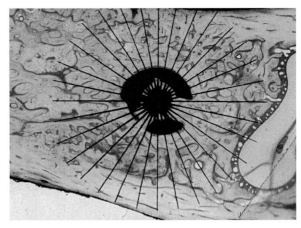

Fig. 15-3 Horizontal section of the implant on to which a grid with 32 radial lines was projected. The evaluation of the osseointegration included the determination of the percentage of direct bone-to-implant contact (magnification ×160). From Melsen & Lang (2001).

None of the implants had lost osseointegration after 11 weeks of orthodontic loading, but loading significantly influenced the turnover of the alveolar bone in the vicinity of the implants. Bone apposition was most frequently found when the calculated strain varied between 3400 and 6600 microstrain. On the other hand, when the strain exceeded 6700 microstrain, the remodeling of the bone resulted in a net loss of bone.

Clearly, the study supported the theory that apposition of bone around an oral implant is the biological response to a mechanical stress below a certain threshold, whereas loss of marginal bone or complete loss of osseointegration may be the result of mechanical stress beyond this threshold. Hence, occlusal forces would have to exeed the physiologic range substantially before occlusal contacts could jeopardize the tissue integrity of an implant.

Several other studies where orthodontic forces have been applied confirmed the apposition or increase in bone density rather than loss of bone surrounding an oral implant (Roberts *et al.* 1984; Wehrbein & Diedrich 1993; Asikainen *et al.* 1997; Akin-Nergiz *et al.* 1998).

Bone reactions to functional loading

A recent study addressed the reaction of peri-implant bone after longstanding functional loading compared to non-loaded controls (Berglundh *et al.* 2005).

After extractions of all mandibular premolars, four AstraTech® implants were placed in one side, and four Brånemark System® fixtures were installed in the contralateral side of the mandible. Three months after abutment connection, fixed dental prostheses (FDPs) were fabricated in gold and cemented on the maxillary canines and premolars (Fig. 15-4). FDPs were also installed on three of the four mandibular implants in both sides. The fourth implant remained unloaded and served as a control (Fig. 15-5).

Radiographs were obtained from each site following implant installation, abutment connection, and FDP placement. All radiographs were repeated after 10 months of functional loading. At this time biopsies were obtained and analyzed histologically.

The radiographic analysis revealed that the largest amount of bone loss occurred following implant

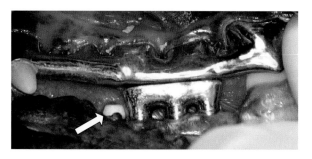

Fig. 15-4 Clinical documentation of the fixed dental prosthesis (FDP) supported by maxillary canines and premolars. In the mandible a FDP is installed on implants to provide masticatory function. The non-loaded control implant is mesial to the FDP (arrow). From Berglundh *et al.* (2005).

installation and abutment connection. This bone loss was more pronounced at Brånemark® than at Astra Tech® implants. However, bone loss as a result of functional loading was small and did not differ from the unloaded control sites (Fig. 15-6).

The histologic analysis showed that implants subjected to 10 months of functional loading had more direct bone-to-implant contact than their unloaded counterparts. This was observed for both implant systems (Fig. 15-7).

Based on radiographic and histologic results this study has demonstrated that *functional loading of implants may enhance osseointegration* (direct bone-to-implant contact) rather than induce marginal bone loss and, hence, such bone loss should not be attributed to loading of implants.

Whenever marginal bone loss is observed around implants in function, the most likely etiologic factor is bacterial in nature (see Chapters 10 and 24).

Excessive occlusal load on implants

The effect of *excessive occlusal load* following placement of titanium implants in the presence of healthy peri-implant mucosal tissues was evaluated in an experimental dog study (Heitz-Mayfield *et al.* 2004). In six Labrador dogs, two TPS (titanium plasma sprayed) implants and two SLA (sandblasted, large grit, acid etched) implants were placed on each side of the mandible (Fig. 15-8a). A total of 45 implants were evaluated. Following 6 months of healing (Fig. 15-8b), gold crowns were placed on implants on the test side of the mandible. The crowns were in supra-occlusal contact with the opposing teeth in order to create excessive occlusal load (Fig. 15-8c). Implants on the control side were not loaded. Plaque control was performed throughout the experimental period. Clinical measurements and standardized radiographs (Fig. 15-8d) were obtained at baseline and 1, 3, and 8 months after loading. At 8 months, all implants were osseointegrated, the dogs were killed, and histologic analyses were performed.

The mean probing depth was 2.5 ± 0.3 and 2.6 ± 0.3 mm at unloaded and loaded implants, respectively. Radiographically, the mean distance from the

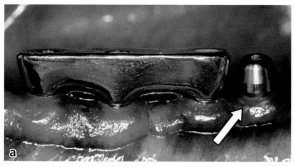 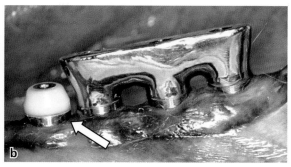

Fig. 15-5 FDPs fabricated of gold and installed on implants for functional loading. Unloaded implant as control (arrows). (a) Astra Tech® implants. (b) Brånemark System®. From Berglundh *et al.* (2005).

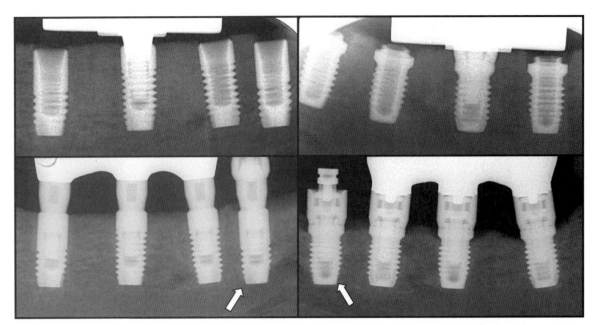

Fig. 15-6 Radiographs obtained from Astra Tech® (left side) and Brånemark® (right side) implants immediately after implant installation (top row) and following 10 months of functional loading (bottom row). Unloaded control implants are indicated with arrows. From Berglundh *et al.* (2005).

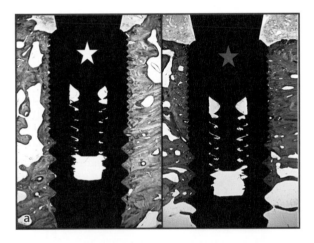

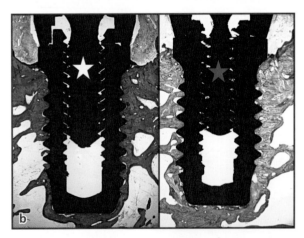

Fig. 15-7 (a) Non-loaded control. Astra Tech® implant after 10 months (white star) and functionally loaded Astra Tech® implant (red star) after 10 months. (b) Non-loaded control. Brånemark® implant after 10 months (white star) and functionally loaded Brånemark® implant (red star) after 10 months. From Berglundh *et al.* (2005).

implant shoulder to the marginal bone level was 3.6 ± 0.4 mm in the control group and 3.7 ± 0.2 mm in the test group. There were no statistically significant changes for any of the parameters from baseline to 8 months in the loaded and unloaded implants. Histologic evaluation (Fig. 15-9) showed a mean mineralized bone-to-implant contact of 73% in the control implants and 74% in the test implants, with no statistically significant difference between test and control implants.

Table 15-1 describes the level of osseointegration in relation to the total length of the implant after 8 months of excessive loading or non-loading. These values were generally slightly below those of the alveolar bone height (Table 15-2) for all sites and surfaces in both test and control implants. The differences varied between 1.1 and 3.7% and were not statistically significant. Likewise, there were no statistically significant differences between the excessively loaded and the unloaded implants in terms of peri-implant bone density either at the implant–bone interface or at a distance of 1 mm from the implant surface (Fig. 15-9) after 8 months.

Since none of the clinical, radiographic or histologic parameters yielded statistically significant differences between non-loaded and excessively loaded implants, the study clearly demonstrated that, in the presence of peri-implant mucosal health, a period of 8 months of *excessive occlusal load* on titanium implants *did not result in loss of osseointegration or marginal bone loss* when compared with non-loaded implants.

Static and cyclic loads on implants

While the study by Berglundh and co-workers (2005) addressed the possible influence of functional loading

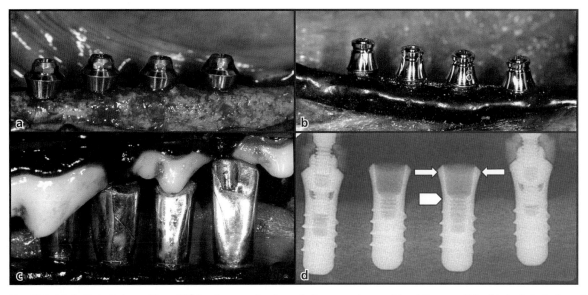

Fig. 15-8 (a) A clinical view of four ITI® implants at the time of placement in one side of the mandible. (b) A clinical view of the ITI® implants after 6 months of non-submerged healing. (c) A clinical view of the test side of the mandible in one dog. Note the four single gold crowns in supra-occlusal contact with the opposing teeth. (d) A standardized radiograph illustrating the level of the implant shoulder (arrows), and the first bone to implant contact visible in the radiograph (arrow head), at the mesial and distal surfaces of the implant. From Heitz-Mayfield *et al.* (2004).

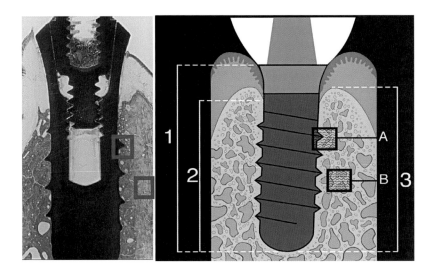

Fig. 15-9 A histologic and diagrammatic representation of the histomorphometric measurements: (1) Implant length = distance from the base of the implant to the implant shoulder. (2) The distance from the base of the implant to the most coronal point of bone-to-implant contact. (3) The distance from the base of the implant to the alveolar bone crest. (A) Percentage of mineralized bone density adjacent to the implant surface. (B) Percentage of mineralized bone density 1 mm distant from the implant surface. From Heitz-Mayfield *et al.* (2004).

Table 15-1 Buccal and lingual percentages of the level of osseointegration (bone-to-implant contact) in relation to the total length of the implant for control and test implants with a TPS or SLA surface after 8 months

	Buccal		Lingual	
	TPS	SLA	TPS	SLA
Control	57.9	60.4	67.5	66.7
	(n = 12)	(n = 11)	(n = 12)	(n = 11)
Test	62.1	59.2	68	68
	(n = 10)	(n = 12)	(n = 10)	(n = 12)

Table 15-2 Buccal and lingual percentages of alveolar bone height in relation to the total length of the implant for control and test implants with a TPS or SLA surface after 8 months

	Buccal		Lingual	
	TPS	SLA	TPS	SLA
Control	61.1	63.8	69.5	68.7
	(n = 12)	(n = 11)	(n = 12)	(n = 11)
Test	64.7	60.3	71.4	70.2
	(n = 10)	(n = 12)	(n = 10)	(n = 12)

on the marginal bone levels of implants applying a flat occlusal plane scheme and physiologic forces, many authors have studied the influence of loading forces exceeding physiologic functional conditions and impacting on the implants in a non-axial direction (Barbier & Schepers 1997; Gotfredsen *et al.* 2001a,b,c; Heitz-Mayfield *et al.* 2004).

The bone tissue reaction to axial versus non-axial load was evaluated using conventional three-unit FDPs in the mandible of beagle dogs for axial loading, while non-axial loading was provoked by installing a distal cantilever of two implants (Barbier & Schepers 1977). Bone remodeling was modest at the implant sites supporting conventional FDPs, while the non-axial load induced by the cantilever FDP yielded a more pronounced bone response including a higher activity of osteoclasts in the peri-implant bone. However, bone levels were not affected. This was interpreted as an adaptive phenomenon within the peri-implant bone as a result of non-axial loading.

Bone reactions around osseointegrated implants to static load was addressed in three studies in dogs (Gotfredsen *et al.* 2001a,b,c). In the first study (Gotfredsen *et al.* 2001a), lateral static load was induced by an orthodontic expansion screw at eight ITI® TPS hollow-screw implants in each dog. After loading period of 24 weeks during which time the screws were activated every 4 weeks from 0.0, 0.2, 0.4, and 0.6 mm, histologic and histometric analysis revealed no marginal bone loss at loaded and unloaded implant sites. Peri-implant bone density and mineralized bone-to-implant contact was higher at the loaded than at unloaded implant sites. This, again, was interpreted that lateral static load resulted in an *adaptive remodeling of the peri-implant bone*.

In the second study (Gotfredsen *et al.* 2001b), two TPS and two turned ITI® hollow-screw implants were subjected to the 24-week loading period in each dog using orthodontic expansion screws. These were, again, activated with 0.6 mm every 4 weeks. The histologic and histometric analysis yielded higher marginal bone levels around TPS implants than around turned implants. Likewise, the peri-implant bone density and mineralized bone-to-implant contact was higher around the roughened TPS than the turned implants. Hence, it was concluded that surface roughness influences the bone reactions to the applied load. This, in turn would indicate that surface roughness may also be a determining factor in the remodeling process triggered by load at the bone-to-implant interface.

The third study (Gotfredsen *et al.* 2001c), addressed the dynamics of applying static load of various durations to ITI® implants in three beagle dogs. Maximal activation of static load was set at 24 weeks on to the implants of the right mandibular side resulting in a total period of load of 46 weeks at sacrifice. At 60 weeks maximal activation of static load was set onto the implants of the left mandibular side resulting in

a total period of load of 10 weeks at sacrifice. Fluorochrome labeling was performed at weeks 62, 64, 66, and 68. The dogs were sacrificed at week 70. Similar distribution of bone markers, bone density, and bone-to-implant contact was observed at 10 and 46 weeks of static lateral loading. However, higher fluorochrome proportions were seen at 10 weeks compared to 46 weeks of lateral loading, suggesting higher adaptive activity at 10 weeks. Nevertheless, the structural adaptation appeared to be similar at the two observation periods.

In all three studies, larger bone-to-implant contact was identified at lateral static load application compared to non-loaded implants. Moreover, lateral static load failed to induce peri-implant bone loss or to enhance peri-implant bone loss. Hence, *lateral static load does not appear to be detrimental* to implants exhibiting peri-implant mucositis or peri-implantitis (Gotfredsen *et al.* 2001a,b,c).

In contrast to the findings of the studies presented are the results from a study in dogs (Hoshaw *et al.* 1994). In that study excessive cyclic axial forces had been applied to implants placed in the tibiae of ten animals. Bone loss was observed to occur around the neck of the Brånemark implants after 1 year and exposed to high cyclic (500 cycles/day) axial tension (10–300 N) for 5 consecutive days (Hoshaw *et al.* 1994). Similar results were reported for a rabbit model (Duyck *et al.* 2001) in which dynamic load to implants resulted in the establishment of marginal crater-like defects, while no effects on osseointegration could be identified at other parts of the implants.

Load and loss of osseointegration

It has been reported (Isidor 1996, 1997) that excessive occlusal load may, under certain circumstances, lead to loss of osseointegration along the entire length of the implant, hereby resulting in implant mobility. In this study, four monkeys received 18 self-tapping screw implants in the mandible after the first molars (n = 7), premolars (n = 8), and incisors (n = 3) had been extracted. Using an opposing maxillary splint in heavy supra-occlusal contacts, *excessive occlusal load*, predominantely in non-axial (lateral) direction was applied to eight implants. Furthermore, cotton ligatures for increased plaque retention were placed around another ten implants resulting first in mucositis and later in peri-implantitis (Lindhe *et al.* 1992; Lang *et al.* 1993). After 18 months of excessive occlusal loading, two of the eight implants were lost. Two implants out of ten revealed partial loss of osseointegration as a result of plaque-induced peri-implantitis (Fig. 15-10a). As for the remaining six implants subjected to excessive load, two implants yielded complete loss of osseointegration with a connective tissue capsule formed around the entire outline of the implants (Fig. 15-10b). Radiographically, the two implants showing complete loss of osseointegration and clinical mobility yielded a peri-implant radiolucency after 18 months of excessive occlusal load. However, no loss of marginal bone height was evident. Also, another two excessively loaded implants (in one monkey) showed no loss of osseointegration whatsoever. Instead, an increase in bone density and the highest percentage of bone-to-implant contact area was seen at these implants in relation to the remaining implants. Neither did this monkey develop ligature induced peri-implantitis (at three implants). Two implants under excessive occlusal load revealed a reduced bone-to-implant contact.

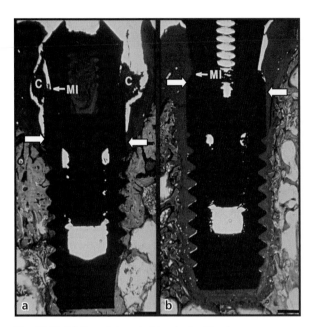

Fig. 15-10 (a) Osseointegrated implant with plaque accumulation. The marginal bone level is located apical to the margin of the implant. (b) Excessively loaded implant with complete loss of osseointegration. The marginal bone level is located near the margin of the implant. Narrow zone of fibrous tissue interposed between implant and bone. MI = margin of implant; white arrows = apical extent of epithelium; C = cotton ligature. (Courtesy of F. Isidor, Århus, Denmark, *Clinical Oral Implants Research* 8, 1–9.)

Thus, the study has demonstrated that excessive occlusal load can, indeed, result in loss of osseointegration characterized by a fibrous connective tissue capsule around the implant as opposed to the marginal bone loss encountered at implants with ligature induced peri-implantitis. It has to be realized, however, that the bone trabecular structure around the implant losing osseointegration as a result of excessive occlusal load (Fig. 15-10b) was much less dense than that of, for example, the implants subjected to experimental peri-implantitis (Fig. 15-10a). In that sense, the described study does not support the concept that occlusal overload may lead to implant losses. Rather, the study supports the fact that marginal bone loss at implants is associated with peri-implant disease.

Masticatory occlusal forces on implants

Closing and occlusal functional force distributions have been studied using one-dimensional (Lundgren *et al.* 1987, 1989; Falk *et al.* 1989, 1990) or three-dimensional piezo-electric force transducers (Meriscke-Stern *et al.* 1996, 2000; Meriscke-Stern 1997, 1998). Eight strain gauge transducers were mounted bilaterally in a maxillary complete denture to occlude with a mandibular implant-supported fixed cantilever prosthesis (Fig. 15-11a) (Lundgren *et al.* 1989).

The study demonstrated that closing and chewing forces *increased* distally along the cantilever beams when occluding with complete dentures. Moreover, on both the preferred and non-preferred chewing sides, significantly larger closing and chewing forces were measured over the cantilever segments than over the implant-supported area (Fig. 15-11b). Also, the distally increasing force distribution pattern could be altered to a distally *decreasing* force distribution pattern by infraoccluding the second cantilever unit by as little as 100 μm. Such slight reductions in

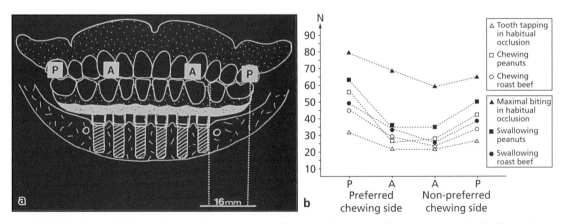

Fig. 15-11 (a) Eight strain gauge transducers placed into a maxillary complete removable prosthesis and occluding against an implant supported fixed mandibular dental prosthesis with cantilever beams of 16 mm. (b) Chewing forces amounting to a maximum biting force of 80 N on the preferred (right) chewing side and 64 N on the non-preferred (left chewing side). While masticating higher forces are applied to the cantilever beams than to the implant-supported part of the mandibular FDP. (Courtesy of D. Lundgren, Göteborg, Sweden, *International Journal of Oral and Maxillofacial Implants* **4**, 277–283.)

posterior occlusal contacts on cantilevers may have to be considered whenever the opposing masticatory unit is a complete removable dental prosthesis. However, maximal biting and chewing forces *decreased* distally along the cantilever beams when occluding with tooth-supported fixed dental prostheses (FDPs) (Fig. 15-12) (Lundgren *et al.* 1987).

From this series of experimental clinical studies it was concluded that forces directed to the implants *per se* are difficult to evaluate using the transducer methodology. Nevertheless, maximal closing forces were always substantially greater than chewing forces. In addition, each subject in the studies referred to developed a preferred chewing side that was associated with higher chewing forces than the non-preferred chewing side (Lundgren *et al.* 1987, 1989; Falk *et al.* 1989, 1990).

More recently, occlusal force distribution patterns have been studied for mandibular overdentures

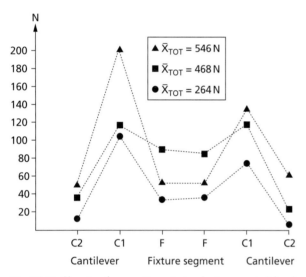

Fig. 15-12 Chewing force patterns in implant-supported fixed dental prosthesis with cantilever beams occluding against tooth-supported FDPs. (Courtesy of D. Lundgren, Göteborg, Sweden, *Journal of Prosthetic Dentistry* **58**, 197–203.)

using three-dimensional piezo-electric transducers that were mounted on to two mandibular implants in the canine region designed to support either a ball-joint-retained or a bar-retained mandibular complete removable prosthesis. Rigid bars provided the best distribution of forces in a vertical direction on to the two mandibular implants (Mericske-Stern *et al.* 1996; Mericske-Stern 1998). Moreover, short distal bar extensions did not negatively influence the force pattern (Mericske-Stern 1997). When ball-joint anchors were used to retain the mandibular overdenture, rather low forces were measured on the implants, particularly in a vertical direction (Mericske-Stern 1998). Vertical forces amounted to 60–140 N, while horizontal forces were much smaller (15–60 N).

Tooth–implant supported reconstructions

In reconstructing patients with inadequate masticatory function, oral implants are often used to increase the patient's chewing comfort (see Chapter 52) and provide additional chewing units in an edentulous posterior region. Occasionally, it may be contemplated to reconstruct a chewing side with a reconstruction supported by both a tooth and an implant (Fig. 15-13). In this way, problems of the location of the mental nerve in an area of a planned implant installation or lack of an adequate bone volume may be overcome.

Combined tooth–implant reconstructions have been associated with numerous clinical problems including root intrusion as a potential clinical hazard of non-rigid connection. Hence, it has been claimed that natural teeth should not be connected to implants beneath a fixed prosthesis. However, experimental studies have clearly established that no detrimental effects on the periodontium of abutment teeth could be demonstrated despite a different biomechanical condition mediated by a periodontal ligament as

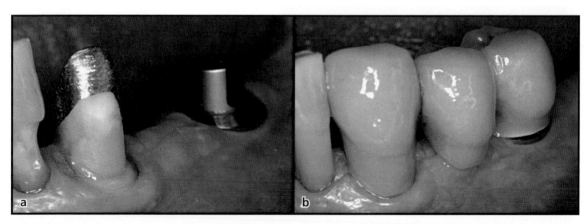

Fig. 15-13 Reconstruction of a chewing side in the left mandible using a fixed dental prosthesis. (a) Prepared abutment tooth 33 after having established adequate abutment height by the installation of a cast post and core prior to seating a three-unit FDP. (b) Tooth–implant-supported three-unit FDP, 10 years after placement.

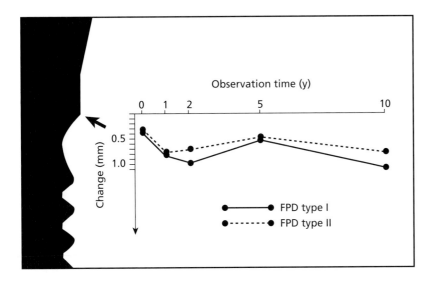

Fig. 15-14 Ten-year randomized controlled clinical trial of three-unit FDPs, either implant–implant (type I) or tooth–implant (type II) supported. No differences in the crestal bone levels after 1, 2, 5, and 10 years in function. (Courtesy of J. Gunne *et al.* *International Journal of Prosthodontics* **12**, 216–221.)

opposed to the ankylotic anchorage of an implant (Biancu *et al.* 1995).

In vivo measurements of vertical forces and bending moments during biting and chewing were carried out on ten three-unit prostheses in the posterior mandibles of five patients. Each patient had two prostheses, one supported by two implants and the other supported by one implant and one tooth. The results demonstrated no major difference in functional load magnitudes related to the support type. Obviously, functional loads were shared between the teeth and the implants (Gunne *et al.* 1997; Rangert *et al.* 1991, 1995). Further studies using finite element analysis yielded no increased risk of stress concentrations at the implant's neck (Gross & Laufer 1997; Laufer & Gross 1998).

Clinical studies reporting life table statistics in combined implant and tooth restorations do not show adverse effects of splinting teeth to implants. No increased risk of tooth intrusion were reported if the implant was rigidly connected to the tooth (Fugazzotto *et al.* 1999; Lindh *et al.* 2001; Naert *et al.* 2001a,b). The results of 843 consecutive patients treated in a private practice (Fugazzotto *et al.* 1999) with 1206 natural tooth–implant supported prostheses utilizing 3096 screw-fixed attachments showed that only 9 intrusion problems were noted after 3–14 years in function. All problems were associated with fractured or lost screws.

Probably the most relevant clinical study was a 10-year randomized controlled prospective study on 23 patients with residual mandibular anterior teeth (Gunne *et al.* 1999). Each patient received two three-unit FDPs either supported by two implants or, on the contralateral side, by one implant and one tooth, thus permitting intraindividual comparison. The distribution of the two types of FDPs in each jaw was randomized. Implant success rates, marginal bone changes, and mechanical complications were studied. The tooth–implant connection did not demonstrate

any negative influences on the overall success rates for the 10-year period when compared to the implant–implant supported FDPs (Fig. 15-14). Hence, it was suggested that a prosthetic construction supported by both a tooth and an implant may be recommended as a predictable and reliable treatment alternative in the posterior mandible (Gunne *et al.* 1999).

Based on the evidence available today it can be stated that a combination of implant and tooth support for FDPs is acceptable (Belser *et al.* 2000). While a recent systematic review (Lang *et al.* 2004) indicated that tooth–implant reconstructions reveal a 5-year survival rate of 94.1%, comparing very well with the 5-year survival rate of implant–implant reconstructions of 95.0% (Pjetursson *et al.* 2004), the 10-year survival of tooth–implant reconstructions (77.8%) appears to be significantly lower than the 10-year survival of implant–implant reconstructions (86.7%). However, owing to the fact that the former 10-year survival rate was based on only 60 (I-T) FDPs and the latter on only 219 (I–I) FDPs, the reliability of such 10-year survival has to be questioned.

The biomechanical aspects of implant–tooth-supported fixed dental prostheses have been presented (Lundgren & Laurell 1994). As the implant is rigidly fixed within the alveolus, and the tooth is surrounded by a periodontal ligament that allows minute movement, rigid FDP designs have been advocated. The movement of the natural tooth abutment was found to affect the load-bearing capacity of the FDP, whenever a long-span FDP was constructed (e.g. a beam length of 24 mm or two premolar or molar pontics). Before occlusal load is applied, the FDP acts as a cantilever construction. Upon loading, an angular deflection of implant–crown unit of approximately 50 μm are noted. Together with bending of the long-span beam an apical deflection of the tooth of approximately 50 μm is allowed, hereby leading to a bilateral (tooth and implant) support of the FDP. If the tooth and implant only support a short-span FDP (e.g. a beam length of 12 mm or one premolar pontic only), however, angular deflection of the implant–crown unit of approximately 50 μm and the bending of the short-span beam are insufficient to achieve a bilateral support of the bridge. The apical deflection of the tooth will not be reached and the implant will cope with the entire occlusal load applied to the FDP. As indicated above, there is no doubt that osseointegration will cope with such functional loads.

References

Adell, R., Lekholm, U., Rockler, B. & Brånemark, P.I. (1981). A 15-year study of osseointegrated implants in the treatment of the edentulous jaw. *International Journal of Oral Surgery* **10**, 387–416.

Akin-Nergiz, N., Nergiz, I., Schulz, A., Arpak, N. & Niedermeier, W. (1998). Reactions of peri-implant tissues to continuous loading of osseointegrated implants. *American Journal of Orthodontics and Dentofacial Orthopedics* **114**, 292–298.

Asikainen, P., Klemetti, E., Vuillemin, T., Sutter, F., Rainio, V. & Kotilainen, R. (1997). Titanium implants and lateral forces. An experimental study with sheep. *Clinical Oral Implants Research* **8**, 465–468.

Balshi, T.J., Ekfeldt, A., Stenberg, T. & Vrielinck, L. (1997). Three-year evaluation of Brånemark implants connected to angulated abutments. *International Journal of Oral and Maxillofacial Implants* **12**, 52–58.

Barbier, L. & Scheppers, E. (1977). Adaptive bone remodelling around oral implants under axial and non-axial loading conditions in the dog mandible. *International Journal of Oral and Maxillofacial Implants* **12**, 215–223.

Belser, U.C., Mericske-Stern, R., Bernard, J.P. & Taylor, T.D. (2000). Prosthetic management of the partially dentate patient with fixed implant restorations. *Clinical Oral Implants Research* **11** (Suppl), 126–145.

Berglundh, T., Abrahamsson, I. & Lindhe, J. (2005). Bone reactions to longstanding functional load at implants: an experimental study in dogs. *Journal of Clinical Periodontology* **32**, 925–932.

Biancu, S., Ericsson, I. & Lindhe, J. (1995). The periodontal ligament of teeth connected to osseointegrated implants. An experimental study in the beagle dog. *Journal of Clinical Periodontology* **22**, 362–370.

Duyck, J., Ronold, H.J., Van Oosterwyck, H., Naert, I., Vander Sloten, J. & Ellingsen, J.E. (2001). The influence of static and dynamic loading on marginal bone reactions around osseointegrated implants: an animal experimental study. *Clinical Oral Implants Research* **12**(3), 207–218.

Ekfeldt, A., Johansson, L.Å. & Isaksson, S. (1997). Implant-supported overdenture therapy: a retrospective study. *International Journal of Prosthodontics* **10**, 366–374.

Falk, H., Laurell, L. & Lundgren, D. (1989). Occlusal force pattern in dentitions with mandibular implant-supported fixed cantilever prostheses occluded with complete dentures. *International Journal of Oral and Maxillofacial Implants* **4**, 55–62.

Falk, H., Laurell, L. & Lundgren, D. (1990). Occlusal interferences and cantilever joint stress in implant-supported prostheses occluding with complete dentures. *International Journal of Oral and Maxillofacial Implants* **5**, 70–77.

Fugazzotto, P.A., Kirsch, A., Ackermann, K.L. & Neuendorff, G. (1999). Implant/tooth-connected restorations utilizing screw-fixed attachments: a survey of 3,096 sites in function for 3 to 14 years. *International Journal of Oral and Maxillofacial Implants* **14**, 819–823.

Fugazzotto, P.A. (2001). A comparison of the success of root resected molars and molar position implants in function in a private practice: results of up to 15-plus years. *Journal of Periodontology* **72**, 1113–1123.

Gotfredsen, K., Berglundh, T. & Lindhe, J. (2001a). Bone reactions adjacent to titanium implants subjected to static load.

A study in the dog (I). *Clinical Oral Implants Research* **12**, 1–8.

Gotfredsen, K., Berglundh, T. & Lindhe, J. (2001b). Bone reactions adjacent to titanium implants with different surface characteristics subjected to static load. A study in the dog (II). *Clinical Oral Implants Research* **12**, 196–201.

Gotfredsen, K., Berglundh, T. & Lindhe, J. (2001c). Bone reactions adjacent to titanium implants subjected to static load of different duration. A study in the dog (III). *Clinical Oral Implants Research* **12**, 552–558.

Gotfredsen, K., Berglundh, T. & Lindhe, J. (2002). Bone reactions at implants subjected to experimental peri-implantitis and static load. A study in the dog. *Journal of Clinical Periodontology* **29**, 144–151.

Gross, M. & Laufer, B.Z. (1997). Splinting osseointegrated implants and natural teeth in rehabilitation of partially edentulous patients. Part I: laboratory and clinical studies. *Journal of Oral Rehabilitation* **24**, 863–870.

Gunne, J., Åstrand, P., Lindh, T., Borg, K. & Olsson, M. (1999). Tooth-implant and implant supported fixed partial dentures: A 10-year report. *International Journal of Prosthodontics* **12**, 216–221.

Gunne, J., Rangert, B., Glantz, P.-O. & Svensson, A. (1997). Functional loads on freestanding and connected implants in three-unit mandibular prostheses opposing complete dentures: an *in vivo* study. *International Journal of Oral and Maxillofacial Implants* **12**, 335–341.

Haanaes, H.R., Stenvik, A., Beyer Olsen, E.S., Tryti, T. & Faehn, O. (1991). The efficacy of two-stage titanium implants as orthodontic anchorage in the preprosthodontic correction of third molars in adults – a report of three cases. *European Journal of Orthodontics* **13**, 287–292.

Heitz-Mayfield, L.J., Schmid, B., Weigel, C., Gerber, S., Bosshardt, D.D., Jonsson, J., Lang, N.P. & Jonsson, J. (2004). Does excessive occlusal load affect osseointegration? An experimental study in the dog. *Clinical Oral Implants Research* **15** (3), 259–268.

Hoshaw, S.J., Brunski, J.B. & Cochran, G.V.B. (1994). Mechanical loading of Brånemark implants affects interfacial bone modeling and remodeling. *International Journal of Oral and Maxillofacial Implants* **9**, 345–360.

Isidor, F. (1996). Loss of osseointegration caused by occlusal load of oral implants. A clinical and radiographic study in monkeys. *Clinical Oral Implants Research* **7**, 143–152.

Isidor, F. (1997). Clinical probing and radiographic assessment in relation to the histologic bone level at oral implants in monkeys. *Clinical Oral Implants Research* **8**, 255–264.

Jemt, T., Lekholm, U. & Adell, R. (1989). Osseointegrated implants in the treatment of partially edentulous patients: a preliminary study on 876 consecutively placed fixtures. *International Journal of Oral and Maxillofacial Implants* **4**, 211–217.

Lang, N.P., Brägger, U, Walther, D., Beamer, B. & Kornman, K. (1993). Ligature-induced peri-implant infection in cynomolgus monkeys. *Clinical Oral Implants Research* **4**, 2–11.

Lang, N.P., Pjetursson, B.E., Tan, K., Brägger, U., Egger, M. & Zwahlen, M. (2004). A systematic review of the survival and complication rates of fixed partial dentures (FPDs) after an observation period of at least 5 years. II. Combined tooth-implant-supported FPDs. *Clinical Oral Implants Research* **15**, 643–653.

Laufer, B.Z. & Gross, M. (1998). Splinting osseointegrated implants and natural teeth in rehabilitation of partially edentulous patients. Part II: principles and applications. *Journal of Oral Rehabilitation* **25**, 69–80.

Lindh, T., Back, T., Nyström, E. & Gunne, J. (2001). Implant versus tooth-implant supported prostheses in the posterior maxilla: a 2-year report. *Clinical Oral Implants Research* **12**, 441–449.

Lindhe, J., Berglundh, T., Ericsson, I., Liljenberg, B. & Marinello, C. (1992). Experimental breakdown of periimplant and periodontal tissues. *Clinical Oral Implants Research* **9**, 1–16.

Lindquist, LW., Rockler, B. & Carlsson, G.E. (1988). Bone resorption around fixtures in edentulous patients treated with mandibular fixed tissue-integrated prostheses. *Journal of Prosthetic Dentistry* **59**, 59–63.

Lundgren, D., Falk, H. & Laurell, L. (1989). Influence of number and distribution of occlusal cantilever contacts on closing and chewing forces in dentitions with implant-supported fixed prostheses occluding with complete dentures. *International Journal of Oral and Maxillofacial Implants* **4**, 277–283.

Lundgren, D. & Laurell, L. (1994). Biomechanical aspects of fixed bridgework supported by natural teeth and endosseous implants. *Periodontology 2000* **4**, 23–40.

Lundgren, D., Laurell, L., Falk, H. & Bergendal, T. (1987). Occlusal force pattern during mastication in dentitions with mandibular fixed partial dentures supported on osseointegrated implants. *Journal of Prosthetic Dentistry* **58**, 197–203.

Melsen, B. & Lang, N.P. (2001). Biological reactions of alveolar bone to orthodontic loading of oral implants. *Clinical Oral Implants Research* **12**, 144–152.

Mericske-Stern, R. (1997). Force distribution on implants supporting overdentures: the effect of distal bar extensions. A 3-D *in vivo* study. *Clinical Oral Implants Research* **8**, 142–151.

Mericske-Stern, R. (1998). Three-dimensional force measurements with mandibular overdentures connected to implants by ball-shaped retentive anchors. A clinical study. *International Journal of Oral and Maxillofacial Implants* **13**, 36–43.

Mericske-Stern, R., Piotti, M. & Sirtes, G. (1996). 3-D *in vivo* force measurements on mandibular implants supporting overdentures. A comparative study. *Clinical Oral Implant Research* **7**, 387–396.

Mericske-Stern, R., Venetz, E., Fahrländer, F. & Bürgin, W. (2000). *In vivo* force measurements on maxillary implants supporting a fixed prosthesis or an overdenture: a pilot study. *Journal of Prosthetic Dentistry* **84**, 535–547.

Naert, I.E., Duyck, J.A., Hosny, M.M. & van Steenberghe, D. (2001a). Freestanding and tooth-implant connected prostheses in the treatment of partially edentulous patients. Part I: An up to 15-years clinical evaluation. *Clinical Oral Implants Research* **12**, 237–244.

Naert, I.E., Duyck, J.A., Hosny, M.M., Quirynen, M. & van Steenberghe, D. (2001b). Freestanding and tooth-implant connected prostheses in the treatment of partially edentu-

lous patients Part II: An up to 15-years radiographic evaluation. *Clinical Oral Implants Research* **12**, 245–251.

Ödman, J., Lekholm, U., Jemt, T., Brånemark, P.I. & Thilander, B. (1988). Osseointegrated titanium implants – a new approach in orthodontic treatment. *European Journal of Orthodontics* **10**, 98–105.

Ödman, J., Lekholm, U., Jemt, T. & Thilander, B. (1994). Osseointegrated implants as orthodontic anchorage in the treatment of partially edentulous adult patients. *European Journal of Orthodontics* **16**, 187–201.

Pjetursson, B.E., Tan, K., Lang, N.P., Brägger, U., Egger, M. & Zwahlen, M. (2004). A systematic review of the survival and complication rates of fixed partial dentures (FPDs) after an observation period of at least 5 years. I. Implant-supported FPDs. *Clinical Oral Implants Research* **15**, 625–642.

Quirynen, M., Naert, I. & van Steenberghe, D. (1992). Fixture design and overload influence marginal bone loss and fixture success in the Brånemark system. *Clinical Oral Implants Research* **3**, 104–111.

Rangert, B., Gunne, J., Glantz, P.-O. & Svensson, A. (1995). Vertical load distribution on a three-unit prosthesis supported by a natural tooth and a single Branemark implant. An in vivo study. *Clinical Oral Implants Research* **6**, 40–46.

Rangert, B., Gunne, J. & Sullivan, D.Y. (1991). Mechanical aspects of a Brånemark implant connected to a natural tooth: an in vitro study. *International Journal of Oral and Maxillofacial Implants* **6**, 177–186.

Roberts, W.E., Smith, R.K., Zilberman, Y., Mozsary, M.D. & Smith, R.S. (1984). Osseous adaptation to continuous loading of rigid endosseous implants. *American Journal of Orthodontics* **84**, 95–111.

Rosenberg, E.S., Torosian, J.P. & Slots, J. (1991). Microbial differences in 2 clinically distinct types of failures of osseointegrated implants. *Clinical Oral Implants Research* **2**, 135–144.

Sanz, M., Alandez, J., Lazzaro, P. Calvo, J.L., Quirynen, M. & van Steenberghe, D. (1991). Histo-pathologic characteristics of peri-implant soft tissues in Brånemark implants with 2 distinct clinical and radiological patterns. *Clinical Oral Implants Research* **2**, 128–134.

Sagara, M., Akagawa, Y., Nikai, H. & Tsuru, H. (1993). The effects of early occlusal loading one-stage titanium alloy implants in beagle dogs: a pilot study. *Journal of Prosthetic Dentistry* **69**, 281–288.

Turley, P.K., Kean, C., Schnur, J., Stefanac, J., Gray, J., Hennes, J. & Poon, L.C. (1988). Orthodontic force application to titanium endosseous implants. *Angle Orthodontist* **58**, 151–162.

Wehrbein, H. & Diedrich, P. (1993). Endosseous titanium implants during and after orthodontic load – an experimental study in the dog. *Clinical Oral Implants Research* **4**, 76–82.

Wehrbein, H., Merz, B.R., Diedrich, P. & Glatzmaier, J. (1996). The use of palatal implants for orthodontic anchorage. Design and clinical application of the Orthosystem. *Clinical Oral Implants Research* **7**, 410–416.

Part 6: Periodontal Pathology

Chapter 16

Non-Plaque Induced Inflammatory Gingival Lesions

Palle Holmstrup

Gingival inflammation, clinically presenting as gingivitis, is not always due to accumulation of plaque on the tooth surface, and non-plaque induced inflammatory gingival reactions often present characteristic clinical features (Holmstrup 1999). They may occur due to several causes, such as specific bacterial, viral or fungal infection without an associated plaque-related gingival inflammatory reaction. Gingival lesions of genetic origin are seen in hereditary gingival fibromatosis, and several mucocutaneous disorders manifest as gingival inflammation. Typical examples of such disorders are lichen planus, pemphigoid, pemphigus vulgaris, and erythema multiforme. Allergic and traumatic lesions are other examples of non-plaque induced gingival inflammation. Dentists, and especially specialists in periodontology, are the key persons in the diagnostic unraveling and treatment of patients affected by such lesions.

This chapter focuses on those non-plaque induced inflammatory gingival lesions of the gingival tissues which are most relevant, either because they are common or because they are important examples for the understanding of the variety of tissue reactions that take place in the periodontium. For further information the reader is referred to oral medicine textbooks. The modifying factors of plaque-related gingivitis such as smoking, sexual hormones, and metabolic anomalies (diabetes) are dealt with in Chapter 12.

Gingival diseases of specific bacterial origin

Infective gingivitis and stomatitis may occur on rare occasions in both immunocompromised and non-immunocompromised individuals, when non-plaque-related pathogens overwhelm innate host resistance (Rivera-Hidalgo & Stanford 1999). The lesions may be due to bacteria and may not be accompanied by lesions elsewhere in the body. Typical examples of such lesions are due to infections with *Neisseria gonorrhoeae* (Scully 1995; Siegel 1996), *Treponema pallidum* (Scully 1995; Ramirez-Amador *et al.* 1996; Siegel 1996; Rivera-Hidalgo & Stanford 1999), streptococci, *Mycobacterium chelonae* (Pedersen & Reibel 1989) or other organisms (Blake & Trott 1959; Littner *et al.* 1982). The gingival lesions manifest as fiery red edematous painful ulcerations, as asymptomatic chancres or mucous patches, or as atypical non-ulcerated, highly inflamed gingivitis. Biopsy supplemented by microbiologic examination reveals the background of the lesions.

Gingival diseases of viral origin

Herpes virus infections

Several viral infections are known to cause gingivitis (Scully *et al.* 1998b). The most important are the herpes viruses: herpes simplex viruses type 1 and 2 and varicella-zoster virus. These viruses usually enter the human body in childhood and may give rise to oral mucosal disease followed by periods of latency and sometimes reactivation. Herpes simplex virus type 1 (HSV-1) usually causes oral manifestations, whereas herpes simplex virus type 2 (HSV-2) is mainly involved in anogenital infections and only occasionally is involved in oral infection (Scully 1989).

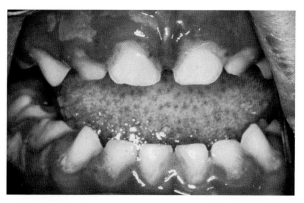

Fig. 16-1 Herpetic gingivostomatitis in a 3-year-old child. Erythematous swelling of attached gingiva with serofibrinous exudate along the gingival margin.

Primary herpetic gingivostomatitis

Herpes simplex infections are among the most common viral infections. Herpes simplex is a DNA virus with low infectiousness, which after entering the oral mucosal epithelium, penetrates a neural ending and, by retrograde transport through the smooth endoplasmatic reticulum (200–300 mm/day), travels to the trigeminal ganglion where it can remain latent for years. The virus has also been isolated in extraneural locations such as the gingiva (Amit *et al.* 1992). Sometimes herpes simplex viruses may also play a role in recurring erythema multiforme. It is presently unknown whether the virus plays a role in other oral diseases, but herpes simplex virus has been found in gingivitis (Ehrlich *et al.* 1983), acute necrotizing gingivitis (Contreras *et al.* 1997), and periodontitis (Parra & Slots 1996).

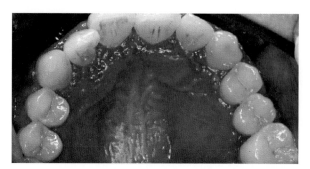

Fig. 16-2 Herpetic gingivostomatitis affecting palatal gingiva. Numerous vesicles and small ulcerations.

When a baby is infected, sometimes from the parent's recurrent herpes labialis, it is often wrongly diagnosed as "teething". With increased hygiene in the industrialized society, more and more primary infections occur at higher ages, i.e. during adolescence or even adulthood. It is estimated in the US that there are about half a million cases per year (Overall 1982). The primary herpetic infection may run an asymptomatic course in early childhood, but may also give rise to severe gingivostomatitis, which usually occurs before adolescence (Fig. 16-1). This manifestation includes painful severe gingivitis with redness, ulcerations with serofibrinous exudate and edema accompanied by stomatitis (Figs. 16-2 and 16-3). The incubation period is 1 week. A characteristic feature is the formation of vesicles, which rupture, coalesce, and leave fibrin-coated ulcers (Scully *et al.* 1991; Miller & Redding 1992). Fever and lymphadenopathy are other classic features. Healing occurs spontaneously without scarring in 10–14 days (Fig. 16-4). During this period pain can render eating difficult.

The virus remains latent in the ganglion cell, probably through integration of its DNA in that of the chromosomal DNA (Overall 1982). Reactivation of the virus resulting in recurrent infections occurs in

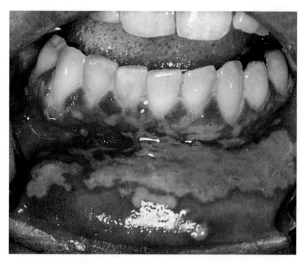

Fig. 16-3 Herpetic gingivostomatitis in a 38-year-old woman. Widespread ulceration of lower lip mucosa and gingiva.

20–40% of individuals with the primary infection (Greenberg 1996) and usually presents in the form of herpes labialis, but recurrent intraoral herpes infections are also seen. Recurrent infections occur in general more than once per year, usually at the same location on the vermilion border and/or the skin adjacent to it, where neural endings are known to be clustering. A large variety of factors trigger reactivation of latent virus. These are trauma, ultraviolet light

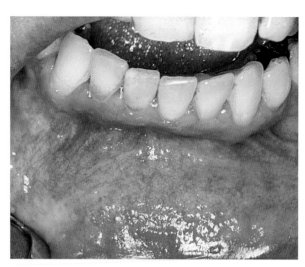

Fig. 16-4 Same patient as shown in Fig. 16-3, 4 weeks later. Healing without loss of tissue or scar formation.

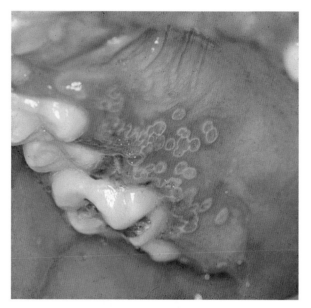

Fig. 16-5 Recurrent intraoral herpes infection. Ruptured vesicles of right palatal gingiva and mucosa.

exposure, fever, menstruation and others (Scully *et al.* 1998b).

While recurrences at the vermilion border are well recognized, recurrent intraoral herpes lesions often remain undiagnosed because they are considered aphthous ulcerations (Lennette & Magoffin 1973; Sciubba 2003), irrespective of the fact that aphthous ulcers do not affect keratinized mucosa. Recurrent intraoral herpes typically presents a less dramatic course than does the primary infection. A characteristic manifestation is a cluster of small painful ulcers in the attached gingiva and hard palate (Yura *et al.* 1986) (Fig. 16-5). The diagnosis can be made on the basis of the patient history and clinical findings supported by isolation of HSV from lesions. A reliable isolation of virus is best obtained from intact vesicular lesions, for instance by aspiration of the vesicle fluid with a small syringe. Isolation and growth of

herpes viruses are elaborate because of their fragility. The virus must be transferred to a special cell line in the laboratory within 24 hours, or stored at –70°C. The herpes virus is detected within 5 days, and while a positive viral culture can be taken as evidence of viral infection, a negative result does not rule out such an infection. Laboratory diagnosis may also involve examination of a blood sample for increased antibody titer against herpes virus. However, this is most relevant in cases of primary infection, because the antibody titer remains elevated for the rest of the lifetime. The histopathologic features of cytologic smears from the gingival lesions are not specific, but the presence of giant cells and intranuclear inclusion bodies may indicate intracellular activity of virus (Burns 1980).

Immunodeficient patients, such as HIV-infected individuals, are at increased risk of acquiring the infection (Holmstrup & Westergaard 1998). In the immunocompromised patient the recurrence of herpes infection, either gingival or elsewhere, may be severe and even life-threatening.

The treatment of herpetic gingivostomatitis includes careful plaque removal to limit bacterial superinfection of the ulcerations, which delays their healing. In severe cases, including patients with immunodeficiency, the systemic use of antiviral drugs such as aciclovir, valaciclovir or famciclovir is recommended (O'Brien & Campoli-Richards 1989; Mindel 1991; Arduino & Porter 2006). Resistance to aciclovir, especially among immunodeficient patients on long-term therapy, is a growing concern (Westheim *et al.* 1987) and explains why other antiviral drugs may be relevant. Prophylactic antiviral treatment before dental treatment has been recommended for patients at risk of experiencing a recurrence as well as to minimize transmission of the disease (Miller *et al.* 2004).

Herpes zoster

Varicella-zoster virus causes varicella (chicken pox) as the primary self-limiting infection. It occurs mainly in children and later reactivation of the virus in adults causes herpes zoster (shingles). Both manifestations can involve the gingiva (Straus *et al.* 1988; Scully 1995). Chicken pox is associated with fever, malaise, and a skin rash. The intraoral lesions are small ulcers usually on the tongue, palate, and gingiva (Miller 1996; Scully *et al.* 1998b). The virus remains latent in the dorsal root ganglion from where it can be reactivated years after the primary infection (Rentier *et al.* 1996). Later reactivation results in herpes zoster, with unilateral lesions following the infected nerve (Miller 1996). The reactivation normally affects the thoracic ganglia in elderly or immunocompromised patients. Reactivation of virus from the trigeminal ganglion occurs in 20% of reported cases (Hudson & Vickers 1971). If the second or third branch of the trigeminal nerve is involved, skin lesions may be associated

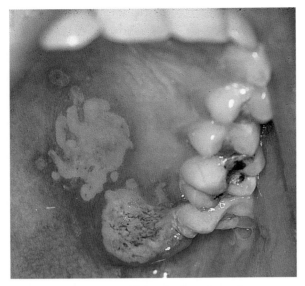

Fig. 16-6 Herpes zoster of left palatal gingiva and mucosa. Irregular fibrin coated ulcerations with severe pain.

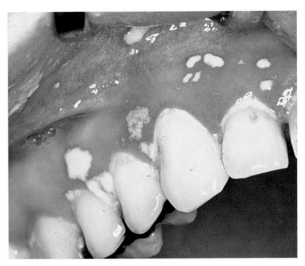

Fig. 16-7 Pseudomembranous candidosis of maxillary gingiva and mucosa in HIV-seropositive patient. The lesions can be scraped off, leaving a slightly bleeding surface.

with intraoral lesions, or intraoral lesions may occur alone (Eisenberg 1978), for instance affecting the palatal gingiva (Fig. 16-6). Initial symptoms are pain and paresthesia, which may be present before lesions occur (Greenberg 1996). The associated pain is usually severe. The lesions, which often involve the gingiva, initiate as vesicles. They soon rupture to leave fibrin-coated ulcers, which often coalesce to irregular forms (Millar & Traulis 1994) (Fig. 16-6). In immunocompromised patients, including HIV-infected individuals, the infection can result in severe tissue destruction with tooth exfoliation and necrosis of alveolar bone and high morbidity (Melbye *et al.* 1987; Schwartz *et al.* 1989). The diagnosis is usually obvious due to the unilateral occurrence of lesions associated with severe pain. Healing of the lesions usually takes place in 1–2 weeks.

Treatment consists of soft or liquid diet, rest, atraumatic removal of plaque, and diluted chlorhexidine rinses. This may be supplemented by antiviral drug therapy.

Gingival diseases of fungal origin

Fungal infection of the oral mucosa includes a range of diseases such as aspergillosis, blastomycosis, candidosis, coccidioidomycosis, cryptococcosis, histoplasmosis, mucormycosis, and paracoccidioidomycosis infections (Scully *et al.* 1998b), but some of the infections are very uncommon and not all of them manifest as gingivitis. The present chapter focuses on candidosis and histoplasmosis, both of which may cause gingival infection.

Candidosis

Various *Candida* species are recovered from the mouth of humans including *C. albicans, C. glabrata, C.*

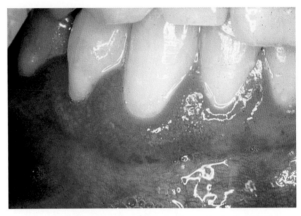

Fig. 16-8 Erythematous candidosis of attached mandibular gingiva of HIV-seropositive patient. The mucogingival junction is invisible.

krusei, C. tropicalis, C. parapsilosis, and *C. guillermondii* (Cannon *et al.* 1995). *C. albicans* is by far the most common. It is a normal commensal of the oral cavity but also an opportunistic pathogen. The prevalence of oral carriage of *C. albicans* in healthy adults ranges from 3–48% (Scully *et al.* 1995), the large variation being due to differences in examined populations and the procedures used. The proportion of *C. albicans* in the total oral yeast population can reach about 50–80% (Wright *et al.* 1985), and by far the most common fungal infection of the oral mucosa is candidosis mainly caused by the organism *C. albicans* (Scully *et al.* 1998b); the proteinase-positive strains of *C. albicans* are associated with disease (Negi *et al.* 1984; Odds 1985) and invasion of keratinized epithelia such as that of the gingiva. Invasion and increased desquamation is due to the hyaluronidase production. Infection by *C. albicans* usually occurs as a consequence of reduced host defense systems (Holmstrup & Johnson 1997), including immunodeficiency (Holmstrup & Samaranayake 1990) (Figs. 16-7 to 16-9), reduced saliva secretion, smoking, and

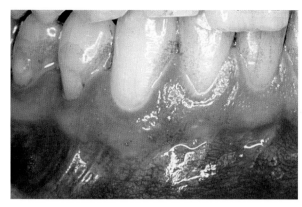

Fig. 16-9 Same patient as shown in Fig. 16-8 after topical antimycotic therapy. The mucogingival junction is visible.

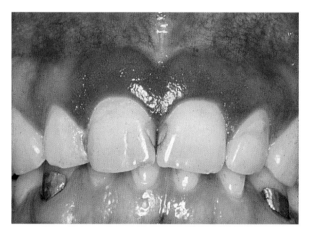

Fig. 16-10 Chronic erythematous candidosis of maxillary attached gingiva of the incisor region.

treatment with corticosteroids, but may be due to a wide range of predisposing factors. The occurrence of oral candidosis may act as a predictor of immune and virologic failure in HIV-infected patients treated with antiviral drugs (Miziara & Weber 2006). Disturbances in the oral microbial flora, such as after therapy with broad-spectrum antibiotics, may also lead to oral candidosis. The predisposing factors are, however, often difficult to identify. Based on their site, infections may be defined as superficial or systemic. Candidal infection of the oral mucosa is usually a superficial infection, but systemic infections are not uncommon in debilitated patients.

In otherwise healthy individuals, oral candidosis rarely manifests in the gingiva. This is surprising, considering the fact that *C. albicans* is frequently isolated from the subgingival flora of patients with severe periodontitis (Slots *et al.* 1988). The most common clinical characteristic of gingival candidal infections is redness of the attached gingiva, often associated with a granular surface (Fig. 16-10).

Various types of oral mucosal manifestations are pseudomembranous candidosis (also known as thrush in neonates), erythematous candidosis, plaque-type candidosis, and nodular candidosis

(Holmstrup & Axéll 1990). Pseudomembranous candidosis shows whitish patches (Fig. 16-7), which can be wiped off the mucosa with an instrument or gauze leaving a slightly bleeding surface. The pseudomembranous type usually has no major symptoms. Erythematous lesions can be found anywhere in the oral mucosa (Fig. 16-10). The intensely red lesions are usually associated with pain, which is sometimes severe. The plaque type of oral candidosis is a whitish plaque, which cannot be removed. There are usually no symptoms and the lesion is clinically indistinguishable from oral leukoplakia. Nodular candidal lesions are infrequent in the gingiva; they are characterized by slightly elevated nodules of white or reddish color (Holmstrup & Axéll 1990).

A diagnosis of candidal infection can be accomplished on the basis of culture, smear, and biopsy. A culture on Nickersons medium at room temperature is easily handled in the dental premises. Microscopic examination of smears from suspected lesions is another easy diagnostic procedure, either performed as direct examination by phase contrast microscopy or as light microscopic examination of periodic-acid-Schiff-stained or Gram-stained smears. Mycelium-forming cells in the form of hyphae or pseudohyphae and blastospores are seen in great numbers among masses of desquamated cells. Since oral carriage of *C. albicans* is common among healthy individuals, positive culture and smear does not necessarily imply candidal infection (Rindum *et al.* 1994). Quantitative assessment of the mycological findings and the presence of clinical changes compatible with the above types of lesions are necessary to obtain a reliable diagnosis, which can also be obtained on the basis of identification of hyphae or pseudohyphae in biopsy specimens from the lesions.

Topical treatment involves application of antifungals, such as nystatin, amphotericin B or miconazole. Nystatin may be used as an oral suspension. Since it is not absorbed it can be used in pregnant or lactating women. Miconazole exists as an oral gel. It should not be given during pregnancy and it can interact with anticoagulants and phenytoin. The treatment of the severe or generalized forms also involves systemic antifungals such as fluconazole.

Linear gingival erythema

Linear gingival erythema (LGE) is regarded as a gingival manifestation of immunosuppression characterized by a distinct linear erythematous band limited to the free gingiva (Consensus Report 1999) (Fig. 16-11). It is characterized by a disproportion of inflammatory intensity for the amount of plaque present. There is no evidence of pocketing or attachment loss. A further characteristic of this type of lesion is that it does not respond well to improved oral hygiene or to scaling (EC Clearinghouse on Oral Problems 1993) and it is now a requirement for the diagnosis to be considered that the lesion persists after removal of

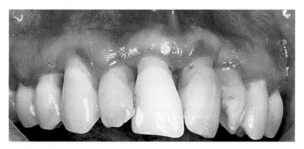

Fig. 16-11 Linear gingival erythema of maxillary gingiva. Red banding along the gingival margin, which does not respond to conventional therapy.

plaque in the initial visit (Umadevi *et al.* 2006). The extent of gingival banding measured by number of affected sites has been shown to depend on tobacco usage (Swango *et al.* 1991). While 15% of affected sites were originally reported to bleed on probing and 11% exhibited spontaneous bleeding (Winkler *et al.* 1988), a key feature of LGE is now considered to be lack of bleeding on probing (Robinson *et al.* 1994).

Some studies of various groups of HIV-infected patients have revealed prevalences of gingivitis with band-shaped patterns in 0.5–49% (Klein *et al.* 1991; Swango *et al.* 1991; Barr *et al.* 1992; Laskaris *et al.* 1992; Masouredis *et al.* 1992; Riley *et al.* 1992; Ceballos-Salobrena *et al.* 1996; Robinson *et al.* 1996). These prevalence values reflect some of the problems with non-standardized diagnosis and selection of study groups. A few studies of unbiased groups of patients have indicated that gingivitis with band-shaped or punctate marginal erythema may be relatively rare in HIV-infected patients, and probably a clinical finding which is no more frequent than in the general population (Drinkard *et al.* 1991; Friedman *et al.* 1991).

It is interesting to note that, whereas there was no HIV-related preponderance of red banding, diffuse and punctate erythema was significantly more prevalent in HIV-infected than in non-HIV-infected individuals in a British study (Robinson *et al.* 1996). Red gingival banding as a clinical feature alone was, therefore, not strongly associated with HIV infection.

There are indications that candidal infection is the background of some cases of gingival inflammation including LGE (Winkler *et al.* 1988; Robinson *et al.* 1994), but studies have revealed a microflora comprising both *C. albicans*, and a number of perio-pathogenic bacteria consistent with those seen in conventional periodontitis, i.e. *Porphyromonas gingivalis*, *Prevotella intermedia*, *Actinobacillus actinomycetemcomitans*, *Fusobacterium nucleatum*, and *Campylobacter rectus* (Murray *et al.* 1988, 1989, 1991). By DNA probe detection, the percentage of positive sites in HIV-associated gingivitis as compared with matched gingivitis sites of HIV-seronegative patients for *A. actinomycetemcomitans* was 23% and 7% respectively, for *P. gingivalis* 52% and 17%, *Pr. intermedia* 63% and 29%, and for *C. rectus* 50% and 14% (Murray *et al.*

1988, 1989, 1991). *C. albicans* has been isolated by culture in about 50% of HIV-associated gingivitis sites, in 26% of unaffected sites of HIV-seropositive patients and in 3% of healthy sites of HIV-seronegative patients. The frequent isolation and the pathogenic role of *C. albicans* may be related to the high levels of the yeasts in saliva and oral mucosa of HIV-infected patients (Tylenda *et al.* 1989).

An interesting histopathologic study of biopsy specimens from the banding zone has revealed no inflammatory infiltrate but an increased number of blood vessels, which explains the red color of the lesions (Glick *et al.* 1990). The incomplete inflammatory reaction of the host tissue may be the background of the lack of response to conventional treatment.

A number of diseases present clinical features resembling those of LGE and which do not resolve after improved oral hygiene and debridement. Examples are (1) oral lichen planus, which is frequently associated with an inflammatory red band of the attached gingiva (Holmstrup *et al.* 1990) and so is sometimes mucous membrane pemphigoid (Pindborg 1992), or (2) erythematous lesions associated with renal insufficiency because of the salivary ammonia production associated with the high levels of urea.

There is little information about treatment based on controlled studies of this type of condition. Conventional therapy plus rinsing with 0.12% chlorhexidine gluconate twice daily has shown significant improvement after 3 months (Grassi *et al.* 1989). It was mentioned above that some cases of LGE might be related to the presence of *Candida* strains; clinical observations suggest that improvement is frequently dependent on successful eradication of intraoral *Candida* strains (Winkler *et al.* 1988). Consequently, attempts to identify the presence of fungal infection either by culture or smear is recommended, followed by antimycotic therapy in *Candida*-positive cases.

Histoplasmosis

Histoplasmosis is a granulomatous disease caused by *Histoplasma capsulatum*, a soil saprophyte found mainly in feces from birds and cats. The infection occurs in the north-eastern, south-eastern, mid Atlantic and central states of the US. It is also found in Central and South America, India, East Asia, and Australia. Histoplasmosis is the most frequent systemic mycosis in the US. It is mediated by airborne spores from the mycelial form of the organism (Rajah & Essa 1993). In the normal host, the course of the infection is subclinical (Anaissie *et al.* 1986). The clinical manifestations include acute and chronic pulmonary histoplasmosis and a disseminated form, mainly occurring in immunocompromised patients (Cobb *et al.* 1989). Oral lesions have been seen in 30% of patients with pulmonary histoplasmosis and in 66% of patients with the disseminated form (Weed & Parkhill 1948; Loh *et al.* 1989). The oral lesions may

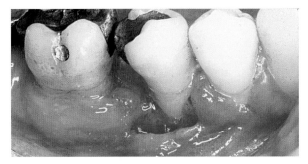

Fig. 16-12 Gingival histoplasmosis with loss of periodontal tissue around second premolar.

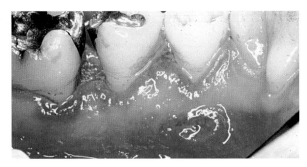

Fig. 16-13 Same patient as shown in Fig. 16-12. Lingual aspect with ulceration in the deeper part of crater-like lesion.

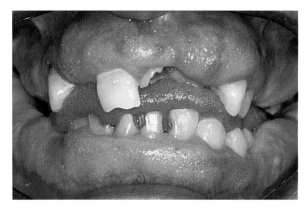

Fig. 16-14 Hereditary gingival fibromatosis. Facial aspect with partial coverage of teeth.

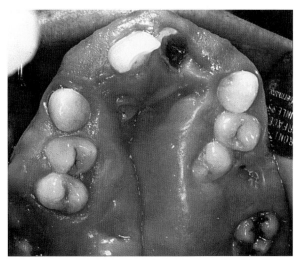

Fig. 16-15 Same patient as shown in Fig. 16-14. The maxillary gingival fibromatosis is severe and has resulted in total disfiguration of the dental arch.

affect any area of the oral mucosa (Chinn *et al.* 1995), including the gingiva, which appears to be one of the most frequent sites affected (Hernandez *et al.* 2004). The lesions are initially nodular or papillary and later may become ulcerative, with loss of gingival tissue, and painful (Figs. 16-12 and 16-13). They are sometimes granulomatous and the clinical appearance may resemble a malignant tumor (Boutros *et al.* 1995). The diagnosis is based on clinical appearance and histopathology and/or culture, and the treatment consists of systemic antifungal therapy.

Gingival lesions of genetic origin

Hereditary gingival fibromatosis

Gingival hyperplasia (synonymous with gingival overgrowth, gingival fibromatosis) may occur as a side effect to systemic medications, including phenytoin, cyclosporine, and nifedipine (Coletta & Graner 2006). These lesions are to some extent plaque-dependent and they are reviewed in Chapter 17. Gingival hyperplasia may also be of genetic origin. Such lesions are known as hereditary gingival fibromatosis (HGF), which is an uncommon condition characterized by diffuse gingival enlargement, sometimes covering major parts of, or the total, tooth surfaces. The lesions develop irrespective of effective plaque removal.

HGF may be an isolated disease entity or part of a syndrome (Gorlin *et al.* 1990), associated with other clinical manifestations, such as hypertrichosis (Horning *et al.* 1985; Cuestas-Carneiro & Bornancini

1988), learning difficulties (Araiche & Brode 1959), epilepsy (Ramon *et al.* 1967), hearing loss (Hartsfield *et al.* 1985), growth retardation (Bhowmick *et al.* 2001), and abnormalities of extremities (Nevin *et al.* 1971; Skrinjaric & Basic 1989). Most cases are related to an autosomal dominant mode of inheritance, but cases have been described with an autosomal recessive background (Emerson 1965; Jorgensen & Cocker 1974; Singer *et al.* 1993). The most common syndrome of HGF includes hypertrichosis, epilepsy and learning difficulties; the two latter features, however, are not present in all cases (Gorlin *et al.* 1990).

Typically, HGF presents as large masses of firm, dense, resilient, insensitive fibrous tissue that cover the alveolar ridges and extend over the teeth, resulting in extensive pseudopockets. The color may be normal or erythematous if inflamed (Figs. 16-14 and 16-15). Depending on extension of the gingival enlargement, patients complain of functional and esthetic problems. The enlargement may result in protrusion of the lips, and they may chew on a considerable hyperplasia of tissue covering the teeth. HGF is seldom present at birth but may be noted at an early age. If the enlargement is present before tooth eruption, the dense fibrous tissue may interfere with or prevent eruption (Shafer *et al.* 1983).

Studies have suggested that an important pathogenic mechanism may be enhanced production of transforming growth factor (TGF-beta 1) reducing the proteolytic activities of HGF fibroblasts, which again favor the accumulation of extracellular matrix (Coletta *et al.* 1999). A locus for autosomal dominant HGF has previously been mapped to a region on chromosome 2 (Hart *et al.* 1998; Xiao *et al.* 2000), although at least two genetically distinct loci seem to be responsible for this type of HGF (Hart *et al.* 2000); a novel locus for maternally inherited human gingival fibromatosis has recently been reported at human chromosome 11p15 (Zhu *et al.* 2006).

The histologic features of HGF include moderate hyperplasia of a slightly hyperkeratotic epithelium with extended rete pegs. The underlying stroma is almost entirely made up of dense collagen bundles with only a few fibroblasts. Local accumulation of inflammatory cells may be present (Shafer *et al.* 1983). Histologic examination may facilitate the differential diagnosis from other genetically determined gingival enlargements such as Fabry disease, which is characterized by telangiectasia.

Treatment of HGF is surgical removal, often in a series of gingivectomies, but relapses are not uncommon. If the volume of the overgrowth is extensive, a repositioned flap to avoid exposure of connective tissue by gingivectomy may better achieve elimination of pseudopockets.

Gingival diseases of systemic origin

Mucocutaneous disorders

Various mucocutaneous disorders present with gingival manifestations, sometimes in the form of desquamative lesions or ulceration of the gingiva. The most important of these diseases are lichen planus, pemphigoid, pemphigus vulgaris, erythema multiforme, and lupus erythematosus.

Lichen planus

Lichen planus is the most common mucocutaneous disease manifesting on the gingiva. The disease may affect skin and oral as well as other mucous membranes in some patients while others may present with either skin or oral mucosal involvement alone. Oral involvement alone is common and concomitant skin lesions in patients with oral lesions have been found in 5–44% of cases (Andreasen 1968; Axéll & Rundquist 1987). The disease may be associated with severe discomfort; it has been shown to possess a premalignant potential, although this is still a controversial issue (Holmstrup 1992), so it is important to diagnose and treat cases and to have regular oral examinations as follow-up (Holmstrup *et al.* 1988; Mattson *et al.* 2002; Mignogna *et al.* 2006).

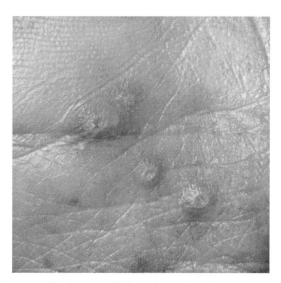

Fig. 16-16 Skin lesions of lichen planus. Papules with delicate white striations.

The prevalence of oral lichen planus (OLP) in various populations has been found to be 0.1–4% (Scully *et al.* 1998a). The disease may afflict patients at any age although it is seldom observed in childhood (Scully *et al.* 1994). Skin lesions are characterized by papules with white striae (Wickham striae) (Fig. 16-16). Itching is a common symptom, and the most frequent locations are the flexor aspects of the arms, the thighs and the neck. In the vast majority of cases the skin lesions disappear spontaneously after a few months, which is in sharp contrast with the oral lesions, which usually remain for years (Thorn *et al.* 1988).

A variety of clinical appearances is characteristic of OLP. These include:

- Papular (Fig. 16-17)
- Reticular (Figs. 16-18 and 16-19)
- Plaque-like (Fig. 16-20)
- Atrophic (Figs. 16-21 to 16-25)
- Ulcerative (Figs 16-22 and 16-27)
- Bullous (Fig. 16-29).

Simultaneous presence of more than one type of lesion is common (Thorn *et al.* 1988). The most characteristic clinical manifestations of the disease and the basis of the clinical diagnosis are white papules (Fig. 16-17) and white striations (Figs 16-18, 16-19, 16-26 and 16-27), which often form reticular patterns (Thorn *et al.* 1988), usually of bilateral occurrence (Ingafou *et al.* 2006). Sometimes atrophic and ulcerative lesions are referred to as erosive (Rees 1989). Papular, reticular, and plaque-type lesions usually do not give rise to significant symptoms, whereas atrophic and ulcerative lesions are associated with moderate to severe pain, especially in relation to oral hygiene procedures and eating. OLP frequently persists for many years (Thorn *et al.* 1988). Any area of the oral mucosa may be affected by OLP, but the

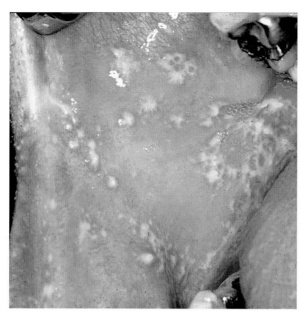

Fig. 16-17 Oral lichen planus. Papular lesion of right buccal mucosa.

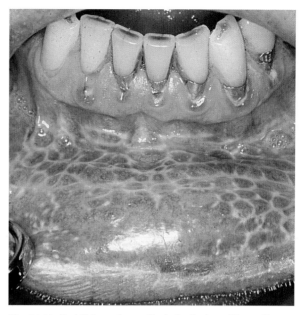

Fig. 16-18 Oral lichen planus. Reticular lesion of lower lip mucosa. The white striations are denoted Wickham striae.

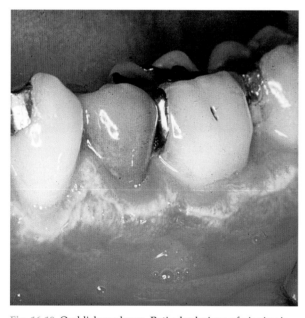

Fig. 16-19 Oral lichen planus. Reticular lesions of gingiva in lower left premolar and molar region.

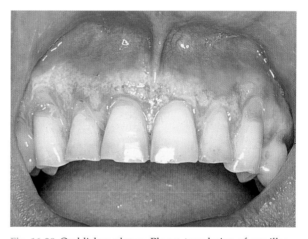

Fig. 16-20 Oral lichen planus. Plaque-type lesion of maxillary gingiva.

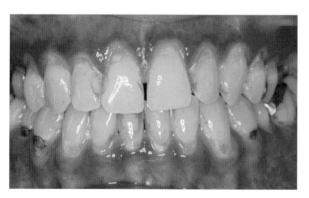

Fig. 16-21 Oral lichen planus. Atrophic lesions of facial maxillary and mandibular gingiva. Such lesions were previously termed desquamative gingivitis.

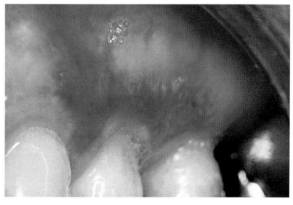

Fig. 16-22 Oral lichen planus. Atrophic and ulcerative lesion of maxillary gingiva. Note that the margin of the gingiva has a normal color in the upper incisor region, which distinguishes the lesions from plaque-induced gingivitis.

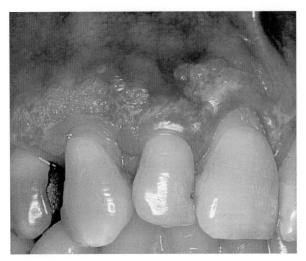

Fig. 16-23 Oral lichen planus. Atrophic and reticular lesion of maxillary gingiva. Several types of lesions are often present simultaneously.

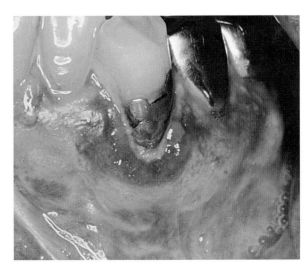

Fig. 16-24 Oral lichen planus. Atrophic and reticular lesion of lower left canine region. Plaque accumulation results in exacerbation of oral lichen planus, and atrophic lesions compromise oral hygiene procedures. This may lead to a vicious circle that the dentist can help in breaking.

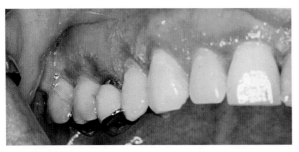

Fig. 16-25 Oral lichen planus. Atrophic and reticular lesion of right maxillary gingiva in a patient using an electric toothbrush, which is traumatic to the marginal gingiva. The physical trauma results in exacerbation of the lesion with atrophic characteristics and pain.

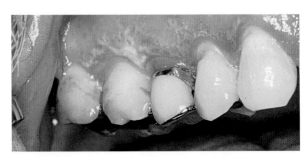

Fig. 16-26 Same patient as shown in Fig. 16-25 after modified toothbrushing procedure with no traumatic action on marginal gingiva.

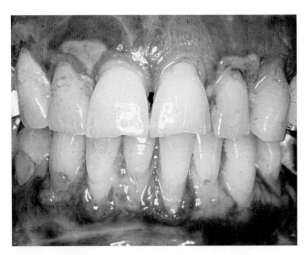

Fig. 16-27 Oral lichen planus. Atrophic and ulcerative/reticular lesions of maxillary and mandibular incisor region. The patient, a 48-year-old woman, suffers from severe discomfort from food, beverages, and toothbrushing.

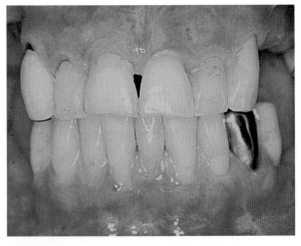

Fig. 16-28 Same patient as shown in Fig. 16-27 after periodontal treatment and extraction of teeth with deep pockets. An individual oral hygiene program, which ensured gentle, meticulous plaque removal has been used by the patient for 3 months. The atrophic/ulcerative lesions are now healed and there are no more symptoms.

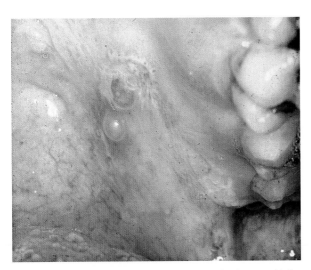

Fig. 16-29 Oral lichen planus. Bullous/reticular lesion of left palatal mucosa.

lesions often change in clinical type and extension over the years. Such changes may imply the development of plaque-type lesions, which are clinically indistinguishable from oral leukoplakia. This may give rise to a diagnostic problem if other lesions more characteristic of OLP have disappeared (Thorn *et al.* 1988).

A characteristic histopathologic feature in OLP is a subepithelial, band-like accumulation of lymphocytes and macrophages characteristic of a type IV hypersensitivity reaction (Eversole *et al.* 1994). The epithelium shows hyperortho- or hyperparakeratinization and basal cell disruption with transmigration of lymphocytes into the basal and parabasal cell layers (Eversole 1995). The infiltrating lymphocytes have been identified as CD4+ and CD8+ cells (Buchner 1984; Walsh *et al.* 1990; Eversole *et al.* 1994). Other characteristic features are Civatte bodies, which are dyskeratotic basal cells. Common immunohistochemical findings of OLP lesions are fibrin in the basement membrane zone, but deposits of IgM, C3, C4, and C5 may also be found. None of these findings are specific to OLP (Schiødt *et al.* 1981; Kilpi *et al.* 1988; Eversole *et al.* 1994).

The subepithelial inflammatory reaction in OLP lesions is presumably due to an as yet unidentified antigen in the junctional zone between epithelium and connective tissue or to components of basal epithelial cells (Holmstrup & Dabelsteen 1979; Walsh *et al.* 1990; Sugerman *et al.* 1994). A lichen planus specific antigen in the stratum spinosum of skin lesions has been described (Camisa *et al.* 1986), but this antigen does not appear to play a significant role in oral lesions since it is rarely identified there. It is still an open question whether OLP is a group of etiologically diverse diseases with common clinical and histopathologic features or a disease entity characterized by a type IV hypersensitivity reaction to an antigen in the basement membrane area. The clinical diagnosis is based on the presence of papular or reticular lesions. The diagnosis may be supported by histo-

pathologic findings of hyperkeratosis, degenerative changes of basal cells, and subepithelial inflammation dominated by lymphocytes and macrophages (Holmstrup 1999).

The uncertain background of OLP results in several borderline cases of so-called oral lichenoid lesions (OLL) for which a final diagnosis is difficult to establish (Thornhill *et al.* 2006). The most common OLLs are probably lesions in contact with dental restorations (Holmstrup 1991) (see later in this chapter). Other types of OLL are associated with various types of medications including antimalarials, quinine, quinidine, non-steroidal anti-inflammatory drugs, thiazides, diuretics, gold salts, penicillamine, beta-blockers, and others (Scully *et al.* 1998a). Graft-versus-host reactions are also characterized by a lichenoid appearance (Fujii *et al.* 1988) and a group of OLLs is associated with systemic diseases, including liver disease (Fortune & Buchanan 1993; Bagan *et al.* 1994; Carrozzo *et al.* 1996). This appears to be particularly evident in Southern Europe and Japan where hepatitis C has been found in 20–60% of OLL cases (Bagan *et al.* 1994; Gandolfo *et al.* 1994; Nagao *et al.* 1995).

Several follow-up studies have demonstrated that OLP is associated with increased development of oral cancer, the frequency of cancer development being in the range of 0.5–2% (Holmstrup *et al.* 1988; Mattson *et al.* 2002; Mignogna *et al.* 2006; Ingafou *et al.* 2006).

The most important part of the therapeutic regimen is an atraumatic meticulous plaque control, which results in significant improvement in many patients (Holmstrup *et al.* 1990) (Figs. 16-25 to 16-28). Individual oral hygiene procedures with the purpose of effective plaque removal without traumatic influence on the gingival tissue should be established for all patients with symptoms. In cases of persistent pain, typically associated with atrophic and ulcerative affections, antifungal treatment may be necessary if the lesions contain yeast, which occurs in 37% of OLP cases (Krogh *et al.* 1987). In painful cases, which have not responded to the treatment above, topical corticosteroids, preferably in a paste or an ointment, should be used three times daily for a number of weeks. However, relapses in such cases are very common, and intermittent episodes of treatment may be needed over an extended period.

Pemphigoid

Pemphigoid is a group of disorders in which autoantibodies towards components of the basement membrane result in detachment of the epithelium from the connective tissue. Bullous pemphigoid predominantly affects the skin, but oral mucosal involvement may occur (Brooke 1973; Hodge *et al.* 1981). If only mucous membranes are affected, the term benign mucous membrane pemphigoid (BMMP) is often used. The term cicatricial pemphigoid is also used to describe subepithelial bullous disease limited to the mouth or eyes and infrequently other mucosal areas.

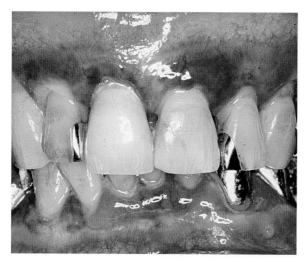

Fig. 16-30 Benign mucous membrane pemphigoid affecting the attached gingiva of both jaws. The lesions are erythematous and resemble atrophic lichen planus lesions. They result in pain associated with oral procedures including eating and oral hygiene.

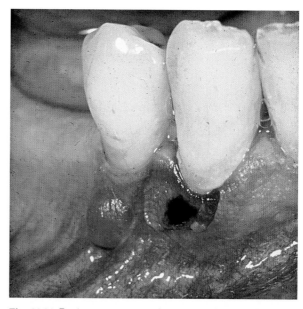

Fig. 16-31 Benign mucous membrane pemphigoid with intact and ruptured gingival bulla.

This term is problematic at least for the oral lesions, because usually oral lesions do not result in scarring, whereas this is a serious risk in ocular lesions (Scully et al. 1998b). It is now evident that BMMP comprises a group of disease entities characterized by an immune reaction involving autoantibodies directed against various basement membrane zone antigens (Scully & Laskaris 1998). These antigens have been identified as hemidesmosome or lamina lucida components (Leonard et al. 1982, 1984; Manton & Scully 1988; Domloge-Hultsch et al. 1992, 1994), and sera from patients with oral lesions have been shown to recognize the alpha6 integrin subunit (Rashid et al. 2006). In addition, complement-mediated cell destructive processes may be involved in the pathogenesis of the disease (Eversole 1994). The trigger mechanisms behind these reactions, however, have not yet been ascertained.

The majority of affected patients are females with a mean age at onset of 50 years or over (Shklar & McCarthy 1971). Oral involvement in BMMP is almost inevitable and usually the oral cavity is the first site of disease activity (Silverman et al. 1986; Gallagher & Shklar 1987). Any area of the oral mucosa may be involved in BMMP, but the main manifestation is desquamative lesions of the gingiva presenting intensely erythematous attached gingiva (Laskaris et al. 1982; Silverman et al. 1986; Gallagher & Shklar 1987) (Fig. 16-30). The inflammatory changes, as always when not caused by plaque, may extend over the entire gingival width and even over the mucogingival junction. Rubbing of the gingiva may precipitate bulla formation (Dahl & Cook 1979). This is denoted a positive Nicholsky sign and is caused by the destroyed adhesion of the epithelium to the connective tissue. The intact bullae are often clear to yellowish or they may be hemorrhagic (Figs. 16-31 and 16-32). This, again, is due to the separation of

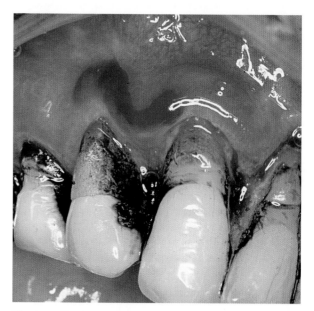

Fig. 16-32 Benign mucous membrane pemphigoid with hemorrhagic gingival bulla. The patient uses chlorhexidine for daily plaque reduction.

epithelium from connective tissue at the junction resulting in exposed vessels inside the bullae. Usually, the bullae rupture rapidly leaving fibrin-coated ulcers. Sometimes, tags of loose epithelium can be found due to rupture of bullae. Other mucosal surfaces may be involved in some patients. Ocular lesions are particularly important because scar formation can result in blindness (Williams et al. 1984) (Fig. 16-33).

The separation of epithelium from connective tissue at the basement membrane area is the main diagnostic feature of BMMP. A non-specific inflammatory reaction is a secondary histologic finding. In addition, immunohistochemical examination can help distinguish BMMP from other vesiculobullous

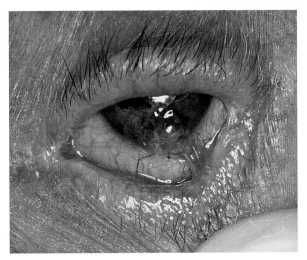

Fig. 16-33 Benign mucous membrane pemphigoid. Eye lesion with scar formation due to coalescence of palpebral and conjunctival mucosa.

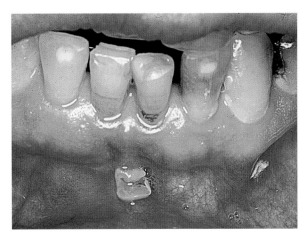

Fig. 16-34 Pemphigus vulgaris. Initial lesion resembling recurrent aphthous stomatitis.

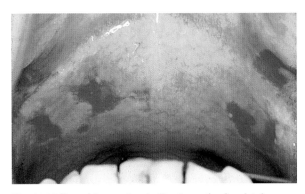

Fig. 16-35 Pemphigus vulgaris. Erosions of soft palatal mucosa. The erosive lesions are due to loss of the superficial part of the epithelium, leaving the connective tissue covered only by the basal cell layers.

diseases, in particular pemphigus, which is life threatening. Deposits of C3, IgG, and sometimes other immunoglobulins as well as fibrin are found at the basement membrane zone in the vast majority of cases (Laskaris & Nicolis 1980; Daniels & Quadra-White 1981; Manton & Scully 1988). It is important to involve peri-lesional tissue in the biopsy because the characteristic features may be lost within lesional tissue (Ullman 1988). Circulating immunoglobulins are found only occasionally in BMMP by indirect immunofluorescence (Laskaris & Angelopoulos 1981).

Therapy consists of professional atraumatic plaque removal and individual instruction in gentle but careful daily plaque control, eventually supplemented with daily use of chlorhexidine and/or topical corticosteroid application if necessary. As for all the chronic inflammatory oral mucosal diseases, oral hygiene procedures are very important and controlling the infection from plaque bacteria may result in considerable reduction of disease activity and symptoms. It is also important to prevent the development of attachment loss due to periodontitis in these patients with difficulties in maintaining oral hygiene (Tricamo *et al.* 2006). However, the disease is chronic in nature and formation of new bullae is inevitable in most patients. Topical corticosteroids, preferably applied as a paste at night, temper the inflammatory reaction.

Pemphigus vulgaris

Pemphigus is a group of autoimmune diseases characterized by formation of intraepithelial bullae in skin and mucous membranes. The group comprises several variants, pemphigus vulgaris (PV) being the most common and most serious form (Barth & Venning 1987).

Individuals of Jewish or Mediterranean background are more often affected by PV than others.

This is an indication of a strong genetic background of the disease (Pisanti *et al.* 1974). The disease may occur at any age, but is typically seen in the middle-aged or elderly. It presents with widespread bulla formation often including large areas of skin, and if left untreated the disease is life threatening. Intraoral onset of the disease with bulla formation is very common and lesions of the oral mucosa including the gingiva are frequently seen. Early lesions may resemble aphthous ulcers (Fig. 16-34), but widespread erosions are common at later stages (Fig. 16-35). Gingival involvement may present as painful desquamative lesions or as erosions or ulcerations, which are remains of ruptured bullae (Fig. 16-36). Such lesions may be indistinguishable from BMMP (Zegarelli & Zegarelli 1977; Sciubba 1996). Since the bulla formation is located in the spinous cell layer, the chance of seeing an intact bulla is even more reduced than in BMMP. Involvement of other mucous membranes is common (Laskaris *et al.* 1982). The ulcers heal slowly, usually without scar formation, and the disease runs a chronic course with recurring bulla formation (Zegarelli & Zegarelli 1977).

Diagnosis is based on the characteristic histological feature of PV that is intraepithelial bulla

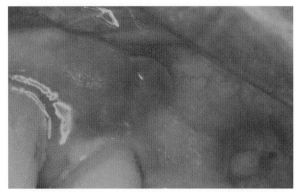

Fig. 16-36 Pemphigus vulgaris. Intact and ruptured gingival bullae.

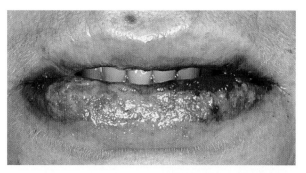

Fig. 16-37 Erythema multiforme with crust formation of the vermilion border of the lower lip.

formation due to destruction of desmosomes resulting in acantholysis. The bullae contain non-adhering free epithelial cells, denoted Tzank cells, which have lost their intercellular bridges (Coscia-Porrazzi *et al.* 1985; Nishikawa *et al.* 1996). Mononuclear cells and neutrophils dominate the associated inflammatory reaction. Immunohistochemistry reveals pericellular epithelial deposits of IgG and C3. Circulating auto-antibodies against interepithelial adhesion molecules are detectable in serum samples of most patients, but at the initial stage of intraoral signs antiepithelial antibody may not be elevated (Melbye *et al.* 1987; Manton & Scully 1988; Lamey *et al.* 1992; Lever & Schaumburg-Lever 1997). The background of bulla formation in PV is damage to the intercellular adhesion caused by autoantibodies to cadherin-type epithelial cell adhesion molecules (desmoglein 1 and 3) (Nousari & Anhalt 1995; Nishikawa *et al.* 1996; Lanza *et al.* 2006). The mechanism by which these molecules trigger the formation of autoantibodies has not yet been established.

Immediate referral of patients with PV to a dermatologist or internal medicine specialist is important because when recognized late the disease can be fatal, although systemic corticosteroid therapy can presently solve most cases. Supplementary local treatment consists of gentle plaque control and professional cleaning as mentioned for the chronic inflammatory oral mucosal diseases above. Sometimes, additional topical corticosteroid application is needed to control the intraoral disease.

Erythema multiforme

Erythema multiforme (EM) is a reactive acute, sometimes recurrent, vesiculobullous disease affecting mucous membranes and skin. A general malaise often precedes the lesions. The disease spectrum comprises a self-limiting, mild, exanthematic, cutaneous variant with minimal oral involvement to a progressive, fulminating, severe variant with extensive mucocutaneous epithelial necrosis. The latter form of the disease has been described as Stevens-Johnson syndrome, with widespread mucous membrane lesions, i.e. oral, ocular and genital, in addition to

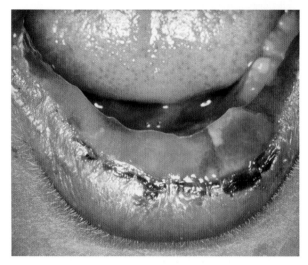

Fig. 16-38 Erythema multiforme with ulceration covered by heavy fibrin exudate.

skin lesions (Lozada-Nur *et al.* 1989; Assier *et al.* 1995; Bystryn 1996; Ayangco & Rogers 2003). The multi-locular entity has to be differentiated from other disorders such as Reiter and Behçet's syndromes, which also affect the eyes, the oral mucosa, and often the genitalia. The pathogenesis of EM remains unknown, but the disease appears to be a cytotoxic immune reaction towards keratinocytes (Ayangco & Rogers 2003) precipitated by a wide range of factors including herpes simplex virus (Lozada & Silverman 1978; Nesbit & Gobetti 1986; Ruokonen *et al.* 1988; Miura *et al.* 1992; Aurelian *et al.* 1998), *Mycoplasma pneumoniae* (McKellar & Reade 1986; Stutman 1987), and various drugs (Bottiger *et al.* 1975; Gebel & Hornstein 1984; Kauppinen & Stubb 1984).

EM may occur at any age but most frequently affects young individuals. It may or may not involve the oral mucosa, but oral involvement occurs in as many as 25–60% of cases (Huff *et al.* 1983); sometimes it is the only involved site. The characteristic oral lesions comprise swollen lips often with extensive crust formation of the vermilion border (Fig. 16-37). The basic lesions, however, are bullae that rupture and leave extensive ulcers usually covered by heavy yellowish fibrinous exudates sometimes described as pseudomembranes (Figs. 16-38 and 16-39). Such

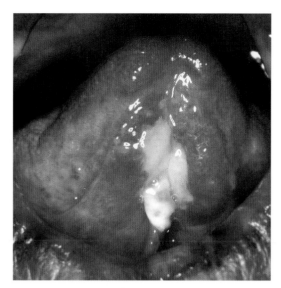

Fig. 16-39 Erythema multiforme. Fibrin-coated ulcerations of ventral surface of tongue and lower lip.

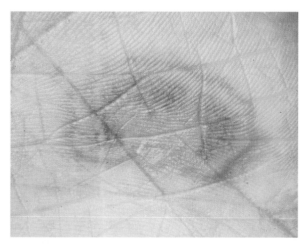

Fig. 16-40 Erythema multiforme. Skin lesion with characteristic iris appearance. Central bulla formation surrounded by a blanched halo within an erythematous zone.

lesions may also involve the buccal mucosa and gingiva (Huff *et al.* 1983; Lozada-Nur *et al.* 1989; Scully *et al.* 1991; Barrett *et al.* 1993). The skin lesions are characteristic due to the iris appearance with a central bulla formation surrounded by a blanched halo within an erythematous zone (Fig. 16-40). Similar intraoral lesions do occur but they are infrequent. The disease is usually self-limiting but recurrences are common. Healing of the lesions may take several weeks (Fabbri & Panconesi 1993).

Histopathology of EM shows intra- or subepithelial separation of epithelium from connective tissue with non-specific inflammation (Reed 1985). Immunohistochemical findings are non-specific and in most instances the diagnosis relies on the clinical findings.

Although periodontal lesions are not the most frequent intraoral manifestation, they can sometimes pose a differential diagnostic problem. The typical crusty ulcerations of the vermilion border and the

heavy fibrin exudates covering intraoral lesions are indicative of EM, sometimes therefore denoted erythema multiforme exudativum. The mucosal ulcerations may take weeks to heal and they are painful (Lozada-Nur *et al.* 1989).

As for any intraoral ulcerations, gentle plaque control and professional cleaning are mandatory. The treatment often involves systemic corticosteroids, but topical treatment may be sufficient in cases with minor lesions.

Lupus erythematosus

Lupus erythematosus (LE) is a group of autoimmune connective tissue disorders in which autoantibodies form to various cellular constituents including nucleus, cytoplasmic membrane and others. All parts of the body may be affected, and the disease is much more prevalent among women than among men. The etiology of LE remains unknown, but deposits of antigen–antibody complexes appear to play a role in the tissue damage characteristic of the disease (Schrieber & Maini 1984). LE includes two major traditional forms: discoid LE (DLE) and systemic LE (SLE) which may involve a range of organ systems including kidney, heart, central nervous system, vascular system, and bone marrow. Recently two new forms, acute and subacute cutaneous LE, have been added to the classification, these forms representing different degrees of disease activity and increased risk of development of SLE (Wouters *et al.* 2004). The prevalence of LE has been estimated at 0.05% (Condemi 1987).

DLE is a mild chronic form, which affects skin and mucous membranes, sometimes involving the gingiva as well as other parts of the oral mucosa (Schiødt 1984a,b). The typical lesion presents a central atrophic area with small white dots surrounded by irradiating fine white striae with a periphery of telangiectasia (Fig. 16-41). The lesions can be ulcerated or clinically indistinguishable from leukoplakia or atrophic oral lichen planus (Fig. 16-42) (Schiødt 1984b). Sometimes patients present brownish gingival lesions, which is a side effect of antimalarial drugs prescribed to these patients as part of their treatment (Fig. 16-43). Eight percent of patients with DLE develop SLE, and ulcerations may be a sign of SLE; SLE demonstrates oral lesions in 25–40% of patients (Schiødt 1984a; Pisetsky 1986; Johnsson *et al.* 1988). The characteristic bordeaux-colored "butterfly" skin lesions are photosensitive, scaly, erythematous macules located on the bridge of the nose and the cheeks (Standefer & Mattox 1986). The systemic type, which can still be fatal because of nephrologic and hematologic complications, also has skin lesions on the face but they tend to spread over the entire body.

Diagnosis is based on clinical and histopathologic findings. The epithelial changes, characteristic of oral LE lesions, are hyperkeratosis, keratin plugging and

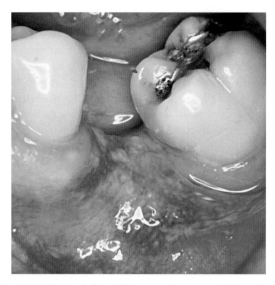

Fig. 16-41 Gingival discoid lupus erythematosus lesion. A central erythematous area with small white dots is surrounded by delicate white striae.

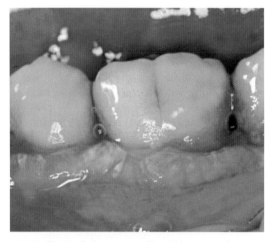

Fig. 16-42 Gingival plaque-type discoid lupus erythematosus lesion resembling frictional keratosis and leukoplakia.

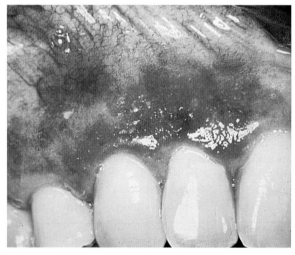

Fig. 16-43 Antimalarial drugs may result in brownish gingival discoloration. This is a patient with discoid lupus erythematosus receiving an antimalarial drug, chloroquine, as part of the treatment regimen.

variation in epithelial thickness, liquefaction degeneration of basal cells, and increased width of the basement membrane. The subepithelial connective tissue harbors inflammation, sometimes resembling OLP but often with a less distinct band-shaped pattern (Schiødt & Pindborg 1984). Immunohistochemical investigation reveals deposits of various immunoglobulins, C3, and fibrin along the basement membrane (Reibel & Schiødt 1986).

Systemic corticosteroid and other anti-inflammatory treatment regimens are required for SLE. Additional topical treatment is sometimes needed for symptomatic intraoral lesions to resolve.

Drug-induced mucocutaneous disorders

A number of drugs cause adverse effects in the oral mucosa. Best known in the periodontal field is gingival hyperplasia related to the intake of phenytoin, cyclosporine, and nifedipine. Because these lesions to some extent are plaque dependent, they are reviewed in Chapter 17. Other types of drugs may give rise to EM as mentioned above.

Several other drugs may be associated with adverse effects that include lesions of the oral mucosa. An example is azathioprine, which is an antimetabolite used for immunosuppression in the treatment of autoimmune and other diseases and to prevent rejection of transplants. Its mode of action is through inhibition of purine base synthesis, resulting in suppression of nucleic acid and protein synthesis, whereby the immune response is inhibited at various stages. Rapidly proliferating tissues such as the bone marrow, the hair follicles, and the gastrointestinal and the oral mucosa may show side effects, e.g. oral ulceration. These ulcerations may include the gingiva. Other examples of drugs frequently resulting in adverse effects in the form of stomatitis are antineoplastic drugs used in cancer chemotherapy. Methotrexate is a cytostatic drug sometimes used in the treatment of leukemia. Epithelial atrophy, superficial sloughing, intense erythema, and ulceration are characteristic findings in the oral mucosa of patients with adverse effects of the chemotherapeutic treatment (Fig. 16-44) (Pindborg 1992). The ulcerative lesions are frequent portals of entry for microorganisms from the mouth, and thereby often sources of serious systemic infection in patients with suppression of the bone marrow and reduced defense systems against infection. Professional plaque removal, mouth rinsing with 0.1% chlorhexidine, and a prophylactic antibiotic regimen are important in such patients (Sonis 1998; Holmstrup & Glick 2002).

Allergic reactions

Allergic manifestations in the oral mucosa are uncommon. Several mechanisms may be involved in allergy, which is an exaggerated immune reaction. Oral mucosal reactions may be type I reactions (immedi-

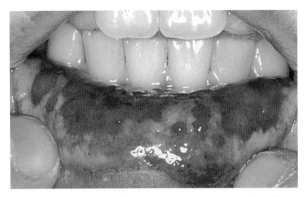

Fig. 16-44 Drug-induced stomatitis sometimes involves the gingiva. This is a mucosal lesion due to azathioprine, which is an antimetabolite used for immunosuppression.

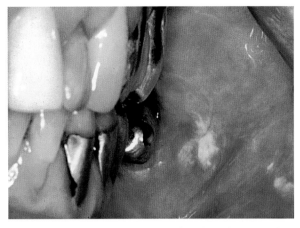

Fig. 16-45 Lichenoid contact lesion of left buccal mucosa due to type IV hypersensitivity to mercury. The lesion is confined to the zone of contact with the amalgam fillings. These lesions usually recover after replacement of the mercury-containing fillings with composites or other materials devoid of allergy-provoking components.

ate type), which is mediated by IgE, or more often they are type IV reactions (delayed type), mediated by T cells. The rare intraoral occurrence may be due to the fact that much higher concentrations of allergen are required for an allergic reaction to occur in the oral mucosa than in skin and other surfaces (Amlot *et al.* 1985; Lüders 1987; Holmstrup 1999). This chapter includes allergies to dental restorative materials, toothpastes, mouthwashes, and food.

Dental restorative materials

The clinical manifestation of type IV allergy (contact allergy) occurs after a period of 12–48 hours following contact with the allergen. The effects on oral mucosa have been denoted contact lesions and prior contact with the allergen resulting in sensitization is prerequisite for these reactions to occur (Holmstrup 1991). Oral mucosal reactions to restorative materials include reactions to mercury, nickel, gold, zinc, chromium, palladium, and acrylics (Ovrutsky & Ulyanow 1976; Zaun 1977; Bergman *et al.* 1980; Council on Dental Materials, Instruments and Equipment Workshop 1984; Fisher 1987). The lesions, which may sometimes affect the gingiva, have clinical similarities with oral lichen planus affections, which is why they are denoted OLL (see earlier in this chapter) or oral leukoplakia (Fig. 16-45). They are reddish or whitish, sometimes ulcerated lesions, but one of the crucial diagnostic observations is that the lesions resolve after removal of the offending material. Additional patch testing to identify the exact allergen gives supplementary information, but for dental amalgam it has been shown that there is no obvious correlation between the result of an epicutaneous patch test and the clinical result after removal of the fillings (Skoglund 1994). A clinical manifestation confined to the area of contact with the offending restorative material and the result after replacing this material indicates the diagnosis (Holmstrup 1999).

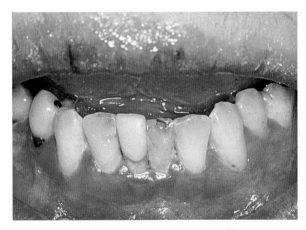

Fig. 16-46 Diffuse gingivitis and cheilitis due to contact allergy to flavor additive in dentifrice.

Reactions to oral hygiene products, chewing gum, and food

Toothpastes, mouthwashes and chewing gum

Contact allergy rarely occurs after the use of toothpastes (Sainio & Kanerva 1995; Skaare *et al.* 1997) and mouthwashes (Sainio & Kanerva 1995). The constituents responsible for the allergic reactions may be flavor additives, for instance carvone and cinnamon (Drake & Maibach 1976) or preservatives (Duffin & Cowan 1985). The flavoring constituents may be used, also, in chewing gum and result in similar forms of gingivostomatitis (Kerr *et al.* 1971). The clinical manifestations of allergy include a diffuse fiery red edematous gingivitis sometimes with ulcerations or whitening (Fig. 16-46). Similar signs may involve the labial, buccal, and tongue mucosa and cheilitis may also be seen. The clinical manifestations, which are characteristic, form the basis of the diagnosis, which may be supported by resolution of the lesions after stopping use of the allergen-containing agent (Holmstrup 1999).

Foods

The gastrointestinal tract is the largest immunologic organ in the body. It is constantly bombarded by a myriad of dietary proteins. Despite the extent of protein exposure, very few patients contract food allergies due to development of oral tolerance to these antigens (Chehade & Mayer 2005). Allergic reactions attributable to food may manifest both as type I and type IV reactions. Type I reaction with severe swelling has been described after intake of food components such as peanuts and pumpkin seed. Birch pollen allergy is associated with some types of oral mucosa allergy, and more than 20% of patients with oral allergy may be hypersensitive to kiwi, peach, apple, chestnut, and salami (Yamamoto *et al.* 1995; Antico 1996; Asero *et al.* 1996; Liccardi *et al.* 1996; Rossi *et al.* 1996; Helbling 1997; Wutrich 1997). Another food allergen resulting in gingivitis or gingivostomatitis is red pepper (Serio *et al.* 1991; Hedin *et al.* 1994). Unless it has been demonstrated that the lesions resolve after removal of the allergen, the diagnosis is difficult to establish.

Other gingival manifestations of systemic conditions

Gastrointestinal diseases

Crohn's disease

Crohn's disease is characterized by chronic granulomatous infiltrates of the wall of the last ileal loops, but any part of the gastrointestinal tract can be affected. The oral cavity is part of the gastrointestinal tract. It is thus not surprising that Crohn's disease can occur from the rectum to the lips.

The number of reports of lesions involving the periodontium is limited (van Steenberghe *et al.* 1976), which is probably related to a tradition by many clinicians of using the term aphthous lesions for any ulcerative disease of the oral mucosa. The oral lesions have striking similarity with those of the intestinal tract as revealed by rectoscopy, i.e. irregular long ulcerations with elevated borders with a cobblestone appearance. Usually, the periodontal lesions appear after the diagnosis has been established on the basis of the intestinal signs, but sometimes the oral lesions are the first findings leading to diagnosis. Characteristic clinical findings are mucosal foldings of the buccal or labial sulcus (Fig. 16-47). Exacerbations of the oral lesions appear in parallel with those of the intestine. An increased risk of periodontal destruction has been reported associated with defective neutrophil function (Lamster *et al.* 1982).

The term orofacial granulomatosis has been used as a collective diagnosis of Crohn's disease, Melkersson-Rosenthal syndrome, and sarcoidosis, because these diseases show the same histopathologic features, i.e. non-caseating, epitheloid cell granulomas in the affected tissue. Rarely, all three diseases

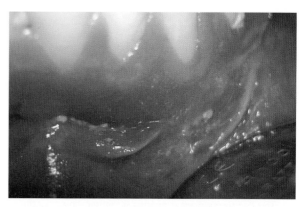

Fig. 16-47 A frequent oral finding in patients with Crohn's disease is mucosal foldings, usually located in the buccal or labial sulcus. Such lesions may be the first clinical finding leading to the diagnosis of the disease. Histopathologic examination of biopsies from these foldings reveal epitheloid cell granulomas. The foldings are characteristic for the other types of orofacial granulomatosis as well.

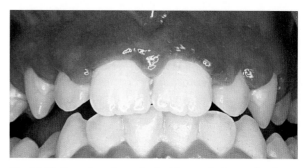

Fig. 16-48 Granulomatous gingival hyperplasia may be due to sarcoidosis, which is one of the orofacial granulomatoses; others are Crohn's disease and Melkersson-Rosenthal syndrome.

may present gingival lesions, characterized by swellings (Pindborg 1992; Mignogna *et al.* 2001); sarcoidosis sometimes causes fiery red granular gingival overgrowth (Fig. 16-48). Among 45 cases of oral sarcoidosis, 13% had gingival lesions (Blinder *et al.* 1997). A recent study of 35 patients with orofacial granulomatosis demonstrated ileal and colonic abnormalities in 54%, and granulomas were revealed in gut biopsies of 64% of the patients. Intestinal abnormality was significantly more likely if the age of onset was less than 30 years (Sanderson *et al.* 2005).

Local treatment consists of intralesional steroid injection (Mignogna *et al.* 2004; El-Hakim & Chauvin 2004) or paste application daily or twice daily during painful exacerbations and meticulous oral hygiene to reduce additional inflammation of the oral cavity. Treatment of any inflammatory condition in the affected oral region, including periodontitis, periapical inflammation, and even mucosal lesions due to hypersensitivity to restorative dental materials, is important for resolution in some cases (Guttman-Yassky *et al.* 2003).

Hematologic disorders

Leukemia

Leukemia is a malignant hematologic disorder with abnormal proliferation and development of leukocytes and their precursors in blood and bone marrow. It can involve any of the subsets of leukocytes, polymorphonuclear leukocytes, lymphocytes or monocytes. Normal hematopoiesis is suppressed and, in most cases of leukemia, the white blood cells appear in the circulating blood in immature forms. The leukemic cell proliferation at the expense of normal hematopoietic cell lines causes bone marrow failure and depressed blood cell count. As a consequence of the inability to produce sufficient functional white blood cells and platelets, death may result from infection or bleeding associated with neutropenia and thrombocytopenia.

The classification of leukemia is based on its course, acute or chronic, and origin of cells involved. The basic forms are: acute lymphocytic leukemia (ALL), acute myelogenous leukemia (AML), chronic lymphocytic leukemia (CLL), and chronic myelogenous leukemia (CML). Acute leukemias have an aggressive course resulting in death within 6 months if untreated. They occur rather seldom and patients are usually either under 20 or over 60 years of age. Chronic leukemias, of which the lymphocytic form is the most common, have less pronounced bone marrow failure and a more indolent course usually lasting several years. They occur during adulthood and normally after the age of 40. Whereas the peripheral granulocyte count is markedly elevated in chronic leukemia, it may be elevated, decreased or normal in acute leukemia (McKenna 2000).

Gingival manifestations in leukemia, which include extensive swelling (Fig. 16-49), ulceration (Fig. 16-50), petechiae (Fig. 16-51), and erythema, are much more common in acute than in chronic forms. Sometimes the manifestations lead to the diagnosis of leukemia; 69% of patients with acute leukemia had oral signs of leukemia on examination and 33% of the patients had gingival swelling (Pindborg 1992). In another study gingival swelling was revealed in 21% of AML patients but in no patients with ALL (Meyer *et al.* 2000). In the latter group, on the other hand, 36% showed both gingival erythema and ulcers. In leukemic children, only 10–17% appear to have gingival swelling (Curtis 1971; Michaud *et al.* 1977). The pronounced gingival swelling seen in leukemic patients is mostly due to plaque-induced inflammation, since stringent plaque control appears to resolve the swelling (Barrett 1984); it may also be due to the presence of leukemic infiltrates, although this has been reported to be an uncommon feature of leukemic patients (Barrett 1984). Gingival bleeding, due to secondary thrombocytopenia, is a common sign in leukemic patients. It has been reported as the initial sign in 17.7% of patients with acute leukemias and in 4.4% of patients with chronic forms (Lynch & Ship 1967).

In general, the periodontal treatment of patients with leukemia is important; it aims at reducing plaque as a source of bacteremia and damage to the periodontal tissues both during disease and during periods of chemotherapy. In such periods, potentially pathogenic bacteria occur in plaque simultaneous with granulocytopenia in these patients (Peterson

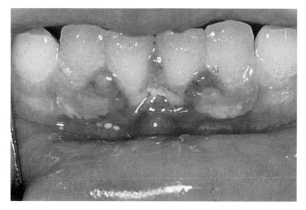

Fig. 16-50 Acute lymphocytic leukemia with gingival ulceration in a child.

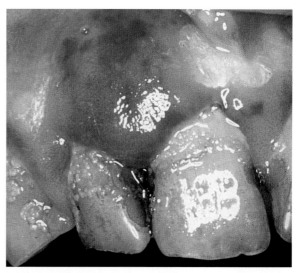

Fig. 16-51 Acute myelogenous leukemia with petechiae and swelling of the gingiva. This patient had several episodes of spontaneous bleeding from the gingiva, which prevented oral hygiene procedures from being undertaken.

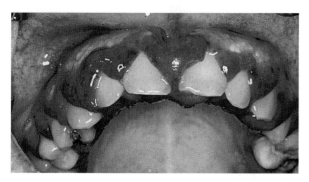

Fig. 16-49 Acute myelogenous leukemia with extensive swelling of the gingiva.

et al. 1990). The reduction of periodontal inflammation may also prevent episodes of gingival bleeding. As with many other patients, chemical plaque control in combination with mechanical debridement appears to be most effective and is the preferred method of periodontal therapy in leukemic patients (Holmstrup & Glick 2002). However, the increased tendency to bleeding in many of these patients may necessitate the use of alternative methods to toothbrushing. A study of professional plaque removal preceding mouthrinsing with 0.1% chlorhexidine in patients with AML showed that the additional initial removal of plaque and calculus was more effective in reducing gingival inflammation than mouthrinsing with chlorhexidine alone (Bergman *et al.* 1992). A 1-day antibiotic prophylaxis regimen with a combination of piperacillin and netilmicin was given prior to and after the mechanical debridement. Periodontal treatment always involves a close cooperation with the medical department or specialist responsible for coordination of the patient's treatment.

Traumatic lesions

The background of traumatic lesions of the oral tissues may be self-inflicted, iatrogenic or accidental. Chemical as well as physical and thermal injuries may affect the periodontium (Armitage 1999).

Chemical injury

Surface etching by various chemical products with toxic properties may result in mucosal reactions including reactions of the gingiva. Chlorhexidine-induced mucosal desquamation (Fløtra *et al.* 1971; Almquist & Luthman 1988) (Fig. 16-52), acetylsalicylic acid burn (Najjar 1977), cocaine burn (Dello Russo & Temple 1982), and slough due to dentifrice detergents are examples of such reactions (Muhler

1970). These lesions are reversible and resolve after quitting the toxic influence. Chemical injury to the gingival tissue may be caused by incorrect use of caustics by the dentist. Paraformaldehyde used for pulp mummification may give rise to inflammation and necrosis of the gingival tissue if the cavity sealing is insufficient (Di Felice & Lombardi 1998). Usually, the diagnosis is obvious from the clinical findings and the patient history.

Physical injury

Oral hygiene agents and inexpedient procedures can be injurious to the gingival tissues. If physical trauma is limited, the gingival response is hyperkeratosis, resulting in a white leukoplakia-like, frictional keratosis (Fig. 16-53). In case of more violent trauma the damage varies from superficial gingival laceration to major loss of tissue resulting in gingival recession (Axéll & Koch 1982; Smukler & Landsberg 1984). Abrasiveness of dentifrice, strong brushing force, and horizontal movement of the toothbrush contribute to the gingival injury even in young patients. Characteristic findings in these patients are extremely good oral hygiene, cervical tooth abrasion, and unaffected tops of the interdental papillae at the site of injury (Figs. 16-54 to 16-57). The condition has been termed traumatic ulcerative gingival lesion (Axéll & Koch 1982). Dental flossing may also cause gingival ulceration and inflammation primarily affecting the top of the interdental papillae (Fig. 16-58). The prevalence of such findings is unknown (Gillette & Van House 1980). Diagnosis of physical injuries is based on the clinical findings. An important differential diagnosis is necrotizing gingivitis (Blasberg *et al.* 1981), see Chapter 20. The latter normally reveals itself as a necrotic gingival margin and interdental

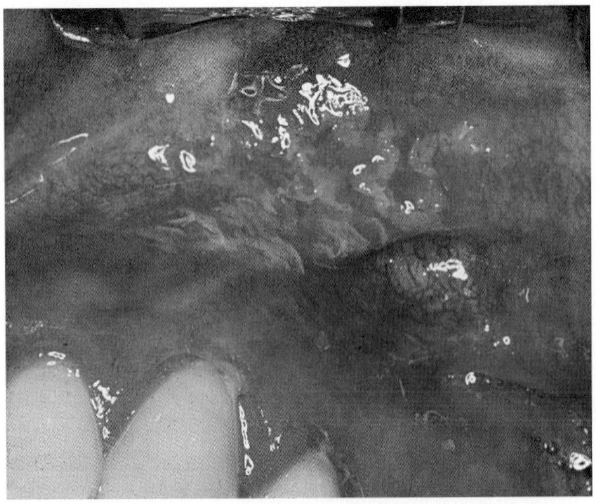

Fig. 16-52 Chlorhexidine-induced mucosal desquamation. This is a reversible type of lesion, which is completely normalized after stopping chlorhexidine use.

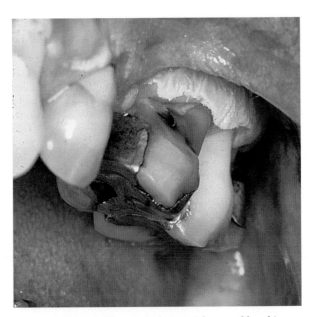

Fig. 16-53 Frictional keratosis due to violent toothbrushing. Note the cervical abrasion of adjacent teeth.

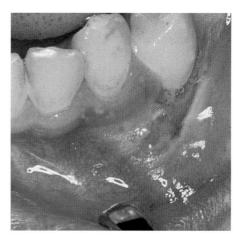

Fig. 16-54 Gingival wounding due to improper toothbrushing. Note the characteristic horizontal extension of the lesion, affecting the most prominent part of the tooth arch.

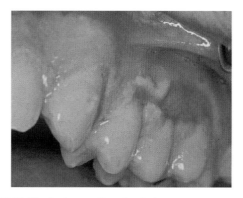

Fig. 16-55 Gingival wounding due to improper toothbrushing. Note the characteristic horizontal extension of the lesion and the uninflamed, unaffected interdental papillae.

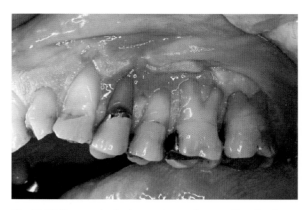

Fig. 16-56 Severe gingival recession and wounding due to improper toothbrushing. Note the unaffected interdental papillae.

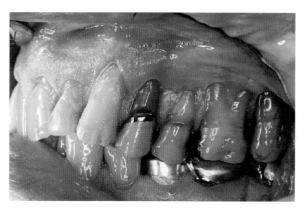

Fig. 16-57 Healing of lesion shown in Fig. 16-56. The damage to the periodontal tissues is severe, leaving extended gingival recession.

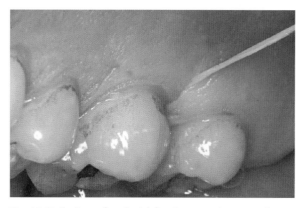

Fig. 16-58 Lesions after dental flossing are common and sometimes result in permanent fissures of the gingival tissue.

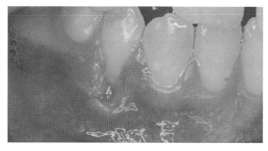

Fig. 16-59 Self-inflicted gingival recession with ulcerated margin due to a 7-year-old boy's scratching with fingernail.

papillae, while brushing trauma leads to ulcerations of a few millimeters of the gingival margin.

Self-inflicted physical injury to the gingival tissues can occur; sometimes the lesions are termed gingivitis artefacta. The lesions often show ulceration of the gingival margin often associated with recession (Figs. 16-59 and 16-60). Such lesions are most common in children and young individuals and two thirds appear to involve female patients. The lesions, which may be hemorrhagic, are usually produced by picking at or scratching the gingiva with a finger or a fingernail; sometimes the lesions are made by instruments (Pattison 1983). The correct diagnosis is often difficult to establish based on clinical findings, and identification of the cause may be impossible.

Thermal injury

Extensive thermal burns of the oral mucosa are very rare, but minor burns particularly from hot

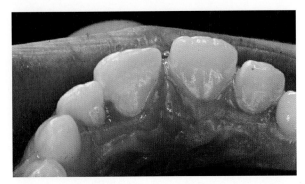

Fig. 16-60 Self-inflicted gingival ulceration of palatal gingiva of the upper right incisor region in the same boy as shown in Fig. 16-59. This lesion was also caused by fingernail scratching.

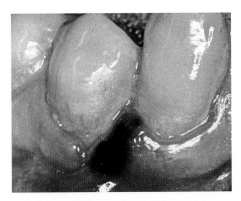

Fig. 16-62 Amalgam tattoo of attached gingiva.

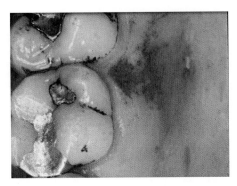

Fig. 16-61 Thermal burn with slight erosion and petechiae of palatal gingiva due to hot coffee intake.

beverages are seen occasionally. Their predilection by site is the palatal and labial mucosa but any part of the oral mucosa can be involved including the gingiva (Colby *et al.* 1961). The area involved is painful and erythematous and may slough a coagulated surface. Vesicles may also occur (Laskaris 1994) and sometimes the lesions present as ulceration, petechia or erosion (Fig. 16-61). Obviously, the history is important for reaching the correct diagnosis. Common causes are hot coffee, pizza, and melted cheese, but dental treatments involving improper

handling of hot hydrocolloid impression material, hot wax or cautery instruments are other causes (Colby *et al.* 1961).

Foreign body reactions

Another type of tissue reaction is established through epithelial ulceration that allows entry of foreign material into gingival connective tissue. This can happen via abrasion or cutting (Gordon & Daley 1997b), a route of tissue injury which is best exemplified by the amalgam tattoo (Buchner & Hansen 1980) (Fig. 16-62). Gingival inflammation associated with foreign bodies has been termed foreign body gingivitis. A clinical study of this condition has shown that it often presents as a red or combined red–white painful chronic lesion frequently misdiagnosed as lichen planus (Gordon & Daley 1997a). An X-ray microanalysis of foreign body gingivitis showed that most of the identified foreign bodies were of dental material origin, usually abrasives (Gordon & Daley 1997b). Another way of introducing foreign substances into the tissues is self-inflicted injury, for instance due to chewing on sticks or self-induced tattooing (Gazi 1986). It is uncertain whether the inflammatory reaction in such cases is due to a toxic or in some instances an allergic reaction.

References

Almquist, H. & Luthman, J. (1988). Gingival and mucosal reactions after intensive chlorhexidine gel treatment with or without oral hygiene measures. *Scandinavian Journal of Dental Research* **96**, 557–560.

Amit, R., Morag, A., Ravid, Z., Hochman, N., Ehrlich, J. & Zakay-Rones, Z. (1992). Detection of herpes simplex virus ingingival tissue. *Journal of Periodontology* **63**, 502–506.

Amlot, P.L., Urbanek, R., Youlten, L.J., Kemeny, M. & Lessof, M.H. (1985). Type I allergy to egg and milk proteins: comparison of skin prick tests with nasal, buccal and gastric provocation tests. *International Archives of Allergy and Applied Immunology* **77**, 171–173.

Anaissie, E., Kantarjian, H., Jones, P., Barlogie, B., Luna, M., Lopez-Berestein, G. & Bodey, G.P. (1986). *Fusarium*: a newly recognized fungal pathogen in immunosuppressed patients. *Cancer* **57**, 2141–2145.

Andreasen, J.O. (1968). Oral lichen planus. 1. A clinical evaluation of 115 cases. *Oral Surgery Oral Medicine Oral Pathology* **25**, 31–42.

Antico, A. (1996). Oral allergy syndrome induced by chestnut (*Castanea sativa*). *Annals of Allergy, Asthma and Immunology* **76**, 37–40.

Araiche, M. & Brode, H. (1959). A case of fibromatosis gingivae. *Oral Surgery* **12**, 1307–1310.

Arduino, P.G. & Porter, S.R. (2006). Oral and perioral herpes simplex virus type 1 (HSV-1) infection: review of its management. *Oral Diseases* **12**, 254–270.

Armitage, G.C. (1999). Development of a classification system for periodontal diseases and conditions. *Annals of Periodontology* **4**, 1–6.

Asero, R., Massironi, F. & Velati, C. (1996). Detection of prognostic factors for oral allergy syndrome in patients with birch pollen hypersensitivity. *Journal of Allergy and Clinical Immunology* **97**, 611–616.

Assier, H., Bastuj-Garin, S., Revuz, J. & Roujeau, J-C. (1995). Erythema multiforme with mucous membrane involvement and Stevens-Johnson syndrome are clinically different disorders with distinct causes. *Archives of Dermatology* **131**, 539–543.

Aurelian, L., Kokuba, H. & Burnett, J.W. (1998). Understanding the pathogenesis of HSV-associated erythema multiforme. *Dermatology* **197**, 219–222.

Axéll, T. & Koch, G. (1982). Traumatic ulcerative gingival lesion. *Journal of Clinical Periodontology* **9**, 178–183.

Axéll, T. & Rundquist, L. (1987). Oral lichen planus – a demographic study. *Community Oral Dentistry and Oral Epidemiology* **15**, 52–56.

Ayangco, L. & Rogers, R.S. 3rd (2003). Oral manifestations of erythema multiforme. *Dermatologic Clinics* **21**, 195–205.

Bagan, J.V., Aguirre, J.M., del Olmo, J.A., Milian, A., Penarrocha, M., Rodrigo, J.M. & Cardona, F. (1994). Oral lichen planus and chronic liver disease: a clinical and morphometric study of the oral lesions in relation to transaminase elevation. *Oral Surgery Oral Medicine Oral Pathology* **78**, 337–342.

Barr, C., Lopez, M.R. & Rua-Dobles, A. (1992). Periodontal changes by HIV serostatus in a cohort of homosexual and bisexual men. *Journal of Clinical Periodontology* **19**, 794–801.

Barrett, A.W., Scully, C. & Eveson, J.W. (1993). Erythema multiforme involving gingiva. *Journal of Periodontology* **64**, 910–913.

Barrett, P.A. (1984). Gingival lesions in leukemia: A classification. *Journal of Periodontology* **55**, 585–588.

Barth, J.H. & Venning, V.A. (1987). Pemphigus. *British Journal of Hospital Medicine* **37**, 326, 330–331.

Bergman, M., Bergman, B. & Söremark, R. (1980). Tissue accumulation of nickel released due to electrochemical corrosion of non-previous dental casting alloys. *Journal of Oral Rehabiltation* **7**, 325–330.

Bergman, O.J., Ellegaard, B., Dahl, M. & Ellegaard, J. (1992). Gingival status during chemical plaque control with or without prior mechanical plaque removal in patients with acute myeloid leukemia. *Journal of Clinical Periodontology* **19**, 169–173.

Bhowmick, S.K., Gidvani, V.K. & Rettig, K.R. (2001). Hereditary gingival fibromatosis and growth retardation. *Endocrine Practice* **7**, 383–387.

Blake, G.C. & Trott, J.R. (1959). Acute streptococcal gingivitis. *Dental Practitioner and Dental Record* **10**, 43–45.

Blasberg, B., Jordan-Knox, A. & Conklin, R.J. (1981). Gingival ulceration due to improper toothbrushing. *Journal of the Canadian Dental Association* **47**, 462–464.

Blinder, D., Yahatom, R. & Taicher, S. (1997). Oral manifestations of sarcoidosis. *Oral Surgery Oral Medicine Oral Pathology Oral Radiology and Endodontics* **83**, 458–461.

Bottiger, L.E., Strandberg, I. & Westerholm, B. (1975). Drug induced febrile mucocutaneous syndrome. *Acta Medica Scandinavica* **198**, 229–233.

Boutros, H.H., Van Winckle, R.B., Evans, G.A. & Wasan, S.M. (1995). Oral histoplasmosis masquerading as an invasive carcinoma. *Journal of Oral Maxillofacial Surgery* **53**, 1110–1114.

Brooke, R.I. (1973). The oral lesions of bullous pemphigoid. *Journal of Oral Medicine* **28**, 36–40.

Buchner, A. & Hansen, L.S. (1980). Amalgam pigmentation (amalgam tattoo) of the oral mucosa. *Oral Surgery Oral Medicine Oral Pathology* **49**, 139–142.

Buechner, S.A. (1984). T cell subsets and macrophages in lichen planus. In situ identification using monoclonal antibodies and histochemical techniques. *Dermatologica* **169**, 325–329.

Burns, J.C. (1980). Diagnostic methods for herpes simplex infection: a review. *Oral Surgery* **50**, 346–349.

Bystryn, J-C. (1996). Erythema multiforme with mucous membrane involvement and Stevens-Johnson syndrome are

clinically different disorders. Comment. *Archives of Dermatology* **132**, 711–712.

Camisa, C., Allen, C.M., Bowen, B. & Olsen, R.G. (1986). Indirect immunofluorescence of oral lichen planus. *Journal of Oral Pathology* **15**, 218–220.

Cannon, R.D., Holmes, A.R, Mason, A.B. & Monk, B.C. (1995). Oral candida: Clearance, colonization, or candidiasis? *Journal of Dental Research* **74**, 1152–1161.

Carrozzo, M., Gandolfo, S., Carbone, M., Colombatto, P., Broccoletti, R., Garzino-Demo, P. & Ghizetti, V. (1996). Hepatitis C virus infection in Italian patients with oral lichen planus: a prospective case control study. *Journal of Oral Pathology and Medicine* **25**, 527–533.

Ceballos-Salobrena, A., Aguirre-Urizar, J.M. & Bagan-Sebastian, J.V. (1996). Oral manifestations associated with human immunodeficiency virus infection in a Spanish population. *Journal of Oral Pathology and Medicine* **25**, 523–526.

Chehade, M. & Mayer, L. (2005). Oral tolerance and its relation to food hypersensitivities. *Journal of Allergy and Clinical Immunology* **115**, 3–12.

Chinn, H., Chernoff, D.N., Migliorati, C.A., Silverman, S. & Green, T.L. (1995). Oral histoplasmosis in HIV-infected patients. *Oral Surgery Oral Medicine Oral Pathology* **79**, 710–714.

Cobb, C.M., Shultz, R.E., Brewer, J.H. & Dunlap, C.L. (1989). Chronic pulmonary histoplasmosis with an oral lesion. *Oral Surgery Oral Medicine Oral Pathology* **67**, 73–76.

Colby, R.A., Kerr, D.A. & Robinson, H.B.G. (1961). *Color Atlas of Oral Pathology*. Philadelphia: JB Lippincott Company, p. 96.

Coletta, R.D. & Graner, E. (2006). Hereditary gingival fibromatosis: a systematic review. *Journal of Periodontology* **77**, 753–764.

Coletta, R.D., Almeida, O.P., Reynolds, M.A. & Sauk, J.J. (1999). Alteration in expression of MMP-1 and MMP-2 but not TIMP-1 and TIMP-2 in hereditary gingival fibromatosis is mediated by TGF-beta 1 autocrine stimulation. *Journal of Periodontal Research* **34**, 457–463.

Condemi, J.J. (1987). The autoimmune diseases. *Journal of the American Medical Association* **258**, 2920–2929.

Consensus Report (1999). *Annals of Periodontology* **4**, 30–31.

Contreras, A., Falkler, W.A., Enwonwu, C.O., Idigbe, E.O., Savage, K.O., Afolabi, M.B., Onwujekwe, D., Rams, T.E. & Slots, J. (1997). Human *Herpesviridae* in acute necrotizing ulcerative gingivitis in children in Nigeria. *Oral Microbiology and Immunology* **12**, 259–265.

Coscia-Porrazzi, L., Maiello, F.M., Ruocco, V. & Pisani, M. (1985). Cytodiagnosis of oral pemphigus vulgaris. *Journal of Acta Cytologica* **29**, 746–749.

Council on Dental Materials, Instruments and Equipment Workshop (1984). Biocompatibility of metals in dentistry – recommendations for clinical implementation. *Journal of the American Dental Association* **109**, 469–471.

Cuestas-Carneiro, R. & Bornancini, C.A. (1988). Hereditary generalized gingival fibromatosis associated with hypertrichosis: report of five cases in one family. *Journal of Oral Maxillofacial Surgery* **46**, 415–420.

Curtis, A.B. (1971). Childhood leukemias: initial oral manifestations. *Journal of the American Dental Association* **83**, 159–164.

Dahl, M.G. & Cook, L.J. (1979). Lesions induced by trauma in pemphigoid. *British Journal of Dermatology* **101**, 469–473.

Daniels, T.E. & Quadra-White, C. (1981). Direct immunofluorescence in oral mucosal disease: a diagnostic analysis of 130 cases. *Oral Surgery Oral Medicine Oral Pathology* **51**, 38–54.

Dello Russo, N.M. & Temple, H.V. (1982). Cocaine effects on gingiva. *Journal of the American Dental Association* **104**, 13.

Di Felice, R. & Lombardi, T. (1998). Gingival and mandibular bone necrosis caused by a paraformaldehyde-containing paste. *Endodontics & Dental Traumatology* **14**, 196–198.

Domloge-Hultsch, N., Anhalt, G.J., Gammon, W.R., Lazarova, Z., Briggaman, R., Welch, M., Jabs, D.A., Huff, C. & Yancey,

K.B. (1994). Antiepiligrin cicatricial pemphigoid. A subepithelial bullous disorder. *Archives of Dermatology* **130**, 1521–1529.

Domloge-Hultsch, N., Gammon, W.R., Briggaman, R.A., Gil, S.G., Carter, W.G. & Yancey, K.B. (1992). Epiligrin, the major human keratinocyte integrin ligand, is a target in both an acquired autoimmune and an inherited subepidermal blistering skin disease. *Journal of Clinical Investigations* **90**, 1628–1633.

Drake, T.E. & Maibach, H.I. (1976). Allergic contact dermatitis and stomatitis caused by cinnamic aldehyde-flavoured toothpaste. *Archives of Dermatology* **112**, 202–203.

Drinkard, C.R., Decker, L., Little, J.W., Rhame, F.S., Balfour, H.H. Jr., Rhodus, N.L., Merry, J.W., Walker, P.O., Miller, C.E., Volberding, P.A. & Melnick, S.L. (1991). Periodontal status of individuals in early stages of human immunodeficiency virus infection. *Community Dentistry and Oral Epidemiology* **19**, 281–285.

Duffin, P. & Cowan, G.C. (1985). An allergic reaction to toothpaste. *Journal of the Irish Dental Association* **32**, 11–12.

EC-Clearinghouse on Oral Problems Related to HIV Infection and WHO Collaborating Centre on Oral Manifestations of the Immunodeficiency Virus (1993). Classification and diagnostic criteria for oral lesions in HIV infection. *Journal of Oral Pathology and Medicine* **22**, 289–291.

Ehrlich, J., Cohen, G.H. & Hochman, N. (1983). Specific herpes simplex virus antigen in human gingiva. *Journal of Periodontology* **54**, 357–360.

Eisenberg, E. (1978). Intraoral isolated herpes zoster. *Oral Surgery Oral Medicine Oral Pathology* **45**, 214–219.

El-Hakim, M. & Chauvin, P. (2004). Orofacial granulomatosis presenting as persistent lip swelling: review of 6 new cases. *Journal of Oral and Maxillofacial Surgery* **62**, 1114–1117.

Emerson, T.G. (1965). Hereditary gingival fibromatosis: a family pedigree of four generations. *Oral Surgery Oral Medicine Oral Pathology* **19**, 1–9.

Eversole, L.R. (1994). Immunopathology of oral mucosal ulcerative, desquamative and bullous diseases. *Oral Surgery Oral Medicine Oral Pathology* **77**, 555–571.

Eversole, L.R. (1995). Oral mucosal diseases. Review of the literature. In: Millard, H.D. & Mason, D.K., eds. *Perspectives on 1993 Second World Workshop on Oral Medicine*. Ann Arbor: University of Michigan, pp. 105–162.

Eversole, L.R., Dam, J., Ficarra, G. & Hwang, C-Y. (1994). Leukocyte adhesion molecules in oral lichen planus: a T cell mediated immunopathologic process. *Oral Microbiology and Immunology* **9**, 376–383.

Fabbri, P. & Panconesi, E. (1993). Erythema multiforme "minus and maius" and drug intake. *Clinics in Dermatology* **11**, 479–489.

Fisher, A.A. (1987). Contact stomatitis. *Clinics in Dermatology* **5**, 709–717.

Fløtra, L., Gjermo, P., Rølla, G. & Wærhaug, J. (1971). Side effects of chlorhexidine mouth washes. *Scandinavian Journal of Dental Research* **79**, 119–125.

Fortune, F. & Buchanan, J.A.G. (1993). Oral lichen planus and coeliac disease. *Lancet* **341**, 1154–1155.

Friedman, R.B., Gunsolley, J., Gentry, A., Dinius, A., Kaplowitz, L. & Settle, J. (1991). Periodontal status of HIV-seropositive and AIDS patients. *Journal of Periodontology* **62**, 623–627.

Fujii, H., Ohashi, M. & Nagura, H. (1988). Immunohistochemical analysis of oral lichen-planus-like eruption in graft-versus-host disease after allogeneic bone marrow transplantation. *American Journal of Clinical Pathology* **89**, 177–186.

Gallagher, G. & Shklar, G. (1987). Oral involvement in mucous membrane pemphigoid. *Clinics in Dermatology* **5**, 18–27.

Gandolfo, S., Carbone, M., Carozzo, M. & Gallo, V. (1994). Oral lichen planus and hepatitis C virus (HCV) infection: is there a relationship? A report of 10 cases. *Journal of Oral Pathology and Medicine* **23**, 119–122.

Gazi, M.I. (1986). Unusual pigmentation of the gingiva. *Oral Surgery Oral Medicine Oral Pathology* **62**, 646–649.

Gebel, K. & Hornstein, O.P. (1984). Drug-induced oral erythema multiforme. Results of a long-term retrospective study. *Dermatologica* **168**, 35–40.

Gillette, W.B. & Van House, R.L. (1980). Ill effects of improper oral hygiene procedure. *Journal of the American Dental Association* **101**, 476–480.

Glick M., Pliskin, M.E., & Weiss, R.C. (1990). The clinical and histologic appearance of HIV-associated gingivitis. *Oral Surgery Oral Medicine Oral Pathology* **69**, 395–398.

Gordon, S.C. & Daley, T.D. (1997a). Foreign body gingivitis: clinical and microscopic features of 61 cases. *Oral Surgery Oral Medicine Oral Pathology* **83**, 562–570.

Gordon, S.C. & Daley, T.D. (1997b). Foreign body gingivitis: identification of the foreign material by energy-dispersive X-ray microanalysis. *Oral Surgery Oral Medicine Oral Pathology* **83**, 571–576.

Gorlin, R.J., Cohen, M.M., & Levis, L.S. (1990). *Syndromes of the Head and Neck*, 3rd edn. New York: Oxford University Press, pp. 847–855.

Grassi, M., Williams, C.A., Winkler, J.R. & Murray, P.A. (1989). Management of HIV-associated periodontal diseases. In: Robertson, P.B. & Greenspan, J.S., eds. Perspectives on Oral Manifestations of AIDS. *Proceedings of First International Symposium on Oral Manifestations of AIDS*. Littleton: PSG Publishing Company, pp. 119–130.

Greenberg, M.S. (1996). Herpes virus infections. *Dental Clinics of North America* **40**, 359–368.

Guttman-Yassky, E., Weltfriend, S. & Bergman, R. (2003). Resolution of orofacial granulomatosis with amalgam removal. *Journal of the European Academy of Dermatology and Venereology* **17**, 344–347.

Hart, T.C., Pallos, D., Bowden, D.W., Bolyard, J., Pettenati, M.J. & Cortelli, J.R. (1998). Genetic linkage of hereditary gingival fibromatosis to chromosome 2p21. *American Journal of Human Genetics* **62**, 876–883.

Hart, T.C., Pallos, D., Bozzo, L., Almeida, O.P., Marazita, M.L., O'Connell, J.R. & Cortelli, J.R. (2000). Evidence of genetic heterogeneity for hereditary gingival fibromatosis. *Journal of Dental Research* **79**, 1758–1764.

Hartsfield, J.K., Bixler, D. & Hazen, R.H. (1985). Gingival fibromatosis with sensoneural hearing loss: an autosomal dominant trait. *American Journal of Medical Genetics* **22**, 623–627.

Hedin, C.A., Karpe, B. & Larsson, Å. (1994). Plasma-cell gingivitis in children and adults. A clinical and histological description. *Swedish Dental Journal* **18**, 117–124.

Helbling, A. (1997). Important cross-reactive allergens. *Schweizerische Medizinische Wochenschrift* **127**, 382–389.

Hernandez, S.L., Lopez, S.A. de Blanc, Sambuelli, R.H., Roland, H., Cornelli, C., Lattanzi, V. & Carnelli, M.A. (2004). Oral histoplasmosis associated with HIV infection: a comparative study. *Journal of Oral Pathology and Medicine* **33**, 445–450.

Hodge, L., Marsden, R.A., Black, M.M., Bhogal, B. & Corbett, M.F. (1981). Bullous pemphigoid: The frequency of mucosal involvement and concurrent malignancy related to indirect immunofluorescence findings. *British Journal of Dermatology* **105**, 65–69.

Holmstrup, P. (1991). Reactions of the oral mucosa related to silver amalgam. *Journal of Oral Pathology and Medicine* **20**, 1–7.

Holmstrup, P. (1992). The controversy of a premalignant potential of oral lichen planus is over. *Oral Surgery Oral Medicine Oral Pathology* **73**, 704–706.

Holmstrup, P. (1999). Non-plaque induced gingival lesions. *Annals of Periodontology* **4**, 20–31.

Holmstrup, P. & Axéll, T. (1990). Classification and clinical manifestations of oral yeast infection. *Acta Odontologica Scandinavica* **48**, 57–59.

Holmstrup, P. & Dabelsteen, E. (1979). Changes in carbohydrate expression of lichen planus affected oral epithelial cell membranes. *Journal of Investigative Dermatology* **73**, 364–367.

Holmstrup, P. & Glick, M. (2002). Treatment of periodontal disease in the immunodeficient patient. *Periodontology 2000* **28**, 190–205.

Holmstrup, P. & Johnson, N.W. (1997). Chemicals in diagnosis and management of selected mucosal disorders affecting the gingiva. In: Lang, N.P., Karring, T. & Lindhe, J., eds. *Proceedings of the 2nd European Workshop.* Berlin: Quintessence, pp. 366–379.

Holmstrup, P. & Samaranayake, L.P. (1990). Acute and AIDS-related oral candidoses. In: Samaranayake, L.P. & MacFarlane, T.W., eds. *Oral Candidosis.* London: Wright, Butterworth & Co. Ltd, pp. 133–155.

Holmstrup, P., Schiøtz, A.W. & Westergaard, J. (1990). Effect of dental plaque control on gingival lichen planus. *Oral Surgery Oral Medicine Oral Pathology* **69**, 585–590.

Holmstrup, P., Thorn, J.J., Rindum, J. & Pindborg, J.J. (1988). Malignant development of lichen-planus-affected oral mucosa. *Journal of Oral Pathology* **17**, 219–225.

Holmstrup, P. & Westergaard, J. (1998). HIV infection and periodontal diseases. *Periodontology 2000* **18**, 37–46.

Horning, G.M., Fisher, J.G., Barker, F., Killoy, W.J. & Lowe, J.W. (1985). Gingival fibromatosis with hypertrichosis. *Journal of Periodontology* **56**, 344–347.

Hudson, C.D. & Vickers, R.A. (1971). Clinicopathologic observations in prodromal herpes zoster of the fifth cranial nerve. *Oral Surgery Oral Medicine Oral Pathology* **31**, 494–501.

Huff, J.C., Weston, W.L. & Tonnesen, M.G. (1983). Erythema multiforme: a critical review of characteristics, diagnostic criteria and causes. *Journal of the American Academy of Dermatology* **8**, 763–775.

Ingafou, M., Leao, J.C., Porter, S.R. & Scully, C. (2006). Oral lichen planus: a retrospective study of 690 British patients. *Oral Diseases* **12**, 463–468.

Jonsson, H., Nived, O. & Sturfelt, G. (1988). The effect of age on clinical and serological manifestations in unselected patients with systemic lupus erythematosus. *Journal of Rheumatology* **15**, 505–509.

Jorgensen, R.J. & Cocker, M.E. (1974). Variation in the inherence and expression of gingival fibromatosis. *Journal of Periodontology* **45**, 472–477.

Kauppinen, K. & Stubb, S. (1984). Drug eruptions: causative agents and clinical types. A series of in-patients during a 10-year period. *Acta Dermatolocica et Venereologica* **64**, 320–324.

Kerr, D.A., McClatchey, K.D. & Regezi, J.A. (1971). Allergic gingivostomatitis (due to gum chewing). *Journal of Periodontology* **42**, 709–712.

Kilpi, A.M., Rich, A.M., Radden, B.G. & Reade, P.C. (1988). Direct immunofluorescence in the diagnosis of oral mucosal disease. *International Journal of Oral Maxillofacial Surgery* **17**, 6–10.

Klein, R.S., Quart, A.M. & Small, C.B. (1991). Periodontal disease in heterosexuals with acquired immuno-deficiency syndrome. *Journal of Periodontology* **62**, 535–540.

Krogh, P., Holmstrup, P., Thorn, J.J., Vedtofte, P. & Pindborg, J.J. (1987). Yeast species and biotypes associated with oral leukoplaki and lichen planus. *Oral Surgery Oral Medicine Oral Pathology* **63**, 48–54.

Lamey P.J., Rees, T.D., Binnie, W.H., Wright, J.M., Rankin, K.V. & Simpson, N.B. (1992). Oral presentation of pemphigus vulgaris and its response to systemic steroid therapy. *Oral Surgery Oral Medicine Oral Pathology* **74**, 54–57.

Lamster, I.B., Rodrick, M.L., Sonis, S.T. & Falchuk, Z.M. (1982). An analysis of peripheral blood and salivary polymorphonuclear leukocyte function, circulating immune complex levels and oral status in patients with inflammatory bowel disease. *Journal of Periodontology* **53**, 231–238.

Lanza, A., Femiano, F., De Rosa, A., Cammarota, M., Lanza, M & Cirillo, N. (2006). The N-terminal fraction of desmoglein 3 encompassing its immunodominant domain is present in human serum: implications for pemphigus vulgaris auto-immunity. *International Journal of Immunopathology and Pharmacology* **19**, 399–407.

Laskaris, G. (1994). *Color Atlas of Oral Diseases.* Stuttgart: Georg Thieme Verlag, p. 66.

Laskaris, G. & Angelopoulos, A. (1981). Cicatricial pemphigoid: direct and indirect immunofluorescent studies. *Oral Surgery Oral Medicine Oral Pathology* **51**, 48–54.

Laskaris, G., Hadjivassiliou, M., Stratigos, J. (1992). Oral signs and symptoms in 160 Greek HIV-infected patients. *Journal of Oral Pathology and Medicine* **21**, 120–123.

Laskaris, G. & Nicolis, G. (1980). Immunopathology of oral mucosa in bullous pemphigoid. *Oral Surgery Oral Medicine Oral Pathology* **50**, 340–345.

Laskaris, G., Sklavounou, A. & Stratigos, J. (1982). Bullous pemphigoid, cicatricial pemphigoid and pemphigus vulgaris: a comparative clinical survey of 278 cases. *Oral Surgery Oral Medicine Oral Pathology* **54**, 656–662.

Lennette, E.H. & Magoffin, R.L. (1973). Virologic and immunologic aspects of major oral ulcerations. *Journal of the American Dental Association* **87**, 1055–1073.

Leonard, J.N., Haffenden, G.P., Ring, N.P., McMinn, R.M., Sidgwick, A., Mowbray, J.F., Unsworth, D.J., Holborow, E.J., Blenkinsopp, W.K., Swain, A.F. & Fry, L. (1982). Linear IgA disease in adults. *British Journal of Dermatology* **107**, 301–316.

Leonard, J.N., Wright, P., Williams, D.M., Gilkes, J.J., Haffenden, G.P., McMinn, R.M. & Fry, L. (1984). The relationship between linear IgA disease and benign mucous membrane pemphigoid. *British Journal of Dermatology* **110**, 307–314.

Lever, W.F. & Schaumburg-Lever, G. (1997). Immunosuppressants and prednisone in pemphigus vulgaris. Therapeutic results obtained in 63 patients between 1961–1978. *Archives of Dermatology* **113**, 1236–1241.

Liccardi, G., D'Amato, M. & D'Amato, G. (1996). Oral allergy syndrome after ingestion of salami in a subject with monosentitization to mite allergens. *Journal of Allergy and Clinical Immunology* **98**, 850–852.

Littner, M.M., Dayan, D., Kaffe, I., Begleiter, A., Gorsky, M., Moskana, D. & Buchner, A. (1982). Acute streptococcal gingivostomatitis. Report of five cases and review of the literature. *Oral Surgery Oral Medicine Oral Pathology* **53**, 144–147.

Loh, F., Yeo, J., Tan, W. & Kumarasinghe, G. (1989). Histoplasmosis presenting as hyperplastic gingival lesion. *Journal of Oral Pathology and Medicine* **18**, 533–536.

Lozada, F. & Silverman, S. Jr. (1978). Erythema multiforme. Clinical characteristics and natural history in fifty patients. *Oral Surgery Oral Medicine Oral Pathology* **46**, 628–636.

Lozada-Nur, F., Gorsky, M. & Silverman, S. Jr. (1989). Oral erythema multiforme: clinical observations and treatment of 95 patients. *Oral Surgery Oral Medicine Oral Pathology* **67**, 36–40.

Lüders, G. (1987). Exogenously induced diseases of the oral mucosa. *Zeitschrift für Hautkrankheiten* **62**, 603–606, 611–612.

Lynch, M.A. & Ship, I.I. (1967). Initial oral manifestations of leukemia. *Journal of the American Dental Association* **75**, 932–940.

Manton, S.M. & Scully, C. (1988). Mucous membrane pemphigoid – an elusive diagnosis. *Oral Surgery Oral Medicine Oral Pathology* **66**, 37–40.

Masouredis, C.M., Katz, M.H., Greenspan, D., Herrera, C., Hollander, H., Greenspan, J.S. & Winkler, J.R. (1992). Prevalence of HIV-associated periodontitis and gingivitis in HIV-infected patients attending an AIDS clinic. *Journal of Acquired Immune Deficiency Syndrome* **5**, 479–483.

Mattson, U., Jontell, M. & Holmstrup, P. (2002). Oral lichen planus and malignant transformation: is a recall of patients justified? *Critical Reviews in Oral Biology and Medicine* **13**, 390–396.

McKellar, G.M. & Reade, P.C. (1986). Erythema multiforme and *Mycoplasma pneumoniae* infection. Report and discussion of a case presenting with stomatitis. *International Journal of Oral Maxillofacial Surgery* **15**, 342–348.

McKenna, S.J. (2000). Leukemia. *Oral Surgery Oral Medicine Oral Pathology Oral Radiology and Endodontics* **89**, 137–139.

Melbye, M., Grossman, R.J., Goedert, J.J., Eyster, M.E. & Biggar, R.J. (1987). Risk of AIDS after herpes zoster. *Lancet* **28**, 728–731.

Meyer, U., Kleinheinz, J., Handschel, J., Kruse-Losler, B., Weingart, D. & Joos, U. (2000). Oral findings in three different groups of immunocompromised patients. *Journal of Oral Pathology and Medicine* **29**, 153–158.

Michaud, M., Baehner, R.L., Bixler, D. & Kafrawy, A.H. (1977). Oral manifestations of acute leukemia in children. *Journal of the American Dental Association* **95**, 1145–1150.

Mignogna, M.D., Fedele, S., Lo Russo, L., Adamo, D. & Satriano, R.A. (2004). Effectiveness of small-volume, intralesional, delayed-release triamcinolone injections in orofacial granulomatosis: a pilot study. *Journal of the American Academy of Dermatology* **51**, 265–268.

Mignogna, M.D., Fedele, S., Lo Russo, L. & Lo Muzio, L. (2001). Orofacial granulomatosis with gingival onset. *Journal of Clinical Periodontology* **28**, 692–696.

Mignogna, M.D., Fedele, S., Lo Russo, L., Mignogna, C., de Rosa, G. & Porter, S.R. (2006) Field cancerization in oral lichen planus. *European Journal of Surgical Oncology*, E-publication ahead of print.

Millar, E.P. & Traulis, M.J. (1994). Herpes zoster of the trigeminal nerve: the dentist's role in diagnosis and management. *Journal of the Canadian Dental Association* **60**, 450–453.

Miller, C.S. (1996). Viral infections in the immunocompetent patient. *Clinics in Dermatology* **14**, 225–241.

Miller, C.S., Cunningham, L.L., Lindroth, J.E. & Avdiushko, S.A. (2004). The efficacy of valacyclovir in preventing recurrent herpes simplex virus infections associated with dental procedures. *Journal of the American Dental Association* **135**, 1311–1318.

Miller, C.S. & Redding, S.W. (1992). Diagnosis and management of orofacial herpes simplex virus infections. *Dental Clinics of North America* **36**, 879–895.

Mindel, A. (1991). Is it meaningful to treat patients with recurrent herpetic infections? *Scandinavian Journal of Infections* **78**, 27–32.

Miura, S., Smith, C.C., Burnett, J.W. & Aurelian, L. (1992). Detection of viral DNA within skin of healed recurrent herpes simplex infection and erythema multiforme lesions. *Journal of Investigative Dermatology* **98**, 68–72.

Miziara, I.D. & Weber, R. (2006). Oral candidosis and oral hairy leukoplakia as predictors of HAART failure in Brazilian HIV-infected patients. *Oral Diseases* **12**, 402–407.

Muhler, J.C. (1970). Dentifrices and oral hygiene. In: Bernier, J.L. & Muhler, J.C., eds. *Improving Dental Practice Through Preventive Measures*. St. Louis: C.V. Mosby Co, pp. 133–157.

Murray, P.A., Grassi, M. & Winkler, J.R. (1989). The microbiology of HIV-associated periodontal lesions. *Journal of Clinical Periodontology* **16**, 636–642.

Murray, P.A., Winkler, J.R., Peros, W.J., French, C.K. & Lippke, J.A. (1991). DNAprobe detection of periodontal pathogens in HIV-associated periodontal lesions. *Oral Microbiology and Immunology* **6**, 34–40.

Murray, P.A., Winkler, J.R., Sadkowski, L., Kornman, K.S., Steffensen, B., Robertson, P. & Holt, S.C. (1988). The microbiology of HIV-associated gingivitis and periodontitis. In: Robertson, P.B. & Greenspan, J.S., eds. Oral manifestations of AIDS. *Proceedings of First International Symposium on Oral Manifestations of AIDS*. Littleton: PSG Publishing Company, pp. 105–118.

Nagao, Y., Sata, M., Tanikawa, K., Itoh, K. & Kameyama, T. (1995). Lichen planus and hepatitis C virus in the northern Kyushu region of Japan. *European Journal of Clinical Investigation* **25**, 910–914.

Najjar, T.A. (1977). Harmful effects of "aspirin compounds". *Oral Surgery Oral Medicine Oral Pathology* **44**, 64–70.

Negi, M., Tsuboi, R., Matsui, T. & Ogawa, H. (1984). Isolation and characterization of proteinase from *Candida albicans*: substrate specificity. *Journal of Investigative Dermatology* **83**, 32–36.

Nesbit, S.P. & Gobetti, J.P. (1986). Multiple recurrence of oral erythema multiforme after secondary herpes simplex: Report of case and review of literature. *Journal of the American Dental Association* **112**, 348–352.

Nevin, N.C., Scally, B.G., Kernohan, D.C. & Dodge, J.A. (1971). Hereditary gingival fibromatosis. *Journal of Mental Deficiency Research* **15**, 130–135.

Nishikawa, T., Hashimoto, T., Shimizu, H., Ebihara, T. & Amagai, M. (1996). Pemphigus from immunofluorescence to molecular biology. *Journal of Dermatological Science* **12**, 1–9.

Nousari, H.C. & Anhalt, G.J. (1995). Bullous skin diseases. *Current Opinion on Immunology* **7**, 844–852.

O'Brien, J.J. & Campoli-Richards, D.M. (1989). Acyclovir. An update of its role in antiviral therapy. *Current Therapeutics* **30**, 81–93.

Odds, F.C. (1985). *Candida albicans* proteinase as a virulence factor in the pathogenesis of Candida infections. *Zentralblatt für Bakteriologie und Hygiene, I. Abt. Orig. A* **260**, 539–542.

Overall, J.C. Jr. (1982). Oral herpes simplex: pathogenesis. Clinical and virologic course, approach to treatment. In: Hooks, J.J. & Jordan, G.W., eds. *Viral Infections in Oral Medicine*. New York: Elsevier/North Holland, pp. 53–78.

Ovrutsky, G.D. & Ulyanow, A.D. (1976). Allergy to chromium using steel dental prosthesis. *Stomatologia (Moscow)* **55**, 60–61.

Parra, B. & Slots, J. (1996). Detection of human viruses in periodontal pockets using polymerase chain reaction. *Oral Microbiology and Immunology* **5**, 289–293.

Pattison, G.L. (1983). Self-inflicted gingival injuries: literature review and case report. *Journal of Periodontology* **54**, 299–304.

Pedersen, A. & Reibel, J. (1989). Intraoral infection with *Mycobacterium chelonae*. *Oral Surgery Oral Medicine Oral Pathology* **67**, 262–265.

Peterson, D.E., Minh, G.E., Reynolds, M.A., Weikel, D.S., Overholser, C.D., DePaola, L.G., Wade, J.C. & Suzuki, J.B. (1990). Effect of granulocytopenia on oral microbial relationships in patients with acute leukemia. *Oral Surgery Oral Medicine Oral Pathology Oral Radiology and Endodontics* **70**, 720–723.

Pindborg, J.J. (1992). *Atlas of Diseases of the Oral Mucosa*, 5th edn. Copenhagen: Munksgaard, p. 246.

Pisanti, S., Sharav, Y., Kaufman, E. & Posner, L.N. (1974). Pemphigus vulgaris: incidence in Jews of different ethnic groups, according to age, sex and initial lesion. *Oral Surgery Oral Medicine Oral Pathology* **38**, 382–387.

Pisetsky, D.S. (1986). Systemic lupus erythematosus. *Medical Clinics of North America* **70**, 337–353.

Rajah, V. & Essa, A. (1993). Histoplasmosis of the oral cavity, oropharynx and larynx. *Journal of Laryngology and Otology* **107**, 58–61.

Ramirez-Amador, V., Madero, J.G., Pedraza, L.E., de la Rosa Garcia, E., Guevara, M.G., Gutierrez, E.R. & Reyes-Teran, G. (1996). Oral secondary syphilis in a patient with human immunodeficiency virus infection. *Oral Surgery Oral Medicine Oral Pathology Oral Radiology and Endodontics* **81**, 652–654.

Ramon, Y., Berman W. & Bubis, J.S. (1967). Gingival fibromatosis combined with cherubism. *Oral Surgery* **24**, 435–448.

Rashid, K.A., Gürcan, H.M. & Ahmed, A.R. (2006). Antigen specificity in subsets of mucous membrane pemphigoid. *Journal of Investigative Dermatology* **126**, 2631–2636.

Reed, R.J. (1985). Erythema multiforme. A clinical syndrome and a histologic complex. *American Journal of Dermatopathology* **7**, 143–152.

Rees, T.D. (1989). Adjunctive therapy. *Proceedings of the World Workshop in Clinical Periodontics*. Chicago: The American Academy of Periodontology, X-1/X-39.

Reibel, J. & Schiødt, M. (1986). Immunohistochemical studies on colloid bodies (Civatte bodies) in oral lesions of discoid lupus erythematosus. *Scandinavian Journal of Dental Research* **94**, 536–544.

Rentier, B., Piette, J., Baudoux, L., Debrus, S., Defechereux, P., Merville, M.P., Sadzot-Delvaux, C. & Schoonbroodt, S. (1996). Lessons to be learned from varicella-zoster virus. *Veterinary Microbiology* **53**, 55–66.

Riley, C., London, J.P. & Burmeister, J.A. (1992). Periodontal health in 200 HIV-positive patients. *Journal of Oral Pathology and Medicine* **21**, 124–127.

Rindum, J.L., Stenderup, A. & Holmstrup, P. (1994). Identification of *Candida albicans* types related to healthy and pathological oral mucosa. *Journal of Oral Pathology and Medicine* **23**, 406–412.

Rivera-Hidalgo, F. & Stanford, T.W. (1999). Oral mucosal lesions caused by infective microorganisms. I. Viruses and bacteria. *Periodontology 2000* **21**, 106–124.

Robinson, P.G., Sheiham, A., Challacombe, S.J. & Zakrzewska, J.M. (1996). The periodontal health of homosexual men with HIV infection: a controlled study. *Oral Diseases* **2**, 45–52.

Robinson, P.G., Winkler, J.R., Palmer, G., Westenhouse, J., Hilton, J.F. & Greenspan, J.S. (1994). The diagnosis of periodontal conditions associated with HIV infection. *Journal of Periodontology* **65**, 236–243.

Rossi, R.E., Monasterolo, G., Operti, D. & Corsi, M. (1996). Evaluation of recombinant allergens Bet v 1 and Bet v 2 (profilin) by Pharmacia CAP system in patients with pollen-related allergy to birch and apple. *Allergy* **51**, 940–945.

Ruokonen, H., Malmstrom, M. & Stubb, S. (1988). Factors influencing the recurrence of erythema multiforme. *Proceedings of the Finnish Dental Society* **84**, 167–174.

Sainio, E.L. & Kanerva, L. (1995). Contact allergens in toothpastes and a review of their hypersensitivity. *Contact Dermatitis* **33**, 100–105.

Sanderson, J., Nunes, C., Escudier, M., Barnard, K., Shirlaw, P., Odell, E., Chinyama, C. & Challacombe, S. (2005). Oro-facial granulomatosis: Crohn's disease or a new inflammatory bowel disease? *Inflammatory Bowel Disease* **11**, 840–846.

Schiødt, M. (1984a). Oral discoid lupus erythematosus. II. Skin lesions and systemic lupus erythematosus in sixty-six patients with 6-year follow-up. *Oral Surgery Oral Medicine Oral Pathology* **57**, 177–180.

Schiødt, M. (1984b). Oral manifestations of lupus erythematosus. *International Journal of Oral Surgery* **13**, 101–147.

Schiødt, M., Holmstrup, P., Dabelsteen, E. & Ullman, S. (1981). Deposits in immunoglobulins, complement, and fibrinogen in oral lupus erythematosus, lichen planus, and leukoplakia. *Oral Surgery Oral Medicine Oral Pathology* **51**, 603–608.

Schiødt, M. & Pindborg, J.J. (1984). Oral discoid lupus erythematosus. I. The validity of previous histopathologic diagnostic criteria. *Oral Surgery Oral Medicine Oral Pathology* **57**, 46–51.

Schrieber, L. & Maini, R.N. (1984). Circulating immune complexes (CIC) in connective tissue diseases (CTD). *Netherland Journal of Medicine* **27**, 327–339.

Schwartz, O., Pindborg, J.J. & Svenningsen, A. (1989). Tooth exfoliation and necrosis of the alveolar bone following trigeminal herpes zoster in HIV-infected patient. *Danish Dental Journal* **93**, 623–627.

Sciubba, J.J. (1996). Autoimmune aspects of pemphigus vulgaris and mucosal pemphigoid. *Advances in Dental Research* **10**, 52–56.

Sciubba, J.J. (2003). Herpes simplex and aphthous ulcerations: presentation, diagnosis and management – an update. *General Dentistry* **51**, 510–516.

Scully, C. (1989). Orofacial herpes simplex virus infections: current concepts in the epidemiology, pathogenesis, and treatment, and disorders in which the virus may be implicated. *Oral Surgery Oral Medicine Oral Pathology* **68**, 701–710.

Scully, C. (1995). Infectious diseases: review of the literature. In: Millard, H.D. & Mason, D.R., eds. *Second World Workshop on Oral Medicine*. Ann Arbor: University of Michigan, pp. 7–16.

Scully, C., Almeida, O.P.D. & Welbury, R. (1994). Oral lichen planus in childhood. *British Journal of Dermatology* **130**, 131–133.

Scully, C., Beyli, M., Ferreiro, M.C., Ficarra, G., Gill, Y., Griffiths, M., Holmstrup, P., Mutlu, S., Porter, S. & Wray, D. (1998a). Update on oral lichen planus: etiopathogenesis and management. *Critical Reviews in Oral Biology and Medicine* **9**, 86–122.

Scully, C., El-Kabir, M. & Samaranayake, L. (1995). Candidosis. In: Millard, H.D. & Mason, E.K., eds. *Perspectives on 1993 Second World Workshop on Oral Medicine*. Ann Arbor: University of Michigan, pp. 27–50.

Scully, C., Epstein, J.B., Porter, S.R. & Cox, M.F. (1991). Viruses and chronic diseases of the oral mucosa. *Oral Surgery Oral Medicine Oral Pathology* **72**, 537–544.

Scully, C. & Laskaris, G. (1998). Mucocutaneous disorders. *Periodontology 2000* **18**, 81–94.

Scully, C., Monteil, R. & Sposto, M.R. (1998b). Infectious and tropical diseases affecting the human mouth. *Periodontology 2000* **18**, 47–70.

Serio, F.G., Siegel, M.A. & Slade, B.E. (1991). Plasma cell gingivitis of unusual origin. A case report. *Journal of Periodontology* **62**, 390–393.

Shafer, W.G., Hine, M.K. & Levy, B.M. (1983). *A Textbook of Oral Pathology*, 4th edn. Philadelphia: W.B. Saunders, pp. 785–786.

Shklar, G. & McCarthy, P.L. (1971). Oral lesions of mucous membrane pemphigoid. A study of 85 cases. *Archives of Otolaryngology* **93**, 354–364.

Siegel, M.A. (1996). Syphilis and gonorrhea. *Dental Clinics of North America* **40**, 369–383.

Silverman, S. Jr, Gorsky, M., Lozada-Nur, F. & Liu, A. (1986). Oral mucous membrane pemphigoid. A study of sixty-five patients. *Oral Surgery Oral Medicine Oral Pathology* **61**, 233–237.

Singer, S.L., Goldblatt, J., Hallam, L.A. & Winters, J.C. (1993). Hereditary gingival fibromatosis with a recessive mode of inheritance. Case reports. *Austrian Dental Journal* **38**, 427–432.

Skaare, A., Kjaerheim, V., Barkvoll, P. & Rolla, G. (1997). Skin reactions and irritation potential of four commercial toothpastes. *Acta Odontologica Scandinavica* **55**, 133–136.

Skoglund, A. (1994). Value of epicutaneous patch testing in patients with oral mucosal lesions of lichenoid character. *Scandinavian Journal of Dental Research* **102**, 216–222.

Skrinjaric, I. & Basic, M. (1989). Hereditary gingival fibromatosis: report on three families and dermatoglyphic analysis. *Journal of Periodontal Research* **24**, 303–309.

Slots, J., Rams, T.E. & Listgarten, M.A. (1988). Yeasts, enteric rods and pseudomonas in the subgingival flora of severe adult periodontitis. *Oral Microbiology and Immunology* **3**, 47–52.

Smukler, H. & Landsberg, J. (1984). The toothbrush and gingival traumatic injury. *Journal of Periodontology* **55**, 713–719.

Sonis, S.T. (1998). Mucositis as a biological process: a new hypothesis for the development of chemotherapy-induced stomatotoxicity. *Oral Oncology* **34**, 39–43

Standefer, J.A. Jr & Mattox, D.E. (1986). Head and neck manifestations of collagen vascular diseases. *Otolaryngologic Clinic of North America* **19**, 181–210.

Straus, S.E., Ostrove, J.M., Inchauspe, G., Felser, J.M., Freifeld, A., Croen, K.D. & Sawyer, M.H. (1988). NIH Conference. Varicella-zoster virus infections. Biology, natural history, treatment and prevention. *Annals of Internal Medicine* **108**, 221–237.

Stutman, H.R. (1987). Stevens-Johnson syndrome and myco-plasma pneumoniae: Evidence for cutaneous infection. *Journal of Pediatrics* **111**, 845–847.

Sugerman, P.B., Savage, N.W. & Seymour, G.J. (1994). Pheno-type and suppressor activity of T-lymphocyte clones extracted from lesions of oral lichen planus. *British Journal of Dermatology* **131**, 319–324.

Swango, P.A., Kleinman, D.V. & Konzelman, J.L. (1991). HIV and periodontal health. A study of military personnel with HIV. *Journal of the American Dental Association* **122**, 49–54.

Thorn, J.J., Holmstrup, P., Rindum, J. & Pindborg, J.J. (1988). Course of various clinical forms of oral lichen planus. A prospective follow-up study of 611 patients. *Journal of Oral Pathology* **17**, 213–218.

Thornhill, M.H., Sankar, V., Xu, X.J., Barrett, A.W., High, A.S., Odell, E.W., Speight, P.M. & Farthing, P.M. (2006). The role of histopathological characteristics in distinguishing amalgam-associated oral lichenoid reactions and oral lichen planus. *Journal of Oral Pathology and Medicine* **35**, 233–240.

Tricamo, M.B., Rees, T.D., Hallmon, W.W., Wright, J.M., Cueva, M.A. & Plemons, J.M. (2006). Periodontal status in patients with gingival mucous membrane pemphigoid. *Journal of Periodontology* **77**, 398–405.

Tylenda, C.A., Larsen, J., Yeh, C-K., Lane, H.E. & Fox, P.C. (1989). High levels of oral yeasts in early HIV-infection. *Journal of Oral Pathology and Medicine* **18**, 520–524.

Ullman, S. (1988). Immunofluorescence and diseases of the skin. *Acta Dermatologica et Venereologica* **140** (Suppl), 1–31.

Umadevi, M., Adeyemi, O., Patel, M., Reichart, P.A. & Robin-son, P.G. (2006). Periodontal diseases and other bacterial infections. *Advances in Dental Research* **1**, 139–145.

van Steenberghe, D., Vanherle, G.V., Fossion, E. & Roelens, J. (1976). Crohn's disease of the mouth: report of a case. *Journal of Oral Surgery* **34**, 635–638.

Walsh, L.J., Savage, N.W., Ishii, T. & Seymour, G.J. (1990). Immunopathogenesis of oral lichen planus. *Journal of Oral Pathology and Medicine* **19**, 389–396.

Weed, L.A. & Parkhill, E.M. (1948). The diagnosis of histoplas-mosis in ulcerative disease of the mouth and pharynx. *American Journal of Clinical Pathology* **18**, 130–140.

Westheim, A.I., Tenser, R.B. & Marks, J.G. (1987). Acyclovir resistance in a patient with chronic mucocutaneous herpes simplex infections. *Journal of the American Academy of Dermatology* **17**, 875–880.

Williams, D.M., Leonard, J.N., Wright, P., Gilkes, J.J., Haffen-den, G.P., McMinn, R.M. & Fry, L. (1984). Benign mucous membrane (cicatricial) pemphigoid revisited: a clinical and immunological reappraisal. *British Dental Journal* **157**, 313–316.

Winkler, J.R., Grassi, M. & Murray, P.A. (1988). Clinical descrip-tion and etiology of HIV-associated periodontal disease. In: Robertson, P.B. & Greenspan, J.S., eds. *Oral Manifestations of AIDS. Proceedings of First International Symposium on Oral Manifestations of AIDS*. Littleton: PSG Publishing Company, pp. 49–70.

Wouters, C.H.P., Diegenant, C, Ceuppens, J.L., Degreef, H. & Stevens, E.A.M. (2004). The circulating lymphocyte profiles in patients with discoid lupus erythematosus and systemic lupus erythematosus suggest a pathogenetic relationship. *British Journal of Dermatology* **150**, 693–700.

Wright, P.S., Clark, P. & Hardie, J.M. (1985). The prevalence and significance of yeasts in persons wearing complete den-tures with soft-lining materials. *Journal of Dental Research* **64**, 122–125.

Wutrich, B. (1997). Oral allergy syndrome to apple after a lover's kiss. *Allergy* **52**, 253–256.

Xiao, S., Wang, X., Qu, B., Yang, M., Liu, G., Bu, L., Wang, Y., Zhu, L., Lei, H., Hu, L., Zhang, X., Liu, J., Zhao, G. & Kong, X. (2000). Refinement of the locus for autosomal dominant hereditary gingival fibromatosis (GINGF) to a 3.8-cM region on 2p21. *Genomics* **68**, 247–252.

Yamamoto, T., Kukuminato, Y., Nui, I., Takada, R., Hirao, M., Kamimura, M., Saitou, H., Asakura, K. & Kataura, A. (1995). Relationship between birch pollen allergy and oral and pha-ryngeal hypersensitivity to fruit. *Journal of Otology Rhinology and Laryngegology of the Society of Japan* **98**, 1086–1091.

Yura, Y., Iga, H., Terashima, K., Yoshida, H., Yanagawa, T., Azuma, M., Hayashi, Y. & Sato, M. (1986). Recurrent intra-oral herpes simplex virus infection. *International Journal of Oral Maxillofacial Surgery* **15**, 457–463.

Zaun, H. (1977). Contact allergies related to dental restorative materials and dentures. *Aktuel Dermatol* **3**, 89–93.

Zegarelli, D. & Zegarelli, E. (1977). Intraoral pemphigus vulgaris. *Oral Surgery Oral Medicine Oral Pathology* **44**, 384–393.

Zhu, Y., Zhang, W., Huo, Z., Zhang, Y., Xia, Y., Li, B., Kong, X. & Hu, L. (2006). A novel locus for maternally inherited human gingival fibromatosis at chromosome 11p15. *Human Genetics*, E-publication ahead of print.

Chapter 17

Plaque-Induced Gingival Diseases

Angelo Mariotti

For almost four millennia the clinical manifestations of gingival diseases have been noted by mankind. Throughout the centuries the notion of cause, effect, and management of these diseases was largely dormant, resulting in a dubious realm of remedies that were dominated by superstition, frequently were subjective, often palliative, sometimes painful, and rarely successful. It was not until the last half of the twentieth century that our views about the nature of gingival diseases began to emerge, where pivotal human experiments showed the unmistakable role of dental biofilms in the initiation and progression of gingival inflammation (Löe *et al.* 1965). During the twenty-first century, we are living in a time of radical shifts of culture and science, one in which evidence-based dentistry increasingly plays a pervasive role in our knowledge regarding gingival diseases.

As more clinical evidence becomes available, the scope and nature of various forms of gingivitis become evident. More specifically, there has been growing acceptance that gingivitis does not represent a single disease but rather a spectrum of diseases that are the outcome of a variety of different processes. It is true that inflammation of the gingiva induced by bacteria is the most common form of gingivitis; however, this has created a bias toward naming all manifestations that affect the gingival tissues (e.g. atrophic, desquamative, neoplastic, etc.) as gingivitis. Although inflammation of the gingival tissues can be induced by a variety of methods (e.g. trauma, chemical agents, temperature extremes, ionizing radiation, viruses, fungi, immune defects, etc.), at this time gingival diseases are considered to be disease entities that are initiated by dental plaque and are restricted to gingival tissues. This chapter will focus on the commonly occurring and diverse family of complex and distinct pathological entities found within the gingiva that are initiated by dental plaque and that can be influenced by systemic conditions, endogenous hormones, genetic factors, drugs, and malnutrition.

Classification criteria for gingival diseases

Categorization of diseases affecting the gingiva requires evaluation of patient signs and symptoms, medical and dental histories, a clinical examination that includes the extent, distribution, duration, and physical description of lesions affecting the gingiva, clinical or relative attachment levels, and radiographs. The universal features of gingival diseases include clinical signs of inflammation, signs and symptoms that are confined to the gingiva, reversibility of the diseases by removal of etiology(ies), the presence of bacteria-laden plaque to initiate and/or exacerbate the severity of the lesion, and a possible role as a precursor to attachment loss around teeth (Table 17-1).

Clinical signs of gingival inflammation involve enlarged gingival contours due to edema or fibrosis (Muhlemann & Son 1971; Polson & Goodson 1985), color transition to a red and/or bluish red hue (Muhlemann & Son 1971; Polson & Goodson 1985),

Table 17-1 Universal features of gingival diseases (Mariotti 1999)

Signs and symptoms that are confined to the gingiva

The presence of dental plaque to initiate and/or exacerbate the severity of the lesion

Clinical signs of inflammation (enlarged gingival contours due to edema or fibrosis, color transition to a red and/or bluish red hue, elevated sulcular temperature, bleeding upon stimulation, increased gingival exudate)

Clinical signs and symptoms associated with stable attachment levels on a periodontium with no loss of attachment or on a stable but reduced periodontium (see Fig. 17-1)

Reversibility of the disease by removing the etiology(ies)

Possible role as a precursor to attachment loss around teeth

Table 17-2 Common clinical changes from gingival health to gingivitis

Parameter	Normal gingiva	Gingivitis
Color	Coral pink (correlated to mucocutaneous pigmentation)	Red/bluish red hue
Contour	Scalloped outline that envelops teeth. Papillary gingiva fills interdental space while marginal gingival forms a knife-edged appearance with tooth surface	Edema blunts marginal tissues leading to loss of knife edge adaptation to tooth and produces bulbous papillary tissues resulting in minimization of tissue scalloping
Consistency	Firm and resilient	Tissue is soft and exhibits pitting edema
Bleeding on provocation	Negative	Positive
Gingival exudate	Minimal	Significantly increased
Sulcular temperature	~34°C	Slight increase

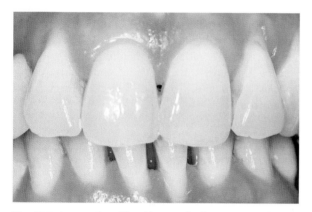

Fig. 17-1 A treated peridontitis case displaying gingival health on a reduced periodontium. If such a case developed inflammation and no further loss of attachment could be demonstrated, the diagnosis of plaque-induced gingivitis would be appropriate.

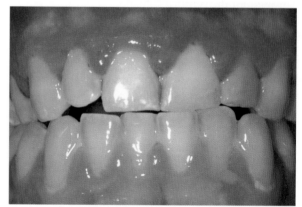

Fig. 17-2 Changes in gingival color and contour associated with plaque-induced gingivitis.

elevated sulcular temperature (Haffajee *et al.* 1992; Wolff *et al.* 1997), bleeding upon probing (Löe *et al.,* 1965; Muhlemann & Son, 1971; Greenstein *et al.* 1981; Engelberger *et al.* 1983), and increased gingival exudates (Löe & Holm-Pedersen 1965; Engelberg 1966; Oliver *et al.* 1969; Rudin *et al.* 1970) (see Table 17-2 and Fig. 17-2). Clinical signs of gingival inflammation indicative of a gingival disease must be associated with stable (i.e. unchanging) attachment levels on a periodontium with no loss of attachment or alveolar bone or on a stable but reduced periodontium.

The classification of gingival diseases relies on the presence of dental plaque and factors that modify the inflammatory status of the gingiva. The modification of plaque-induced gingivitis can occur by local or systemic factors. Local factors include tooth anatomic factors (Fig. 17.3), dental restorations (Fig. 17.4) and appliances (Fig. 17.5), root fractures (Fig. 17.6), and cervical root resorption (Fig. 17.7) (Blieden 1999), whereas, systemic factors involve the endocrine system, hematologic diseases, drugs, or malnutrition (Mariotti 1999). Table 17-3 presents a classification of plaque-induced gingival diseases (Mariotti 1999).

Table 17-3 Plaque-induced gingival diseases (modified from Mariotti 1999)

Associated with bacterial plaque only	Associated with a periodontium that exhibits no attachment loss	Plaque-induced gingivitis
	Associated with a stable but reduced periodontium	
Associated with bacterial plaque and modified by systemic factors	Associated with endogenous sex steroid hormones	Puberty-associated gingivitis Menstrual cycle-associated gingivitis Pregnancy-associated gingivitis Pregnancy-associated pyogenic granuloma
	Associated with medications	Drug-influenced gingival enlargements Oral contraceptive-associated gingivitis
	Associated with systemic diseases	Diabetes mellitus-associated gingivitis Leukemia-associated gingivitis
	Associated with malnutrition	Ascorbic acid deficiency gingivitis

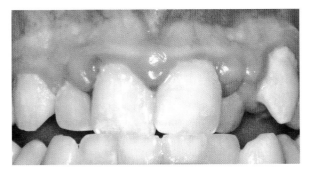

Fig. 17-3 Gingival inflammation as a result of tooth anatomic factors (malocclusion).

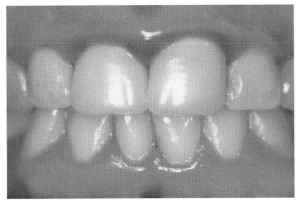

Fig. 17-4 Gingival inflammation associated with violation of the biologic width and overhanging restorations retaining plaque.

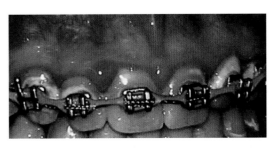

Fig. 17-5 The presence of appliances, such as braces, allows for the accumulation of plaque resulting in gingival inflammation.

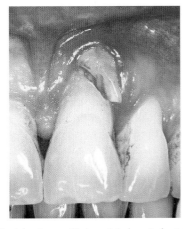

Fig. 17-6 Root fracture with associated periodontal destruction and gingival inflammation.

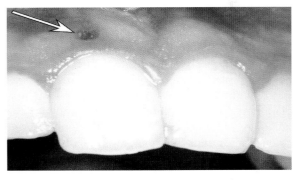

Fig. 17-7 Early cervical resorption and associated inflammation.

Plaque-induced gingivitis

Plaque-induced gingivitis is inflammation of the gingiva resulting from bacteria located at the gingival margin. The relationship of plaque to gingival inflammation has often been postulated as the cause for gingivitis, but it was not until the elegant experimental human gingivitis studies that a plaque bacterial etiology was confirmed (Löe et al. 1965). Epidemiological data have shown plaque-induced gingivitis to be prevalent at all ages of dentate

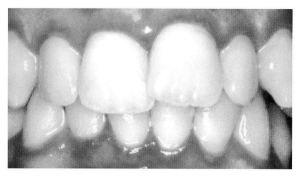

Fig. 17-8 Typical generalized marginal and papillary gingivitis.

populations (US Public Health Service 1965, 1972, 1987; Stamm 1986; Bhat 1991; Albandar 2002; Gjermo *et al.* 2002; Baelum & Schutz 2002; Sheiham & Netuveli 2002; Corbet *et al.* 2002) and this disease has been considered to be the most common form of periodontal disease (Page 1985). In children, the prevalence of plaque-induced gingivitis continues to increase until it reaches a zenith at puberty (Parfitt 1957; Hugoson *et al.* 1981; Stamm 1986). The initial changes from health to plaque-induced gingivitis may not be detectable clinically (Page & Schroeder 1976), but as plaque-induced gingivitis progresses to more advanced forms of this disease, clinical signs and symptoms become more obvious.

Plaque-induced gingivitis begins at the gingival margin and can spread throughout the remaining gingival unit. Clinical signs of gingival inflammation involving changes to gingival contour, color and consistency (Muhlemann & Son 1971; Polson & Goodson 1985), are associated with a stable periodontium which exhibits no loss of periodontal attachment or alveolar bone (Fig. 17-8). In children, gingivitis is not as intense as that found in young adults with similar amounts of dental plaque (Matsson 1978; Matsson & Goldberg 1985). This age-related difference in the development and severity of gingivitis may be associated with the quantity and/or quality of dental plaque, response of the immune system, and/or morphological differences in the periodontium between children and adults (Bimstein & Matsson 1999). More specifically, dental plaque of children usually contains lower concentrations of putative periodontal pathogens and the thicker junctional epithelium is coupled with increased vascularity in the gingival connective tissues and a developing immune system (Bimstein & Matsson 1999). In contrast to children and young adults, gingival inflammation in senior adult populations is more pronounced even when similar amounts of dental plaque are present (Fransson *et al.* 1996). The reason for the difference in senior adults may be the result of age-related differences in cellular inflammatory response to plaque (Fransson *et al.* 1996, 1999).

The intensity of the clinical signs and symptoms of gingivitis will vary between individuals (Tatakis & Trombelli 2004; Trombelli *et al.* 2004) as well as

between sites within a dentition. The common clinical findings of plaque-induced gingivitis include erythema, edema, bleeding, sensitivity, tenderness, and enlargement (Löe *et al.* 1965; Suzuki 1988). Radiographic analysis and/or probing attachment levels of individuals with plaque-induced gingivitis will not indicate loss of supporting structures. Histopathologic changes include proliferation of basal junctional epithelium leading to apical and lateral cell migration, vasculitis of blood vessels adjacent to the junctional epithelium, progressive destruction of the collagen fiber network with changes in collagen types, cytopathologic alteration of resident fibroblasts, and a progressive inflammatory/immune cellular infiltrate (Page & Schroeder 1976). Although the composition of bacterial flora associated with plaque-induced gingivitis differs from the flora associated with gingival health, there are no specific bacterial flora that are pathognomonic for plaque-induced gingivitis (Ranney 1993).

Gingival diseases associated with endogenous hormones

Since the nineteenth century, evidence has accumulated to support the concept that tissues of the periodontium are modulated by androgens, estrogens, and progestins. The majority of information concerning sex hormone-induced effects have been gender-specific observations in the gingiva. Much of the evidence that has been documented concerning the effects of sex steroid hormones on the periodontium has come from observing the changes in gingival tissues during distinct endocrinological events (e.g. menstrual cycle, pregnancy, etc.). Although a significant amount of data have shown the gingiva to be a target for sex steroid hormones, the etiology for the changes has not been thoroughly elucidated. The principal explanations for sex steroid hormone-induced changes in the gingiva have pointed to changes of microbiota in dental plaque, immune function, vascular properties, and cellular function in the gingiva (Mariotti 1994, 2005). The actions of sex steroid hormones in the periodontium are multifactorial (Mariotti 1994). Theoretically, sex steroid hormones will affect the host by influencing cellular (i.e. in the blood vessels, epithelium, and connective tissue) and immune function and, together with hormone-selected bacterial populations that occupy the gingival sulcus, induce specific changes in gingival tissues that become clinically observable (Mariotti 1994).

Puberty-associated gingivitis

Puberty is not a single episode but a complex process of endocrinologic events that produce changes in the physical appearance and behavior of adolescents. The incidence and severity of gingivitis in adolescents are influenced by a variety of factors, including

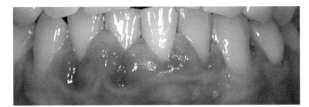

Fig. 17-9 Gingival inflammation can result from an increased secretion of sex steroid hormones during puberty.

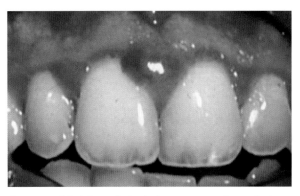

Fig. 17-10 A heightened gingival response to plaque during pregnancy results in pregnancy-associated gingivitis.

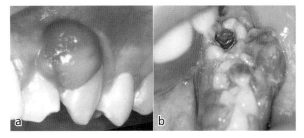

Fig. 17-11 (a) Pyogenic granuloma of pregnancy. (b) Large pyogenic granuloma of pregnancy interfering with occlusal function.

plaque levels, dental caries, mouth breathing, crowding of the teeth, and tooth eruption (Stamm 1986); however, the dramatic rise in steroid hormone levels during puberty in both sexes has a transient effect on the inflammatory status of the gingiva (Mariotti 1994). Several studies have demonstrated an increase in gingival inflammation in circumpubertal age individuals of both sexes without a concomitant increase in plaque levels (Parfitt 1957; Sutcliffe 1972; Hefti *et al.* 1981) (Fig. 17-9). Although puberty-associated gingivitis has many of the clinical features of plaque-induced gingivitis, this disease will develop frank signs of gingival inflammation in the presence of relatively small amounts of plaque during the circumpubertal period.

Menstrual cycle-associated gingivitis

Following menarche, there is a periodicity of sex steroid hormone secretion over a 25- to 30-day period: the menstrual cycle. A clinical case report of significant and observable inflammatory changes in the gingiva during the menstrual cycle has been described (Muhlemann 1948); however, women rarely exhibit overt gingival changes that fluctuate in conjunction with the menstrual cycle (Mariotti 1994). The more common gingival inflammatory changes involve less dramatic signs of inflammation in the gingiva during ovulation (Machtei *et al.* 2004). More specifically, gingival exudate increased approximately 20% during ovulation in roughly three quarters of women tested (Hugoson 1971), while observable signs of gingival inflammation have been shown to be clinically insignificant (Machtei *et al.* 2004). Since these changes in crevicular fluid flow and gingival color are not readily observable, most young women with gingival inflammation induced by the menstrual cycle will present with a very mild form of the disease.

Pregnancy-associated gingival diseases

Some of the most remarkable endocrine and oral alterations accompany pregnancy due to the prominent increase in plasma hormone levels over several months. During human gestation, pregnancy-associated gingivitis is characterized by an increase in the prevalence and severity of gingivitis during the second and third trimester of pregnancy (Löe &

Silness 1963; Löe 1965; Hugoson 1971; Arafat 1974b) (Fig. 17-10). Both longitudinal and cross-sectional studies have found the prevalence and severity of gingival inflammation significantly higher in the pregnant versus the post-partum subject even though plaque scores remained the same between the two groups (Löe & Silness 1963; Hugoson 1971; Moss *et al.* 2005). In addition, gingival probing depths are deeper (Löe & Silness 1963; Hugoson 1971; Miyazaki *et al.* 1991), bleeding on probing or toothbrushing is increased (Arafat 1974b; Miyazaki *et al.* 1991), and gingival crevicular fluid flow is elevated (Hugoson 1971) in pregnant women. The features of pregnancy-associated gingivitis are similar to plaque-induced gingivitis, except for the propensity to develop frank signs of gingival inflammation in the presence of relatively little plaque during pregnancy.

Pregnancy-associated pyogenic granuloma or "pregnancy tumor" was described over a century ago (Coles 1874); this is not a tumor but an exaggerated inflammatory response during pregnancy to an irritation resulting in a solitary polyploid capillary hemangioma which can easily bleed upon mild provocation (Sills *et al.* 1996) (Fig 17-11). Pregnancy-associated pyogenic granuloma presents clinically as a painless protuberant, mushroom-like, exophytic mass that is attached by a sessile or pedunculated base and arises from the gingival margin or more commonly from an interproximal space (Sills *et al.* 1996). Pregnancy-associated pyogenic granuloma has been reported to occur in 0.5–5.0% of pregnant women (Ziskin & Nesse 1946; Maier & Orban 1949;

Arafat 1974a; Kristen 1976). It is more common in the maxilla (Sills *et al.* 1996) and may develop as early as the first trimester (Sills *et al.* 1996), ultimately regressing or completely disappearing following parturition (Ziskin & Nesse 1946).

Gingival diseases associated with medications

In the past century, an astonishing array of medications for the alleviation of human diseases has lead to the creation of new side effects in the oral cavity. Drugs that specifically affect the gingival tissues have principally caused an increase in either inflammation and/or size.

Drug-influenced gingival enlargement

Esthetically disfiguring overgrowth of gingiva is a significant side effect which may be associated with (Hassell & Hefti 1991; Seymour *et al.* 1996; Seymour 2006):

- Anticonvulsant (e.g. phenytoin, sodium valproate, etc.)
- Immunosuppressant (e.g. cyclosporine A) (Fig. 17-12)
- Calcium channel blocking agents (e.g. nifedipine, verapamil, etc.).

The common clinical characteristics of drug-influenced gingival enlargements (Table 17-4) include patient variations in the pattern of enlargement (i.e. genetic predisposition) (Hassell & Hefti 1991; Seymour *et al.* 1996), a tendency to occur more often in anterior gingiva (Hassell & Hefti 1991; Seymour *et al.* 1996), a higher prevalence in younger age groups (Esterberg & White 1945; Rateitschak-Pluss *et al.* 1983; Hefti *et al.* 1994), onset within 3 months of use (Hassell 1981; Hassell & Hefti 1991; Seymour 1991; Seymour & Jacobs 1992) that is usually first observed in the papilla (Hassell & Hefti 1991); although it can be found in a periodontium with or without bone loss, it is not associated with attachment loss or tooth mortality (Hassell & Hefti 1991; Seymour *et al.* 1996).

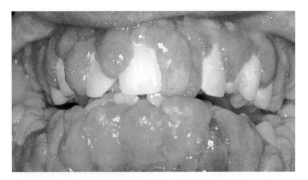

Fig. 17-12 Severe enlargement of the gingiva associated with cyclosporine medication in a kidney transplant patient.

Furthermore, all of these drugs produce clinical lesions and histologic characteristics that are indistinguishable from one another (Hassell & Hefti 1991; Seymour *et al.* 1996).

The influence of plaque on the induction of gingival enlargements by drugs in humans has not been fully elucidated (Hassell & Hefti 1991); however, it does appear that the severity of the lesion is affected by the oral hygiene of the patient (Steinberg & Steinberg 1982; Addy *et al.* 1983; Hassell *et al.* 1984; Tyldesley & Rotter 1984; Daley *et al.* 1986; McGaw *et al.* 1987; Modeer & Dahllof 1987; Yahia *et al.* 1988; Barclay *et al.* 1992).

The first description of a drug causing an enlargement of the gingiva was reported in 1939 and was associated with the use of phenytoin (Kimball 1939). Phenytoin, which is used on a chronic regimen for the control of epileptic seizures, induces gingival enlargements in approximately 50% of patients using this agent (Angelopoulous & Goaz 1972). One prominent theory of the etiology of phenytoin-associated gingival enlargements suggests that the accumulation of genetically distinct populations of gingival fibroblasts results in the accumulation of connective tissues resulting from reduced catabolism of the collagen molecule (Hassell & Hefti 1991).

Calcium channel blockers have also been identified as agents that affect enlargement of the gingiva. Calcium channel blockers are a class of drugs that exert effects principally at voltage-gated Ca^{2+} channels located in the plasma membrane and are commonly prescribed as antihypertensive, anti-arrhythmic and anti-anginal agents. In 1984, calcium channel

Table 17-4 Characteristics of drug-influenced gingival enlargement (Mariotti 1999)

Variation in interpatient and intrapatient pattern
Predilection for anterior gingiva
Higher prevalence in children
Onset within 3 months
Change in gingival contour leading to modification of gingival size
Enlargement first observed at the interdental papilla
Change in gingival color
Increased gingival exudate
Bleeding upon provocation
Found in gingiva with or without bone loss but is not associated with attachment loss
Pronounced inflammatory response of gingiva in relation to the plaque present
Reductions in dental plaque can limit the severity of lesion
Must be using phenytoin, cyclosporine A or certain calcium channel blockers; the plasma concentrations to induce the lesion have not been clearly defined in humans

blockers were first linked to gingival enlargements (Ramon *et al.* 1984) and the prevalence of gingival lesions associated with these drugs has been estimated to be approximately 20% (Barclay *et al.* 1992), with nifedipine being the primarily calcium channel blocker associated with gingival enlargement (Ellis *et al.* 1999). Presently, the cause(s) of gingival enlargement by calcium channel blockers are still under investigation but these drugs may directly influence gingival connective tissues by stimulating an increase of gingival fibroblasts as well as an increase in the production of the connective tissue matrix (Fu *et al.* 1998).

The final drug class that has been associated with increases in gingival mass is cyclosporine A (CsA), which is a powerful immunoregulating drug used primarily in the prevention of organ transplant rejection (Seymour & Jacobs 1992). The clinical features of cyclosporine-influenced gingival enlargement were first described in 1983 (Rateitschak-Pluss *et al.* 1983) and cyclosporine appears to affect between 25 and 30% of the patients taking this medication (Hassell & Hefti 1991; Seymour *et al.* 1987). Hypotheses explaining why cyclosporine A affects the gingiva are diverse but a leading theory suggests that the principal metabolite of cyclosporine A, hydroxycyclosporine (M-17), in conjunction with the parent compound, stimulates fibroblast proliferation (Mariotti *et al.* 1998). This increase in cell number coupled with a reduction in the breakdown of gingival connective tissues (Hassell & Hefti 1991) has been speculated to be the cause of excessive extracellular matrix accumulation in cyclosporine A associated gingival enlargements.

Oral contraceptive-associated gingivitis

Oral contraceptive agents are one of the most widely utilized classes of drugs in the world. Today, as a result of the early onset of menarche, changing social mores and increased emphasis on family planning, the use of oral contraceptives in adolescents and young adults has increased to reduce unwanted pregnancies. Clinical case reports have described gingival enlargement induced by oral contraceptives in otherwise healthy females with no history of gingival overgrowth (Lynn 1967; Kaufman 1969; Sperber 1969). In all cases, the increased gingival mass was reversed when oral contraceptive use was discontinued or the dosage reduced. Early clinical studies demonstrated that women using hormonal contraceptive drugs had a higher incidence of gingival inflammation in comparison to women who did not use these agents (Lindhe & Bjorn 1967; El-Ashiry *et al.* 1970; Pankhurst *et al.* 1981) and that long-term use of oral contraceptives may affect periodontal attachment levels (Knight & Wade 1974). All studies prior to the 1980s recording changes to gingival tissues by oral contraceptives were completed when contraceptive concentrations were at much higher levels than

are currently available today. A recent clinical study evaluating the effects of low-dose oral contraceptives on gingival inflammation in young women found no effect of these hormonal agents on gingival tissues (Preshaw *et al.* 2001). Furthermore, cross-sectional data from NHANES III have failed to show a relationship between low-dose oral contraceptive use and increased levels of gingivitis (Taichman & Eklund 2005). From these data it appears that current low-dose compositions of oral contraceptives are probably not as harmful to the periodontium as the early formulations.

Gingival diseases associated with systemic diseases

Diabetes mellitus-associated gingivitis

Diabetes mellitus (DM) is a chronic systemic disease characterized by disorders in insulin production, metabolism of carbohydrate, fat, and protein, and the structure and function of blood vessels. DM most commonly appears as one of two recognized clinical entities: type 1 DM (insulin-dependent DM or juvenile onset) and type 2 DM (non-insulin-dependent DM or adult onset). DM-associated gingivitis is a consistent feature found in children with poorly controlled type 1 DM (Cianciola *et al.* 1982; Gusberti *et al.* 1983; Ervasti *et al.* 1985). The features of gingivitis associated with DM are similar to plaque-induced gingivitis, except that the level of diabetic control is more of an important aspect than plaque control in the severity of the gingival inflammation (Cianciola *et al.* 1982; Gusberti *et al.* 1983; Ervasti *et al.* 1985). In adults with DM, it is difficult to detect the effects of this endocrine disease on gingival diseases since most studies have evaluated gingival inflammation in association with attachment loss (AAP 1999); however, young adults with type I DM developed an earlier and more pronounced inflammatory response compared to non-diabetic controls in experimental gingivitis studies (Salvi *et al.* 2005). These data suggest that the gingival inflammatory response in adult diabetics is an overt response to the dental biofilm. In addition to the effects of DM on the gingiva, reports in the literature have suggested that reductions in gingival inflammation of diabetic patients will also reduce the amount of insulin needed to control blood glucose levels (Mealey & Oates 2006). This has been a controversial premise given the competing results of numerous studies; however, a meta-analysis of interventional studies suggest that control of gingival inflammation will not substantially affect glycemic control in diabetic patients (Janket *et al.* 2005).

Leukemia-associated gingivitis

Leukemia is a progressive, malignant hematologic disorder characterized by an abnormal proliferation and development of leukocytes and precursors of leukocytes in the blood and bone marrow. Leukemia

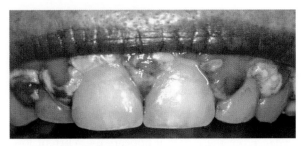

Fig. 17-13 Gingival changes associated with acute monocytic leukemia. Note the acute candidosis superimposed upon the infiltrative gingival changes.

is classified on the duration (acute or chronic) and the type of cell involved (myeloid or lymphoid) and the number of cells in the blood (leukemic or aleukemic). There are noticeable correlations of leukemias with age. For example, acute lymphoblastic leukemia comprise 80% of all childhood leukemias while acute myelogenous leukemia usually affects adults. Oral manifestations have primarily been described in acute leukemias and consist of cervical adenopathy, petechiae, mucosal ulcers, as well as gingival inflammation and enlargement (Fig. 17-13) (Lynch & Ship 1967). Signs of inflammation in the gingiva include swollen, glazed, and spongy tissues which are red to deep purple in appearance (Dreizen *et al.* 1984). Gingival bleeding is a common sign in patients with leukemia and is the initial oral sign and/or symptom in 17.7% and 4.4% of patients with acute and chronic leukemias, respectively (Lynch & Ship 1967). Gingival enlargement has also been reported, initially beginning at the interdental papilla followed by marginal and attached gingiva (Dreizen *et al.* 1984). Although local irritants can predispose and exacerbate the gingival response in leukemia, they are not prerequisites for lesions to form in the oral cavity (Dreizen *et al.* 1984).

Linear gingival erythema

Infection with the human immunodeficiency virus (HIV) produces an irreversible and progressive immunosuppression that renders a person susceptible to a variety of oral diseases. In humans, HIV depletes CD4+ lymphocytes (T helper cells) which leads to the development of a variety of fungal, viral, and bacterial oral infections (Connor & Ho 1992).

Oral manifestations of HIV infection have been used to stage HIV disease (Justice *et al.* 1989; Royce *et al.* 1991; Prevention CDC 1992), identify prophylactic treatment of other serious infections (Force USPHST 1993), and indicate disease prognosis (Dodd *et al.* 1991; Katz *et al.* 1992). In the gingiva, manifestations of HIV infection were formerly known as HIV-associated gingivitis but currently are designated as linear gingival erythema (LGE). LGE is distinguished by a 2–3 mm marginal band of intense erythema in the free gingiva (Winkler *et al.* 1988). This band of gingival erythema may extend into the attached

gingiva as a focal or diffuse erythema and/or extend beyond the mucogingival line into the alveolar mucosa (Winkler *et al.* 1988). LGE may be localized to one or two teeth but it is more commonly a generalized gingival condition.

The etiology of this gingival lesion is not well understood; however, research has begun to investigate the relationship of periodontal pathogens and the local host response in regard to how HIV infection affects the gingiva. Although LGE does not respond to conventional scaling, root planing, and plaque control (Winkler & Murray 1987; Grassi *et al.* 1988; Winkler *et al.* 1988, 1989), the anaerobic microflora from subgingival sites of HIV-infected patients with gingivitis seems to be essentially the same as seen in non-infected patients (Moore *et al.* 1993). Despite the similarities in anaerobic microflora between infected and uninfected individuals, organisms not generally associated with gingivitis in HIV-negative patients, such as *Candida* species, have been identified with LGE (Lamster *et al.* 1998). In addition, LGE lesions have been shown to have reduced proportions of T cells and macrophages and an increased number of IgG plasma cells and PMNs (Gomez *et al.* 1995). These host cell responses and unusual microbiota may be responsible for the refractory nature of this lesion to conventional periodontal treatment of gingivitis.

With the advent of antiretroviral therapy for HIV-positive patients, the prevalence of HIV-specific lesions has been dramatically reduced; even so, plaque accumulation with reduced CD4+ counts will still account for a pronounced gingival inflammatory response (Kroidl *et al.* 2005).

Gingival diseases associated with malnutrition

Although some nutritional deficiencies can significantly exacerbate the response of the gingiva to plaque bacteria, the precise role of nutrition in the initiation or progression of periodontal diseases remains to be elucidated. The studies that have attempted to investigate the relationship of nutrition to periodontal disease have examined the periodontal status of individuals in developed and in developing countries and have failed to show a relationship between periodontal disease and nutrition (Russell 1962; Waerhaug 1967; Wertheimer *et al.* 1967). While there is a paucity of information available regarding the effects of a specific, single nutritional deficiency on human periodontal tissues, severe vitamin C deficiency or scurvy has been one of the earliest nutritional deficiencies to be examined in the oral cavity (Lind 1953). Even though scurvy is unusual in areas with an adequate food supply, certain populations on restricted diets (e.g. infants from low socioeconomic families) are at risk of developing this condition (Oeffinger 1993). The classic clinical signs of scurvy describe the gingiva as being bright red,

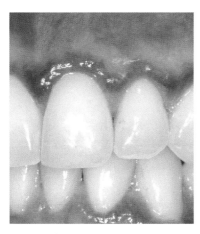

Fig. 17-14 Gingival changes associated with vitamin C deficiency. Note the absence of dental plaque and the distances of the color changes from marginal gingiva.

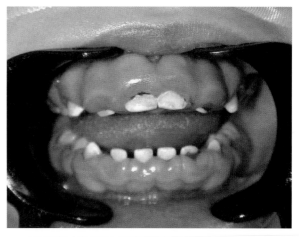

Fig. 17-15 Generalized, benign, non-inflammatory, fibrotic enlargement of gingival tissues.

swollen, ulcerated, and susceptible to hemorrhage (van Steenberghe 1997). Although there is no dispute about the necessity of dietary ascorbic acid for periodontal health, in the absence of frank scurvy the effect of declining ascorbic acid levels on the gingiva can be difficult to detect clinically (Woolfe *et al*. 1980) and when it is detected usually has characteristics that are similar to plaque-induced gingivitis (Fig. 17-14).

Gingival diseases associated with heredity

Benign, non-inflammatory fibrotic enlargement of the maxillary and/or mandibular gingiva associated with a familial aggregation has been designated by such terms as gingivomatosis elephantiasis, familial elephantiasis, juvenile hyaline fibromatosis, congenital familial fibromatosis, idiopathic fibromatosis, idiopathic gingival fibromatosis, hereditary gingival hyperplasia, and hereditary gingival fibromatosis. Although there have been over 100 reports of gingival enlargements associated with heredity in the literature over the past century, our knowledge concerning the natural history of this disease is extremely limited and the etiology of this rare condition has not been determined.

Hereditary gingival fibromatosis appears to be a slowly progressive gingival enlargement that develops upon eruption of the permanent dentition; however, gingival enlargement can also occur in the primary dentition (Emerson 1965; Jorgenson & Cocker 1974; Lai *et al*. 1995; Miyake *et al*. 1995). The disease can be localized or generalized and may ultimately cover the occlusal surfaces of teeth. The enlarged gingiva is non-hemorrhagic and firm but there can be an overlay of gingival inflammation which can augment the enlargement (Fig. 17-15). The histologic features of hereditary gingival fibromatosis include dense fibrotic connective tissue as well as epithelial hyperplasia with elongated and increased rete pegs (Johnson *et al*. 1986; Clark 1987).

Hereditary gingival fibromatosis can be inherited as a simple Mendelian trait in some chromosomal disorders, and as a malformation syndrome (Witkop 1971; Jones *et al*. 1977; Skrinjaric & Bacic 1989; Takagi *et al*. 1991; Goldblatt & Singer 1992; Hallet *et al*. 1995). Currently, a mutation in the *son of sevenless-1* gene has been implicated as a genetic factor responsible for hereditary gingival fibromatosis (Hart *et al*. 2002). Recent research into the cellular responses of this disease suggest an accumulation of specific populations of gingival fibroblasts that result in an abnormal accumulation of connective tissues (Huang *et al*. 1997; Tipton *et al*. 1997; Lee *et al*. 2006).

Gingival diseases associated with ulcerative lesions

Necrotizing ulcerative gingivitis (NUG) has been observed for centuries and has been recognized by numerous names including trench mouth and Vincent's infection. At this time, acute necrotizing ulcerative gingivitis is a term used to describe the clinical onset of the disease and should not be used as a diagnostic classification since some forms of NUG may be recurrent or possibly chronic.

NUG is most often distinguished by a sudden onset. The clinical signs of NUG include intense gingival pain that usually is responsible for the patient seeking professional care, papillary necrosis, that has been described as a "punched out" appearance of the gingival papilla, and gingival bleeding that requires little or no provocation (Fig. 17-16) (Grupe & Wilder 1956; Goldhaber & Giddon 1964; Johnson & Engel 1986). Although these three signs must be present to diagnosis NUG, other signs and symptoms may be present but do not necessarily occur in all individuals with this disease. These signs and symptoms include fever, malaise, lymphadenopathy, metallic taste, and malodor (Schluger 1943; Wilson 1952; Murayama *et al*. 1994). Systemic reactions of acute NUG are usually more severe in children. Significant destruction of the gingival connective tissue is possible with NUG but

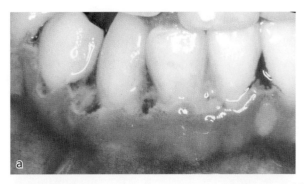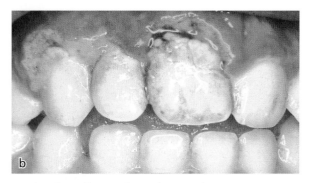

Fig. 17-16 Necrotizing ulcerative gingivitis. (a) Destruction of the interdental papilla, pseudomembrane and spontaneous bleeding. (b) Although usually confined to the papilla, occasionally the marginal tissues are involved.

when attachment loss occurs this condition should be considered as a necrotizing ulcerative periodontitis (NUP).

The etiology of NUG has been associated with a bacterial infection. The four zones of the NUG gingival lesion include the bacterial zone (the superficial area that consists of various bacteria and some spirochetes), neutrophil-rich zone (follows the bacterial zone and contains leukocytes and bacteria including spirochetes), necrotic zone (consists of disintegrated cells and connective tissue elements with many large and intermediate spirochetes) and the spirochetal infiltration zone (the deepest zone that is infiltrated with no other bacteria but intermediate and large spirochetes) (Listgarten 1965). The cultivable flora of NUG that predominates includes *Provetella intermedia* and *Fusobacterium* species while microscopically *Treponema* and *Selenomonas* species are observed (Loesche *et al*. 1982; Rowland *et al*. 1993b). Additional factors such as smoking (AAP 1996), psychological stress (Moulton *et al*. 1952; Cohen-Cole *et al*. 1983), malnutrition (Grupe & Wilder 1956; Goldhaber & Giddon 1964; Johnson & Engel 1986), and immune suppression (Moulton *et al*. 1952; Rowland *et al*. 1993a) can predispose an individual to NUG.

NUG can affect any age group but is considered to be a disease of young adults in industrialized countries (Melnick *et al*. 1988). In developing countries, NUG is a disease found in children from families with a low socioeconomic status (Melnick *et al*. 1988). The onset of NUG in children is associated with inappropriate nutritional intake, especially low protein consumption (Sheiham 1966; Taiwo 1995). In addition, viral infections such as measles can induce NUG in malnourished children (Enwonwu 1972; Osuji 1990). Even though NUG has occurred in epidemic patterns, this disease is not considered communicable (Rosebury 1942).

Treatment of plaque-induced gingival diseases

Personal and professional mechanical oral hygiene measures are critical aspects for the treatment of plaque-induced gingival diseases. Proper oral hygiene reduces the build-up of dental plaque on tooth surfaces and diminishes the incidence of various types of gingival diseases (Garmyn *et al*. 1998). For effective, self-care, mechanical plaque control, the appropriate use of manual (Jepsen 1998) or powered (van der Weijden *et al*. 1998) toothbrushes combined with interdental mechanical cleaning (Kinane 1998) is essential. Dentifrices also have important roles in the reduction of dental plaque. First of all, dentifrices can be used to help in the removal of dental plaque by enhancing the mechanical scrubbing and cleaning power of the toothbrush (Mariotti & Burrell 2006). Secondly, since dentifrices are also drug-delivery systems; agents (e.g. tricolsan) present in a toothpaste will provide a pharmacologic advantage by reducing the bacteria found in dental biofilms and/or inflammation in gingival tissues (DeVizio & Davies 2004). Additionally, adjunctive, self-applied, locally delivered, pharmacologic agents (e.g. chlorhexidine) can also be an effective option for individuals with physical or medical limitations that constrain their ability to perform adequate home care.

Professional intervention is required as an adjunct to self-performed hygiene when plaque-retaining factors, such as dental calculus, defective restorations or anatomic factors, prevent an individual from effectively removing dental plaque. In instances where systemic factors modify the gingival response to dental biofilms, a combined treatment plan with the appropriate medical professional can be effective in addressing the root causes of the gingival inflammation.

The significance of gingivitis

The presence of gingival inflammation was at one time considered a normal variant of health but in the mid-twentieth century that concept changed dramatically when it was hypothesized that sites with untreated gingivitis were destined to progress to destructive periodontal disease. Although this concept was supported by some clinical studies showing an association between gingivitis and bone loss (Marshall-Day *et al*. 1955), longitudinal studies examining the natural history of periodontal disease failed to show complete conversion of chronic gingivitis to periodontitis (Löe *et al.* 1986). Gingival inflammation is probably a necessary precursor for periodontitis (Löe & Morrison 1986; Page & Kornman 1997) but this does not mean that all sites which exhibit gingival inflammation progress to periodontitis (Schätzle *et al.* 2003).

If the majority of the adult population exhibit some form of gingivitis how does one determine which inflamed sites within particular individuals are susceptible to conversion to destructive periodontal disease? There has been an awareness that differences in the inflammatory responsiveness to dental plaque cannot be fully accounted for by the quantity or quality of the plaque (Tatakis & Trombelli 2004). More specifically, there seems to be a differential gingival inflammatory response that is independent of the amount or rate of accumulation of dental plaque (Trombelli *et al.* 2004). Hence, the

predilection of inflamed gingival sites to convert to destructive forms of periodontal disease may be dependent on the susceptibility and responsiveness of the individual to gingivitis (van der Velden *et al.* 1985a,b; Abbas *et al.* 1986; Winkel *et al.* 1987; Dietrich *et al.* 2006). In other words, these data suggest that specific types of inflammatory responses in the gingiva are necessary to initiate destruction of connective tissue attachment apical to the cemento-enamel junction. As we learn more about different gingival inflammatory phenotypes our notions about the initiation of periodontal destruction continue to emerge.

Acknowledgment

The author thanks Professor Noel Claffey for supplying some of the photographs in this chapter.

References

AAP (1996). Tobacco use and the periodontal patient. *Journal of Periodontology* **67**, 51–56.

AAP (1999). Diabetes and periodontal diseases. *Journal of Periodontology* **70**, 935–949.

Abbas, F., van der Velden, U., Moorer, W.R., Everts, V., Vroom, T.M. & Scholte, G. (1986). Experimental gingivitis in relation to susceptibility to periodontal disease. II. Phase-contrast microbiological features and some host-response observations. *Journal of Clinical Periodontology* **13**, 551–557.

Addy, V., McElnay, J.C., Eyre, D.G., Campbell, N. & D'Arcy, P.F. (1983). Risk factors in phenytoin-induced gingival hyperplasia. *Journal of Periodontology* **54**, 373–377.

Albandar, J.M. (2002). Periodontal diseases in North America. *Periodontology 2002* **29**, 31–69.

Angelopoulous, A.P. & Goaz, P.W. (1972). Incidence of diphenylhydantoin gingival hyperplasia. *Oral Surgery Oral Medicine Oral Pathology* **34**, 898–906.

Arafat, A. (1974a). The prevalence of pyogenic granuloma in pregnant women. *Journal of the Baltimore College of Dental Surgery* **29**, 64–70.

Arafat, A.H. (1974b). Periodontal status during pregnancy. *Journal of Periodontology* **45**, 641–643.

Baelum, V. & Schutz, F. (2002). Periodontal disease in Africa. *Periodontology 2000* **29**, 79–103.

Barclay, S., Thomason, J.M., Idle, J.R. & Seymour R.A. (1992). The incidence and severity of nefedipine-induced gingival overgrowth. *Journal of Clinical Periodontology* **19**, 311–314.

Bhat, M. (1991). Periodontal health of 14–17-year-old US school-children. *Journal of Public Health Dentistry* **51**, 5–11.

Bimstein, E. & Matsson, L. (1999). Growth and development considerations in the diagnosis of gingivitis and periodontitis in children. *Pediatric Dentistry* **21**, 186–191.

Blieden, T.M. (1999). Tooth-related issues. *Annals of Periodontology* **4**, 91–97.

Cianciola, L.J., Park, B.H., Bruck, E., Mosovich, L. & Genco, R.J. (1982). Prevalence of periodontal disease in insulin-dependent diabetes mellitus (juvenile diabetes). *Journal of the American Dental Association* **104**, 653–660.

Clark, D. (1987). Gingival fibromatosis and its related syndromes. A review. *Journal of the Canadian Dental Association* **2**, 137–140.

Cohen-Cole, S., Cogen, R.B., Stevens, A.W., Kirk, K., Gaitan, E., Bird, J., Cooksey, R. & Freeman, A. (1983). Psychiatric, psychosocial, and endocrine correlates of acute and necrotizing

ulcerative gingivitis (trench mouth): a perliminary report. *Psychiatric Medicine* **1**, 215–225.

Coles, O. (1874). On the condition of the mouth and teeth during pregnancy. *American Journal of Dental Science* **8**, 361–369.

Connor, R.J. & Ho, D.D. (1992). Etiology of AIDS: biology of human retroviruses. In: DeVita, T., Hellman, S., Rosenberg, S.A., eds. *AIDS: Etiology, Diagnosis, Treatment and Prevention*. Philadelphia: J.B. Lippincott, pp. 13–38.

Corbet, E.F., Zee, K.Y. & Lo, E.C.M. (2002). Periodontal disease in Asia and Oceania. *Periodontology 2000* **29**, 122–152.

Daley, T.D., Wysocki, G.P. & Day, C. (1986). Clinical and pharmacologic correlations in cyclosporine-induced gingival hyperplasia. *Oral Surgery Oral Medicine Oral Pathology* **62**, 417–421.

DeVizio, W. & Davies, R. (2004). Rationale for the daily use of a dentifrice containing triclosan in the maintenance of oral health. *Compendium of Continuing Education in Dentistry* **25** (suppl 7), 54–57.

Dietrich, T., Krall Kaye, E., Nunn, M.E., van Dyke, T. & Garcia, R.I. (2006). Gingivitis susceptibility and its relation to periodontitis in men. *Journal of Dental Research* **85**, 1134–1137.

Dodd, C.L., Greenspan, D., Katz, M.H., Westenhouse, J.L., Feigal, D.W. & Greenspan J.S. (1991). Oral candidiasis in HIV infection: pesudomembranous and erthymatous candidiasis show similar rates of progression to AIDS. *AIDS* **5**, 1339–1343.

Dreizen, S., McCredie, K.B. & Keating, M.J. (1984). Chemotherapy-associated oral hemorrhages in adults with acute leukemia. *Oral Surgery Oral Medicine Oral Pathology* **57**, 494–498.

El-Ashiry, G.M., El-Kafrawy, A.H., Nasr, M.F. & Younis, N. (1970). Comparative study of the influence of pregnancy and oral contraceptives on the gingivae. *Oral Surgery Oral Medicine Oral Pathology* **30**, 472–475.

Ellis, J.S., Seymour, R.A., Steele, J.G., Robertson, P., Butler, T.J. & Thomason, J.M. (1999). Prevalence of gingival overgrowth induced by calcium channel blockers: a community-based study. *Journal of Periodontology* **70**, 63–67.

Emerson, T. (1965). Hereditary gingival hyperplasia. A family pedigree of four generations. *Oral Surgery Oral Medicine Oral Pathology* **19**, 1–9.

Engelberg, J. (1966). Permeability of the dento-gingival blood vessels. I. Application of the vascular labelling method and gingival fluid measurements. *Periodontal Research* **1**, 180–191.

Engelberger, T., Hefti, A., Kallenberger, A. & Rateitschak, K.H. (1983). Correlations among papilla bleeding index, other clinical indices and histologically determined inflammation of gingival papilla. *Journal of Clinical Periodontology* **10**, 579–589.

Enwonwu, C.O. (1972). Epidemiological and biochemical studies of necrotizing ulcerative gingivits and noma (cancrum oris) in Nigerian children. *Archives of Oral Biology* **17**, 1357–1371.

Ervasti, T., Knuutila, M., Pohjamo, L. & Haukipuro, K. (1985). Relation between control of diabetes and gingival bleeding. *Journal of Periodontology* **56**, 154–157.

Esterberg, H.L. & White, P.H. (1945). Sodium dilantin gingival hyperplasia. *Journal of the American Dental Association* **32**, 16–24.

Force USPHST (1993) Recommendations for prophylaxis against *Pneumocystis carinii* pneumonia for persons infected with human immunodeficiency virus. U.S. Public Health Service Task Force on Antipneumocystis Prophylaxis in Patients with Human Immunodeficiency Virus Infection. *Journal of Acquired Immune Deficiency Syndromes* **6**, 46–55.

Fransson, C., Berglundh, T. & Lindhe, J. (1996). The effect of age on the development of gingivitis. Clinical, microbiological and histologic findings. *Journal of Clinical Periodontology* **23**, 379–385.

Fransson, C., Mooney, J., Kinane, D.F. & Berglundh, T. (1999) Differences in the inflammatory response in young and old human subjects during the course of experimental gingivitis. *Journal of Clinical Periodontology* **26**, 453–460.

Fu, E., Nieh, S., Hsiao, C.T., Hsieh, Y.D., Wikesjo, U.M.E. & Shen E.C. (1998). Nifedipine-induced gingival overgrowth in rats: brief review and experimental study. *Journal of Periodontology* **69**, 765–771.

Garmyn, P., van Steenberghe, D. & Quirynen, M. (1998). Efficacy of plaque control in the maintenance of gingival health: plaque control in primary and secondary prevention. In: Lang, N.P., Attström, R. & Löe, H., eds. *Proceedings of the European Workshop on Mechanical Plaque Control*. Chicago: Quintessence Publishing Co., Inc., pp. 107–120.

Gjermo, P., Rösing, C.K., Susin, C. & Oppermann, R. (2002). Periodontal disease in Central and South America. *Periodontology 2000* **29**, 70–78.

Goldblatt, J. & Singer, S.L. (1992). Autosomal recessive gingival fibromatosis with distinct facies. *Clinical Genetics* **42**, 306–308.

Goldhaber, P. & Giddon, D.B. (1964). Present concepts concerning etiology and treatment of acute necrotizing ulcerative gingivitis. *International Dental Journal* **14**, 468–496.

Gomez, R.S., Colsta, J.E., Loyola, A.M., Araùjo, N.S. & Araùjo, V.C. (1995). Immunohistochemical study of linear gingival erythema from HIV-positive patients. *Journal of Periodontal Research* **30**, 355–359.

Grassi, M., Williams, C.A. & Winkler, J.R. (1988). Management of HIV-associated periodontal diseases. In: Robertson, P.B. & Greenspan, J.S. eds. *Perspectives of Oral Manifestations of AIDS*. Proceedings of first international symposium on oral manifestations of AIDS. Littleton, MA: PSG Publishing, pp. 119–130.

Greenstein, G., Caton, J. & Polson, A.M. (1981). Histologic characteristics associated with bleeding after probing and visual signs of inflammation. *Journal of Periodontology* **52**, 420–425.

Grupe, H.E. & Wilder, L.S. (1956). Observations of necrotizing gingivitis in 870 military trainees. *Journal of Periodontology* **27**, 255–261.

Gusberti, F.A., Syed, S.A., Bacon, G., Grossman, N. & Loesche, W.J. (1983). Puberty gingivitis in insulin-dependent diabetic children. I. Cross-sectional observations. *Journal of Periodontology* **54**, 714–720.

Haffajee, A.D., Socransky, S.S. & Goodson, J.M. (1992). Subgingival temperature (I) Relation to baseline clinical parameters. *Journal of Clinical Periodontology* **19**, 401–408.

Hallet, K.B., Bankier, A., Chow, C.W., Bateman, J. & Hall, R.K. (1995). Gingival fibromatosis and Klippel-Trenaunay-Weber syndrome. Case report. *Oral Surgery Oral Medicine Oral Pathology* **79**, 678–682.

Hart, T.C., Zhang, Y., Gorry, M.C., Hart, P.S., Cooper, M., Marazita, M.L., Marks, J.M., Cortelli, J.R. & Pallos, D. (2002). A mutation in the SOS 1 gene causes hereditary gingival fibromatosis type 1. *American Journal of Human Genetics* **70**, 943–954.

Hassell, T., O'Donnell, J., Pearlman, J., Tesini, D., Murphy, T. & Best, H. (1984). Phenytoin induced gingival overgrowth in institutionalized epileptics. *Journal of Clinical Periodontology* **11**, 242–253.

Hassell, T.M. (1981). Phenytoin: gingival overgrowth. In: Myers, H.M. ed. *Epilepsy and the Oral Manifestations of Phenytoin Therapy*. Basel: S. Karger AG, pp. 116–202.

Hassell, T.M. & Hefti, A.F. (1991). Drug-induced gingival overgrowth: old problem, new problem. *Critical Reviews in Oral Biology and Medicine* **2**, 103–137.

Hefti, A., Engelberger, T. & Buttner, M. (1981). Gingivitis in Basel schoolchildren. *Helvetica Odontologica Acta* **25**, 25–42.

Hefti, A., Eshenaur, A.E., Hassell, T.M. & Stone, C. (1994). Gingival overgrowth in cyclosporine A treated multiple sclerosis patients. *Journal of Periodontology* **65**, 744–749.

Huang, J.S., Ho, K.Y., Chen, C.C., Wu, Y.M. & Wang C.C. (1997) Collagen synthesis in idiopathic and dilatin-induced gingival fibromatosis. *Kao Hsiung I Hsueh Tsa Chih* **13**, 141–148.

Hugoson, A. (1971). Gingivitis in pregnant women. A longitudinal clinical study. *Odontologisk Revy* **22**, 65–84.

Hugoson, A., Koch, G. & Rylander, H. (1981). Prevalence and distribution of gingivitis-periodontitis in children and adolescents. Epidemiological data as a base for risk group selection. *Swedish Dental Journal* **5**, 91–103.

Janket, S.J., Wightman, A., Baird, A.E., van Dyke, T.E. & Jones, J.A. (2005). Does periodontal treatment improve glycemic control in diabetic patients? A meta-analysis of intervention studies. *Journal of Dental Research* **84**, 1154–1159.

Jepsen, S. (1998). The role of manual toothbrushes in effective plaque control: advantages and limitations. In: Lang, N.P., Attström, R. & Löe, H., eds. *Proceedings of the European Workshop on Mechanical Plaque Control*. Quintessence Publishing Co., Inc. Chicago, pp. 121–137.

Johnson, B., el-Guindy, M., Ammons, W., Narayanan, A. & Page, R. (1986). A defect in fibroblasts from an unidentified syndrome with gingival hyperplasia as the predominant feature. *Journal of Periodontal Research* **21**, 403–413.

Johnson, B.D. & Engel, D. (1986). Acute necrotizing ulcerative gingivitis. A review of diagnosis, etiology and treatment. *Journal of Periodontology* **57**, 141–150.

Jones, G., Wilroy Jr., R.S. & McHaney, V. (1977). Familial gingival fibromatosis associated with progressive deafness in five generations of a family. *Birth Defects Original Article Series* **13**, 195–201.

Jorgenson, R.J. & Cocker, M.E. (1974). Variation in the inheritance and expression of gingival fibromatosis. *Journal of Periodontology* **45**, 472–477.

Justice, A.C., Feinstein, A.R. & Wells, C.K. (1989). A new prognostic staging system for the acquired immunodeficiency syndrome. *The New England Journal of Medicine* **320**, 1388–1393.

Katz, M.H., Greenspan, D., Westenhouse, J., Hessol, N.A., Buchbinder, S.P., Lifson, A.R., Shiboski, S., Osmond, D., Moss, A. & Samuel, M. (1992). Progression to AIDS in HIV-infected homosexual and bisexual men with hairy leukoplakia and oral candidiasis. *AIDS* **6**, 95–100.

Kaufman, A.Y. (1969). An oral contraceptive as an etiologic factor in producing hyperplastic gingivitis and a neoplasm of the pregnancy tumor type. *Oral Surgery Oral Medicine Oral Pathology* **28**, 666–670.

Kimball, O. (1939). The treatment of epilepsy with sodium diphenyl-hydantoinate. *Journal of the American Medical Association* **112**, 1244–1245.

Kinane, D.F. (1998). The role of interdental cleaning in effective plaque control: need for interdental cleaning in primary and secondary prevention. In: Lang, N.P., Attström, R. & Löe, H., eds. *Proceedings of the European Workshop on Mechanical Plaque Control.* Chicago: Quintessence Publishing Co., Inc., pp. 156–168.

Knight, G.M. & Wade, A.B. (1974). The effects of hormonal contraceptives on the human periodontium. *Journal of Periodontal Research* **9**, 18–22.

Kristen, V.K. (1976). Veranderungen der Mundschleimhaut wahrend Schwangerschaft und kontrazeptiver Hormonbehandlung. *Fortschritte der Medizin* **94**, 52–54.

Kroidl, A., Schaeben, A., Oette, M., Wettstein, M., Herfordt, A. & Haussinger, D. (2005). Prevalence of oral lesions and periodontal diseases in HIV-infected patients on antiretroviral therapy. *European Journal of Medical Research* **18**, 448–453.

Lai, L.L., Wang, F.L. & Chan, C.P. (1995). Hereditary gingival fibromatosis: a case report. *Chang Gung Medical Journal / Chang Gung Memorial Hospital* **18**, 403–408.

Lamster, I.B., Grbic, J.T., Mitchell-Lewis, D.A., Begg, M.D. & Mitchell, A. (1998). New concepts regarding the pathogenesis of periodontal disease in HIV infection. *Annals of Periodontology* **3**, 62–75.

Lee, E.J., Jang, S.I., Pallos, D., Kather, J. & Hart T.C. (2006). Characterization of fibroblasts with son of sevenless-1 mutation. *Journal of Dental Research* **85**, 1050–1055.

Lind, J. (1953). The diagnostics, or signs. In: Stewart, C.P., Guthrie, D., eds. *Lind's Treatise on Scurvy.* Edinburgh: Edinburgh University Press, pp. 113–128.

Lindhe, J. & Bjorn, A-L. (1967). Influence of hormonal contraceptives on the gingiva of women. *Journal of Periodontal Research* **2**, 1–6.

Listgarten, M.A. (1965). Electron microscopic observations on the bacterial flora of acute necrotizing ulcerative gingivitis. *Journal of Periodontology* **36**, 328–339.

Löe, H. (1965). Periodontal changes in pregnancy. *Journal of Periodontology* **36**, 209–216.

Löe, H., Ånerud, Å., Boysen, H. & Morrison E. (1986). Natural history of periodontal disease in man. Rapid, moderate and no loss of attachment in Sri Lankan laborers 14 to 46 years of age. *Journal of Clinical Periodontology* **13**, 431–440.

Löe, H. & Holm-Pedersen, P. (1965). Absence and presence of fluid from normal and inflamed gingiva. *Periodontics* **3**, 171–177.

Löe, H. & Morrison, E. (1986). Periodontal health and disease in young people: screening for priority care. *International Dental Journal* **36**, 162–167.

Löe, H. & Silness, J. (1963). Periodontal disease in pregnancy. I. Prevalence and severity. *Acta Odontologica Scandinavica* **21**, 533–551.

Löe, H., Theilade, E. & Jensen, S.B. (1965). Experimental gingivitis in man. *Journal of Periodontology* **36**, 177–187.

Loesche, W.J., Syed, S.A., Laughon, B.E. & Stall, J. (1982). The bacteriology of acute necrotizing ulcerative gingivitis. *Journal of Periodontology* **53**, 223–230.

Lynch, M.A. & Ship, I.I. (1967). Initial oral manifestations of leukemia. *Journal of the American Dental Association* **75**, 932–940.

Lynn, B.D. (1967). "The pill" as an etiologic agent in hypertrophic gingivitis. *Oral Surgery Oral Medicine Oral Pathology* **24**, 333–334.

Machtei, E.E., Mahler, D., Sanduri, H. & Peled, M. (2004). The effect of menstrual cycle on periodontal health. *Journal of Periodontology* **75**, 408–412.

Mackler, S.B. & Crawford, J.J. (1973). Plaque development and gingivitis in the primary dentition. *Journal of Periodontology* **44**, 18–24.

Maier, A.W. & Orban, B. (1949). Gingivitis in pregnancy. *Oral Surgery Oral Medicine Oral Pathology* **2**, 334–373.

Mariotti, A. (1994). Sex steroid hormones and cell dynamics in the periodontium. *Critical Reviews in Oral Biology and Medicine* **5**, 27–53.

Mariotti, A. (1999). Dental plaque-induced gingival diseases. *Annals of Periodontology* **4**, 7–19.

Mariotti, A. (2005). Estrogen and extracellular matrix influences human gingival fibroblast proliferation and protein production. *Journal of Periodontology*, **76**, 1391–1397.

Mariotti, A. & Burrell, K.H. (2006). Mouthrinses and dentifrices. In: Ciancio, S.G., ed. *ADA/PDR Guide to Dental Therapeutics*, 4th edn. Chicago: ADA Publishing Division, pp. 263–271.

Mariotti, A., Hassell, T., Jacobs, D., Manning, C.J. & Hefti, A.F. (1998). Cyclosporin A and hydroxycyclosporine (M-17) affect the secretory phenotype of human gingival fibroblasts. *Journal of Oral Pathology and Medicine* **27**, 260–261.

Marshall-Day, C.D., Stephen, R.G. & Quigley, L.F., Jr. (1955). Periodontal disease: prevalence and incidence. *Journal of Periodontology* **18**, 291–299.

Matsson, L. (1978). Development of gingivitis in pre-school children and young adults. A comparative experimental study. *Journal of Clinical Periodontology* **5**, 24–34.

Matsson, L. & Goldberg, P. (1985). Gingival inflammatory reaction in children at different ages. *Journal of Clinical Periodontology* **12**, 98–103.

McGaw, T., Lam, S. & Coates, J. (1987). Cyclosporin-induced gingival overgrowth: correlation with dental plaque scores, gingivitis scores, and cyclosporine levels in serum and saliva. *Oral Surgery Oral Medicine Oral Pathology* **64**, 293–297.

Mealey, B.L. & Oates, T.W. (2006). Diabetes mellitus and periodontal diseases. *Journal of Periodontology* **77**, 1289–1303.

Melnick, S.L., Roseman, J.M., Engel, D. & Cogen, R.B. (1988). Epidemiology of acute necrotizing ulcerative gingivitis. *Epidemiologic Reviews* **10**, 191–211.

Miyake, I., Tokumaru, H., Sugino, H., Tanno, M. & Yamamoto, T. (1995). Juvenile hyaline fibromatosis. Case report with five years' follow up. *The American Journal of Dermatopathology* **17**, 584–590.

Miyazaki, H., Yamashita, Y., Shirahama, R., Goto-Kimura, K., Shimada, N., Sogame, A. and Takehara, T. (1991). Periodontal condition of pregnant women assessed by CPITN. *Journal of Clinical Periodontology* **18**, 751–754.

Modeer, T. & Dahllof, G. (1987). Development of phenytoin-induced gingival overgrowth in non-institutionalized epileptic children subjected to different plaque control programs. *Acta Odontologica Scandinavica* **45**, 81–85.

Moore, L.V.H., Moore, W.E.C., Riley, C., Brooks, C.N., Burmeister, J.A. & Smibert, R.M. (1993). Periodontal microflora of HIV positive subjects with gingivitis or adult periodontitis. *Journal of Periodontology* **64**, 48–56.

Moss, K.L., Beck, J.D. & Offenbacher, S. (2005). Clinical risk factors associated with incidence and progression of periodontal conditions in pregnant women. *Journal of Clinical Periodontology* **32**, 492–498.

Moulton, R., Ewen, S. & Thieman, W. (1952). Emotional factors in periodontal disease. *Oral Surgery Oral Medicine Oral Pathology* **5**, 833–860.

Muhlemann, H.R. (1948). Eine Gingivitis intermenstrualis. *Schweizerische Monatsschrift für Zahnheilkunde* **58**, 865–885.

Muhlemann, H.R. & Son, S. (1971). Gingival sulcus bleeding – a leading symptom in initial gingivitis. *Helvetica Odontologica Acta* **15**, 107–113.

Murayama, Y., Kurihara, H., Nagai, A., Dompkowski, D. & Van Dyke, T.E. (1994). Acute necrotizing ulcerative gingivitis: risk factors involving host defense mechanisms. *Periodontology 2000* **6**, 116–124.

Oeffinger, K.C. (1993). Scurvy: more than historical relevance. *American Family Physician* **48**, 609–613.

Oliver, R.C., Holm-Pedersen, P. & Löe, H. (1969). The correlation between clinical scoring, exudate measurements and microscopic evaluation of inflammation in the gingiva. *Journal of Periodontology* **40**, 201–209.

Osuji, O.O. (1990). Necrotizing ulcerative gingivitis and cancrum oris (noma) in Ibadan, Nigeria. *Journal of Periodontology* **61**, 769–772.

Page, R.C. (1985). Oral health status in the United States: Prevalence of inflammatory periodontal diseases. *Journal of Dental Education* **49**, 354–364.

Page, R.C. & Kornman, K.S. (1997). The pathogenesis of human periodontitis: an introduction. *Periodontology 2000* **14**, 9–11.

Page, R.C. & Schroeder, H.E. (1976). Pathogenesis of inflammatory periodontal disease. *Laboratory Investigation* **33**, 235–249.

Pankhurst, C.L., Waite, I.M., Hicks, K.A., Allen, Y. & Harkness, R.D. (1981). The influence of oral contraceptive therapy on the periodontium – duration of drug therapy. *Journal of Periodontology* **52**, 617–620.

Parfitt, G.J. (1957). A five year longitudinal study of the gingival condition of a group of children in England. *Journal of Periodontology* **28**, 26–32.

Polson, A.M. & Goodson, J.M. (1985). Periodontal diagnosis. Current status and future needs. *Journal of Periodontology* **56**, 25–34.

Preshaw, P.M., Knutson, M.A. & Mariotti, A. (2001). Experimental gingivitis in women using oral contraceptives. *Journal of Dental Research* **80**, 2011–2015.

Prevention CDC (1992). 1993 revised classification system for HIV infection and expanded surveillance case definition for AIDS among adolescents and adults. *Morbidity and Mortality Weekly Report. Recommendations and Reports* **41**, 1–19.

Ramon, Y., Behar, S., Kishon, Y. & Engelberg, I.S. (1984). Gingival hyperplasia caused by nifedipine – a preliminary report. *International Journal of Cardiology* **5**, 195–204.

Ranney, R.R. (1993). Classification of periodontal diseases. *Periodontology 2000* **2**, 13–25.

Rateitschak-Pluss, E.M., Hefti, A., Lortscher, R. & Thiel, G. (1983). Initial observation that cyclosporin-A induces gingival enlargement in man. *Journal of Clinical Periodontology* **10**, 237–246.

Rosebury, T. (1942). Is Vincent's infection a communicable disease? *Journal of the American Dental Association* **29**, 823–834.

Rowland, R.W., Escobar, M.R., Friedman, R.B. & Kaplowitz, L.G. (1993a). Painful gingivitis may be an early sign of infection with the human immunodeficiency virus. *Clinical Infectious Diseases* **16**, 233–236.

Rowland, R.W., Mestecky, J., Gunsolley, J.C. & Cogen, R.B. (1993b). Serum IgG and IgM levels to bacterial antigens in necrotizing ulcerative gingivitis. *Journal of Periodontology* **64**, 195–201.

Royce, R.A., Luckman, R.S., Fusaro, R.E. & Winkelstein Jr., W. (1991). The natural history of HIV-1 infection: staging classification of disease. *AIDS* **5**, 355–364.

Rudin, H.J., Overdiek, H.F. & Rateitschak, K.H. (1970). Correlation between sulcus fluid rate and clinical and histological inflammation of the marginal gingiva. *Helvetica Odontologica Acta* **14**, 21–26.

Russell, A.L. (1962). Periodontal disease in well- and malnourished populations. A preliminary report. *Archives of Environmental Health* **5**, 153–157.

Salvi, G.E., Kandylaki, M., Troendle, A., Persson, G.R. & Lang, N.P. (2005) Experimental gingivitis in type I diabetics: a controlled clinical and microbiological study. *Journal of Clinical Periodontology* **32**, 310–316.

Schätzle, M., Löe, H., Bürgin, W., Ånerud, Å., Boysen, H. & Lang, N.P. (2003). Clinical course of chronic periodontitis. I. Role of gingivitis. *Journal of Clinical Periodontology* **30**, 887–901.

Schluger, S. (1943). The etiology and treatment of Vincent's infection. *Journal of the American Dental Association* **39**, 524–532.

Seymour, R.A. (1991). Calcium channel blockers and gingival overgrowth. *British Dental Journal* **170**, 376–379.

Seymour, R.A. (2006). Effects of medications on the periodontal tissues in health and disease. *Periodontology 2000* **40**, 120–129.

Seymour, R.A. & Jacobs, D.J. (1992). Cyclosporin and the gingival tissues. *Journal of Clinical Periodontology* **19**, 1–11.

Seymour, R.A., Smith, D.G. & Rogers, S.R. (1987). The comparative effects of azathioprine and cyclosporin on some gingival health parameters of renal transplant patients. A longitudinal study. *Journal of Clinical Periodontology* **14**, 610–613.

Seymour, R.A., Thomason, J.M. & Ellis, J.S. (1996). The pathogenesis of drug-induced gingival overgrowth. *Journal of Clinical Periodontology* **23**, 165–175.

Sheiham, A. (1966). An epidemiological survey of acute ulcerative gingivitis in Nigerians. *Archives of Oral Biology* **11**, 937–942.

Sheiham, A. & Netuveli, G.S. (2002). Periodontal diseases in Europe. *Periodontology 2000* **29**, 104–121.

Sills, E.S., Zegarelli, D.J., Hoschander, M.M. & Strider, W.E. (1996). Clinical diagnosis and management of hormonally responsive oral pregnancy tumor (pyogenic granuloma). *Journal of Reproductive Medicine* **41**, 467–470.

Skrinjaric, I. & Bacic, M. (1989). Hereditary gingival fibromatosis: report on three families and dermatoglyphic analysis. *Journal of Periodontolgy* **24**, 303–309.

Sperber, G.H. (1969). Oral contraceptive hypertrophic gingivitis. *Journal of the Dental Association of South Africa* **24**, 37–40.

Stamm, J.W. (1986). Epidemiology of ginigivitis. *Journal of Clinical Periodontology* **13**, 360–366.

Steinberg, S.C. & Steinberg, A.D. (1982). Phenytoin-induced gingival overgrowth control in severly retarded children. *Journal of Periodontology* **53**, 429–433.

Sutcliffe, P. (1972). A longitudinal study of gingivitis and puberty. *Journal of Periodontal Research* **7**, 52–58.

Suzuki, J.B. (1988). Diagnosis and classification of the periodontal diseases. *Dental Clinics of North America* **32**, 195–216.

Taichman, S.L. & Eklund, S.A. (2005). Oral contraceptives and periodontal disease: rethinking the association based upon analysis of National Health and Nutrition Examination Survey data. *Journal of Periodontology* **76**, 1374–1385.

Taiwo, J.O. (1995). Severity of necrotizing ulcerative gingivitis in Nigerian children. *Periodontal Clinical Investigations* **17**, 24–27.

Takagi, M., Yamamoto, H., Mega, H., Hsieh, K.J., Shioda, S. & Enomoto, S. (1991). Heterogeneity in the gingival fibromatoses. *Cancer* **68**, 2202–2212.

Tatakis, D.N, & Trombelli, L. (2004). Modulation of clinical expression of plaque-induced gingivitis. I. Background review and rationale. *Journal of Clinical Periodontology* **31**, 229–238.

Tipton, D.A., Howell, K.J. & Dabbous, M.K. (1997). Increased proliferation, collagen, and fibronectin production by hereditary gingival fibromatosis fibroblasts. *Journal of Periodontology* **68**, 524–530.

Trombelli, L., Tatakis, D.N., Scapoli, C., Bottega, S., Orlandini, E. & Tosi, M. (2004). Modulation of clinical expression of plaque-induced gingivitis. II. Indentification of "high responder" and "low responder" subjects. *Journal of Clinical Periodontology* **31**, 239–252.

Tyldesley, W.R. & Rotter, E. (1984). Gingival hyperplasia induced by cyclosporin-A. *British Dental Journal* **157**, 305–309.

US Public Health Service NCfHS (1965). Periodontal Disease in Adults, United States 1960–1962. Washington DC: Government Printing Office.

US Public Health Service NCfHS (1972). Periodontal Diseases and Oral Hygiene among Children, United States. Washington DC: Government Printing Office.

US Public Health Service NIoDR (1987). Oral Health of United States Adults; National Findings. Bethseda MD: NIDR.

van der Velden, U., Abbas, F. & Hart, A.A. (1985a). Experimental gingivitis in relation to susceptibilty to periodontal disease. I. Clinical observations. *Journal of Clinical Periodontology* **12**, 61–68.

van der Velden, U., Winkel, E.G. & Abbas, F. (1985b). Bleeding/plaque ratio. A possible prognostic indicator for periodontal breakdown. *Journal of Clinical Periodontology* **12**, 861–866.

van der Weijden, G.A., Timmerman, M.F., Danser, M.M. & van der Velden, U. (1998). The role of electric toothbrushes: advantages and limitations. In: Lang, N.P., Attström, R. & Löe, H. eds. *Proceedings of the European Workshop on Mechanical Plaque Control*. Chicago: Quintessence Publishing Co., Inc., pp. 138–155.

van Steenberghe, D. (1997). Systemic disorders and the periodontium. In: Lindhe, J., Karring, T. & Lang, N.P. eds. *Clinical Periodontology and Implant Dentistry*, 3rd edn. Copenhagen: Munksgaard, pp. 332–355.

Waerhaug, J. (1967). Prevalence of periodontal disease in Ceylon. Association with age, sex, oral hygiene, socio-economic factors, vitamin deficiencies, malnutrition, betel and tobacco consumption and ethnic group. Final report. *Acta Odontologica Scandinavica* **25**, 205–231.

Wertheimer, F.W., Brewster, R.H. & White, C.L. (1967). Periodontal disease and nutrition in Thailand. *Journal of Periodontology* **38**, 100–104.

Wilson, J.R. (1952). Etiology and diagnosis of bacterial gingivitis including Vincent's disease. *Journal of the American Dental Association* **44**, 671–679.

Winkel, E.G., Abbas, F., van der Velden, U., Vroom, T.M., Scholte, G. & Hart, A.A. (1987). Experimental gingivitis in relation to age in individuals not susceptible to periodontal destruction. *Journal of Clinical Periodontology* **14**, 499–507.

Winkler, J.R., Grassi, M. & Murray, P.A. (1988). Clinical description and etiology of HIV-associated periodontal diseases. In: Robertson, P.B. & Greenspan, J.S., eds. *Perspectives of Oral Manifestations of AIDS*. Proceedings of first international symposium on oral manifestations of AIDS. Littleton, MA: PSG Publishing, pp. 49–70.

Winkler, J.R. & Murray, P.A. (1987). Periodontal disease. A potential intraoral expression of AIDS may be rapidly progressive periodontitis. *Journal of the Canadian Dental Association* **15**, 20–24.

Winkler, J.R., Murray, P.A., Grassi, M. & Hammerle, C. (1989). Diagnosis and management of HIV-associated periodontal lesions. *Journal of the American Dental Association* Suppl, 25S–34S.

Witkop, C.J., Jr. (1971). Heterogeneity in gingival fibromatosis. *Birth Defects Original Article Series* **7**, 210–221.

Wolff, L.F., Koller, N.J., Smith, Q.T., Mathur, A. & Aeppli, D. (1997). Subgingival temperature: relation to gingival crevicular fluid enzymes, cytokines, and subgingival plaque microorganisms. *Journal of Clinical Periodontology* **24**, 900–906.

Woolfe, S.N., Hume, W.R. & Kenney, E.B. (1980). Ascorbic acid and periodontal disease: a review of the literature. *The Journal of the Western Society of Periodontology/Periodontal Abstracts* **28**, 44–56.

Yahia, N., Seibel, W., McCleary, L., Lesko, L. & Hassell, T. (1988). Effect of toothbrushing on cyclosporine-induced gingival overgrowth in beagles. *Journal of Dental Research* **67**, 332.

Ziskin, D.E. & Nesse, G.J. (1946). Pregnancy gingivitis: history, classification, etiology. *American Journal of Orthodontics and Oral Surgery* **32**, 390–432.

Chapter 18

Chronic Periodontitis

Denis F. Kinane, Jan Lindhe, and Leonardo Trombelli

Chronic periodontitis is considered to start as *plaque-induced gingivitis* (see Chapter 17), a reversible condition that, left untreated, may develop into *chronic periodontitis*. Chronic periodontitis lesions include loss of attachment and bone and are regarded as irreversible. In this chapter, various aspects of chronic periodontitis will be described, including its links to plaque-induced gingivitis.

Clinical features of chronic periodontitis

The clinical features of chronic periodontitis include symptoms such as (1) color, texture and volume alterations of the marginal gingiva, (2) bleeding on probing (BoP) from the gingival pocket area, (3) reduced resistance of the soft marginal tissues to probing (increased pocket depth or periodontal pocketing), (4) loss of probing attachment level, (5) recession of the gingival margin, (6) loss of alveolar bone (even or angular pattern), (7) root furcation exposure, (8) increased tooth mobility, (9) drifting and eventually exfoliation of teeth.

Figure 18-1 illustrates the clinical status of a 30-year-old male with severe chronic periodontitis. The clinical examination revealed that (1) most approximal and lingual/palatal sites exhibited BoP, (2) most teeth showed increased mobility, and (3) gingival recession had occurred at a large number of buccal and interproximal sites. Tooth 16 had erupted beyond the occlusal plane. Teeth 37 and 38 had tilted mesially. The altered position of the molars had evidently compromised the occlusion. Forces elicited during function may have caused the maxillary incisors to tilt in a buccal direction and multiple open spaces,

diastemata, had developed in the front tooth segment of the maxilla.

Figure 18-2 presents the radiographic status of the same patient. In the radiographs it can be observed that a large number of teeth have lost substantial amounts of bone support. At teeth 17, 16, 27, 37, 36, and 47 the furcation areas have lost their periodontal tissue support and are open for "through and through" probing.

Overall characteristics of chronic periodontitis

- Chronic periodontitis is prevalent in adults but may occur in children.
- The amount of destruction of the periodontal tissues seen in a given patient is commensurate with oral hygiene and plaque levels, local predisposing factors, smoking, stress, and systemic risk factors.
- The subgingival biofilm harbors a variety of bacterial species; the composition of the biofilm may vary between subjects and sites.
- Subgingival calculus is invariably present at diseased sites.
- Chronic periodontitis is classified as localized when <30% of sites are affected and generalized when this level is exceeded.
- Severity of chronic periodontitis at the site level may be classified based on the degree of probing attachment loss (PAL) as *mild* (PAL = 1–2 mm), *moderate* (PAL = 3–4 mm), and *severe* (PAL ≥ 5 mm).
- Although chronic periodontitis is initiated and sustained by microbial plaque, host factors deter-

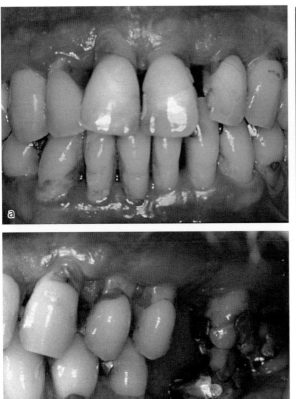
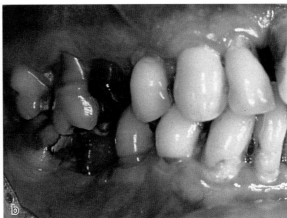
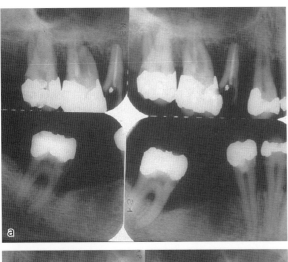

Fig. 18-1 A 30-year-old male patient with chronic periodontitis, clinical status prior to treatment.

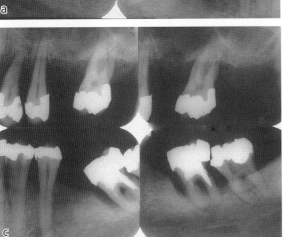
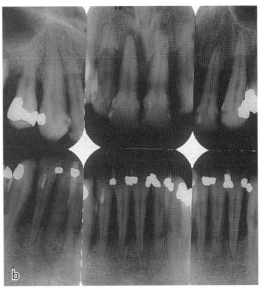

Fig. 18-2 Same patient as in Fig. 18-1. Radiographs from the initial examination.

mine the pathogenesis and (rate of) progression of the disease.

- The rate of progression of chronic periodontitis is in most cases slow to moderate; periods of rapid tissue destruction may, however, occur.
- Additional periodontal tissue breakdown is likely to occur in diseased sites that are left untreated.

Gingivitis as a risk for chronic periodontitis

Findings from epidemiologic studies (cross-sectional as well as longitudinal) indicate that gingival inflammation is invariably a component of chronic periodontitis and that gingivitis precedes the onset of periodontitis (see Chapter 11). The interpretation of data from early cross-sectional studies led to the belief that untreated gingivitis always progressed to chronic periodontitis. More recent studies have demonstrated, however, that this is not the case. Gingivitis lesions may remain stable for many years, and may never progress to become periodontitis lesions that include features such as attachment and bone loss. The two conditions have been considered, therefore, as separate disease entities with the explanation being that the bacterial plaque challenge will induce overt gingivitis but that the degree of response of the host (the susceptibility) will determine whether or not chronic periodontitis will develop. In a review paper, Kinane and Attström (2005) evaluated epidemiologic and experimental data on gingivitis and chronic periodontitis. The independence of these two conditions was called into question. It was proposed that gingivitis and periodontitis most likely represented different aspects of the same disease, namely chronic periodontitis.

Gingivitis becomes manifest after only days or weeks of plaque accumulation (Löe et al. 1965) while destructive chronic periodontitis is a condition that in the majority of cases requires far longer periods (years) of plaque and calculus exposure to develop (Lindhe et al. 1975; Löe et al. 1978). The proportion of untreated gingival lesions in a given subject or in a population that converts to destructive periodontitis lesions is at present unknown. Furthermore, the factors that cause the conversion are not well understood (Schätzle et al. 2003).

Findings from epidemiologic studies and prospective clinical trials have indicated that the presence of gingivitis may be regarded as a risk factor for chronic periodontitis. In a 2-year longitudinal study of 15–24-year-old Chinese adolescents from a rural district, it was observed that the percentage of sites that bled on probing at a baseline examination was related to overall attachment loss after 2 years of monitoring (Suda et al. 2000). This suggests that gingival inflammation was a risk indicator for additional attachment loss in this cohort. The role of gingivitis in the pathogenesis of chronic periodontitis was further elucidated by Schätzle et al. (2004) in longitudinal studies

on the initiation and progression of periodontal disease in a Norwegian population. The results demonstrated that gingival sites, which during a 20-year interval never showed signs of inflammation, experienced modest loss of attachment (1.86 mm). For sites which presented with mild inflammation at each examination, the corresponding attachment loss was 2.25 mm, while at sites with severe gingival inflammation, the mean loss of attachment was 3.23 mm. Moreover, while teeth surrounded with healthy gingival tissues were maintained during the study period, teeth with gingivitis lesions were 46 times more likely to be lost.

The above data indicate that gingival inflammation may represent a relevant risk factor not only for destructive chronic periodontitis but also for tooth loss. This conclusion is in agreement with results documenting the absence of gingivitis as a good indicator for long-term maintenance of periodontal health in a subject (Joss et al. 1994) as well as at a site (Lang et al. 1990) level.

Susceptibility to chronic periodontitis

As stated above plaque-induced gingivitis and chronic periodontitis represent different aspects of the same disease (Kinane & Attström 2005). An important question is whether both gingivitis and chronic periodontitis are affected by the same subject response (the host response) to plaque. If this is the case, the corollary is that susceptibility to gingivitis will reflect susceptibility to chronic periodontitis and may have prognostic utility.

Even in the very first reports from studies called "Experimental gingivitis in man" (Löe et al. 1965; Theilade et al. 1966) (see Chapters 11 and 17), evidence was presented that suggested that the onset and severity of the inflammatory response of the gingiva to plaque accumulation differed markedly among participants. The differences were, however, at that time attributed to differences in plaque accumulation rates (quantitative plaque differences) and/or differences in bacterial species present in plaque (qualitative plaque differences). More recent studies utilizing the "Experimental gingivitis" model have documented that significant differences in the inflammatory response occurred in different subjects although their plaque accumulation was quantitatively and/or qualitatively similar (Trombelli et al. 2004, 2005). It was suggested that the intensity of the inflammatory response to the plaque challenge may represent an individual trait (Tatakis & Trombelli 2004). Thus, an individual's susceptibility to gingivitis may be dependent on host-related factors, possibly of genetic origin (Shapira et al. 2005; Scapoli et al. 2005).

With the use of the "Experimental gingivitis" model it was also demonstrated that the susceptibility to gingivitis differed between two groups of patients consistent with different susceptibilities to periodontitis (Abbas *et al.* 1986; Winkel *et al.* 1987). Thus, the group with greater periodontitis susceptibility had also a greater susceptibility to gingivitis. Furthermore, in more recent studies it was documented that subjects with a history of aggressive periodontitis presented significantly more gingivitis in response to *de novo* plaque accumulation when compared to periodontally healthy subjects matched for extent and rate of supragingival plaque accumulation (Trombelli *et al.* 2006).

Prevalence of chronic periodontitis

From epidemiologic studies (see Chapter 7) it was concluded that chronic periodontitis is the most commonly occurring form of periodontal disease. While most subjects over 50 years of age have suffered moderate amounts of periodontal tissue destruction, advanced forms of chronic periodontitis are seen in only a small (<10%) subset of the population. Both age of onset of chronic periodontitis and subsequent rate of progression of the disease vary between individuals and are probably influenced by genetics (see Chapter 13) and environmental risk factors (see Chapters 7 and 12). Findings from examination of dizygotic and monozygotic twins (Michalowicz *et al.* 1991, 2000) indicated that (1) between 38% (regarding probing attachment loss) and 82% (regarding gingivitis) of the population variance could be attributed to genetic factors (Michalowicz *et al.* 1991), and (2) chronic periodontitis has about 50% heritability (Michalowicz *et al.* 2000).

On a population basis chronic periodontitis is often classified according to number (prevalence) of diseased sites (extent) and severity of tissue breakdown (probing attachment loss) at such sites. For the extent of chronic periodontitis, the low category would involve one to ten diseased (probing attachment loss) sites, the medium category would involve 11–20 sites, while the high category would involve more than 20 diseased sites. The amount of PAL at a given site may be used to describe the severity of chronic periodontitis. The severity may be considered as mild (PAL = 1–2 mm), moderate (PAL= 3–4 mm) or severe (PAL ≥ 5 mm). It has been documented that the extent and severity of chronic periodontitis are useful predictors of future disease progression.

Clinical (probing) attachment loss of 1–2 mm at one or several sites can be found in nearly all members of an adult population. The prevalence of subjects with one or more sites with PAL ≥ 3 mm increases with age. Furthermore the number of diseased sites in any one individual increases with age, as does the population prevalence (extent and severity) of chronic periodontitis with age.

Progression of chronic periodontitis

Chronic periodontitis is generally a slowly progressing form of periodontal disease that at any stage may undergo exacerbation resulting in additional loss of attachment and bone.

Tissue destruction in chronic periodontitis does not affect all teeth evenly, but has site predilection. In other words, in the same dentition some teeth may be severely affected with periodontal tissue destruction while other teeth are almost free of signs of attachment and bone loss. Figure 18-3 illustrates the clinical condition of a subject with chronic periodontitis. Clinically (Fig. 18-3a) it can be observed that most teeth exhibit advanced recession of the soft tissue margin. In the corresponding radiographs (Fig. 18-3b) it is noted that the mesial surface of tooth 16 has a normal periodontal tissue support, while the neighboring tooth, i.e. the first premolar (tooth 14), has lost several millimeters of bone support on the distal aspect. The mesial surface of tooth 14, on the

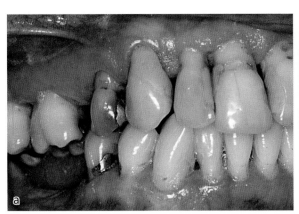
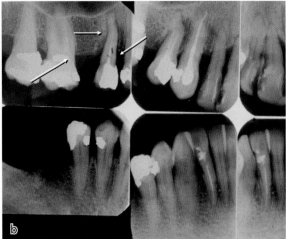

Fig. 18-3 (a) The clinical condition in quadrants 1 and 3 of a subject with chronic periodontitis. Most teeth in both quadrants exhibit advanced recession of the soft tissue margin. (b) Corresponding radiographs: the mesial surface of tooth 16 (arrow) has a normal periodontal tissue support, while the neighboring tooth, tooth 14, has lost several millimeters of bone support on the distal aspect (arrow). The mesial surface of tooth 14 has a comparatively normal tissue support (arrow).

other hand, has a comparatively normal tissue support.

When considering changes in attachment level over time, it is also peculiar that only relatively few sites in a subject with chronic periodontitis undergo marked, additional tissue destruction during any given observation period. Based on data from a series of longitudinal studies, Socransky *et al.* (1984) proposed that chronic periodontitis progressed in episodes of exacerbation and remission. They termed this the "burst hypothesis" of disease progression. Findings from other similar studies, however, indicated that the progression of chronic periodontitis may be a continuous, slowly destructive process rather than exhibiting a "burst" pattern. The current consensus is that the progression of chronic periodontitis in most subjects and at most sites is a continuous process but that periods of exacerbation occasionally may occur. Clinically, the progressive nature of the disease can only be confirmed by repeated examinations over time but it is a safe assumption that untreated lesions of chronic periodontitis will progress and cause additional attachment and bone loss. Flemmig (1999) reported a mean additional PAL of ≥3 mm in up to 27% of subjects in untreated populations during a 1-year period. When progression was studied on a site basis, the overall annualized incidence ranged from 0.3–4.2% (Flemmig 1999). This indicates that the number of sites that actually exhibited progression within a given time varied considerably between subjects.

It is important to realize that factors associated with the initiation of chronic periodontitis may also influence disease progression. Furthermore, the extent and severity of disease within an individual, i.e. number of sites with attachment loss, bone loss, and/or deep pockets, are good predictors of future disease occurrence. In fact the best predictor of disease progression is previous disease experience.

Risk factors for chronic periodontitis

The term "risk factor" means an aspect of lifestyle, an environmental exposure, or an inborn or inherited characteristic, which on the basis of epidemiologic evidence is known to be associated with a given disease. Risk factors may be part of the causal chain of a disease and/or may predispose the host to develop a disease. An individual presenting with one or more risk factors has an increased probability of contracting the disease or of the disease being made worse.

Bacterial plaque

Bacterial aspects of periodontal disease are dealt with in Chapters 8 and 9. From the data presented it is obvious that a cumulative risk for a given microbiota can be estimated. It is not clear, however, if the specific microbiota is the principal disease-causing factor or whether it reflects the disease process. Specific microorganisms have been considered as potential periodontal pathogens but it is clear that, although pathogens are necessary, their mere presence may not be enough for the progressive disease to occur. Microbial plaque (biofilm) is a crucial factor in inflammation of the periodontal tissues, but the progression of gingivitis to periodontitis is largely governed by host-based risk factors (Michalowicz 1994; Shapira *et al.* 2005). Microbial biofilms of particular compositions will initiate chronic periodontitis (Marsh 2005) in certain individuals whose host response and cumulative risk factors predispose them to periodontal tissue destruction and attachment loss.

Age

Although the prevalence of periodontal disease increases with age it is unlikely that becoming older in itself greatly increases susceptibility to periodontal disease. It is more likely that the cumulative effects of disease over a lifetime, i.e. deposits of plaque and calculus, and the increased number of sites capable of harboring such deposits, as well as attachment and bone loss experience, explain the increased prevalence of disease in older people.

Smoking

The association between periodontal disease and smoking is dealt with in detail in Chapter 12. Only a brief discussion of smoking as a risk factor for chronic periodontitis is thus given here. The literature consistently indicates a positive association between smoking and chronic periodontitis across the many cross-sectional and longitudinal studies performed over the years (Kinane & Chestnutt 2000) and the risk attributable to tobacco for chronic periodontitis is between 2.5 and 7.0. It is not only the risk of developing the disease that is enhanced by smoking, but also the response to periodontal therapy is impaired in smokers. A further feature in smokers is that their signs and symptoms of both gingivitis and chronic periodontitis, mainly gingival redness and bleeding on probing (BOP), are masked by the dampening of inflammation seen for smokers as compared to non-smokers.

Systemic disease

It is difficult to determine the precise role any systemic disease may play in the pathogenesis of chronic periodontitis. There are several reasons for this. Firstly, in epidemiologic studies attempting to evaluate the effect of systemic disease, control groups should be carefully matched in respect of age, sex, oral hygiene, and socioeconomic status. Many studies, particularly before the etiologic importance of dental plaque was recognized, failed to include such controls. Secondly, because of the chronic nature of periodontal disease, longitudinal studies spanning several years are preferable in individuals both with and without systemic disease. Unfortunately, most of the available data are derived from cross-sectional studies (Kinane 1999).

A reduction in number or function of polymorphonuclear leukocytes (PMNs) generally results in increased rate and severity of periodontal tissue destruction (Wilton *et al.* 1988). Many drugs, such as phenytoin, nifedipine, and cyclosporine, predispose to gingival overgrowth in response to plaque and thus may modify pre-existing chronic periodontitis (Ellis *et al.* 1999). Changes in circulating hormone levels may increase severity of plaque-induced gingival inflammation but typically do not result in any increased susceptibility to periodontitis. Hormonal changes following menopause have been associated with osteoporosis but studies are lacking to link this disease or an estrogen deficient state to a higher susceptibility to periodontal disease. Immunosuppressive drug therapy and any disease resulting in suppression of inflammatory and immune processes (such as HIV infection) may predispose the individual to exaggerated periodontal tissue destruction (Barr *et al.* 1992).

Nutritional deficiencies in animals have been shown to affect the periodontal tissues. Epidemiologic data do not support the suggestion that such deficiencies play an important role in chronic periodontal disease although nutritional influences on inflammation are now accepted and are now actively being researched (Ritchie & Kinane 2005). Gingival bleeding is the most consistent oral feature of vitamin C deficiency or scurvy but there is also some evidence to suggest that avitaminosis-C may aggravate established chronic periodontitis.

The periodontal features of *histiocytosis X* and other conditions in the rare histiocytoses disease group may present as necrotizing ulcerative periodontitis (Kinane 1999). Diabetes appears to be one of the most fascinating systemic diseases that interacts with periodontitis. On the one hand periodontitis severity and prevalence are increased in subjects with long-duration diabetes and more so in poorly controlled diabetics, than non-diabetics. On the other hand, periodontitis may also exacerbate diabetes as it may decrease glycemic control (Thorstenson 1995).

Despite the paucity of high quality data on individuals both with and without systemic disease the following general conclusions can be drawn (Kinane 1999):

- The *blood cells* have a vital role in supplying oxygen, hemostasis and protection to the tissues of the periodontium. Systemic hematological disorders can thus have profound effects on the periodontium by denying any of these functions necessary for the integrity of the periodontium.
- The *polymorphonuclear leukocyte* (PMN cell) is undoubtedly crucial to the defense of the periodontium. To exert this protective function several activities of PMNs must be integrated, namely chemotaxis, phagocytosis, and killing or neutraliza-

tion of the ingested organism or substance. Individuals with either quantitative (neutropenia) or qualitative (chemotactic or phagocytic) PMN deficiencies, exhibit severe destruction of the periodontal tissues, which is strong evidence that PMNs are an important component of the host's protective response to the subgingival biofilm. Quantitative deficiencies are generally accompanied by destruction of the periodontium of all teeth, whereas qualitative defects are often associated with localized destruction affecting only the periodontium of certain teeth (i.e. chronic periodontitis may be modified).

- *Leukemias* which give excessive numbers of leukocytes in the blood and tissues also cause a greatly depleted bone marrow function with concomitant anemia, thrombocytopenia, neutropenia, and reduced range of specific immune cells which give some characteristic periodontal features: anemic gingival pallor; gingival bleeding; gingival ulceration. Leukemic features are further complicated by the potential for the proliferating leukocytes to infiltrate the gingiva and result in gingival enlargement. In broad terms leukemias result in gingival pathologies, whereas periodontal bone loss is the consequence of neutrophil functional defects or deficient numbers and other severe functional defects such as deficiency of leukocyte adhesion receptors.
- *Diabetes mellitus:* there are numerous confounding variables which must be considered in determining the true relationship between periodontitis and diabetes. The current consensus is that diabetics are at increased risk of periodontal disease, and whilst periodontitis can be successfully treated, both disease susceptibility and the outcome of therapy are influenced by poor metabolic control. Thus, it may be of benefit to the dentist to have knowledge of the control status of diabetes in an individual patient, as in the longer term metabolic control could indicate the probable outcome of periodontal therapy. In addition, it is now accepted that periodontal therapy can improve metabolic control in diabetics, meaning that the relationship is two-way and periodontal therapy is beneficial to the control of both diseases.
- *Medications* such as phenytoin, cyclosporine, and nifedipine may predispose to gingival overgrowth in patients with gingivitis.
- *Genetic traits*, which result in diseases that modify the periodontal structures or change the immune or inflammatory responses, can result in gross periodontal destruction in the affected individual; although the destruction seen may imitate periodontitis, this is not etiopathologically chronic periodontitis.

Stress

Stressful life events and negative emotions have been shown to modulate several physiologic systems, including the endocrine and the immune system, leading to health changes (Kiecolt-Glaser *et al.* 2002; LeResche & Dworkin 2002). The association between stress and disease is particularly strong for infectious diseases, inflammatory conditions, and impaired wound healing (Kiecolt-Glaser *et al.* 2002; LeResche & Dworkin 2002; Broadbent *et al.* 2003). Specific periodontal conditions have been associated with psychosocial variables, including chronic periodontitis (Green *et al.* 1986; Linden *et al.* 1996; Genco *et al.* 1999; Wimmer *et al.* 2002; Pistorius *et al.* 2002), necrotizing ulcerative gingivitis (Shields 1977; Cohen-Cole *et al.* 1983; Horning & Cohen 1995), chronic and experimental gingivitis (Minneman *et al.* 1995; Deinzer *et al.* 1998; Waschul *et al.* 2003). In adults, the reported contribution of psychosocial factors to enhanced gingivitis expression (Deinzer *et al.* 1998) may relate to the stress-associated increase in plaque accumulation (Deinzer *et al.* 2001). However, the possible association of other psychosocial variables, such as personality traits and coping behavior, which are associated with either susceptibility or resistance to stress, with changes in the inflammatory response of the gingiva to *de novo* plaque accumulation, remains uncertain (Trombelli *et al.* 2005).

Most of the literature on stress and periodontal conditions is quite old, and reports of acute necrotizing ulcerative gingivitis (or trench mouth) were made on stressed soldiers on the front line during World War I. It is understood that stress may be immunosuppressive and that acute necrotizing ulcerative gingivitis may occur in the immunosuppressed (also in HIV patients), but there is insufficient data as yet to substantiate the assumption that psychosocial factors are indeed of etiologic importance in chronic periodontitis.

Genetics

There is convincing evidence from twin studies for a genetic predisposition to the periodontal diseases. The twin studies have indicated that risk of chronic periodontitis has a high inherited component. A great deal of research is underway attempt-

ing to identify the genes and polymorphisms associated with all forms of periodontitis. It is likely that chronic periodontitis involves many genes, the composition of which may vary across individuals and races. Much attention has focused on polymorphisms associated with the genes involved in cytokine production (Shapira *et al.* 2005). Such polymorphisms have been linked to an increased risk for chronic periodontitis but these findings have yet to be corroborated (Kinane & Hart 2003; Kinane *et al.* 2005).

Scientific basis for treatment of chronic periodontitis

Chronic periodontitis is initiated and sustained by microorganisms living in biofilm communities which are present in supra- and subgingival plaque in the form of uncalcified and calcified biofilms. Prevention of initiation or primary prevention of periodontitis is clearly related to preventing formation and/or eradication of the microbial biofilm and it follows that prevention of gingivitis is a primary preventive measure for chronic periodontitis. Initial periodontal therapy or basic treatment of periodontitis involves the removal of both sub- and supragingival plaque. The clinical outcome is largely dependent on the skill of the operator in removing subgingival plaque and the skill and motivation of the patient in practicing adequate home care. A further variable is the innate susceptibility of the patient which is related to the way in which their innate, inflammatory, and immune systems operate in response to the microbial challenge. In addition, local and systemic risk factors can influence the quantity and quality of both the microbial challenge and the host response to these pathogens. The relative contribution of these risk factors has yet to be fully determined but their influence would be limited if the periodontium were kept free of microbial plaque. Thus, sub- and supragingival debridement and the quality of the patient's home care are of vital importance in preventing inflammation that manifests as both gingivitis and periodontitis.

References

Abbas, F., van der Velden, U., Hart A.A., Moorer, W.R., Vroom, T.M. & Scholte, G. (1986). Bleeding/plaque ratio and the development of gingival inflammation. *Journal of Clinical Periodontology* **13**, 774–782.

Barr, C., Lopez, M.R. & Rua-Dobbs, A. (1992). Periodontal changes by HIV serostatus in a cohort of homosexual and bisexual men. *Journal of Clinical Periodontology* **19**, 794–801.

Broadbent, E., Petrie, K.J., Alley, P.G. & Booth, R.J. (2003). Psychological stress impairs early wound repair following surgery. *Psychosomatic Medicine* **65**, 865–869.

Cohen-Cole, S.A., Cogen, R.B., Stevens, A.W. Jr., Kirk, K., Gaitan, E., Bird, J. & Cooksey, R. (1983). Psychiatric, psychosocial, and endocrine correlates of acute necrotizing ulcerative gingivitis (trench mouth): a preliminary report. *Psychiatric Medicine* **1**, 215–225.

Deinzer, R., Ruttermann, S., Mobes, O. & Herforth, A. (1998). Increase in gingival inflammation under academic stress. *Journal of Clinical Periodontology* **25**, 431–433.

Deinzer, R., Hilpert, D., Bach, K., Schawacht, M. & Herforth, A. (2001). Effects of academic stress on oral hygiene – a potential link between stress and plaque-associated disease? *Journal of Clinical Periodontology* **28**, 459–464.

Ellis, J.S., Seymour, R.A., Steele, J.G., Robertson, P., Butler, T.J. & Thomason, J.M. (1999). Prevalence of gingival overgrowth induced by calcium channel blockers: a community-based study. *Journal of Periodontology* **70**, 63–67.

Flemmig, T.F. (1999). Periodontitis. *Annals of Periodontology* **4**, 32–38.

Genco, R.J., Ho, A.W., Grossi, S.G., Dunford, R.G. & Tedesco, L.A. (1999). Relationship of stress, distress and inadequate coping behaviors to periodontal disease. *Journal of Periodontology* **70**, 711–723.

Green, L.W., Tryon, W.W., Marks, B. & Huryn, J. (1986). Periodontal disease as a function of life events stress. *Journal of Human Stress* **12**, 32–36.

Horning, G.M. & Cohen, M.E. (1995) Necrotizing ulcerative gingivitis, periodontitis, and stomatitis: clinical staging and predisposing factors. *Journal of Periodontology* **66**, 990–998.

Joss, A., Adler, R. & Lang, N.P. (1994). Bleeding on probing. A parameter for monitoring periodontal conditions in clinical practice. *Journal of Clinical Periodontology* **21**, 402–408.

Kiecolt-Glaser, J.K., McGuire, L., Robles, T.F. & Glaser, R. (2002). Psychoneuroimmunology and psychosomatic medicine: back to the future. *Psychosomatic Medicine* **64**, 15–28.

Kinane, D.F. (1999). Periodontitis modified by systemic factors. *Annals of Periodontology* **4**, 54–64.

Kinane, D.F. & Chestnutt, I. (2000). Smoking and periodontal disease. *Critical Reviews in Oral Biology and Medicine* **11**, 356–365.

Kinane, D.F. & Hart, T.C. (2003). Genes and gene polymorphisms associated with periodontal disease. *Critical Reviews in Oral Biology and Medicine* **14**, 430–449.

Kinane, D.F. & Attström, R. (2005). Advances in the pathogenesis of periodontitis. Group B consensus report of the fifth European Workshop in Periodontology. *Journal of Clinical Periodontology* **32**, Suppl 6, 130–131.

Kinane, D.F., Shiba, H. & Hart, T.C. (2005). The genetic basis of periodontitis. *Periodontology 2000* **39**, 91–117.

LeResche, L. & Dworkin, S.F. (2002). The role of stress in inflammatory disease, including periodontal disease: review of concepts and current findings. *Periodontology 2000* **30**, 91–103.

Lang, N.P., Adler, R., Joss, A. & Nyman S. (1990). Absence of bleeding on probing. An indicator of periodontal stability. *Journal of Clinical Periodontology* **17**, 714–721.

Linden, G.J., Mullally, B.H. & Freeman, R. (1996). Stress and the progression of periodontal disease. *Journal of Clinical Periodontology* **23**, 675–680.

Lindhe, J., Hamp, S. & Löe H. (1975). Plaque induced periodontal disease in beagle dogs. A 4-year clinical, roentgenographical and histometrical study. *Journal of Periodontal Research* **8**, 1–10.

Löe, H., Theilade, E. & Jensen, S.B. (1965). Experimental gingivitis in man. *Journal of Periodontology* **36**, 177–187.

Löe, H., Anerud, A., Boysen, H. & Smith, M. (1978), The natural history of periodontal disease in man. The rate of periodontal destruction before 40 years of age. *Journal of Periodontology* **49**, 607–620.

Marsh, P.D. (2005). Dental plaque: biological significance of a biofilm and community life-style. *Journal of Clinical Periodontology* **32** (Suppl 6), 7–15.

Michalowicz, B.S., Aeppli, D., Virag, J.G., Klump, D.G., Hinrichs, J.E., Segal, N.L., Bouchard, T.J. & Philstrom, B.L. (1991). Periodontal findings in adult twins. *Journal of Periodontology* **62**, 293–299.

Michalowicz, B.S. (1994). Genetic and heritable risk factors in periodontal disease. *Journal of Periodontology* **65**, 479–488.

Michalowicz, B.S., Diehl, S.R., Gunsolley, J.C., Sparks, B.S., Brooks, C.N., Koertge, T.E., Califano, J.V., Burmeister, J.A. & Schenkein, H.A. (2000). Evidence of a substantial genetic basis for risk of adult periodontitis. *Journal of Periodontology* **71**, 1699–1707.

Minneman, M.A., Cobb, C., Soriano, F., Burns, S. & Schuchman, L. (1995). Relationships of personality traits and stress to gingival status or soft-tissue oral pathology: an exploratory study. *Journal of Public Health Dentistry* **55**, 22–27.

Pistorius, A., Krahwinkel, T., Willershausen, B. & Boekstegen, C. (2002). Relationship between stress factors and periodontal disease. *European Journal of Medical Research* **7**, 393–398.

Ritchie, C. & Kinane, D.F. (2005). Nutrition, inflammation, and periodontal disease. *Nutrition* **19**, 475–476.

Scapoli, C., Tatakis, D.N., Mamolini, E. & Trombelli, L. (2005). Modulation of clinical expression of plaque-induced gingivitis: interleukin-1 gene cluster polymorphisms. *Journal of Periodontology* **76**, 49–56.

Schätzle, M., Löe, H., Burgin, W., Ånerud, Å., Boysen, H. & Lang, N.P. (2003). Clinical course of chronic periodontitis. I. Role of gingivitis. *Journal of Clinical Periodontology* **30**, 887–901.

Schätzle, M., Löe, H., Lang, N.P., Burgin, W., Ånerud, Å. & Boysen, H. (2004). The clinical course of chronic periodontitis. *Journal of Clinical Periodontology* **31**, 1122–1127.

Shapira, L., Wilensky, A. & Kinane, D.F. (2005). Effect of genetic variability on the inflammatory response to periodontal infection. *Journal of Clinical Periodontology* **32** (Suppl 6), 72–86

Shields, W.D. (1977). Acute necrotizing ulcerative gingivitis. A study of some of the contributing factors and their validity in an army population. *Journal of Periodontology* **48**, 346–349.

Socransky, S.S., Haffajee, A.D., Goodson, J.M. & Lindhe, J. (1984). New concepts of destructive periodontal disease. *Journal of Clinical Periodontology* **11**, 21–32.

Suda, R., Cao, C., Hasegawa, K., Yang, S., Sasa, R. & Suzuki, M. (2000). 2-year observation of attachment loss in a rural Chinese population. *Journal of Periodontology* **71**, 1067–1072.

Tatakis, D.N. & Trombelli, L. (2004). Modulation of clinical expression of plaque-induced gingivitis. I. Background review and rationale. *Journal of Clinical Periodontology* **31**, 229–238.

Theilade, E., Wright, W.H., Börglum-Jensen, S. & Löe, H. (1966). Experimental gingivitis in man. II. A longitudinal clinical and bacteriological investigation. *Journal of Periodontal Research* **1**, 1–13.

Thorstensson, H. (1995) Periodontal disease in adult insulin-dependent diabetics. *Swedish Dental Journal* **107** (Suppl), 1–68.

Trombelli, L., Scapoli, C., Tatakis, D.N. & Grassi, L. (2005). Modulation of clinical expression of plaque-induced gingivitis: effects of personality traits, social support and stress. *Journal of Clinical Periodontology* **32**, 1143–1150.

Trombelli, L., Scapoli, C., Tatakis, D.N. & Minenna, L. (2006). Modulation of clinical expression of plaque-induced gingivitis: response in aggressive periodontitis subjects. *Journal of Clinical Periodontology* **33**, 79–85.

Trombelli, L., Tatakis, D.N., Scapoli, C., Bottega, S., Orlandini, E. & Tosi, M. (2004). Modulation of clinical expression of plaque-induced gingivitis. II. Identification of "high responder" and "low responder" subjects. *Journal of Clinical Periodontology* **31**, 239–252.

Waschul, B., Herforth, A., Stiller-Winkler, R., Idel, H., Granrath, N. & Deinzer, R. (2003). Effects of plaque, psychological stress and gender on crevicular Il-1beta and Il-1ra secretion. *Journal of Clinical Periodontology* **30**, 238–248.

Wilton, J.M.A., Griffiths, G.S. & Curtis, M.A. (1988). Detection of high-risk groups and individuals for periodontal diseases. *Journal of Clinical Periodontology* **15**, 339–346.

Winkel, E.G., Abbas, F., van der Velden, U., Vroom, T.M., Scholte, G. & Hart, A.A. (1987). Experimental gingivitis in relation to age in individuals not susceptible to periodontal destruction. *Journal of Clinical Periodontology* **14**, 499–507.

Wimmer, G., Janda, M., Wieselmann-Penkner, K., Jakse, N., Polansky, R. & Pertl, C. (2002). Coping with stress: its influence on periodontal disease. *Journal of Periodontology* **73**, 1343–1351.

Chapter 19

Aggressive Periodontitis

Maurizio S. Tonetti and Andrea Mombelli

Periodontitis is an infection that can have many different clinical presentations. This has led to the recognition of different clinical syndromes. Until recently, the question of whether or not these dissimilar clinical presentations represented different forms of disease has been open to discussion. Today several lines of evidence support the existence of truly different forms of periodontitis. These include:

1. The growing clinical consensus of differential prognosis and need for specific treatment approaches for the various syndromes
2. Heterogeneity in etiology with possible therapeutic implications
3. Heterogeneity in genetic and environmental susceptibility.

At the 1999 international classification workshop, the different forms of periodontitis were reclassified into three major forms (chronic, aggressive, and necrotizing forms of periodontitis) and into periodontal manifestations of systemic diseases. This chapter deals with aggressive, type 1, periodontitis. Until recently, this group of diseases was defined primarily based on the age of onset/diagnosis and was thus named early onset periodontitis (EOP). Features of this form of disease, however, can present themselves at any age and this form of periodontitis is not necessarily confined to individuals under the arbitrarily chosen age of 35.

Aggressive periodontitis (AgP) comprises a group of rare, often severe, rapidly progressive forms of periodontitis often characterized by an early age of clinical manifestation and a distinctive tendency for cases to aggregate in families. At the above mentioned classification workshop, AgP was characterized by the following major common features (Lang *et al*. 1999):

- Non-contributory medical history
- Rapid attachment loss and bone destruction
- Familial aggregation of cases.

Frequently AgP presents early in the life of the individual; this implies that etiologic agents have been able to cause clinically detectable levels of disease over a relatively short time. This fact is central to the current understanding of these diseases, since it implies infection with a highly virulent microflora and/or a high level of subject susceptibility to periodontal disease. AgP, however, can occur at any age. Diagnosis of AgP requires exclusion of the presence of systemic diseases that may severely impair host defenses and lead to premature tooth loss (periodontal manifestations of systemic diseases).

The existence of specific forms of AgP has also been recognized based on specific clinical and laboratory features: localized aggressive periodontitis (LAP, formerly known as localized juvenile periodontitis or LJP) and generalized aggressive periodontitis (GAP, formerly termed generalized juvenile periodontitis (GJP) or generalized early onset periodontitis, G-EOP) (Tonetti & Mombelli 1999).

In spite of its rare occurrence AgP has been the focus of many investigations aimed at understanding its etiology and pathogenesis. Difficulties in gathering sufficiently large populations, however, have resulted in few clinical studies addressing both diagnostic and therapeutic procedures for these subjects. Utilization of both clinical and advanced diagnostic procedures as well as a variety of treatment approaches remains largely anecdotal and based on the specific experience of individual clinicians rather than on well documented scientific evidence.

Classification and clinical syndromes

In the absence of an etiologic classification, aggressive forms of periodontal disease have been defined based on the following primary features (Lang *et al.* 1999):

- Non-contributory medical history
- Rapid attachment loss and bone destruction
- Familial aggregation of cases.

Secondary features that are considered to be generally but not universally present are:

- Amounts of microbial deposits inconsistent with the severity of periodontal tissue destruction
- Elevated proportions of *Actinobacillus actinomycetemcomitans* (recently renamed *Aggregatibacter actinomycetemcomitans*) and, in some Far East populations, *Porphyromonas gingivalis*
- Phagocyte abnormalities
- Hyper-responsive macrophage phenotype, including elevated production of prostaglandin E_2 (PGE_2) and interleukin-1β (IL-1β) in response to bacterial endotoxins
- Progression of attachment loss and bone loss may be self-arresting.

The international classification workshop identified clinical and laboratory features deemed specific enough to allow subclassification of AgP into localized and generalized forms (Lang *et al.* 1999; Tonetti & Mombelli 1999). The following features were identified:

- *Localized aggressive periodontitis* (LAP) (Fig. 19-1):
  - Circumpubertal onset
  - Localized first molar/incisor presentation with interproximal attachment loss on at least two permanent teeth, one of which is a first molar, and involving no more than two teeth other than first molars and incisors
  - Robust serum antibody response to infecting agents
- *Generalized aggressive periodontitis* (GAP) (Fig. 19-2):
  - Usually affecting persons under 30 years of age, but patients may be older
  - Generalized interproximal attachment loss affecting at least three permanent teeth other than first molars and incisors
  - Pronounced episodic nature of the destruction of attachment and alveolar bone
  - Poor serum antibody response to infecting agents.

Diagnosis of one of these AgP forms requires the absence of systemic diseases that may severely impair host defenses and lead to premature exfoliation of teeth. In such instances the appropriate clinical diagnosis will be periodontal manifestation of systemic disease.

GAP represents the most heterogeneous group and includes the most severe forms of periodontitis. They comprise forms originally described as generalized juvenile periodontitis (emphasis on a possible relationship with LAP), severe periodontitis (emphasis on the advanced destruction in comparison with patient age), or rapidly progressing periodontitis (emphasis on the fast rate of progression of lesions in these forms). Each of these GAP forms, however, remains highly heterogeneous in terms of clinical presentation and response to therapy. The European Workshop on Periodontology has therefore suggested that, while a better etiologic classification remains unavailable, these forms should be considered as a group to be further defined by the use of various clinical descriptors of the disease based on clinical, microbiologic, and immunologic parameters (Attström & Van der Velden 1993). Further rationale for an imprecise classification of these GAP forms comes from the fact that, given the severity of the disease and the heterogeneity of clinical presentation, each of these rare cases deserves individual consideration.

Subjects often present with attachment loss that does not fit the specific diagnostic criteria established for AgP or chronic periodontitis; this occurrence has been termed *incidental attachment loss*. It includes: recession associated with trauma or tooth position; attachment loss associated with impacted third molars; attachment loss associated with removal of impacted third molars, etc. It may include initial clinical presentations of periodontitis. Patients with this clinical diagnosis should be considered as a high-risk group for AgP or chronic periodontitis.

Besides clinical presentation, a variety of radiographic, microbiologic, and immunologic parameters are currently being used, along with the assessment of environmental exposures such as cigarette smoking, to further describe the AgP affecting the individual subject. These descriptors are important in treatment selection and to establish long-term prognosis. They will be further discussed in the section on diagnosis later in this chapter.

It is also important to underline that, in the present state of uncertainty regarding both the causative agents and the genetic and environmental susceptibility to AgP, it is possible that, in spite of the lines of evidence presented above, LAP and GAP may simply represent phenotypic variations of a single disease entity. Conversely, it is possible that different AgP forms may manifest themselves with a common clinical presentation. This aspect is of great diagnostic and therapeutic importance.

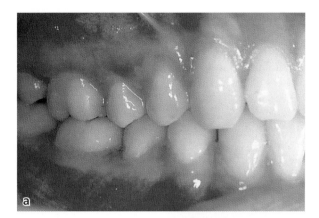
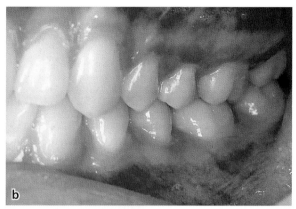
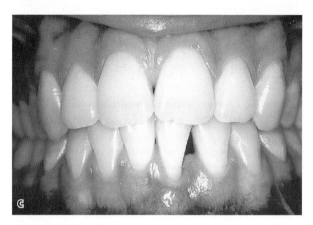
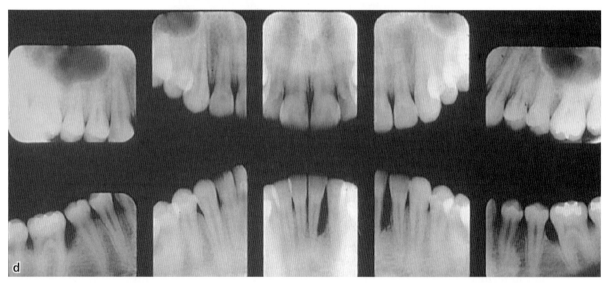

Fig. 19-1 (a–c) Clinical appearance of the periodontal tissues of a 15-year-old girl suffering from localized aggressive periodontitis. Note the proper oral hygiene conditions and the scalloped outline of the gingival margin. In the lower anterior region, the interdental papilla between teeth 31 and 32 has been lost. (d) Intraoral radiographs show the presence of localized angular bony defects, associated with clinical attachment level loss, at the mesial aspect of tooth 46, 36 and at the distal aspect of tooth 31. No significant bone loss and/or attachment loss was detectable in other areas of the dentition. Diagnosis: localized aggressive periodontitis (LAP). (e–g) Clinical appearance of the 14-year-old sister of the proband depicted in (a–d). Note that in spite of the excellent oral hygiene status, bleeding on probing was provoked in the mesial of the molars, where deep pockets were present. (h) Angular bone loss is evident on the mesial of 16, 26 and 46.

Some case reports have indicated that some subjects may experience periodontitis affecting the primary dentition, followed by LAP and later by GAP (Shapira *et al.* 1994). One investigation indicated that the primary dentition of LAP patients presented

bone loss at primary molars in 20–52% of cases, suggesting that at least some LAP cases may initially affect the primary dentition (Sjodin *et al.* 1989, 1993). Furthermore, in LAP subjects an association between the number of lesions and the age of the subject has

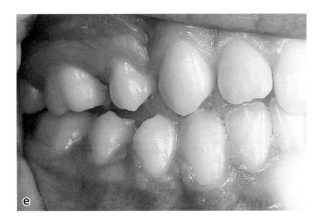
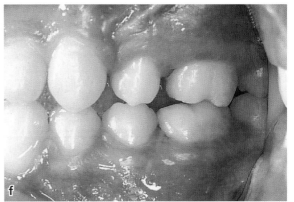

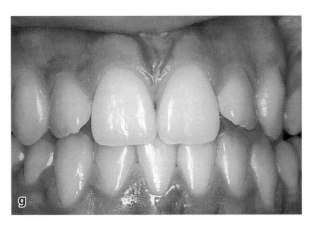

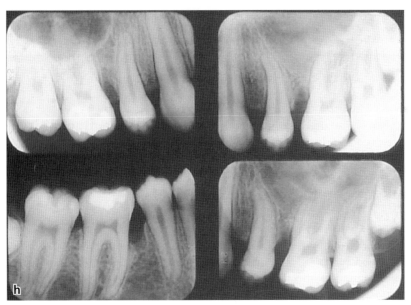

Fig. 19-1 *Continued*

been described, suggesting an age-dependent shift from localized to generalized forms of AgP (Hormand & Frandsen 1979; Burmeister *et al.* 1984).

Epidemiology

Given the recent definition of AgP and the fact that it does not represent just a new term for the previously defined EOP, epidemiologic studies available relate primarily to EOP. Relatively few investigations employing different epidemiologic techniques have estimated the prevalence and the progression of EOP in the primary and permanent dentition(s) of children and young adults. All available investigations, however, indicate that early onset (aggressive) forms of periodontal diseases are detectable in all age and ethnic groups (Papapanou 1996). Wide variation in prevalence, however, has been reported, with some

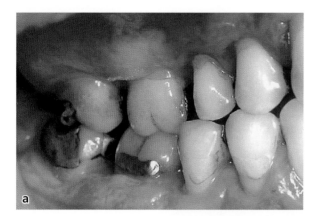
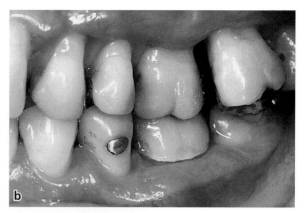
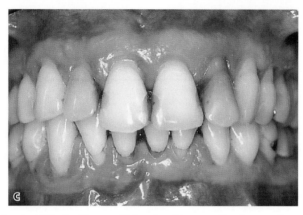

Fig. 19-2 (a–c) Clinical presentation in 1990 of a 32-year-old female with generalized severe bone loss and clinical attachment loss, recession of the gingival margin and presence of deep periodontal pockets. Presence of local factors, and intense inflammation and edema of the gingival margin are evident. (d–f). Previous radiographic examinations were available from 1984 and 1987. Comparison of the radiographs obtained over the 6-year period from 1984 to 1990 indicates that most of the periodontal destruction occurred during the last 3 years. The patient had been smoking 20 cigarettes/day for more than 10 years. Diagnosis: generalized aggressive periodontitis (GAP) in a cigarette smoker.

studies showing up to 51.5% affected individuals. These differences are probably due to differences in the employed epidemiologic methodologies and definition of EOP.

Primary dentition

Little evidence is available concerning the prevalence of AgP affecting the primary dentition. In the few studies from industrialized countries, marginal alveolar bone loss has been found to affect the primary dentition of 5–11-year-olds with frequencies ranging from 0.9–4.5% of subjects (Sweeney *et al.* 1987; Bimstein *et al.* 1994; Sjodin & Mattson 1994). In this respect, it should be emphasized that periodontitis affecting the primary dentition does not necessarily mean presence of an aggressive form of periodontitis, but may indicate a chronic form of disease with relative abundance of local factors (plaque and calculus). A clinical case of localized periodontitis affecting the primary dentition is illustrated in Fig. 19-3. More severe cases affecting the primary dentition and leading to tooth exfoliation early in life are usually interpreted as periodontal manifestations of systemic (hematologic) diseases, such as leukocyte adhesion deficiency (see Chapter 7 and Fig. 19-4).

Permanent dentition

In the permanent dentition of 13–20-year-old individuals, the majority of studies have reported a prevalence of periodontitis of less than 1% (usually 0.1–0.2% in Caucasian populations). The risk of developing periodontitis at such an early age, however, does not seem to be shared equally in the population: among US schoolchildren 5–17 years of age, the prevalence of periodontitis has been estimated to range from about 0.2% for white subjects to about 2.6% for black subjects (Löe & Brown 1991). Furthermore, in these young age groups higher prevalence of periodontitis has been reported in studies from some developing countries (see Chapter 7).

Longitudinal studies of disease progression in adolescents indicate that subjects with signs of destructive periodontitis at a young age are prone to further deterioration. Such deterioration appears to be more pronounced at initially affected sites, and in patients diagnosed with LAP and from low socioeconomic groups. Deterioration of the periodontal status involves both an increase in extent (number of lesions within the dentition) and in severity of lesions (further alveolar bone loss at initially diseased sites) (Fig. 19-5)

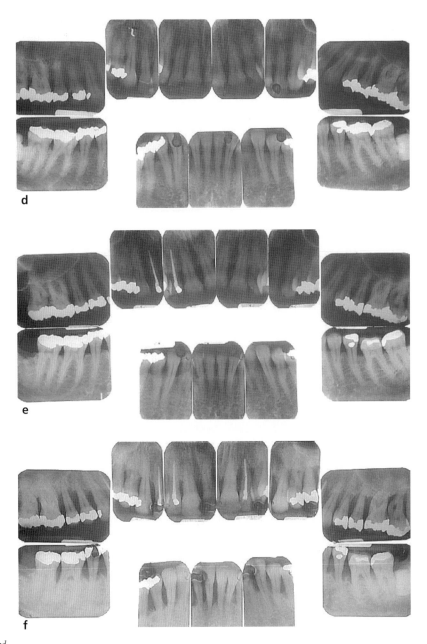

d

e

f

Fig. 19-2 *Continued*

(Clerehugh *et al.* 1990; Lissau *et al.* 1990; Albandar *et al.* 1991a,b; Albandar 1993; Aass *et al.* 1994).

Some epidemiologic investigations have reported high prevalence of attachment loss in adolescents and young adults that did not fit the characteristics of recognized periodontitis clinical syndromes. Such occurrences have been termed *incidental attachment loss*, and have been reported in 1.6–26% of the subjects. This group is thought to comprise both initial forms of periodontitis (including AgP) and a variety of defects, such as recession due to traumatic toothbrushing, attachment loss associated with removal of impacted third molars, etc.

Conclusion

A small but significant proportion of children and young adults is affected by some form of periodon-

titis. A substantial proportion of these subjects is thought to be affected by AgP. Given the severity of these forms of periodontal disease and their tendency to progress, early detection of periodontitis, and AgP in particular, should be a primary concern of both practitioners and public health officers. The whole population, including children and young adults, should receive a periodontal screening as part of their routine dental examination.

Screening

Given the low prevalence of AgP patients within the population, cost-effective detection of cases requires utilization of a sensitive screening approach, i.e. the application of a diagnostic approach able to correctly identify most of the cases with disease. The objective of screening is the detection in a population of

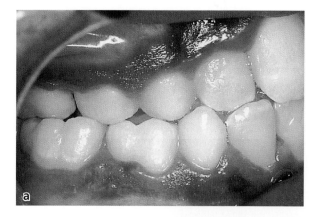
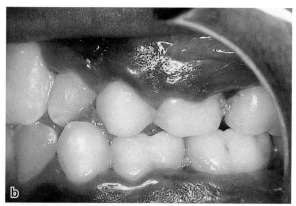
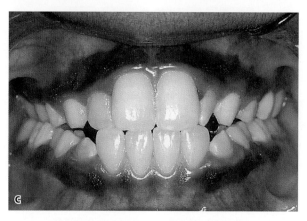
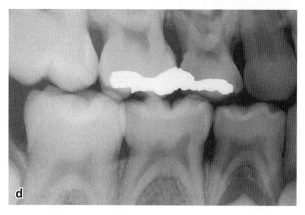
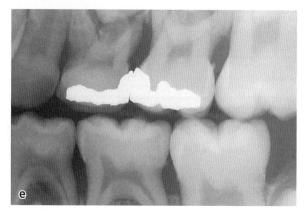

Fig. 19-3 Seven-year-old African American female presenting with radiographic alveolar bone loss and probing attachment loss at the primary molars and permanent first molars and incisors. (a–c) Clinical photographs, buccal view. (d–e) Bite-wing radiographs. Clinical presentation shows moderate plaque accumulation, localized gingival inflammation, with ulceration of the gingival margin and loss of the interdental papilla mesial of #65. In the primary molar regions there were 4–6 mm pockets with bleeding on probing. Bone loss and attachment loss were limited to the molar region. The mesial aspects of the first permanent molars are also initially involved. Radiographic subgingival calculus is evident. Note that the upper left posterior sextant seems to be more severely affected than the other posterior segments. Diagnosis: localized aggressive (type 1) periodontitis.

possibly diseased subjects that would require a more comprehensive examination. In periodontology, the most sensitive diagnostic test for the detection of periodontitis is the measurement of attachment loss by probing. Application of this diagnostic procedure in the mixed dentition and in teeth that are not fully erupted, however, may be difficult.

In younger subjects, therefore, a currently utilized screening approach is the measurement of the distance between the alveolar crest and the cemento-enamel junction on bite-wing radiographs. An advantage of this approach relates to the fact that in most industrialized countries bite-wing radiographs of children and young adolescents in mixed dentition are routinely taken for caries prevention programs; these radiographs should therefore be screened not only for carious lesions but also for the presence of marginal alveolar bone loss.

Recent investigations have attempted to determine the "normal" distance between the cemento-enamel junction and the alveolar crest of primary and permanent molars in 7–9-year-old children (Sjodin &

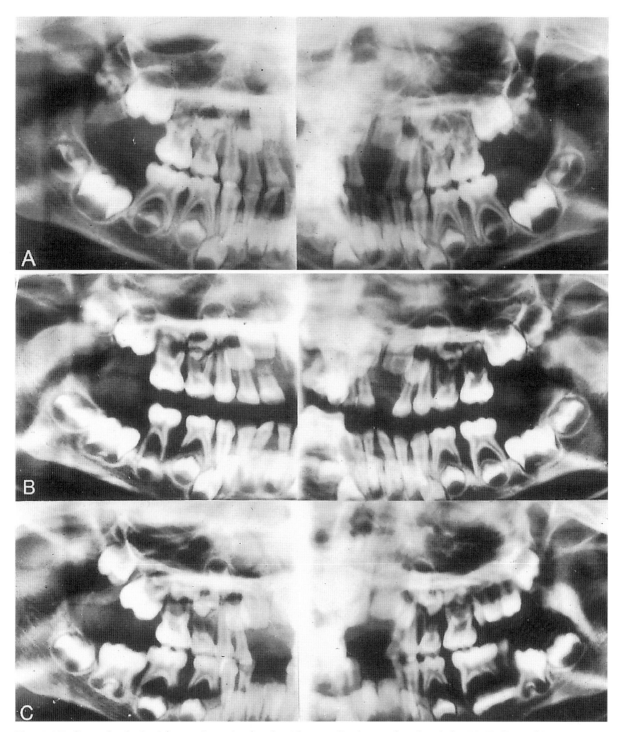

Fig. 19-4 Radiographs obtained from a Caucasian female with generalized pre-pubertal periodontitis. Radiographic situation in (A) April 1978 when she was 4–5 years old, (B) December 1978, and (C) August 1979. The radiographs illustrate the extent of alveolar bone loss that occurred over the 15-month period. Note the widespread bone loss. During infancy, this patient had severe, recurrent skin and ear infections sustained by *Staphylococcus aureus* and *Pseudomonas aeruginosa*, respectively. Delayed healing was also observed following minor injuries. White cell counts revealed a persistent leukocytosis, with absolute neutrophil counts always above 8000/mm³. Gingival biopsy indicated that the inflammatory infiltrate consisted almost completely of plasma cells and lymphocytes. No neutrophils were present, in spite of the abundance of these cells in the circulation. This history and clinical manifestation appears to be consistent with the diagnosis of periodontal manifestations of systemic disease in a subject with leukocyte adhesion deficiency (LAD). From Page *et al.* (1983b) with permission from the American Academy of Periodontology.

Mattson 1992; Needleman *et al.* 1997). Median distances at primary molars were 0.8–1.4 mm. These values were in agreement with those previously reported for primary molars of 3–11-year-old children (Bimstein & Soskolne 1988). The cemento-

enamel junction of permanent molars was 0–0.5 mm apical to the alveolar crest in 7–9-year-olds. These values were age-dependent, and related to the state of eruption of the tooth. In general, however, it should be noted that the majority of children present with

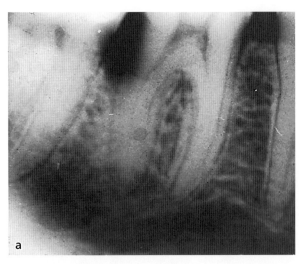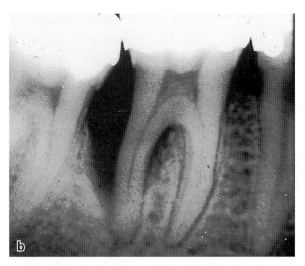

Fig. 19-5 Radiographs illustrating bone loss at the distal aspect of the mandibular first molar in a 15-year-old girl (a) and progression of disease 1 year later (b).

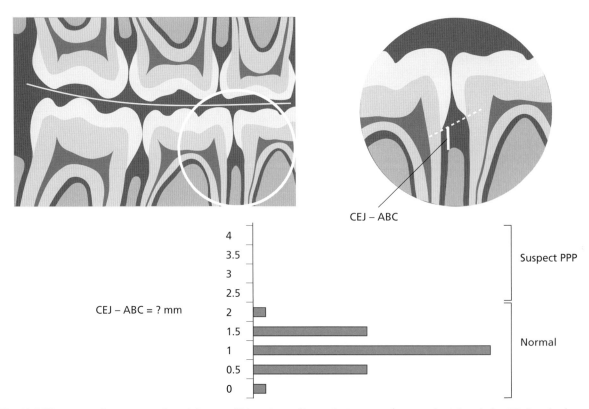

Fig. 19-6 Diagrammatic representation of the use of bite-wing radiographs to screen for prepubertal periodontitis in mixed dentition. The distance from the cemento-enamel junction (CEJ) and the alveolar bone crest (ABC) is measured from a line connecting the CEJ of the two adjacent teeth. Measurements are taken for each mesial and distal surface. Normal CEJ-ABC distances for 7–9 year olds are less than 2.0 mm. If the measurement exceeds this value, prepubertal periodontitis should be suspected, and a comprehensive periodontal examination should be performed.

distances significantly smaller than the 2–3 mm considered normal for the completely erupted dentitions of adults. In children, significantly greater distances have been detected at sites with caries, fillings or open contacts, indicating that these factors may contribute to bone loss in similar ways to those in adult patients. Furthermore, presence of one of these local factors may suggest a local cause of bone loss, other than periodontitis. A distance of 2 mm between the cemento-enamel junction and the alveolar crest, in the absence of the above-mentioned local factors, argues therefore for a suspected diagnosis of periodontitis (Figs. 19-6 and 19-7) (Sjodin & Mattson 1992). This tentative diagnosis will have to be confirmed by a complete periodontal examination. In utilizing bite-wing radiographs for the screening of

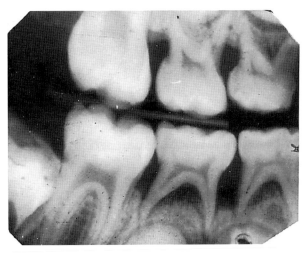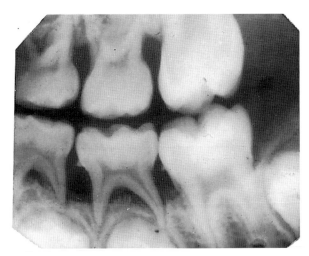

Fig. 19-7 Bite-wing radiographs illustrating advanced bone loss at primary molars, and initial involvement of the mesial aspect of the first molar in a child with early onset periodontitis. Note the marginal pattern of bone loss, which is significantly different from the pattern expected in association with the normal exfoliation of deciduous teeth. Subgingival calculus can also be observed.

patients, clinicians should be aware that radiographic marginal bone loss (in the presence of probing attachment loss) is a highly specific diagnostic sign of periodontitis. Its sensitivity, however, is lower than that of periodontal probing because initial intrabony lesions may not appear on radiographs as a result of the masking effects of intact cortical plates (Suomi *et al.* 1968; Lang & Hill 1977). Some initial cases of periodontitis may therefore remain undetected.

In older adolescents and adults, periodontal probing is a more appropriate screening examination than the use of radiographs. It is important to differentiate between clinical use of periodontal probing to perform a complete periodontal examination, and its use as a screening tool. Using probing to detect attachment loss during a screening examination requires circumferential probing to evaluate all sites around the tooth. In a screening examination, however, attachment loss values for all sites are usually not recorded. Furthermore, the screening examination can be stopped once evidence of attachment loss has been detected, and therefore the need for a comprehensive examination has been established. The American Academy of Periodontology has recently endorsed a simplified screening examination for this purpose. This examination is based on a modification of the Community Periodontal Index of Treatment Needs (CPITN) (Ainamo *et al.* 1982; American Academy of Periodontology & American Dental Association 1992).

Once a case has been detected by a screening examination, a comprehensive periodontal examination will be necessary to establish a proper diagnosis. At this stage, once a case of periodontitis has been confirmed, a differential diagnosis between aggressive (type 1) periodontitis and chronic (type 2) periodontitis needs to be made in accordance with the criteria mentioned above and keeping in mind that

cases which do not fit the AgP criteria should be diagnosed as chronic periodontitis.

Conclusion

Screening periodontal examinations should be performed as part of every dental visit. Marginal bone loss assessed on bite-wing radiographs, though less sensitive than periodontal probing, may be used as a screening tool in subjects with primary and mixed dentitions. Attachment loss evaluated by periodontal probing is the most sensitive screening approach currently available; it should be used in older adolescents and adults. Differential diagnosis between AgP and chronic periodontitis is made based on exclusion of AgP.

Etiology and pathogenesis

As a group, aggressive forms of periodontitis are characterized by severe destruction of the periodontal attachment apparatus at an early age. This early manifestation of clinically detectable lesions is generally interpreted as being the expression of highly virulent causative agents or high levels of susceptibility of the individual patient, or a combination of the two.

Bacterial etiology

The evidence implicating bacteria in the etiology of periodontitis has been described in Chapter 9. The most abundant evidence regarding a bacterial etiology of AgP comes from studies of LAP. Evidence relating to other forms of AgP (GAP) will be discussed only when specifically different from LAP.

Acceptance of bacterial etiology of aggressive forms of periodontitis has been particularly difficult since clinical presentation of cases frequently shows little visible plaque accumulation, and proximal caries, another dental disease of bacterial origin affecting younger individuals, seems much less prevalent in LAP patients than in age-, gender-, and race-matched controls (Fine *et al.* 1984; Sioson *et al.* 2000). Of great importance, in this respect, were microscopic studies demonstrating the presence of a layer of bacterial deposits on the root surface of advanced AgP lesions (Listgarten 1976; Westergaard *et al.* 1978). Early studies attempting the identification of the involved bacteria using culture techniques were performed by Newman *et al.* and by Slots (Newman *et al.* 1976; Slots 1976; Newman & Socransky 1977). In these studies, Gram-negative organisms comprised approximately two thirds of the isolates from deep periodontal pockets. In contrast, these organisms averaged only about one third of the isolates in control sites with normal gingiva. A substantial part of the isolates was not identifiable at that time due to methodological limitations and ambiguous classification schemes. Dominant microorganisms in LAP included *Actinobacillus actinomycetemcomitans* (*A.a.*, now termed *Aggregatibacter actinomycetemcomitans*), *Capnocytophaga* sp., *Eikenella corrodens*, saccharolytic Bacteroides-like organisms now classified as *Prevotella* sp., and motile anaerobic rods today labeled *Campylobacter rectus*. Gram-positive isolates were mostly streptococci, actinomycetes, and peptostreptococci. *A.a.*, *Capnocytophaga* sp., and *Prevotella* sp. were also shown to be the most prominent members of the subgingival microbiota of periodontitis lesions in the primary dentition. The microbial patterns observed in periodontal lesions of the primary dentition seemed, however, to be more complex than the ones found in LAP patients.

One of these organisms, *A. actinomycetemcomitans*, a short, facultatively anaerobic, non-motile, Gram-negative rod, received particular attention and was increasingly viewed as a key microorganism in LAP. This view was principally based on four lines of evidence (Socransky & Haffajee 1992):

1. Association studies, linking the organism to the disease: *A.a.* was isolated in periodontal lesions from more than 90% of LAP patients and was much less frequent in periodontally healthy individuals (Table 19-1) (for more recent investigations, see also Ashley *et al.* 1988; Van der Velden *et al.* 1989; Albandar *et al.* 1990; Gunsolley *et al.* 1990; Slots *et al.* 1990; Asikainen *et al.* 1991; Aass *et al.* 1992; Ebersole *et al.* 1994; Listgarten *et al.* 1995). In some studies it was possible to demonstrate elevated levels of *A.a.* in sites showing evidence of recent or ongoing periodontal tissue destruction (Haffajee *et al.* 1984; Mandell 1984; Mandell *et al.* 1987).

2. Demonstration of virulence factors: *A.a.* was shown to produce several potentially pathogenic substances, including a leukotoxin, was capable of translocating across epithelial membranes, and could induce disease in experimental animals and non-oral sites (for review see Zambon *et al.* 1988; Slots & Schonfeld 1991).

3. Findings of immune responses towards this bacterium: investigators repeatedly reported significantly elevated levels of serum antibodies to *A.a.* in LAP patients (Listgarten *et al.* 1981; Tsai *et al.* 1981; Altman *et al.* 1982; Ebersole *et al.* 1982, 1983; Genco *et al.* 1985; Vincent *et al.* 1985; Mandell *et al.* 1987; Sandholm *et al.* 1987). Such patients were furthermore shown to produce antibodies locally against this organism at diseased sites (Schonfeld

Table 19-1 Classical studies on the distribution of *A.a.* in LAP, gingivitis, adult periodontitis, and in normal non-diseased subjects

Study	Diagnosis	No. of subjects (sites)	% *A.a.*-positive subjects	% *A.a.*-positive sites
Slots *et al.* 1980	LAP	10 (34)	90	79
	Adult periodontitis	12 (49)	50	35
	Normal juveniles	10 (60)	20	3
	Normal adults	11 (66)	36	17
Mandell & Socransky 1981	LAP	6 (18)	100	79
	Adult periodontitis	25 (50)	0	–
	Gingivitis	23 (46)	0	–
Zambon *et al.* 1983	LAP	29	97	–
	Adult periodontitis	134	21	–
	Normal juveniles/adults	142	17	–
Eisenmann *et al.* 1983	LAP	12 (12)	100	100
	Normal juveniles	10 (10)	60	60
Moore *et al.* 1985	LAP	14 (31)	36	5
Asikainen *et al.* 1986	LAP	19 (38)	89	68

See text for a selection of more recent investigations.

& Kagan 1982; Ebersole *et al.* 1985b; Tew *et al.* 1985).

4. Clinical studies showing a correlation between treatment outcomes and levels of *A.a.* after therapy: unsuccessful treatment outcomes were linked to a failure in reducing the subgingival load of *A.a.* (Slots & Rosling 1983; Haffajee *et al.* 1984; Christersson *et al.* 1985; Kornman & Robertson 1985; Mandell *et al.* 1986, 1987; Preus 1988).

In consideration of these findings, *A.a.* was one of the few oral microorganisms recognized by many to be a true infectious agent, and LAP as an infection essentially caused by *A.a.* Accepting such a concept has far-reaching consequences with regards to strategies for prevention and therapy. For example, if *A.a.* is a real exogenous pathogen for LAP, or AgP in general, avoidance of exposure to the organism becomes a relevant issue in prevention (the mere presence of *A.a.* would be an indication for intervention), and the elimination of *A.a.* may be a valid treatment goal. Consequently, highly sensitive tests to detect the bacterium would be useful diagnostic tools. Several studies have, in fact, provided evidence for transmission of *A.a.* between humans, e.g. from parent to child or between spouses (DiRienzo *et al.* 1990, 1994b; Preus *et al.* 1992; Petit *et al.* 1993a,b; Poulsen *et al.* 1994; Von Troil-Lindén *et al.* 1995). Other studies have indicated that *A.a.* can be eliminated with appropriate mechanical treatment and adjunctive antibiotic therapy (Rams *et al.* 1992; Pavicic *et al.* 1994).

However, the view of LAP as an *A.a.* infection did not remain undisputed. It was contested by citing cross-sectional studies showing a high general *A.a.* prevalence in certain populations, particularly from developing countries (Eisenmann *et al.* 1983; Dahlén *et al.* 1989; McNabb *et al.* 1992; Al-Yahfoufi *et al.* 1994; Gmür & Guggenheim 1994). It was also argued that *A.a.* could be detected in subgingival plaque samples from sites with and without disease, and that there were patients with LAP who apparently neither showed presence of *A.a.* in the oral flora nor had elevated antibody titers to the organism (Loesche *et al.* 1985; Moore 1987). A systematic review with the purpose of determining to what extent adjunctive microbiological testing could distinguish between chronic and aggressive periodontitis concluded that the presence or absence of *A.a.* (as well as of four other suspected periodontal pathogens) could not discriminate between subjects with aggressive periodontitis from those with chronic periodontitis (Mombelli *et al.* 2002). Although a diagnosis of AgP was more likely in a subject positive for *A.a.* than in an individual negative for this organism, any *A.a.*-positive individual with periodontitis was three times more likely to be suffering from chronic than from aggressive periodontitis.

If a putative pathogen can be detected frequently in subjects without a given clinical diagnosis, this suggests that not all humans are equally susceptible and/or that there is variation in virulence and pathogenic potential. Strong evidence has been produced in recent years demonstrating that the virulence of *A.a.* is in fact variable, and proving the existence of at least one particularly virulent subpopulation of *A.a.*

Using monoclonal antibody technology, five serotypes (a, b, c, d, e) of *A.a.* can be distinguished. Each of these serotypes represents a separate evolutionary lineage. A serotype-dependent pattern of association with LAP was found in the United States, where serotype b strains were more often isolated from patients with localized juvenile periodontitis than from other subjects (Zambon *et al.* 1983b, 1996). A higher frequency of serotype b strains was also reported from Finnish subjects with periodontitis (Asikainen *et al.* 1991, 1995). Differing results were, however, reported from other parts of the world, suggesting that there may be specific distribution patterns in ethnically distinct populations (Chung *et al.* 1989; Gmür & Baehni 1997; Höltta *et al.* 1994). Using restriction fragment length polymorphism (RFLP) analysis, DiRienzo *et al.* (1994a,b) could discriminate twelve genotypes of *A.a.* One of them (RFLP type II) was uniquely associated with periodontal disease. Others, however, were linked to healthy periodontal conditions.

Several properties of *A.a.* are regarded as important determinants of virulence and pathogenic potential (Table 19-2). All Gram-negative bacteria are enveloped by two membranes, of which the outer is rich in endotoxin. This identifying feature of Gram-negative bacteria consists of a lipid and a polysaccharide part and is therefore frequently termed lipopolysaccharide (LPS). LPS is set free when bacterial cells die or multiply. *A.a.* can also secrete membrane vesicles that can serve as transport vehicles to spread endotoxin as well as other pathogenic substances produced by the bacterium. The LPS of *A.a.* can activate host cells, and macrophages in

Table 19-2 Determinants of virulence and pathogenic potential of *A. actinomycetemcomitans*

Factor	Significance
Leukotoxin	Destroys human polymorphonuclear leukocytes and macrophages
Endotoxin	Activates host cells to secrete inflammatory mediators (prostaglandins, interleukin-1β, tumor necrosis factor-α)
Bacteriocin	May inhibit growth of beneficial species
Immunosuppressive factors	May inhibit IgG and IgM production
Collagenases	Cause degradation of collagen
Chemotactic inhibition factors	May inhibit neutrophil chemotaxis

particular, to secrete inflammatory mediators such as prostaglandins, interleukin-1β and tumor necrosis factor-α. It is also highly immunogenic, since high titers of antibodies against its antigenic determinant are frequently detected in infected individuals. Additional virulence factors interfering with fibroblast proliferation have been identified for certain strains of *A.a.* Immunosuppressive properties of *A.a.*, as well as collagenolytic activity and inhibition of neutrophil chemotaxis, have been demonstrated (for review see Fives-Taylor *et al.* 1996). The key element of virulence and pathogenicity of *A.a.*, however, is considered to be the production of a leukotoxin, playing an important role in the evasion of local host defenses. The leukotoxin produced by *A.a.* exhibits cytotoxic specificity and destroys human polymorphonuclear leukocytes and macrophages, but neither epithelial and endothelial cells nor fibroblasts. It belongs to the family of the RTX (Repeats in ToXin) toxins, which are pore-forming lytic toxins (for details see Lally *et al.* 1996).

Leukotoxin production varies significantly among strains of *A.a.* (Brogan *et al.* 1994; Kolodrubetz *et al.* 1989; Spitznagel *et al.* 1991; Zambon *et al.* 1983a). The strain-specific difference in leukotoxin production seems to be regulated at the level of transcription (Spitznagel *et al.* 1991). Brogan *et al.* (1994) detected a 530 bp deletion in the promoter region of the leukotoxin operon and found that strains with this feature produced 10–20 times more leukotoxin. Subsequent analysis showed that the occurrence of such highly toxigenic strains coincided with the high frequency of serotype b in patients with localized juvenile periodontitis, and that these strains actually constituted a specific clone of serotype b, now referred to as the JP2 clone (the initial isolate of this clone is strain JP2, from an African American child with prepubertal periodontitis) (Tsai *et al.* 1984). Extensive further research (Poulsen *et al.* 1994; Haubek *et al.* 1995, 1996, 1997, 2001; Tinoco *et al.* 1997; Bueno *et al.* 1998; He *et al.* 1999; Macheleidt *et al.* 1999; Mombelli *et al.* 1999; Contreras *et al.* 2000; Haraszthy *et al.* 2000; Tan *et al.* 2001; Cortelli *et al.* 2005) has clearly identified the JP2 clone as a common isolate in patients of North and West African descent suffering from aggressive periodontitis, even if they lived in another geographical region (e.g. North and South America or Europe). The disease association of RFLP type II reflects the fact that the JP2 clone represents a subpopulation of strains showing the RFLP type II pattern.

Our current knowledge with regards to the genetic and phenotypic diversity of *A.a.*, and its distribution in various populations and cohorts, with or without a clinical diagnosis of LAP, suggests that *A.a.* may be considered an opportunistic pathogen, or even a commensal bacterial species as a whole. However, at least one distinct subpopulation, the JP2 clone, displays the properties of a true pathogen in at least one group of humans of North and West African descent (Kilian *et al.* 2006). Prevention of vertical transmis-

sion of such virulent clones may a be feasible measure to prevent AgP (Van Winkelhoff & Boutaga 2005).

Generalized aggressive periodontitis (GAP), formerly named generalized early onset periodontitis (G-EOP) and rapidly progressive periodontitis (RPP), has been frequently associated with the detection of *Porphyromonas gingivalis*, *Bacteroides forsythus* and *A.a.* In contrast to *A.a.*, which is facultatively anaerobic, *P. gingivalis* and *B. forsythus* are fastidious strict anaerobes. *P. gingivalis* produces several potent enzymes, in particular collagenases and proteases, endotoxin, fatty acids, and other possibly toxic agents (Shah 1993). A relationship between the clinical outcome of therapy and bacterial counts has also been documented for *P. gingivalis*, and non-responding lesions often contain this organism in elevated proportions. High local and systemic immune responses against this bacterium have been demonstrated in patients with GAP (Tolo & Schenck 1985; Vincent *et al.* 1985; Ebersole *et al.* 1986; Murray *et al.* 1989).

Bacterial damage to the periodontium

Disease-associated bacteria are thought to cause destruction of the marginal periodontium via two related mechanisms: (1) the direct action of the microorganisms or their products on the host tissues, and/or (2) as a result of their eliciting tissue-damaging inflammatory responses (see Chapter 11) (Tonetti 1993). The relative importance of these two mechanisms in AgP remains speculative. Human investigations have indicated that *Aggregatibacter actinomycetemcomitans* is able to translocate across the junctional epithelium and invade the underlying connective tissue (Saglie *et al.* 1988). These data support the hypothesis that direct bacterial invasion may be responsible for some of the observed tissue breakdown. Data from chronic periodontitis, however, seem to indicate that two thirds of attachment loss and alveolar bone resorption is preventable through the action of non-steroidal anti-inflammatory drugs, and therefore tissue destruction seems to be driven by the inflammatory process (Williams *et al.* 1985, 1989). Apical spread of bacteria loosely adhering to the hard, non-shedding surface of the tooth is thought to be controlled through a first line of defense consisting of mechanisms such as the high turnover of junctional epithelium keratinocytes, the outward flow of crevicular fluid, and the directed migration of polymorphonuclear leukocytes through the junctional epithelium; the efficiency of these innate immune mechanisms is highly enhanced by the presence of specific antibodies and complement fragments in the gingival crevicular fluid (Page 1990) (Table 19-3) (see Chapter 11).

Host response to bacterial pathogens

Both local and systemic host responses to AgP-associated microflora have been described. Local

Table 19-3 Host defense mechanisms in the gingival sulcus (modified from Page 1990)

Intact epithelial barrier and epithelial attachment

Salivary flushing action, agglutinins, antibodies

Sulcular fluid flushing action, opsonins, antibodies, complement and other plasma components

Local antibody production

High levels of tissue turnover

Presence of normal flora or beneficial species

Emigrating PMNs and other leukocytes

---

inflammatory responses have been characterized by an intense recruitment of polymorphonuclear leukocytes (PMNs) both within the tissues and into the periodontal pocket. Such a preponderance of PMNs underlines the importance of these cells in the local defense against bacterial aggression and their potential role in host-mediated tissue destruction. B cells and antibody-producing plasma cells represent a significant component of the mononuclear cell-dominated connective tissue lesion (Liljenberg & Lindhe 1980). Plasma cells have been shown to be predominantly IgG-producing cells, with a lower proportion of IgA-producing cells (Mackler *et al.* 1977, 1978; Waldrop *et al.* 1981; Ogawa *et al.* 1989). Local IgG$_4$-producing cells, in particular, seem to be elevated. Another important component of the local inflammatory infiltrate are T cells. Subset analysis of local T cells has indicated a depressed T-helper to T-suppressor ratio as compared to both healthy gingiva and peripheral blood. These findings have been interpreted to suggest the possibility of altered local immune regulation (Taubman *et al.* 1988, 1991). Peripheral blood mononuclear cells from AgP patients have been reported to exhibit a reduced autologous mixed lymphocyte reaction, as well as a higher than normal response to B cell mitogens (for review see Engel 1996). Local inflammatory responses are characterized by high levels of PGE$_2$, IL-1α and IL-1β in both crevicular fluid and tissue (Masada *et al.* 1990; Offenbacher *et al.* 1993). PGE$_2$ production, in particular, has been shown to be highly elevated in AgP subjects when compared to periodontally healthy individuals and chronic periodontitis patients.

Specific antibodies against AgP-associated microorganisms (Lally *et al.* 1980; Steubing *et al.* 1982; Ebersole *et al.* 1984, 1985a,b) and cleaved complement fragments (Schenkein & Genco 1977; Patters *et al.* 1989) have also been detected in crevicular fluid from AgP lesions. Of interest is the evidence indicating that crevicular fluid titers of antibodies against AgP-associated microorganisms are frequently higher than in the serum of the same patient (Ebersole *et al.* 1984, 1985a,b). This observation, together with sub-

stantial *in vitro* and *ex vivo* data, strongly suggests that substantial fractions of these antibodies are locally produced in the inflammatory infiltrate (Steubing *et al.* 1982; Hall *et al.* 1990, 1991, 1994). Substantial titers of antibodies against *A.a.* and *P. gingivalis* have also been detected in the serum of AgP patients. Furthermore, in some patients, titers of antibodies reactive with *A.a.* have been shown to be as high as the ones against *Treponema pallidum* present in tertiary syphilis (0.1–1 g/ml); this clearly indicates the extent of host response that can be mounted against these periodontal pathogens (for a review see Ebersole 1990, 1996).

Recent investigations have identified the immunodominant *A. actinomycetemcomitans* antigen to be the serotype-specific carbohydrate; furthermore, it has been shown that the vast majority of antibodies reactive with this carbohydrate in AgP patients consist of IgG$_2$ (Califano *et al.* 1992). High titers and high avidity of *A.a.*-specific IgG$_2$ have been demonstrated in LAP patients, where high antibody titers are thought to be associated with the host's ability to localize attachment loss to few teeth; conversely, GAP patients are frequently seronegative for *A.a.* or display low titers and avidity. Anti-*A.a.* serotype polysaccharide IgG$_2$, therefore, are considered to be protective against widespread AgP (Tew *et al.* 1996).

Of importance are findings reporting antibody response to *P. gingivalis* in GAP forms. Patients suffering from these forms of disease frequently show both low levels of serum antibodies against *P. gingivalis* and low levels of antibody avidity, indicating a specific inability of some GAP patients to cope effectively with these bacteria. Importantly, however, both titers and avidity of antibodies reacting with *P. gingivalis* can be improved as a result of therapy.

Another important aspect of host response towards AgP microorganisms has been the recognition that PMNs of some LAP and GAP patients present decreased migration and antibacterial functions (Genco *et al.* 1980, 1986; Van Dyke *et al.* 1982, 1986, 1988). These abnormalities are frequently minor in the sense that they are usually not associated with infections other than periodontitis. A key report has indicated that PMN abnormalities in LAP patients seem to cluster in families much in the same way as AgP does (Fig. 19-8) (Van Dyke *et al.* 1985). This evidence has been interpreted as a suggestion that the LAP-associated PMN defect may be inherited. Other recent reports have indicated that PMN abnormalities in LAP patients may be, at least in part, the result of a hyper-inflammatory state resulting in the presence of pro-inflammatory cytokines in the serum of some AgP patients (Shapira *et al.* 1994; Agarwal *et al.* 1996).

Genetic aspects of host susceptibility

Several family studies have indicated that the prevalence of AgP is disproportionately high among certain

(a)

Localized aggressive periodontitis in siblings of 22 families

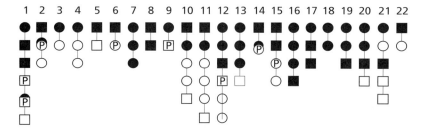

Prevalence of LAP
67% of siblings (> 12 yrs), uncorrected
34% of siblings (> 12 yrs), corrected for proband bias

Key:

○ Female, normal   Ⓟ Pre-pubertal female

□ Male, normal   ☐P Pre-pubertal male

● Female, LAP   ⊚ Pre-pubertal female, LAP developed during study

■ Male, LAP   ⊡ Pre-pubertal male, LAP developed during study

(b)

Neutrophil chemotaxis in LAP families

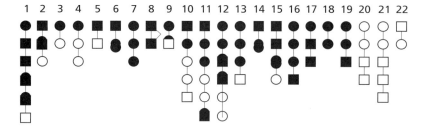

Fig. 19-8 (a) Patients suffering from LAP in 22 families are represented by solid black figures. In each family the proband is on the left. (b) Diagrammatic representation of sibships involved in study group. Numbers are the same as in (a). Solid black figures represent patients exhibiting depressed neutrophil chemotaxis. In this group, after correcting for sampling bias, 40% of subjects present with abnormal chemotaxis. Subjects in sibship 8 are identical twins. From Van Dyke *et al.* (1985).

families, where the percentage of affected siblings may reach 40–50% (Saxen & Nevanlinna 1984; Beaty *et al.* 1987; Long *et al.* 1987; Boughman *et al.* 1992; Marazita *et al.* 1994; Llorente & Griffiths 2006). Such a dramatic familial aggregation of cases indicates that genetic factors may be important in susceptibility to AgP. Genetic studies in these families suggest that the pattern of disease transmission is consistent with mendelian inheritance of a gene of major effect (Saxen & Nevanlinna 1984; Beaty *et al.* 1987; Boughman *et al.* 1992; Hart *et al.* 1992; Marazita *et al.* 1994). This means that the observed familial pattern can be partly accounted for by one or more genes that could predispose individuals to develop AgP.

Segregation analyses have indicated that the likely mode of inheritance is autosomal dominant (Fig. 19-9a) (Saxen & Nevanlinna 1984; Beaty *et al.* 1987; Hart *et al.* 1992; Marazita *et al.* 1994). Most of these investigations, however, were carried out in African-American populations; it is therefore possible that other modes of inheritance may exist in different populations. Segregation analysis can provide information about the mode of inheritance of a genetic

trait but does not provide information about the specific gene(s) involved. The chromosomal location of a gene of major effect for a trait such as AgP susceptibility can be determined by linkage analysis. An investigation utilizing this methodology reported linkage of LAP to the vitamin D binding locus on region q of chromosome 4 in a large family of the Brandywine population (Boughman *et al.* 1986). These results, however, were not confirmed in a subsequent study utilizing a different population (Hart *et al.* 1993). A recent study has linked localized AgP with the q25 region of chromosome 1 in an area close to the cyclo-oxygenase 2 (COX-2) gene (Li *et al.* 2004). Another has established evidence of linkage with the q13–14 region of chromosome 2 that contains the IL-1 gene complex (Scapoli *et al.* 2005). Such data are currently considered to support the existence of genetic heterogeneity in LAP forms, and of distinct forms of AgP. Therefore, it is currently maintained that although formal genetic studies of AgP support the existence of a gene of major effect, it is unlikely that all forms of AgP are due to the same genetic variant (Hart 1996; Loos *et al.* 2005). This notion is consistent

(a) Major gene locus: AgP susceptibility gene

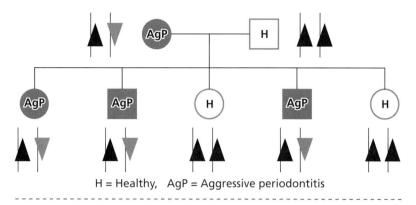

H = Healthy,   AgP = Aggressive periodontitis

(b) Modifying gene locus: IgG$_2$ response

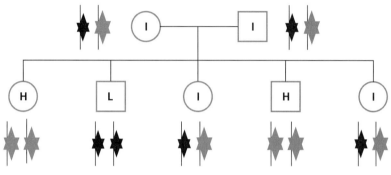

H = high IgG$_2$ titer,   I = intermediate IgG$_2$ titer,   L = low IgG$_2$ titer

(c) Clinical disease expression

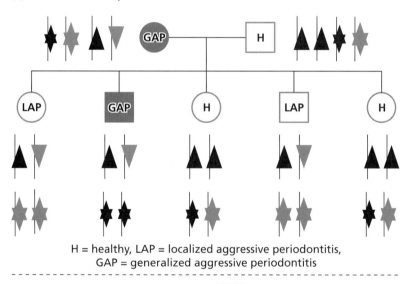

H = healthy, LAP = localized aggressive periodontitis,
GAP = generalized aggressive periodontitis

Key   ◯ female   ▢ male

▲ normal allele   ▽ AgP allele   ✦ low IgG$_2$ response allele   ✦ high IgG$_2$ response allele

Fig. 19-9 (a) Genetic predisposition to AgP is determined by a single gene of major effect, inherited as an autosomal dominant trait. (b) Modifying genes may control immune responses that determine the clinical extent and severity of periodontal destruction in AgP. Here an allele controlling IgG$_2$ levels is inherited as a codominant trait. (c) Independent inheritance of major locus and modifying locus illustrating how LAP and GAP may segregate within the same family. The propensity to develop AgP is dependent upon inheritance of a major susceptibility gene. The clinical phenotype is dependent upon host ability to produce IgG$_2$ in response to periodontopathic bacteria. High IgG$_2$ titers limit disease extension. Intermediate and low IgG$_2$ titers are less effective in limiting intermediate disease progression. From Schenkein (1994), as modified by Hart (1996), with permission from the American Academy of Periodontology.

with the fact that numerous diseases and syndromes with similar clinical appearance are known to result from different genetic polymorphisms.

A recent study providing an additional line of evidence for a genetic component to aggressive peri-

odontitis has shown that quantitative measures of periodontal parameters show substantial levels of hereditability in AgP patients (Diehl *et al.* 2005).

Based on current knowledge that AgP subjects present high prevalence of PMN function defects,

Table 19-4 Genes known to affect human PMN function or host response to LPS load and/or thought to be among the candidate genes of major effect in EOP susceptibility

Condition	OMIM*	Transmission	Chromosome location	Comments
Bactericidal permeability increasing protein (BPIP)	109195	AD	20q11–12	BPIP is associated with PMN granules and is bactericidal to Gram organisms. It binds to LPS with high affinity. BPIP is 45% homologous to LPS binding protein
Lipopolysaccharide binding protein (LBP)	151990	AD	20q11–12	Produced during acute phase of infection: binds to LPS and functions as a carrier for LPS; functions in monocyte response
Monocyte differentiation antigen (CD14)	158126	AD	5q31	Receptor for LBP-LPS complex
Prostaglandin synthase 2 (PTGS2)	600262	AR	1q25.2–3	Major role in regulation of prostaglandin synthesis. Dramatic induction of PTGS2 mRNA occurs in normal peripheral blood leukocytes in response to LPS
PMN actin dysfunction (NAD)	257150	AR	?	Carriers (heterozygotes) have a 50% decrease in actin filament assembly; affected individuals (homozygotes) have recurrent bacterial infections. PMN severely defective in migration and particle ingestion; basic defect due to failure of PMN actin polymerization
Myeloperoxidase deficiency (MPO)	254600	AR	17q12–21	Absence of MPO. MPO is a dimeric protein that catalyzes the production of oxidating agents with microbicidal activity against a wide range of microbes. Several variants have been described
IgE elevation with PMN chemotaxis defect	147060	AD	?	Impaired lymphocyte response to *Candida* antigen; recurrent bacterial infections
Fc receptor gamma IIA polymorphism (FCGR2A)	146790	AD	1q21-q23	Allelic variants of the Fc-gamma receptor 2A confer distinct phagocytic capacities providing a possible mechanism for hereditary susceptibility to infection. The H131 allele is the only FGR2A that recognizes IgG_2 efficiently, and optimal IgG_2 handling occurs only in the homozygous state for H131. The allelic variant R131 has low binding of IgG_2
Immunoglobulin G_2m allotypes	N/A	?	N/A	Specific allotypes associated with IgG_2 response to specific bacterial antigens. Subjects lacking specific allotypes may be selectively unable to mount efficient antibody response against specific antigens

* Online Mendelian Inheritance in Man (OMIM). Modified from Hart (1996).

that they have been shown to produce high levels of inflammatory mediators in response to LPS stimulation, and of the relevance of connective tissue homeostasis in periodontitis, several loci have been proposed as genes conferring increased susceptibility to AgP. Hart (1996) compiled a list of candidate genes (Table 19-4) associated with increased susceptibility to AgP.

A series of studies has been performed to assess whether or not specific polymorphisms in these candidate genes were associated with AgP (for a recent review see Shapira *et al.* 2005 and Loos *et al.* 2005).

Significant associations have been observed for genes encoding for proteins that are associated with neutrophil function (Fu *et al.* 2002; Loos *et al.* 2003; Kaneko *et al.* 2004; Jordan *et al.* 2005; Nibali *et al.* 2006; de Souza & Colombo 2006), with inflammation and with the host ability to effectively deal with exposure to bacterial components such as endotoxin (Suzuki *et al.* 2004; Scapoli *et al.* 2005; Brett *et al.* 2005; Noack *et al.* 2006), and with connective tissue homeostasis (Suzuki *et al.* 2004; Park *et al.* 2006; Soedarsono *et al.* 2006). It should be emphasized, however, that the validity of the conclusions of the majority of these studies suffers from small sample sizes, study of a single or few specific polymorphisms in the gene, as well as failure to account for ethnic variations and correction for environmental factors (e.g. cigarette smoking) (Tonetti & Claffey 2005). These three factors may be responsible for false-positive associations and bigger studies need to be performed to establish consistent associations.

Besides genes of major effect that may determine susceptibility to AgP, other genes may act as modifying genes and influence clinical expression of the disease. In this respect, particular interest has been focused on the impact of genetic control on antibody responses against specific AgP-associated bacteria and against *A.a.* in particular. These studies have indicated that the ability to mount high titers of specific antibodies is race-dependent and probably protective (Gunsolley *et al.* 1987, 1988). This has been shown to be under genetic control as a co-dominant trait, independent of the risk for AgP. In individuals susceptible to AgP, therefore, the ability to mount high titers of antibodies (IgG_2 in particular) may be protective and prevent extension of disease to a generalized form (Schenkein 1994; Diehl *et al.* 2003) (Fig. 19-9b,c). Allelic variations in the Fc receptor for IgG_2 immunoglobulins have also been suggested to play a role in suboptimal handling of *A.a.* infections. PMN expressing the R131 allotype of FcγRIIa (i.e. an Fc receptor containing an arginine instead of a histidine at amino acid 131) show decreased phagocytosis of *A.a.* (Wilson & Kalmar 1996).

Environmental aspects of host susceptibility

Recent evidence has indicated that, besides genetic influences, environmental factors may affect the clinical expression of AgP. In a large study, cigarette smoking was shown to be a risk factor for patients with generalized forms of AgP (Schenkein *et al.* 1995). Smokers with GAP had more affected teeth and greater mean levels of attachment loss than patients with GAP who did not smoke (Table 19-5). Environmental exposure to cigarette smoking, therefore, seems to add significant risk of more severe and

prevalent disease to this group of already highly susceptible subjects. The mechanism(s) for this observation are not completely understood, but findings from the same group indicate that IgG_2 serum levels as well as antibody levels against *A.a.* are significantly depressed in subjects with GAP who smoke. Since these antibodies are considered to represent a protective response against *A.a.*, it is possible that depression of IgG_2 in smokers may be associated with the observed increase in disease extent and severity in these subjects.

Current concepts

Aggressive forms of periodontitis are currently considered to be multifactorial diseases developing as a result of complex interactions between specific host genes and the environment. Inheritance of AgP susceptibility is probably insufficient for the development of disease: environmental exposure to potential pathogens endowed with specific virulence factors is also a necessary step. Host inability to effectively deal with the bacterial aggression and to avoid inflammatory tissue damage results in the initiation of the disease process. Interactions between the disease process and environmental (e.g. cigarette smoking) and genetically controlled (e.g. IgG_2 response to *A.a.*) modifying factors are thought to contribute to determining the specific clinical manifestation of disease (Figs. 19–9a-c and 19-10).

Diagnosis

Clinical diagnosis

Clinical diagnosis is based on information derived from a specific medical and dental history and from the clinical examination of the periodontium. Limitations that will be discussed in this section, however, frequently require supplementation of clinical and anamnestic parameters with other, more advanced aids to properly diagnose, plan treatment for and monitor these diseases. The purpose of clinical diagnosis is the identification of patients suffering from AgP and of factors that have an impact on how the case should be treated and monitored.

In the diagnosis of AgP the initial question that the clinician should ask is:

• Is there periodontitis?

This may sound like a trivial question, but in fact many cases of AgP are currently not identified because of a failure to detect signs of periodontitis. Conversely, some clinicians attribute to periodontitis pathological changes associated with other unrelated and sometimes self-limiting processes. Correctly answering this question requires systematic collection of clinical information regarding the following items:

Table 19-5 Effect of smoking on extent and severity of GAP

Smoking status	Mean percentage of sites with PAL ≥5 mm*	Mean PAL (mm)*
Smokers	49.0 ± 3.9	2.78 ± 0.2
Non-smokers	36.8 ± 3.8	2.14 ± 0.2

* Values adjusted for age and mean plaque index, subject as unit of analysis. Smokers showed significantly greater extent and severity of periodontal disease than non-smokers after correcting for age and oral hygiene level.
Modified from Schenkein *et al.* (1995).

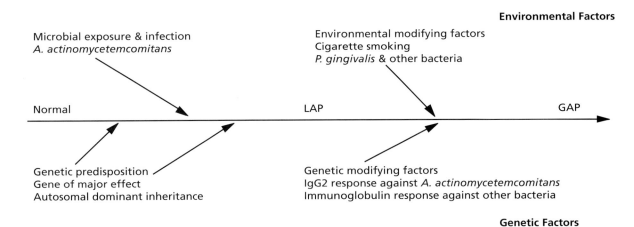

Fig. 19-10 Diagrammatic representation of the current understanding of the eco-genetic interactions leading to development of LAP and GAP in African-American populations. (See text for explanation.)

- Is there loss of periodontal support (loss of clinical attachment and marginal resorption of alveolar bone)?
- Is the loss of attachment accompanied by pocket formation or mostly the result of recession?
- Is there a plausible cause for attachment loss other than periodontitis?
- Is there another process imitating periodontal disease by pseudopocket formation?

From a clinical standpoint, it is important to realize that clinically detectable loss of attachment may occur as a result of pathological events other than periodontitis. Examples are traumatic injuries, removal or presence of impacted teeth (Kugelberg 1992), tooth position, orthodontic tooth movement, advanced decay, subgingival margins of restorations, etc. This means that the clinician must recognize different causes for attachment loss and must rule out other causes of attachment loss by a combination of careful clinical examination and assessment of the dental history. Orthodontic considerations are necessary to evaluate attachment loss without pocket formation (recession). In such instances the appropriate clinical diagnosis may be *incidental attachment loss*.

After establishing the presence of periodontitis, the clinician should determine which clinical diagnosis best describes the disease in the individual patient: chronic, aggressive or necrotizing periodontitis. Since the current classification is based on the combination of clinical presentation, rate of disease progression, and pattern of familial aggregation of cases in the absence of a systemic cause for the clinical observations, the next questions should address these parameters:

- Does the patient have a systemic condition that would in itself explain the presence of periodontitis?

As indicated, the diagnosis of chronic, aggressive or necrotizing periodontitis implies presence of peri-

odontal destruction in the absence of systemic diseases that may severely impair host defense. A well constructed and well taken medical history is fundamental for identifying the presence of systemic involvements accompanied with periodontitis (see Chapter 7). Careful questioning regarding recurrent infections, their familiarity, presence of severe diseases or their symptoms and signs should be part of the evaluation of all periodontal patients. Consultation with the attending physician and evaluation of laboratory parameters are frequently necessary. Understanding of the medical condition that may be associated with periodontitis is fundamental. Some conditions are relatively frequent disorders such as poorly controlled diabetes mellitus; others are rare inherited disorders such as the palmo-plantar keratosis (Papillon-Lefèvre and Heim-Munk syndromes) or hypophosphatasia. Some are inborn defects such as the leukocyte adhesion deficiencies (LAD); others are acquired following exposure to pharmacological agents such as drug-induced granulocytopenia. Positive confirmed history of a significant systemic condition results in the diagnosis of *periodontal manifestation of systemic disease*.

In such instances, the periodontitis is likely to represent an oral manifestation of the systemic disease. Examples of significant conditions are AIDS, leukemia, neutropenia, diabetes or rare genetic diseases such as histiocytosis X, Papillon-Lefèvre syndrome or Chediak-Steinbrinck-Higashi syndrome (see Chapter 11 and Fig. 19-4).

In the absence of significant systemic components, the next questions relate to the exclusion of the rare but clearly identified necrotizing/ulcerative forms. The question will then be:

- Does the patient have signs or symptoms of necrotizing periodontitis?

If the answer to both of the previous questions is negative, differential diagnosis between chronic or aggressive periodontitis will be required. In this respect it is important to observe that chronic periodontitis has been defined as the common form of periodontitis whose diagnosis is done by excluding the presence of aggressive periodontitis (Armitage 1999). Diagnosis of AgP is made by verification of the satisfaction by the individual cases of the primary and secondary features described in the international classification workshop (see discussion above).

In this respect it must be recognized that the features include both clinical and laboratory aspects. In the diagnosis of a case, clinical and history parameters are initially utilized to suspect the presence of AgP, while laboratory tests are frequently utilized to confirm the diagnosis. In this respect, it is important to realize that periodontal diagnosis based only on periodontal probing and dental radiography does not classify causes; rather, it describes destruction patterns.

A tentative clinical diagnosis of AgP is made based on the following criteria:

- Absence of significant systemic conditions
- Rapid attachment loss and bone destruction
- Familial aggregation of cases
- Lack of consistency between clinically visible bacterial deposits and severity of periodontal breakdown.

A rapid rate of destruction of the periodontium is a major criterion for the diagnosis of AgP. It is aimed at identifying subjects characterized by high virulence of the microflora and/or high levels of susceptibility. Although correct application of this criterion requires availability of clinical or radiographic data from more than one time point, presence of severe destruction in relation to the age of the subject is frequently considered to be sufficient information to infer rapid progression.

Establishing the presence of familial aggregation of cases is based on a combination of history and clinical examination of family members of the affected individual. At this stage there is inadequate evidence to establish the best approach to obtain a significant estimation of familial aggregation. A recent study, in particular, questioned the reliability of family history as a way to establish familial aggregation (Llorente & Griffiths 2006).

It is maintained that in the majority of AgP cases the amount of periodontal destruction seems to be higher than that expected from the mere accumulation of local factors. This observation, however, may not be true for all cases. In general, a discrepancy between local factors and the amount of periodontal tissue breakdown is considered to be an indication for either infection with particularly virulent microorganisms, or presence of a highly susceptible host. This information may be consequential in determining surgical goals of therapy, the impact of antibiotics, and the possible impact of sub-optimal hygiene as a risk factor for disease recurrence.

The international classification workshop consensus indicated that not all listed primary and secondary features need to be present in order to assign an AgP diagnosis and that the diagnosis may be based on clinical, radiographic, and historical data alone. It also indicated that laboratory testing, although helpful, might not be essential in making an AgP diagnosis.

Once an AgP diagnosis has been made based on the criteria above, differential diagnosis between LAP and GAP needs to be made. In this respect specific clinical features have been suggested. A diagnosis of LAP is made based on evidence of circumpubertal onset and localized first molar/incisor presentation with interproximal attachment loss on at least two permanent teeth, one of which is a first molar, and involving no more than two teeth other than first molars and incisors. A diagnosis of GAP takes into account the fact that this form of disease usually affects persons under 30 years of age (but patients may be older) and that it presents with generalized interproximal attachment loss affecting at least three permanent teeth other than first molars and incisors. Furthermore this pathology is characterized by a pronounced episodic nature of the destruction of attachment and alveolar bone. The differential diagnosis may benefit from additional laboratory investigations of the individual host response to the infecting organisms.

In order to properly describe the specific AgP case, modifying factors should also be explored by addressing the question of the presence of modifying or contributory factors such as smoking or drug abuse. Such additional information is relevant since these factors may explain a specific presentation of disease in terms of its extent and severity. Furthermore, these factors, unlike genetic factors, are amenable to modification through appropriate intervention. Therapy should therefore include an approach aimed at controling the impact of these factors.

Even though differential diagnosis between AgP and chronic periodontitis and differentiation between LAP and GAP is mostly based on history and clinical presentation, it must be emphasized that clinical parameters alone cannot further discriminate between forms of disease with similar clinical appearance. Inferences regarding a specific etiology are speculative under such circumstances and require further laboratory testing for confirmation.

In the previous classification system, age at onset or age at diagnosis was considered helpful to further characterize specific clinical syndromes. LAP, in particular, is thought to occur in adolescents, 13–14 years old to 25 years, while GAP is generally found in adolescents or young adults of less than 30–35 years. It should be realized, however, that (1) some cases may present initial LAP at an earlier age, (2) LAP may start before puberty and affect the primary dentition, (3) patterns of periodontal destruction compatible with LAP may be initially detected at an age older than 25, and (4) there may be a tendency toward spreading from a localized to a generalized pattern of AgP in older subjects of these groups.

Another difficulty is related to the fact that periodontal destruction is often diagnosed when the attachment loss is already fairly advanced. In general, distinct alterations in the morphology of the periodontium and substantial tissue damage are necessary for establishing a clear diagnosis. Milder or initial stages of disease or sites at risk for future periodontal breakdown cannot be detected based on clinical parameters. This makes it difficult to intercept and treat initial forms of AgP. Furthermore, such difficulty makes it extremely important to examine the other members of the family of the proband as well: siblings may present with clinically undetectable disease in spite of the presence of the putative pathogens. A common strategy employed to overcome the insufficient ability of clinical parameters to detect early disease is to closely monitor high-risk patients such as the siblings of the probands. It is in this respect important to underline that "incidental attachment loss" may, in some cases, represent an initial manifestation of AgP. In such a case an isolated periodontal lesion characterized by attachment loss with pocketing may represent the only clinically evident AgP lesion. Such subjects should, therefore, be considered at high risk for the development of AgP and require close monitoring and possibly further microbiologic diagnosis.

Microbiologic diagnosis

The presence of specific microorganisms is considered as one of the secondary features of AgP. A systematic review has, however, clearly indicated that the presence or absence of suspected periodontal pathogens such as *A.a.* on the species level cannot fully discriminate subjects with AgP from subjects with chronic periodontitis. Although it is more than ten times more likely that *A.a.*-negative patients suffer from chronic than from aggressive periodontitis, any *A.a.*-positive individual with periodontitis is three times more likely to be suffering from chronic than from aggressive periodontitis (Mombelli *et al.* 2002). The noted limitations in discriminating power to distinguish AgP from ChP should not be interpreted to mean that a test aiming at the detection of target microorganisms is completely useless in any clinical situation. Treatment studies suggest that *A.a.* is particularly difficult to suppress with conventional mechanical therapy (Mombelli *et al.* 1994a, 2000), longitudinal and retrospective studies have indicated an increased risk for periodontal breakdown in positive sites (Fine 1984; Slots *et al.* 1986; Bragd *et al.* 1987; Slots & Listgarten 1988; Rams *et al.* 1996), and results of treatment seemed to be better if *A.a.* could not be detected any more at follow up (Bragd *et al.* 1987; Carlos *et al.* 1988; Haffajee *et al.* 1991; Grossi *et al.* 1994; Haffajee & Socransky 1994). Therefore, even

if microbiologic testing alone cannot distinguish between chronic and aggressive periodontitis, access to microbiologic data may improve the outcome of periodontal therapy. This should be taken into account particularly with regards to the highly leukotoxic variant of *A.a.*, which shows a stronger association with AgP than *A.a.* as a whole. In discussing the diagnostic potential of a test, one should also consider that the main difference between clinical groups may not be the prevalence but rather the amount of putative pathogens found in positive samples (Gunsolley *et al.* 1990).

Microbiologic data may be useful to establish a differential diagnosis in patients clinically diagnosed with AgP. Knowledge of whether a clinical condition is associated with *A.a.*, and/or with other periodontal pathogens, such as *P. gingivalis*, has an impact on the need to supplement conventional therapy with antibiotics and on the choice of the antimicrobial drug (see Chapter 42). Microbiologic information can be useful at different stages of the treatment plan, i.e. as a part of the initial diagnosis, at re-evaluation or during the recall phase. The need for microbiologic information before therapy depends on the general strategy for treatment. Many clinicians prefer to remove bacterial deposits mechanically in a first treatment phase without the adjunctive use of systemic antibiotics. As microbiologic findings have no influence on the way this initial treatment is performed, microbiologic testing may be postponed until the first phase is completed. One should keep in mind, however, that the reduction in bacterial load might increase the possibility of false-negative results when an insensitive microbiologic test is used. If the specific clinical diagnosis is LAP, then the clinician can assume even without a microbiologic test that the treatment should be directed towards a maximal suppression of *A.a.* This is due to the fact that the great majority of LAP patients are infected with this organism. This is different for all other forms of AgP, where such a close association of one microbial species with the disease cannot be assumed, and therefore microbial testing should be performed.

Since *A.a.* and *P. gingivalis* can be transmitted from periodontal patients to family members, microbial testing of spouses, children or siblings of AgP patients may be indicated to intercept early disease in susceptible individuals.

Evaluation of host defenses

Several forms of AgP have been associated with impairment of host defenses. Classic studies have indicated that in some populations both LAP and GAP forms are associated with high incidence of phagocyte functional disturbances, such as depressed neutrophil chemotaxis and other phagocyte antibacterial dysfunctions. In many of these patients, AgP was the only infection that was associated with the reduced phagocyte function(s); this observation is important in two respects. First, AgP-associated phagocyte defects are frequently insignificant in terms of increasing susceptibility to infections other than periodontitis. Furthermore, it is likely that such "mild" leukocyte defects may go unnoticed until laboratory testing is performed in conjunction with periodontal diagnosis. Reports of such phagocyte defects relate mostly to AgP subjects from African American groups; systematic evaluations of PMN and monocyte functions associated with clinical diagnosis of AgP in European Caucasians failed to confirm a high prevalence of abnormalities (Kinane et al. 1989a,b). Testing for these host defense parameters, therefore, may be more restricted to specific populations. Another important aspect is that, so far, no specific study has attempted to associate treatment response or incidence of recurrent disease with the presence of the above-mentioned abnormalities.

More recent investigations have indicated that specific patterns of host response to bacterial pathogens are associated with different forms of AgP; this early evidence may be extremely helpful for the development of clinically useful tests to estimate the risk of developing AgP. In this respect two findings deserve to be mentioned:

1. AgP patients present significantly higher levels of crevicular fluid PGE_2 than chronic periodontitis patients or healthy subjects. This finding may indicate that monocytes from these patients respond to bacterial and inflammatory stimuli with very high levels of local release of inflammatory mediators. These may induce an exuberant inflammatory reaction associated with high levels of activation of tissue-degrading matrix-metalloproteinases.
2. GAP patients have a decreased ability to mount high titers of specific IgG_2 antibodies to A.a. These subjects exhibit a tendency towards progressive periodontal destruction leading to tooth loss over a relatively short period of time. LAP patients, on the other hand, seem to have better prognosis and do not express this trait. Since there are indications that at least some LAP cases may progress into generalized forms, early detection of patients infected with A.a. but producing low levels of specific antibodies may allow early identification of a high-risk group for development of GAP. Serum antibody titers (IgG_2 in particular) and/or avidity to A.a. may be particularly useful in the differential diagnosis of GAP and LAP syndromes and in the early detection of the LAP cases with high risk for progression into the more widespread forms of disease.

Genetic diagnosis

Given the disproportionately high incidence of AgP in the families of affected individuals, evaluation of siblings of the proband and other family members is a requirement. Clinical determination of different disease forms in the family should be followed by construction of a pedigree of the AgP trait. Such diagnosis may bring considerable information regarding the level of risk eventually shared within the family. Furthermore, it helps to establish the need for monitoring clinically unaffected individuals.

All the evidence gathered during the diagnostic process should contribute to the definition of a specific diagnosis. An example of such diagnosis is illustrated in Fig. 19-11: LAP in a 22-year-old systemically healthy African American female patient, associated with A.a. infection without detectable levels of P. gingivalis, inconsistency between local factors and amount of clinically detectable breakdown, absence of demonstrable leukocyte defects, no known contributory factors, and no siblings displaying clinically detectable periodontitis.

Principles of therapeutic intervention

Treatment of AgP should only be initiated after completion of a careful diagnosis by a specifically trained periodontist. The severity of some of the AgP forms suggests that specialists, possibly working in association with highly specialized centers, could best perform both diagnosis and treatment of these rare forms of periodontitis. The roles of the general practitioner, the pedodontist or the orthodontist, however, are fundamental in the detection of possible cases to be referred for further evaluation and therapy.

Successful treatment of AgP is considered to be dependent on early diagnosis, directing therapy towards elimination or suppression of the infecting microorganisms and providing an environment conducive to long-term maintenance. The differential element of treatment of AgP, however, relates to specific efforts to affect the composition and not only the quantity of the subgingival microbiota.

Elimination or suppression of the pathogenic flora

A.a. elimination has been associated with successful therapy; conversely, recurrent lesions have been shown to still harbor this organism. Several investigators have reported that scaling and root planing of juvenile periodontitis lesions could not predictably suppress A.a. below detection levels (Slots & Rosling 1983; Christersson et al. 1985; Kornman & Robertson 1985). Soft tissue curettage and access flap therapy also had limited success in eliminating A.a. (Christersson et al. 1985).

A.a. is also difficult to eliminate by conventional mechanical therapy in adult periodontitis patients, and it is therefore not surprising to observe the presence of this microorganism in the subgingival microflora of many non-responding periodontitis patients (Bragd et al. 1985; van Winkelhoff et al. 1989; Renvert

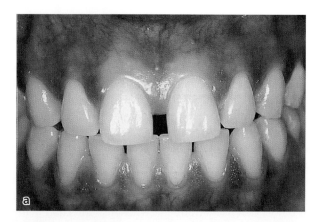

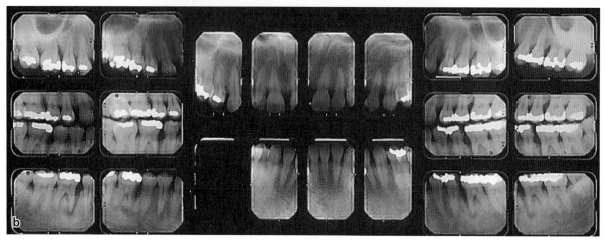

Fig. 19-11 (a,b) Clinical and radiographic presentation of a 22-year-old African-American female. Clinical attachment loss and alveolar bone loss are localized on the mesial aspect of the first molars, where deep, vertical defects are apparent. (c–e) Detailed views of the defect on the mesial aspect of 26. No other tooth appears to be affected. Microbiology (DNA probe analysis of *A. actinomycetemcomitans*, *P. gingivalis* and *P. intermedia*) confirmed the presence of high levels (>104 bacteria/sample) of *A. actinomycetemcomitans* in all four deep lesions. *Pr. intermedia* was also detectable in three of four sites, while *P. gingivalis* was undetectable. The patient did not display abnormal leukocyte functions; furthermore, she had a non-contributory medical history, and did not smoke. She had a younger brother (15 years old) and an older sister (27 years old); on clinical examination, the periodontium of both of them appeared to be within normal limits. The following diagnosis was made: "LAP in a 22-year-old systemically healthy African-American female; associated with *A. actinomycetemcomitans* infection without clinically detectable levels of *P. gingivalis*; absence of demonstrable leukocyte defects; no known contributory factors; no cigarette smoking; no siblings displaying clinically detectable AgP".

et al. 1990a,b; Rodenburg *et al.* 1990; Mombelli *et al.* 1994a). Similar, but less systematic observations have also been reported for the ability to suppress the microflora associated with some GAP forms, where high subgingival loads of *P. gingivalis*, *B. forsythus*, *A.a.*, and other highly virulent bacteria are frequently detected.

Use of antibiotics has been suggested as a rational complement to mechanical debridement in these cases. Regimens, including the adjunctive administration of tetracyclines or metronidazole, have been tested for the treatment of LAP and other forms of AgP (see Chapter 42).

The choice of antibiotic can either be empiric (based on published information on the efficacy of the regimen in similar populations) or guided by information about the nature of the involved pathogenic microorganism(s) and/or their antibiotic susceptibility profile. Both approaches have been

suggested but currently there is no direct evidence that microbiologic diagnosis and targeted selection of the antibiotic regimen provides an additional benefit compared to empiric use.

With regards to empiric use, effectiveness is based on outcomes of a series of trials that have specifically assessed the clinical outcomes following administration of a specific antibiotic regimen or placebo in combination with mechanical instrumentation of the root surface and oral hygiene instructions. The approach is supported by a meta-analysis (Haffajee *et al.* 2003) indicating significantly greater clinical improvements following systemic antibiotic administration upon completion of subgingival instrumentation. Metronidazole in combination with amoxicillin may suppress *A.a.* more effectively than single antibiotic regimes and has thus become increasingly popular. Substantial evidence indicates that subgingival *A.a.* can be eliminated or suppressed for a

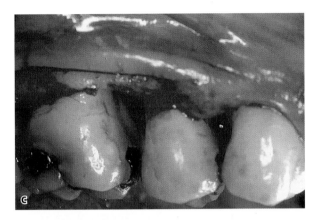

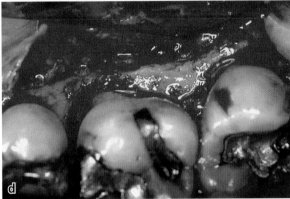

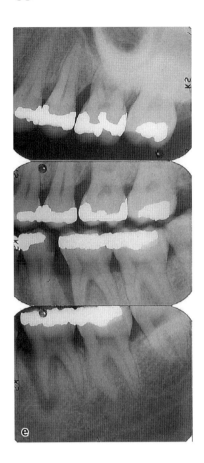

Fig. 19-11 *Continued*

prolonged period by mechanical debridement supplemented with systemic metronidazole plus amoxicillin.

Systemic antibiotics should only be administered as an adjunct to mechanical debridement because in undisturbed subgingival plaque the target organisms are effectively protected from the antibiotic agent due to the biofilm effect (see Chapter 42).

Antibiotics have been used in essentially two ways for the treatment of AgP: (1) in combination with intensive instrumentation over a short period of time after achievement of adequate plaque control in a pretreatment motivation period; or (2) as a staged approach after completion of the initial therapy.

A recent randomized controlled clinical trial (Guerrero *et al.* 2005) has provided evidence of a significant benefit arising from a treatment approach consisting of: (1) achievement of adequate supragingival plaque control (less than 25% of tooth sites with detectable plaque); (2) subgingival instrumentation with a combination of hand and mechanical instruments delivered intensively over a 2-day period; (3) an adjunctive systemic antibiotic regimen consisting of metronidazole (500 mg, tid for 7 days) combined with amoxicillin (500 mg, tid for 7 days). The results of the placebo arm showed highly significant improvements in clinical parameters including reductions of probing depth and improvement of clinical attachment levels throughout the dentition. The

adjunctive antibiotic provided additional benefits in the deeper pockets in terms of all parameters.

As part of the second option, treatment is started with an initial phase of mechanical therapy, including systematic scaling and planing of all accessible root surfaces and the introduction of meticulous oral hygiene. After a period of 4–6 weeks, the case is reassessed clinically. Based on persistence of periodontal lesions, a second phase of therapy is planned. Decisions are made as to how to gain access to deep lesions with appropriate surgical procedures and concerning the administration of antimicrobial agents. Microbial samples from the deepest pocket in each quadrant may provide additional information about the presence and relative importance of putative pathogens. Systemic antimicrobial therapy with the appropriate agent is usually initiated immediately upon completion of the surgical interventions or immediatedly after another round of mechanical instrumentation to ensure that subgingival plaque deposits have been reduced as much as possible and to disrupt the subgingival biofilm.

Microbiologic testing, if performed, may be repeated at 1–3 months after completion of therapy to verify the elimination or marked suppression of the putative pathogen(s). After resolution of the periodontal infection, the patient should be placed on an individually tailored maintenance care program, including continuous evaluation of the occurrence and of the risk of disease progression. Optimal plaque control by the patient is of paramount importance for a favorable clinical and microbiologic response to therapy. Recurrence of disease is an indication for a repetition of microbiologic tests, for re-evaluation of the host immune response, and re-assessment of the local and systemic modifying factors. Further therapy should be targeted against putative periodontal pathogens and should take into account the systemic immune responses of the subject.

References

Aass, A., Preus, H. & Gjermo, P. (1992). Association between detection of oral *Actinobacillus actinomycetemcomitans* and radiographic bone loss in teenagers. *Journal of Periodontology* **63**, 682–685.

Aass, A., Tollefsen, T. & Gjermo, P. (1994). A cohort study of radiographic alveolar bone loss during adolescence. *Journal of Clinical Periodontology* **21**, 133–138.

Agarwal, S., Huang, J.P., Piesco, N., Suzuki, J.B. Riccelli, A.E. & Johns, L.P. (1996). Altered neutrophil function in localized juvenile periodontitis: intrinsic or induced? *Journal of Periodontology* **67**, 337–344.

Ainamo, J., Barmes, D., Beagrie, B., Cutress, T., Martin, J. & Sardo-Infirri, J. (1982). Development of the World Health Organization (WHO) Community Periodontal Index of Treatment Needs (CPITN). *International Dental Journal* **32**, 281–291.

Al-Yahfoufi, Z., Albandar, J., Olsen, I. & Gjermo, P. (1990). Associations between six DNA probe-detected periodontal bacteria and alveolar bone loss and other clinical signs of periodontitis. *Acta Odontologica Scandinavica* **48**, 415–423.

Al-Yahfoufi, Z., Mombelli, A., Wicki, A. & Lang, N.P. (1994). The occurrence of *Actinobacillus actinomycetemcomitans*, *Porphyromonas gingivalis* and *Prevotella intermedia* in an Arabic population with minimal periodontal disease. *Microbial Ecology in Health and Disease* **7**, 217–224.

Albandar, J.M. (1993). Juvenile periodontitis – pattern of progression and relationship to clinical periodontal parameters. *Journal of Clinical Periodontology* **21**, 185–189.

Albandar, J., Baghdady, V. & Ghose, L. (1991a). Periodontal disease progression in teenagers with no preventive dental care provisions. *Journal of Clinical Periodontology* **18**, 300–304.

Albandar, J.M., Buischi, Y.A. & Barbosa, M.F. (1991b). Destructive forms of periodontal disease in adolescents. A 3-year longitudinal study. *Journal of Periodontology* **62**, 370–376.

Albandar, J.M., Olsen, I. & Gjermo, P. (1990). Associations between six DNA probe-detected periodontal bacteria and alveolar bone loss and other clinical signs of periodontitis. *Acta Odontologica Scandinavica* **48**, 415–423.

Altman, L.C., Page, R.C. & Ebersole, J.L. (1982). Assessment of host defenses and serum antibodies to suspected periodontal pathogens in patients with various types of periodontitis. *Journal of Periodontal Research* **17**, 495–497.

American Academy of Periodontology (1996). Position Paper: Periodontal disease in children and adolescents. *Journal of Periodontology* **67**, 57–62.

American Academy of Periodontology & American Dental Association (1992). Periodontal screening and recording: an early detection system.

Armitage, G. (1999). Development of a classification system for periodontal diseases and conditions. *Annals of Periodontology* **4**, 1–6.

Ashley, F.P., Gallagher, J. & Wilson, R.F. (1988). The occurrence of *Actinobacillus actinomycetemcomitans*, *Bacteroides gingivalis*, *Bacteroides intermedius* and spirochaetes in the subgingival microflora of adolescents and their relationship with the amount of supragingival plaque and gingivitis. *Oral Microbiology and Immunology* **3**, 77–82.

Asikainen, S. (1986). Occurrence of *Actinobacillus actinomycetemcomitans* and spirochetes in relation to age in localized juvenile periodontitis. *Journal of Periodontology* **57**, 537–541.

Asikainen, S., Chen, C. & Slots, J. (1995). *Actinobacillus actinomycetemcomitans* genotypes in relation to serotypes and periodontal status. *Oral Microbiology and Immunology* **10**, 65–68.

Asikainen, S., Lai, C.-H., Alaluusua, S. & Slots, J. (1991). Distribution of *Actinobacillus actinomycetemcomitans* serotypes in periodontal health and disease. *Oral Microbiology and Immunology* **6**, 115–118.

Attström, R. & Van der Velden, U. (1993). Summary of session 1. In: Lang, N. & Karring, T., eds. *Proceedings of the 1st European Workshop in Periodontology*. Berlin: Quintessence, pp. 120–126.

Baer, P. (1971). The case of periodontosis as a clinical entity. *Journal of Periodontology* **42**, 516–520.

Beaty, T.H., Boughman, J.A., Yang, P., Astemborski, J.A. & Suzuki, J.B. (1987). Genetic analysis of juvenile periodontitis in families ascertained through an affected proband. *American Journal of Human Genetics* **40**, 443–452.

Bimstein, E. & Soskolne, A. (1988). A radiographic study of interproximal alveolar bone crest between the primary molars in children. *ASDC Journal of Dentistry for Children* **55**, 348–350.

Bimstein, E., Treasure, E., Williams, S. & Dever, J. (1994). Alveolar bone loss in 5-year old New Zealand children: its prevalence and relationship to caries prevalence, socio-economic status and ethnic origin. *Journal of Clinical Periodontology* **21**, 447–450.

Boughman, J.A., Astemborski, J.A. & Suzuki, J.B. (1992). Phenotypic assessment of early onset periodontitis in sibships. *Journal of Clinical Periodontology* **19**, 233–239.

Boughman, J.A., Halloran, S.L., Roulston, D., Schwartz, S., Suzuki, J.B., Weitkamp, L.R., Wenk, R.E., Wooten, R. & Cohen, M.M. (1986). An autosomal-dominant form of juvenile periodontitis: its localization to chromosome 4 and linkage to dentinogenesis imperfecta and Gc. *Journal of Craniofacial Genetics and Developmental Biology* **6**, 341–350.

Bragd, L., Dahlén, G., Wikström, M. & Slots, J. (1987). The capability of *Actinobacillus actinomycetemcomitans*, *Bacteroides gingivalis* and *Bacteroides intermedius* to indicate progressive periodontitis; a retrospective study. *Journal of Clinical Periodontology* **14**, 95–99.

Bragd, L., Wikström, M. & Slots, J. (1985). Clinical and microbiological study of "refractory" adult periodontitis. *Journal of Dental Research* **64**, 234.

Brett, P.M., Zygogianni, P., Griffiths, G.S., Tomaz, M., Parkar, M., D'Aiuto, F. & Tonetti, M. (2005). Functional gene polymorphisms in aggressive and chronic periodontitis. *Journal of Dental Research* **84**,1149–1153.

Brogan, J.M., Lally, E.T., Poulsen, K., Kilian, M. & Demuth, D.R. (1994). Regulation of *Actinobacillus actinomycetemcomitans* leukotoxin expression: analysis of the promoter regions of leukotoxic and minimally leukotoxic strains. *Infection and Immunity* **62**, 501–508.

Bueno, L.C., Mayer, M.P. & DiRienzo, J.M. (1998). Relationship between conversion of localized juvenile periodontitis-susceptible children from health to disease and *Actinobacillus actinomycetemcomitans* leukotoxin promoter structure. *Journal of Periodontology* **69**, 998–1007.

Burmeister, J.A., Best, A.M., Palcanis, K.G., Caine, F.A. & Ranney, R.R. (1984). Localized juvenile periodontitis and generalized severe periodontitis: clinical findings. *Journal of Clinical Periodontology* **11**, 181–192.

Califano, J.V., Schenkein, H.A. & Tew, J.G. (1992). Immuno-dominant antigens of *Actinobacillus actinomycetemcomitans* serotype b in early onset periodontitis patients. *Oral Microbiology and Immunology* **7**, 65–70.

Carlos, J.P., Wolfe, M.D., Zambon, J.J. & Kingman, A. (1988). Periodontal disease in adolescents: some clinical and microbiologic correlates of attachment loss. *Journal of Dental Research* **67**, 1510–1514.

Christersson, L.A., Slots, J., Rosling, B.G. *et al.* (1985). Microbiological and clinical effects of surgical treatment of localized juvenile periodontitis. *Journal of Clinical Periodontology* **12**, 465–476.

Chung, H., Chung, C., Son, S. & Nisengard, R.J. (1989). *Actinobacillus actinomycetemcomitans* serotypes and leukotoxicity in Korean localized juvenile periodontitis. *Journal of Periodontology* **60**, 506–511.

Clerehugh, V., Lennon, M. & Worthington, H. (1990). 5 year results of a longitudinal study of early onset periodontitis in 14 to 19-year old adolescents. *Journal of Clinical Periodontology* **17**, 702–708.

Contreras, A., Rusitanonta, T., Chen, C., Wagner, W.G., Michalowicz, B.S. & Slots, J. (2000). Frequency of 530-bp deletion in *Actinobacillus actinomycetemcomitans* leukotoxin promoter region. *Oral Microbiology and Immunology* **15**, 338–340.

Cortelli, J.R., Cortelli, S.C., Jordan, S., Haraszthy, V.I. & Zambon, J.J. (2005). Prevalence of periodontal pathogens in Brazilians with aggressive or chronic periodontitis. *Journal of Clinical Periodontology* **32**, 860–866.

Dahlén, G., Firoze, M., Baelum, V. & Fejerskov, O. (1989). Black-pigmented *Bacteroides* species and *Actinobacillus actinomycetemcomitans* in subgingival plaque of adult Kenyans. *Journal of Clinical Periodontology* **16**, 305–310.

de Souza, R.C. & Colombo, A.P. (2006). Distribution of FcgammaRIIa and FcgammaRIIIb genotypes in patients with generalized aggressive periodontitis. *Journal of Periodontology* **77**, 1120–1128.

Diehl, S.R., Wu, T., Burmeister, J.A., Califano, J.V., Brooks, C.N., Tew, J.G. & Schenkein, H.A. (2003). Evidence of a substantial genetic basis for IgG2 levels in families with aggressive periodontitis. *Journal of Dental Research* **82**, 708–712.

Diehl, S.R., Wu, T., Michalowicz, B.S., Brooks, C.N., Califano, J.V., Burmeister, J.A. & Schenkein, H.A. (2005). Quantitative measures of aggressive periodontitis show substantial heritability and consistency with traditional diagnoses. *Journal of Periodontology* **76**, 279–288.

DiRienzo, J.M., Cornell, S., Kazoroski, L. & Slots, J. (1990). Probe-specific DNA fingerprinting applied to the epidemiology of localized juvenile periodontitis. *Oral Microbiology and Immunology* **5**, 49–56.

DiRienzo, J.M. & McKay, T.L. (1994a). Identification and characterization of genetic cluster groups of *Actinobacillus actinomycetemcomitans* isolated from the human oral cavity. *Journal of Clinical Microbiology* **32**, 75–81.

DiRienzo, J.M., Slots, J., Sixou, M., Sol, M.A., Harmon, R. & McKay, T. (1994b). Specific genetic variants of *Actinobacillus actinomycetemcomitans* correlate with disease and health in a regional population of families with localized juvenile periodontitis. *Infection and Immunity* **62**, 3058–3065.

Ebersole, J.L. (1990). Systemic humoral immune response in periodontal disease. *Critical Reviews in Oral Biology and Medicine* **1**, 283–331.

Ebersole, J. (1996). Immune responses in periodontal diseases. In: Wilson, T. & Kornman, K., eds. *Fundamentals of Periodontics*. Chicago: Quintessence Publishing Co, pp. 109–158.

Ebersole, J., Cappelli, D. & Sandoval, M. (1994). Subgingival distribution of *A. actinomycetemcomitans* in periodontitis. *Journal of Clinical Periodontology* **21**, 65–75.

Ebersole, J., Taubman, M. & Smith, D. (1985a). Local antibody responses in periodontal diseases. *Journal of Periodontology* **56**, 51–56.

Ebersole, J.L., Taubman, M.A. & Smith, D.J. (1985b). Gingival crevicular fluid antibody to oral microorganisms. II. Distribution and specificity of local antibody responses. *Journal of Periodontal Research* **20**, 349–356.

Ebersole, J.L., Taubman, M.A., Smith, D.A. *et al.* (1983). Human immune response to oral microorganisms. II. Serum antibody responses to antigens from *Actinobacillus actinomycetemcomitans*. *Journal of Clinical Immunology* **3**, 321–331.

Ebersole, J.L., Taubman, M.A., Smith, D.J. & Frey, D.E. (1986). Human immune response to oral microorganisms: patterns of antibody levels to *Bacteroides* species. *Infection and Immunity* **51**, 507–513.

Ebersole, J.L., Taubman, M.A., Smith, D.J., Genco, R.J. & Frey, D.E. (1982). Human immune responses to oral microorganisms. I. Association of localized juvenile periodontitis (LJP) with serum antibody responses to *Actinobacillus actinomycetemcomitans*. *Clinical Experimental Immunology* **47**, 43–52.

Ebersole, J.L., Taubman, M.A., Smith, D.J. & Goodson, J.M. (1984). Gingival crevicular fluid antibody to oral microorganisms. I. Method of collection and analysis of antibody. *Journal of Periodontal Research* **19**, 124–132.

Eisenmann, A.C., Eisenmann, R., Sousa, O. & Slots, J. (1983). Microbiological study of localized juvenile periodontitis in Panama. *Journal of Periodontology* **54**, 712–713.

Engel, D. (1996). Lymphocyte function in early-onset periodontitis. *Journal of Periodontology* **67**, 332–336.

Fine, D.H. (1994). Microbial identification and antibiotic sensitivity testing, an aid for patients refractory to periodontal therapy. *Journal of Clinical Periodontology* **21**, 98–106.

Fine, D.H., Goldberg, D. & Karol, R. (1984). Caries levels in patients with juvenile periodontitis. *Journal of Periodontology* **55**, 242–246.

Fives-Taylor, P., Meyer, D. & Mintz, K. (1996). Virulence factors of the periodontopathogen *Actinobacillus actinomycetemcomitans*. *Journal of Periodontology* **67**, 291–297.

Fu, Y., Korostoff, J.M., Fine, D.H. & Wilson, M.E. (2002). Fc gamma receptor genes as risk markers for localized aggressive periodontitis in African-Americans. *Journal of Periodontology* **73**, 517–523.

Genco, R.J., Van, D.T.E., Park, B., Ciminelli, M. & Horoszewicz, H. (1980). Neutrophil chemotaxis impairment in juvenile periodontitis: evaluation of specificity, adherence, deformability, and serum factors. *Journal of the Reticuloendothelial Society* **28**, 81s–91s.

Genco, R.J., VanDyke, T.E., Levine, M.J., Nelson, R.D. & Wilson, M.E. (1986). Molecular factors influencing neutrophil defects in periodontal disease (1985 Kreshover lecture). *Journal of Dental Research* **65**, 1379–1391.

Genco, R.J., Zambon, J.J. & Murray, P.A. (1985). Serum and gingival fluid antibodies as adjuncts in the diagnosis of *Actinobacillus actinomycetemcomitans*-associated periodontal disease. *Journal of Periodontology* **56**, 41–50.

Gmür, R. & Baehni, P.C. (1997). Serum immunoglobulin G responses to various *Actinobacillus actinomycetemcomitans* serotypes in a young ethnographically heterogenous periodontitis patient group. *Oral Microbiology and Immunology* **12**, 1–10.

Gmür, R. & Guggenheim, B. (1994). Interdental supragingival plaque – A natural habitat of *Actinobacillus actinomycetemcomitans*, *Bacteroides forsythus*, *Campylobacter rectus* and *Prevotella nigrescens*. *Journal of Dental Research* **73**, 1421–1428.

Grossi, S.G., Zambon, J.J., Ho, A.W., Koch, G., Dunford, R.G., Machtei, E.E., Norderyd, O.M. & Genco, R.J. (1994). Assessment of risk for periodontal disease. I. Risk indicators for attachment loss. *Journal of Periodontology* **65**, 260–267.

Guerrero, A., Griffiths, G.S., Nibali, L., Suvan, J., Moles, D.R., Laurell, L. & Tonetti, M.S. (2005). Adjunctive benefits of systemic amoxicillin and metronidazole in non-surgical treatment of generalized aggressive periodontitis: a randomized placebo-controlled clinical trial. *Journal of Clinical Periodontology* **32**, 1096–1107.

Gunsolley, J.C., Burmeister, J.A., Tew, J.G., Best, A.M. & Ranney, R.R. (1987). Relationship of serum antibody to attachment level patterns in young adults with juvenile periodontitis or generalized severe periodontitis. *Journal of Periodontology* **58**, 314–320.

Gunsolley, J.C., Ranney, R.R., Zambon, J.J., Burmeister, J.A. & Schenkein, H.A. (1990). *Actinobacillus actinomycetemcomitans* in families afflicted with periodontitis. *Journal of Periodontology* **61**, 643–648.

Gunsolley, J.C., Tew, J.G., Gooss, C.M., Burmeister, J.A. & Schenkein, H.A. (1988). Effects of race and periodontal status on antibody reactive with *Actinobacillus actinomycetemcomitans* strain. *Journal of Periodontal Research* **23**, 303–307.

Haffajee, A.D. & Socransky, S.S. (1994). Microbial etiological agents of destructive periodontal diseases. *Periodontology 2000* **5**, 78–111.

Haffajee, A.D., Socransky, S.S. & Ebersole, J.L. (1984). Clinical, microbiological and immunological features associated with the treatment of active periodontosis lesions. *Journal of Clinical Periodontology* **11**, 600–618.

Haffajee, A.D., Socransky, S.S. & Gunsolley, J.C. (2003). Systemic anti-infective periodontal therapy. A systematic review. *Annals of Periodontology* **8**, 115–181.

Haffajee, A.D., Socransky, S.S., Smith, C. & Dibart, S. (1991). Relation of baseline microbial parameters to future periodontal attachment loss. *Journal of Clinical Periodontology* **18**, 744–750.

Hall, E.R., Falkler, W.A. Jr., Martin, S.A. & Suzuki, J.B. (1991). The gingival immune response to *Actinobacillus actinomycetemcomitans* in juvenile periodontitis. *Journal of Periodontology* **62**, 792–798.

Hall, E.R., Falkler, W.A. Jr. & Suzuki, J.B. (1990). Production of immunoglobulins in gingival tissue explant cultures from juvenile periodontitis patients. *Journal of Periodontology* **61**, 603–608.

Hall, E.R., Martin, S.A., Suzuki, J.B. & Falkler, W.A. Jr. (1994). The gingival immune response to periodontal pathogens in juvenile periodontitis. *Oral Microbiology and Immunology* **9**, 327–334.

Hammond, B.F., Lillard, S.E. & Stevens, R.H. (1987). A bacteriocin of *Actinobacillus actinomycetemcomitans*. *Journal of Periodontology* **55**, 686–691.

Haraszthy, V.I., Hariharan, G., Tinoco, E.M., Cortelli, J.R., Lally, E.T., Davis, E. & Zambon, J.J. (2000). Evidence for the role of highly leukotoxic *Actinobacillus actinomycetemcomitans* in the pathogenesis of localized juvenile and other forms of early-onset periodontitis. *Journal of Periodontology* **71**, 912–922.

Hart, T. (1996). Genetic risk factors for early onset periodontitis. *Journal of Periodontology* **67**, 355–366.

Hart, T., Marazita, M., McCanna, K., Schenkein, H. & Diehl, S. (1993). Re-evaluation of the chromosome 4q candidate region for early onset periodontitis. *Human Genetics* **91**, 416–422.

Hart, T.C., Marazita, M.L., Schenkein, H.A. & Diehl, S.R. (1992). Re-interpretation of the evidence for X-linked dominant inheritance of juvenile periodontitis. *Journal of Periodontology* **63**, 169–173.

Haubek, D., Dirienzo, J.M., Tinoco, E.M., Westergaard, J., Lopez, N.J., Chung, C.P., Poulsen, K. & Kilian, M. (1997). Racial tropism of a highly toxic clone of *Actinobacillus actinomycetemcomitans* associated with juvenile periodontitis. *Journal of Clinical Microbiology* **35**, 3037–3042.

Haubek, D., Ennibi, O.K., Poulsen, K., Poulsen, S., Benzarti, N. & Kilian, M. (2001). Early-onset periodontitis in Morocco is associated with the highly leukotoxic clone of *Actinobacillus actinomycetemcomitans*. *Journal of Dental Research* **80**, 1580–1583.

Haubek, D., Poulsen, K., Asikainen, S. & Kilian, M. (1995). Evidence for absence in northern Europe of especially virulent clonal types of *Actinobacillus actinomycetemcomitans*. *Journal of Clinical Microbiology* **33**, 395–401.

Haubek, D., Poulsen, K., Westergaard, J., Dahlen, G. & Kilian, M. (1996). Highly toxic clone of *Actinobacillus actinomycetemcomitans* in geographically widespread cases of juvenile periodontitis in adolescents of African origin. *Journal of Clinical Microbiology* **34**, 1576–1578.

He, T., Nishihara, T., Demuth, D.R. & Ishikawa, I. (1999). A novel insertion sequence increases the expression of leukotoxicity in *Actinobacillus actinomycetemcomitans* clinical isolates. *Journal of Periodontology* **70**, 1261–1268.

Hölttä, P., Alaluusua, S., Saarela, M. & Asikainen, S. (1994). Isolation frequency and serotype distribution of mutans streptococci and *Actinobacillus actinomycetemcomitans*, and clinical periodontal status in Finnish and Vietnamese children. *Scandinavian Journal of Dental Research* **102**, 113–119.

Hormand, J. & Frandsen, A. (1979). Juvenile periodontitis. Localization of bone loss in relation to age, sex, and teeth. *Journal of Clinical Periodontology* **6**, 407–416.

Jordan, W.J., Eskdale, J., Lennon, G.P., Pestoff, R., Wu, L., Fine, D.H. & Gallagher, G. (2005). A non-conservative, coding single-nucleotide polymorphism in the N-terminal region of lactoferrin is associated with aggressive periodontitis in an African-American, but not a Caucasian population. *Genes and Immunity* **6**, 632–635.

Kaneko, S., Kobayashi, T., Yamamoto, K., Jansen, M.D., van de Winkel, J.G. & Yoshie, H. (2004). A novel polymorphism of FcalphaRI (CD89) associated with aggressive periodontitis. *Tissue Antigens* **63**, 572–577.

Kilian, M., Frandsen, E.V., Haubek, D. & Poulsen, K. (2006). The etiology of periodontal disease revisited by population genetic analysis. *Periodontology 2000* **42**, 158–179.

Kolodrubetz, D., Dailey, T., Ebersole, J. & Kraig, E. (1989). Cloning and expression of the leukotoxin gene from *Actinobacillus actinomycetemcomitans*. *Infection and Immunity* **57**, 1465–1469.

Kinane, D.F., Cullen, C.F., Johnston, F.A. & Evans, C.W. (1989a). Neutrophil chemotactic behaviour in patients with early onset forms of periodontitis. I. Leading front analysis in Boyden chambers. *Journal of Clinical Periodontology* **16**, 242–246.

Kinane, D.F., Cullen, C.F., Johnston, F.A. & Evans, C.W. (1989b). Neutrophil chemotactic behaviour in patients with early onset forms of periodontitis. II. Assessment using the under agarose technique. *Journal of Clinical Periodontology* **16**, 247–251.

Kornman, K.S. & Robertson, P.B. (1985). Clinical and microbiological evaluation of therapy for juvenile periodontitis. *Journal of Periodontology* **56**, 443–446.

Kugelberg, C.F. (1992). Third molar surgery. *Current Opinions in Oral and Maxillofacial Surgery and Infections* **2**, III, 9–16.

Lally, E., Baehni, P. & McArthur, W. (1980). Local immunoglobulin synthesis in periodontal disease. *Journal of Periodontal Research* **15**, 159–164.

Lally, E.T., Kieba, I.R., Golub, E.E., Lear, J.D. & Tanaka, J.C. (1996). Structure/function aspects of *Actinobacillus actinomycetemcomitans* leukotoxin. *Journal of Periodontology* **67**, 298–308.

Lang, N.P., Bartold, P.M., Cullinam, M., Jeffcoat, M., Mombelli, A., Murakami, S., Page, R., Papapanou, P., Tonetti, M. & Van Dyke, T. (1999). International Classification Workshop. Consensus report: Aggressive periodontitis. *Annals of Periodontology* **4**, 53.

Lang, N. & Hill, R. (1977). Radiographs in periodontics. *Journal of Clinical Periodontology* **4**, 16–28.

Li, Y., Xu, L., Hasturk, H., Kantarci, A., DePalma, S.R. & Van Dyke, T.E. (2004). Localized aggressive periodontitis is linked to human chromosome 1q25. *Human Genetics* **114**, 291–297.

Liljenberg, B. & Lindhe, J. (1980). Juvenile periodontitis: some microbiological, histopathologic and clinical characteristics. *Journal of Clinical Periodontology* **7**, 748–761.

Lissau, I., Holst, D. & Friis-Hasché, E. (1990). Dental health behaviors and periodontal disease indicators in Danish youths. *Journal of Clinical Periodontology* **17**, 42–47.

Listgarten, M.A. (1976). Structure of the microbial flora associated with periodontal health and disease in man. *Journal of Periodontology* **47**, 1–18.

Listgarten, M.A., Lai, C.H. & Evian, C.I. (1981). Comparative antibody titers to *Actinobacillus actinomycetemcomitans* in juvenile periodontitis, chronic periodontitis, and periodontally healthy subjects. *Journal of Clinical Periodontology* **8**, 155–164.

Listgarten, M.A., Wong, M.Y. & Lai, C.H. (1995). Detection of *Actinobacillus actinomycetemcomitans, Porphyromonas gingivalis,* and *Bacteroides forsythus* in an *A. actinomycetemcomitans*-positive patient population. *Journal of Periodontology* **66**, 158–164.

Llorente, M.A. & Griffiths, G.S. (2006). Periodontal status among relatives of aggressive periodontitis patients and reliability of family history report. *Journal of Clinical Periodontology* **33**, 121–125.

Löe, H. & Brown, L.J. (1991). Early onset periodontitis in the United States of America. *Journal of Periodontology* **62**, 608–616.

Loesche, W.J., Syed, S.A., Schmidt, E. & Morrison, E.C. (1985). Bacterial profiles of subgingival plaques in periodontitis. *Journal of Clinical Periodontology* **56**, 447–456.

Long, J., Nance, W., Waring, P., Burmeister, J. & Ranney, R. (1987). Early onset periodontitis: a comparison and evaluation of two modes of inheritance. *Genetic Epidemiology* **4**, 13–24.

Loos, B.G., Leppers-Van de Straat, F.G., Van de Winkel, J.G. & Van der Velden, U. (2003). Fcgamma receptor polymorphisms in relation to periodontitis. *Journal of Clinical Periodontology* **30**, 595–602.

Loos, B.G., John, R.P. & Laine, M.L. (2005). Identification of genetic risk factors for periodontitis and possible mechanisms of action. *Journal of Clinical Periodontology* **32** (Suppl 6), 154–174.

Macheleidt, A., Muller, H.P., Eger, T., Putzker, M., Fuhrmann, A. & Zoller, L. (1999). Absence of an especially toxic clone among isolates of *Actinobacillus actinomycetemcomitans* recovered from army recruits. *Clinical Oral Investigations* **3**, 161–167.

Mackler, B.F., Frostad, K.B., Robertson, R.B. & Levy, B.M. (1977). Immunoglobulin bearing lymphocytes and plasma cells in human periodontal disease. *Journal of Periodontal Research* **12**, 37–45.

Mackler, B.F., Waldrop, T.C., Schur, P., Robertson, P.B. & Levy, B.M. (1978). IgG subclasses in human periodontal disease. I. Distribution and incidence of IgG subclasses bearing lymphocytes and plasma cells. *Journal of Periodontal Research* **13**, 109–119.

Mandell, R.L. (1984). A longitudinal microbiological investigation of *Actinobacillus actinomycetemcomitans* and *Eikenella corrodens* in juvenile periodontitis. *Infection and Immunity* **45**, 778–780.

Mandell, R.L., Ebersole, L.J. & Socransky, S.S. (1987). Clinical immunologic and microbiologic features of active disease sites in juvenile periodontitis. *Journal of Clinical Periodontology* **14**, 534–540.

Mandell, R.L. & Socransky, S.S. (1981). A selective medium for *Actinobacillus actinomycetemcomitans* and the incidence of the organism in juvenile periodontitis. *Journal of Periodontology* **52**, 593–598.

Mandell, R.L., Tripodi, L.S., Savitt, E., Goodson, J.M. & Socransky, S.S. (1986). The effect of treatment on *Actinobacillus actinomycetemcomitans* in localized juvenile periodontitis. *Journal of Periodontology* **57**, 94–99.

Marazita, M., Burmeister, J. & Gunsolley, J. (1994). Evidence for autosomal dominant inheritance and race-specific heterogeneity in early-onset periodontitis. *Journal of Periodontology* **65**, 623–630.

Masada, M.P., Persson, R., Kenney, J.S., Lee, S.W., Page, R.C. & Allison, A.C. (1990). Measurement of interleukin-1 alpha and beta in gingival crevicular fluid: implications for pathogenesis of periodontal disease. *Journal of Periodontal Research* **25**, 156–163.

McNabb, H., Mombelli, A., Gmür, R., Mathey-Dinç, S. & Lang, N.P. (1992). Periodontal pathogens in shallow pockets in immigrants from developing countries. *Oral Microbiology and Immunology* **7**, 267–272.

Mombelli, A., Casagni, F. & Madianos, P.N. (2002). Can presence or absence of periodontal pathogens distinguish between subjects with chronic and aggressive periodontitis? A systematic review. *Journal of Clinical Periodontology* **29** Suppl 3, 10–21.

Mombelli, A., Gmür, R., Lang, N.P., Corbet, E.F. & Frey, J. (1999). *A. actinomycetemcomitans* in Chinese adults. Serotype distribution and analysis of the leukotoxin gene promoter locus. *Journal of Clinical Periodontology* **26**, 505–510.

Mombelli, A., Gmür, R., Gobbi, C. & Lang, N.P. (1994). *Actinobacillus actinomycetemcomitans* in adult periodontitis. II. Characterization of isolated strains and effect of mechanical periodontal treatment. *Journal of Periodontology* **65**, 827–834.

Mombelli, A., Schmid, B., Rutar, A. & Lang, N.P. (2000). Persistence patterns of *Porphyromonas gingivalis, Prevotella intermedia/nigrescens,* and *Actinobacillus actinomycetemcomitans* after mechanical therapy of periodontal disease. *Journal of Periodontology* **71**, 14–21.

Mombelli, A., Wicki, A. & Lang, N.P. (1994). The occurrence of *Actinobacillus actinomycetemcomitans, Porphyromonas gingivalis* and *Prevotella intermedia* in an Arabic population with minimal periodontal disease. *Microbial Ecology in Health and Disease* **7**, 217–224.

Moore, W.E.C. (1987). Microbiology of periodontal disease. *Journal of Periodontal Research* **22**, 335–341.

Moore, W.E.C., Holdeman, L.V., Cato, E.P., Good, I.J., Smith, E.P., Palcanis, K.G. & Ranney, R.R. (1985). Comparative bacteriology of juvenile periodontitis. *Infection and Immunity* **48**, 507–519.

Murray, P.A., Burstein, D.A. & Winkler, J.R. (1989). Antibodies to *Bacteroides gingivalis* in patients with treated and untreated periodontal disease. *Journal of Periodontology* **60**, 96–103.

Needleman, H., Nelson, L., Allred, E. & Seow, K. (1997). Alveolar bone height of primary and first permanent molars in healthy 7 to 9-year-old children. *ASDC Journal of Dentistry for Children* **64** (3), 188–196.

Newman, M.G. & Socransky, S.S. (1977). Predominant cultivable microbiota in periodontosis. *Journal of Periodontal Research* **12**, 120.

Newman, M.G., Socransky, S.S., Savitt, E.D., Propas, D.A. & Crawford, A. (1976). Studies of the microbiology of periodontosis. *Journal of Periodontology* **47**, 373–379.

Nibali, L., Parkar, M., Brett, P., Knight, J., Tonetti, M.S. & Griffiths, G.S. (2006). NADPH oxidase (CYBA) and FcgammaR polymorphisms as risk factors for aggressive periodontitis: a case-control association study. *Journal of Clinical Periodontology* **33**, 529–539.

Noack, B., Gorgens, H., Hoffmann, T. & Schackert, H.K. (2006). CARD15 gene variants in aggressive periodontitis. *Journal of Clinical Periodontology* **33**, 779–783.

Offenbacher, S., Heasman, P. & Collins, J. (1993). Modulation of host PGE2 secretion as a determinant of periodontal disease. *Journal of Periodontology* **64**, 432–444.

Ogawa, T., Tarkowski, A., McGhee, M.L., Moldoveanu, Z., Mestecky, J., Hirsch, H.Z., Koopman, W.J., Hamada, S., McGhee, J.R. & Kiyono, H. (1989). Analysis of human IgG and IgA antibody secreting cells from localized chronic inflammatory tissue. *Journal of Immunology* **142**, 1140–1158.

Online Mendelian Inheritance in Man, OMIM. (1996). Center for Medical Genetics, Johns Hopkins University (Baltimore, MD) and National Center for Biotechnology Information,

National Library of Medicine (Bethesda, MD). World Wide Web URL: http://www3.ncbi.nlm.nih.gov/omim/

Page, R.C. (1990). Risk factors involving host defense mechanisms. In: Bader, J.D., ed. *Risk Assessment in Dentistry.* Chapel Hill: University of North Carolina Dental Ecology, pp. 94–104.

Page, R.C., Altman, L.C., Ebersole, J.L., Vandesteen, G.E., Dahlberg, W.H., Williams, B.L. & Osterberg, S.K. (1983a). Rapidly progressive periodontitis. A distinct clinical condition. *Journal of Periodontology* **54**, 197–209.

Page, R.C., Bowen, T., Altman, L., Edward, V., Ochs, H., Mackenzie, P., Osterberg, S., Engel, L.D. & Williams, B.L. (1983b). Prepubertal periodontitis. I. Definition of a clinical disease entity. *Journal of Periodontology* **54**, 257–271.

Papapanou, P. (1996). Periodontal diseases: epidemiology. *Annals of Periodontology* **1**, 1–36.

Park, K.S., Nam, J.H. & Choi, J. (2006). The short vitamin D receptor is associated with increased risk for generalized aggressive periodontitis. *Journal of Clinical Periodontology* **33**, 524–528.

Patters, M., Niekrash, C. & Lang, N. (1989). Assessment of complement cleavage during experimental gingivitis in man. *Journal of Clinical Periodontology* **16**, 33–37.

Pavicic, M.J.A.M.P., van Winkelhoff, A.J., Douqué, N.H., Steures, R.W.R. & de Graaff, J. (1994). Microbiological and clinical effects of metronidazole and amoxicillin in *Actinobacillus actinomycetemcomitans*-associated periodontitis. *Journal of Clinical Periodontology* **21**, 107–112.

Petit, M.D.A., van Steenbergen, T.J.M., de Graaff, J. & van der Velden, U. (1993a). Transmission of *Actinobacillus actinomycetemcomitans* in families of adult periodontitis patients. *Journal of Periodontal Research* **28**, 335–345.

Petit, M.D.A., van Steenbergen, T.J.M., Scholte, L.H.M., van der Velden, U. & de Graaff, J. (1993b). Epidemiology and transmission of *Porphyromonas gingivalis* and *Actinobacillus actinomycetemcomitans* among children and their family members – a report of four surveys. *Journal of Clinical Periodontology* **20**, 641–650.

Poulsen, K., Theilade, E., Lally, E.T., Demuth, D.R. & Kilian, M. (1994). Population structure of *Actinobacillus actinomycetemcomitans*: A framework for studies of disease-associated properties. *Microbiology* **140**, 2049–2060.

Preus, H.R. (1988). Treatment of rapidly destructive periodontitis in Papillon-Lefèvre syndrome. Laboratory and clinical observations. *Journal of Clinical Periodontology* **15**, 639–643.

Preus, H.R., Russell, D.T. & Zambon, J.J. (1992). Transmission of *Actinobacillus actinomycetemcomitans* in families of adult periodontitis patients. *Journal of Dental Research* **71**, 606.

Rams, T.E., Feik, D. & Slots, J. (1992). Ciprofloxacin/metronidazole treatment of recurrent adult periodontitis. *Journal of Dental Research* **71**, 319.

Rams, T.E., Listgarten, M.A. & Slots, J. (1996). The utility of 5 major putative periodontal pathogens and selected clinical parameters to predict periodontal breakdown in adults on maintenance care. *Journal of Clinical Periodontology* **23**, 346–354.

Renvert, S., Wikström, M., Dahlén, G., Slots, J. & Egelberg, J. (1990a). Effect of root debridement on the elimination of *Actinobacillus actinomycetemcomitans* and *Bacteroides gingivalis* from periodontal pockets. *Journal of Clinical Periodontology* **17**, 345–350.

Renvert, S., Wikström, M., Dahlén, G., Slots, J. & Egelberg, J. (1990b). On the inability of root debridement and periodontal surgery to eliminate *Actinobacillus actinomycetemcomitans* from periodontal pockets. *Journal of Clinical Periodontology* **17**, 351–355.

Rodenburg, J.P., van Winkelhoff, A.J., Winkel, E.G., Goene, R.J., Abbas, F. & de Graff, J. (1990). Occurrence of *Bacteroides gingivalis*, *Bacteroides intermedius* and *Actinobacillus actinomycetemcomitans* in severe periodontitis in relation to age and treatment history. *Journal of Clinical Periodontology* **17**, 392–399.

Saglie, F.R., Marfany, A. & Camargo, P. (1988). Intragingival occurrence of *Actinobacillus actinomycetemcomitans* and *Bacteroides gingivalis* in active destructive periodontal lesions. *Journal of Periodontology* **59**(4), 259–265.

Sandholm, L., Tolo, K. & Olsen, I. (1987). Salivary IgG, a parameter of periodontal disease activity? High responders to *Actinobacillus actinomycetemcomitans* Y4 in juvenile and adult periodontitis. *Journal of Clinical Periodontology* **14**, 289–294.

Saxen, L. & Nevanlinna, H.R. (1984). Autosomal recessive inheritance of juvenile periodontitis: test of a hypothesis. *Clinical Genetics* **25**, 332–335.

Scapoli, C., Trombelli, L., Mamolini, E. & Collins, A. (2005). Linkage disequilibrium analysis of case-control data: an application to generalized aggressive periodontitis. *Genes and Immunity* **6**, 44–52.

Schenkein, H. (1994). Genetics of early onset periodontal disease. In: Genco, R., Hamada, S., Lehner, T, McGhee, J. & Mergenhagen, S., eds. *Molecular Pathogenesis of Periodontal Disease.* Washington, DC: American Society for Microbiology, pp. 373–383.

Schenkein, H.A. & Genco, R.J. (1977). Gingival fluid and serum in periodontal diseases. II. Evidence for cleavage of complement component C3, C3 proactivator (factor B) and C4 in gingival fluid. *Journal of Periodontology* **48**, 778–784.

Schenkein, H.A., Gunsolley, J.C., Koertge, T.E., Schenkein, J.G. & Tew, J.G. (1995). Smoking and its effects on early-onset periodontitis. *Journal of the American Dental Association* **126**, 1107–1113.

Schenkein, H. & Van-Dyke, T. (1994). Early onset periodontitis. Systemic aspects of etiology and pathogenesis. *Periodontology 2000* **6**, 7–25.

Schonfeld, S.E. & Kagan, J.M. (1982). Specificity of gingival plasma cells for bacterial somatic antigens. *Journal of Periodontal Research* **17**, 60–69.

Shah, H.N. (1993). *Biology of the Species Porphyromonas gingivalis.* Boca Raton: CRC Press.

Shapira, L., Smidt, A., Van, D.T.E., Barak, V., Soskolne, A.W., Brautbar, C., Sela, M.N. & Bimstein, E. (1994). Sequential manifestation of different forms of early-onset periodontitis. A case report. *Journal of Periodontology* **65**, 631–635.

Shapira, L., Warbington, M. & Van Dyke, T.E. (1994). TNF-alpha and IL-1 beta in serum of LJP patients with normal and defective neutrophil chemotaxis. *Journal of Periodontal Research* **29**, 371–373.

Shapira, L., Wilensky, A. & Kinane, D.F. (2005). Effect of genetic variability on the inflammatory response to periodontal infection. *Journal of Clinical Periodontology* **32** (Suppl 6), 67–81.

Sioson, P.B., Furgang, D., Steinberg, L.M. & Fine, D.H. (2000). Proximal caries in juvenile periodontitis patients. *Journal of Periodontology* **71**, 710–716.

Sjodin, B. & Mattson, L. (1992). Marginal bone level in the normal primary dentition. *Journal of Clinical Periodontology* **19**, 672–678.

Sjodin, B. & Mattson, L. (1994). Marginal bone loss in the primary dentition. A survey of 7 to 9 year olds in Sweden. *Journal of Clinical Periodontology* **21**, 313–319.

Sjodin, B., Crossner, C.G., Unell, L. & Ostlund, P. (1989). A retrospective radiographic study of alveolar bone loss in the primary dentition in patients with localized juvenile periodontitis. *Journal of Clinical Periodontology* **16**, 124–127.

Sjodin, B., Matsson, L., Unell, L. & Egelberg, J. (1993). Marginal bone loss in the primary dentition of patients with juvenile periodontitis. *Journal of Clinical Periodontology* **20**, 32–36.

Slots, J. (1976). The predominant cultivable organisms in juvenile periodontitis. *Scandinavian Journal of Dental Research* **84**, 1.

Slots, J., Bragd, L., Wikström, M. & Dahlén, G. (1986). The occurrence of *Actinobacillus actinomycetemcomitans*, *Bacteroides gingivalis* and *Bacteroides intermedius* in destructive periodontal disease in adults. *Journal of Clinical Periodontology* **13**, 570–577.

Slots, J., Feik, D. & Rams, T.E. (1990). *Actinobacillus actinomycetemcomitans* and *Bacteroides intermedius* in human periodontitis: age relationship and mutual association. *Journal of Clinical Periodontology* **17**, 659–662.

Slots, J. & Listgarten, M.A. (1988). *Bacteroides gingivalis, Bacteroides intermedius* and *Actinobacillus actinomycetemcomitans* in human periodontal diseases. *Journal of Clinical Periodontology* **15**, 85–93.

Slots, J., Reynolds, H.S. & Genco, R.J. (1980). *Actinobacillus actinomycetemcomitans* in human periodontal disease: a cross-sectional microbiological investigation. *Infection and Immunity* **29**, 1013–1020.

Slots, J. & Rosling, B.G. (1983). Suppression of the periodontopathic microflora in localized juvenile periodontitis by systemic tetracycline. *Journal of Clinical Periodontology* **10**, 465–486.

Slots, J. & Schonfeld, S.E. (1991). *Actinobacillus actinomycetemcomitans* in localized juvenile periodontitis. In: Hamada, S., Holt, S.C. & McGhee, J.R., eds. *Periodontal Disease. Pathogens and Host Immune Responses.* Tokyo: Quintessence, pp. 53–64.

Socransky, S.S. & Haffajee, A.D. (1992). The bacterial etiology of destructive periodontal disease: current concepts. *Journal of Periodontology* **63**, 322–331.

Soedarsono, N., Rabello, D., Kamei, H., Fuma, D., Ishihara, Y., Suzuki, M., Noguchi, T., Sakaki, Y., Yamaguchi, A. & Kojima, T. (2006). Evaluation of RANK/RANKL/OPG gene polymorphisms in aggressive periodontitis. *Journal of Periodontal Research* **41**, 397–404.

Spitznagel, J., Kraig, E. & Kolodrubetz, D. (1991). Regulation of leukotoxin in leukotoxic and nonleukotoxic strains of *Actinobacillus actinomycetemcomitans*. *Infection and Immunity* **59**, 1394–1401.

Steubing, P., Mackler, B., Schur, P. & Levy, B. (1982). Humoral studies of periodontal disease. I. Characterisation of immunoglobulins quantitated from cultures of gingival tissue. *Clinical Immunology and Immunopathology* **22**, 32–43.

Suomi, J., Plumbo, J. & Barbano, J. (1968). A comparative study of radiographs and pocket measurements in periodontal disease evaluation. *Journal of Periodontology* **39**, 311–315.

Suzuki, A., Ji, G., Numabe, Y., Muramatsu, M., Gomi, K., Kanazashi, M., Ogata, Y., Shimizu, E., Shibukawa, Y., Ito, A., Ito T., Sugaya, A., Arai, T., Yamada, S., Deguchi, S. & Kamoi, K. (2004). Single nucleotide polymorphisms associated with aggressive periodontitis and severe chronic periodontitis in Japanese. *Biochemical and Biophysical Research Communications* **317**, 887–892

Sweeney, E.A., Alcoforado, G.A.P., Nyman, S. & Slots, J. (1987). Prevalence and microbiology of localized prepubertal periodontitis. *Oral Microbiology and Immunology* **2**, 65–70.

Tan, K.S., Woo, C.H., Ong, G. & Song, K.P. (2001). Prevalence of *Actinobacillus actinomycetemcomitans* in an ethnic adult Chinese population. *Journal of Clinical Periodontology* **28**, 886–890.

Taubman, M.A., Stoufi, E.D., Seymour, G.J., Smith, D.J. & Ebersole, J.L. (1988). Immunoregulatory aspects of periodontal diseases. *Advances in Dental Research* **2**, 328–333.

Taubman, M.A., Wang, H-Y., Lundqvist, C.A., Seymour, G.J., Eastcott, J.W. & Smith, D.J. (1991). The cellular basis of host responses in periodontal diseases. In: Hamada, S., Holt, S.C. & McGhee, J.R., eds. *Periodontal Disease: Pathogens and Host Immune Responses.* Tokyo: Quintessence Publishing Co, pp. 199–208.

Tew, J.G., Marshall, D.R. & Burmeister, J.A. (1985). Relationship between gingival crevicular fluid and serum antibody titers in young adults with generalized and localized periodontitis. *Infection and Immunity* **49**, 487–493.

Tew, J.G., Zhang, J.B., Quinn, S., Tangada, S., Nakashima, K., Gunsolley, J.C. Schenkein, H.A. & Califano, J.V. (1996). Antibody of the IgG2 subclass, *Actinobacillus actinomycetem-comitans*, and early onset periodontitis. *Journal of Periodontology* **67**, 317–322.

Tinoco, E.M.B., Stevens, R., Haubek, D., Lai, C.H., Balachandran, S. & Preus, H. (1997). Relationship of serotype, leukotoxin gene type and lysogeny in *Actinobacillus actinomycetemcomitans* to periodontal disease status. *European Journal of Oral Sciences* **105**, 310–317.

Tolo, K. & Schenck, K. (1985). Activity of serum immunoglobulins G, A, and M to six anaerobic, oral bacteria in diagnosis of periodontitis. *Journal of Periodontal Research* **20**, 113–121.

Tonetti, M. (1993). Etiology and pathogenesis. In: *Proceedings of the 1st European Workshop on Periodontology*, Lang, N.P. & Karring, T., eds. Berlin: Quintessenz Verlags-GmbH, pp. 54–89.

Tonetti, M. & Mombelli, A. (1999). Early onset periodontitis. *Annals of Periodontology* **4**, 39–53.

Tonetti, M.S., Claffey, N., on behalf of the European Workshop in Periodontology group C. (2005). Advances in the progression of periodontitis and proposal of definitions of a periodontitis case and disease progression for use in risk factor research. *Journal of Clinical Periodontology* **32** (Suppl 6), 205–208.

Tsai, C.C., McArthur, W.P., Baehni, P.C. *et al.* (1981). Serum neutralizing activity against *Actinobacillus actinomycetemcomitans* leukotoxin in juvenile periodontitis. *Journal of Clinical Periodontology* **8**, 338–348.

Tsai, C.C., Shenker, B.J., DiRienzo, J.M., Malmud, D. & Taichman, N.S. (1984). Extraction and isolation of a leukotoxin from *Actinobacillus actinomycetemcomitans* with polymyxin B. *Infection and Immunity* **43**, 700–705.

van der Velden, U., Abbas, F., Van Steenbergen, T.J.M., De Zoete, O.J., Hesse, M., De Ruyter, C., De Laat, V.H.M. & De Graaff, J. (1989). Prevalence of periodontal breakdown in adolescents and presence of *Actinobacillus actinomycetemcomitans* in subjects with attachment loss. *Journal of Periodontology* **60**, 604–610.

Van Dyke, T.E., Horozewicz, H.U. & Genco, R.J. (1982). The polymorphonuclear leukocyte (PMNL) locomotor defect in juvenile periodontitis. *Journal of Periodontology* **53**, 682–687.

Van Dyke, T.E., Offenbacher, S., Kalmar, J. & Arnold, R.R. (1988). Neutrophil defects and host-parasite interactions in the pathogenesis of localized juvenile periodontitis. *Advances in Dental Research* **2**, 354–358.

Van Dyke, T.E., Schweinebraten, M., Cianciola, L.J., Offenbacher, S. & Genco, R.J. (1985). Neutrophil chemotaxis in families with localized juvenile periodontitis. *Journal of Periodontal Research* **20**, 503–514.

Van Dyke, T.E., Zinney, W., Winkel, K., Taufiq, A., Offenbacher, S. & Arnold, R.R. (1986). Neutrophil function in localized juvenile periodontitis. Phagocytosis, superoxide production and specific granule release. *Journal of Periodontology* **57**, 703–708.

van Winkelhoff, A.J. & Boutaga, K. (2005). Transmission of periodontal bacteria and models of infection. *Journal of Clinical Periodontology* **32** (Suppl 6), 16–27.

van Winkelhoff, A.J., Rodenburg, J.P., Goene, R.J., Abbas, F., Winkel, E.G. & de Graaff, J. (1989). Metronidazole plus amoxycillin in the treatment of *Actinobacillus actinomycetemcomitans* associated periodontitis. *Journal of Clinical Periodontology* **16**, 128–131.

Vincent, J.W., Suzuki, J.B., Falkler, W.A. & Cornett, W.C. (1985). Reaction of human sera from juvenile periodontitis, rapidly progressive periodontitis, and adult periodontitis patients with selected periodontopathogens. *Journal of Periodontology* **56**, 464–469.

Von Troil-Lindén, B., Torkko, H., Alaluusua, S., Wolf, J., Jousimies-Somer, H. & Asikainen, S. (1995). Periodontal findings in spouses: A clinical, radiographic and microbiological study. *Journal of Clinical Periodontology* **22**, 93–99.

Waldrop, T.C., Mackler, B.F. & Schur, P. (1981). IgG and IgG subclasses in human periodontosis (juvenile periodontitis). Serum concentrations. *Journal of Periodontology* **52**, 96–98.

Watanabe, K. (1990). Prepubertal periodontitis: a review of diagnostic criteria, pathogenesis, and differential diagnosis. *Journal of Periodontal Research* **25**, 31–48.

Westergaard, J., Frandsen, A. & Slots, J. (1978). Ultrastructure of the subgingival microflora in juvenile periodontitis. *Scandinavian Journal of Dental Research* **86**, 421–429.

Williams, R.C., Jeffcoat, M.K., Howell, T.H. *et al.* (1989). Altering the course of human alveolar bone loss with the nonsteroidal anti-inflammatory drug fluorbiprofen. *Journal of Periodontology* **60**, 485–490.

Williams, R.C., Jeffcoat, M.K., Kaplan, M.L., Goldhaber, P., Johnson, H.G. & Wechter, W.J. (1985). Fluorbiprofen: a potent inhibitor of alveolar bone resorption in beagles. *Science* **227**, 640–642.

Wilson, M.E. & Kalmar, J.R. (1996) FcRIIa (CD32): a potential marker defining susceptibility to localized juvenile periodontitis. *Journal of Periodontology* **67**, 323–331.

Zambon, J.J., Christersson, L.A. & Slots, J. (1983). *Actinobacillus actinomycetemcomitans* in human periodontal disease. Prevalence in patient groups and distribution of biotypes and serotypes within families. *Journal of Periodontology* **54**, 707–711.

Zambon, J.J., DeLuca, C., Slots, J. & Genco, R.J. (1983a). Studies of leukotoxin from *Actinobacillus actinomycetemcomitans* using the promyelocytic HL-60 cell line. *Infection and Immunity* **40**, 205–212.

Zambon, J.J., Slots, J. & Genco, R.J. (1983b). Serology of oral *Actinobacillus actinomycetemcomitans* and serotype distribution in human periodontal disease. *Infection and Immunity* **41**, 19–27.

Zambon, J.J., Haraszthy, V.I., Hariharan, G., Lally, E.T. & Demuth, D.R. (1996). The microbiology of early-onset periodontitis: association of highly toxic *Actinobacillus actinomycetemcomitans* strains with localized juvenile periodontitis. *Journal of Periodontology* **67**, 282–290.

Zambon, J.J., Umemoto, T., De Nardin, E., Nakazawa, F., Christersson, L.A. & Genco, R.J. (1988). *Actinobacillus actinomycetemcomitans* in the pathogenesis of human periodontal disease. *Advances in Dental Research* **2**, 269–274.

Chapter 20

Necrotizing Periodontal Disease

Palle Holmstrup and Jytte Westergaard

Nomenclature

Necrotizing gingivitis (NG), necrotizing periodontitis (NP), and necrotizing stomatitis (NS) are the most severe inflammatory periodontal disorders caused by plaque bacteria. The necrotizing diseases usually run an acute course and therefore the term acute is often included in the diagnoses. They are rapidly destructive and debilitating, and they appear to represent various stages of the same disease process (Horning & Cohen 1995). A distinction between NG and NP has not always been made in the literature, but parallel to the use of the term gingivitis, NG should be limited to lesions only involving gingival tissue with no loss of periodontal attachment (Riley *et al.* 1992). Most often, however, the disease results in loss of attachment (MacCarthy & Claffey 1991), and a more correct term in cases with loss of attachment is NP, provided the lesions are confined to the periodontal tissues including gingiva, periodontal ligament, and alveolar bone. Further progression to include tissue beyond the mucogingival junction is characteristic of necrotizing stomatitis and distinguishes this disease from NP (Williams *et al.* 1990).

The necrotizing periodontal diseases have had several names, including ulceromembranous gingivitis, acute necrotizing ulcerative gingivitis (ANUG), Vincent's gingivitis or Vincent's gingivostomatitis, necrotizing gingivostomatitis, and trench mouth (Pickard 1973; Johnson & Engel 1986; Horning & Cohen 1995). Vincent first described the mixed fusospirochetal microbiota of the so-called "Vincent's angina", characterized by necrotic areas in the tonsils (Vincent 1898). A similar mixed microbiota has been isolated from NG lesions, but Vincent's angina and NG usually occur independently of each other, and should be regarded as separate disease entities.

NS has features in common with the far more serious *cancrum oris*, also denoted noma. This is a destructive and necrotizing, frequently fatal, stomatitis in which the same mixed fusospirochetal flora dominates. It occurs almost exclusively in certain developing countries, mostly in children suffering from systemic diseases including malnutrition (Enwonwu 1972, 1985). It has been suggested that cancrum oris always develops from pre-existing NG (Emslie 1963) but this connection has not been confirmed (Pindborg *et al.* 1966, 1967; Sheiham 1966).

In the literature, a distinction between NG, NP, and NS is seldom made. However, the reader should be aware of this uncertainty and the consequences of the lack of distinction between the three diagnoses in reports. The uncertainty is reflected in the present chapter by the use of the term necrotizing periodontal disease (NPD) as a common denominator for necrotizing gingivitis, necrotizing periodontitis, and necrotizing stomatitis.

Prevalence

During World War II, up to 14% of Danish military personnel encountered NPD (Pindborg 1951a). Large numbers of civilians also suffered from the disease (King 1943; Stammers 1944). After World War II, the prevalence of NPD declined substantially and it is now rare in industrialized countries. It occurs particularly among young adults. In the 1960s NPD was found in 2.5% of 326 US students during their first college year, but over the next year more students became affected, with a total of 6.7% demonstrating the disease during their first two college years (Giddon et al. 1964). Among 9203 students in Chile, 6.7% showed at least one necrotic ulcerated lesion on the papillae (Lopez et al. 2002), and the presence of necrotizing lesions was associated with the occurrence of clinical attachment loss (Lopez & Bælum 2004). Other studies in industrialized countries have reported prevalence of 0.5% or less (Barnes et al. 1973; Horning et al. 1990). In Scandinavia, the disease is now very rare among otherwise healthy individuals, with a prevalence of 0.001% among young Danish military trainees (personal communication, F. Prætorius). NPD can be observed in all age groups but there are geographic differences in the age distribution.

The disease seems to occur slightly more often among HIV-infected individuals. Studies among groups of HIV-infected individuals have revealed prevalences of NPD between 0% and 27.7% (Reichart et al. 2003; Holmstrup & Westergaard 1994). However, most studies have included cohorts of individuals connected with hospitals or dental clinics. Studies conducted outside these environments have shown relatively low prevalence figures. NP was found in 1% of 200 HIV-seropositive individuals in Washington, DC (Riley et al. 1992), and the prevalence may not, in fact, differ so much from that of the general population (Drinkard et al. 1991; Friedman et al. 1991; Barr et al. 1992); this is particularly true after introduction of antiretroviral therapy (Tappuni & Flemming 2001).

In developing countries, the prevalence of NPD is higher than in the industrialized countries, and the disease frequently occurs in children. This is practically never seen in western countries. In Nigerian villages, between 1.7% and 26.9% of 2–6-year-old children were found with NPD (Sheiham 1966). In India, 54–68% of NPD cases occurred in children below 10 years of age (Migliani & Sharma 1965; Pindborg et al. 1966).

Clinical characteristics

Development of lesions

NG is an inflammatory destructive gingival condition, characterized by ulcerated and necrotic papillae and gingival margins resulting in a characteristic punched-out appearance. The ulcers are covered by a yellowish white or grayish slough, which has been termed "pseudomembrane". However, the sloughed material has no coherence, and bears little resemblance to a membrane. It consists primarily of fibrin and necrotic tissue with leukocytes, erythrocytes, and masses of bacteria. Consequently, the term is misleading and should not be used. Removal of the sloughed material results in bleeding and ulcerated underlying tissue becomes exposed.

The necrotizing lesions develop rapidly and are painful, but in the initial stages, when the necrotic areas are relatively few and small, pain is usually moderate. Severe pain is often the chief reason for patients to seek treatment. Bleeding is readily provoked. This is due to the acute inflammation and necrosis with exposure of the underlying connective tissue. Bleeding may start spontaneously as well as in response to even gentle touch. In early phases of the disease lesions are typically confined to the top of a few interdental papillae (Fig. 20-1). The first lesions are often seen interproximally in the mandibular anterior region, but they may occur in any interproximal space. In regions where lesions first appear, there are usually also signs of pre-existing chronic gingivitis, but the papillae are not always edematous at this stage and gingival stippling may be maintained. Usually, however, the papillae swell rapidly and develop a rounded contour; this is particularly evident in the facial aspect. The zone between the marginal necrosis and the relatively unaffected gingiva usually exhibits a well demarcated narrow erythematous zone, sometimes referred to as the linear erythema. This is an expression of hyperemia due to dilation of the vessels in the gingi-

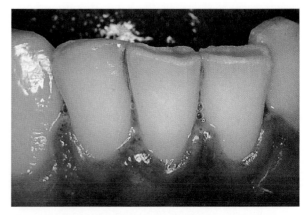

Fig. 20-1 Necrotizing gingivitis with initial punched out defects at the top of the interdental papillae of the mandibular incisor region. Courtesy of Dr. Finn Prætorius.

val connective tissue in the periphery of the necrotic lesions (see Fig. 20-17a).

A characteristic and pronounced *foetor ex ore* is often associated with NPD, but can vary in intensity and in some cases is not very noticeable. Strong *foetor ex ore* is not pathognomonic of NPD as it can also be found in other pathologic conditions of the oral cavity such as chronic destructive periodontal disease.

Interproximal craters

The lesions are seldom associated with deep pocket formation, because extensive gingival necrosis often coincides with loss of crestal alveolar bone. The gingival necrosis develops rapidly and within a few days the involved papillae are often separated into one facial and one lingual portion with an interposed necrotic depression, a negative papilla, between them. The central necrosis produces considerable tissue destruction and a regular crater is formed. At this stage of the disease, the disease process usually involves the periodontal ligament and the alveolar bone, and loss of attachment is now established. The diagnosis of the disease process is consequently NP.

Along with the papilla destruction, the necrosis usually extends laterally along the gingival margin at the oral and/or facial surfaces of the teeth. Necrotic areas originating from neighboring interproximal spaces frequently merge to form a continuous necrotic area (Figs. 20-2 and 20-3). Superficial necrotic lesions only rarely cover a substantial part of the attached gingiva, which becomes reduced in width as the result of disease progression. The palatal and lingual marginal gingiva is less frequently involved than the corresponding facial area. Frequently, gingiva of semi-impacted teeth and in the posterior maxillary region are affected (Figs. 20-4 and 20-5). Progression of the interproximal process often results in destruction of most interdental alveolar bone (Fig. 20-6). In more advanced cases, pain is often considerable and may be associated with a markedly increased salivary flow. As a result of pain it is often difficult for

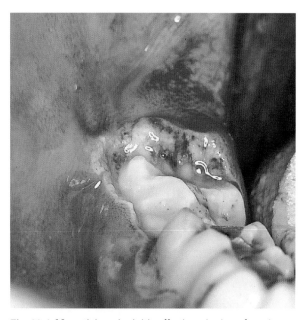

Fig. 20-4 Necrotizing gingivitis affecting gingiva of semi-impacted right mandibular third molar. Courtesy of Dr. Finn Prætorius.

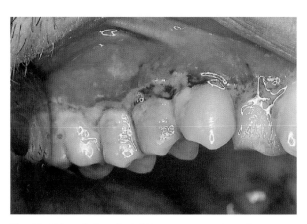

Fig. 20-2 Necrotizing gingivitis progressing along the gingival margin of the right maxilla. The interproximal necrotizing processes have merged.

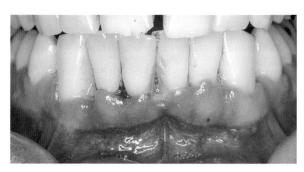

Fig. 20-3 Necrotizing periodontitis with more advanced lesions of interdental papillae and gingival margin.
Note the irregular morphology of the gingival margin as determined by the progressive loss of the interdental papillae.

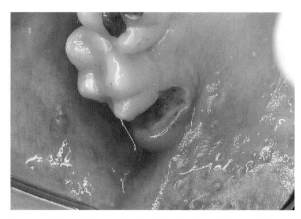

Fig. 20-5 Necrotizing periodontitis affecting right maxillary second molar periodontium. Note the extensive punched out lesion.

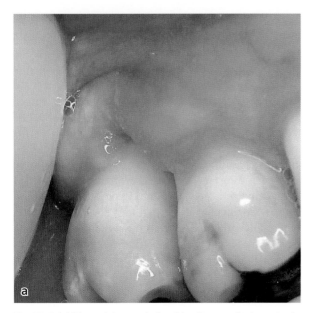
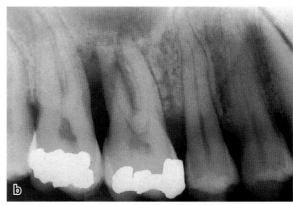

Fig. 20-6 (a) Necrotizing periodontitis often results in major loss of interdental tissue including alveolar bone of the molar regions as demonstrated in the radiograph (b).

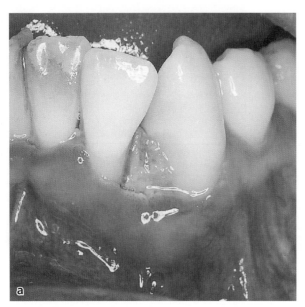
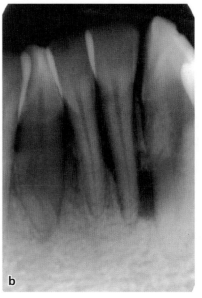

Fig. 20-7 (a) Necrotizing periodontitis with sequestration of alveolar bone between left mandibular lateral incisor and canine. (b) The extension of the sequestrum as seen in the radiograph covers the interdental septum almost to the apices of the roots.

the patients to eat, and a reduced food intake may be critical to HIV-infected patients because they may already lose weight in association with their HIV infection.

Sequestrum formation

The disease progression may be rapid and result in necrosis of small or large parts of the alveolar bone. Such a development is particularly evident in severely immunocompromised patients including HIV-seropositive individuals. The necrotic bone, denoted a sequestrum, is initially irremovable but after some time becomes loosened, whereafter it may be removed with forceps. Analgesia may not be required. A sequestrum may not only involve interproximal bone

but also include adjacent facial and oral cortical bone (Fig. 20-7).

Involvement of alveolar mucosa

When the necrotic process progresses beyond the mucogingival junction, the condition is denoted NS (Figs. 20-8 and 20-9) (Williams et al. 1990). The severe tissue destruction characteristic of this disease is related to seriously compromised immune functions typically associated with HIV infection and malnutrition (Fig. 20-10). Importantly, it may be life-threatening. NS may result in extensive denudation of bone, resulting in major sequestration with the development of oro-antral fistula and osteitis (SanGiacomo et al. 1990; Felix et al. 1991).

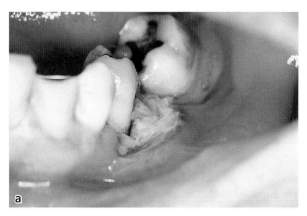 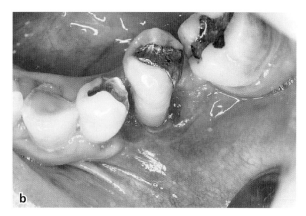

Fig. 20-8 (a) Necrotizing stomatitis affecting periodontium of left mandibular premolar region and adjacent alveolar mucosa. (b) After treatment and healing, no attached gingiva remains.

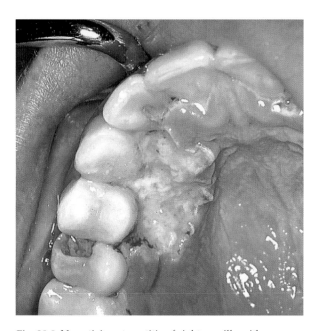

Fig. 20-9 Necrotizing stomatitis of right maxilla with extensive necrotic ulcer of palatal mucosa.

Swelling of lymph nodes

Swelling of the regional lymph nodes may occur in NPD but is particularly evident in advanced cases. Such symptoms are usually confined to the submandibular lymph nodes, but the cervical lymph nodes may also be involved. In children with NPD, swelling of lymph nodes and increased bleeding tendency are often the most pronounced clinical findings (Jiménez & Baer 1975).

Fever and malaise

Fever and malaise is not a consistent characteristic of NPD. Some investigations indicate that elevated body temperature is not common in NG and that, when present, the elevation of body temperature is usually moderate (Grupe & Wilder 1956; Goldhaber & Giddon 1964; Shields 1977; Stevens *et al.* 1984). A small decrease in body temperature in NG has even

been described. The disagreement on this point may, in fact, be due to misdiagnosis of primary herpetic gingivostomatitis as NG (see below).

Oral hygiene

The oral hygiene in patients with NPD is usually poor. Moreover, brushing of teeth and contact with the acutely inflamed gingiva is painful. Therefore, large amounts of plaque on the teeth are common, especially along the gingival margin. A thin, whitish film sometimes covers parts of the attached gingiva (Fig. 20-11). This film is a characteristic finding in patients who have neither eaten nor performed oral hygiene for days. It is composed of desquamated epithelial cells and bacteria in a meshwork of salivary proteins. The film is easily removed.

In general, the clinical characteristics of NPD in HIV-seropositive patients do not essentially differ from those in HIV-seronegative patients. However, the lesions in HIV-seropositive patients may not be associated with large amounts of plaque and calculus. Thus, the disease activity in these patients sometimes shows limited correlation with etiologic factors as determined by the amount of bacterial plaque (Holmstrup & Westergaard 1994). Further, lesions of NPD in HIV-seropositive patients have sometimes been revealed in gingival tissue affected by Kaposi's sarcoma (Fig. 20-12).

Acute and recurrent/chronic forms of necrotizing gingivitis and periodontitis

In most instances the course of the diseases is acute, characterized by the rapid destruction of the periodontal tissue. However, if inadequately treated or left untreated, the acute phase may gradually subside. The symptoms then become less unpleasant to the patient, but the destruction of the periodontal tissues continues, although at a slower rate, and the necrotic tissues do not heal completely. Such a condition has been termed chronic necrotizing gingivitis, or periodontitis in the case of attachment loss (Fig. 20-13).

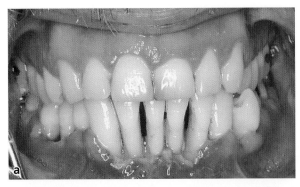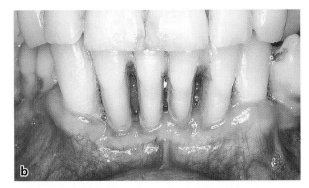

Fig. 20-10 (a) Necrotizing stomatitis affecting the mandible of an HIV-seropositive patient. (b) Two years after treatment the result of treatment is satisfactory, and there has been no recurrence.

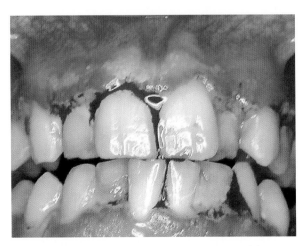

Fig. 20-11 A whitish film sometimes covers parts of the attached gingiva in patients with NPD as demonstrated in the maxillary gingiva. The film is composed of desquamated epithelial cells which have accumulated because the patient has not eaten or performed oral hygiene for days.

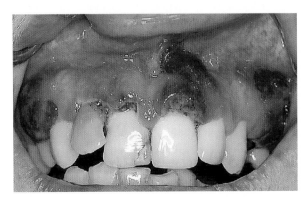

Fig. 20-12 Necrotizing periodontitis affecting Kaposi's sarcoma of left maxillary central incisor gingiva in an HIV-infected patient. The sarcoma affected almost the entire maxillary gingiva after 9 months.

The necrotizing lesions persist as open craters, frequently with a content of subgingival calculus and bacterial plaque. Although the characteristic ulcerative, necrotic areas of the acute phase usually disappear, acute exacerbations with intervening periods of quiescence may also occur. In recurrent acute phases, subjective symptoms again become more prominent

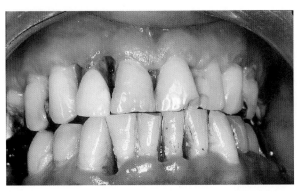

Fig. 20-13 Chronic necrotizing periodontitis with edematous gingiva particularly of mandible. The slightly active necrotizing processes at the bottom of the negative papillae are not visible.

and necrotic ulcers reappear. Some authors prefer the term recurrent rather than chronic to describe this category of necrotizing disease (Johnson & Engel 1986). Plaque and necrotic debris are often less conspicuous in these phases than in the acute forms, because they are located in pre-existing interdental craters. Several adjoining interdental craters may fuse, resulting in total separation of facial and oral gingivae, which form two distinct flaps. Recurrent forms of NG and NP may produce considerable destruction of supporting tissues. The most pronounced tissue loss usually occurs in relation to the interproximal craters.

Diagnosis

The diagnosis of NG, NP, and NS is based on clinical findings as described above. The patient has usually noticed pain and bleeding from the gingiva, particularly upon touch. The histopathology of the necrotizing diseases is not pathognomonic for NG, and biopsy is certainly not indicated in the heavily infected area.

Differential diagnosis

NPD may be confused with other diseases of the oral mucosa. Primary herpetic gingivostomatitis (PHG) is

Table 20-1 Important characteristics for differential diagnosis between NPD and PHG

	NPD	PHG
Etiology	Bacteria	Herpes simplex virus
Age	15–30 years	Frequently children
Site	Interdental papillae. Rarely outside the gingiva	Gingiva and the entire oral mucosa
Symptoms	Ulcerations and necrotic tissue and a yellowish white plaque	Multiple vesicles which disrupt, leaving small round fibrin-covered ulcerations
	Foetor ex ore Moderate fever may occur	*Foetor ex ore* Fever
Duration	1–2 days if treated	1–2 weeks
Contagious	–	+
Immunity	–	Partial
Healing	Destruction of periodontal tissue remains	No permanent destruction

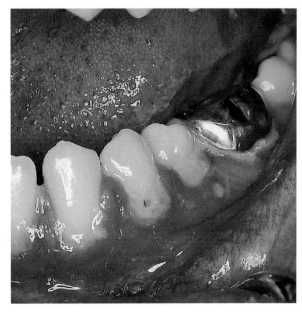

Fig. 20-14 Primary herpetic gingivostomatitis. Note that the ulcers affect the gingival margin but not primarily interdental papillae. A circular ulcer of the second premolar gingiva is highly suggestive of the diagnosis.

not infrequently mistaken for NPD (Klotz 1973). The important differential diagnostic criteria for the two diseases are listed in Table 20-1. It should be noted that in the USA and in northern Europe, NPD occurs very rarely in children, whereas PHG is most commonly found in children. If the body temperature is markedly raised, to 38°C or more, PHG should be suspected. NG and NP has a marked predilection for the interdental papillae, while PHG shows no such limitation and may occur anywhere on the free or the attached gingiva, or in the alveolar mucosa (Fig. 20-14). In PHG erythema is of a more diffuse character and may cover the entire gingiva and parts of the alveolar mucosa. The vesicular lesions in PHG, which disrupt and produce small ulcers surrounded by diffuse erythema, occur both on the lips and tongue as well as on the buccal mucosa. PHG and NPD may occur simultaneously in the same patient, and in such cases there may be mucosal lesions outside the gingiva, and fever and general malaise tend to occur more frequently than with NPD alone.

Oral mucosal diseases that have been confused with NPD include desquamative gingivitis, benign mucous membrane pemphigoid, erythema multiforme exudativum, streptococcal gingivitis, gonococcal gingivitis, and others. All of these are clinically quite distinct from NPD.

In some forms of leukemia, especially acute leukemia, necrotizing ulcers may occur in the oral mucosa and are not infrequently seen in association with the gingival margin, apparently as an exacerbation of an existing chronic inflammatory condition. The clinical appearance can resemble NPD lesions, and the symptoms they produce may be the ones that first make the patient seek professional consultation. In acute leukemia the gingiva often appears bluish red and

edematous with varying degrees of ulceration and necrosis. Generally, the patient has more marked systemic symptoms than with ordinary NPD, but can feel relatively healthy for a while. The dentist should be aware of the possibility that leukemias present such oral manifestations, which require medical examination of the patient, whereas biopsy is usually not indicated.

Histopathology

Histopathologically, NG lesions are characterized by ulceration with necrosis of epithelium and superficial layers of the connective tissue and an acute, nonspecific inflammatory reaction (Fig. 20-15). An important aspect is the role of the microorganisms in the lesions, because they have been demonstrated not only in the necrotic tissue components but also in vital epithelium and connective tissue.

Sometimes the histologic findings demonstrate the formation of regular layers with certain characteristics (Listgarten 1965) but there may be variations in regularity. The surface cover of yellowish white or grayish slough can be observed clinically; under the light microscope it appears to be a meshwork of fibrin with degenerated epithelial cells, leukocytes and erythrocytes, bacteria, and cellular debris. At the ultrastructural level, bacteria of varying sizes and forms including small, medium-sized, and large spirochetes have been revealed between the inflammatory cells, the majority of which are neutrophilic granulocytes. Moreover, in presumably vital parts of the surface epithelium, compact masses of spirochetes and short, fusiform rods have been found intercellularly.

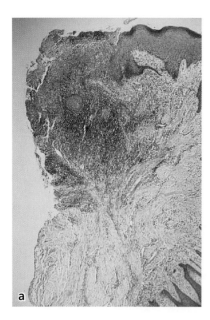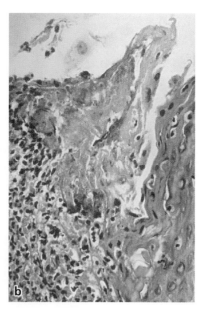

Fig. 20-15 Photomicrograph of gingival tissue affected by necrotizing gingivitis. (a) Upper right part of gingival biopsy shows gingival oral epithelium whereas upper left is ulcerated surface. Underneath the ulcer the connective tissue is heavily infiltrated by inflammatory cells. (b) Higher magnification of margin of ulcer shows necrotic tissue infiltrated with neutrophils. Right border is covered by epithelium. Courtesy of Dr. Finn Prætorius.

The vital connective tissue in the bottom of the lesion is covered by necrotic tissue, characterized by disintegrated cells, many large and medium-sized spirochetes, and other bacteria which, judging from their size and shape, may be fusobacteria. In the superior part of the vital connective tissue, characterized by intact tissue components, the tissue is infiltrated by large and medium-sized spirochetes, but no other microorganisms have been seen. In the vital connective tissue the vessels are dilated. They also proliferate to form granulation tissue, and the tissue is heavily infiltrated by leukocytes. As always in acute processes the inflammatory infiltrate is dominated by neutrophils (Figs. 20-15b and 20-16). In the deeper tissue, the inflammatory process also comprises large numbers of monocytes and plasma cells (Listgarten 1965; Heylings 1967).

Microbiology

Microorganisms isolated from necrotizing lesions

Microbial samples from NPD lesions have demonstrated a constant and a variable part of the flora. The "constant flora" primarily contained *Treponema* sp., *Selenomonas* sp., *Fusobacterium* sp., and *B. melaninogenicus* ss *intermedius* (*Prevotella intermedia*), and the "variable flora" consisted of a heterogeneous array of bacterial types (Loesche *et al.* 1982). Although the characteristic bacterial flora of spirochetes and fusobacteria has been isolated in large numbers from the necrotic lesions in several studies, their presence is not evidence of a primary etiologic importance. Their presence could equally well result from secondary overgrowth. Moreover, the microorganisms associated with NG are also harbored by healthy mouths and mouths with gingivitis or periodontitis (Johnson & Engel 1986). An important role for *Treponema* sp. and *B. intermedius* (*P. intermedia*) has been suggested

by studies of antibodies in NPD patients to such bacteria, compared to levels in age- and sex-matched controls with healthy gingiva or simple gingivitis (Chung *et al.* 1983).

There is little available information about the microbiology of HIV-associated NPD. *Borrelia*, Gram-positive cocci, β-hemolytic streptococci and *Candida albicans* have been isolated from the lesions (Reichart & Schiødt 1989). It has also been proposed that human cytomegalovirus (HCMV) may play a role in the pathogenesis of NPD (Sabiston 1986). This virus has been found in the digestive tract of HIV-patients (Kanas *et al.* 1987; Langford *et al.* 1990), and a case of oral HCMV infection with similarities to necrotizing periodontitis has been reported (Dodd *et al.* 1993). An increased frequency of HCMV and other herpes viruses found in necrotizing lesions among Nigerian children supports a contributory role of the viruses (Contreras *et al.* 1997), although it remains to be demonstrated in future studies whether cytomegalovirus does play a causal role.

Pathogenic potential of microorganisms

Our knowledge of the pathogenic mechanisms by which the bacterial flora produces the tissue changes characteristic of NPD is limited. One reason is that it has been difficult to establish an acceptable animal experimental model. However, several of the pathogenic mechanisms which have been associated with chronic gingivitis and periodontitis may also be of etiologic importance in the necrotizing forms of the diseases.

An important aspect in the pathogenesis of periodontitis is the capacity of the microorganisms to invade the host tissues. Among the bacteria isolated from necrotizing lesions, spirochetes and fusiform bacteria can, in fact, invade the epithelium (Heylings 1967). The spirochetes can also invade the vital

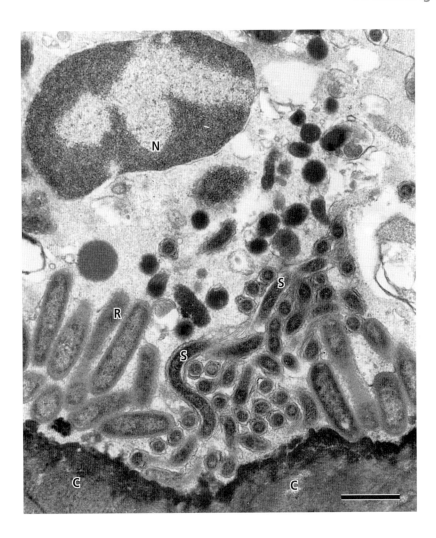

Fig. 20-16 Electronmicrograph demonstrating phagocytosing neutrophil (N) close to the surface of a sequestrum (C), covered by numerous microorganisms including spirochetes (S) and rods (R). Bar = 1 μm.

connective tissue (Listgarten 1965). The pathogenic potential is further substantiated by the fact that both fusobacteria and spirochetes can liberate endotoxins (Mergenhagen *et al.* 1961; Kristoffersen & Hofstad 1970).

A number of observations indicate that the effects of endotoxins are more prominent in NPD than in chronic gingivitis and periodontitis. The large masses of Gram-negative bacteria liberate endotoxins in close contact with connective tissue. Endotoxins may produce tissue destruction both by direct toxic effects and indirectly, by activating and modifying tissue responses of the host (Wilton & Lehner 1980). Through a direct toxic effect, endotoxins may lead to damage of cells and vessels. Necrosis is a prominent feature in the so-called "Shwartzman reaction", which is caused by endotoxins. Indirectly, endotoxins can contribute to tissue damage in several ways: they can function as antigens and elicit immune reactions; they can activate complement directly through the alternative pathway and thereby liberate chemotoxins; but they can also activate macrophages, B and T lymphocytes, and influence the host's immune reactions by interfering with cytokines produced by these cells. Studies have shown that endotoxins can stimulate catabolic processes with degradation of

both connective tissue and bone induced by the released cytokines. The extent to which such reactions contribute to host defense or to tissue damage is not yet known.

An aspect which has been of major concern, especially in wartime, is the communicability of the disease. Several reports have considered this aspect but it has been concluded that the necrotizing diseases are not transmissible by ordinary means of contact (Johnson & Engel 1986). Attempts to transmit the disease from one animal to another, or to produce necrotic lesions in experimental animals, have failed to yield conclusive results (MacDonald *et al.* 1963). Several suspect microorganisms and several combinations of microorganisms can produce similar lesions in experimental animals. A combination of four different bacteria, none of them fusobacteria or spirochetes, has been found to possess such properties and there are indications that among the four bacterial species, *Bacteroides melaninogenicus* was the true pathogen (MacDonald *et al.* 1956, 1963). *B. melaninogenicus* may, under certain conditions, produce an enzyme which degrades native collagen (Gibbons & MacDonald 1961). It is still not clear, however, whether this microorganism is of particular importance in the pathogenesis of NPD. NG lesions have also been induced in dogs pretreated with steroids and inoculated with a fusiform–spirochete culture from dogs which had gingival lesions similar to the NG lesions seen in humans (Mikx & van Campen 1982). The lesions produced in experimental animals may not be identical to those which occur in humans. It is also important to note that even if necrotic lesions can be transmitted by transmission of infectious material or bacterial cultures, this does not necessarily mean that the disease is truly contagious.

It is obvious from the above observations and assumptions that a fundamental question remains to be answered, and at this point it may be stated that the necrotizing periodontal diseases belong to those diseases to which Pasteur referred when he said: "there are some bacteria that cause a disease, but there are some diseases that bring about a condition that is ideal for the growth of some bacteria" (Wilson 1952). If the microorganisms mentioned above play a role in the etiology of the disease, then, presumably, the disease is an opportunistic infection. Consequently, the pathogenic characteristics of the microorganisms are normally overcome by the host defenses, and disease occurs when the host defenses are impaired. The isolated microorganisms do possess biologic activities which may contribute to the pathogenesis, but the exact role of the various microorganisms has not yet been clarified (Johnson & Engel 1986).

Host response and predisposing factors

It is particularly evident for HIV-infected patients that the disease is associated with diminished host resistance; among other predisposing factors, the basic mechanism may include altered host immunity. Changes in leukocyte function and the immune system have been observed in some studies, although the biologic reason for, and significance of, these findings are unclear (Johnson & Engel 1986).

Significantly increased IgG and IgM antibody titers to intermediate-sized spirochetes and higher IgG titers to *B. melaninogenicus* ssp *intermedius* have been found in NG patients as compared to age- and sex-matched healthy and gingivitis control groups (Chung *et al.* 1983). These results, however, are in disagreement with other data showing no differences in serum antibody levels to bacterial antigens (Wilton *et al.* 1971).

Total leukocyte counts have been found to be similar for patients and controls. NG patients, however, displayed marked depression in polymorphonuclear leukocyte chemotaxis and phagocytosis as compared with control individuals. Reduced mitogen-induced proliferation of peripheral blood lymphocytes has also been found in NG patients. It was suggested that elevated blood steroids may account for the reduced chemotactic and phagocytic responses (Cogen *et al.* 1983).

For many years it has been known that a number of predisposing factors may interact with the host defense systems and render the patient susceptible to NPD. Usually, a single one of these factors is not sufficient to establish disease. The various factors, which have been focused upon, comprise systemic diseases, including HIV infection and malnutrition, poor oral hygiene, pre-existing gingivitis and history of previous NPD, psychologic stress and inadequate sleep, smoking and alcohol use, Caucasian background, and young age.

A recent analysis of suspected predisposing factors among American patients with NPD has shown that HIV seropositivity overwhelmed all other factors in importance when present (Horning & Cohen 1995). Among the HIV-seronegative patients the ranked importance of the predisposing factors was: history of previous NPD; poor oral hygiene; inadequate sleep; unusual psychologic stress; poor diet; recent illness; social or greater alcohol use; smoking; Caucasian background; and age under 21 years. The various predisposing factors mentioned below are obviously not equally important in industrialized and developing countries, but many of these factors are known to relate to impaired immunity.

Systemic diseases

Systemic diseases which impair immunity predispose to NPD. This is why NPD occurs more frequently in HIV-infected individuals and in patients with other leukocyte diseases including leukemia (Melnick *et al.* 1988). Examples of other diseases predisposing to NPD are measles, chicken pox, tuberculosis, herpetic gingivostomatitis, and malaria, but malnutrition is also important. Whereas these examples of predisposing factors are rare in western patients, they are evident in developing countries, where they often predispose to NPD and noma in children (Emslie 1963; Pindborg *et al.* 1966, 1967; Sheiham 1966; Enwonwu 1972, 1985). It is important to note that NPD is sometimes an early signal of impending serious illness (Enwonwu 1972).

HIV infection

In Africa, the general population shows a high HIV-seropositive prevalence rate, ranging up to 33% in some populations. In Europe, prevalence figures have been established for areas in the UK, where the prevalence figures were 0.1–0.2% (Nicoll *et al.* 2000). In South Africa NPD in otherwise systemically healthy individuals was correlated with HIV infection, with a predictive value of 69.6% (Shangase *et al.* 2004). In industrialized countries, a significant portion of patients with NPD are HIV-infected patients, and no characteristics have been revealed that distinguish NPD in HIV-seropositive from that in HIV-seronegative patients. A history of frequent relapses and poor response to traditional or drug therapy may be suggestive (Greenspan *et al.* 1986; Horning & Cohen 1995). Suspicion of HIV infection is also supported by the simultaneous presence of oral candidosis, "hairy leukoplakia", or Kaposi's tumor, but these lesions are far from always present in HIV-infected patients.

HIV infection attacks the T-helper cells of the body, causing a drastic change in the T-helper(CD4+)/T-suppressor(CD8+) ratio with severe impairment of the host's resistance to infection. Depleted peripheral T-helper lymphocyte counts correlate closely with the occurrence of NG as demonstrated in a study of 390 US HIV-seropositive soldiers (Thompson *et al.* 1992). Furthermore, a complete absence of T cells in gingival tissue of HIV-infected patients with periodontitis has been reported (Steidley *et al.* 1992). The lack of local immune effector and regulatory cells in HIV-seropositive patients could in fact explain the characteristic and rapidly progressive nature of periodontitis in these patients. Moreover, a protective effect has been encountered with antiviral treatment of the HIV infection against NPD (Tappuni & Fleming 2001) as well as against HIV-associated gingivitis and periodontitis (Masouredis *et al.* 1992). NP has been revealed as a marker for immune deterioration, with a 95% predictive value that CD4+ cell counts were below 200 cells/mm^3, and, if untreated, a cumulative probability of death within 24 months (Glick *et al.* 1994). As a consequence of this finding, if possible all NPD patients should be recommended to have a test for HIV infection.

Malnutrition

In developing countries malnutrition has often been mentioned as a predisposing factor to NPD (Enwonwu 1972; Osuji 1990). Malnutrition results in lowered resistance to infection and protein malnutrition has been emphasized as the most common public health problem affecting underprivileged Nigerian children who are most often affected by NPD (Enwonwu 1985, 1994). In response to periodontal pathogens, phagocytes elaborate destructive oxidants, proteinases, and other factors. Periodontal damage may occur as the result of the balance between these factors, the antioxidants and host-derived antiproteinases. Malnutrition is characterized by marked tissue depletion of the key antioxidant nutrients, and impaired acute-phase protein response to infections. This is due to impairment in the production and cellular action of the cytokines. Other features of malnutrition include inverted helper/suppressor T lymphocyte ratio, histaminemia, hormonal imbalance with increased blood and saliva levels of free cortisol, and defective mucosal integrity. Malnutrition usually involves concomitant deficiencies of several essential macro- and micronutrients, and therefore has the potential to adversely influence the prognosis of periodontal infections (Enwonwu 1994).

Poor oral hygiene, pre-existing gingivitis, and history of previous NPD

Many of the early studies of NPD showed that a low standard of oral hygiene contributed to the establishment of the disease (Johnson & Engel 1986). This has been supported by recent studies in the USA and Nigeria (Taiwo 1993; Horning & Cohen 1995). Consequently, NPD is usually established on the basis of preexisting chronic gingivitis (Pindborg 1951b). It should be emphasized, however, that plaque accumulation as seen in NPD patients may also be enhanced by the discomfort experienced with oral hygiene practices due to the disease. Based on questionnaires and personal interviews, 28% of NPD patients have been found with a history of previous painful gingival infection and 21% had gingival scars suggestive of previous NPD (Horning & Cohen 1995).

Psychologic stress and inadequate sleep

Just as other ulcerative gastrointestinal conditions have been shown to have psychogenic origins, psychologic stress has often and for many years been mentioned as a predisposing factor (Johnson & Engel 1986). Epidemiologic investigations seem to indicate a more frequent occurrence of necrotizing diseases in periods when the individuals are exposed to psychologic stress (Pindborg 1951a,b; Giddon *et al.* 1963; Goldhaber & Giddon 1964). New recruits and deploying military personnel, college students during examination periods, patients with depression or other emotional disorders, and patients feeling inadequate at handling life situations are more susceptible to NPD (Pindborg 1951a,b; Moulton *et al.* 1952; Giddon *et al.* 1963; Cohen-Cole *et al.* 1983). Urine levels of corticosteroids have been used as a physiologic measure of stress, and increased free cortisol levels have been encountered in the urine of NPD patients as compared with controls. The NPD patients showed significantly higher levels of trait anxiety, depression, and emotional disturbance than did control individuals (Cohen-Cole *et al.* 1983). The role of anxiety and psychologic stress in the pathogenesis of NG has been borne out by both psychiatric and biochemical investigations (Moulton *et al.* 1952; Shannon *et al.* 1969; Maupin & Bell 1975). There are several ways by which psychologic stress factors may interfere with host susceptibility. Host tissue resistance may be changed by mechanisms acting through the autonomic nervous system and endocrine glands resulting in elevation of corticosteroid and catecholamine levels. This may reduce gingival microcirculation and salivary flow and enhance nutrition of *Prevotella intermedia*, but also depress neutrophil and lymphocyte functions which facilitate bacterial invasion and damage (Johnson & Engel 1986; Horning & Cohen 1995).

Inadequate sleep, often as the result of lifestyle choices or job requirements, has been mentioned by many patients with NPD (Horning & Cohen 1995).

Smoking and alcohol use

Smoking has been listed as a predisposing factor to NPD for many years and presumably predisposes to other types of periodontitis as well (The American Academy of Periodontology 1996). Two studies from the 1950s found that 98% of the patients were smokers (Pindborg 1951a; Goldhaber 1957). More recent data have confirmed this by finding only 6% non-smokers among NPD patients in contrast to 63% in a matched control group (Stevens *et al.* 1984). The amount smoked also appears important since 41% of subjects with NG smoked more than 20 cigarettes daily whereas only 5% of controls smoked that much (Goldhaber & Giddon 1964).

The relationship between tobacco usage and NPD appears to be complex. It has often been stated that smokers in general have poorer oral hygiene than non-smokers but studies have shown that there is little difference in the level of plaque accumulation in smokers versus non-smokers. Also, there have been no conclusive studies to show that smoking adversely affects periodontal tissues by altering the microbial composition of plaque (The American Academy of Periodontology 1996). Smoking could lead to increased disease activity by influencing host response and tissue reactions. As examples, smokers have depressed numbers of T-helper lymphocytes, and tobacco smoke can also impair chemotaxis and phagocytosis of oral and peripheral phagocytes (Eichel & Shahrik 1969; Kenney *et al.* 1977; Ginns *et al.* 1982; Costabel *et al.* 1986; Lannan *et al.* 1992; Selby *et al.* 1992). Nicotine-induced secretion of epinephrine resulting in gingival vasoconstriction has been proposed as one possible mechanism by which smoking may influence tissue susceptibility (Schwartz & Baumhammers 1972; Kardachi & Clarke 1974; Bergström & Preber 1986). The exact mechanism of tobacco smoking predisposing to NPD, however, remains to be determined.

Social or heavy drinking has been admitted by NPD patients and its role as a predisposing factor has been accounted for by its numerous physiologic effects which add to other factors as general sources of debilitation (Horning & Cohen 1995).

Caucasian background

A number of American studies have demonstrated a 95% preponderance of Caucasian patients with NPD including a study in which the referring population was 41% African American (Barnes *et al.* 1973; Stevens *et al.* 1984; Horning & Cohen 1995), but a proportion of 49% of African Americans in another study casts doubt on race as a predisposing factor alone, and the mechanism for this factor is unknown.

Young age

In industrialized countries, young adults appear to be the most predisposed to NPD. The disease can occur at any age, the reported mean age for NPD being between 22 and 24 years. This may reflect a number of factors such as military population age, wartime stress, and probably is related to the involvement of other factors such as smoking (Horning & Cohen 1995).

Treatment

The treatment of the necrotizing periodontal diseases is divided into two phases: acute and maintenance phase treatment.

Acute phase treatment

The aim of the acute phase treatment is to eliminate disease activity as manifest by ongoing tissue necrosis developing laterally and apically. A further aim is to avoid pain and general discomfort which may severely compromise food intake. Among patients suffering from systemic diseases resulting in loss of weight, further weight loss due to reduced food intake should be avoided by rapid therapeutic intervention.

At the first consultation scaling should be attempted, as thoroughly as the condition allows. Ultrasonic scaling may be preferable to the use of hand instruments. With minimal pressure against the soft tissues, ultrasonic cleaning may accomplish the removal of soft and mineralized deposits. The continuous water spray combined with adequate suction usually allows good visibility. How far it is possible to proceed with debridement at the first visit usually depends on the patient's tolerance of pain during instrumentation. Obviously toothbrushing in areas with open wounds does not promote wound healing. Therefore, patients should be instructed in substituting toothbrushing with chemical plaque control in such areas until healing is accomplished.

Hydrogen peroxide and other oxygen-releasing agents also have a long-standing tradition in the initial treatment of NPD. Hydrogen peroxide (3%) is still used for debridement in necrotic areas and as a mouth rinse (equal portions 3% H_2O_2 and warm water). It has been thought that the apparently favorable effects of hydrogen peroxide may be due to mechanical cleaning, and the influence on anaerobic bacterial flora of the liberated oxygen (Wennström & Lindhe 1979; MacPhee & Cowley 1981). Further adjunctive local oxygen therapy of NDP showed a more rapid clinical restitution with less periodontal destruction than in a group without oxygen therapy (Gaggl *et al.* 2006).

Twice daily rinsing with a 0.2% chlorhexidine solution is a very effective adjunct to reduce plaque formation, particularly when toothbrushing is not performed. It also assists self-performed oral hygiene during the first weeks of treatment. Its effect is discussed elsewhere in this book. For an optimal effect of this medicament, it should be used only in conjunction with and in addition to systematic scaling and root planing. The chlorhexidine solution does not penetrate subgingivally and the preparation is readily inactivated by exudates, necrotic tissues, and masses of bacteria (Gjermo 1974). The effectiveness of chlorhexidine mouth rinses is therefore dependent upon a simultaneous, thorough mechanical, debridement.

In some cases of NPD the patient's response to debridement is minimal or the general health is affected to such an extent that the supplementary use of systemic antibiotics or chemotherapeutics is indicated. This also applies to patients with malaise, fever, and lassitude. The choice of drug aims at a direct action on bacteria which are the cause of the inflammatory process in NPD. Supplementary treatment with metronidazole 250 mg three times daily has been found effective against spirochetes and appears to be the first choice in the treatment of NPD (Proctor & Baker 1971; Shinn 1976; Loesche et al. 1982). The adjunctive use of metronidazole in HIV-associated NPD is reported to be extremely effective in reducing acute pain and promoting rapid healing (Scully et al. 1991). Acute pain usually disappears after a few hours (Fig. 20-17).

Antibiotics such as penicillins and tetracyclines are also effective. Penicillin (1 million i.u. three times daily) should be used as an adjunct to scaling as for metronidazole until the ulcers are healed. Topical application of antibiotics is not indicated in the treatment of NPD, because intralesional bacteria are frequent, and topical application does not result in sufficient intralesional concentration of antibiotics.

It is important to emphasize that many HIV-seropositive patients with NPD at their initial visit are not aware of their serostatus. If HIV infection is a suspected predisposing factor, the patient can be referred to her or his physician for further examination. Some patients may prefer referral to a hospital department. Information on HIV-serostatus is frequently not available at initiation of therapy, but the lack of information has no serious implications for the choice of treatment or for the handling of the patient. As a consequence of a lack of information on HIV-serostatus of patients seeking dental treatment in general, all procedures in the dental office must always include precautions to protect against transmission of the virus to the dentist, to the dental auxiliaries, and to other patients.

If the dentist asks the patient about his or her possible chance of having contracted HIV infection this should be done with great care, because HIV infection has serious implications for the patient. Consequently, a successful outcome depends on a

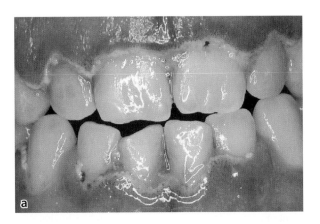
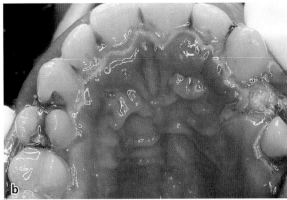
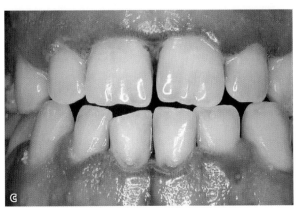
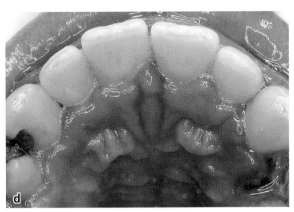

Fig. 20-17 Necrotizing periodontitis with severe pain. The entire gingival margin is the seat of a necrotic ulcer. (a) Facial aspect. (b) Palatal aspect. (c,d) The patient was treated with scaling supplemented with metronidazole and the next day the patient was free of symptoms and the clinical features were significantly improved.

confidential relationship between patient and dentist. In the case of a new patient, such a relationship is first established after at least a couple of appointments in the clinic.

In HIV-infected patients antibiotic prophylaxis in relation to scaling does not usually appear to be necessary. Bacteria recovered from venipuncture 15 minutes after scaling were not detectable in samples obtained at 30 minutes (Lucartoto *et al.* 1992). Neither does removal of sequestra always appear to require antibiotic cover (Robinson 1991). HIV-infected patients are susceptible to candidal infections (Holmstrup & Samaranayake 1990) and if oral candidosis is present or occurs throughout the period of antibiotic treatment, treatment with appropriate antimycotic drugs such as miconazole may be necessary.

Patients with NPD should be seen almost daily as long as the acute symptoms persist. Appropriate treatment alleviates symptoms within a few days. Thereafter the patient should return in approximately 5 days. Systematic subgingival scaling should be continued with increasing intensity as the symptoms subside. Correction of restoration margins and polishing of restorations and root surfaces should be completed after healing of ulcers. When the ulcerated areas are healed, local treatment is supplemented with oral hygiene instruction and patient motivation. Instruction in gentle but effective toothbrushing and approximal cleaning is mandatory. In many cases the extensive tissue destruction results in residual soft tissue defects that are difficult for the patient to keep clean. Oral hygiene in these areas often requires the use of interproximal devices and soft, smaller brushes. Sometimes healing is delayed in HIV-infected patients and intensive professional control may be necessary for prolonged periods of time.

Patients with NPD are not always easily motivated to carry out a proper program of oral hygiene. They frequently have poor oral hygiene habits and possibly a negative attitude to dental treatment in general. As a result, some patients discontinue treatment as soon as pain and other acute symptoms are alleviated. Motivation and instruction should be planned to prevent this happening, and should be reinforced during later visits. Patients with severely impaired immune function, for instance due to HIV infection, may suffer from other infections or diseases during the period of treatment. This may complicate the treatment, because patients may be hospitalized.

Maintenance phase treatment

When the acute phase treatment has been completed, necrosis and acute symptoms in NPD have disappeared. The formerly necrotic areas are healed and the gingival craters are reduced in size, although some defects usually persist. Bacterial plaque readily accumulates in such areas, and the craters, therefore, predispose to recurrence of NPD or to further destruction because of a persisting chronic inflammatory process, or both. These sites, therefore, may require surgical correction. Shallow craters can be removed by simple gingivectomy, while the elimination of deep defects may require flap surgery. Treatment of necrotizing gingivitis has not been completed until all gingival defects have been eliminated and optimal conditions for future plaque control have been established. If possible, elimination of predisposing factors is also very important to prevent recurrence. Due to delayed healing in HIV-infected patients, periodontal surgery is not recommended in these patients. Instead, intensive approximal cleaning is necessary to prevent recurrence of disease.

References

American Academy of Periodontology (1996). Tobacco use and the periodontal patient. *Journal of Periodontology* **67**, 51–56.

Barnes, G.P., Bowles, W.F. & Carter, H.G. (1973). Acute necrotizing ulcerative gingivitis: a survey of 218 cases. *Journal of Periodontology* **44**, 35–42.

Barr, C., Lopez, M.R. & Rua-Dobles, A. (1992). Periodontal changes by HIV serostatus in a cohort of homosexual and bisexual men. *Journal of Clinical Periodontology* **19**, 794–801.

Bergström, J. & Preber, H. (1986). The influence of cigarette smoking on the development of experimental gingivitis. *Journal of Periodontal Research* **21**, 668–676.

Chung, C.P., Nisengard, R.J., Slots, J. & Genco, R.J. (1983). Bacterial IgG and IgM antibody titers in acute necrotizing ulcerative gingivitis. *Journal of Periodontology* **54**, 557–562.

Cogen, R.B., Stevens, A.W. Jr., Cohen-Cole, S., Kirk, K. & Freeman, A. (1983). Leukocyte function in the etiology of acute necrotizing gingivitis. *Journal of Periodontology* **54**, 402–407.

Cohen-Cole, S.A., Cogen, R.B., Stevens, A.W. Jr., Kirk, K., Gaitan, E., Bird, J., Cooksey, A. & Freeman, A. (1983). Psychiatric, psychosocial and endocrine correlates of acute nec-

rotizing ulcerative gingivitis (trench mouth): a preliminary report. *Psychiatric Medicine* **1**, 215–225.

Contreras, A., Falkler, W.A. Jr., Enwonwu, C.O., Idigbe, E.O., Savage, K.O., Afolabi, M.B., Onwujekwe, D., Rams, T.E. & Slots, J. (1997). Human Herpesviridae in acute necrotizing ulcerative gingivitis in children in Nigeria. *Oral Microbiology and Immunology* **12**, 259–265.

Costabel, U., Bross, K.J., Reuter, C., Rühle, K.H. & Matthys, H. (1986). Alterations in immunoregulatory T-cell subsets in cigarette smokers. A phenotypic analysis of bronchoalveolar and blood lymphocytes. *Chest* **90**, 39–44.

Dodd, C.L., Winkler, J.R., Heinic, G.S., Daniels, T.E., Yee, K. & Greenspan, D. (1993). Cytomegalovirus infection presenting as acute periodontal infection in a patient infected with the human immunodeficiency virus. *Journal of Clinical Periodontology* **20**, 282–285.

Drinkard, C.R., Decher, L., Little, J.W., Rhame, F.S., Balfour, H.H. Jr., Rhodus, N.L., Merry, J.W., Walker, P.O., Miller, C. E., Volberding, P.A. & Melnick, S.L. (1991). Periodontal status of individuals in early stages of human immunodeficiency virus infection. *Community Dentistry and Oral Epidemiology* **19**, 281–285.

Eichel, B. & Shahrik, H.A. (1969). Tobacco smoke toxicity: Loss of human oral leukocyte function and fluid cell metabolism. *Science* **166**, 1424–1428.

Emslie, R.D. (1963). Cancrum oris. *Dental Practitioner* **13**, 481–495.

Enwonwu, C.O. (1972). Epidemiological and biochemical studies of necrotizing ulcerative gingivitis and noma (cancrum oris) in Nigerian children. *Archives of Oral Biology* **17**, 1357–1371.

Enwonwu, C.O. (1985). Infectious oral necrosis (cancrum oris) in Nigerian children: a review. *Community Dentistry and Oral Epidemiology* **13**, 190–194.

Enwonwu, C.O. (1994). Cellular and molecular effects of malnutrition and their relevance to periodontal diseases. *Journal of Clinical Periodontology* **21**, 643–657.

Felix, D.H., Wray, D., Smith, G.L. & Jones, G.A. (1991). Oro-antral fistula: an unusual complication of HIV-associated periodontal disease. *British Dental Journal* **171**, 61–62.

Friedman, R.B., Gunsolley, J., Gentry, A., Dinius, A., Kaplowitz, L. & Settle, J. (1991). Periodontal status of HIV-seropositive and AIDS patients. *Journal of Periodontology* **62**, 623–627.

Gaggl, A.J., Rainer, H., Grund, E. & Chiari, F.M. (2006). Local oxygen therapy for treating acute necrotizing periodontal disease in smokers. *Journal of Periodontology* **77**, 31–38.

Gibbons, R.J. & MacDonald, J.B. (1961). Degradation of collagenous substrates by *Bacteroides melaninogenicus*. *Journal of Bacteriology* **81**, 614–621.

Giddon, D.B., Goldhaber, P. & Dunning, J.M. (1963). Prevalence of reported cases of acute necrotizing ulcerative gingivitis in a university population. *Journal of Periodontology* **34**, 366–371.

Giddon, D.B., Zackin, S.J. & Goldhaber, P. (1964). Acute necrotizing ulcerative gingivitis in college students. *Journal of the American Dental Association* **68**, 381–386.

Ginns, L.C., Goldenheim, P.D., Miller, L.G., Burton, R.C., Gillick, L., Colvin, R.B., Goldstein, G., Kung, P.C., Hurwitz, C. & Kazemi, H. (1982). T-lymphocyte subsets in smoking and lung cancer. Analyses of monoclonal antibodies and flow cytometry. *American Review of Respiratory Disease* **126**, 265–269.

Gjermo, P. (1974). Chlorhexidine in dental practice. *Journal of Clinical Periodontology* **1**, 143–152.

Glick, M., Muzyka, B.C., Salkin, L.M. & Lurie, D. (1994). Necrotizing ulcerative periodontitis: a marker for immune deterioration and a predictor for the diagnosis of AIDS. *Journal of Periodontology* **65**, 393–397.

Goldhaber, P. (1957). A study of acute necrotizing ulcerative gingivitis. *Journal of Dental Research* **35**, 18.

Goldhaber, P. & Giddon, D.B. (1964). Present concepts concerning the etiology and treatment of acute necrotizing ulcerative gingivitis. *International Dental Journal* **14**, 468–496.

Greenspan, D., Greenspan, J.S., Pindborg, J.J. & Schiödt, M. (1986). *Aids and the Dental Team*. Copenhagen: Munksgaard.

Grupe, H.E. & Wilder, L.S. (1956). Observations of necrotizing gingivitis in 870 military trainees. *Journal of Periodontology* **27**, 255–261.

Heylings, R.T. (1967). Electron microscopy of acute ulcerative gingivitis (Vincent's type). Demonstration of the fusospirochaetal complex of bacteria within prenecrotic gingival epithelium. *British Dental Journal* **122**, 51–56.

Holmstrup, P. & Samaranayake, L.P. (1990). Acute and AIDS-related oral candidoses. In: Samaranayake, L.P. & MacFarlane, T.W., eds. *Oral Candidosis*. London: Wright, pp. 133–156.

Holmstrup, P. & Westergaard, J. (1994). Periodontal diseases in HIV-infected patients. *Journal of Clinical Periodontology* **21**, 270–280.

Horning, G.M. & Cohen, M.E. (1995). Necrotizing ulcerative gingivitis, periodontitis, and stomatitis: clinical staging and predisposing factors. *Journal of Periodontology* **66**, 990–998.

Horning, G.M., Hatch, C.L. & Lutskus, J. (1990). The prevalence of periodontitis in a military treatment population. *Journal of the American Dental Association* **121**, 616–622.

Jiménez, M.L. & Baer, P.N. (1975). Necrotizing ulcerative gingivitis in children: a 9-year clinical study. *Journal of Periodontology* **46**, 715–720.

Johnson, B.D. & Engel, D. (1986). Acute necrotizing ulcerative gingivitis. A review of diagnosis, etiology and treatment. *Journal of Periodontology* **57**, 141–150.

Kanas, R.J., Jensen, J.L., Abrams, A.M. & Wuerker, R.B. (1987). Oral mucosal cytomegalovirus as a manifestation of the acquired immune deficiency syndrome. *Oral Surgery, Oral Medicine, Oral Pathology* **64**, 183–189.

Kardachi, B.J. & Clarke, N.G. (1974). Aetiology of acute necrotizing ulcerative gingivitis: a hypothetical explanation. *Journal of Periodontology* **45**, 830–832.

Kenney, E.B., Kraal, J.H., Saxe, S.R. & Jones, J. (1977). The effect of cigarette smoke on human oral polymorphonuclear leukocytes. *Journal of Periodontal Research* **12**, 227–234.

King, J.D. (1943). Nutritional and other factors in "trench mouth" with special reference to the nicotinic acid component of the vitamin B2 complex. *British Dental Journal* **74**, 113–122.

Klotz, H. (1973). Differentiation between necrotic ulcerative gingivitis and primary herpetic gingivostomatitis. *New York State Dental Journal* **39**, 283–294.

Kristoffersen, T. & Hofstad, T. (1970). Chemical composition of lipopolysaccharide endotoxins from oral fusobacteria. *Archives of Oral Biology* **15**, 909–916.

Langford, A., Kunze, R., Timm, H., Ruf, B. & Reichart, P. (1990). Cytomegalovirus associated oral ulcerations in HIV-infected patients. *Journal of Oral Pathology & Medicine* **19**, 71–76.

Lannan, S., McLean, A., Drost, E., Gillooly, M., Donaldson, K., Lamb, D. & MacNee, W. (1992). Changes in neutrophil morphology and morphometry following exposure to cigarette smoke. *International Journal of Experimental Pathology* **73**, 183–191.

Listgarten, M.A. (1965). Electron microscopic observations on the bacterial flora of acute necrotizing ulcerative gingivitis. *Journal of Periodontology* **36**, 328–339.

Loesche, W.J., Syed, S.A., Laughon, B.E. & Stoll, J. (1982). The bacteriology of acute necrotizing ulcerative gingivitis. *Journal of Periodontology* **53**, 223–230.

Lopez, R. & Bælum, V. (2004). Necrotizing ulcerative gingival lesions and clinical attachment loss. *European Journal of Oral Sciences* **112**, 105–107.

Lopez, R, Fernandez, O., Jara, G. & Bælum, V. (2002). Epidemiology of necrotizing ulcerative gingival lesions in adolescents. *Journal of Periodontal Research* **37**, 439–444.

Lucartoto, F.M., Franker, C.K. & Maza, J. (1992). Postscaling bacteremia in HIV-associated gingivitis and periodontitis. *Oral Surgery, Oral Medicine, Oral Pathology* **73**, 550–554.

MacCarthy, D. & Claffey, N. (1991). Acute necrotizing ulcerative gingivitis is associated with attachment loss. *Journal of Clinical Periodontology* **18**, 776–779.

MacDonald, J.B., Socransky, S.S. & Gibbons, R.J. (1963). Aspects of the pathogenesis of mixed anaerobic infections of mucous membranes. *Journal of Dental Research* **42**, 529–544.

MacDonald, J.B., Sutton, R.M., Knoll, M.L., Medlener, E.M. & Grainger, R.M. (1956). The pathogenic components of an experimental fusospirochaetal infection. *Journal of Infectious Diseases* **98**, 15–20.

MacPhee, T. & Cowley, G. (1981). *Essentials of Periodontology*, 3rd edn. Oxford: Blackwell Science, pp. 157–177.

Masouredis, C.M., Katz, M.H., Greenspan, D., Herrera, C., Hollander, H., Greenspan, J.S. & Winkler, J.R. (1992). Prevalence of HIV-associated periodontitis and gingivitis and gingivitis in HIV-infected patients attending an AIDS clinic. *Journal of Acquired Immune Deficiency Syndromes* **5**, 479–483.

Maupin, C.C. & Bell, W.B. (1975). The relationship of 17-hydroxycorticosteroid to acute necrotizing ulcerative gingivitis. *Journal of Periodontology* **46**, 721–722.

Melnick, S.L., Roseman, J.M., Engel, D. & Cogen, R.B. (1988). Epidemiology of acute necrotizing ulcerative gingivitis. *Epidemiologic Reviews* **10**, 191–211.

Mergenhagen, S.E., Hampp, E.G. & Scherp, H.W. (1961). Preparation and biological activities of endotoxin from oral bacteria. *Journal of Infectious Diseases* **108**, 304–310.

Migliani, D.C. & Sharma, O.P. (1965). Incidence of acute necrotizing gingivitis and periodontosis among cases seen at the Government Hospital, Madras. *Journal of All India Dental Association* **37**, 183.

Mikx, F.H. & van Campen, G.J. (1982). Microscopical evaluation of the microflora in relation to necrotizing ulcerative gingivitis in the beagle dog. *Journal of Periodontal Research* **17**, 576–584.

Moulton, R., Ewen, S. & Thieman, W. (1952). Emotional factors in periodontal disease. *Oral Surgery, Oral Medicine, Oral Pathology* **5**, 833–860.

Nicoll, A., Gill, O.N., Peckham, C.S., Ades, A.E., Parry, J., Mortimer, P., Goldberg, D., Noone, A., Bennett, D. & Catchpole, M. (2000). The public health applications of unlinked anonymous seroprevalence monitoring for HIV in the United Kingdom. Review Article. *International Journal of Epidemiology* **29**, 1–10.

Osuji, O.O. (1990). Necrotizing ulcerative gingivitis and cancrum oris (noma) in Ibadan, Nigeria. *Journal of Periodontology* **61**, 769–772.

Pickard, H.M. (1973). Historical aspects of Vincent's disease. *Proceedings of the Royal Society of Medicine* **66**, 695–698.

Pindborg, J.J. (1951a). Gingivitis in military personnel with special reference to ulceromembranous gingivitis. *Odontologisk Revy* **59**, 407–499.

Pindborg, J.J. (1951b). Influence of service in armed forces on incidence of gingivitis. *Journal of the American Dental Association* **42**, 517–522.

Pindborg, J.J., Bhat, M., Devanath, K.R., Narayana, H.R. & Ramachandra, S. (1966). Occurrence of acute necrotizing gingivitis in South Indian children. *Journal of Periodontology* **37**, 14–19.

Pindborg, J.J., Bhat, M. & Roed-Petersen, B. (1967). Oral changes in South Indian children with severe protein deficiency. *Journal of Periodontology* **38**, 218–221.

Proctor, D.B. & Baker, C.G. (1971). Treatment of acute necrotizing ulcerative gingivitis with metronidazole. *Journal of the Canadian Dental Association* **37**, 376–380.

Reichart, P.A., Khongkhunthian, P. & Bendick, C. (2003). Oral manifestations in HIV-infected individuals from Thailand and Cambodia. *Medical Microbiology and Immunology* **92**, 157–160.

Reichart, P.A. & Schiødt, M. (1989). Non-pigmented oral Kaposi's sarcoma (AIDS): report of two cases. *International Journal of Oral & Maxillofacial Surgery* **18**, 197–199.

Riley, C., London, J.P. & Burmeister, J.A. (1992). Periodontal health in 200 HIV-positive patients. *Journal of Oral Pathology & Medicine* **21**, 124–127.

Robinson, P. (1991). The management of HIV. *British Dental Journal* **170**, 287.

Sabiston, C.B. Jr. (1986). A review and proposal for the etiology of acute necrotizing gingivitis. *Journal of Clinical Periodontology* **13**, 727–734.

SanGiacomo, T.R., Tan, P.M., Loggi, D.G. & Itkin, A.B. (1990). Progressive osseous destruction as a complication to HIV-periodontitis. *Oral Surgery, Oral Medicine, Oral Pathology* **70**, 476–479.

Schwartz, D.M. & Baumhammers, A. (1972). Smoking and periodontal disease. *Periodontal Abstracts* **20**, 103–106.

Scully, C., Laskaris, G., Pindborg, J.J., Porter, S.R. & Reichardt, P. (1991). Oral manifestations of HIV infection and their management. I. More common lesions. *Oral Surgery, Oral Medicine, Oral Pathology* **71**, 158–166.

Selby, C., Drost, E., Brown, D., Howie, S & MacNee, W. (1992). Inhibition of neutrophil adherence and movement by acute-cigarette smoke exposure. *Experimental Lung Research* **18**, 813–827.

Shangase, L., Feller, L. & Blignaut, E. (2004). Necrotizing ulcerative gingivitis/periodontitis as indicators of HIV-infection. *Journal of the South African Dental Association* **9**(3), 105–108.

Shannon, I.L., Kilgore, W.G. & O'Leary, T.J. (1969). Stress as a predisposing factor in necrotizing ulcerative gingivitis. *Journal of Periodontology* **40**, 240–242.

Sheiham, A. (1966). An epidemiological survey of acute ulcerative gingivitis in Nigerians. *Archives of Oral Biology* **11**, 937–942.

Shields, W.D. (1977). Acute necrotizing ulcerative gingivitis. A study of some of the contributing factors and their validity in an army population. *Journal of Periodontology* **48**, 346–349.

Shinn, D.L. (1976). Vincent's disease and its treatment. In: *Metronidazole*. Proceedings of the International Metronidazole Conference. pp. 334–340. Montreal, Quebec, Canada, May 26–28.

Stammers, A. (1944). Vincent's infection observations and conclusions regarding the etiology and treatment of 1017 civilian cases. *British Dental Journal* **76**, 147–209.

Steidley, K.E., Thompson, S.H., McQuade, M.J., Strong, S.L., Scheidt, M.J. & van Dyke, T.E. (1992). A comparison of T4:T8 lymphocyte ratio in the periodontal lesion of healthy and HIV-positive patients. *Journal of Periodontology* **63**, 753–756.

Stevens, A. Jr., Cogen, R.B., Cohen-Cole, S. & Freeman, A. (1984). Demographic and clinical data associated with acute necrotizing ulcerative gingivitis in a dental school population (ANUG-demographic and clinical data). *Journal of Clinical Periodontology* **11**, 487–493.

Taiwo, J.O. (1993). Oral hygiene status and necrotizing ulcerative gingivitis in Nigerian children. *Journal of Periodontology* **64**, 1071–1074.

Tappuni, A.R. & Flemming, G.J.P. (2001). The effect of antiretroviral therapy on the prevalence of oral manifestations in HIV-infected patients; a UK study. *Oral Surgery, Oral Medicine, Oral Pathology, Oral Radiology and Endodontics* **92**, 623–628.

Thompson, S.H., Charles, G.A. & Craig, D.B. (1992). Correlation of oral disease with the Walter Reed staging scheme for HIV-1-seropositive patients. *Oral Surgery, Oral Medicine, Oral Pathology* **73**, 289–292.

Vincent, H. (1898). Sur une forme particulière d'engine différoïde (engine à bacilles fusiformes). *Archives Internationales de Laryngologie* **11**, 44–48.

Wennström, J. & Lindhe, J. (1979). Effect of hydrogen peroxide on developing plaque and gingivitis in man. *Journal of Clinical Periodontology* **6**, 115–130.

Williams, C.A., Winkler, J.R., Grassi, M. & Murray, P.A. (1990). HIV-associated periodontitis complicated by necrotizing stomatitis. *Oral Surgery, Oral Medicine, Oral Pathology* **69**, 351–355.

Wilson, J.R. (1952). Etiology and diagnosis of bacterial gingivitis including Vincent's disease. *Journal of the American Dental Association* **44**, 19–52.

Wilton, J.M.A., Ivanyi, L. & Lehner, T. (1971). Cell-mediated immunity and humoral antibodies in acute ulcerative gingivitis. *Journal of Periodontal Research* **6**, 9–16.

Wilton, J.M.A. & Lehner, T. (1980). Immunological and microbial aspects of periodontal disease. In: Thompson, R.A., ed. *Recent Advances in Clinical Immunology*, No. 2. Edinburgh: Churchill Livingstone, pp. 145–181.

Chapter 21

Periodontal Disease as a Risk for Systemic Disease

Ray C. Williams and David W. Paquette

Throughout the history of mankind, there has been the belief that diseases which affect the mouth, such as periodontal disease, can have an effect on the rest of the body. Over the centuries, writings from the ancient Egyptians, Hebrews, Assyrians, Greeks, and Romans, to name a few, have all noted the importance of the mouth in overall health and wellbeing. Thus, one could say that the concept linking systemic disease and periodontitis can be traced back to the beginning of recorded history and medicine (O'Reilly & Claffey 2000).

This chapter examines the evidence which has emerged since the early 1990s implicating periodontal disease as a risk factor for several systemic conditions such as cardiovascular disease, adverse pregnancy outcomes, diabetes, and pulmonary disease. But first, it is helpful for the student of dentistry to understand the historical perspective under which this relationship emerged. The concept of "focal infection" which emerged around 1900 has resurfaced and has stimulated much new interest and research into the role of periodontitis as a risk for systemic disease.

Early twentieth century concepts

At the beginning of the twentieth century, medicine and dentistry were searching for reasons to explain why people became afflicted with a wide range of systemic diseases. Medicine at that time had very little insight into what caused diseases such as arthritis, pneumonia, and pancreatitis. Through the writings and lectures of principally two individuals, Willoughby D. Miller, a microbiologist in Philadelphia, and William Hunter, a London physician, the concept that oral bacteria and infection were likely causes of most systemic illnesses suddenly became

very popular (O'Reilly & Claffey 2000). For the next 40 years, physicians and dentists would embrace the idea that infections, especially those originating in the mouth, caused most human suffering and illness. This era, which came to be known as the "era of focal infection", can be attributed primarily to Willoughby D. Miller and William Hunter (O'Reilly & Claffey 2000).

Willoughby Miller was an instructor at the University of Pennsylvania School of Dental Medicine around the turn of the twentieth century. Miller had earlier trained in microbiology in Berlin in Robert Koch's institute. Koch was a pioneer in microbiology and the father of the modern "germ theory" of disease. While under the influence of Robert Koch, Miller too became intensely interested in the role of "germs" or bacteria in causing diseases. Miller returned to the US following his training, convinced that the bacteria residing in the mouth could cause or be attributed to most systemic diseases in patients. In a paper published in 1891, entitled "The human mouth as a focus of infection", Miller argued that the oral flora caused ostitis, osteomyelitis, septicemia, pyemia, disturbances of the alimentary tract, noma, dyptheria, tuberculosis, syphilis, and thrush (Miller 1891). Clearly from this one publication, one can appreciate just how extensively the mouth and oral infection were blamed for causing systemic disease (O'Reilly & Claffey 2000).

While attending one of Miller's lectures at the International Congress of Hygiene in London, William Hunter, a physician from the London Fever Hospital, noted that he and Miller were in strong agreement about the systemic impact of oral infections or oral sepsis. Shortly after, Hunter was invited to speak at the opening of the Strathcona Medical Building at McGill University in Montreal in 1910. In his address to the audience, he blamed poor dentistry and the resulting oral sepsis for causing most of mankind's systemic disease. Hunter remarked that the crowns, bridges and partial dentures he saw in his patients in London were built on teeth surrounded by a "mass of sepsis". Indeed, this oral sepsis could explain why most individuals developed chronic diseases (Hunter 1900; O'Reilly & Claffey 2000). It is likely that Hunter was referring to the untreated periodontal diseases, caries, and defective restorations he was noting in his adult patients at the London Fever Hospital. But whatever Hunter thought he observed in the mouths of his sick patients, his speech at McGill University and his subsequent publication on the role of sepsis and antisepsis in medicine (Hunter 1910) ushered in an era of belief that periodontitis, caries, and poor oral hygiene were the primary cause of systemic illness. The term "oral sepsis" used by Hunter was replaced with the term "focal infection" in 1911 (Billings 1912). Focal infection implied that there was a nidus of infection somewhere in the body, such as periodontitis, which could affect distant sites and organs via the bloodstream. Throughout the 1920s and 1930s, dentists and physicians believed that the bacteria on the teeth and the resultant infectious diseases, such as caries, gingivitis, and periodontitis, were a focus of infection that led to a wide variety of systemic problems. It became popular during this period to extract teeth as a means of ridding the body of oral bacteria and preventing and/or treating diseases affecting the joints, as well as diseases of the heart, liver, kidneys, and pancreas (Cecil & Angevine 1938; O'Reilly & Claffey 2000).

However, by 1940, medicine and dentistry were realizing that there was much more to explain a patient's general systemic condition than bacteria in the mouth. Dentists and physicians realized that (1) extracting a person's teeth did not necessarily make the person better or make their disease go away, (2) people with very healthy mouths and no obvious oral infection developed systemic disease, and (3) people who had no teeth and thus no apparent oral infection still developed systemic diseases (Galloway 1931; Cecil & Angevine 1938).

By 1950, it was apparent to medicine and dentistry that oral infections, such as dental caries, gingivitis, and periodontitis, could not explain why individuals developed a wide range of systemic diseases. By this time medicine was making strides in discovering the true etiologies of many diseases, and dentistry was making great strides in the prevention as well as the treatment of caries and periodontal disease. Thus, the era of focal infection as a primary cause of systemic diseases came to an end (O'Reilly & Claffey 2000).

Throughout the second half of the twentieth century, several researchers and clinicians continued to question whether oral infection (and inflammation) might in some way contribute to a person's overall health, but the reasons given were mostly speculative. Clinicians continued to propose that bacteria and bacterial products within the periodontal pocket, and which could enter the bloodstream from the mouth, could surely in some way be harmful to the body as a whole (Thoden van Velzen *et al.* 1984). However, it was not until the last decade of the twentieth century that dentistry and medicine again began to examine the relationship of periodontitis as a risk for systemic disease. The student of dentistry thus needs to appreciate the intense focus on oral infection as a "likely" cause of many systemic diseases from 1900–1950, then the era of retreat from the focal infection theories of disease causation from 1950 to around 1989, and now the new look at emerging science that suggests periodontitis as a possible risk factor for several systemic diseases, including cardiovascular disease, adverse pregnancy outcomes, diabetes mellitus, and bacterial pneumonia.

Periodontitis as a risk for cardiovascular disease

In 1989 Kimmo Mattila and co-workers in Finland conducted a case–control study on patients who had experienced an acute myocardial infarction and compared these patients to control subjects selected from the community. A dental examination was performed on all of the subjects studied and a dental index computed. The dental index used by Mattila was the sum of scores from the number of carious lesions, missing teeth and periapical lesions, and probing depth measures to indicate periodontitis and the presence or absence of pericoronitis. Mattila and his group reported a highly significant association between poor dental health, as measured by the dental index, and acute myocardial infarction. The association was independent of other risk factors for heart attack such as age, total cholesterol, high density lipoprotein (HDL) triglycerides, C peptide, hypertension, diabetes, and smoking (Mattila *et al.* 1989).

Mattila's findings initiated a great deal of interest in the scientific community. Might it be possible that there was a significant association between periodontitis and cardiovascular disease? Physicians and dentists noted the following commonalities. Patients with periodontal disease share many of the same risk factors as patients with cardiovascular disease, including age, gender (predominantly male), lower socioeconomic status, stress, and smoking (Beck *et al.* 1998). Additionally, a large proportion of patients with periodontal disease also exhibit cardiovascular disease (Umino & Nagao 1993). These observations suggest that periodontal disease and atherosclerosis share similar or common etiologic pathways. Scannapieco and colleagues (2003a) conducted a systematic review of the evidence supporting or refuting any relationship. In response to the focused questions, "Does periodontal disease influence the initiation/progression of atherosclerosis and therefore cardiovascular disease, stroke and peripheral vascular disease?" the investigators identified 31 human

Table 21-1 Summary of select case–control and cohort observational studies supporting an association between periodontal disease and cardiovascular disease

Reference	Study design	Population	Periodontal outcome or exposure	Cardiovascular outcome	Findings and conclusions
Matilla et al. 1989	Case–control	Finland; 100 cases and 102 controls	Dental Severity Index (sum of scores for caries, periodontal disease, periapical pathosis and pericoronitis)	Evidence of myocardial infarction (MI) from EKG and elevated enzyme levels (creatinine phosphokinase isoenzyme MB)	Dental health significantly worse in patients with MI versus controls after adjusting for smoking, social class, smoking, serum lipids, and diabetes
Beck et al. 2001	Cohort	United States; 6017 subjects (ARIC Study)	Severe periodontitis defined as clinical attachment loss ≥3 mm at ≥30% of sites	Carotid artery intima media wall thickness (IMT) ≥1 mm	Periodontitis may influence atheroma formation (OR = 1.3)
Beck et al. 2005	Cohort	United States; 15 792 subjects (ARIC Study)	Serum antibodies to periodontal pathogens	Carotid artery IMT ≥1 mm	Presence of antibody to C. rectus was associated with carotid atherosclerosis (OR = 2.3)
Hung et al. 2004	Cohort	United States; 41 407 males from the HPFS and 58 974 females from the NHS	Self-reported tooth loss at baseline	Incident fatal and non-fatal MI or stroke	For males with tooth loss, the relative risk for coronary heart disease was 1.36. For females with tooth loss, the relative risk was 1.6
Engebretson et al. 2005	Cohort	United States; 203 subjects from INVEST	Radiographic alveolar bone loss	Carotid plaque thickness via ultrasonography	Severe periodontal bone loss was independently associated with carotid atherosclerosis (OR = 3.64)
Desvarieux et al. 2005	Cohort	United States; 1056 subjects from INVEST	Subgingival bacterial burden	Carotid artery IMT ≥1 mm	Severe periodontal bone loss was independently associated with carotid atherosclerosis (OR = 3.64)
Pussinen et al. 2004	Cohort	Finland; 6950 subjects in the Mobile Clinic Health Survey	Serum antibodies to P. gingivalis or A. actinomycetemcomitans	Incident fatal or non-fatal stroke	Seropositive subjects had an OR of 2.6 for stroke
Abnet et al. 2005	Cohort	China; 29 584 rural subjects	Tooth loss	Incidence of fatal MI or stroke	Tooth loss was associated with an increased odds for death from MI (RR = 1.29) and stroke (RR = 1.1)

studies. Table 21-1 lists selected influential studies identified in the review plus additional recent observational studies discussed below. Although the authors did not perform a meta-analysis due to differences in reported outcomes, the authors noted relative (not absolute) consistency and concluded, "Periodontal disease may be modestly associated with atherosclerosis, myocardial infarction and cardiovascular events." An accompanying consensus report approved by the American Academy of Peri-

odontology recommends, "Patients and health care providers should be informed that periodontal intervention may prevent the onset or progression of atherosclerosis-induced diseases."

Since Scannapieco's review and consensus report, other meta-analyses on the cardiovascular–periodontal disease association have been conducted and published. Meurman and co-workers (2004) reported a 20% increase in the risk for cardiovascular disease among patients with periodontal disease (95% CI

1.08–1.32), and an even higher risk ratio for stroke varying from 2.85 (95% CI 1.78–4.56) to 1.74 (CI 1.08–2.81). Similarly, Vettore and co-workers reported relative risk estimates of 1.19 (95% CI 1.08–1.32) and 1.15 (95% CI 1.06–1.25) respectively (Khader *et al.* 2004; Vettore 2004). These meta-analyses of the available observational human data suggest a modest but statistically significant increase in the risk for cardiovascular disease with periodontal disease.

Recent findings from several worldwide population studies also should be noted. These studies include the Atherosclerosis Risk in Communities Study (ARIC), the Health Professional Follow-up Study (HPFS), the Nurses Health Study (NHS), and the Oral Infections and Vascular Disease Epidemiology Study (INVEST) conducted in the United States. Other studies have involved populations from Sweden, Finland, and China.

Periodontal probing data were collected on 6017 persons, 52–75 years of age, participating in the ARIC study (Beck *et al.* 2001, 2005; Elter *et al.* 2004). The investigators assessed both the presence of clinical cardiovascular disease (MI or revascularization procedure) and subclinical atherosclerosis (carotid artery intima media wall thickness (IMT) using B-mode ultrasound) as dependent variables in the population. Individuals with both high attachment loss (≥10% of sites with attachment loss >3 mm) and high tooth loss exhibited elevated odds of prevalent cardiovascular disease as compared to individuals with low attachment loss and low tooth loss (OR = 1.5, 95% CI 1.1–2.0 and OR = 1.8, CI 1.4–2.4 respectively) (Elter *et al.* 2004). A second logistic regression analysis indicated a significant association between severe periodontitis and thickened carotid arteries after adjusting for covariates like age, gender, diabetes, lipids, hypertension, and smoking (Beck *et al.* 2001). Accordingly, the odds ratio for severe periodontitis (i.e. 30% or more of sites with ≥3 mm clinical attachment loss) and subclinical carotid atherosclerosis was 1.31 (95% CI 1.03–1.66). In a third report, these investigators quantified serum IgG antibody levels specific for 17 periodontal organisms using a whole bacterial checkerboard immunoblotting technique (Beck *et al.* 2005). Analyzing mean carotid IMT (≥1 mm) as the outcome and serum antibody levels specific as exposures for this same population, the investigators noted the presence of antibody to *Campylobacter rectus* increased the risk for subclinical atherosclerosis two-fold (OR = 2.3, 95% CI 1.83–2.84). In particular, individuals with both high *C. rectus* and *Peptostreptococcus micros* antibody titers had almost twice the prevalence of carotid atherosclerosis as compared to those with only a high *C. rectus* antibody (8.3% versus 16.3%). Stratification by smoking indicated that all microbial models significant for smokers were also significant for never smokers except for *Porphyromonas gingivalis*. Thus, clinical signs of periodontitis are associated with cardiovascular disease and subclinical atherosclerosis in the ARIC population, and exposures to specific periodontal pathogens significantly increase the risk for atherosclerosis in smoking and non-smoking subjects.

Self-reported periodontal disease outcomes and incident cardiovascular disease were assessed in two extant databases, HPFS (n = 41 407 males followed for 12 years) and NHS (n = 58 974 females followed for 6 years) (Hung *et al.* 2004). After controlling for important cardiovascular risk factors, males with a low number of teeth (≤10 at baseline) had a significantly higher risk of cardiovascular disease (RR = 1.36; 95% CI 1.11–1.67) as compared to males with a higher number of teeth (25 or more). For females with the same reported extent of tooth loss, the relative risk for cardiovascular disease was 1.64 (95% CI 1.31–2.05) as compared to women with at least 25 teeth. The relative risks for fatal cardiovascular disease events increased to 1.79 (95% CI 1.34–2.40) for males and 1.65 (95% CI 1.11–2.46) for females with tooth loss respectively. In a second report, the investigators evaluated the association between self-reported periodontal disease and serum elevations in cardiovascular disease biomarkers cross-sectionally in a subset of HPFS participants (n = 468 males) (Joshipura *et al.* 2004). Serum biomarkers included C-reactive protein (CRP), fibrinogen, factor VII, tissue plasminogen activator (t-PA), LDL cholesterol, von Willebrand factor, and soluble TNF receptors 1 and 2. In multi-variate regression models controlling for age, cigarette smoking, alcohol intake, physical activity, and aspirin intake, self-reported periodontal disease was associated with significantly higher levels of CRP (30% higher among periodontal cases compared with non-cases), t-PA (11% higher), and LDL cholesterol (11% higher). These analyses reveal significant associations between self-reported number of teeth at baseline and risk of cardiovascular disease and between self-reported periodontal disease and serum biomarkers of endothelial dysfunction and dyslipidemia.

One population study called INVEST has been planned *a priori* and conducted exclusively to evaluate the association between cardiovascular disease and periodontal outcomes in a cohort population. It was reported that for a group of 203 stroke-free subjects (ages 54–94) at baseline, mean carotid plaque thickness (measured with B-mode ultrasound) was significantly greater among dente subjects with severe periodontal bone loss (≥50% measured radiographically) as compared to those with less bone loss (<50%) (Engebretson *et al.* 2005). These investigators noted a clear dose–response relationship when they graphed subject tertiles of periodontal bone loss versus carotid plaque thickness. The investigators next collected subgingival plaque from 1056 subjects and tested for the presence of 11 known periodontal bacteria using DNA techniques (Desvarieux *et al.* 2005). The investigators found that cumulative periodontal bacterial burden was significantly related to carotid IMT after adjusting for cardiovascular disease risk factors. Whereas mean IMT values were similar across burden tertiles for putative (orange complex) and health-associated bacteria, IMT values rose with each tertile of etiologic bacterial burden (*Actinobacillus acinomycetemcomitans* (recently renamed *Aggregatibacter acinomycetemcomitans*), *P. gingivalis*, *Treponema denticola* and *Tannerella forsythia*). Similarly, white blood cell values (but not serum CRP) increased across these burden tertiles. These data from INVEST provide evidence of a direct relationship between periodontal microbiology and subclinical atherosclerosis independent of CRP.

Consistent associations between periodontal outcomes and atherosclerosis have been recently demonstrated among populations in Europe and Asia. For 131 adult Swedes, mean carotid IMT values were significantly higher in subjects with clinical and/or radiographic evidence of periodontal disease compared to periodontally healthy controls (Soder *et al.* 2005). Multiple logistic regression analysis identified periodontal disease as a principal independent predictor of carotid atherosclerosis with an odds ratio of 4.64 (95% CI 1.64–13.10). Pussinen *et al.* (2004) monitored antibody responses for *A. actinomycetemcomitans* and *P. gingivalis* among 6950 Finnish subjects for whom cardiovascular disease outcomes over 13 years were available (Mobile Clinic Health Survey). Compared with the subjects who were seronegative for these pathogens, seropositive subjects had an odds ratio of 2.6 (95% CI 1.0–7.0) for a secondary stroke. In a second report on 1023 males (Kuopio Ischemic Heart Disease Study), Pussinen and co-workers (2005) observed that cases with myocardial infarction or cardiovascular disease death were more often seropositive for *A. actinomycetemcomitans* than those controls who remained healthy (15.5% versus 10.2%). In the highest tertile of *A. actinomycetemcomitans* antibodies, the relative risk for MI or coronary heart disease death was 2.0 (95% CI 1.2–3.3) compared with the lowest tertile. For *P. gingivalis* antibody responses, the relative risk was of 2.1 (95% CI 1.3–3.4). Abnet and co-workers (2005) recently published findings from a cohort study of 29 584 healthy, rural Chinese adults monitored for up to 15 years. Tooth loss was evaluated as an exposure outcome for periodontal disease, and mortality from heart disease or stroke were modeled as dependent variables. Individuals with greater than the age-specific median number of teeth lost exhibited a significantly increased risk of death from MI (RR = 1.28, 95% CI 1.17–1.40) and stroke (RR = 1.2, 95% CI 1.02–1.23). These elevated risks were present in male and females irrespective of smoking status. Collectively, these findings indicate consistent associations for periodontal disease and pathogenic exposures with cardiovascular disease for European and Asian populations.

Biologic rationale

Many investigators have asked the question: what is the biologic rationale to explain how periodontitis may be related to cardiovascular disease? Scientists have noted that a patient who has, for example, 28 teeth with pocket depths of 6–7 mm and bone loss, has a large overall surface area of infection and inflammation (Waite & Bradley 1965). In patients with moderate periodontitis, the surface area could be the size of the palm of the hand or larger. In addition, the subgingival bacteria in periodontal pockets exists in a highly organized biofilm. Since periodontal infections result in low-grade bacteremias and endotoxemias in affected patients (Sconyers *et al.* 1973; Silver *et al.* 1980), systemic effects on vascular physiology via these exposures appear biologically plausible. Four specific pathways have been proposed to explain the plausibility of a link between cardiovascular disease and periodontitis (Fig. 21-1). These pathways (acting independently or collectively) include: (1) direct bacterial effects on platelets, (2) autoimmune responses, (3) invasion and/or uptake of bacteria in endothelial cells and macrophages, and (4) endocrine-like effects of pro-inflammatory mediators. In support of the first pathway, two oral bacteria, *P. gingivalis* and *Streptococcus sanguis* express virulence factors called "collagen-like platelet aggregation associated proteins" (PAAP) that induce platelet aggregation *in vitro* and *in vivo* (Hertzberg & Meyer 1996, 1998). Secondly, autoimmune mechanisms may play a role since antibodies that cross react with periodontal bacteria and human heat shock proteins have been identified (Hinode *et al.* 1998; Sims *et al.* 2002). Deshpande *et al.* (1998) have thirdly demonstrated that *P. gingivalis* can invade aortic and heart endothelial cells via fimbriae. Several investigative groups have independently identified specific oral pathogens in atheromatous tissues (Chui 1999; Haraszthy *et al.* 2000). In addition, macrophages incubated *in vitro* with *P. gingivalis* and LDL uptake the bacteria intracellularly and transform into foam cells (Giacona *et al.* 2004). In the last potential pathway, systemic pro-inflammatory mediators are up-regulated for endocrine-like effects in vascular tissues, and studies consistently demonstrate elevations in CRP and fibrinogen among periodontally diseased subjects (Slade *et al.* 2000; Wu *et al.* 2000a,b).

Experiments with animal models demonstrate that specific infections with periodontal pathogens accelerate atherogenesis. For example, inbred heterozygous and homozygous apoE-deficient mice exhibit increased aortic atherosclerosis when challenged orally or intravenously with invasive strains of *P. gingivalis* (Li *et al.* 2002; Lalla *et al.* 2003; Chi *et al.* 2004; Gibson *et al.* 2004). While *P. gingivalis* challenges increased aortic atherosclerosis in apoE-deficient mice in a hypercholesterolemic background only, normocholesterolemic pigs were recently shown to develop both coronary and aortic lesions with *P. gingivalis* challenges (Brodala *et al.* 2005). This finding suggests that *P. gingivalis* bacteremia may exert an atherogenic stimulus independent of high cholesterol

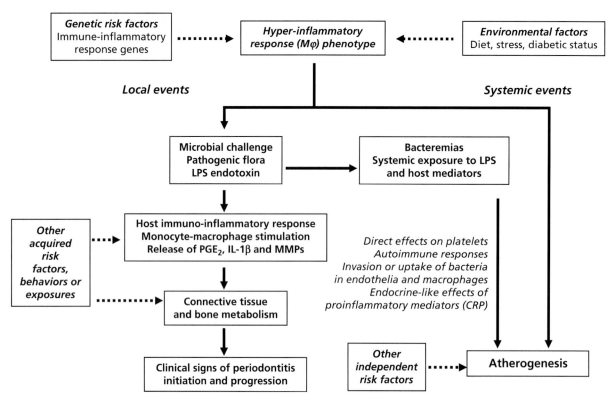

Fig. 21-1 Proposed model and mechanisms linking periodontal disease and cardiovascular disease.

levels in pigs. It is worth noting that a wide range of *P. gingivalis* doses was used in these animal studies. While the clinically relevant dose for human subjects is unknown at present, it probably varies greatly (Daly *et al.* 2001; Haynes & Stanford 2003; Ide *et al.* 2004). Importantly, *P. gingivalis* challenges enhance atherosclerosis despite these different routes of administration and dosing regimens in both species. *P. gingivalis* 16 ribosomal DNA was detected by polymerase chain reaction (PCR) in atheromas from some but not all of these mutant mice and the pigs. These experiments suggest that both the host response and the virulence of the specific *P. gingivalis* strains appear to be important variables in these infection–atherogenesis models. Collectively, when one looks at the body of evidence gathered so far since 1989, there appears to be a compelling association between periodontitis and coronary heart disease.

Periodontitis as a risk for adverse pregnancy outcomes

In 1996, following a landmark report by Offenbacher and colleagues (1996), there has been much interest and research into whether periodontitis may be a possible risk factor for adverse pregnancy outcomes. Adverse pregnancy outcomes that have been linked to periodontal disease include preterm birth, low birthweight, miscarriage or early pregnancy loss, and pre-eclampsia. Pre-eclampsia and preterm births are major causes of maternal and prenatal morbidity and mortality.

Preterm infants who are born with low birthweights represent a major social and economic public health problem, even in industrialized nations. Although there has been an overall decline in infant mortality in the US over the past 40 years, preterm low birthweight remains a significant cause of perinatal mortality and morbidity. A 47% decrease in the infant mortality rate to a level of 13.1 per 1000 live births occurred between 1965 and 1980. But from 1980 to 2000, the percentage of low birthweight infants increased by 11.8% and that of very low birthweight infants increased by 24.3% in the US; among survivors, low birthweight is a major contributor to long-term disability.

Preterm low birthweight deliveries represent approximately 10% of annual births in industrialized nations and account for two-thirds of overall infant mortality. Approximately one-third of these births are elective while two-thirds are spontaneous preterm births. About a half of the spontaneous preterm births are due to premature rupture of membranes and the other half are due to preterm labor. For the spontaneous preterm births, 10–15% occur before 32 weeks gestation, result in very low birthweight (<1500 g) and often cause long-term disability, such as chronic respiratory diseases and cerebral palsy (Offenbacher *et al.* 1996, 1998; Champagne *et al.* 2000; Scannapieco *et al.* 2003c; Xiong *et al.* 2006).

Among the known risk factors for preterm low birthweight deliveries are young maternal age (<18 years), drug, alcohol and tobacco use, maternal stress, genetic background, and genitourinary tract infections. Although 25–50% of preterm low birthweight deliveries occur without any known etiology, there is increasing evidence that infection may play a significant role in preterm delivery (Hill 1998; Goldenberg *et al.* 2000; Sobel 2000; Williams *et al.* 2000; Scannapieco *et al.* 2003c; Xiong *et al.* 2006).

One of the more important acute exposures that has been implicated in preterm birth is an acute maternal genitourinary tract infection at some point during the pregnancy. Bacterial vaginosis (BV) is a Gram-negative, predominantly anaerobic infection of the vagina, usually diagnosed from clinical signs and symptoms. It is associated with a decrease in the normal lactobacillus-dominated flora and an increase in anaerobes and facultative species including *Gardenerella vaginalis*, *Mobiluncus curtsii*, *Prevotella bivia*, and *Bacteroides ureolyticus*. Bacterial vaginosis is a relatively common condition that occurs in about 10% of all pregnancies. It may ascend from the vagina to the cervix and even result in inflammation of the maternal fetal membranes (chorioamnionitis). Extending beyond the membranes, the organisms may appear in the amniotic fluid compartment that is shared with the fetal lungs and/or involve placental tissues and result in exposure to the fetus via the bloodstream. Despite the observed epidemiologic linkage of bacterial vaginosis with preterm birth, the results from randomized clinical trials to determine the effects of treating bacterial vaginosis with systemic antibiotics on incident preterm birth are equiv-

ocal (Goldenberg *et al.* 2000). Still, there are compelling data linking maternal infection and the subsequent inflammation to preterm birth. It appears that inflammation of the uterus and membranes represents a common effector mechanism that results in preterm birth, and, thus, either clinical infection or subclinical infection is a likely stimulus for increased inflammation.

In the early 1990s, it was hypothesized that oral infections, such as periodontitis, could represent a significant source of both infection and inflammation during pregnancy. It was noted that periodontal disease is a Gram-negative anaerobic infection with the potential to cause Gram-negative bacteremias in persons with periodontal disease. It was hypothesized that periodontal infections, which serve as reservoirs for Gram-negative anaerobic organisms, lipopolysaccharide (LPS, endotoxin), and inflammatory mediators including prostaglandin E_2 (PGE$_2$) and tumor necrosis factor-α (TNF-α), may be a potential threat to the fetal–placental unit (Fig. 21-2) (Collins *et al.* 1994a,b).

As a first step in testing this hypothesis, Greg Collins in Offenbacher's laboratory conducted a series of experiments in the pregnant hamster animal model. It had been noted earlier by Lanning *et al.* (1983) that pregnant hamsters challenged with *Escherichia coli* LPS had malformation of fetuses, spontaneous abortions, and low fetal weight. The work by Lanning and co-workers clearly demonstrated that

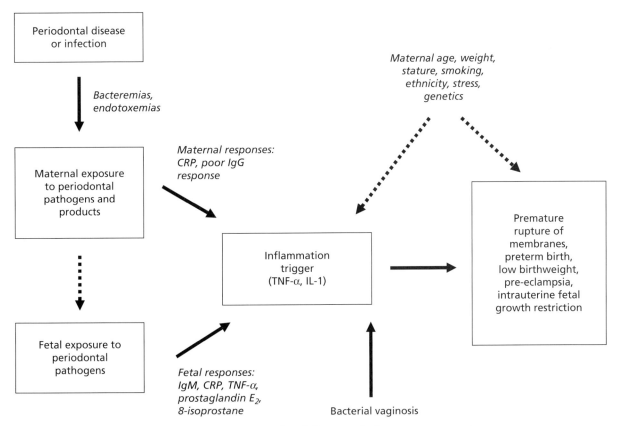

Fig. 21-2 Proposed model for relationship between periodontal disease and adverse pregnancy outcomes.

infections in pregnant animals could elicit many pregnancy complications including spontaneous abortion, preterm labor, low birthweight, fetal growth restriction, and skeletal abnormalities. It was not clear, however, if these findings from *E. coli* would be similar if endotoxin from oral anaerobes was studied. First of all, LPS from Gram-negative enteric organisms differs in structure and biological activity from oral LPS. Thus, Collins needed to demonstrate that LPS from oral organisms had similar effects on fetal outcomes when administered to pregnant animals. Secondly, the oral cavity represents a distant site of infection. Although pneumonia has been a recognized example of a distant site of infection triggering maternal obstetric complications, it was important to demonstrate that distant, non-disseminating infections with oral pathogens could elicit pregnancy complications in animal models. Thirdly, oral infections are chronic in nature. Increased obstetric risk is generally associated with acute infections that occur during pregnancy. Thus, in concept, maternal adaptation to a chronic infectious challenge was assumed to afford protection to the fetus, even during acute flare-ups that may occur during pregnancy.

Collins' landmark hamster studies (Collins *et al.* 1994a,b) demonstrated that chronic exposure to oral pathogens like *P. gingivalis* in a chamber model (Genco & Arko 1994) does not in fact afford protection, but actually enhances the fetal–placental toxicity of exposure during pregnancy. Thus during pregnancy the mother does not become "tolerant" of infectious challenge from oral organisms. Collins and Offenbacher also wanted to demonstrate that the low-grade infections with low numbers of oral pathogens were not of sufficient magnitude to induce maternal malaise or fever. They noted however a measurable local increase of PGE_2 and TNF-α in chamber fluid with *P. gingivalis* as well as a 15–18% decrease in fetal weight. Further, the magnitude of the PGE_2 and TNF-α response was inversely related to the weight of the fetuses, mimicking the intra-amniotic changes seen in humans with preterm low birthweight. LPS dosing experiments demonstrated that higher levels of LPS could induce fever and weight loss in pregnant animals and resulted in more severe pregnancy outcomes including spontaneous abortions and malformations. These more noteworthy outcomes were not seen in the low-challenge oral infection models, but rather resulted in a consistent decrease in fetal weight. Previous sensitization or exposures to these pathogens prior to pregnancy enhanced the severity of the fetal growth restriction when a secondary exposure occurred during pregnancy.

Collins and colleagues (1994b) next studied infection and pregnancy in the hamster by experimentally inducing periodontal disease in the animal model. Four groups of animals were fed either control chow or plaque-promoting chow for an 8-week period to induce experimental periodontitis prior to mating.

Two additional groups of animals (i.e. one control chow and one plaque-promoting chow) received exogenous *P. gingivalis* via oral gavage. Animals fed the plaque-promoting diet beginning 8 weeks prior to mating developed periodontitis. These animals also had litters with a mean fetal weight of 1.25 ± 0.07 g that was 81% of the weight of the control groups. Animals receiving both plaque-promoting diet and *P. gingivalis* gavage also had significantly smaller fetuses. The mean fetal weight for this group was 1.20 ± 0.19 g which represented a significant 22.5% reduction in fetal weight compared to controls. Exogenous *P. gingivalis* challenge by gastric gavage did not appear to promote either more severe periodontal disease or more severe fetal growth restriction. This experiment indicated that experimentally induced periodontitis in the hamster could also alter fetal weight in the hamster.

More recently this group has focused on a possible role for *Campylobacter rectus* in contributing to adverse pregnancy outcomes (Madianos *et al.* 2001). In recent animal studies utilizing the BALB/C mouse model, Yeo *et al.* (2005) have reported that maternal *Campylobacter rectus* infection mediates fetal growth restriction in pregnant mice. More recently, Bobetsis and colleagues (Offenbacher *et al.* 2005) found that maternal *C. rectus* infection induced placental inflammation and decidual hyperplasia as well as a concomitant increase in fetal brain IFN-γ. Maternal infection with *C. rectus* increased mouse pup mortality and also affected the hippocampal region of the neonatal brain, suggesting that maternal infection with *C. rectus* may also affect perinatal neurological growth and development (Offenbacher *et al.*, 2005).

In what is now viewed as a landmark human study, Offenbacher and colleagues (1996) conducted a case–control study on 124 pregnant or postpartum women (Table 21-2). Preterm low birthweight cases were defined as a mother whose infant had a birthweight of less than 2500 g and also had one or more of the following: gestational age <37 weeks, preterm labor or preterm premature rupture of membranes. Controls were all mothers whose infant had a normal birthweight. Assessments included a broad range of known obstetric risk factors such as tobacco usage, drug use, and alcohol consumption, level of prenatal care, parity, genitourinary tract infections, and weight gain during pregnancy. Each subject received a full-mouth periodontal examination to determine clinical attachment levels. Mothers of preterm low birthweight (PLBW) cases and first birth PLBW cases had significantly more advanced periodontal disease as measured with attachment loss than the respective mothers of normal birthweight controls. Multi-variate logistic regression models, controlling for other known risk factors and co-variates, demonstrated that periodontitis was a statistically significant risk factor for preterm low birthweight, with adjusted odds ratios of 7.9 and 7.5 for all PLBW cases and primiparous PLBW cases respectively. This research

Table 21-2 Summary of case–control observational studies on periodontal disease and adverse pregnancy outcomes

Reference	Population	Periodontal outcome or exposure	Adverse pregnancy outcome	Findings and conclusions
Offenbacher et al. 1996	United States; 93 cases and 31 controls	≥60% of sites with clinical attachment levels ≥3 mm	Birthweight <2500 g, gestational age <37 weeks, preterm labor and/or premature rupture of membranes	Significant association between periodontal disease and preterm low birthweight (LBW) (OR = 7.5)
Davenport et al. 2002	United Kingdom; 236 cases and 507 controls	Mean pocket depth (mm)	Preterm delivery <37 weeks and birthweight <2499 g	No association detected for periodontal disease and preterm LBW (OR = 0.83)
Goepfert et al. 2004	United States; 59 cases and 44 controls	Clinical attachment levels ≥5 mm	Spontaneous preterm birth <32 weeks	Significantly higher risk for preterm birth for mothers with periodontal disease (OR = 3.4)
Radnai et al. 2004	Hungary; 41 cases and 44 controls	One or more sites with probing depth ≥4 mm and bleeding on probing ≥50%	Premature labor, spontaneous rupture of membranes and/or the birthweight of the newborn ≤2499 g	Significant association between periodontal disease and preterm LBW (OR = 5.4)
Jarjoura et al. 2005	United States; 83 cases and 120 controls	Five or more sites with clinical attachment levels ≥3 mm	Preterm delivery <37 weeks	Significant association between periodontal disease and preterm delivery (OR = 2.75, 95% CI 1.01–7.54)
Moliterno et al. 2005	Brazil; 76 cases and 75 controls	Four or more sites with pocket depth >4 mm and clinical attachment levels ≥3 mm	Preterm delivery <37 weeks and birthweight <2500 g	Significantly higher risk for preterm LBW for mothers with periodontal disease (OR = 3.48)
Buduneli et al. 2005	Turkey; 53 cases and 128 controls	Mean pocket depth (mm)	Preterm delivery <37 weeks or birthweight <2500 g	No statistically significant differences between the cases and controls with regard clinical periodontal parameters
Moore et al. 2005	United Kingdom; 61 cases and 93 controls	Number of sites with pocket depth ≥5 mm	Preterm delivery <37 weeks	No association between periodontal disease and preterm birth
Bosnjak et al. 2006	Croatia; 17 cases and 64 controls	>60% of sites with clinical attachment levels ≥4 mm	Spontaneous preterm birth <37 weeks	Significant association between periodontal disease and preterm birth (OR = 8.13)
Skuldbol et al. 2006	Denmark; 21 cases and 33 controls	Pocket depth ≥4 mm and bleeding on probing	Preterm delivery <35 weeks	No difference in mean periodontal parameters between the two groups; no association between periodontal disease and preterm birth
Radnai et al. 2006	Hungary; 77 cases and 84 controls	One or more sites with probing depth ≥4 mm and bleeding on probing ≥50%	Preterm delivery <37 weeks and birthweight <2500 g	Significant association between periodontal disease and preterm LBW (OR = 3.32)
Contreras et al. 2006	Colombia; 130 cases and 243 controls	Pocket depth and clinical attachment loss ≥4 mm and bleeding on probing	Pre-eclampsia: blood pressure ≥140/90 mmHg and ≥2+ proteinuria	Significant association for periodontal disease and pre-eclampsia (OR = 3.0)

was the first to demonstrate an association between periodontal infection and adverse pregnancy outcomes in humans (Offenbacher *et al.* 1996).

Offenbacher and co-workers proceeded to conduct a prospective cohort study, entitled Oral Conditions and Pregnancy (OCAP), which was designed to determine whether maternal periodontal disease was predictive of preterm (<37 weeks) or very preterm (<32 weeks) birth. One thousand and twenty pregnant women were periodontally examined antepartum (<26 weeks gestation) and postpartum. Again, logistic regression models were developed using maternal exposure to either periodontal disease at enrollment or disease progression during pregnancy (clinical attachment loss ≥2 mm at one or more sites) as independent variables and adjusting for known risk factors (e.g. previous preterm delivery, race, smoking, social domain variables, and other infections). Overall, the incidence of preterm was 11.2% among periodontally healthy women, compared with 28.6% in women with moderate–severe periodontal disease (adjusted risk ratio or RR = 1.6, 95% CI 1.1–2.3). Antepartum moderate–severe periodontal disease was associated with an increased incidence of spontaneous preterm births (15.2% versus 24.9%, adjusted RR = 2.0, 95% CI 1.2–3.2). Similarly, the unadjusted rate of very preterm delivery was 6.4% among women with periodontal disease progression, significantly higher than the 1.8% rate among women without disease progression (adjusted RR = 2.4, 95% CI 1.1–5.2). This second study by the Offenbacher group implicated maternal periodontal disease exposure and progression as independent risk factors for PTB outcomes (Offenbacher *et al.* 2001, 2006; Lieff *et al.* 2004).

A subsequent analysis of OCAP data further indicates that maternal periodontal disease is associated with small-for-gestational-age births (Boggess *et al.* 2006). Defining "small-for-gestational-age" as birthweight less than the tenth percentile for gestational age, Boggess *et al.* (2006) reported that its prevalence was significantly higher among women with moderate or severe periodontal disease, compared with those with health or mild disease (13.8% versus 3.2%). Indeed, mothers with moderate or advanced periodontal disease were 2.3 times (RR, 95% CI 1.1–4.7) more likely to have small-for-gestational-age infants as compared to mothers with periodontal health even after adjusting for age, smoking, drugs, marital/insurance status, and pre-eclampsia (i.e. pregnancy-related hypertension with proteinuria or edema).

Jeffcoat and co-workers (2001a,b) also found a positive association between maternal periodontal disease and preterm birth in a comparable US cohort study involving 1313 pregnant subjects. Complete periodontal, medical, and behavioral assessments were made between 21 and 24 weeks gestation for each subject. Gestational ages of the infants were determined following delivery, and logistic regression modeling was performed to assess any relation-

ship between periodontal disease and preterm birth while making adjustments for other known risk factors. Notably, subjects with severe or generalized periodontal disease had an adjusted OR of 4.45 (95% CI 2.16–9.18) for preterm delivery (<37 weeks) as compared with periodontally healthy subjects. The adjusted OR increased with advancing prematurity to 5.28 (95% CI 2.05–13.60) before 35 weeks gestational age and to 7.07 (95% CI 1.70–27.4) before 32 weeks gestational age. Hence, mothers with severe periodontal disease were four to seven times more likely to deliver a preterm infant relative to mothers with periodontal health.

Two other observational studies involving US populations report a consistent association for maternal periodontal disease and preterm low birthweight. One case–control study, involved 59 women with early spontaneous preterm births (<32 weeks of gestation), 36 women with early indicated preterm births (<32 weeks of gestation), and 44 controls with uncomplicated births at term (≥37 weeks) (Goepfert *et al.* 2004). Severe periodontal disease (clinical attachment loss ≥5 mm) was more common in the spontaneous preterm birth group (49%) as compared to the indicated preterm and term control groups (25% and 30% respectively). The odds for severe periodontal disease and spontaneous preterm birth were 3.4 (95% CI 1.5–7.7). For the second observational study involving 83 preterm cases (<37 weeks gestation) and 120 term delivery controls, preterm birth was associated with severe periodontitis, i.e. five or more sites with clinical attachment loss ≥3 mm, adjusted OR = 2.75, (95% CI 1.1–7.54) (Jarjoura *et al.* 2005).

This relationship has been explored in other cross-sectional and cohort populations around the globe (Tables 21-2 and 21-3). Bosnjak *et al.* (2006) reported an adjusted OR of 8.13 (95% CI 2.73–45.9) for maternal periodontal disease and preterm birth for a Croatian population (17 preterm cases and 64 controls). Similarly, a Finnish study (Oittinen *et al.* 2005) involving 130 consecutively enrolled pregnant mothers found that those with periodontal disease were 5.5 times (95% CI 1.4–21.2) more likely to have preterm deliveries or adverse pregnancy outcomes. Two case–control studies involving Hungarian subjects found positive associations between maternal early localized periodontitis (more than one site with probing depth ≥4 mm and bleeding on probing ≥50%) and preterm low birth weight (OR = 5.4, 95% CI 1.7–17.3; OR = 3.32, 95% CI 1.64–6.69) (Radnai *et al.* 2004, 2006). Another observational study with 96 Spanish pregnant women found a higher severity of periodontal disease (percentage of sites with probing depths ≥4 mm) among those having low birthweight infants relative to those with normal weight infants (Moreu *et al.* 2005). Moliterno and co-workers (2005) measured periodontal disease and birth outcomes for 150 Brazilian mothers and reported a significant association between periodontitis and low birthweight with an OR of 3.48 (95% CI 1.17–10.36). Chilean

Table 21-3 Summary of cohort observational studies on periodontal disease and adverse pregnancy outcomes

Reference	Population	Periodontal outcome or exposure	Adverse pregnancy outcome	Findings and conclusions
Offenbacher et al. 2001, 2006; Lieff et al. 2004	United States; 1020 subjects	Moderate–severe disease: four or more sites with pocket depths ≥5 mm and clinical attachment levels ≥2 mm; progressive disease: one or more sites with clinical attachment loss ≥2 mm	Preterm delivery <37 weeks; very preterm <32 weeks	Moderate–severe periodontal disease (RR = 1.6) and progressive disease (RR = 2.4) are significant risk factors for preterm delivery
Jeffcoat et al. 2001	United States; 1313 subjects	Severe or generalized disease: ≥90 sites with clinical attachment levels ≥3 mm	Preterm delivery <37 weeks	Severe or generalized periodontal disease is associated with preterm delivery (OR = 4.5)
Lopez et al. 2002b	Chile; 639 subjects	Four or more teeth showing one or more sites with pocket depth ≥4 mm and with clinical attachment level ≥3 mm	Preterm delivery <37 weeks and birthweight <2500 g	Significant association between periodontal disease and preterm LBW (RR = 3.5)
Boggess et al. 2003	United States; 763 subjects	Severe disease: ≥15 sites with pocket depths ≥4 mm; progressive disease: four or more sites with increases in pocket depth ≥2 mm and resulting in pockets ≥4 mm in depth	Pre-eclampsia: blood pressure >140/90 mm Hg and ≥1+ proteinuria	Significantly higher risk for pre-eclampsia among women with severe (OR = 2.4) or progressive (OR = 2.1) periodontal disease
Holbrook et al. 2004	Iceland; 96 subjects	Pocket depth ≥4 mm	Preterm delivery <37 weeks or birthweight <2500 g	No association between periodontal disease and preterm LBW
Moore et al. 2004	United Kingdom; 3738 subjects	Percentage of sites with pocket depth >4 or 5 mm	Preterm delivery <37 weeks or birthweight <2500 g	No association between periodontal disease case definitions and preterm delivery or LBW
Moreu et al. 2005	Spain; 96 subjects	Percentage sites with pocket depths ≥3 mm	Preterm delivery <37 weeks and birthweight <2500 g	Higher severity of periodontal disease among those having LBW infants
Rajapakse et al. 2005	Sri Lanka; 227 subjects	Pocket depth, bleeding and plaque scores > median value in the total cohort	Preterm delivery < 37 weeks and birthweight <2500 g	No association between periodontal disease and preterm delivery (OR = 2.3)
Boggess et al. 2006	United States; 1017 subjects	Moderate–severe disease: ≥15 sites with pocket depths ≥4 mm	Small-for-gestational-age births: birthweight <10% for gestational age	Association between periodontal disease and small-for-gestational-age births (RR = 2.3)
Meurman et al. 2006	Finland; 207 subjects	Community Periodontal Index for Treatment Needs	Preterm delivery <37 weeks, birthweight <2500 g, caesarean section, gestational diabetes or hypertension, pre-eclampsia or infant Apgar score <7	No association between poor periodontal health and pregnancy or delivery complications

mothers with periodontal disease appear to be 3.5 times (RR, 95% CI 1.5–7.9) more likely to have a preterm low birthweight infant versus mothers with periodontal health (Lopez *et al.* 2002a).

A smaller number of observational studies involving populations in Europe and Asia have failed to detect any significant association between maternal periodontal disease and adverse pregnancy outcomes (Davenport *et al.* 2002; Holbrook *et al.* 2004; Buduneli *et al.* 2005; Moore *et al.* 2005; Rajapakse *et al.* 2005; Skuldbol *et al.* 2006; Meurman *et al.* 2006). One prospective study finding no association was conducted at Guy's and St. Thomas' Hospital Trust in London and involved a large cohort of 3738 pregnant subjects (Moore *et al.* 2004). Regression analysis indicated no significant relationships between the severity of periodontal disease (periodontal pocketing or clinical attachment loss) and either preterm birth or low birthweight. The investigators did note a correlation between poorer periodontal health and mothers who experienced a late miscarriage. A subsequent analysis on non-smokers within this same population confirmed no associations between poor periodontal health and either preterm birth or low birthweight (Farrell *et al.* 2006). Again, non-smoking mothers who experienced late miscarriages exhibited a higher mean probing depth as compared with the subjects with term births. This same group of investigators performed genetic testing (restriction fragment length polymerase techniques) on a sub-cohort of 48 preterm cases and 82 control subjects (Moore *et al.* 2004). There were no significant associations reported for the tested cytokine polymorphisms (interleukin-1β+3953 and TNF-α-308 allelic variants), prematurity, and the severity of periodontal disease. In addition, the combination of genotype and periodontal disease did not increase the risk of preterm delivery in this subcohort. These studies reporting no association are a small proportion of the total available evidence collected to date and suggest that differences in the susceptibility to periodontal disease-associated prematurity may occur in certain global populations.

Association of periodontal disease and pre-eclampsia

Pre-eclampsia is a common hypertensive disorder of pregnancy that independently contributes to maternal and infant morbidity and mortality. Accordingly, atherosclerotic-like changes in placental tissues involving oxidative and inflammatory events are thought to initiate the development of pre-eclampsia (Ramos *et al.* 1995). Boggess and co-workers (2003) hypothesized that maternal exposure to periodontal disease or infection may be associated with the development of pre-eclampsia. Using data collected as part of the OCAP study, the investigators conducted logistic regression analyses on outcomes collected from 763 women who were enrolled at less than 26 weeks gestation and who delivered live infants.

Pre-eclampsia (defined here as blood pressure >140/90 mmHg on two separate occasions, and ≥1+ proteinuria on catheterized urine specimen) affected 5.1% of subjects. The adjusted OR for severe periodontal disease at delivery (≥15 sites with pocket depths ≥4 mm in depth) and pre-eclampsia was 2.4 (95% CI 1.1–5.3). For women exhibiting periodontal disease progression during pregnancy (four or more sites with increases in pocket depth ≥2 mm and resulting in pockets ≥4 mm in depth) the adjusted OR was 2.1 (95% CI 1.0–4.4). After adjusting for other risk factors, such as maternal age, race, smoking, gestational age at delivery, and insurance status, the results from this cohort study indicate that severe and progressive maternal periodontal disease during pregnancy is associated with an increased risk for pre-eclampsia.

This same hypothesis was tested in a case–control study conducted in Colombia and including 130 pre-eclamptic (blood pressure ≥149/90 mmHg and ≥2+ proteinuria) and 243 non-pre-eclamptic women recruited between 26 and 36 weeks of pregnancy (Contreras *et al.* 2006). In addition to sociodemographic data, obstetric risk factors, and clinical periodontal outcomes, Contreras and co-workers examined the maternal subgingival microbial flora with sampling and anaerobic culture techniques. Sixty-four percent of pre-eclamptic women had chronic periodontitis (pocket depth and clinical attachment loss ≥4 mm and bleeding on probing) (OR = 3.0, 95% CI 1.91–4.87) versus 37% of controls. Notably, a higher proportion of pre-eclamptic women were infected subgingivally with periodontal pathogens including *P. gingivalis* (OR = 1.77, 95% CI 1.12–2–8), *T. forsythia* (OR = 1.8, 95% CI 1.06–3.00), and *Eikenella corrodens* (OR = 1.8, 95% CI 1.14–2.84). This case–control report demonstrates a consistent relationship between exposure to periodontal disease or subgingival pathogens and pre-eclampsia in pregnant women.

Xiong and co-workers (2006) have recently reviewed all of the existing evidence to date that examines the influence of periodontitis on adverse pregnancy outcomes. Twenty-two studies (13 case–control and 9 cohort) focused on preterm low birthweight, low birthweight, preterm birth, birthweight by gestational age, miscarriage or pregnancy loss, and pre-eclampsia. Fifteen studies suggested an association between periodontal disease and increased risk of adverse pregnancy outcome (odds ratio ranging from 1.10 to 20.0) while seven found no evidence of an association (odds ratio ranging from 0.78 to 2.54). This report concludes that more methodologically vigorous studies are needed and those studies are currently being conducted.

Periodontitis as a risk for diabetic complications

Similar to cardiovascular disease, diabetes mellitus is a common, multifactorial disease process involving genetic, environmental, and behavioral risk factors. Affecting up to 5% of the general population and over 124 million persons worldwide (King *et al.* 1998), this chronic condition is marked by defects in glucose metabolism that produce hyperglycemia in patients. Diabetes mellitus is broadly classified under two major types (American Diabetes Association Expert Committee on the Diagnosis and Classification of Diabetes Mellitus 1997). In patients with type I diabetes, (formerly called insulin-dependent diabetes mellitus), the defect occurs at the level of the pancreatic beta cells that are destroyed. Consequently type 1 diabetics produce insufficient levels of the hormone insulin for homeostasis. In contrast, patients with type 2 diabetes (formerly called non-insulin-dependent diabetes mellitus), exhibit the defect at the level of the insulin molecule or receptor. Cells in type 2 diabetics cannot respond or are resistant to insulin stimulation.

Diabetes mellitus is usually diagnosed via laboratory fasting blood glucose levels that are greater than 7 mmol/L (126 mg/dL). Additionally, casual or non-fasting blood glucose values are elevated above 11.1 mmol/L (200 mg/dL). Thirdly, diabetic patients exhibit abnormal glucose tolerance tests (i.e. blood glucose levels greater than 8.3 mmol/L (150 mg/dL) at 2 hours following a 100 g glucose load). Elevated glycated hemoglobin levels (HbA1 and HbA1c) comprise a fourth laboratory parameter and one that provides a 30–90-day record of the patient's glycemic status. Classic signs and symptoms of diabetes include polyuria, polydipsia, polyphagia, pruritis, weakness, and fatigue. End-stage diabetes mellitus is characterized by problems with several organ systems including micro- and macrovascular disease (atherosclerosis), retinopathy, nephropathy, neuropathy, and periodontal disease.

Although environmental exposures, viral infection, autoimmunity, and insulin resistance are currently considered to play principal roles in the etiology of diabetes mellitus (Yoon 1990; Atkinson & Maclaren 1990), pathogenesis of the disease and end-organ damage relies heavily on the formation and accumulation of advanced glycation end-products (AGEs) (Brownlee 1994). Accordingly, the chronic hyperglycemia in diabetes results in the non-enzymatic and irreversible glycation of body proteins. These AGEs, in turn, bind to specific receptors for advanced glycation end-products (RAGEs) on monocytes, macrophages, and endothelial cells, and alter intracellular signaling (transduction) pathways (Esposito *et al.* 1992; Kirstein *et al.* 1992). With AGE–RAGE binding, monocytes and macrophages are stimulated to proliferate, up-regulate pro-inflammatory cytokines, and produce oxygen free radicals (Vlassara *et al.* 1988; Yan *et al.* 1994; Yui *et al.* 1994). While oxygen free radicals directly damage host tissues, pro-inflammatory cytokines like IL-1, IL-6 and TNF-α exacerbate this damage via a cascade of catabolic events and the recruitment of other immune cells (T and B lymphocytes). Patients with

diabetes exhibit elevated levels of AGEs in tissues including those of the periodontium (Brownlee 1994; Schmidt *et al.* 1996). Diabetics also present with elevated serum and gingival crevicular fluid levels of pro-inflammatory cytokines (Nishimura *et al.* 1998; Salvi *et al.* 1998). Furthermore, monocytes isolated from diabetics and stimulated with LPS secrete higher concentrations of pro-inflammatory cytokines and prostaglandins (Salvi *et al.* 1998). Chronic hyperglycemia, the accumulation of AGEs and the hyper-inflammatory response may promote vascular injury and altered wound healing via increased collagen cross-linking and friability, thickening of basement membranes, and altered tissue turnover rates (Weringer & Arquilla 1981; Lien *et al.* 1984; Salmela *et al.* 1989; Cagliero *et al.* 1991). Lastly, diabetic patients exhibit impairments in neutrophil chemotaxis, adherence, and phagocytosis (Bagdade *et al.* 1978; Manouchehr-Pour *et al.* 1981; Kjersem *et al.* 1988), and thus are at high risk for infections like periodontitis.

Numerous epidemiologic surveys demonstrate an increased prevalence of periodontitis among patients with uncontrolled or poorly controlled diabetes mellitus. For example, Cianciola *et al.* (1982) reported that 13.6% and 39% of type 1 diabetics, 13–18 and 19–32 years of age respectively, had periodontal disease. In contrast, none of the non-diabetic sibling controls and 2.5% of the non-diabetic, unrelated controls exhibited clinical evidence of periodontitis. In a classic study, Thorstensson and Hugoson (1993) examined the severity of periodontitis in patients with diabetes mellitus and compared severity of periodontitis with the duration a patient had been diagnosed with diabetes. In looking at three age cohorts, 40–49 years, 50–59 years, and 60–69 years, the 40–49 years age group diabetics had more periodontal pockets ≥6 mm and more extensive alveolar bone loss than non-diabetics. In this same age group, there were also more subjects with severe periodontal disease experience among the diabetics than among the non-diabetics. In noting that the younger age diabetics had more periodontitis than the older age diabetics, these authors reported that early onset of diabetes is a much greater risk factor for periodontal bone loss than mere disease duration.

Safkan-Seppala and Ainamo (1992) conducted a cross-sectional study of 71 type 1 diabetics diagnosed with the condition for an average of 16.5 years. Diabetics identified with poor glycemic control demonstrated significantly more clinical attachment loss and radiographic alveolar bone resorption as compared to well controlled diabetics with the same level of plaque control. Two longitudinal cohort studies monitoring type 1 diabetics for 5 and 2 years respectively documented significantly more periodontitis progression among diabetics overall and among those whose diabetes was poorly controlled (Seppala *et al.* 1993; Firatli 1997).

Investigators from the State University of New York at Buffalo have published a number of papers documenting the periodontal status of Pima Indians, a population with a high prevalence of type 2 diabetes mellitus. Shlossman *et al.* (1990) first documented the periodontal status of 3219 subjects from this unique population. Diagnosing type 2 diabetes with glucose tolerance tests, the investigators found a higher prevalence of clinical and radiographic periodontitis for diabetics versus non-diabetics independent of age. This investigative group next focused on a cross-sectional analysis of 1342 dental subjects (Emrich *et al.* 1991). A logistic regression analysis indicated that type 2 diabetics were 2.8 times more likely to exhibit clinical attachment loss and 3.4 times more likely to exhibit radiographic alveolar bone loss indicative of periodontitis relative to non-diabetic controls. In a larger study of 2273 Pima subjects, 60% of type 2 diabetics were affected with periodontitis versus 36% of non-diabetic controls (Nelson *et al.* 1990). When a cohort of 701 subjects with little or no evidence of periodontitis at baseline were followed for approximately 3 years, diabetics were 2.6 times more likely to present with incident alveolar bone resorption as compared to non-diabetics. Taylor *et al.* (1998a,b) similarly reported higher odds ratios of 4.2 and 11.4 for the risk of progressive periodontitis among diabetic Pima Indians in general and poorly controlled diabetics (i.e. with glycated hemoglobin levels >9%) respectively.

The studies cited above review the evidence that diabetes is a modifier or risk factor for periodontitis. Of tremendous importance also are the data that have emerged indicating that the presence of periodontitis or periodontal inflammation can increase the risk for diabetic complications, principally poor glycemic control. Taylor *et al.* (1996) tested this hypothesis using longitudinal data on 88 Pima subjects. Severe periodontitis at baseline as defined clinically or radiographically was significantly associated with the risk of worsening glycemic control (glycated hemoglobin >9%) by six-fold over a 2-year period. Other significant co-variates in the regression modeling included subject age, smoking, and baseline severity and duration of type 2 diabetes. Collin and co-workers (1998) studied older adults in Finland and found that people with advanced periodontitis were more likely to have higher HbAlc levels than those who had no or moderate periodontitis at follow-up.

With the emerging evidence reviewed earlier in this chapter that periodontal disease is a significant risk factor for cardiovascular disease, Saremi *et al.* (2005) conducted a longitudinal trial to examine the effect of periodontal disease on overall mortality and cardiovascular disease-related mortality in 600 subjects with type 2 diabetes. In subjects with severe periodontitis, the death rate from ischemic heart disease was 2.3 times as high as the rate in subjects with no or mild periodontitis after accounting for other known risk factors. The death rate from diabetic nephropathy was 8.5 times higher in those with severe periodontitis. When deaths from renal and

cardiac causes were analyzed together, the mortality rate from cardiorenal disease was 3.5 times higher in patients with severe periodontitis. These findings further suggest that periodontal disease is a risk for cardiovascular and renal mortality in people with diabetes (Janket *et al.* 2003; Scanniapieco *et al.* 2003a; Mealey & Rose 2005; Saremi *et al.* 2005; Mealey & Oates 2006).

Periodontitis as a risk for respiratory infections

There is emerging evidence that in certain at risk populations, periodontitis and poor oral health may be associated with several respiratory conditions. Respiratory diseases contribute considerably to morbidity and mortality in human populations. Lower respiratory infections were ranked as the third most common cause of death worldwide in 1990, and chronic obstructive pulmonary disease (COPD) was ranked sixth (Scannapieco 1999; Scannapieco *et al.* 2003).

Bacterial pneumonia is either community-acquired or hospital-acquired (nosocomial). Community-acquired pneumonia is usually caused by bacteria that reside on the oropharyngeal mucosa, such as *Streptococcus pneumoniae* and *Haemophilus influenzae*. Hospital-acquired pneumonia is often caused by bacteria within the hospital or health care environment, such as Gram-negative bacilli, *Pseudomonas aeruginosa*, and *Staphylococcus aureus* (Scannapieco 1999; Mealey & Klokkvold 2006). As many as 250 000 to 300 000 hospital-acquired respiratory infections occur in the US each year with an estimated mortality rate of about 30%. Pneumonia also contributes to a significant number of other deaths by acting as a complicating or secondary factor with other diseases or conditions.

COPD is another common severe respiratory disease characterized by chronic obstruction to airflow with excess production of sputum resulting from chronic bronchitis and/or emphysema. Chronic bronchitis is the result of irritation to the bronchial airway causing an expansion of the propagation of mucus-secreting cells within the airway epithelium. These cells secrete excessive tracheobronchial mucus sufficient to cause cough with expectoration for at least 3 months of the year over 2 consecutive years. Emphysema is the distention of the air spaces distal to the terminal bronchiole with destruction of the alveolar septa (Scannapieco 1999).

Beginning in 1992 with a report by Scannapieco's group at SUNY-Buffalo (Scannapieco *et al.* 1992), several investigators have hypothesized that oral and/or periodontal infection may increase the risk for bacterial pneumonia or COPD. It seems plausible from all the evidence reviewed in this chapter that the oral cavity may have a critical role in respiratory infections. For example, oral bacteria from the periodontal pocket can be aspirated into the lung to cause aspiration pneumonia. The teeth may also serve as a reservoir for respiratory pathogen colonization and subsequent nosocomial pneumonia. Typical respiratory pathogens have been shown to colonize the dental plaque of hospitalized intensive care and nursing home patients. Once established in the mouth, these pathogens may be aspirated into the lung to cause infection. Also, periodontal disease-associated enzymes in saliva may modify mucosal surfaces to promote adhesion and colonization by respiratory pathogens, which are then aspirated into the lungs. These same enzymes may also destroy salivary pellicles on pathogenic bacteria to hinder their clearance from the mucosal surface. Lastly, cytokines originating from periodontal tissues may alter respiratory epithelium to promote infection by respiratory pathogens (Scannapieco 1999).

Data from a longitudinal study of more than 1100 men revealed that alveolar bone loss was associated with the risk of COPD. Over a 25-year period, 23% of subjects were diagnosed with COPD. Subjects who had more severe bone loss at the baseline dental examination had a significantly increased risk of subsequently developing COPD compared with subjects with less bone loss (Hayes *et al.* 1998). Scannapieco and co-workers (1998) found that individuals with poor oral hygiene were at increased risk for chronic respiratory diseases such as bronchitis and emphysema. Scannapieco and Ho (2001) reported that patients with a history of COPD had significantly more periodontal attachment loss (1.48 ± 1.35 mm) than subjects without COPD (1.17 ± 1.09 mm). However, two recent systematic reviews of all of the current evidence indicate that at present there is not sufficient evidence to say that there is an association between periodontal disease and COPD (Scannapieco *et al.* 2003; Azarpazhooh & Leake 2006). There is emerging evidence for an association between hospital-acquired (nosocomial) bacterial pneumonia and periodontal disease. It is thought that potential respiratory pathogens, usually from the gastrointestinal tract, can colonize the oral cavity, where they are subsequently aspirated, leading to pneumonia (Mealey & Klokkevold 2006).

Effects of treatment of periodontitis on systemic diseases

This chapter has examined the evidence, gathered by many investigators since the early 1990s, which suggests that periodontitis may be a risk for certain systemic conditions such as cardiovascular disease, adverse pregnancy outcomes, diabetes mellitus, and pulmonary disease. Collectively, the findings gathered from investigators world-wide are very compelling. It would certainly appear that periodontal disease is strongly associated with systemic conditions.

Students of dentistry will next ask, "If you treat periodontitis, do you prevent the onset or reduce the severity of these systemic complications?" It is clear that dentistry must now focus on intervention studies to determine whether treating periodontitis will have a beneficial effect on systemic diseases. This is not an easy task and some studies will take considerable time before we know the answer. However, there are initial data which examine intervention and the impact of periodontal treatment on several systemic conditions and the results are promising.

Regarding cardiovascular disease, evidence in human subjects demonstrating the beneficial effects of periodontal therapy on cardiovascular disease outcomes is limited and indirect at present. D'Aiuto and co-workers (2004) demonstrated that periodontitis patients treated with scaling and root planing exhibited significant serum reductions in the cardiovascular disease biomarker, CRP, and IL-6. In particular, patients who clinically responded to periodontal therapy in terms of pocket depth reductions were four times more likely to exhibit serum decreases in CRP relative to patients with a poor clinical periodontal response. Elter and colleagues (2006) also reported decreases in these serum biomarkers plus improved endothelial functions (i.e. flow-mediated dilation of the brachial artery) for 22 periodontitis patients treated with "complete mouth disinfection" (i.e. scaling and root planing, periodontal flap surgery, and extraction of hopeless teeth within a 2-week interval). Similarly, Seinost and co-workers (2005) tested endothelial function in 30 patients with severe periodontitis versus 31 periodontally healthy control subjects. Prior to interventions, flow-mediated dilation was significantly lower in patients with periodontitis than in control subjects. Periodontitis patients with favorable clinical responses to non-surgical periodontal therapy (i.e. scaling and root planing, topical and peroral antimicrobials plus mechanical retreatment) exhibited concomitant improvements in flow-mediated dilatation of the brachial artery and serum CRP concentrations. While the effects of periodontal therapy on cardiovascular disease events in patients have yet to be determined, the available pilot data suggest that periodontal therapies can improve surrogate cardiovascular disease outcomes like serum biomarkers and endothelial dysfunction.

In considering adverse pregnancy outcomes, four published intervention studies provide early evidence that preventive and treatment interventions aimed at reducing maternal periodontal infection and inflammation may reduce the likelihood of preterm low birthweight infants, while one study did not find an effect. Mitchell-Lewis and co-workers (2000) conducted a non-randomized pilot trial involving 164 US inner-city minority pregnant women. One group received full mouth debridement (scaling with hand and/or ultrasonic instruments) plus tooth polishing and oral hygiene instructions. The second group received no periodontal intervention. No differences in clinical periodontal status were observed between preterm low birthweight cases and women with normal birth outcomes, but preterm low birthweight mothers had significantly higher levels of subgingival pathogens like *T. forsythia* and *C. rectus*. Strikingly, while 18.9% of women receiving no periodontal intervention delivered preterm low birthweight infants, only 13.5% of the treated women had preterm low birthweight infants.

A second pilot trial conducted in the US involved 366 women with periodontitis recruited between 21 and 25 weeks gestation (Jeffcoat *et al.* 2003). Subjects were stratified for risk factors (previous spontaneous PTB at <35 weeks, body mass index <19.8 or bacterial vaginosis as assessed by Gram stain) and randomized to one of three treatment groups as follows: (1) dental prophylaxis plus placebo capsule; (2) scaling and root planing plus placebo capsule; or (3) scaling and root planing plus metronidazole capsule (250 mg tid for 1 week). An additional group of 723 pregnant women meeting the same criteria for periodontitis but receiving no intervention served as the negative control. Women treated with scaling and root planing plus placebo capsules exhibited the lowest incidence rate for PTB <35 weeks (0.8%). Those treated with dental prophylaxis plus placebo capsules or scaling and root planing plus metronidazole capsules exhibited intermediate incidence rates for preterm deliveries (4.9% and 3.3% respectively). In contrast, the rate of PTB for the untreated reference group was 6.3%. This trial supported the hypothesis that mechanical periodontal therapy alone may reduce PTB in pregnant women with periodontitis.

Lopez and co-workers (2002a, 2005) have reported results from two intervention studies conducted in Chile demonstrating consistent, significant, and beneficial effects of mechanical periodontal therapy on preterm low birthweight outcomes. In the first trial, the investigators enrolled 351 pregnant women with clinical evidence of periodontitis (four or more teeth with one or more site exhibiting pocket depth ≥4 mm and clinical attachment loss ≥3 mm) and randomized them to immediate mechanical periodontal therapy (scaling and root planing) versus delayed (postpartum) treatment. The total incidence of PLBW in this cohort of periodontitis subjects was 6.26%. For women treated for periodontal disease, the incidence of PLBW was only 1.84%, while the incidence was 10.11% in untreated women. When a multivariate logistic regression analysis was performed controlling for other risk factors, delayed periodontal disease treatment was the strongest factor related to PLBW with an OR of 4.70 (95% CI 1.29–17.13). In the second trial, 870 pregnant women with gingivitis (≥25% of sites bleeding on probing but no clinical attachment loss ≥2 mm) were randomly assigned to immediate versus postpartum periodontal treatment (supra- and subgingival scaling, tooth polishing, and daily rinsing with 0.12% chlorhexidine gluconate). Those receiving immediate periodontal treatment also received maintenance therapy plus oral hygiene instructions every 2–3 weeks until delivery. Accordingly, the incidence of preterm low birthweight in the immediate treatment group was 2.14% versus 6.71% for the control group (OR = 3.26, 95% CI 1.56–6.83). After adjusting for other known risk factors, women with gingivitis receiving delayed intervention were almost three times more likely to deliver preterm as compared to women who received periodontal treatment (OR = 2.76, 95% CI 1.29–5.88). One trial did not find an effect of scaling and root planing on adverse pregnancy outcomes (Michalowicz *et al.* 2006). Overall, these clinical trials suggest that mechanical intervention in pregnant mothers with gingivitis or periodontitis can reduce the incidence of preterm low birthweight.

Clinicians and investigators working with patients who have diabetes mellitus have studied whether periodontal treatment can improve glycemic control. Several investigators have sought to answer this question using periodontal mechanical treatment as the intervention (Seppala & Ainamo 1994; Aldridge *et al.* 1995; Smith *et al.* 1996; Christgau *et al.* 1998; Stewart *et al.* 2001). Some of these studies have failed to detect an improvement in glycated hemoglobin level with scaling and root planing alone, while others have shown an improvement.

Kiran and co-workers conducted a study of patients with well controlled type 2 diabetes who had gingivitis or mild periodontitis. Prophylaxis and scaling and root planing, without systemic antibiotic therapy, was examined for the effect on periodontal disease and glycemic control. Control diabetic subjects with periodontal disease received no treatment. The treated subjects had a 50% reduction in the prevalence of gingival bleeding 3 months after treatment. In addition these subjects had a significant improvement in glycemic control, with a reduction in the mean HbA1c value of 0.8%. The control subjects who were not treated had no change in periodontal status or glycemic control (Kiran *et al.* 2005).

Grossi *et al.* (1997) reported positive findings from an intervention trial featuring 113 Pima Indians with type 2 diabetes and periodontitis who received both mechanical and antimicrobial treatment. At baseline, participants were treated with scaling and root planing plus one of five antimicrobial regimens: (1) water (placebo) rinse and peroral doxycycline (100 mg qid for 2 weeks), (2) 0.12% chlorhexidine rinse and peroral doxycycline, (3) povidone–iodine rinse and peroral doxycycline, (4) 0.12% chlorhexidine rinse and peroral placebo, or (5) povidone–iodine rinse and peroral placebo. Subjects were evaluated using clinical, microbiologic, and laboratory parameters prior to therapy and at 3 and 6 months. All treatment groups on average demonstrated clinical and microbiological improvements; however, those groups treated with adjunctive peroral tetracycline exhibited significant and greater reductions in pocket depth and subgingival detection rates for *P. gingivalis* as compared to the groups receiving peroral placebo.

Most strikingly, diabetic subjects receiving mechanical therapy plus peroral tetracycline demonstrated significant, 10% reductions in their glycated hemoglobin levels. Two small, uncontrolled cohort studies with type 1 diabetic–periodontitis patients each similarly reported improvements in glycemic control with combination mechanical–antimicrobial therapy (Williams & Mahan 1960; Miller *et al.* 1992).

At present it is still not clear what can be expected from treating or reducing periodontal disease in diabetic subjects on glycemic control. There are enough available data to at least say that the effect of periodontal disease treatment on reducing HbAlc levels in subjects with diabetes has promise. There is such great variability among patients in the studies to date that it appears that some diabetic subjects had little change in glycemic control while others had major improvement. Nonetheless, it is very clear that periodontal health is a major goal for subjects with diabetes (Mealey & Oates 2006).

Last, the evidence for the effect of periodontal intervention on bacterial pneumonia shows promise. There are a number of studies which examine the effect of treating oral infection in reducing the risk of pneumonia in high-risk populations. DeRiso and colleagues (1996) studied subjects admitted to a surgical intensive care unit. When subjects received a chlorhexidine rinse twice a day compared to control subjects receiving a placebo rinse, the incidence of pneumonia was reduced 60% in the chlorhexidine treated group compared to the control group. Fourrier and colleagues (2000) found a similar 60% reduction in pneumonia with the use of a 0.2% chlorhexidine gel.

In a landmark study, Yoneyama and co-workers (2002) examined the role of supervised toothbrushing plus providone–iodine on the incidence of pneumonia in a group of elders living in nursing homes in Japan. When these subjects had their mouths cleaned, with supervision, there was a 39% reduction in pneumonia over a 2-year period compared to the control group. Recent reviews of the evidence clearly indicate that when bacterial plaque is reduced in the mouth in at-risk subjects, the risk of pneumonia is reduced. These findings are limited at present to special-care populations. Little evidence exists that poor oral hygiene and periodontal disease increase the risk for community-acquired pneumonia (Azarpazhooh & Leake 2006; Scannapieco *et al.* 2003b).

Dentistry has come a long way since 1900 when Willoughby Miller and William Hunter proclaimed that oral disease caused most systemic disease. A century later we are developing a scientifically based understanding of how in fact periodontitis may be a risk for certain systemic diseases. As these more recent observations are confirmed and clarified, dentistry will have a new responsibility in caring for patients who may develop or who have periodontitis. It is no longer just teeth that are at risk.

References

Abnet, C.D., Qiao, Y.L., Dawsey, S.M., Dong, S.W., Taylor, P.R. & Mark, S.D. (2005). Tooth loss is associated with increased risk of total death and death from upper gastrointestinal cancer, heart disease, and stroke in a Chinese population-based cohort. *International Journal of Epidemiology* **34**, 467–474.

Aldridge, J.P., Lester, V., Watts, T.L.P., Collins, A., Viberti, G. & Wilson, R.F. (1995). Single-blind studies of the effects of improved periodontal health on metabolic control in Type I diabetes mellitus. *Journal of Clinical Periodontology* **22**, 271–275.

American Diabetes Association Expert Committee on the Diagnosis and Classification of Diabetes Mellitus (1997). Committee Report. *Diabetes Care* **20**, 1183–1197.

Atkinson, M.A. & Maclaren, J.K. (2006). What causes diabetes? *Scientific American* **164**, 95–123.

Azarpazhooh, A. & Leake, J.L. (2006). Systematic review of the association between respiratory diseases and oral health. *Journal of Periodontology* **77**, 1465–1482.

Bagdade, J.D., Stewart, M. & Waters, E. (1978). Impaired granulocyte adherence. A reversible defect in host defense in patients with poorly controlled diabetes. *Diabetes* **27**, 677–681.

Beck, J.D., Eke, P., Lin, D., Madianos, P., Cooper, D., Moss, K., Elter, J., Heiss, G. & Offenbacher, S. (2005). Associations between IgG antibody to oral organisms and carotid intima-medial thickness in community-dwelling adults. *Atherosclerosis* **183**, 342–348.

Beck, J., Elter, J., Heiss, G., Couper, D., Mauriello, S. & Offenbacher, S. (2001). Relationship of periodontal disease to carotid artery intimal-media wall thickness: the Atherosclerosis Risk in Communities (ARIC) Study. *Arteriosclerosis, Thrombosis and Vascular Biology* **21**, 1816–1822.

Beck, J.D., Offenbacher, S., Williams, R.C., Gibbs, P. & Garcia, K. (1998). Periodontitis: a risk factor for coronary heart disease? *Annals of Periodontology* **3**, 127–141.

Billings, F. (1912). Chronic focal infections and their etiologic relations to arthritis and nephritis. *Archives of Internal Medicine* **9**, 484–498.

Boggess, K.A., Beck, J.D., Murtha, A.P., Moss, K. & Offenbacher, S. (2006). Maternal periodontal disease in early pregnancy and risk for a small-for-gestational-age infant. *American Journal of Obstetrics and Gynecology* **194**, 1316–1322.

Boggess, K.A., Lieff, S., Murtha, A.P. *et al.* (2003). Maternal periodontal disease is associated with an increased risk for preeclampsia. *Obstetrics and Gynecology* **101**, 227–231.

Bosnjak, A., Relja, T., Vucicevic-Boras, V., Plasaj, H. & Plancak, D. (2006). Pre-term delivery and periodontal diseases: a case-control study from Croatia. *Journal of Clinical Periodontology* **33**, 710–716.

Brodala, N., Bellinger, D.A., Damrongsri, D., Offenbacher, S., Beck, J., Madianos, P., Sotres, D., Chang, Y.L., Koch, G. & Nichols, T.C. (2005). *Porphyromonas gingivalis* bacteremia induces coronary and aortic atherosclerosis in normocholesterolemic and hypercholesterolemic pigs. *Arteriosclerosis, Thrombosis and Vascular Biology* **25**, 1446–1451.

Brownlee, M. (1994). Glycation and diabetic complications. *Diabetes* **43**, 836–841.

Buduneli, N., Baylas, H., Buduneli, E. *et al.* (2005). Periodontal infections and pre-term low birth weight: a case-control study. *Journal of Clinical Periodontology* **32**, 174–181.

Cagliero, E., Roth, T., Roy, S. & Lorenzi, M. (1991). Characteristics and mechanisms of high-glucose-induced over expression of basement membrane components in cultured human endothelial cells. *Diabetes* **40**, 102–110.

Cecil, R.L. & Angevine, D.M. (1938). Clinical and experimental observations on focal infection with an analysis of 200 cases of rheumatoid arthritis. *Annals of Internal Medicine* **12**, 577–584.

Champagne, C.M.E., Madianos, P.N., Lieff, S., Murtha, A.P., Beck, J.D. & Offenbacher, S. (2000) Periodontal medicine; emerging concepts in pregnancy outcomes. *Journal of the International Academy of Periodontology* **2**, 9–13.

Chi, H., Messas, E., Levine, R.A., Graves, D.T. & Amar, S. (2004). Interleukin-1 receptor signaling mediates atherosclerosis associated with bacterial exposure and/or a high-fat diet in a murine apolipoprotein E heterozygote model: pharmacotherapeutic implications. *Circulation* **110**, 1678–1685.

Chiu, B. (1999). Multiple infections in carotid atherosclerotic plaques. *American Heart Journal* **138**, 534–536.

Christgau, M., Pallitzsch, K.D., Schmalz, G., Kreiner, U. & Frenzel, S. (1998). Healing response to non-surgical periodontal therapy in patients with diabetes mellitus: clinical, microbiological and immunologic results. *Journal of Clinical Periodontology* **25**, 112–124.

Cianciola, L.J., Park, B.H., Bruk, E., Mosovich, L. & Genco, R.J. (1982). Prevalence of periodontal disease in insulin-dependent diabetes mellitus (juvenile diabetes). *Journal of the American Dental Association* **104**, 653–660.

Collin, H.L., Uusitupa, M., Niskanen, L. *et al.* (1998). Periodontal findings in elderly patients with non-insulin dependent diabetes. *Journal of Periodontology* **69**, 962–966.

Collins, J.G., Smith, M.A., Arnold, R.R. & Offenbacher, S. (1994a). Effects of *E. coli* and *P. gingivalis* lipopolysaccharide on pregnancy outcome in the golden hamster. *Infection and Immunity* **62**, 4652–4655.

Collins, J.G., Windley, H.W., Arnold, R.R. & Offenbacher, S. (1994b) Effects of a *Porphyromonas gingivalis* infection on inflammatory mediator response and pregnancy outcomes in hamsters. *Infection and Immunity* **62**, 4356–4361.

Contreras, A., Herrera, J.A., Soto, J.E. *et al.* (2006). Periodontitis is associated with preeclampsia in pregnant women. *Journal of Periodontology* **77**, 182–188.

D'Aiuto, F., Ready, D. & Tonetti, M.S. (2004). Periodontal disease and C-reactive protein-associated cardiovascular risk. *Journal of Periodontal Research* **39**, 236–241.

Daly, C.G., Mitchell, D.H., Highfield, J.E., Grossberg, D.E. & Stewart, D. (2001). Bacteremia due to periodontal probing: a clinical and microbiological investigation. *Journal of Periodontology* **72**, 210–214.

Davenport, E.S., Williams, C.E., Sterne, J.A. *et al.* (2002). Maternal periodontal disease and preterm low birthweight: case-control study. *Journal of Dental Research* **81**, 313–318.

DeRiso, A.J., Ladowski, J.S., Dillon, T.A., Justice, J.W. & Peterson, A.C. (1996). Chlorhexidine gluconate 0.12% oral rinse reduces the incidence of total nosocomical respiratory infection and nonprophylactic systemic antibiotic use in patients undergoing heart surgery. *Chest* **109**, 1556–1561.

Deshpande, R.G., Khan, M.B. & Genco, C.A. (1998). Invasion of aortic and heart endothelial cells by *Porphyromonas gingivalis*. *Infection & Immunity* **66**, 5337–5343.

Desvarieux, M., Demmer, R.T., Rundek, T., Boden-Albala, B., Jacobs, D.R., Jr, Sacco, R.L. & Papapanou, P.N. (2005). Periodontal microbiota and carotid intima-media thickness: the Oral Infections and Vascular Disease Epidemiology Study (INVEST). *Circulation* **111**, 576–582.

Elter, J.R., Champagne, C.M., Offenbacher, S. & Beck, J.D. (2004). Relationship of periodontal disease and tooth loss to prevalence of coronary heart disease. *Journal of Periodontology* **75**, 782–790.

Elter, J.R., Hinderliter, A.L., Offenbacher, S., Beck, J.D., Caughey, M., Brodala, N. & Madianos, P.N. (2006). The effects of periodontal therapy on vascular endothelial function: a pilot trial. *American Heart Journal* **151**, 47.

Emrich, L.J., Shlossman, M. & Genco, R.J. (1991). Periodontal disease in non-insulin dependent diabetes mellitus. *Journal of Periodontology* **62**,123–131.

Engebretson, S.P., Lamster, I.B., Elkind, J.S., Rundek, T., Serman, N.J., Demmer, R.T., Sacco, R.L., Papapanou, P.N. & Desvarieux, M. (2005). Radiographic measures of chronic periodontitis and carotid artery plaque. *Stroke* **36**, 561–566.

Esposito, C., Gerlach, H., Brett, J., Stern, D. & Vlassara, H. (1992). Endothelial receptor-mediated binding of glucose-modified albumin is associated with increased monolayer permeability and modulation of cell surface coagulant properties. *Journal of Experimental Medicine* **170**, 1388–1407.

Farrell, S., Ide, M. & Wilson, R.F. (2006). The relationship between maternal periodontitis, adverse pregnancy outcome and miscarriage in never smokers. *Journal of Clinical Periodontology* **33**, 115–120.

Firatli, E. (1997). The relationship between clinical periodontal status and insulin-dependent diabetes mellitus. Results after 5 years. *Journal of Periodontology* **68**, 136–140.

Fourrier, F., Cau-Pottier, E., Boutigny, H., Roussel-Delvallez, M., Jourdain, M. & Chopin, C. (2000). Effects of dental plaque antiseptic decontamination in bacterial colonization and nosocomial infections in critically ill patients. *Intensive Care Medicine* **26**, 1239–1247.

Fourrier, F., Duvivier, B., Boutigny, H., Roussel-Delvallez, M. & Chopin, C. (1998). Colonization of dental plaque: a source of nosocomial infections in intensive care unit patients. *Critical Care Medicine* **26**(2), 301–308.

Galloway, C.E. (1931). Focal infection. *American Journal of Surgery* **14**, 643–645.

Genco, C.A. & Arko, R.J. (1994). Animal chamber models for study of host–parasite interactions. *Methods in Enzymology* **235**, 120–140.

Giacona, M.B., Papapanou, P.N., Lamster, I.B., Rong, L.L., D'Agati, V.D., Schmidt, A.M. & Lalla, E. (2004). *Porphyromonas gingivalis* induces uptake by human macrophages and promotes foam cell formation *in vitro*. *FEMS Microbiology Letters* **241**, 95–101.

Gibson, F.C., 3rd, Hong, C., Chou, H.H., Yumoto, H., Chen, J., Lien, E., Wong, J. & Genco, C.A. (2004). Innate immune recognition of invasive bacteria accelerates atherosclerosis in apolipoprotein E-deficient mice. *Circulation* **109**, 2801–2806.

Goepfert, A.R., Jeffcoat, M.K., Andrews, W.W. *et al.* (2004). Periodontal disease and upper genital tract inflammation in early spontaneous preterm birth. *Obstetrics and Gynecology* **104**, 777–783.

Goldenberg, R., Hauth, J.C. & Andrews, W.W. (2000). Intrauterine infection and preterm delivery. *New England Journal of Medicine* **3434**, 1500–1507.

Grossi, S.G., Skrepcinski, F.B., DeCaro, T., Robertson, D.C., Ho, A.W., Dunford, R.G. & Genco, R.J. (1997). Treatment of periodontal disease in diabetics reduces glycated hemoglobin. *Journal of Periodontology* **68**, 713–719.

Haraszthy, V.I., Zambon, J.J., Trevisan, J., Zeid, M. & Genco, R.J. (2000). Identification of periodontal pathogens in atheromatous plaques. *Journal of Periodontology* **71**, 1554–1560.

Hayes, C., Sparrow, D., Cohen, M., Vokonas, P. & Garcia, R. (1998). Periodontal disease and pulmonary function: The VA longitudinal study. *Annals of Periodontology* **3**, 257–261.

Haynes, W.G. & Stanford, C. (2003). Periodontal disease and atherosclerosis: from dental to arterial plaque. *Arteriosclerosis, Thrombosis and Vascular Biology* **23**, 1309–1311.

Herzberg, M.C. & Meyer, M.W. (1996). Effects of oral flora on platelets: possible consequences in cardiovascular disease. *Journal of Periodontology* **67**, 1138–1142.

Herzberg, M.E. & Meyer, M.W. (1998). Dental plaque, platelets and cardiovascular disease. *Annals of Periodontology* **3**, 152–160.

Hill, G.B. (1998). Preterm birth: associations with genital and possibly oral microflora. *Annals of Periodontology* 3, 222–232.

Hinode, D., Nakamura, R., Grenier, D. *et al.* (1998).Cross-reactivity of specific antibodies directed to heat shock proteins from periodontopathogenic bacteria and of human origin. *Oral Microbiology and Immunology* 13, 55–58.

Holbrook, W.P., Oskarsdottir, A. & Fridjonnson, T. *et al.* (2004). No link between low-grade periodontal disease and preterm birth: a pilot study in a healthy Caucasian population. *Acta Odontologica Scandinavica* 62, 177–179.

Hung, H.C., Joshipura, K.C., Colditz, G., Manson, J.E., Rimm, E.B., Speizer, F.E. & Willet, W.C. (2004). The association between tooth loss and coronary heart disease in men and women. *Journal of Public Health Dentistry* 64, 209–215.

Hunter, W. (1900). Oral sepsis as a cause of disease. *British Medical Journal* 1, 215–261.

Hunter, W. (1910). The role of sepsis and antisepsis in medicine. *Lancet* 1, 79–86.

Ide, M., Jagdev, D., Coward, P.Y., Crook, M., Barclay, G.R. & Wilson, R.F. (2004). The short-term effects of treatment of chronic periodontitis on circulating levels of endotoxin, C-reactive protein, tumor necrosis factor-alpha, and interleukin-6. *Journal of Periodontology* 75, 420–428.

Janket, S., Baird, A.E., Chuang, S. & Jones, J.A. (2003). Meta-analysis of periodontal disease and risk of coronary heart disease and stroke. *Oral Surgery, Oral Medicine, Oral Pathology, Oral Radiology, and Endodontics* 95, 559–563.

Jarjoura, K., Devine, P.C. & Perez-Delboy, A. *et al.* (2005). Markers of periodontal infection and preterm birth. *American Journal of Obstetrics and Gynecology* 192, 513–519.

Jeffcoat, M.K., Geurs, N., Reddy, M.S., Cliver, S.O., Goldenberg, R.L. & Hauth, J.C. (2001a). Periodontal infection and preterm birth. *Journal of the American Dental Association* 132, 875–880.

Jeffcoat, M.K., Geurs, N.C., Reddy, M.S., Cliver, S., Goldenberg, R. & Hauth, J. (2001b). Periodontal infections and preterm birth: results of a prospective study. *Journal of Dental Research* 80, 956 (abstract 1222).

Jeffcoat, M.K., Hauth, J.C., Geurs, N.C. *et al.* (2003). Periodontal disease and preterm birth: results of a pilot intervention study. *Journal of Periodontology* 74, 1214–1218.

Joshipura, K.J., Wand, H.C., Merchant, A.T. & Rimm, E.B. (2004). Periodontal disease and biomarkers related to cardiovascular disease. *Journal of Dental Research* 83, 151–155.

Khader, Y.S., Albashaireh, Z.S. & Alomari, M.A. (2004). Periodontal diseases and the risk of coronary heart and cerebrovascular diseases: a meta-analysis. *Journal of Periodontology* 75, 1046–1053.

King, H., Aubert, R.E. & Herman, W.H. (1998). Global burden of diabetes 1995–2025; prevalence, numerical estimates and projections. *Diabetes Care* 21, 1414–1431.

Kiran, M., Arpak, N., Unsal, E. *et al.* (2005). The effect of improved periodontal health on metabolic control in Type 2 diabetes mellitus. *Journal of Periodontology* 32, 266–272.

Kirstein, M., Aston, C., Hintz, R. & Vlassara, H. (1992). Receptor-specific induction of insulin-like growth factor 1 in human monocytes by advanced glycosylation end product-modified proteins. *Journal of Clinical Investigation* 90, 439–446.

Kjersem, H., Hilsted, J., Madsbad, S., Wandall, J.H., Johnsen, J.S. & Borregaard, N. (1998). Polymorphonuclear leucocyte dysfunction during short-term metabolic changes from normal to hyperglycemia in type 2 (insulin dependent) diabetic patients. *Infection* 16, 215–221.

Lalla, E., Lamster, I.B., Hofmann, M.A., Bucciarelli, L., Kerud, A.P., Tucker, S., Lu, Y., Papapanou, P.N. & Schmidt, A.M. (2003). Oral infection with a periodontal pathogen accelerates early atherosclerosis in apolipoprotein E-null mice. *Arteriosclerosis, Thrombosis and Vascular Biology* 23, 1405–1411.

Lanning, J.C., Kilbelink, D.R. & Chen, L.T. (1983). Teratogenic effects of endotoxin in the golden hamster. *Teratogenesis, Carcinogenesis & Mutagenesis* 3, 145–149.

Li, L., Messas, E., Batista, E.L., Jr., Levine, R.A. & Amar, S. (2002). *Porphyromonas gingivalis* infection accelerates the progression of atherosclerosis in a heterozygous apolipoprotein E-deficient murine model. *Circulation* 105, 861–867.

Lieff, S., Boggess, K.A., Murtha, A.P. *et al.* (2004). The oral conditions and pregnancy study: periodontal status of a cohort of pregnant women. *Journal of Periodontology* 75, 116–126.

Lien, Y.H., Stern, R., Fu, J.C.C. & Siegel, R.C. (1984). Inhibition of collagen fibril formation *in vitro* and subsequent cross-linking by glucose. *Science* 225, 1489–1491.

Lopez, N.J., Da Silva, I., Ipinza, J. & Gutierrez, J. (2005). Periodontal therapy reduces the rate of preterm low birth weight in women with pregnancy-associated gingivitis. *Journal of Periodontology* 76, 2144–2153.

Lopez, N.J., Smith, P.C. & Gutierrez, J. (2002a). Periodontal therapy may reduce the risk of preterm low birth weight in women with periodontal disease: a randomized controlled trial. *Journal of Periodontology* 73, 911–924.

Lopez, N.J., Smith, P.C. & Gutierrez, J. (2002b). Higher risk of preterm birth and low birth weight in women with periodontal disease. *Journal of Dental Research* 81, 58–63.

Madianos, P.N., Lieff, S. & Murtha, A.P. *et al.* (2001). Maternal periodontitis and prematurity. Part II: Maternal infection and fetal exposure. *Annals of Periodontology* 6, 175–182.

Manouchehr-Pour, M., Spagnuolo, P.J., Rodman, H.M. & Bissada, N.F. (1981). Impaired neutrophil chemotaxis in diabetic patients with severe periodontitis. *Journal of Dental Research* 60, 729–730.

Mattila, K., Nieminen, M., Valtonen, V., Rasi, V., Kesaniemi, Y., Syrjala, S., Jungul, P., Isoluoma, M., Hietaniemi, K., Jokinen, M. & Huttunen, J. (1989). Association between dental health and acute myocardial infarction. *British Medical Journal* 298, 779–782.

Mealey, B.L. & Klokkvold, P.R. (2006). Periodontal medicine: impact of periodontal infection on systemic health. In: Newman, M.G. *et al.* eds. *Carranza's Clinical Periodontology*. Saunders, pp. 312–329.

Mealey, B.L. & Oates, T.W. (2006). Diabetes mellitus and periodontal disease. *Journal of Periodontology* 77, 1289–1303.

Mealey, B.L. & Rose, L.F. (2005). Periodontal inflammation and diabetes mellitus. *Connections* 1, 1–8.

Meurman, J.H., Furuholm, J., Kaaja, R., Rintamaki, H. & Tikkanen, U. (2006). Oral health in women with pregnancy and delivery complications. *Clinical Oral Investigations* 10, 96–101.

Meurman, J.H., Sanz, M. & Janket, S.J. (2004). Oral health, atherosclerosis and cardiovascular disease. *Critical Reviews in Oral Biology and Medicine* 15, 403–413.

Michalowicz, B.S., Hodges, J.S. & DiAngelis, A.J. *et al.* (2006). Treatment of periodontal disease and the risk of preterm birth. *New England Journal of Medicine* 355, 1885–1894.

Miller, L.S., Manwell, M.A., Newbold, D., Redding, M.E., Rasheed, A., Blodgett, J. & Kornman, K.S. (1992). The relationship between reduction in periodontal inflammation and diabetes control: a report of 9 cases. *Journal of Clinical Periodontology* 63, 843–848.

Miller, W.D. (1891). The human mouth as a focus of infection. *Dental Cosmos* 33, 689–713.

Mitchell-Lewis, D.A., Papapanou, P.N., Engebretson, S., Grbic, J., Herrera-Abreu, M., Celenti, R., Chen, J.C. & Lamster, I.B. (2000). Periodontal intervention decreases the risk of preterm low birthweight. *Journal of Dental Research* 79, abstract 3712.

Moliterno, L.F., Monteiro, B., Figueredo, C.M. & Fischer, R.G. (2005). Association between periodontitis and low birthweight: a case-control study. *Journal of Clinical Periodontology* 32, 886–890.

Moore, S., Ide, M., Coward, P.Y. *et al.* (2004). A prospective study to investigate the relationship between periodontal disease and adverse pregnancy outcome. *British Dental Journal* **197**, 251–258.

Moore, S., Ide, M., Randhawa, M. *et al.* (2004). Relationship between maternal periodontal disease and low-birth-weight pre-term infants. *BJOG: an International Journal of Obstetrics and Gynaecology* **111**, 125–132.

Moore, S., Randhawa, M. & Ide, M. (2005). A case-control study to investigate an association between adverse pregnancy outcome and periodontal disease. *Journal of Clinical Periodontology* **32**, 1–5.

Moreu, G., Tellez, L. & Gonzalez-Jaranay, M. (2005). Relationship between maternal periodontal disease and low-birth-weight pre-term infants. *Journal of Clinical Periodontology* **32**, 622–627.

Nelson, R.G., Shlossman, M., Budding, L.M., Pettitt, D.J., Saad, M.F., Genco, R.J. & Knowler, W.C. (1990). Periodontal disease and NIDDM in Pima Indians. *Diabetes Care* **13**, 836–840.

Nishimura, F., Takahashi, K., Kurihara, M., Takashiba, S. & Murayama, Y. (1998). Periodontal disease as a complication of diabetes mellitus. *Annals of Periodontology* **3**, 20–29.

Offenbacher, S., Boggess, K.A., Murtha, A.P. *et al.* (2006). Progressive periodontal disease and risk of very preterm delivery. *Obstetrics and Gynecology* **107**, 29–36.

Offenbacher, S., Jared, H.L., O'Reilly, P.G., Wells, S.R., Salvi, G.E., Lawrence, H.P., Socransky, S.S. & Beck, J.D. (1998). Potential pathogenic mechanisms of periodontitis-associated pregnancy complication. *Annals of Periodontology* **3**, 233–250.

Offenbacher, S., Katz, V., Fertik, G., Collins, J., Boyd, D., Maynor, G., McKaig, R. & Beck, J. (1996). Periodontal infection as a possible risk factor for preterm low birthweight. *Journal of Periodontology* **67**, 1103–1113.

Offenbacher, S., Lieff, S., Boggess, K.A. *et al.* (2001). Maternal periodontitis and prematurity. Part I: obstetric outcome of prematurity and growth restriction. *Annals of Periodontology* **6**, 164–174.

Offenbacher, S., Riche, E.L., Barros, S.P. *et al.* (2005). Effects of maternal *Campylobacter rectus* infection on murine placenta, fetal and neonatal survival, and brain development. *Journal of Periodontology* **76**, 2133–2143.

Oittinen, J., Kurki, T., Kekki, M. *et al.* (2005). Periodontal disease and bacterial vaginosis increase the risk for adverse pregnancy outcome. *Infectious Diseases in Obstetrics and Gynecology* **13**, 213–216.

O'Reilly, P.G. & Claffey, W.M. (2000). A history of oral sepsis as a cause of disease. *Periodontology 2000* **23**, 13–18.

Pussinen, P.J., Alfthan, G., Rissanen, H., Reunanen, A., Asikainen, S. & Knekt, P. (2004). Antibodies to periodontal pathogens and stroke risk. *Stroke* **35**, 2020–2023.

Pussinen, P.J., Nyyssonen, K., Alfthan, G., Salonen, R., Laukkanen, J.A. & Salonen, J.T. (2005). Serum antibody levels to *Actinobacillus actinomycetemcomitans* predict the risk for coronary heart disease. *Arteriosclerosis, Thrombosis and Vascular Biology* **25**, 833–838.

Radnai, M., Gorzo, I., Nagy, E. *et al.* (2004). A possible association between preterm birth and early periodontitis. A pilot study. *Journal of Clinical Periodontology* **31**, 736–741.

Radnai, M., Gorzo, I., Urban, E. *et al.* (2006). Possible association between mother's periodontal status and preterm delivery. *Journal of Clinical Periodontology* **33**, 791–796.

Rajapakse, P.S., Nagarathne, M., Chandrasekra, K.B. & Dasanayake, A.P. (2005). Periodontal disease and prematurity among non-smoking Sri Lankan women. *Journal of Dental Research* **84**, 274–277.

Ramos, J.G., Martins-Costa, S., Edelweiss, M.I. & Costa, C.A. (1995). Placental bed lesions and infant birth weight in hypertensive pregnant women. *Brazilian Journal of Medical and Biological Research* **28**, 447–455.

Safkan-Seppala, B. & Ainamo, J. (1992). Periodontal conditions in insulin-dependent diabetes mellitus. *Journal of Clinical Periodontology* **19**, 24–29.

Salmela, P.I., Oikarinen, A., Pirtiaho, H., Knip, M., Niemi, M. & Ryhänen, L. (1989). Increased non-enzymatic glycosylation and reduced solubility of skin collagen in insulin-dependent diabetic patients. *Diabetics Research* **11**, 115–120.

Salvi, G.E., Beck, J.D. & Offenbacher, S. (1998). PGE₂, Il-1beta, and TNF-alpha responses in diabetics as modifiers of periodontal disease expression. *Annals of Periodontology* **3**, 40–50.

Saremi, A., Nelson, R.G., Tulloch-Reid, M. *et al.* (2005). Periodontal disease and mortality in Type 2 diabetes. *Diabetes Care* **28**, 27–32.

Scannapieco, F.A. (1999). Role of oral bacteria in respiratory infection. *Journal of Periodontology* **70**, 793–802.

Scannapieco, F.A., Bush, R.B. & Paju, S. (2003a). Associations between periodontal disease and risk for atherosclerosis, cardiovascular disease, and stroke. A systematic review. *Annals of Periodontology* **8**, 38–53.

Scannapieco, F.A., Bush, R.B. & Paju, S. (2003b). Associations between periodontal disease and risk for nosocomial bacterial pneumonia and chronic obstructive pulmonary disease: a systematic review. *Annals of Periodontology* **8**, 54–69.

Scannapieco, F.A., Bush, R.B. & Paju, S. (2003c). Periodontal disease as a risk for adverse pregnancy outcomes. *Annals of Periodontology* **8**, 70–78.

Scannapieco, F.A. & Ho, A.W. (2001). Potential associations between chronic respiratory disease and periodontal disease: Analysis of National Health and Nutrition Examination Survey III. *Journal of Periodontology* **72**, 50–56.

Scannapieco, F.A., Papandonatos, G.D. & Dunford, R.G. (1998). Associations between oral conditions and respiratory disease in a national sample survey populations. *Annals of Periodontology* **3**, 251–256.

Scannapieco, F.A., Stewart, E.M. & Mylotte, J.M. (1992). Colonization of dental plaque by respiratory pathogens in medical intensive care patients. *Critical Care Medicine* **20**, 740–745.

Schmidt, A.M., Weidman, E., Lalla, E., Yan, S.D., Hori, O., Cao, R., Brett, J.G. & Lamster, I.B. (1996). Advanced glycation end products (AGEs) induce oxidant stress in the gingiva: a potential mechanism underlying accelerated periodontal disease associated with diabetes. *Journal of Periodontal Research* **31**, 508–515.

Sconyers, J.R., Crawford, J.J. & Moriarty, J.D. (1973). Relationship of bacteremia to toothbrushing in patients with periodontitis. *Journal of the American Dental Association* **87**, 616–622.

Seinost, G., Wimmer, G., Skerget, M., Thaller, E., Brodmann, M., Gasser, R., Bratschko, R.O. & Pilger, E. (2005). Periodontal treatment improves endothelial dysfunction in patients with severe periodontitis. *American Heart Journal* **361**, 1149–1158.

Seppälä, B. & Ainamo, J. (1994). A site-by-site follow-up study on the effect of controlled versus poorly controlled insulin-dependent diabetes mellitus. *Journal of Clinical Periodontology* **20**, 161–165.

Seppälä, B., Seppälä, M. & Ainamo, J. (1993). A longitudinal study on insulin-dependent diabetes mellitus and periodontal disease. *Journal of Clinical Periodontology* **20**, 161–165.

Shlossman, M., Knowler, W.C., Pettit, D.J. & Genco, R.J. (1990). Type 2 diabetes mellitus and periodontal disease. *Journal of the American Dental Association* **121**, 532–536.

Silver, J.G., Martin, A.W. & McBride, B.C. (1980). Experimental transient bacteremias in human subjects with varying degrees of plaque accumulation and gingival inflammation. *Journal of Clinical Periodontology* **4**, 92–99.

Sims, T.J., Lernmark, A., Mancl, L.A. *et al.* (2002). Serum IgG to heat shock proteins and *Porphyromonas gingivalis* antigens in diabetic patients with periodontitis. *Journal of Clinical Periodontology* **29**, 551–562.

Skuldbol, T., Johansen, K.H., Dahlen, G., Stoltze, K. & Holmstrup, P. (2006). Is pre-term labor associated with periodontitis in a Danish maternity ward? *Journal of Clinical Periodontology* **33**, 177–183.

Slade, G.D., Offenbacher, S., Beck, J.D., Heiss, G. & Pankow, J.S. (2000). Acute-phase inflammatory response to periodontal disease in the US population. *Journal of Dental Research* **79**, 49–57.

Smith, G.T., Greenbaum, C.J., Johnson, B.D. & Persson, G.R. (1996). Short-term responses to periodontal therapy in insulin-dependent diabetic patients. *Journal of Periodontology* **67**, 794–802.

Sobel, J.D. (2000). Bacterial vaginosis. *Annual Review of Medicine* **51**, 349–356.

Söder, P.O., Söder, B., Nowak, J. & Jogestrad, T. (2005). Early carotid atherosclerosis in subjects with periodontal diseases. *Stroke* **36**, 1195–1200.

Stewart, J.E., Wager, K.A., Friedlander, A.H. & Zadeh, H.H. (2001). The effect of periodontal treatment on glycemic control in patients with Type 2 diabetes mellitus. *Journal of Clinical Periodontology* **28**, 306–310.

Taylor, G.W., Burt, B.A., Becker, M.P., Genco, R.J., Shlossman, M., Knowler, W.C. & Pettit, D.J. (1996). Severe periodontitis and risk for poor glycemic control in patients with non-insulin-dependent diabetes mellitus. *Journal of Periodontology* **67** (10 Suppl), 1085–1093.

Taylor, G.W., Burt, B.A., Becker, M.P., Genco, R.J., Shlossman, J., Knowler, W.E. & Pettit, D.J. (1998a). Non-insulin dependent diabetes mellitus and alveolar bone loss progression over 2 years. *Journal of Periodontology* **69**, 76–83.

Taylor, G.W., Burt, B.A., Becker, M.P., Genco, R.J. & Shlossman, M. (1998b). Glycemic control and alveolar bone loss progression in Type 2 diabetics. *Annals of Periodontology* **3**, 30–39.

Thoden van Velzen, T., Abraham-Inpijin, L. & Moore, W.R. (1984). Plaque and systemic disease: reappraisal of the focal concept. *Journal of Clinical Periodontology* **11**, 209–220.

Thorstensson, H. & Hugoson, A. (1993). Periodontal disease experience in adult long-duration insulin-dependent diabetics. *Journal of Clinical Periodontology* **20**, 352–358.

Umino, M. & Nagao, M. (1993). Systemic diseases in elderly dental patients. *International Dental Journal* **43**, 213–218.

Vettore, M.V. (2004). Periodontal disease and cardiovascular disease. *Evidence-Based Dentistry* **5**, 69.

Vlassara, H., Brownlee, M., Manogue, K.R., Dinarello, C.A. & Pasagian, A. (1988). Cachetin/TNF and IL-1 induced by glucose-modified proteins: role in normal tissue remodeling. *Science* **240**, 1546–1548.

Waite, D.E. & Bradley, R.E. (1965). Oral infections. *Journal of the American Dental Association* **71**, 587–592.

Weringer, E.J. & Arquilla, E.R. (1981). Wound healing in normal and diabetic Chinese hamsters. *Diabetologia* **21**, 394–401.

Williams, C.E., Davenport, E.S., Sterne, J.A., Sivapathasundaram, V., Fearne, J.M. & Curtis, M.A. (2000). Mechanisms of risk in preterm low birthweight infants. *Periodontology 2000* **23**, 142–150.

Williams, R. & Mahan, C. (1960). Periodontal disease and diabetes in young adults. *Journal of the American Medical Association* **172**, 776–778.

Wu, T., Trevisan, M., Genco, R., Falkner, K., Dorn, J. & Sempos, C. (2000a). An examination of the relation between periodontal health status and cardiovascular risk factors: serum total and HDL cholesterol, C-reactive protein and plasma fibrinogen. *American Journal of Epidemiology* **151**, 273–282.

Wu, T., Trevisan, M., Genco, R.J., Dorn, J.P., Falkner, K.L. & Sempos, C.T. (2000b). Periodontal disease and risk of cerebrovascular disease. The first national health and nutrition examination survey and its follow-up study. *Archives of Internal Medicine* **160**, 2749–2755.

Xiong, X., Buekens, P., Fraser, W.D., Beck, J. & Offenbacher, S. (2006). Periodontal disease and adverse pregnancy outcomes: a systematic review. *BJOG: an International Journal of Obstetrics and Gynaecology* **113**, 135–143.

Yan, S.D., Schmidt, A.M., Anderson, G.M., Zhang, J., Brett, J., Zou, Y.S., Pinsky, D. & Stern, D. (1994). Enhanced cellular oxidant stress by the interaction of advanced glycation end products with their receptors/binding proteins. *Journal of Biological Chemistry* **269**, 9889–9897.

Yeo, A., Smith, M.A., Lin, D. *et al.* (2005). Campylobacter rectus mediates growth restriction in pregnant mice. *Journal of Periodontology* **76**, 551–557.

Yoneyama, T., Yoshita, M., Ohrui, T. *et al.* (2002). Oral care reduces pneumonia in older patients in nursing homes. *Journal of the American Geriatrics Society* **50**, 430–433.

Yoon, J.W. (1990). The role of viruses and environmental factors in the induction of diabetes. *Current Topics in Microbiology and Immunology* **164**, 95–123.

Yui, S., Sasaki, T., Araki, N., Horiuchi, S. & Yamazaki, M. (1994). Introduction of macrophage growth by advanced glycation end products of the Maillard reaction. *Journal of Immunology* **152**, 1943–1949.

Chapter 22

The Periodontal Abscess

Mariano Sanz, David Herrera, and Arie J. van Winkelhoff

Introduction

Odontogenic abscesses include a broad group of acute infections that originate from the tooth and/or the periodontium. Such abscesses are associated with an array of symptoms, including a localized purulent inflammation in the periodontal tissues that causes pain and swelling. Abscesses are one of the main causes for patients to seek emergency care in the dental clinic. Depending on the origin of the infection the lesions can be classified as periapical, periodontal, and pericoronary abscesses.

Classification

Different classifications have been suggested for periodontal abscesses: chronic or acute; single or multiple; gingival or periodontal; occurring in the supporting periodontal tissues or in the gingiva. A classification has been proposed (Meng 1999) and includes *gingival abscesses* (in previously healthy sites and caused by impactation of foreign bodies), *periodontal abscesses* (either acute or chronic, in relation to a periodontal pocket), and *pericoronal abscesses* (at incompletely erupted teeth). This classification was included at the revised classification system for periodontal diseases developed at *The International Workshop for a Classification of Periodontal Diseases and Conditions* organized by the American Academy of Periodontology in 1999, and for the first time, periodontal abscesses were included as an independent entity.

The most rational classification of periodontal abscesses is, however, the one based on its aetiology. Depending on the cause of the acute infectious process, two types of abscesses may occur:

- *Periodontitis-related abscess*, when the acute infection originates from bacteria present at the subgingival biofilm in a deepened periodontal pocket

- *Non-periodontitis-related abscess*, when the acute infection originates from bacteria originating from another local source, such as a foreign body impaction or from alterations in the integrity of the root leading to bacteria colonization.

In a periodontitis patient a periodontal abscess represents a period of active tissue breakdown and is the result of an extension of the infection into the still intact periodontal tissues. This abscess formation is usually due to the marginal closure of a deep periodontal pocket and lack of proper drainage. Therefore, the existence of deep, tortuous pockets and deep concavities associated with furcation lesions favors the development of these acute conditions. Once the acute inflammatory process is started, there is a local accumulation of neutrophils, formation of pus, and tissue breakdown. The retention of pus in the pocket may further compromise the drainage and the lesion may progress rapidly.

There are different mechanisms behind the formation of a *periodontitis-related abscess*:

- *Exacerbation of a chronic lesion.* Such abscesses may develop in a deepened periodontal pocket without any obvious external influence, and may occur in: (a) an untreated periodontitis patient, or (b) as a recurrent infection during supportive periodontal therapy.
- *Post-therapy periodontal abscesses.* There are various reasons why an abscess may occur during the course of active therapy:
  ○ Post-scaling periodontal abscess (Dello Russo 1985). When these lesions occur immediately after scaling or after a routine professional prophylaxis they are usually related to the presence of small fragments of remaining calculus that obstruct the pocket entrance once the oedema in the gingiva has disappeared (Dello Russo 1985; Carranza 1990). This type of

abscess formation can also occur when small fragments of calculus have been forced into the deep, previously uninflamed portion of the periodontal tissues (Dello Russo 1985).

 ○ Post-surgery periodontal abscess. When an abscess occurs immediately following periodontal surgery, it is often the result of an incomplete removal of subgingival calculus or to the presence of foreign bodies in the periodontal tissues, such as sutures, regenerative devices, or periodontal pack (Garrett *et al.* 1997).

 ○ Post-antibiotic periodontal abscess. Treatment with systemic antibiotics without subgingival debridement in patients with advanced periodontitis may also cause abscess formation (Helovuo & Paunio 1989; Helovuo *et al.* 1993; Topoll *et al.* 1990). In such patients, the subgingival biofilm may protect the residing bacteria from the action of the antibiotic, resulting in a super-infection leading to an acute process with the ensuing inflammation and tissue destruction. Helovuo *et al.* (1993) followed patients with untreated periodontitis who were given broad-spectrum antibiotics (penicillin, erythromycin) for non-oral reasons. They showed that 42% of these patients developed marginal abscesses within 4 weeks of antibiotic therapy.

Non-periodontitis-related abscess formation may also occur in relation to a periodontal pocket, but in such cases, there is always an external local factor that explains the acute inflammatory process. Such factors may include:

- Impaction of foreign body in the gingival sulcus or periodontal pocket (Gillette & Van House 1980; Abrams & Kopczyk 1983). It may be related to oral hygiene practices (toothbrush, toothpicks, etc.) (Gillette & Van House 1980; Abrams & Kopczyk 1983), orthodontic devices, food particles, etc.
- Root morphology alterations. In this instance local anatomic factors, such as an invaginated root (Chen *et al.* 1990), a fissured root (Goose 1981), an external root resorption, root tears (Haney *et al.* 1992; Ishikawa *et al.* 1996) or iatrogenic endodontic perforations (Abrams *et al.* 1992), may be the cause of the abscess formation.

Prevalence

The prevalence of periodontal abscesses was studied in emergency dental clinics (Ahl *et al.* 1986; Galego-Feal *et al.* 1996), in general dental clinics (Lewis *et al.* 1990), in periodontitis patients before treatment (Gray *et al.* 1994), and in periodontitis patients during supportive periodontal therapy (SPT) (Kaldahl *et al.* 1996; McLeod *et al.* 1997).

Among all dental conditions in need of emergency treatment, periodontal abscesses represent between 8% and 14% (Ahl *et al.* 1986; Galego-Feal *et al.* 1996). Gray *et al.* (1994) monitored periodontal patients in a military clinic and found that periodontal abscesses had a prevalence of 27.5%. In this population, 13.5% of the patients undergoing active periodontal treatment had experienced abscess formation, while untreated patients showed a higher figure, 59.7%. McLeod *et al.* (1997) followed 114 patients in SPT and identified 42 patients (27.5%) that had suffered from acute episodes of periodontal abscess.

In a prospective longitudinal treatment study, by Kaldahl *et al.* (1996), the occurrence of periodontal abscesses during 7 years of periodontal maintenance was also studied. From the 51 patients included, 27 abscesses were detected. Twenty-three of the abscesses occurred at teeth in quadrants treated only by coronal scaling, three in areas treated by root planing, and only one in areas treated by surgical therapy. Sixteen out of 27 abscess sites had an initial probing pocket depth >6 mm, while in eight sites the probing depth was 5–6 mm.

Abscesses often occur in molar sites, representing more than 50% of all sites affected by abscess formation (Smith & Davies 1986; McLeod *et al.* 1997; Herrera *et al.* 2000a). The most likely reason for this high prevalence of abscesses in molars could be presence of pockets involving the furcation and the complex anatomy and root morphology of such teeth. However, in a recently published study in Colombian patients, the lower anterior incisors were the most frequently affected teeth (Jaramillo *et al.* 2005).

The occurrence of a periodontal abscess may be important not only due to its relatively high prevalence, but also on how these acute infections may influence the prognosis of the affected teeth. Since abscesses sometimes develop during SPT in teeth with remaining deep periodontal pockets and a reduced periodontal support, the additional periodontal destruction occurring during the acute periodontal process may be the main indication for its extraction (Chace & Low 1993; McLeod *et al.* 1997).

Pathogenesis and histopathology

The periodontal abscess lesion contains bacteria, bacterial products, inflammatory cells, tissue breakdown products, and serum. The precise pathogenesis of this lesion is still obscure. It is hypothesized that the occlusion of the periodontal pocket lumen, due to trauma or tissue tightening, will prevent drainage and result in extension of the infection from the pocket into the soft tissues of the pocket wall, resulting in the formation of the abscess. The entry of bacteria into the soft tissue pocket wall could be the event that initiates the formation of a periodontal abscess, however it is the accumulation of leukocytes and the formation of an acute inflammatory infiltrate what will be the main cause of the connective tissue

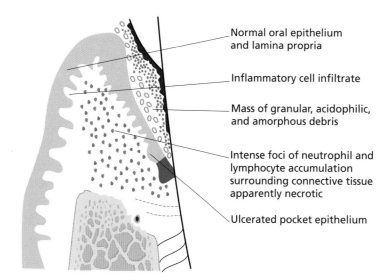

Normal oral epithelium
and lamina propria

Inflammatory cell infiltrate

Mass of granular, acidophilic,
and amorphous debris

Intense foci of neutrophil and
lymphocyte accumulation
surrounding connective tissue
apparently necrotic

Ulcerated pocket epithelium

Fig. 22-1 Schematic drawing showing the histopathology of a periodontal abscess.

destruction, encapsulation of the bacterial mass, and formation of pus. The inflammatory cells and their extracellular enzymes are, therefore, the main cause of this destruction of connective tissue. Both the lowered tissue resistance and the virulence and number of bacteria will determine the course of this acute infection.

The histopathology of this lesion demonstrates, in its first phases, the central area of the abscess filled with neutrophils, in close vicinity with remains of tissue destruction and soft tissue debris. At a later stage, a pyogenic membrane, composed of macrophages and neutrophils, is organized. The rate of tissue destruction within the lesion will depend on the growth of bacteria inside the foci and their virulence, as well as on the local pH. An acidic environment will favor the activity of lysosomal enzymes and promote tissue destruction (DeWitt *et al.* 1985).

De Witt *et al.* (1985) studied biopsies sampled from 12 abscesses. The biopsies were taken immediately apical to the centre of the abscess and processed for histologic examination. They observed that the sites examined had a normal oral epithelium and lamina propria, but an inflammatory cell infiltrate resided lateral to the pocket epithelium. There were foci of neutrophil and lymphocyte accumulations in areas characterized by massive tissue destruction and a mass of granular, acidophilic, and amorphous debris present in the pocket (Fig. 22-1). Gram-negative bacteria were seen invading both the pocket epithelium and the compromised connective tissue in seven out of nine biopsies evaluated by electron microscopy.

Microbiology

In review articles and textbooks it is usually cited that that purulent oral infections are polymicrobial, and mainly caused by endogenous bacteria (Tabaqhali 1988). However, very few studies have investigated the specific microbiota of periodontal abscesses. Newman & Sims (1979) studied nine abscesses and

found that 63.1% of the microbiota was comprised of strict anaerobes. Topoll *et al.* (1990) analysed 20 abscesses in 10 patients who had taken antibiotics prior to the study. They reported that 59.5% of the microbiota was made up of strict anaerobes. Herrera *et al.* (2000a) reported that 45.1% of the bacteria in the abscess material included anaerobes.

These studies have shown that the microbiota of periodontal abscess is not different from the microbiota of chronic periodontitis lesions. This microflora is polymicrobial and dominated by non-motile, Gram-negative, strict anaerobic, rod-shaped species. From this group, *Porphyromonas gingivalis* is probably the most virulent and relevant microorganism. The occurrence of *P. gingivalis* in periodontal abscesses ranges from 50–100% (Newman & Sims 1979; van Winkelhoff *et al.* 1985; Topoll *et al.* 1990; Hafström *et al.* 1994; Herrera *et al.* 2000a; Jaramillo *et al.* 2005). Using a polymerase chain reaction technique, Ashimoto *et al.* (1998) found *P. gingivalis* in all of the seven cases of abscesses they investigated. Other anaerobic species that are usually found include *Prevotella intermedia*, *Prevotella melaninogenica*, *Fusobacterium nucleatum*, and *Tannerella forsythia*. Spirochetes (*Treponema* species) are also found in most cases (Ashimoto *et al.* 1998). The majority of the Gram-negative anaerobic species are non-fermentative and display moderate to strong proteolytic activity. Strict anaerobic, Gram-positive bacterial species in periodontal abscesses include *Micromonas micros*, *Actinomyces* spp., and *Bifidobacterium* spp. Facultative anaerobic Gram-negative bacteria that can be isolated from periodontal abscesses include *Campylobacter* spp., *Capnocytophaga* spp., and *Aggregatibacter actinomycetemcomitans* (Hafström *et al.* 1994). The presence of Gram-negative enteric rods has also been reported (Jaramillo *et al.* 2005).

Diagnosis

The diagnosis of a periodontal abscess should be based on the overall evaluation and interpretation of

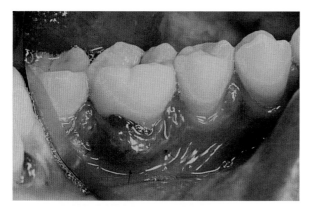

Fig. 22-2 Periodontal abscess associated with a lower right first molar. Observe the association between the abscess formation and the furcation lesion in this molar.

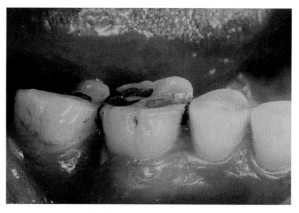

Fig. 22-4 Periodontal abscess associated with a lower right first molar. Observe the spontaneous suppuration expressed through the gingival margin.

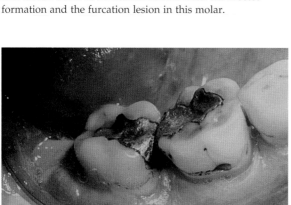

Fig. 22-3 Periodontal abscess associated with a mandibular second molar. There is diffuse swelling affecting all the buccal surface of the molar.

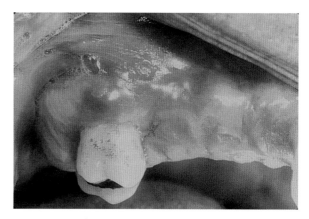

Fig. 22-5 Periodontal abscess associated with an upper right third molar. This lesion is associated with tooth extrusion and mobility.

the patient's chief complaint, together with the clinical and radiological signs found during the oral examination (Corbet 2004).

The most prominent symptom of a periodontal abscess is the presence of an ovoid elevation of the gingival tissues along the lateral side of the root (Fig. 22-2). Abscesses located deep in the periodontium may be more difficult to identify by this swelling of the soft tissue, and may present as diffuse swellings or simply as a red area (Fig. 22-3). Another common finding is suppuration, either from a fistula or, most commonly, from the pocket (Fig. 22-4). This suppuration may be spontaneous or occur after applying pressure on the outer surface of the gingiva.

The clinical symptoms usually include pain (from light discomfort to severe pain), tenderness of the gingiva, swelling, and sensitivity to percussion of the affected tooth. Other related symptoms are tooth elevation and increased tooth mobility (Fig. 22-5).

During the periodontal examination, the abscess is usually found at a site with a deep periodontal pocket. Signs associated with periodontitis such as bleeding on probing, suppuration and sometimes increased tooth mobility are also present (Smith & Davies 1986; Hafström *et al.* 1994; Herrera *et al.* 2000a). The radiographic examination may reveal either a normal appearance of the interdental bone or evident bone loss, ranging from just a widening of the periodontal ligament space to pronounced bone loss involving most of the affected root (Fig. 22-6).

In some patients the occurrence of a periodontal abscess may be associated with elevated body temperature, malaise, and regional lymphadenopathy (Smith & Davies 1986; Carranza 1990; Ibbott *et al.* 1993; Herrera *et al.* 2000a). Herrera *et al.* (2000a) reported laboratory data from blood and urine in patients immediately after the diagnosis of a periodontal abscess and reported that in 30% of the patients there was an elevated number of blood leukocytes. The absolute number of blood neutrophils and monocytes was also increased in 20–40% of the patients.

Differential diagnosis

The differential diagnosis of periodontal abscesses should always be made with other abscesses that can occur in the oral cavity. Acute infections, such as periapical abscesses, lateral periapical cysts, vertical root fractures, endo-periodontal abscesses, may have a similar appearance and symptomatology as a periodontal abscess, although with a clearly different

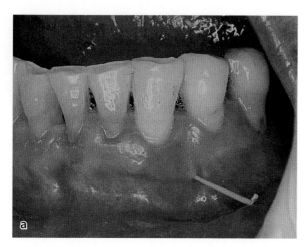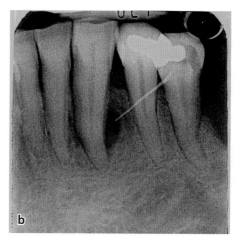

Fig. 22-6 (a) Periodontal abscess associated with a lower left canine. The fistulous tract opening is demonstrated with a gutta-percha point. (b) Radiologic image of the lower canine from (a). The differentiation from a periapical abscess was by the positive tooth vitality and absence of caries or restoration in the canine and the presence of a deep periodontal pocket in the lingual aspect of this tooth.

aetiology. Signs and symptoms indicating a more likely periodontal origin include: a history of periodontal disease or previous periodontal therapy; clinical signs of deep periodontal pockets releasing pus; frequently a vital pulp response; and radiographic findings of crestal bone loss, frequently associated with angular bone defects and furcations. On the contrary signs and symptoms indicating a more likely periapical (endodontic) origin will include: a history of caries, restorative or endodontic therapy; clinical signs of questionable or lack of response to pulp tests; presence of advanced caries lesions or restorations and the presence of a sinus tract; the radiographic findings will usually evidence the presence of a periapical radiolucency associated with either a carious or restored tooth or an endodontically treated tooth showing more or less endodontic filling or endodontic or post perforations.

Other lesions may appear in the oral cavity with a similar appearance as a periodontal abscess. Parrish *et al.* (1989) described three cases of osteomyelitis in periodontitis patients, initially diagnosed as periodontal abscesses. Different tumors may also have the appearance of a periodontal abscess. Such tumors include gingival squamous cell carcinoma (Torabinejad & Rick 1980; Kirkham *et al.* 1985), a metastatic carcinoma from pancreatic origin (Selden *et al.* 1998), a metastatic head and neck cancer (Elkhoury *et al.* 2004), and an eosinophilic granuloma diagnosed by rapid bone destruction after periodontal therapy (Girdler 1991). In cases where the abscess does not respond to conventional therapy, a biopsy and pathologic diagnosis are recommended (see also Chapter 16).

Treatment

The treatment of the periodontal abscess usually includes two stages: (1) the management of the acute lesion, and (2) the appropriate treatment of the origi-

nal and/or residual lesion, once the emergency situation has been controlled.

For the treatment of the acute lesion, different alternatives have been proposed ranging from: (1) incision and drainage, (2) scaling and root planing, (3) periodontal surgery, and (4) the use of different systemically administered antibiotics. Some authors have recommended a pure mechanical treatment with either surgical drainage through the pocket, or scaling and planing of the root surface and compression and debridement of the soft tissue wall (Ahl *et al.* 1986; Ammons 1996). This mechanical therapy may cause irreversible damage to healthy periodontal tissues adjacent to the lesion. Such damage may particularly occur when the swelling is diffuse or is associated with marked tissue tension. In order to avoid this damage to healthy periodontal tissue other authors recommend the use of systemically administered antibiotics as the only initial treatment in abscesses with marked swelling, tension, and pain. In such instances, once the acute condition has receded, mechanical debridement, including root planing, should be performed.

The clinical evidence of the efficacy of these different therapeutic approaches is scarce, since only few clinical studies have assessed the efficacy of abscess therapy. Smith and Davies (1986) studied 62 abscesses in 55 patients. Their proposed treatment included incision, drainage, and systemic metronidazole (200 mg, tid for 5 days) and after the acute phase, regular periodontal treatment. Hafström *et al.* (1994) recommended supragingival debridement, together with systemic tetracycline therapy for 2 weeks, and reported good clinical outcomes when drainage and irrigation were added to the protocol. Similar good results were obtained in a controlled parallel study in which two systemic antibiotic regimes (amoxicillin/clavulanate, 500 + 125 mg, tid for 8 days; and azithromycin, 500 mg, once per day for 3 days) were used as the only treatment during the phase of initial

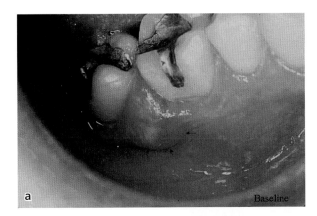 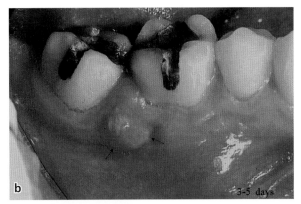

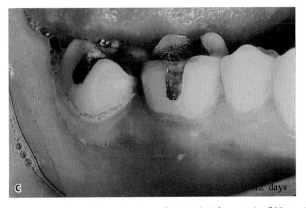

Fig. 22-7 (a) Treatment of a periodontal abscess with systemic antibiotics (azithromycin, 500 mg for 3 days) without any mechanical therapy. Baseline situation. (b) 5 days after antibiotic therapy. (c) 12 days after antibiotic therapy, just before the final periodontal instrumentation.

therapy. This was followed by regular periodontal treatment once the acute phase was resolved (Herrera *et al.* 2000b). The study showed that the short-term clinical outcome with the use of both antibiotics regimens was successful and the infectious process and abscess symptomatology was controlled just by using systemic antibiotics without concomitant or prior debridement (Fig. 22-7). There was a rapid reduction of the pain, significant resolution of the oedema, redness, and swelling, and the suppuration almost entirely disappeared. Periodontal outcome measurements, such as bleeding and periodontal probing depth, were also significantly reduced. Short-term microbiological results demonstrated a reduction of the microbiota in the abscess, as well as the number of selected periodontal pathogens (Herrera *et al.* 2000b). However, none of the antibiotic therapies were able to resolve the infection entirely. This implies that mechanical debridement, sometimes including a surgical approach, is an essential measure in the definitive treatment of this lesion. Moreover, two different studies have provided information on the antibiotic susceptibility profiles of periodontal pathogens isolated from periodontal abscesses and have reported the presence of resistant strains (Herrera *et al.* 2000b; Jaramillo *et al.* 2005).

Table 22-1 shows a number of different antibiotics that may be used in the treatment of a periodontal abscess. Doses and regimes recommended may differ between different countries. In principle, a high dose of the antibiotic delivered during a short period of time, is recommended. If the patient is recovering properly, the antibiotic should not be given for more than a 5-day period.

Complications

Tooth loss

Periodontal abscesses have been suggested as the main cause for tooth extraction during the phase of supportive periodontal therapy (SPT) (Chace & Low 1993). A tooth with a history of repeated abscess formation is considered to be a tooth with a questionable prognosis (Becker *et al.* 1984). In a retrospective study, 45% of teeth with periodontal abscesses in a SPT population were extracted (McLeod *et al.* 1997). Another retrospective study including 455 of teeth with a questionable prognosis showed that 55 (12%) were lost after a mean of 8.8 years, and that the main reason for tooth extraction was periodontal abscess formation (Chace & Low 1993). Smith and Davies (1986) evaluated 62 teeth with abscesses; 14 (22.6%) teeth were extracted as initial therapy, and 9 (14.5%) after the acute phase. Out of the 22 teeth treated and subsequently monitored, 14 had to be extracted during the following 3 years.

Table 22-1 Antimicrobial agents that may be used in the treatment of periodontal abscesses

Antimicrobial agent	Effective against	Properties
Penicillin V	Streptococci, some strict anaerobes	Poorly absorbed, affected by β-lactamases, bactericidal
Amoxicillin	Most Gram-positive oral species, many Gram-negative	Well absorbed, affected by β-lactamases but can be protected by clavulanic acid, bactericidal
Cephalexin	Anaerobes, streptococci, strict anaerobes, facultative	Well absorbed, affected by β-lactamases, not against methicillin-resistant staphylococci, bactericidal
Ceftibuten	Gram-negative rods, broad-spectrum against Gram-negative and Gram-positive bacteria	Resistant to most β-lactamases, bactericidal, not effective against staphylococci, pseudomonads
Clindamycin	Gram-positive cocci including staphylococci	Bacteriostatic or bactericidal depending on local concentration and susceptibility of the pathogen, drug of choice in case of rapid local spread
Metronidazole	Gram-positive and Gram-negative anaerobes	Well absorbed, not effective against facultative bacteria, bactericidal
Azithromycin	Most anaerobes, Gram-positive and negative bacteria, many strict anaerobes	Good tissue concentration, bacteriostatic for most pathogens

Dissemination of the infection

A number of publications, mainly case reports, have described different systemic infections in different parts of the body, in which the suspected source of infection was a periodontal abscess. Two possible sources of dissemination have been described:

• Dissemination of the bacteria inside the tissues during therapy. A case of pulmonary actinomycosis was related to the treatment of a periodontal abscess, which was ultrasonically scaled 1 month earlier (Suzuki & Delisle 1984). A case of brain abscess was observed in a healthy patient with a periodontal abscess who was treated with drainage and curettage without systemic antibiotic 2 weeks earlier. The microbiology of the lesions demonstrated, among other bacteria, *Prevotella*

melaninogenica and other *Bacteroides* sp. (Gallaguer *et al.* 1981). A retrospective study on total knee arthroplasty infections (Waldman *et al.* 1997) discovered that 9 out of 74 infections had been previously treated for an oral infection, including the drainage of a periodontal abscess.
• Bacterial dissemination through the blood stream due to bacteremia from an untreated abscess. Cellulitis in breast cancer patients have been reported following gingivitis or an abscess (Manian 1997), due to transient bacteremia and reduced host defenses (radiation therapy and axillary dissection). A periodontal abscess was associated with the development of a cervical necrotizing fasciitis (Chan & McGurk 1997). A necrotizing cavernositis was thought to be related to a severe periodontal infection, including three periodontal abscesses (Pearle & Wendel 1993).

References

Abrams, H., Cunningham, C. & Lee, S. (1992). Periodontal changes following coronal/root perforation and formocresol pulpotomy. *Journal of Endodontics* **18**, 399–402.
Abrams, H. & Kopczyk, R.A. (1983). Gingival sequela from a retained piece of dental floss. *Journal of the American Dental Association* **106**, 57–58.
Ahl, D.R., Hilgeman, J.L. & Snyder, J.D. (1986). Periodontal emergencies. *Dental Clinics of North America* **30**, 459–472.
Ammons, W.F.J. (1996). Lesions in the oral mucous membranes. Acute lesions of the periodontium. In: Wilson, T.G. & Korman, K.S., eds. *Fundamentals of Periodontics*. Singapore: Quintessence, pp. 435–440.
Ashimoto, A., Tanaka, T., Ryoke, K. & Chen, C. (1998). PCR detection of periodontal/endodontic pathogens associated with abscess formation. *Journal of Dental Research* **77**, 854.
Becker, W., Berg, L. & Becker, B.E. (1984). The long term evaluation of periodontal treatment and maintenance in 95 patients. *The International Journal of Periodontics and Restorative Dentistry* **2**, 55–70.

Carranza, F.J. (1990). *Glickman's Clinical Periodontology*, 7th edn. Philadelphia: W.B. Saunders Company.
Chace, R.J. & Low, S.B. (1993). Survival characteristics of periodontally-involved teeth: a 40-year study. *Journal of Periodontology* **64**, 701–705.
Chan, C.H. & McGurk, M. (1997). Cervical necrotising fasciitis – a rare complication of periodontal disease. *British Dental Journal* **183**, 293–296.
Chen, R.-J., Yang, J.-F. & Chao, T.-C. (1990). Invaginated tooth associated with periodontal abscess. *Oral Surgery Oral Medicine Oral Pathology* **69**, 659.
Corbet, E.F. (2004). Diagnosis of acute periodontal lesions. *Periodontology 2000* **34**, 204–216.
Dello Russo, M.M. (1985). The post-prophylaxis periodontal abscess: etiology and treatment. *The International Journal of Periodontics and Restorative Dentistry* **1**, 29–37.
DeWitt, G.V., Cobb, C.M. & Killoy, W.J. (1985). The acute periodontal abscess: microbial penetration of the tissue wall.

The International Journal of Periodontics and Restorative Dentistry **1**, 39–51.

Elkhoury, J., Cacchillo, D.A., Tatakis, D.N., Kalmar, J.R., Allen, C.M. & Sedghizadeh, P.P. (2004). Undifferentiated malignant neoplasm involving the interdental gingiva: a case report. *Journal of Periodontology* **75**, 1295–1299.

Galego-Feal, P., García-Quintans, A., Gude-Sampedro, F. & García-García, A. (1996). Tramadol en el tratamiento del dolor de origen dentario en un servicio de urgencias hospitalario. *Emergencias* **8**, 480–484.

Gallaguer, D.M., Erickson, K. & Hollin, S.A. (1981). Fatal brain abscess following periodontal therapy: a case report. *The Mount Sinai Journal of Medicine* **48**, 158–160.

Garrett, S., Polson, A.M., Stoller, N.H., Drisko, C.L., Caton, J. G., Harrold, C.Q., Bogle, G., Greenwell, H., Lowenguth, R. A., Duke, S.P. & DeRouen, T.A. (1997). Comparison of a bioabsorbable GTR barrier to a non-absorbable barrier in treating human class II furcation defects. A multi-center parallel design randomized single-blind study. *Journal of Periodontology* **68**, 667–675.

Gillette, W.B. & Van House, R.L. (1980). Ill effects of improper oral hygiene procedures. *Journal of the American Dental Association* **101**, 476–481.

Girdler, N.M. (1991). Eosinophilic granuloma presenting as a chronic lateral periodontal abscess: a lesson in diagnosis? *British Dental Journal* **170**, 250.

Goose, D.H. (1981). Cracked tooth syndrome. *British Dental Journal* **150**, 224–225.

Gray, J.L., Flanary, D.B. & Newell, D.H. (1994). The prevalence of periodontal abscess. *Journal of the Indiana Dental Association* **73**, 18–23.

Hafström, C.A., Wikström, M.B., Renvert, S.N. & Dahlén, G.G. (1994). Effect of treatment on some periodontopathogens and their antibody levels in periodontal abscesses. *Journal of Periodontology* **65**, 1022–1028.

Haney, J.M., Leknes, K.N., Lie, T., Selvig, K.A. & Wikesjö, U. (1992). Cemental tear related to rapid periodontal breakdown: a case report. *Journal of Periodontology* **63**, 220–224.

Helovuo, H., Hakkarainen, K. & Paunio, K. (1993). Changes in the prevalence of subgingival enteric rods, staphylococci and yeasts after treatment with penicillin and erythromycin. *Oral Microbiology and Immunology* **8**, 75–79.

Helovuo, H. & Paunio, K. (1989). Effects of penicillin and erythromycin on the clinical parameters of the periodontium. *Journal of Periodontology* **60**, 467–472.

Herrera, D., Roldán, S., González, I. & Sanz, M. (2000a). The periodontal abscess. I. Clinical and microbiological findings. *Journal of Clinical Periodontology* **27**, 387–394.

Herrera, D., Roldán, S., O'Connor, A. & Sanz, M. (2000b). The periodontal abscess: II. Short-term clinical and microbiological efficacy of two systemic antibiotics regimes. *Journal of Clinical Periodontology* **27**, 395–404.

Ibbott, C.G., Kovach, R.J. & Carlson-Mann, L.D. (1993). Acute periodontal abscess associated with an immediate implant site in the maintenance phase: a case report. *International Journal of Oral and Maxillofacial Implants* **8**, 699–702.

Ishikawa, I., Oda, S., Hayashi, J. & Arakawa, S. (1996). Cervical cemental tears in older patients with adult periodontitis. Case reports. *Journal of Periodontology* **67**, 15–20.

Jaramillo, A., Arce, R.M., Herrera, D., Betancourth, M., Botero, J.E. & Contreras, A. (2005). Clinical and microbiological characterization of periodontal abscesses. *Journal of Clinical Periodontology* **32**, 1213–1218.

Kaldahl, W.B., Kalwarf, K.L., Patil, K.D., Molvar, M.P. & Dyer, J.K. (1996). Long-term evaluation of periodontal therapy: I. Response to 4 therapeutic modalities. *Journal of Periodontology* **67**, 93–102.

Kirkham, D.B., Hoge, H.W. & Sadegui, E.M. (1985). Gingival squamous cell carcinoma appearing as a benign lesion: report of a case. *Journal of the American Dental Association* **111**, 767–768.

Lewis, M., Meechan, C., MacFarlane, T.W., Lamey, P.-J. & Kay, E. (1990). Presentation and antimicrobial treatment of acute orofacial infections in general dental practice. *British Journal of Oral and Maxillofacial Surgery* **28**, 359–366.

Manian, F.A. (1997). Cellulitis associated with an oral source of infection in breast cancer patients: report of two cases. *Scandinavian Journal of Infectious Diseases* **29**, 421–422.

McLeod, D.E., Lainson, P.A. & Spivey, J.D. (1997). Tooth loss due to periodontal abscess: a retrospective study. *Journal of Periodontology* **68**, 963–966.

Meng, H.X. (1999). Periodontal abscess. *Annals of Periodontology* **4**, 79–83.

Newman, M.G. & Sims, T.N. (1979). The predominant cultivable microbiota of the periodontal abscess. *Journal of Periodontology* **50**, 350–354.

Parrish, L.C., Kretzschmar, D.P. & Swan, R.H. (1989). Osteomyelitis associated with chronic periodontitis: a report of three cases. *Journal of Periodontology* **60**, 716–722.

Pearle, M.S. & Wendel, E.F. (1993). Necrotizing cavernositis secondary to periodontal abscess. *Journal of Urology* **149**, 1137–1138.

Selden, H.S., Manhoff, D.T., Hatges, N.A. & Michel, R.C. (1998). Metastatic carcinoma to the mandible that mimicked pulpal/periodontal disease. *Journal of Endodontics* **24**, 267–270.

Smith, R.G. & Davies, R.M. (1986). Acute lateral periodontal abscesses. *British Dental Journal* **161**, 176–178.

Suzuki, J.B. & Delisle, A.L. (1984). Pulmonary actinomycosis of periodontal origin. *Journal of Periodontology* **55**, 581–584.

Tabaqhali, S. (1988). Anaerobic infections in the head and neck region. *Scandinavian Journal of Infectious Diseases* **57**, 24–34.

Topoll, H.H., Lange, D.E. & Müller, R.F. (1990). Multiple periodontal abscesses after systemic antibiotic therapy. *Journal of Clinical Periodontology* **17**, 268–272.

Torabinejad, M. & Rick, G.M. (1980). Squamous cell carcinoma of the gingiva. *Journal of the American Dental Association* **100**, 870–872.

van Winkelhoff, A.J., Carlee, A. & de Graaff, J. (1985). *Bacteroides endodontalis* and other black-pigmented *Bacteroides* species in odontogenic abscesses. *Infection and Immunity* **49**, 494–497.

Waldman, B.J., Mont, M.A. & Hungerford, D.S. (1997). Total knee arthroplasty infections associated with dental procedures. *Clinical Orthopaedics and Related Research* **343**, 164–172.

Chapter 23

Lesions of Endodontic Origin

Gunnar Bergenholtz and Domenico Ricucci

Introduction

In the study of pathogenesis and causality of periodontal disease processes, lesions of endodontic origin are significant as they frequently extend and manifest themselves in the attachment apparatus. Not only do these lesions produce signs and symptoms of inflammation in apical areas of teeth, they may also induce tissue destruction along the lateral aspects of roots and in furcations of two- and multi-rooted teeth. In either instance, the lesions are maintained by noxious elements that derive from the pulpal space along openings to the periodontal tissues. Channels connecting the two tissue compartments include foramina at the apex and lateral ramifications termed accessory canals.

Microorganisms residing in necrotic areas of a more or less broken down pulp usually maintain these lesions. Lesions of endodontic origin may also appear or prevail following endodontic treatment. In these cases, treatment measures, aimed at either preventing the establishment of a root canal infection or getting rid of an already manifest infection, have been unsuccessful. As root canal infections have been assumed to have an impact on both the progression of periodontitis and the potential to achieve optimal results of periodontal therapy, the first part of this chapter describes the specific features and dynamic events that are associated with lesions of the pulp and the manner by which they may interfere with the periodontium.

The fact that the periodontium and the dental pulp are anatomically interconnected also implies that exchange of noxious agents may also occur in the opposite direction, that is from the external environment to the pulp. A prerequisite for this is that those communication pathways that are normally secured by healthy periodontal tissue have been uncovered. This will occur as periodontal disease advances. The lesion of the pulp that may follow may involve both pain and tissue destruction. Resorptive processes and treatment measures aimed at managing periodontal disease enhance this potential as the accompanying exposure of dentinal tubules, by loss of cementum, establishes yet another passage across the body of the tooth structure. In fact, a common complication to periodontitis and periodontal therapy is an ailment commonly termed root dentin hypersensitivity, a condition associated with the direct exposure of root dentin to the oral environment (Gillam & Orchardson 2006).

The second part of this chapter is concerned with the consequences for the vital pulp of root surface exposure by periodontal disease and periodontal therapy. It also covers aspects of the mechanisms and management of root dentin hypersensitivity.

Disease processes of the dental pulp

Causes

The dental pulp is normally well protected from injurious influences by an intact hard tissue encasement and by a healthy periodontium. The healthy condition of the pulp, however, is regularly challenged under clinical conditions. While some adverse influences are of minor significance and cause only negligible tissue injury and minimal discomfort to the patient, others threaten the pulp's vital functions and can result in infectious complications, with effects both locally and systemically. Lesions of the pulp may have either a direct infectious background or may be induced by non-infectious injury. Both causes will be covered here in some detail.

Of non-infectious impairments, accidental trauma causing rupture of the neurovascular supply at the apex and major internal bleeding represents a distinct threat to the vitality of the pulp. Hence, concussions, sub-luxations, and various forms of tooth displacements may result in widespread ischemia leading to complete necrosis of the tissue. As the potential for tissue regeneration is slim in the fully developed tooth (Kristerson & Andreasen 1984), such pulp tissue necrosis, although not primarily infected, acts as a target for microbial invasion. The infecting microorganisms usually originate from the oral cavity. Following their penetration of cracks in the enamel and the dentinal tubules, multiplication in the necrotic pulp results in the development of inflammatory lesions of the periodontal tissues (Bergenholtz 1974; Sundqvist 1976).

Most pulpal conditions are initiated and maintained by infectious elements that access the pulp following loss of hard tissue integrity. Tooth destruction by caries is by far the most common source of bacterial exposure and is especially threatening when the lesion has reached the vicinity of the pulp tissue proper (see further below). Also fractures of teeth and dental restorative work bring an inherent risk for detrimental bacterial effects, should a restoration fail to seal completely the defect in the tooth substance (see review by Bergenholtz 2000). Most risky are extensive restorative works like full coverage crowns, which often require substantial sacrifice of healthy tooth tissue. Clearly in the short term, before the permanent restoration is cemented, the tissue exposure is subject to bacterial leakage along the margins of the temporary restoration, especially if it is poorly adapted to the remaining tooth substance. Yet, even though the pulp may have survived the initial stress of the cutting trauma and the leakage of bacterial elements, the injury induced usually results in considerable repair phenomena (scars). Such tissue changes involve hard tissue depositions and soft tissue fibrosis, which occur at the expense of vascularity and nerve tissue support (Bender & Seltzer 1972). Tissue alterations of this nature logically result in impaired immune defense function and, thus, reduce the potential for the pulp to resist future bacterial challenges.

Clinical follow-ups of teeth supplied with single crowns or included as abutments in bridge works have indeed demonstrated that pulp tissue necrosis is not a rare complication and may affect 10–20% of the observed teeth over a 10–15-year period (Bergenholtz & Nyman 1984; Karlsson 1986; Saunders & Saunders 1998; Cheung et al. 2005). In fact, the incidence of loss of pulpal vitality has been reported to

increase over the course of time (Bergenholtz & Nyman 1984; Cheung et al. 2005). A similar increasing rate of pulpal infections has also been reported for young permanent teeth suffering traumatic ischemic injuries where pulps have been partly or completely replaced by hard tissue repair (Jacobsen & Kerekes 1977; Robertson et al. 1998).

Conclusion

Injurious elements that may put the vital functions of the pulp at risk include deep caries, accidental trauma, and dental restorative procedures. A single insult, such as a traumatic injury, may cause an immediate breakdown of the tissue by severing the neurovascular supply. In other instances tissue breakdown is preceded by a direct bacterial exposure or following tissue repair to non-infectious and infectious insults.

Progression and dynamic events

Although any injury may have serious implications for the vitality of the pulp, its ability to withstand insults, especially of a microbial nature, is far better if an intervening layer of dentin remains than if the tissue is directly exposed through the hard tissue barrier. In the former case even a thin dentin wall, although permeable, usually allows the pulp to mount an appropriate inflammatory response to offset bacterial threats. The common observation that the pulp rarely suffers breakdown underneath a caries lesion confined to dentin is strong evidence of the pulp's defense potential (Reeves & Stanley 1966; Massler 1967; Kamal et al. 1997; see also review by Björndal & Mjör 2001). The mechanisms involved relate both to innate and adaptive immune responses (Hahn et al. 2003; Dommisch et al. 2005; Durand et al. 2006; for a review see also Jontell et al. 1997) as well as to changes in dentin that constrict its permeability (for reviews see Pashley 1996; Bergenholtz 2000).

Experimental evidence to this effect derives from observations in both humans (Lundy & Stanley 1969; Warfvinge & Bergenholtz 1986) and animals (Lervik & Mjör 1977; Warfvinge & Bergenholtz 1986; Taylor et al. 1988). In some of these studies test cavities were prepared deep into dentin and were left unrestored to the oral environment (Lundy & Stanley 1969; Taylor et al. 1988). In other experimental series, similar cavities were challenged with soft carious dentin (Mjör & Tronstad 1972; Lervik & Mjör 1977) or components of dental plaque bacteria (Bergenholtz & Lindhe 1975; Warfvinge & Bergenholtz 1986). Reflecting the permeability of dentin to microbial elements, inflammatory sequels consisting of increased vascular permeability, migration of polymorphonuclear leukocytes (PMNs) (Bergenholtz & Lindhe 1975; Warfvinge & Bergenholtz 1986), and nerve fiber sproutings (Taylor et al. 1988) rapidly emerged in the pulp adjacent to the exposed dentinal tubules. The

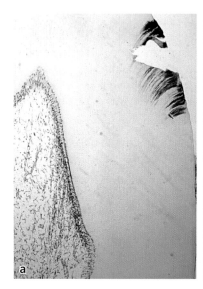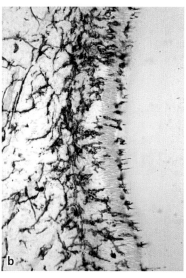

Fig. 23-1 (a) Defense response of a human dental pulp to superficial caries in dentin (defect and dark stain at upper right hand corner) as represented by increased accumulation of Class II molecule-expressing cells of a dendritic morphology. (b) Extensions of cytoplasmatic processes into the dentinal tubules are numerous. Images kindly provided by Dr. Takashi Okiji.

adapative immune defense is also activated at very early stages as indicated by an increased presence of antigen-presenting cells (Jontell *et al.* 1997). Indeed, dendritic cells appear soon in an area of the pulp next to both cavity preparations (Ohshima *et al.* 1995) and superficial caries (Kamal *et al.* 1997) (Fig. 23-1). Yet, over the course of time, these responses subside and reparative dentin and soft tissue repair emerge, along with a reduction of immunocompetent cells, at the site of the previous inflammatory event (Lundy & Stanley 1969; Lervik & Mjör 1977; Warfvinge & Bergenholtz 1986; Kamal *et al* 1997). In the experiments involving unrestored human teeth (Lundy & Stanley 1969), patients experienced pain and increased sensitivity of the exposed dentin along with the initial inflammatory episode. As repair and healing progressed the pain symptoms disappeared.

An important point is that although inflammatory responses develop rapidly and early to bacterial challenges, microorganisms *per se* are rarely able to penetrate the dentinal barrier and enter the pulp tissue, so long as it retains vital functions. Staining for bacteria in the histologic analysis of Lundy and Stanley (1969), for example, revealed that in no case, observed after 2–240 days, were organisms traced in the pulp tissue proper, while the exposed dentinal tubules were invaded to a varying extent. This finding once again demonstrates that dentin and pulp in concert are able to oppose bacterial threats.

By contrast, direct exposure of the pulp to the oral environment puts its vital functions at risk as bacteria in the oral cavity now may gain direct access to the tissue. Even a minuscule exposure is critical, unless properly treated, as there is little self-healing capacity by virtue of epithelium that can bridge the defect. Defense mechanisms may therefore prevent bacterial invasion of the pulpal space for only a limited period of time.

Three clinical cases, displayed in Figs. 23-2 to 23-4, demonstrate how pulpal inflammatory processes

may typically develop and progress to the adjoining periodontal tissues. In these cases, caries has advanced to expose the tissue at an earlier point in time.

In the first example (Fig. 23-2) an inflammatory lesion is present at the site where caries has exposed the pulpal tissue. A rather thick layer of reparative dentine has formed at the roof of the pulp chamber next to the exposure indicating a repair response to previous irritation (Fig. 23-2a). Note that, except for the lesion area, the pulp displays normal tissue morphology with intact odontoblast layers lining the periphery of the tissue. Bacteria have accumulated (blue stains in dentin) near the exposure site (Fig. 23-2c). The high magnification in Fig. 23-2d reveals numerous bacterial profiles in the pulp as well, where they are opposed by infiltrating PMNs in the lesion area. In this particular case the inflammatory process was clearly localized and both radiographic (Fig. 23-2a) and histologic examination gave no indication of interference with the periodontium.

A more advanced pulpal lesion is demonstrated in Fig. 23-3, where the inflammatory response to the distally located caries process in the lower molar has extended to the furcation area along a wide accessory canal (23-3b). Intrafurcal alveolar bone is resorbed and has been replaced by inflammatory tissue displaying proliferating epithelium (23-3c). There is also an apical radiolucency at the distal root, while the apical region of the mesial root seems unaffected (23-3a).

A third case (Fig. 23-4) shows necrosis of the coronal pulp following what has obviously been a rather long-standing caries process in a lower first molar. There are radiographic signs of apical periodontitis on both the distal and the mesial roots and a widened periodontal ligament space in the furcation (Fig. 23-4A). At the mesial aspect of the tooth, gingival tissue has proliferated into the pulp chamber (Fig. 23-4B). Figure 23-4C displays an area of the pulpal space at the entrance of the distal root canal,

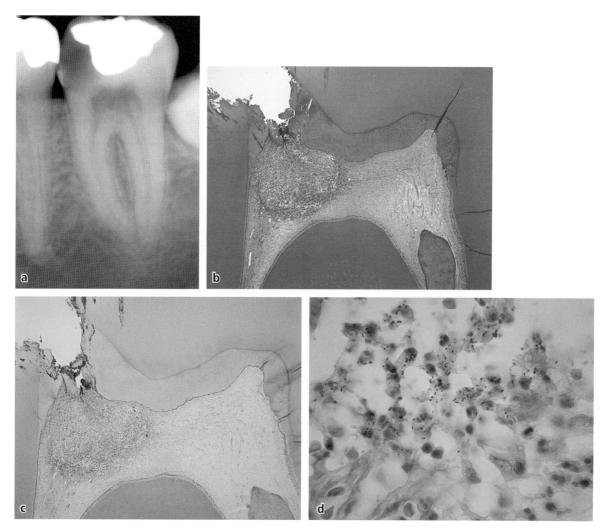

Fig. 23-2 (a) Second lower molar from a 30-year-old man with deep caries at the mesial aspect. Before extraction of the tooth the patient had presented with typical signs of pulpitis including percussion sensitivity and radiating pain. (b) A localized inflammatory response is present in the pulp adjacent to the site of caries penetration without spreading. In a section stained for bacteria (c) organisms are seen at the exposure site (blue stain) as well as in the inflammatory tissue lesion *per se* (d) (see also text).

where the pulp is necrotic and where bacterial organisms have aggregated on the canal walls in a biofilm structure. Further down in the middle portion of the root, numerous PMNs meet the bacterial front and are engaged in phagocytic activities (Fig. 23-4D and inset). In more apical portions of the canal, numerous widened blood vessels are seen along with an infiltrated pulp connective tissue (Fig. 23-4E). The most apical portion of the pulp shows normal tissue structure (Fig. 23-4G), which also applies to the soft tissue attached to the root tip (Fig. 23-4F and inset) representing the apical radiolucency at the distal root in Fig. 23-4A.

Conclusion

The cases selected demonstrate an important function of the inflammatory defense in general that also applies to the dental pulp, which is to confine infectious elements and limit spread to other body compartments. The cases also demonstrate that a pulpal lesion has its prime focus at the source of the bacterial

exposure. Hence, it is only following extension due to breakdown of the pulp and advancement of the bacterial front that periodontal tissue involvement is imminent. In some cases this may occur at a rather early stage of the pulp tissue lesion if an accessory canal is open to the marginal periodontium such as in the case in Fig. 23-3. In the absence of accessory canals extensive breakdown of the pulp is first required before the periodontal tissues may become engaged.

Accessory canals

Accessory canals are lateral ramifications off the root canal system that connect the neurovascular system of the pulp with that of the periodontal ligament. Such anastomoses are formed during the early phases of tooth development, but may become blocked or reduced in width during the completion of root formation. Patent communications of varying sizes, numbers and locations, however, may remain in the fully developed tooth and serve as additional

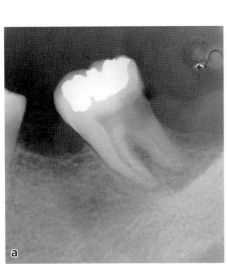

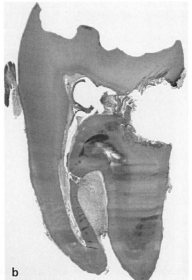

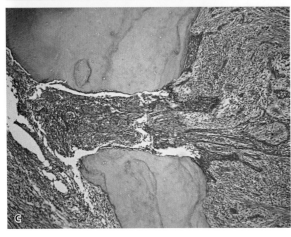

Fig. 23-3 Tooth specimen of a 48-year-old man, who presented with spontaneous pain, pain on mastication, percussion, and tooth mobility. An extensive inflammatory tissue destruction of the coronal pulp extends into the furcal area along an accessory canal. More apically, the pulp of the mesial root has retained normal tissue structures. There was no clinical swelling or remarkable pocket probing depth in this case indicating periodontal involvement (see text).

pathways for the neurovascular supply of the pulp beyond that of the main apical foramen.

Accessory canals can be observed in all groups of teeth. In fact, careful examinations of large numbers of extracted teeth, rendered transparent and injected with contrasting medium in the pulp chamber to allow three-dimensional visualizations, have revealed accessory canals in cervical and middle-root areas as well as in the apical root portions (DeDeus 1975; Vertucci 1984). Clearly the majority is found apically, whereas the prevalence tapers off in the middle and cervical root segments (DeDeus 1975; Vertucci 1984). In a study of 1140 extracted human teeth from adult subjects, De Deus (1975) reported accessory canals in 27% of the examined teeth. These canals were distributed at various levels of the root as depicted in Fig. 23-5.

Molars harbor accessory canals more frequently than premolars and anterior teeth. Patent canals are especially common in the furcation areas, where they have been found in between 20% and 60% of examined teeth (Lowman *et al.* 1973; Vertucci & Williams 1974; Gutmann 1978; Vertucci 1984). Vertucci (2005) has distinguished between different directions of entry by which accessory canals go into the furcation

of mandibular molars. In some cases they run more or less vertically from the pulpal chamber. They may also extend off either root canal in a horizontal direction of which 80% derive from the distal root canal (Vertucci 2005) (Fig. 23-6).

When accessory canals do occur, the potential dissemination of inflammatogenic elements from a diseased pulp to the periodontium is obvious. There is no documentation yet available to indicate how often such lesions develop. Although clinical observations demonstrate occurrence (Figs. 23-3, 23-7, 23-8), the rate at which endodontic lesions appear in the marginal periodontium from accessory and furcation canals seems to be low, as indicated by lack of reports of this being a significant clinical problem. It is to be expected that the wider accessory canals are, the greater is the likelihood for overt lesions to develop. Diameters of furcation canals in mandibular molars for example have been reported to vary from just a few microns to 720 microns (Vertucci 2005). Consequently, thin accessory canals, with the potential to mediate some release of infectious substances, may not cause more than a minor periodontal reaction that goes clinically undetected.

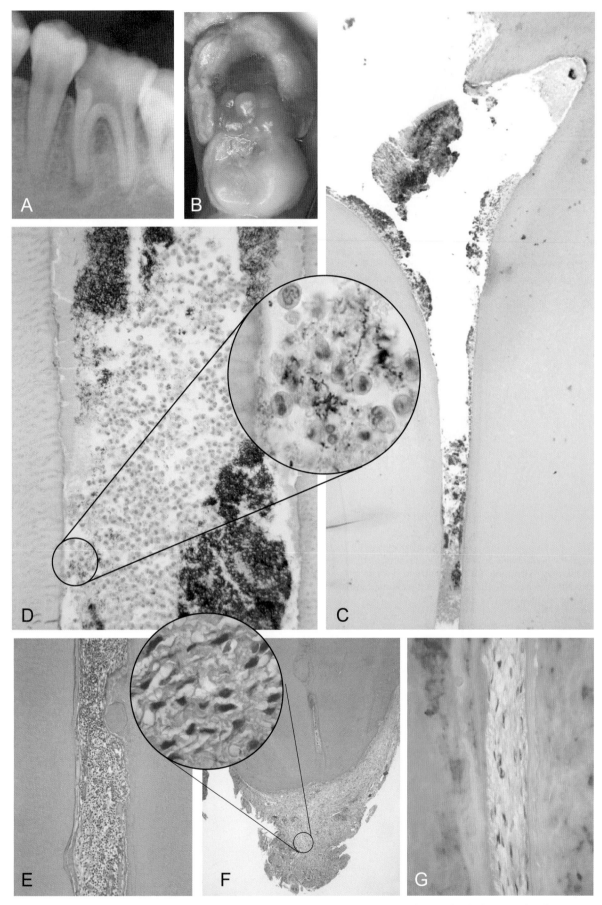

Fig. 23-4 Tooth specimen of a 19-year-old female with extensive caries in a 1st lower molar that has led to partial pulp tissue breakdown, bacterial invasion, and establishment of an inflammatory defense line inside the pulpal space (see text). From Ricucci & Bergenholtz (2004), images appeared in *Endodontic Topics* 2004, **8**, 68–67.

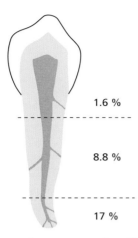

Fig. 23-5 Frequency of accessory canals at different levels of the root. The data are average values obtained from DeDeus (1975). Observations were made after teeth had been rendered transparent and the root canal system filled with India ink. The figures given for the coronal portion include those of bi- and trifurcations of two- and multi-rooted teeth.

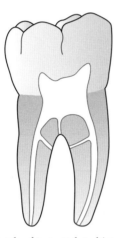

Fig. 23-6 Furcal canals of two- and multirooted teeth, when present, may extend into the periodontium from the pulpal space either in a horizontal or vertical direction or both. Drawing adapted from Vertucci (2005).

Conclusion

Although they occur, the large majority of teeth lack accessory canals in their cervical and middle root regions. This fact may explain why pulpal inflammatory lesions rarely are seen extended to the marginal periodontium. Most often they become centered around root apices only. When present with a diameter similar to that of the apical foramen, accessory canals can certainly mediate lesions of endodontic origin in the marginal periodontium. In endodontically treated teeth iatrogenic root perforations, carried out in conjunction with root canal instrumentation or post preparations, may serve as yet another pathway for dissemination of noxious elements to the periodontium (see Chapter 40).

Periodontal tissue lesions to root canal infection

The ultimate outcome of an inflammatory breakdown of the pulp is microbial take over of the pulpal space (Fig. 23-9). As host defense mechanisms are unable to reach far into root canals of necrotic pulps in order to combat the infection and pave the way for regeneration of pulpal tissue, an inflammatory defense zone is established in the periodontal tissues at exits of accessory canals and apical foramina. Hence, lesions of this nature remain as chronic processes unless subjected to treatment. Because the inflammatory process most frequently becomes positioned near root apices, the term apical periodontitis is commonly employed. As lesions may also develop along the lateral aspects of roots, the expression endodontic lesion will be used throughout this text to denote a periodontal lesion in any position that is sustained by noxious elements of endodontic origin.

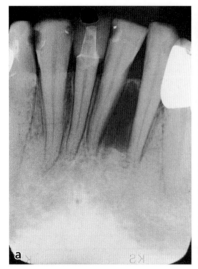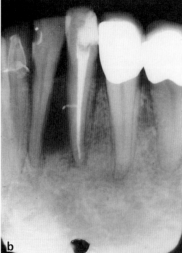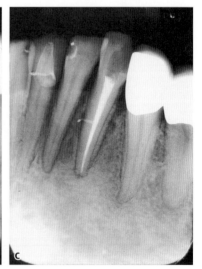

Fig. 23-7 (a) A lateral, alveolar bone destruction is observed between the roots of teeth #31 and #32. (b) The lesion in this case turned out to be associated with an accessory canal (filled in conjunction with the root filling procedure) emanating from an infected root canal in tooth #32. (c) Two-year recall of the endodontic treatment demonstrates near complete resolution of the bone lesion. Courtesy of Dr. Conrad Jacobsson.

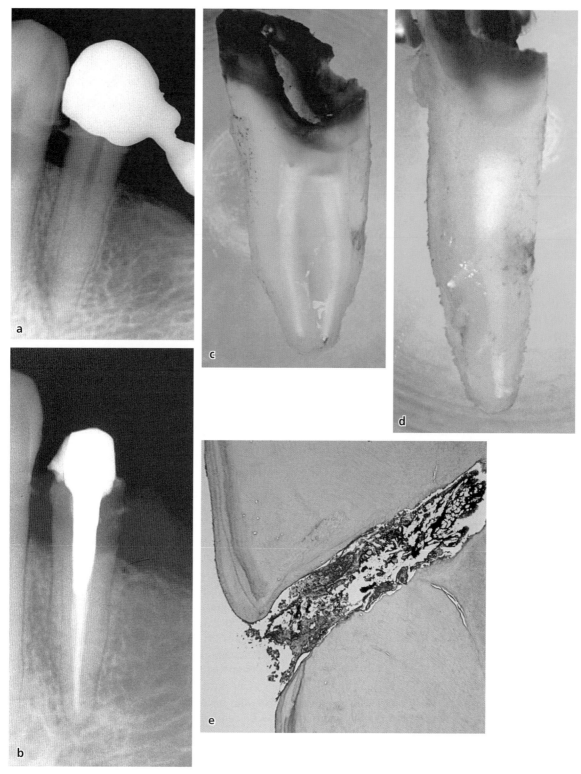

Fig. 23-8 Radiographs of a lower premolar molar; (a) prior to endodontic treatment, (b) prior to extraction due to extensive caries 11 years after endodontic treatment. (c, d) Cleared specimens show numerous accessory canals filled with root filling material. (e) Histologic examination shows that accessory canals are only partially filled (black material interspersed with inflammatory tissue).

The bacterial organisms that are able to initiate and maintain endodontic lesions have been studied in great detail over the years, primarily by sampling infected root canals followed by laboratory processing and phenotypic identification. The purpose of such studies has been to identify organisms that are prevalent and which can be linked to more or less aggressive forms of apical periodontitis (see below). In recent years molecular identification methods, including the polymerase chain reaction (PCR), have been used to supplement the picture (for reviews see Siqueira & Rocas 2005a; Spratt 2004). Indeed it has

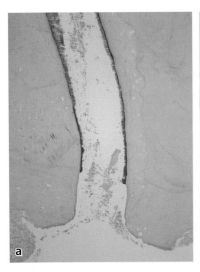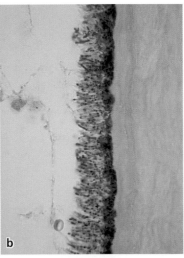

Fig. 23-9 (a) Tooth specimen with complete absence of pulp tissue. (b) Filaments and coccoid organisms are seen attached in a biofilm to the root canal walls. From Dr Ricucci's collection, images previously published by Svensäter & Bergenholtz (2004).

been demonstrated that many more species are involved than previously anticipated and the concept that only a limited group of 20–30 common isolates are associated with these lesions is currently being reassessed (Siqueria & Rocas 2005a,b; Siqueria *et al.* 2005). Yet, the microbiota in primary endodontic infections show features similar to that of deep periodontal pockets (Kerekes & Olsen 1990) and anaerobes usually have a dominant role. Spirochetes (Dahle *et al.* 1996; Rocas & Siqueria 2005; Foschi *et al.* 2005) and fungi (Waltimo *et al.* 1997; Peciuliene *et al.* 2001; Egan *et al.* 2002) may also reside in infected root canals and may contribute to the maintenance of these lesions. By contrast persistent infections subsequent to endodontic treatments seem less dominated by anaerobes and cultivation studies have demonstrated high prevalences of Gram-positive facultatives (Molander *et al.* 1998; Sundqvist *et al.* 1998; Chavez de Paz *et al.* 2003; Gomes *et al.* 2004; Forschi *et al.* 2005).

Although not comprehensively studied, root canal infections most likely involve attachment of bacterial organisms to the root canal walls and the development of microbial communities in biofilms (Fig. 23-9) (Svensäter & Bergenholtz 2004). Organization in biofilms affords these organisms better protection against host defense mechanisms in comparison to their planktonic counterparts, but they are detached from such sites and dispersed for colonization at other body sites. Root canal bacteria usually have limited potential to survive in the periodontal tissue lesion *per se* although bacterial organisms can be found in acute abscesses (Oguntebi *et al.* 1982; Williams *et al.* 1983; Lewis *et al.* 1986). It should also be mentioned that case reports have indicated that *Actinomyces*-related species occasionally may invade the tissue lesion and aggregate in clusters or nests that elude host tissue elimination (Sundqvist & Reuterving 1980; Happonen *et al.* 1986). Yet in most instances bacteria are confined to the root canal space (Nair 1987). While the front line may be established at the orifice of the canal (Fig. 23-10), the host tissue–

bacterial interface zone usually becomes localized well inside the root canal exits (Nair 1987) (Fig. 23-11). In what may be a rare situation (Siqueira & Lopes 2001), bacterial organisms in primary endodontic infections may overcome the host defense and aggregate as a biofilm on the outer root surface (Lomcali *et al.* 1996) (Fig. 23-12). Such structures have also been observed on root ends of teeth which have not responded favorably to endodontic treatment (Tronstad *et al.* 1990).

The shape and character of the periodontal tissue response to a root canal infection may vary. Often lesions assume a limited and stable extension around root apices and/or at orifices of accessory canals. The inflammatory process may then remain unchanged in size for years, although cyst transformation can result in substantial destruction of alveolar bone (Fig. 23-13). However, the initial expansion of an emerging lesion or acute exacerbation of a chronic lesion, can result in rapid and extensive destruction of the attachment apparatus. In certain cases the periodontal tissue support can be lost to an extent that the gingival sulcus is involved, from where drainage of pus occurs to the oral environment (Fig. 23-14). Such an apical marginal communication along the root surface may later become a permanent pathway for pus that will be released periodically along what is simply a fistulous tract.

The character of the infecting microbiota, its metabolic activity, and the virulence factors it produces, together with the capacity of the host defense to confine and neutralize the bacterial elements, are important parameters that decide the course of the inflammatory process. Hence, growing and multiplying organisms with capacities to invade the periodontal tissues and evade host defense mechanisms mediate acute manifestations of endodontic lesions. Single organisms are normally unable to cause these lesions, which are maintained by groups of organisms; virulent strains of *Porphyromonas*, *Prevotella*, *Fusobacterium* and *Peptostreptococcus* spp. have been implicated by culture studies (Dahlén 2002). Recent

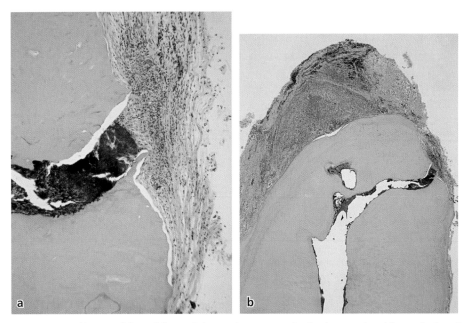

Fig. 23-10 (a) Demonstration of bacterial front (blue stain) near the root canal exit of a root tip with attached periapical tissue lesion (low magnification in (b)). From Ricucci & Bergenholtz (2004).

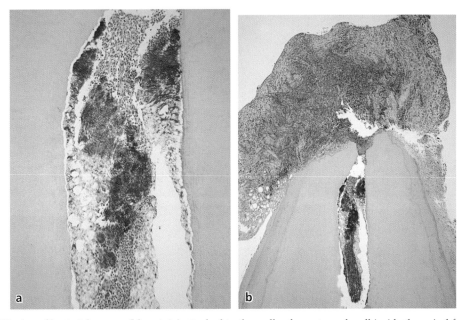

Fig. 23-11 (a) Display of bacterial masses (blue stain) attached to the walls of a root canal well inside the apical foramen. A band of inflammatory cells appear to be in combat with the infection. (b) A low magnification overview of the root with attached periapical tissue lesion. From Ricucci & Bergenholtz (2004).

reports utilizing PCR methodology have inferred that a variety of other species, unrecognized by culture, may be of prime importance (Rocas & Siqueria 2005; Sakamoto *et al.* 2006). Given the recent surge in use of molecular methods to map the structure of the endodontic microbiota, it is likely that, in the future, a clearer understanding will be gained of the key organisms which cause acute manifestations of endodontic infections.

The endodontic microbiota associated with asymptomatic lesions is apparently less aggressive. This condition is likely to be linked to the harsh nutri-

tional supply that usually prevails in root canals and which puts the organisms in a low state of metabolic activity. Nutrients are available primarily from tissue components of the necrotic pulp. In the absence of inflammatory exudate entering the root canal along apical foramina and accessory canals, organisms will consequently have little drive to grow, multiply, and invade the periodontal tissue compartment. When this condition of relative starvation is broken by increase of the nutritional supply, an acute endodontic lesion may occur. Suppressed virulent strains can then be revived and become the dominant organisms

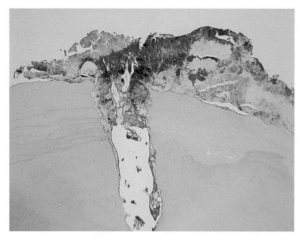

Fig. 23-12 Accumulation of bacterial mass (blue stain) at the external root surface of a tooth with an infected necrotic pulp. From Ricucci & Bergenholtz (2004).

at the expense of the less virulent members of the microbial community. Consequently, acute exacerbations of asymptomatic endodontic lesions may occur, for example, when saliva and gingival exudates gain access to the root canal space following a direct exposure of root canals to the oral environment. Similarly during endodontic treatment, inadvertent enlargement of the apical foramen increases the passageway for protein-rich inflammatory exudate into the root canal space.

While acute manifestations of endodontic lesions are characterized by expanding bone resorption, exudation and influx of phagocytic cells, a balanced host–parasite relationship will be established sooner or later (Stashenko 1990; Nair 1997; Stashenko et al. 1998). Microscopically, the established lesion is characterized by a richly vascularized granulation tissue, which is infiltrated, to a varying degree, by inflammatory cells (Fig. 23-15). PMNs play a most

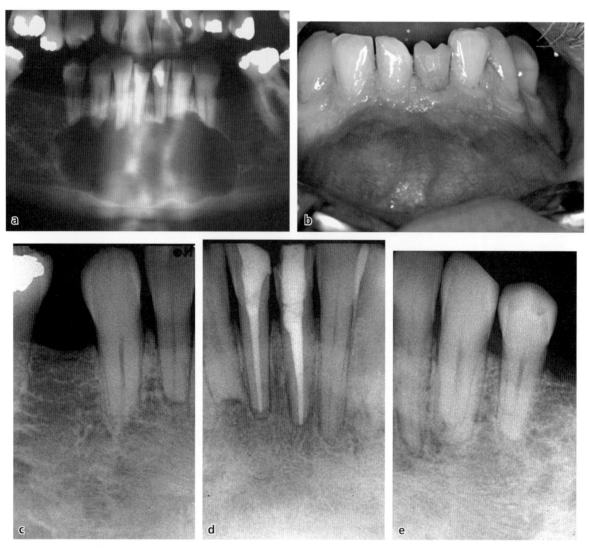

Fig. 23-13 Extensive destruction of alveolar bone as a result of cyst transformation of a periapical lesion emanating from tooth #31. (a) Note root resorption of neighboring teeth. (b) Buccal protrusion of the process was non-painful to palpation. All teeth responded vital to pulp testing except for the root filled teeth #31 and #41. The latter tooth, however, had a vital pulp as revealed on accessing the root canal. Treatment, carried out in collaboration with Dr. Ulf Lekholm, included placement of an oburator for drainage, decompression, and saline irrigation of the cyst cavity over 6 months. Following its reduction, teeth #31 and #41 received completion of endodontic treatment and a residue of the process was excised surgically. (c–e) Complete resolution of the process 10 months post surgery.

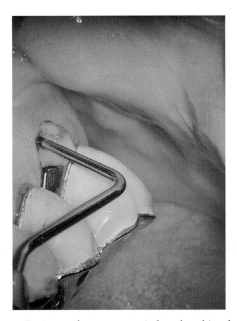

Fig. 23-14 Drainage of pus upon periodontal probing from a lesion of endodontic origin associated with an upper molar.

important role in confining the infection to the pulpal space (Stashenko *et al.* 1995) and constitute an important cellular front line (Fig. 23-11). The remainder of the lesion will be composed of a mixed cellular response (Fig. 23-15c) typical of a longstanding infectious process where various immunocompetent cells (*viz.* dendritic cells, macrophages, T and B cells) are prevalent (Torabinejad & Kettering 1985; Babal *et al.* 1987; Okiji *et al.* 1994; Stashenko *et al.* 1998; Marton & Kiss 2000). With increasing distances from the root canal apertures, the established lesion harbors a decreasing number of inflammatory cells and an increasing amount of fibrovascular elements representing attempts at repair. More peripherally there is a much stronger expression of fibroblastic activity and formation of new vessels. In the most peripheral portions of the lesion, a collagen-rich connective tissue normally separates it from the surrounding bone tissue (Bergenholtz *et al.* 1983) (Fig. 23-15a,d).

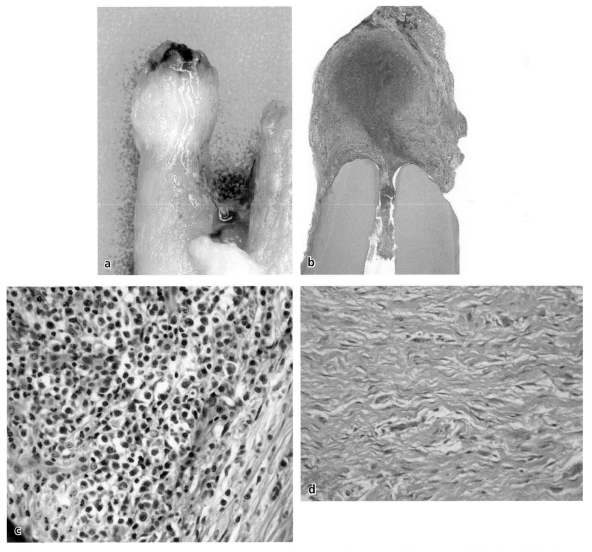

Fig. 23-15 Series of images demonstrating features of apical inflammatory lesions caused by root canal infection. (a) A soft lesion attached to the tip of the palatal root of an extracted upper molar. (b) The longitudinally cut tissue section through the root tip shows an overview of the lesion. The outer collagen-rich connective tissue confines the soft tissue lesion and attaches it to the root surface. (c) A typical mixed inflammatory cell infiltrate at the center of a lesion. (d) In the most peripheral portion the connective of an established lesion is rich in collagen and devoid of inflammatory cells. Microphotograph in (c) is from an apical lesion in a monkey.

In non-symptomatic endodontic lesions, the relative distribution of cellular and tissue elements may show great variation and some, but far from every lesion, may also contain proliferating epithelial cells (Nair 1997). The origin of epithelial strands is thought to be the epithelial rests of Malassez (Ten Cate 1972) that are stimulated to divide and proliferate by the release of pro-inflammatory cytokines and growth factors during the process of inflammation (Thesleff 1987; Lin *et al.* 1996; Suzuki *et al.* 2002). In the lesion, they appear to take a random course, but sometimes they may also attach to the root surface (Fig. 23-16) and eventually block the root canal exit for bacterial advancement into the periapical tissue compartment (Nair & Schroeder 1985). Their contribution to periodontal pocket formation upon an endodontic lesion, developing in close proximity to the epithelial sulcus of the marginal periodontium, remains obscure.

Conclusion

Inflammatory processes of the periodontium associated with necrotic dental pulps have an infectious etiology similar to periodontal disease. An essential difference between the two disease entities is their different source of infection. While periodontal disease is maintained by bacterial accumulations in the dentogingival region, endodontic lesions are directed towards infectious elements released from the pulpal space. The bacterial organisms in endodontic infections are usually confined to the root canal space. They may also be found in the soft tissue lesion *per se* either as clusters or as bacterial aggregations on the external root surface. Endodontic lesions rarely involve the marginal periodontium, unless abscessed. Cyst transformation may occur but even then marginal involvement is not common. In its established form, the endodontic lesion is clearly localized and constitutes an immunologically active protection zone which is important in preventing the dissemination of endodontic pathogens to the surrounding tissues (Stashenko 1990).

Effects of periodontal disease and periodontal therapy on the condition of the pulp

Influences of periodontal disease

The formation of bacterial plaque on detached root surfaces following periodontal disease has the potential to induce inflammation in the pulp along the very same pathways as an endodontic infection can affect the periodontium in the opposite direction. Thus, bacterial products and substances released by the inflammatory process in the periodontium may gain access to the pulp via exposed accessory canals and apical foramina, as well as dentinal tubules.

A clear association between progressive periodontal disease and pulpal involvement, however, does not exist. While inflammatory alterations as well as localized inflammatory cell infiltrates and necrosis of pulp tissue have been observed adjacent to accessory canals in teeth exposed by periodontal disease (Seltzer *et al.* 1963; Rubach & Mitchell 1965), a number of clinical studies has failed to confirm a direct relationship between progression of periodontitis and pulp tissue changes (Mazur & Massler 1964; Czarnecki & Schilder 1979; Torabinejad & Kiger 1985). In the cases in these studies, the pulp was observed to remain fully functional without overt inflammatory changes even though the periodontal tissue breakdown was severe. As already pointed out, an important reason for the lack of pulp tissue involvement, is that patent accessory canals are not invariably present and especially not in the cervical root portions. Another is that cementum obviously exerts protection. It is only when the cementum layer has been damaged, by, for example, instrumentation in periodontal therapy, wear from tooth cleaning, external root resorption, and root surface caries, that dentinal tubules can serve as pathways for microbial elements to the pulp (Figs. 23-17 to 23-19).

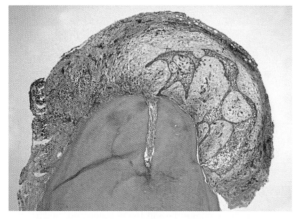

Fig. 23-16 Display of a periapical inflammatory process with proliferating epithelium partially attached to the root surface.

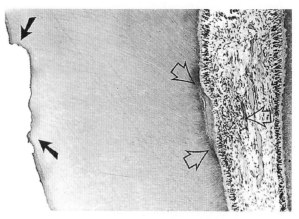

Fig. 23-17 Histologic section of a monkey tooth exposed to experimental periodontal tissue breakdown. Beneath resorptive defects in the external root surface a minor inflammatory cell infiltrate and a small rim of reparative dentin have been formed in the pulp. From Bergenholtz & Lindhe (1978).

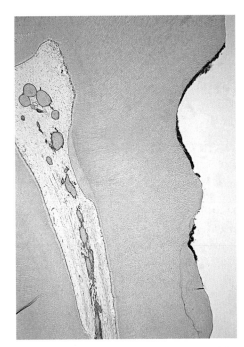

Fig. 23-18 Histologic section of a human tooth with bacterial accumulations on the external root surface. There are obvious defects in the root surface. Pulp tissue is minimally affected, however, except for numerous mineralization processes both in the tissue proper and at the inner root canal wall.

The fact that tissue changes develop infrequently and even so only locally in the pulp of teeth subjected to periodontitis was underscored by an experimental study in monkeys (Bergenholtz & Lindhe 1978). Following a ligature-induced breakdown of the attachment apparatus, it was found that the majority of the root specimens examined (70%) exhibited no inflammatory changes, despite the fact that approximately 30–40% of the periodontal attachment was lost. The remaining roots (30%) displayed only small inflammatory cell infiltrates and/or formations of reparative dentin in the pulp subjacent to root areas exposed by the periodontal tissue destruction. These tissue changes were associated with root surface resorption (Fig. 23-17), supporting the view that dentinal tubules have to be uncovered before external irritants can be transmitted to the pulp. Consequently, the lack of correlation found in clinical observations between periodontal disease and pulp tissue alterations, may simply depend on the fact that few open pathways exist to the pulp in many periodontally involved teeth. Furthermore, as described above, once the dentin/pulp complex has been exposed to bacterial elements, repair and healing will often be instituted

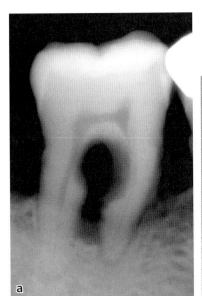

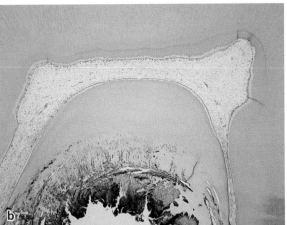

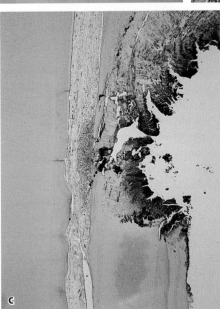

Fig. 23-19 (a) Tooth with extensive caries in the furcation region of a lower molar. (b) Note the overall normal tissue morphology of the pulp except for an area at the mid-root portion of the distal root, where caries process has reached the pulp (c).

soon after the initial inflammatory events, leaving the remaining tissue unaffected.

In the study by Bergenholtz and Lindhe (1978), destructive periodontal disease was produced experimentally during a comparatively short period (5–7 months), while in humans a similar degree of destruction of periodontal tissue normally requires several years. It has been reported that the pulp of teeth with longstanding periodontal disease develops fibrosis and various forms of intra-pulpal mineralizations (Bender & Seltzer 1972; Lantelme *et al.* 1976) (Fig. 23-18). If there is an association, it seems reasonable to assume that tissue changes of this nature represent the accumulated response of the pulp to the relatively weak, but repeatedly occurring, insults to the tissue over time, for example by microbial elements reaching the pulp over root surface exposures. Nonetheless the pulp can obviously remain healthy for as long as periodontal disease has not arrived at a terminal stage, when plaque accumulation and associated inflammatory lesions interfere with the neurovascular supply of the tissue through the main apical foramen (Fig. 23-20).

Conclusion

Available documentation suggests that the vital functions of the pulp are rarely threatened by periodontal disease influences. In teeth with moderate breakdown of the attachment apparatus, the pulp usually remains healthy. Breakdown of the pulp presumably does not occur until the periodontal disease process has reached a terminal stage, i.e. when plaque and the periodontal inflammatory process have progressed to the main apical foramina, whereby a retrograde destructive inflammatory pulpal lesion is initiated (Langeland *et al.* 1974) (Fig. 23-20). Consequently, as long as the blood supply through the apical foramen remains intact, the pulp is usually capable of withstanding injurious elements released by the lesion in the periodontium.

Influence of periodontal treatment measures on the pulp

Pocket/root debridement in periodontal therapy by hand instrumentation (scaling and root planing, S/RP) or ultrasonics is indispensable in the treatment of periodontal disease. However, this treatment is associated with a number of undesired side effects. Except for recession of gingival tissues resulting in exposures of root surfaces, the instrumentation *per se* may also inadvertently remove root cementum and the superficial parts of dentin. Thereby a large number of dentinal tubules will become exposed to the oral environment as treated root surfaces are normally left unprotected. Subsequent contact with microbial elements in the oral cavity is potentially harmful to the pulp as bacterial invasion of the exposed dentinal tubules may occur (Adriaens *et al.* 1988). While

localized inflammatory lesions may be initiated in the pulp, the experimental study by Bergenholtz and Lindhe (1978) did not observe increased incidence of pulpal lesions in teeth subjected to S/RP in comparison to non-treated teeth subjected to periodontal tissue breakdown alone. In the study, root surfaces denuded of root cementum were left open to the oral environment for up to 30 days. The finding that plaque accumulation on root dentin exposed by one session of S/RP does not seriously threaten the vitality of the pulp has been confirmed in similarly designed experimental studies (Nilvéus & Selvig 1983; Hattler & Listgarten 1984). Yet, root dentin hypersensitivity may follow such treatment measures, causing an uncomfortable problem which is difficult to manage (see below).

During the maintenance phase of periodontal therapy, there are reasons to restrict repeated instrumentations, as some additional dentin always will be removed. Such therapy can result in weakening of the tooth structure and also in extensive reparative dentin formation in the pulp (Fig. 23-21).

Conclusion

Results of clinical observations and animal experiments support the view that pocket/root debridement procedures normally do not threaten the vitality of the pulp. Localized inflammatory alterations may occur adjacent to instrumented root surfaces followed by tissue repair in the form of hard tissue depositions on the root canal walls.

Root dentin hypersensitivity

Symptoms and incidence

Patients who have received pocket/root debridement in periodontal therapy may frequently experience sensitivity of the treated teeth to evaporative, tactile, thermal, and osmotic stimuli (Fischer *et al.* 1991; Kontturi-Närhi 1993; Chabanski *et al.* 1996; Tammaro *et al.* 2000; for review see Gillam & Orchardson 2006). Usually, the symptoms, when they occur, develop and peak during the first week, and then subside or disappear within the subsequent weeks; they are, although uncomfortable, most often a temporary and sustainable problem (Schuurs *et al.* 1995; Chabanski *et al* 1996; Gillam *et al.* 1999; Fardal *et al.* 2002). Occasionally, the condition may become a chronic pain problem and may persist for months or years. Patients appear to be especially at risk after periodontal surgery. In a comprehensive questionnaire survey, severe painful symptoms were reported to prevail in 26% of the subjects 6 months to 5 years after the completion of treatment, while 16%, treated non-surgically, reported pain symptoms (Kontturi-Närhi 1993). In a clinical trial comprising 35 patients, Tammaro *et al.* (2000) observed that the incidence of sensitive teeth increased following non-surgical

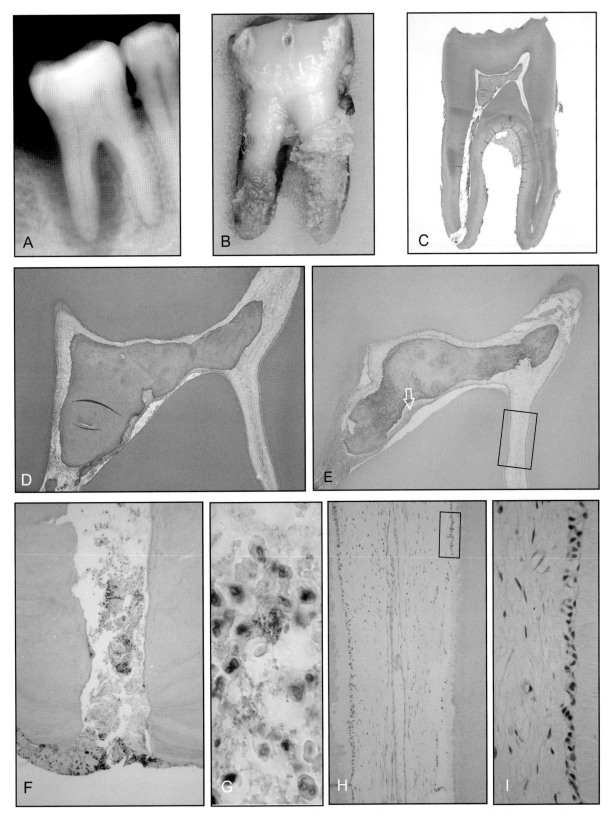

Fig. 23-20 (A) Extensive periodontal tissue breakdown circumscribing the distal root of a lower molar. (B, F) Plaque and calculus cover the root surface to the apical foramen. (C–G) The pulp is necrotic and infected all the way to the extensive hard tissue deposition in the coronal pulp (to arrow in E). Microphotographs enlarging marked area in (E) (H, I) indicate that the pulp tissue of the mesial root is completely unaffected and displays normal tissue morphology. Tooth responded vital to pulp testing.

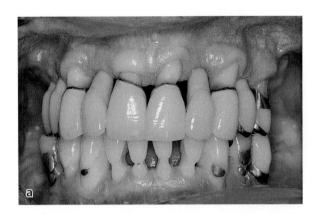 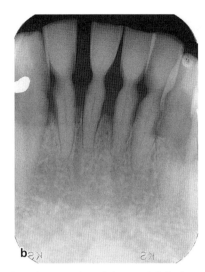

Fig. 23-21 (a) Clinical photograph of a patient, who has been in the maintenance phase for periodontal disease. While there are excellent gingival conditions and no pocket probing depths, there is substantial loss of cervical root dentin. (b) One of the lower incisors later had a horizontal fracture, but without a pulpal exposure due to fill of reparative dentin in the coronal portion of the pulp chamber. Courtesy of Dr. Sture Nyman.

periodontal instrumentation in comparison to non-instrumented teeth after initiating a self-performed oral hygiene program in patients with moderate to advanced periodontal disease. While affecting a majority of the patients, pain was generally reported to be minor. Only a few teeth in a small number of the patients developed highly sensitive root surfaces.

The main initial symptom is sharp pain of rapid onset that disappears once the stimulus is removed. In more severe, long-standing cases, shorter or longer periods of lingering, dull or aching pain may be provoked. These symptoms of a pulpitis character may not only be localized to the tooth (teeth) in question but to both quadrants of the jaw. Even a minimal contact with a toothbrush may elicit intense pain – a condition which is not only uncomfortable but one that is likely to hinder proper oral hygiene measures.

Mechanisms

The painful condition has been given many names, including dentine sensitivity, cervical dentine hypersensitivity, root dentine sensitivity, and root dentine hypersensitivity, reflecting some of the confusion that still exists regarding its etiologic background (Gillam & Orchardson 2006). The fact that root surfaces become sensitive to a variety of externally derived stimuli after periodontal instrumentation is not surprising as dentinal tubules become uncovered to the oral environment and subject to hydrodynamic forces. Hence, a variety of pain-evoking stimuli including evaporative, tactile, thermal, and osmotic stimuli may elicit sudden fluid shifts in the exposed tubules, thereby inducing a painful sensation according to the hydrodynamic theory of dentin sensitivity (Brännström 1966; Pashley 1996). This mechanism

alone can certainly explain the sensitivity patients experience immediately after the instrumentation procedure and during a short period afterwards, while it does not make clear why the symptoms increase over time and why pain may prevail in certain patients and in certain teeth.

The increase in pain intensity may have one or both of the following two explanations. Firstly, the smear layer formed on the root surface by the S/RP procedure will be dissolved within a few days (Kerns et al. 1991). This in turn will increase the hydraulic conductance of the involved dentinal tubules (Pashley 1996) and thus decrease the peripheral resistance to fluid flow across dentin. Thereby pain sensations are more readily evoked. Secondly, open dentinal tubules serve as pathways for diffusive transport of bacterial elements in the oral cavity to the pulp, which may cause a localized inflammatory pulpal response (Bergenholtz & Lindhe 1975, 1978). Indeed, experiments in dogs have shown that dentin exposures left unprotected greatly enhance the sensitivity of responding nerve fibers (Närhi et al. 1994). A large number of intradental A-delta fibers, normally inactive, then become able to respond (Närhi et al. 1996). It has furthermore been shown that the receptive field of each individual fiber gets wider (Närhi et al. 1996). In addition, sprouting of new terminal branches from pulpal axons may occur in the area subjacent to the root surface defect (Taylor et al. 1988). As already stated, sprouting of nerves is a temporary event and will subside if inflammation disappears; a feature which is consistent with their involvement in root dentin hypersensitivity (Byers & Närhi 1999). In other words, an essential component of the increasing root sensitivity patients experience after an instrumentation procedure is likely to be related to a peripheral sensitization of pulpal nociceptors leading to what is termed primary hyperalgesia.

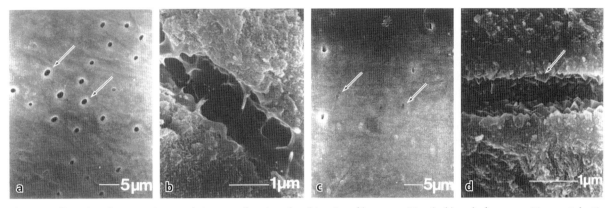

Fig. 23-22 Scanning electron microscopic images of root surface biopsies of hypersensitive (a, b) and of non-sensitive root dentin areas of human teeth (c, d). Numerous wide tubular apertures are seen in (a). These tubules show no evidence of hard tissue deposition after being opened longitudinally (b). By contrast, most tubules are occluded in (c) and below the surface rhombohedral crystals of from 0.1–0.3 μm are present. Images kindly provided by Dr. Masahiro Yoshiyama and published with permission of the *Journal of Dental Research*.

The fact that root dentin hypersensitivity often disappears a few weeks after the instrumentation procedure is best explained by the development of a natural occlusion of the exposed dentinal tubules. The deposition of mineral crystals in the tubular lumen may play an important role (Yoshiyama *et al.* 1989, 1990) (Fig. 23-22), firstly by inactivating the hydrodynamic mechanism for dentinal pain and secondly, by restricting the potential for an inward diffusion of bacterial elements to the pulp. The observation of few open tubules in non-sensitive root dentin (Hiatt & Johansen 1972; Absi *et al.* 1987; Yoshiyama *et al.* 1989; Cuenin *et al.* 1991; Oyama & Matsumoto 1991; Kontturi-Närhi 1993), while hypersensitive root areas show large numbers of tubular apertures on their surfaces (Absi *et al.* 1987; Yoshiyama *et al.* 1989; Cuenin *et al.* 1991; Oyama & Matsumoto 1991; Kontturi-Närhi 1993), supports this view.

The fact that only certain individuals become seriously affected may be related to local factors in the oral cavity, as well as to the level of the subjects' pain perception. Certain dietary factors, in particular fruit juices, yoghurt, and wines, have been implicated in the causation of root dentin hypersensitivity (Addy *et al.* 1987). By their acidity and ability to etch dentin these substances may dissolve the occlusions of the dentinal tubules or prevent them from forming. It needs be recognized that pain is not only an expression of injury and noxious stimuli, but also a psychobiologic phenomenon having both a physiologic and psychologic basis for its perception and reaction to it. Indeed, a variety of emotional elements may influence the subjective interpretation of pain. Anxiety, fear, and depression are factors that are known to affect pain perception as well as the subject's ability to identify coping methods (Eli 2003).

An important consideration in the deliberation of the mechanisms behind enhanced and lingering pain symptoms of root dentin hypersensitivity is the potential of central nervous system sensitization (for review see Sessle 2006). It is now well documented

that frequent and repeated pain stimulations result in structural and functional changes that allow the brain to respond more rapidly and more effectively to the same stimuli. Such an increase of the excitability of central neurons has a downside in that pain may continue as a memory function even if the peripheral cause has been eliminated. Thus, it is possible that central sensitization phenomena explain failure of treatment attempts in some patients.

Principles for management

In patients suffering from severe root dentin hypersensitivity, active treatment is urgent. However, the methods presently available provide an unpredictable remedy and at best only temporary relief is attained (Ikola 2001; Gillam & Orchardson 2006). Since tubular patency of the exposed dentin seems to play a crucial role in the pathogenesis of root dentin hypersensitivity most procedures hitherto attempted are logically aimed at inducing blockage of the peripheral openings. Some agents commonly employed, primarily for dentist-applied treatment, act by causing an astringent or coagulating effect on the tubular content. Such chemicals include strontium chloride, sodium monofluorophosphate, sodium fluoride, calcium hypophosphate, calcium hydroxide, potassium nitrate, potassium oxalates, glutaraldehyde, ferric oxalate, and stannous fluoride. Other methods aim to produce a physical block for example by the use of grafting procedures and laser applications (for reviews see Zappa 1994; Gangarosa 1994; Ikola 2001; Gillam & Orchardson 2006).

There may be several explanations why such treatments sometimes fail to remedy the problem. One is likely to be of a technical nature in that it is often difficult to attain a completely dry dentin surface during the application of, for example, an astringent solution. Hence, the release of gingival fluid from the sulcus is not easily restrained by compressed air or other methods. Consequently, upon application of the agent, protein from the gingival exudate might primarily be brought to coagulation rather than the tubular content. The precipitate is then easily removed upon subsequent tooth cleaning measures leaving the tubules unoccluded. Most agents furthermore may only cause a superficial block that may be dissolved over the course of time. Also topical applications do not address the pain mechanisms associated with either peripheral or central sensitization of nociceptors. Agents able to decrease the excitability of intradental nerves have, therefore, been proposed based on the assumption that potassium ions released from formulations containing potassium salts (e.g. chlorides, nitrates, citrate, and oxalates) may penetrate dentinal tubules and temper intradental nerve activity (Markowitz & Kim 1992; Orchardson & Peacock 1994). Toothpastes with potassium-containing preparations as active ingredients have indeed shown promise in clinical trials by giving better relief of pain in selected teeth in comparison to toothpastes without active substance (Sowinski et al. 2001; Wara-Aswapati et al. 2005). Experiments employing electrophysiological recordings in dogs, however, have shown that the effect of topical application of potassium salt is weak and becomes abolished after irrigation (Ikola 2001). More research appears necessary to confirm a clear treatment effect of potassium salts in gels, mouthwashes, and toothpastes (Orchardson & Gillam 2000). This also applies to any other treatment mode. It needs be recognized that demonstrating a significant treatment effect of a given compound in clinical trials is fraught with several difficulties. One is to assemble a sufficient number of patients that are reasonably identical in terms of duration and level of pain. Another is that the pain condition may go into natural remission at any time. A large placebo effect also operates in studies of this nature (Holland et al. 1997; Yates et al. 1998; Orchardson & Gillam 2000).

Any treatment approach to root dentin hypersensitivity should be preceded by a careful analysis of conditions that may be the cause of, or contributory to, the symptoms. Cracked teeth including cusp fractures, fractured or leaky restorations, caries, as well as a variety of other exposures of dentin to the oral environment may cause pulpal pain sensations to the very same stimuli which elicit root dentin hypersensitivity. An area of exposed dentin may be more sensitive if there is irritation of the pulp from other areas of the tooth, for example from the margin of a restoration that is not sealed from the oral environment (Närhi et al. 1994). Particular care should be taken to eliminate traumatic occlusion to alleviate any activation of pulpal nociceptors. Furthermore, dietary counseling should be given to patients who admit excessive consumption of citrus fruits, apples, or any other food or drinks that are acidic in nature.

Self-performed plaque control is important for the prevention and treatment of root dentin hypersensi-

tivity. It has been observed clinically that, with time, teeth in patients with excellent oral hygiene habits develop hard, smooth, and insensitive root surfaces. Electron microscopic examination of the dentin of such root surfaces has revealed that mineral deposits obliterate the tubular openings (Hiatt & Johansen 1972). However, when severe symptoms of root hypersensitivity have emerged, it is difficult to motivate the patient to maintain the degree of plaque control that is necessary to allow for a natural occlusion of the dentinal tubules. In such situations, an agent which has a capacity to block the tubular openings, may be beneficial at least temporarily, so that proper oral hygiene measures can be reinforced. In severe cases, where no remedy is achieved with any advice or treatment approach, pulpectomy and root filling are a last resort.

Any pain treatment should take into consideration the potential of preventing the condition from emerging in the first place. However, no well proven protocol has as yet been established whereby root dentine hypersensitivity can be effectively prevented. Attempts to block the exposed dentinal tubules immediately following S/RP should be an obvious approach. In fact a couple of placebo-controlled studies have shown promise in that significantly fewer sensitive teeth were attained subsequent to instrumentation when 6% ferric oxalate (Wang et al. 1993) and 3% potassium oxalate (Pillon et al. 2004) were applied topically. The long-term outcome of such procedures awaits confirmation.

Conclusion

Root dentin hypersensitivity frequently develops as an uncomfortable and sometimes difficult ailment to treat subsequent to scaling and root planing procedures in periodontal therapy. Although the exact mechanism is not well established, the condition is clearly related to open dentinal tubules that allow hydrodynamic mechanisms to elicit painful sensations upon external stimulation. Both peripheral and central sensitizations are likely to contribute to the more intense and lingering pain symptoms some patients experience after root dentin exposure.

Diagnosis and treatment planning should consider contributory etiologic factors including overconsumption of acidic food items. Root dentin hypersensitivity should also be checked against other conditions causing similar pain symptoms and rule out cracked teeth, leaky restoration margins, caries in the tooth or in neighboring teeth, as well as trauma from occlusion. A large number of treatment methods are available for both in-office and over-the-counter applications. Some aim to block tubular patency of the exposed root dentin and others attempt to decrease excitability of intradental nerves for reduced pain transmission. Unpredictable treatment results are to be expected and only temporary relief may be attained.

References

Absi, E.G., Addy, M. & Adams, D. (1987). Dentine hypersensitivity. A study of the patency of dentinal tubules in sensitive and non-sensitive cervical dentin. *Journal of Clinical Periodontology* **14**, 280–284.

Addy, M., Absi, E.G. & Adams, D. (1987). Dentine hypersensitivity. The effects *in vitro* of acids and dietary substances on root-planed and burred dentine. *Journal of Periodontology* **14**, 274–279.

Adriaens, P.A., De Boever, J.A. & Loesche, W.J. (1988). Bacterial invasion in root cementum and radicular dentin of periodontally diseased teeth in humans. *Journal of Periodontology* **59**, 222–230.

Babal, P., Soler, P., Brozman, M., Jakubovsky, J., Beyly, M. & Basset, F. (1987). *In situ* characterization of cells in periapical granuloma by monoclonal antibodies. *Oral Surgery Oral Medicine Oral Pathology* **64**, 348–352.

Bender, I.B. & Seltzer, S. (1972). The effect of periodontal disease on the pulp. *Oral Surgery Oral Medicine Oral Pathology* **33**, 458–474.

Bergenholtz, G. (1974). Micro-organisms from necrotic pulp of traumatized teeth. *Odontologisk Revy* **25**, 347–358.

Bergenholtz G. (2000). Evidence for bacterial causation of adverse pulpal responses in resin-based dental restorations. *Critical Reviews in Oral Biology and Medicine* **11**, 467–480.

Bergenholtz, G., Lekholm, U., Liljenberg, B. & Lindhe, J. (1983). Morphometric analysis of chronic inflammatory periapical lesions in root filled teeth. *Oral Surgery Oral Medicine Oral Pathology* **55**, 295–301.

Bergenholtz, G. & Lindhe, J. (1975). Effect of soluble plaque factors on inflammatory reactions in the dental pulp. *Scandinavian Journal of Dental Research* **83**, 153–158.

Bergenholtz, G. & Lindhe J. (1978). Effect of experimentally induced marginal periodontitis and periodontal scaling on the dental pulp. *Journal of Clinical Periodontology* **5**, 59–73.

Bergenholtz, G. & Nyman, S. (1984). Endodontic complications following periodontal and prosthetic treatment of patients with advanced periodontal disease. *Journal of Periodontology* **55**, 63–68.

Björndal, L. & Mjör, I.A. (2001). Pulp-dentin biology in restorative dentistry. Part 4: Dental caries–characteristics of lesions and pulpal reactions. *Quintessence International* **32**, 717–736.

Brännström, M. (1966). Sensitivity of dentine. *Oral Surgery Oral Medicine Oral Pathology* **21**, 517–526.

Byers, M.R. & Närhi, M.V.O. (1999). Dental injury models: Experimental tools for understanding neuroinflammatory interactions and polymodal nociceptor functions. *Critical Reviews in Oral Biology and Medicine* **10**, 4–39.

Chabanski, M.B, Gillam, D.G. & Newman, H.N. (1996). Prevalence of cervical dentine sensitivity in a population of patients referred to a specialist Periodontology Department. *Journal of Clinical Periodontology* **23**, 989–992.

Chavez De Paz, L.E., Dahlén, G., Molander, A., Möller, Å. & Bergenholtz, G. (2003). Bacteria recovered from teeth with apical periodontitis after antimicrobial endodontic treatment. *International Endodontic Journal* **36**, 500–508.

Cheung, G.S., Lai, S.C. & Ng, R.P. (2005). Fate of vital pulps beneath a metal-ceramic crown or a bridge retainer. *International Endodontic Journal* **38**, 521–530.

Cuenin, M.F., Scheidt, M.J., ONeal, R.B., Strong, S.L., Pashley, D.H., Horner, J.A. & Van Dyke, T.E. (1991). An *in vivo* study of dentin sensitivity: The relation of dentin sensitivity and the patency of dentin tubules. *Journal of Periodontology* **62**, 668–673.

Czarnecki, R.T. & Schilder, H. (1979). A histological evaluation of the human pulp in teeth with varying degrees of periodontal disease. *Journal of Endodontics* **5**, 242–253.

Dahle, U.R., Tronstad, L. & Olsen, I. (1996). Characterization of new periodontal and endodontic isolates of spirochetes. *European Journal of Oral Sciences* **104**, 41–47.

Dahlén, G. (2002). Microbiology and treatment of dental abscesses and periodontal-endodontic lesions. *Periodontology 2000* **28**, 206–239.

DeDeus, Q.D. (1975). Frequency, location, and direction of the lateral secondary and accessory canals. *Journal of Endodontics* **1**, 361–366.

Dommisch, H., Winter, J., Acil, Y., Dunsche, A., Tiemann, M. & Jepsen S. (2005). Human beta-defensin (hBD-1, -2) expression in dental pulp. *Oral Microbiology and Immunology* **20**,163–166.

Durand, S.H., Flacher, V., Romeas, A., Carrouel, F., Colomb, E., Vincent, C., Magloire, H., Couble, M.L., Bleicher, F., Staquet, M.J., Lebecque, S. & Farges, J.C. (2006). Lipoteichoic acid increases TLR and functional chemokine expression while reducing dentin formation in in vitro differentiated human odontoblasts. *Journal of Immunology* **176**, 2880–2887.

Egan, M.W., Spratt, D.A., Ng, Y.L., Lam, J.M., Moles, D.R. & Gulabivala, K. (2002). Prevalence of yeasts in saliva and root canals of teeth associated with apical periodontitis. *International Endodontic Journal* **35**, 321–329.

Eli, I. (2003). The multidisciplinary nature of pain. In: Bergenholtz, G., Hörsted-Bindslev, P. & Reit, C., eds. *Textbook of Endodontology*. Blackwell Munksgaard, pp. 57–65.

Fardal, Ø., Johannessen, A.C. & Linden, G.J. (2002). Patient perceptions of periodontal therapy completed in a periodontal practice. *Journal of Periodontology* **73**, 1060–1066.

Fischer, C., Wennberg, A., Fischer, R.G. & Attström, R. (1991). Clinical evaluation of pulp and dentine sensitivity after supragingival and subgingival scaling. *Endodontics and Dental Traumatology* **7**, 259–263.

Foschi, F., Cavrini, F., Montebugnoli, L., Stashenko, P., Sambri, V. & Prati, C. (2005). Detection of bacteria in endodontic samples by polymerase chain reaction assays and association with defined clinical signs in Italian patients. *Oral Microbiology and Immunology* **20**, 289–295.

Gangarosa Sr, L.P. (1994). Current strategies of dentist-applied treatment in the management of hypersensitive dentine. *Archives of Oral Biology* **39** (Suppl), 101S–106S.

Gillam, D.G. & Orchardson, R. (2006). Advances in the treatment of root dentine sensitivity-mechanisms and treatment principles. *Endodontic Topics* **13**, 13–33.

Gillam, D.G., Seo, H.S., Bulman, J.S. & Newman, H.N. (1999). Perceptions of dentine hypersensitivity in a general practice population. *Journal of Oral Rehabilitation* **26**, 710–714.

Gomes, B.P., Pinheiro, E.T., Gade-Neto, C.R., Sousa, E.L., Ferraz, C.C., Zaia, A.A., Teixeira, F.B. & Souza-Filho, F.J. (2004). Microbiological examination of infected dental root canals. *Oral Microbiology and Immunology* **19**, 71–76.

Gutmann, J.L. (1978). Prevalence, location and patency of accessory canals in the furcation region of permanent molars. *Journal of Periodontology* **49**, 21–26.

Hahn, C.L., Best, A.M. & Tew, J.G. (2003). Cytokine induction by *Streptococcus mutans* and pulpal pathogenesis. *Infection and Immunity* **68**, 6785–6789.

Happonen, R.-P., Söderling, E., Viander, M., Linko-Kettunen, L. & Pelliniemi, L.J. (1986). Immunocytochemical demonstration of *Actinomyces* species and *Arachnia propionica* in periapical infections. *Journal of Oral Pathology* **14**, 405–413.

Hattler, A.B. & Listgarten, M.A. (1984). Pulpal response to root planing in a rat model. *Journal of Endodontics* **10**, 471–476.

Hiatt, W.H. & Johansen, E. (1972). Root preparation. I. Obturation of dentinal tubules in treatment of root hypersensitivity. *Journal of Periodontology* **43**, 373–380.

Holland, G.R., Närhi, M., Addy, M., Gangarosa, L. & Orchardson R. (1997). Guidelines for the design and conduct of clinical trials on dentine hypersensitivity. *Journal of Clinical Periodontology* **24**, 808–813.

Ikola, S. (2001). Dentin hypersensitivity and its treatment methods. Thesis. Institute of Dentistry, University of Turku.

Jacobsen, I. & Kerekes, K. (1977). Long-term prognosis of traumatized permanent anterior teeth showing calcifying processes in the pulp cavity. *Scandinavian Journal of Dental Research* **85**, 588–598.

Jontell, M., Okiji, T., Dahlgren, U. & Bergenholtz G. (1997). Immune defense mechanisms of the dental pulp. *Critical Reviews in Oral Biology and Medicine* **9**, 179–200.

Kamal, A.M., Okiji, T., Kawashima, N. & Suda, H. (1997). Defense responses of dentin/pulp complex to experimentally induced caries in rat molars: an immunohistochemical study on kinetics of pulpal Ia antigen-expressing cells and macrophages. *Journal of Endodontics* **23**, 115–120.

Karlsson, S. (1986) A clinical evaluation of fixed bridges, 10 years following insertion. *Journal of Oral Rehabilitation* **13**, 423–432.

Kerekes, K. & Olsen, I. (1990). Similarities in the microfloras of root canals and deep periodontal pockets. *Endodontics and Dental Traumatology* **6**, 1–5.

Kerns, D.G., Scheidt, M.J., Pashley, D.H., Horner, J.A., Strong, S.L. & Van Dyke, T.E. (1991). Dentinal tubule occlusion and root hypersensitivity. *Journal of Periodontology* **62**, 421–428.

Kontturi-Närhi, V. (1993). Dentin hypersensitivity. Factors related to the occurrence of pain symptoms. Academic Dissertation, University of Kuopio.

Kristerson, L. & Andreasen, J.O. (1984). Influence of root development on periodontal and pulpal healing after replantation of incisors in monkeys. *International Journal of Oral Surgery* **13**, 313–323.

Langeland, K., Rodrigues, H. & Dowden, W. (1974). Periodontal disease, bacteria and pulpal histopathology. *Oral Surgery Oral Medicine Oral Pathology* **37**, 257–270.

Lantelme, R.L., Handelman, S.L. & Herbison, R.J. (1976). Dentin formation in periodontally diseased teeth. *Journal of Dental Research* **55**, 48–51.

Lervik, T. & Mjör, I.A. (1977). Evaluation of techniques for the induction of pulpitis. *Journal de Biologie Buccale* **5**, 137–148.

Lewis, M.A.O., McFarlane, T.W. & McGowan, D.A. (1986). Quantitative bacteriology of acute dento-alveolar abscesses. *Journal of Medical Microbiology* **21**, 101–104.

Lomcali, G., Sen, B.H. & Cankaya, H. (1996) Scanning electron microscopic observations of apical root surfaces of teeth with apical periodontitis. *Endodontics and Dental Traumatology* **12**, 70–76.

Lin, L.M., Wang, S.L., Wu-Wang, C., Chang, K.M. & Leung, C. (1996). Detection of epidermal growth factor receptor in inflammatory periapical lesions. *International Endodontic Journal* **29**, 179–184.

Lowman, J.V., Burke, R.S. & Pelleu, G.B. (1973). Patent accessory canals: Incidence in molar furcation region. *Oral Surgery Oral Medicine Oral Pathology* **36**, 580–584.

Lundy, T. & Stanley, H.R. (1969). Correlation of pulpal histopathology and clinical symptoms in human teeth subjected to experimental irritation. *Oral Surgery Oral Medicine Oral Pathology* **27**,187–201.

Markowitz, K. & Kim, S. (1992). The role of selected cations in the desensitization of intradental nerves. *Proceedings of the Finnish Dental Society* **88** (Suppl I), 39–54.

Marton, I.J. & Kiss, C. (2000). Protective and destructive immune reactions in apical periodontitis. *Oral Microbiology and Immunology* **15**, 139–150.

Massler, M. (1967). Pulpal reactions to dental caries. *International Dental Journal* **17**, 441–460.

Mazur, B. & Massler, M. (1964). Influence of periodontal disease on the dental pulp. *Oral Surgery Oral Medicine Oral Pathology* **17**, 592–603.

Mjör, I.A. & Tronstad, L. (1972). Experimentally induced pulpitis. *Oral Surgery Oral Medicine Oral Pathology* **34**, 102–108.

Molander, A., Reit, C., Dahlén, G. & Kvist, T. (1998). Microbiological status of root-filled teeth with apical periodontitis. *International Endodontic Journal* **31**, 1–7.

Nair, P.N.R. (1987). Light and electron microscopic studies of root canal flora and periapical lesions. *Journal of Endodontics* **13**, 29–39.

Nair, P.N.R. (1997). Apical periodontitis a dynamic encounter between root canal infection and host response. *Periodontology 2000* **13**, 121–148.

Nair, P.N.R. & Schroeder, H.E. (1985). Epithelial attachment at diseased human tooth-apex. *Journal of Periodontal Research* **20**, 293–300.

Närhi, M., Yamamoto, H., Ngassapa, D. & Hirvonen, T. (1994). The neurophysiological basis and the role of the inflammatory reactions in dentine hypersensitivity. *Archives of Oral Biology* **39** (Suppl), 23S–30S.

Närhi, M., Yamamoto, H. & Ngassapa, D. (1996). Function of intradental nociceptors in normal and inflamed teeth. *Proceedings of the International Conference on Dentin/Pulp Complex* 1995. Berlin: Quintessence, pp. 136–140.

Nilvéus, R. & Selvig, K.A. (1983). Pulpal reactions to the application of citric acid to root-planed dentin in beagles. *Journal of Periodontal Research* **18**, 420–428.

Oguntebi, B., Slee, A.M., Tanzer, J.M. & Langeland, K. (1982). Predominant microflora associated with human dental periapical abscesses. *Journal of Clinical Microbiology* **15**, 964–966.

Ohshima, H., Sato, O., Kawahara, I., Maeda, T. & Takano Y. (1995). Responses of immunocompetent cells to cavity preparation in rat molars: an immunohistochemical study using OX6-monoclonal antibody. *Connective Tissue Research* **32**, 303–311.

Okiji, T., Kawashima, N., Kosaka, T., Kobayashi, C. & Suda, H. (1994). Distribution of Ia antigen-expressing nonlymphoid cells in various stages of induced periapical lesions in rat molars. *Journal of Endodontics* **20**, 27–31.

Orchardson, R. & Gillam, D.G. (2000). The efficacy of potassium salts as agents for treating dentin hypersensitivity. *Journal of Orofacial Pain* **14**, 9–19.

Orchardson, R. & Peacock, J.M. (1994). Factors affecting nerve excitability and conduction as a basis for desensitizing dentine. *Archives of Oral Biology* **39** (Suppl), 81S–86S.

Oyama, T. & Matsumoto, K. (1991). A clinical and morphological study of cervical hypersensitivity. *Journal of Endodontics* **17**, 500–502.

Pashley, D.H. (1996). Dynamics of the pulpo-dentin complex. *Critical Reviews in Oral Biology and Medicine* **7**, 104–133.

Peciuliene, V., Reynaud, A.H., Balciuniene, I. & Haapasalo, M. (2001). Isolation of yeasts and enteric bacteria in root-filled teeth with chronic apical periodontitis. *International Endodontic Journal* **34**, 429–434.

Pillon, F.L., Romani, I.G. & Schmidt, E.R. (2004). Effect of a 3% potassium oxalate topical application on dentinal hypersensitivity after subgingival scaling and root planing. *Journal of Periodontology* **75**, 1461–1464.

Reeves, R. & Stanley, H.R. (1966). The relationship of bacterial penetration and pulpal pathosis in carious teeth. *Oral Surgery Oral Medicine Oral Pathology* **22**, 59–65.

Ricucci, D. & Bergenholtz, G. (2004). Histologic features of apical periodontitis in human biopsies. *Endodontic Topics* **8**, 68–87.

Robertson, A., Andreasen, F.M., Bergenholtz, G., Andreasen, J.O. & Norén, J.G. (1998). Incidence of pulp necrosis subsequent to pulp canal obliteration from trauma of permanent incisors. *Journal of Endodontics* **22**, 557–560.

Rocas, I.N. & Siqueira, J.F. Jr. (2005). Occurrence of two newly named oral treponemes – *Treponema parvum* and *Treponema putidum* – in primary endodontic infections. *Oral Microbiology and Immunology* **20**, 372–375.

Rubach, W.C. & Mitchell, D.F. (1965). Periodontal disease, accessory canals and pulp pathosis. *Journal of Periodontology* **36**, 34–38.

Sakamoto, M., Rocas, I.N., Siqueira, J.F. Jr. & Benno, Y. (2006). Molecular analysis of bacteria in asymptomatic and symptomatic endodontic infections. *Oral Microbiology and Immunology* **21**, 112–122.

Saunders, W.P. & Saunders, E.M. (1998). Prevalence of periradicular periodontitis associated with crowned teeth in an adult Scottish subpopulation. *British Dental Journal* **185**, 137–140.

Schuurs, A.H., Wesselink, P.R., Eijkman, M.A. & Duivenvoorden, H.J. (1995). Dentists' views on cervical hypersensitivity and their knowledge of its treatment. *Endodontics and Dental Traumatology* **11**, 240–244.

Seltzer, S., Bender, I.B. & Ziontz, M. (1963). The interrelationship of pulp and periodontal disease. *Oral Surgery Oral Medicine Oral Pathology* **16**, 1474–1490.

Sessle, B.J. (2006). Mechanisms of oral somatosensory and motor functions and their clinical correlate. *Journal of Oral Rehabilitation* **33**, 243–261.

Siqueira, J.F. Jr. & Lopes, H.P. (2001). Bacteria on the apical root surfaces of untreated teeth with periradicular lesions: a scanning electron microscopy study. *International Endodontic Journal* **34**, 216–220.

Siqueira, J.F. Jr. & Rocas, I.N. (2005a). Exploiting molecular methods to explore endodontic infections: Part 1 – current molecular technologies for microbiological diagnosis. *Journal of Endodontics* **31**, 411–423.

Siqueira, J.F. Jr. & Rocas, I.N. (2005b). Exploiting molecular methods to explore endodontic infections: Part 2 – Redefining the endodontic microbiota. *Journal of Endodontics* **31**, 488–498.

Siqueira, J.F. Jr., Rocas, I.N., Cunha, C.D. & Rosado, A.S. (2005). Novel bacterial phylotypes in endodontic infections. *Journal of Dental Research* **84**, 565–569.

Sowinski, J., Ayad, F., Petrone, M., DeVizio, W., Volpe, A., Ellwood, R. & Davies, R. (2001). Comparative investigations of the desensitising efficacy of a new dentifrice. *Journal of Clinical Periodontology* **28**, 1032–1036.

Spratt, D.A. (2004). Significance of bacterial identification by molecular biology methods. *Endodontic Topics* **9**, 5–14.

Stashenko, P. (1990). Role of immune cytokines in the pathogenesis of periapical lesions. *Endodontics and Dental Traumatology* **6**, 89–96.

Stashenko, P., Teles, R. & D'Souza, R. (1998). Periapical inflammatory responses and their modulation. *Crititical Reviews in Oral Biology and Medicine* **9**, 498–521.

Stashenko, P., Wang, C.Y., Riley, E., Wu, Y., Ostroff, G. & Niederman, R. (1995). Reduction of infection-stimulated periapical bone resorption by the biological response modifier PGG Glucan. *Journal of Dental Research* **74**, 323–330.

Sundqvist, G. (1976). Bacteriologic studies of necrotic dental pulps. Umeå University Odontological Dissertation #7.

Sundqvist, G., Figdor, D., Persson, S. & Sjögren, U. (1998). Microbiologic analysis of teeth with failed endodontic treatment and the outcome of conservative re-treatment. *Oral Surgery Oral Medicine Oral Pathology Oral Radiology Endodontics* **85**, 86–93.

Sundqvist, G. & Reuterving, C.O. (1980). Isolation of *Actinomyces israelii* from periapical lesion. *Journal of Endodontics* **6**, 602–606.

Suzuki, T., Kumamoto, H., Ooya, K. & Motegi, K. (2002). Expression of inducible nitric oxide synthase and heat shock proteins in periapical inflammatory lesions. *Journal of Oral Pathology and Medicine* **31**, 488–493.

Svensäter, G. & Bergenholtz, G. (2004). Biofilms in endodontic infections. *Endodontic Topics* **9**, 27–36.

Tammaro, S., Wennström, J. & Bergenholtz, G. (2000). Root dentin sensitivity following non-surgical periodontal treatment. *Journal of Clinical Periodontology* **27**, 690–697.

Taylor, P.E., Byers, M.R. & Redd, P.E. (1988). Sprouting of CGRP nerve fibers in response to dentin injury in rat molars. *Brain Research* **461**, 371–376.

Ten Cate, A.R. (1972). The epithelial cell rests of Malassez and the genesis of the dental cyst. *Oral Surgery Oral Medicine Oral Pathology* **34**, 956–964.

Thesleff, I. (1987). Epithelial cell rests of Malassez bind epidermal growth factor intensely. *Journal of Periodontal Research* **22**, 419–421.

Torabinejad, M. & Kettering, J.D. (1985). Identification and relative concentration of B and T lymphocytes in human chronic periapical lesions. *Journal of Endodontics* **11**, 122–125.

Torabinejad, M. & Kiger, R.D. (1985). A histologic evaluation of dental pulp tissue of a patient with periodontal disease. *Oral Surgery Oral Medicine Oral Pathology* **59**, 198–200.

Tronstad, L., Barnett, F. & Cervone, F. (1990) Periapical bacterial plaque in teeth refractory to endodontic treatment. *Endodontics and Dental Traumatology* **6**, 73–77.

Vertucci, F.J. (1984). Root canal anatomy of the human permanent teeth. *Oral Surgery Oral Medicine Oral Pathology* **58**, 589–599.

Vertucci, F.J. (2005). Root canal morphology and its relationship to endodontic procedures. *Endodontic Topics* **10**, 3–29.

Vertucci, F.J. & Williams, R.G. (1974). Furcation canals in the human mandibular first molar. *Oral Surgery Oral Medicine Oral Pathology* **38**, 308–314.

Waltimo, T.M., Siren, E.K., Torkko, H.L., Olsen, I. & Haapasalo, M.P. (1997). Fungi in therapy-resistant apical periodontitis. *International Endodontic Journal* **30**, 96–101.

Wang, H.L., Yeh, C.T., Smith, F., Burgett, F.G., Richards, P., Shyr, Y. & O'Neal, R. (1993). Evaluation of ferric oxalate as an agent for use during surgery to prevent post-operative root hypersensitivity. *Journal of Periodontology* **64**, 1040–1044.

Wara-Aswapati, N., Krongnawakul, D., Jiraviboon, D., Adulyanon, S., Karimbux, N. & Pitiphat, W. (2005). The effect of a new toothpaste containing potassium nitrate and triclosan on gingival health, plaque formation and dentine hypersensitivity. *Journal of Clinical Periodontology* **32**, 53–58.

Warfvinge, J. & Bergenholtz, G. (1986). Healing capacity of human and monkey dental pulps following experimentally induced pulpitis. *Endodontics and Dental Traumatology* **2**, 256–262.

Williams, B.L., McCann, G.F. & Schoenknecht, F.D. (1983). Bacteriology of dental abscesses of endodontic origin. *Journal of Clinical Microbiology* **18**, 770–774.

Yates, R., Owens, R., Jackson, R., Newcombe, R.G. & Addy, M. (1998). A split mouth placebo-controlled study to determine the effect of amorphous calcium phosphate in the treatment of dentine hypersensitivity. *Journal of Clinical Periodontology* **25**, 687–692.

Yoshiyama, M., Masada, A., Uchida, A. & Ishida, H. (1989). Scanning electron microscopic characterization of sensitive vs. insensitive human radicular dentin. *Journal of Dental Research* **68**, 1498–1502.

Yoshiyama, M., Noiri, Y., Ozaki, K., Uchida, A., Ishikawa, Y. & Ishida, H. (1990). Transmission electron microscopic characterization of hypersensitive human radicular dentin. *Journal of Dental Research* **69**, 1293–1297.

Zappa, U. (1994). Self-applied treatments in the management of dentine hypersensitivity. *Archives of Oral Biology* **39** (Suppl), 107S–112S.

Part 7: Peri-implant Pathology

Chapter 24

Peri-implant Mucositis and Peri-implantitis

Tord Berglundh, Jan Lindhe, and Niklaus P. Lang

Definitions

Peri-implant disease

Inflammatory processes in the tissues surrounding an implant (Albrektsson & Isidor 1994).

Peri-implant mucositis

Reversible inflammatory process in the soft tissues surrounding a functioning implant.

Peri-implantitis

Inflammatory process additionally characterized by loss of peri-implant bone.
  See Fig. 24-1.

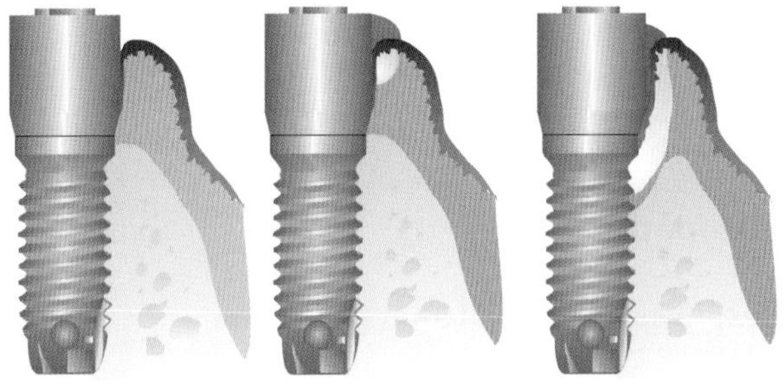

Ridge mucosa

The edentulous, hard tissue portion of the alveolar process is covered by a mucosa that is about 2–4 mm thick (see also Chapter 3). The mucosa is lined by a keratinized epithelium and is comprised of a connective tissue that is rich in fibroblasts, collagen fibers, and vascular structures (e.g. Türk 1965; Krajicek *et al.* 1984; Liljenberg *et al.* 1996). The connective tissue is continuous with the cortical bone crest via the periosteum. A few scattered inflammatory cells can be observed adjacent to the basement membrane in the connective tissue papillae between the rete pegs of the epithelium.

Peri-implant mucosa

Following implant installation, a transmucosal passage is formed around the abutment portion of

Fig. 24-1 Schematic drawing illustrating healthy peri-implant mucosa, peri-implant mucositis, and peri-implantitis.

the device. The ridge mucosa at such sites adapts to the new functional demands and a peri-implant mucosa becomes established. The mucosa surrounding implants and the gingiva surrounding teeth have many features in common. Both types of tissues are lined with a keratinized oral epithelium; at clinically healthy sites this is continuous with a thin non-keratinized barrier or junctional epithelium that faces the implant or the tooth surface. In the connective tissue immediately lateral to these thin epithelial linings small infiltrates of inflammatory cells (neutrophils, macrophages, T cells, B cells) are frequently seen (Liljenberg *et al.* 1997). The inflammatory cells represent the host's defense against bacterial products and hence they may be considered as one important component of the biological seal that separates the peri-implant and periodontal attachment tissues from the oral cavity (see also Chapters 3 and 11).

Peri-implant mucositis

Clinical features

The clinical features of peri-implant mucositis are in many respects similar to those of in gingivitis at teeth and include classical symptoms of inflammation, such as swelling and redness (see Chapter 17). Differences in the morphology of the peri-implant mucosa and the lack of light transmission through the metal of the device, however, may mask visible signs of inflammation. Assessment of peri-implant mucositis must therefore always include assessment of bleeding following probing (Fig. 24-2).

Prevalence

Bleeding on probing (BoP) is a good discriminating indicator of peri-implant mucositis. The prevalence of this disease remains difficult to estimate since data on BoP at implants are infrequently reported (Berglundh *et al.* 2002). In a study on 25 subjects treated with implant-supported fixed prosthesis, Lekholm *et al.* (1986) reported that BoP occurred at 80% of the implants. Roos-Jansåker *et al.* (2006a,b,c) examined 987 implants in 216 patients and reported that more than 73% of all implants exhibited BoP. Higher frequencies of BoP at implants were presented by Fransson *et al.* (2007) in a study on 82 subjects. It was reported that BoP occurred in more than 90% of implant sites.

Histopathology

Response to early plaque formation

The response of the gingiva and the peri-implant mucosa to early and more long-standing periods of plaque formation was analyzed both in studies in man and in experiments in animals. Pontoriero *et al.* (1994) engaged 20 partially edentulous human subjects in a clinical "Experimental gingivitis in man" (Löe *et al.* 1965) study. All subjects had been treated for advanced periodontal disease and thereafter had been restored with implants in one or several segments of the dentition. During a 6-month period fol-

lowing the prosthetic rehabilitation, the subjects were enrolled in a meticulous maintenance program that included regularly repeated supportive measures. A baseline examination was subsequently performed including assessment of plaque, soft tissue inflammation, probing pocket depth (PPD), soft tissue recession, and composition of oral biofilms. The participants refrained from all oral hygiene measures for 3 weeks. It was observed that during this interval plaque build-up (amount and composition) and the soft tissue response to the microbial challenge, e.g. inflammation and PPD change, developed in a similar manner in the tooth and implant segments of the dentition.

Zitzmann *et al.* (2001) studied the response to plaque formation in the soft tissues at implant and tooth sites in humans. Twelve subjects with healthy periodontal and peri-implant conditions were asked to refrain from tooth/implant cleaning for a period of 3 weeks (Fig. 24-3). Clinical examinations were performed and soft tissue biopsies were harvested prior to and at the end of the plaque accumulation period. The tissues were examined using histologic techniques. It was demonstrated that plaque build-up was associated with clinical signs of soft tissue inflammation. Furthermore, the initially minute lesions in the gingiva and in the peri-implant mucosa markedly increased in size after 3 weeks of plaque build-up: from 0.03 mm^2 at baseline to 0.3 mm^2 (gingiva) and 0.2 mm^2 (peri-implant mucosa). In addition, the proportion of B cells and neutrophils increased more in the lesion in the gingiva than in its counterpart in the peri-implant mucosa.

Experimental model

In a carefully supervised experiment in the dog, Berglundh *et al.* (1992) compared the reaction of the gingiva and the peri-implant mucosa to 3 weeks of *de novo* plaque formation. The mandibular premolars in one side of the mandible were extracted, leaving the premolars on the contralateral side as controls. After 3 months of socket healing, implants were inserted in the edentulous ridge. The animals were placed in a plaque-control program to allow for ideal healing of the mucosa at the implants and to prevent

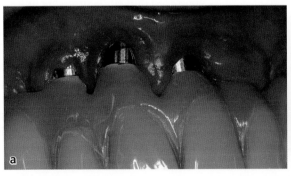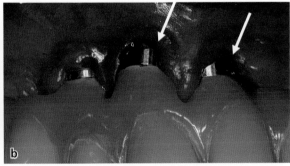

Fig. 24-2 (a) Clinical symptoms of peri-implant mucositis including varying signs of redness and swelling. (b) Probing resulted in bleeding from the margin of the mucosa.

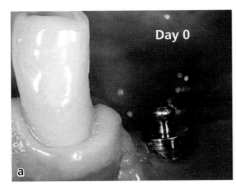 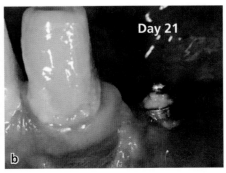

Fig. 24-3 (a) Clinical photograph from sites with healthy gingiva and peri-implant mucosa. (b) The sites illustrated in (a) following 3 weeks of plaque formation.

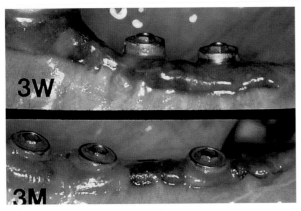 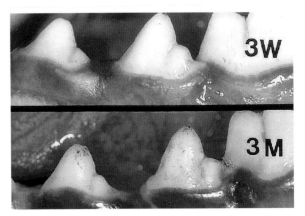

Fig. 24-4 A clinical view illustrating 3 weeks (3 W) and 3 months (3 M) of undisturbed plaque formation on the implants and the teeth of a beagle dog.

gingivitis from occurring in the tooth segments of the dentition. After this healing period, the dogs were examined and samples from the minute biofilms that were present on the implant and the tooth surfaces were harvested. The plaque-control program was terminated and the animals given a soft diet, that allowed gross plaque formation. Re-examinations, including clinical assessment (Fig. 24-4), sampling of plaque from teeth and implants as well as biopsy, were performed after 3 weeks.

During the course of the study, it was observed that similar amounts of plaque formed on the tooth and implant segments of the dentition. The composition of the two developing plaques was also similar. It was therefore concluded that early microbial colonization on titanium implants followed the same pattern as that on teeth (Leonhardt *et al.* 1992).

Both the gingiva and the peri-implant mucosa responded to this microbial colonization with the establishment of overt inflammatory lesions, i.e. infiltrates of leukocytes in the connective tissue. The lesions in the gingiva and in the peri-implant mucosa were matched both with respect to size and location. Hence, both lesions were consistently found in the marginal portion of the soft tissues and between the keratinized oral epithelium and the junctional or barrier epithelium (Fig. 24-2).

Response to long-standing plaque formation

With increasing duration of plaque build-up (3 months) in the dog model described above, the lesions in the peri-implant mucosa seemed to have expanded and to have progressed further "apically" while the gingival lesions remained unchanged (Ericsson *et al.* 1992) (Fig. 24-5). Furthermore, the lesion in the peri-implant mucosa contained a much smaller number of fibroblasts than the corresponding infiltrate in the gingiva. In any inflammatory lesion of long standing, periods of breakdown and periods of repair interchange. It was suggested, therefore, that in the gingival lesion, the amount of tissue breakdown that occurred during the 3 month interval was more or less fully compensated by tissue build-up that took place during a subsequent phase of repair. In the lesion within the peri-implant mucosa, the tissue breakdown was not fully recovered by reparative events. This reduced build-up may have been the reason for the resulting additional propagation and spread of the lesion in the peri-implant mucosa.

In a similar dog experiment Abrahamsson *et al.* (1998) studied soft tissue lesions after 5 months of plaque formation at three different implant systems. They observed that the response of the peri-implant mucosa to long-standing plaque formation appeared

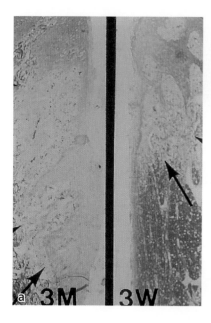 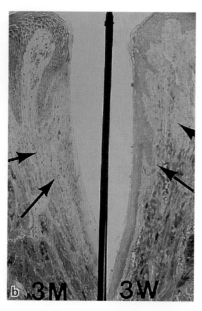

Fig. 24-5 Microphotographs illustrating the establishment of inflammatory cell infiltrates (ICT) in the peri-implant mucosa (a) and the gingiva (b) (3 W = 3 weeks; 3 M = 3 months). Note, in the microphotographs representing 3 months, the infiltrate in the peri-implant mucosa extends much deeper into the tissue than is the case in the gingiva.

to be independent of the implant system that harbored the biofilm.

Peri-implantitis

Clinical features

Peri-implantitis represents a clinical condition that includes the presence of (1) an inflammatory lesion in the peri-implant mucosa and (2) loss of peri-implant bone. The assessment of the diagnosis *peri-implantitis* must consequently require detection of both bleeding on probing (BoP) as well as bone loss in radiographs. Peri-implantitis initially affects the marginal part of the peri-implant tissues and the implant may remain stable and in function for varying periods of time. Implant mobility is therefore not an essential symptom for peri-implantitis but may occur in a final stage of disease progression and indicates complete loss of integration.

As pointed out for the clinical characteristics of peri-implant mucositis, various factors such as the morphology of the peri-implant mucosa and position of the implant may also influence the clinical appearance of inflammation in peri-implantitis. Probing is therefore a prerequisite in the examination of peri-implant tissues and should include assessment of both BoP and probing pocket depth (PPD).

The clinical appearance of peri-implantitis may, hence, vary and may not always be associated with overt signs of pathology. Two different cases are illustrated in Figs. 24-6 and 24-7. While plaque and calculus together with clinical signs of inflammation are present in the case in Fig. 24-6, the case in Fig. 24-7a does not reveal such symptoms. Probing the site in Fig. 24-7a, however, resulted in a PPD of about 10 mm and BoP (Fig. 24-7b).

Crater-formed defects around implants are frequently found in radiographs obtained from sites with peri-implantitis (Fig. 24-8). Bone loss in such

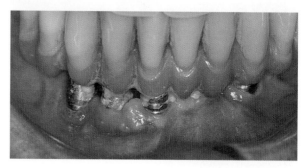

Fig. 24-6 Clinical symptoms of peri-implantitis. Note the large amounts of plaque and calculus and visible signs of inflammation in the peri-implant mucosa.

sites appears also to be symmetric, i.e. similar amount of bone loss occur at mesial, distal, buccal, and lingual aspects of the implants. On the other hand, the morphology of the osseous defect may vary depending on the horizontal dimension of the alveolar ridge. Thus, in sites where the buccal–lingual width of the ridge exceeds that of the peri-implantitis lesion, a buccal and lingual bone wall may remain. Conversely, in sites with a narrow ridge the buccal and lingual bone will be resorbed and lost during progression of peri-implantitis.

Conclusion

Symptoms of peri-implantitis relate to the infectious/inflammatory nature of the lesion. Thus, there is radiographic evidence of bone loss and the bone loss often has the shape of a crater. Swelling and redness of the mucosa as well as bleeding on gentle probing occur. Suppuration is also a frequent finding. The implant may remain stable over long periods.

Prevalence

Previous estimates of the prevalence of peri-implantitis were based on reports describing varying

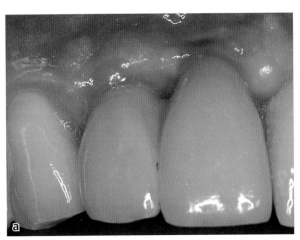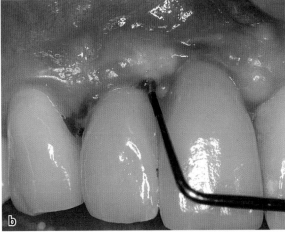

Fig. 24-7 Clinical photograph from two implant-supported crowns in the lateral (12) and central (11) incisor positions. (a) No or minor signs of inflammation in the surrounding mucosa. (b) Probing resulted in bleeding and suppuration from the implant site in the lateral incisor position.

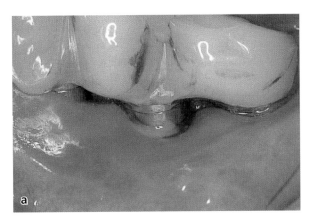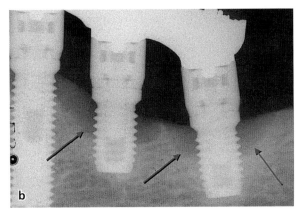

Fig. 24-8 Clinical (a) and radiographic (b) characteristics of two implant sites with peri-implantitis in the left side of the mandible. Note the presence of swelling and suppuration in the peri-implant mucosa (a) and the crater-formed bone destruction around the implants in the radiograph (arrows) (b).

frequencies of implant failures that were associated with high plaque scores or severe signs of inflammation (van Steenberge *et al.* 1993; Weyant & Burt 1993; Weyant 1994; Esposito *et al.* 1998). Other criteria were used by Mombelli and Lang (1998) and Brägger *et al.* (2001) and it was suggested that the prevalence of peri-implantitis may vary between 5 and 10% among implants.

The difficulty of retrieving information on the prevalence of peri-implantitis was confirmed in a systematic review by Berglundh *et al.* (2002). They evaluated the incidence of biologic and technical complications in implant therapy reported in prospective longitudinal studies of at least 5 years. From the 1310 titles and abstracts provided by the search in databases, 159 studies were selected for full-text analysis, out of which 51 studies were used for meta-analysis. Implant loss was the most frequently reported type of complication, while information regarding peri-implantitis and pronounced bone loss was only provided in 40–50% of the studies. The limited information on the incidence of peri-implan-

titis was explained by the fact that the term peri-implantitis, with the definition by Albrektsson and Isidor (1994) referred to above, was included in only a few studies. The inability to use information on the incidence of peri-implantitis and the occurrence of pronounced bone loss at implants was also due to the lack of data describing frequency distributions of various probing depths and amount of radiographic bone loss.

It is important to use appropriate terms in clinical reports to avoid confusion. Peri-implantitis is a clinical condition and should not be mistaken for implant failure. If left untreated, however, peri-implantitis may progress and lead to implant loss. The term failure should thus be avoided and terms referring to peri-implant disease (peri-implant mucositis and peri-implantitis) should be used for implants in function. Implant loss is consequently the term to use for implants that were lost or removed. In a consensus report from the 4th European Workshop on Periodontology, Lang *et al.* (2002) suggested that authors should avoid the terms implant success and failure and report data on implant survival in combination with incidence of complications. It was also recommended that data should be provided on a subject basis. The majority of publications in implant dentistry, however, describe results based on number or proportions of implants. This information is of limited value for the clinician and, hence, data that relate the outcome of treatment for the patient under examination should be required.

Recently subject-based data on peri-implantitis were presented. Fransson *et al.* (2005) evaluated the prevalence of subjects with progressive bone loss at implants with a function time of at least 5 years. Radiographs of 1346 patients who had attended annual follow-up visits at the Brånemark Clinic, Göteborg, Sweden were retrieved. 662 subjects fulfilled the inclusion criteria. Implants that had suffered bone loss amounting to three or more threads of an implant were identified. Progressive bone loss at implants in the study was defined as bone loss occurring between the 1-year examination and the 5 or more years of follow-up examination. It was reported that 27.8% (184) of the 662 included subjects had one or more implants with "progressive" bone loss. A logistic regression analysis revealed that the individuals in this group carried a significantly larger number of implants than the subjects in whom no implants with progressive loss were detected (6 vs. 4.8). Furthermore, >30% of the subjects in the group with progressive bone loss had three or more identified implants and about 33% of all such implants in this group exhibited extensive bone loss. Out of the total 3413 implants included in the study, 423 implants (12.4%) demonstrated progressive bone loss. Fransson *et al.* (2005) concluded that the prevalence of progressive bone loss at implants assessed from subject-based data is higher than that evaluated from implant-based data. In a subsequent clinical study Fransson *et al.* (2007) reported that about 94% of the implants with "progressive" bone loss exhibited BoP. Thus, according to the definition of peri-implantitis presented in this chapter, the findings in the study by Fransson *et al.* (2005) suggest that the prevalence of subjects with peri-implantitis within this implant population was about 28%.

Roos-Jansåker *et al.* (2006b) examined 216 implant-treated patients (Brånemark System®) after 9–14 years of function and reported that 16% of the subjects and 6.6% of the implants had peri-implantitis. Roos-Jansåker *et al.* (2006b), however, used a modified definition of peri-implantitis and suggested that a certain amount of bone loss (≥1.8 mm compared with the 1-year data) together with the finding of BoP was required for the diagnosis *peri-implantitis*. It should be pointed out, however, that the prevalence of implants with peri-implantitis in the study by Roos-Jansåker *et al.* (2006b) would be >43% if normal criteria for peri-implantitis, i.e. bone loss and BoP, were applied.

Conclusion

The majority of clinical studies reported in the literature did not provide sufficient data on the prevalence of peri-implant mucositis and peri-implantitis. Results from recent publications, however, indicate that both peri-implant mucositis and peri-implantitis are common disorders. The prevalence of subjects with peri-implantitis in more recent studies varied between 25 and 45%.

Histopathology

Microscopic examinations of tissues harvested from peri-implantitis sites in humans consistently revealed that the mucosa contained large inflammatory cell infiltrates. Sanz *et al.* (1991) analyzed soft tissue biopsies from six patients with peri-implantitis and reported that 65% of the connective tissue portion was occupied by an inflammatory lesion. Piattelli *et al.* (1998) described some pathological features of tissues harvested from 230 retrieved implants. It was reported that at sites where implants were removed due to peri-implantitis, "an inflammatory infiltrate, composed of macrophages, lymphocytes and plasma cells, was found in the connective tissue around the implants". In a study including 12 human peri-implantitis lesions, Berglundh *et al.* (2004) found that the mucosa contained very large lesions in which numerous plasma cells, lymphocytes, and macrophages were present (Fig. 24-9). It was furthermore observed that the inflammatory cell infiltrate consistently extended to an area apical to the pocket epithelium and that the apical part of the soft tissue lesion frequently reached the bone tissue. Berglundh *et al.* (2004) also reported that numerous neutrophil granulocytes (PMN cells) were present in the lesions. Such cells occurred not only in the pocket epithelium and associated areas of the lesions, but also in perivascular compartments in the center of the infiltrate, i.e. distant from the implant surface. In the apical part of the lesion the inflamed connective tissue appeared to be in direct contact with the biofilm on the implant surface. Gualini and Berglundh (2003) included six subjects in a study and used immunohistochemical techniques to analyze the composition of peri-implantitis. PMN cells were found in large numbers in the central portions of the infiltrate. This finding was in agreement with observations made by Hultin *et al.* (2002). They analyzed the exudate that could be harvested from implant sites in 17 patients with peri-implantitis and reported the presence of large numbers of PMN cells.

Experimental models

In order to study the ability of the peri-implant mucosa to respond to long-standing plaque exposure and to manage the associated inflammatory lesions, an experimental periodontitis/peri-implantitis model was developed in the dog (Lindhe *et al.* 1992) and in

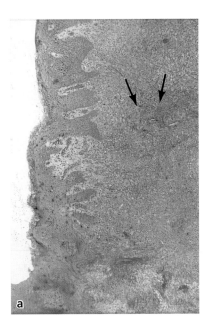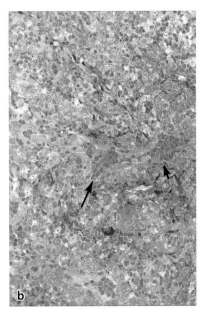

Fig. 24-9 (a) Microphotograph illustrating a human peri-implantitis lesion. Note the large inflammatory infiltrate lateral to the pocket epithelium. The implant was positioned to the left. (b) Arrows indicate vascular units illustrated in a larger magnification.

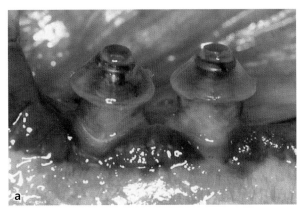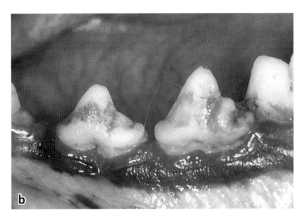

Fig. 24-10 (a) A clinical view describing features of experimental peri-implantitis in the beagle dog. (b) A clinical view describing features of experimental periodontitis in the beagle dog.

the monkey (Lang *et al.* 1993; Schou *et al.* 1993). Although the experiments had somewhat varying design, the outcome of the studies was almost identical and, hence, only the result from the dog model will be reported.

In the *dog model*, the premolars were extracted in one side of the mandible, fixtures (Brånemark system®) were inserted and abutment connection performed 3 months later as described above (Berglundh *et al.* 1991). During the healing phase a strict plaque control regimen was maintained and healthy tissue conditions were thereby established in all tooth and implant sites to be monitored. On a given day, the periodontitis and peri-implantitis lesions were induced. This was accomplished by (1) terminating the plaque control regimen and (2) placing cotton floss ligatures around the neck of both the premolar teeth and the implants. The ligatures were forced into a position apical to the soft tissue margins. A "pocket" between the tooth/gingiva and implant/mucosa was thereby created, a submarginal microbiota rapidly formed, and inflammatory lesions

developed in the neighboring tissues. Radiographs obtained after 6 weeks of the experiment revealed that a substantial amount of bone tissue had been lost at both teeth and implant sites. The ligatures were removed. After another 4 weeks, the animals were re-examined (Fig. 24-10), radiographs obtained, bacteria sampled, and biopsies of tooth and implant sites harvested.

It was observed that the plaque that had formed in the deep "pockets" was similar at tooth and implant sites and was dominated by Gram-negative and anaerobic species (Leonhardt *et al.* 1992). This observation is consistent with findings indicating that, in humans, the microbiota at teeth and implants has many features in common but also that the microbiota at healthy and diseased sites – tooth sites as well as implant sites – is very different. Thus, implants and teeth that are surrounded by healthy soft tissues are associated with biofilms including small amounts of Gram-positive coccoid cells and rods. Sites with extensive periodontal and peri-implant inflammation harbor biofilms with large numbers of

Gram-negative anaerobic bacteria (for review see Mombelli 1999).

The histopathologic examination of the biopsy samples from the dog study (Lindhe *et al.* 1992) revealed that there were marked differences in the size and location of the inflammatory lesions of the two sites. Thus, while the lesions in the periodontal sites (Fig. 24-11) were consistently separated from the alveolar bone by a zone, about 1 mm high, of uninflamed connective tissue, the lesion in the peri-implant tissue in most situations extended into and involved the marrow spaces of the alveolar bone. It

was concluded that the pattern of spread of inflammation was different in periodontal and peri-implant tissues. The lesions in plaque-associated periodontitis were limited to the connective tissue, while in the peri-implant tissues the lesions extended to the alveolar bone (Fig. 24-12).

It was suggested that the peri-implant tissues, in variance with the periodontal tissues, are poorly organized to resolve progressive, plaque-associated lesions. The validity of this conclusion was substantiated in subsequent studies (Marinello *et al.* 1995; Ericsson *et al.* 1996; Persson *et al.* 1996; Gotfredsen *et al.* 2002), using similar models but allowing for different periods of tissue breakdown.

It was also reported that peri-implantitis lesions, which initially were experimentally induced by ligatures as reported above, could spontaneously progress after the removal of the ligatures. Thus, Zitzmann *et al.* (2004) prepared 21 sites with ligature-induced experimental peri-implantitis in five Labrador dogs. After the lesions had become established, the ligatures were removed and the sites were monitored for an additional 12-month interval. It was observed that in 16 sites the aggressive peri-implantitis conditions persisted and caused continuous bone loss. In the remaining five sites, however, the lesions became encapsulated and no further breakdown of peri-implant bone took place. Using a similar model, Berglundh *et al.* (2007) evaluated progression of peri-implantitis at implants with different surface roughness. Experimental peri-implantitis was induced at implants with either a sandblasted acid-etched surface (SLA) or a polished surface. The ligatures were removed when about 40% of the height of the supporting bone had been lost and plaque accumulation continued during an additional 5 months. It was reported that following ligature removal the progression of bone loss was larger at SLA than at

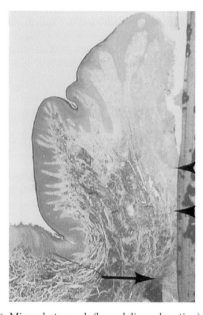

Fig. 24-11 Microphotograph (buccal–lingual section) illustrating a periodontitis lesion. Note the apical extension of the infiltrate (arrow) but also the presence of a zone of normal connective tissue between the infiltrate and the bone crest (arrow).

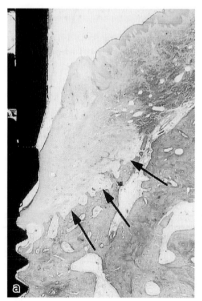
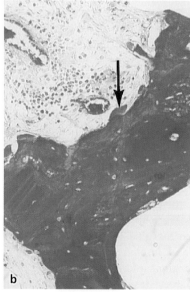

Fig. 24-12 (a) Ground section illustrating a peri-implantitis lesion. The implant is positioned to the left and the apical portions of the infiltrate (arrows) extend into contact with the bone. (b) Close-up of (a) illustrating the presence of inflammatory cells and osteoclasts (arrow) on the bone surface.

polished sites. The histologic examination revealed that both bone loss and the size of the inflammatory lesion in the connective tissue were larger in SLA than in polished implant sites. The area of plaque was also larger at implants with a SLA surface than at implants with a polished surface. It was concluded that the progression of peri-implantitis, if left untreated, is more pronounced at implants with a moderately rough surface than at implants with a polished surface.

Conclusion

Peri-implantitis lesions are poorly encapsulated, extend to the marginal bone tissue and may, if they are allowed to progress, lead to the loss of the implant. The large numbers of neutrophils in the peri-implantitis lesion and the absence of an epithelial lining between the lesion and the biofilm, indicate that the peri-implantitis lesions have features that are different from those of periodontitis lesions. Progres-

sion of peri-implantitis is more pronounced at implants with rough than at smooth surfaces.

Summary

Studies in man and experiments in animals have documented that *de novo* formation of a biofilm on the implant surface initiates a host response that involves the establishment of an inflammatory lesion in the peri-implant mucosa (peri-implant mucositis). This lesion is initially located in the connective tissue immediately lateral to the barrier epithelium and is, in many respects, similar to that which develops in the gingiva when plaque forms on adjacent tooth surfaces. In the continued presence of a submarginal biofilm, the lesion in the marginal mucosa around implants may occasionally spread in an "apical" direction to involve the hard tissue, compromise osseointegration, cause varying degrees of marginal bone loss (peri-implantitis), and eventually the loss of the implant.

References

Abrahamsson, I., Berglundh, T. & Lindhe, J. (1998). Soft tissue response to plaque-formation at different implant systems. A comparative study in the dog. *Clinical Oral Implants Research* 9, 73–79.

Albrektsson, T. & Isidor, F. (1994). Consensus report: Implant therapy. In: Lang, N.P. & Karring, T., eds. *Proceedings of the 1st European Workshop on Periodontology*. Berlin: Quintessence, pp. 365–369.

Berglundh, T., Lindhe, J., Ericsson, I, Marinello, C.P., Liljenberg, B. & Thomsen, P. (1991). The soft tissue barrier at implants and teeth. *Clinical Oral Implants Research* 2, 81–90.

Berglundh, T., Lindhe, J., Ericsson, I, Marinello, C.P. & Liljenberg, B. (1992). Soft tissue reactions to de novo plaque formation at implants and teeth. An experimental study in the dog. *Clinical Oral Implants Research* 3, 1–8.

Berglundh, T., Persson, L. & Klinge, B. (2002). A systematic review on the incidence of biological and technical complications in implant dentistry reported in prospective longitudinal studies of at least 5 years. *Proceedings from the 4th European Workshop on Periodontology. Journal of Clinical Periodontology* 29 (Suppl), 197–212.

Berglundh, T., Gislason, Ö., Lekholm, U., Sennerby, L. & Lindhe, J. (2004). Histopathological observations on human periimplantitis lesions. *Journal of Clinical Periodontology* 31, 341–347.

Berglundh, T., Gotfredsen, K., Zitzmann, N., Lang, N.P. & Lindhe, J. (2007). Spontaneous progression of ligature induced periimplantatitis at implants with different surface roughness. An experimental study in dogs. *Clinical Oral Implants Research,* 18, 655–661.

Brägger, U., Aeschlimann, S., Bürgin, W., Hämmerle, C. & Lang, N.P. (2001). Biological and technical complications and failures with fixed partial dentures (FPD) on implants and teeth after four to five years of function. *Clinical Oral Implants Research* 12, 26–34.

Ericsson, I., Berglundh, T., Marinello, C.P., Liljenberg, B. & Lindhe, J. (1992). Long-standing plaque and gingivitis at implants and teeth in the dog. *Clinical Oral Implants Research* 3, 99–103.

Ericsson, I., Persson, L.G., Berglundh, T., Edlund, T. & Lindhe, J. (1996). The effect of antimicrobial therapy on peri-implantitis lesions. An experimental study in the dog. *Clinical Oral Implants Research* 7, 320–328.

Esposito, M., Hirsch, J.M., Lekholm, U. & Thomsen, P. (1998). Biological factors contributing to failures of osseointegrated oral implants. (I) Success criteria and epidemiology. *European Journal of Oral Sciences* 106, 527–551.

Fransson, C., Lekholm, U., Jemt, T. & Berglundh T. (2005). Prevalence of subjects with progressive loss at implants. *Clinical Oral Implants Research* 16, 440–446.

Fransson, C., Wennström, J. & Berglundh T. (2007). Clinical characteristics at implants with a history of progressive bone loss. *Clinical Oral Implants Research*, in press.

Gotfredsen, K., Berglundh, T. & Lindhe, J. (2002). Bone reactions at implants subjected to experimental peri-implantitis and static load. An experimental study in the dog. IV. *Journal of Clinical Periodontology* 29, 144–151.

Gualini, F. & Berglundh, T. (2003). Immunohistochemical characteristics of inflammatory lesions at implants. *Journal of Clinical Periodontology*, 30, 14–18.

Hultin, M., Gustafsson, A., Hallström, H., Johansson, L-Å, Ekfeldt, A. & Klinge, B. (2002). Microbiological findings and host response in patients with peri-implantitis. *Clinical Oral Implants Research* 13, 349–358.

Krajicek, D.D., Dooner, J. & Porter, K. (1984). Observations on the histologic features of the human edentulous ridge. Part I: Mucosal epithelium. *Journal of Prosthetic Dentistry* 52, 526–531.

Lang, N.P., Brägger, U., Walther, D., Beamer, B. & Kornman, K. (1993). Ligature-induced peri-implant infection in cynomolgus monkeys. *Clinical Oral Implants Research* 4, 2–11.

Lang, N.P., Karring, T. & Meredith, N. (2002). Consensus report. Group E summary. *Proceedings from the 4th European Workshop on Periodontology. Journal of Clinical Periodontology* 29 (Suppl), 232–234.

Lekholm, U., Adell, R., Lindhe, J., Brånemark, P.I., Eriksson, B., Rockler, B., Lindvall, A.M. & Yoneyama, T. (1986). Marginal tissue reactions at osseointegrated titanium fixtures. (II) A cross-sectional retrospective study. *International Journal of Oral & Maxillofacial Implants* 15, 53–61.

Leonhardt, Å., Berglundh, T., Ericsson, I. & Dahlén, G. (1992). Putative periodontal pathogens on titanium implants and teeth in experimental gingivitis and periodontitis in beagle dogs. *Clinical Oral Implants Research* 3, 112–119.

Liljenberg, B., Gualini, F., Berglundh, T., Tonetti, M. & Lindhe, J. (1996). Some characteristics of the ridge mucosa before and after implant installation. A prospective study in humans. *Journal of Clinical Periodontology* **23**, 1008–1013.

Liljenberg, B., Gualini, F., Berglundh, T., Tonetti, M. & Lindhe, J. (1997). Composition of plaque associated lesions in the gingiva and the periimplant mucosa in partially edentulous subjects. *Journal of Clinical Periodontology* **24**, 119–123.

Lindhe, J., Berglundh, T., Ericsson, I., Liljenberg, B. & Marinello, C.P. (1992). Experimental breakdown of periimplant and periodontal tissues. A study in the beagle dog. *Clinical Oral Implants Research* **3**, 9–16.

Löe, H., Theilade E. & Jensen S.B. (1965). Experimental gingivitis in man. *Journal of Periodontology* **36**, 177–187.

Marinello, C.P., Berglundh, T., Ericsson, I., Klinge, B., Glantz, P.O. & Lindhe, J. (1995). Resolution of ligature-induced peri-implantitis lesions in the dog. *Journal of Clinical Periodontology* **22**, 475–480.

Mombelli, A. (1999). Prevention and therapy of peri-implant infections. In: Lang, N.P., Karring, T. & Lindhe, J., eds. *Proceedings of the 3rd European Workshop on Periodontology*. Berlin: Quintessence, pp. 281–303.

Mombelli, A. & Lang, N.P. (1998). The diagnosis and treatment of periimplantitis. *Periodontology* **17**, 63–76.

Persson, L.G., Ericsson, I., Berglundh, T. & Lindhe, J. (1996). Guided bone generation in the treatment of periimplantitis, *Clinical Oral Implants Research* **7**, 366–372.

Piattelli, A., Scarano, A. & Piattelli, M. (1998). Histologic observations on 230 retrieved dental implants: 8 years' experience (1989–1996). *Journal of Periodontology* **69**, 178–184.

Pontoriero, R., Tonelli, M.P., Carnevale, G., Mombelli, A., Nyman, S. & Lang, N.P. (1994). Experimentally induced peri-implant mucositis. A clinical study in humans. *Clinical Oral Implants Research* **5**, 254–259.

Roos-Jansåker, A.M., Lindahl, C., Renvert, H. & Renvert, S. (2006a). Nine- to fourteen-year follow-up of implant treatment. Part I: implant loss and associations to various factors. *Journal of Clinical Periodontology* **33**, 283–289.

Roos-Jansåker, A.M., Lindahl, C., Renvert, H. & Renvert, S. (2006b). Nine- to fourteen-year follow-up of implant treatment. Part II: presence of peri-implant lesions. *Journal of Clinical Periodontology* **33**, 290–295.

Roos-Jansåker, A.M., Renvert, H., Lindahl, C. & Renvert, S. (2006c) Nine- to fourteen-year follow-up of implant treatment. Part III: factors associated with peri-implant lesions. *Journal of Clinical Periodontology* **33**, 296–301.

Sanz, M., Aladez, J., Lazaro, P., Calvo, J.L., Quirynen, M. & van Steenberghe, D. (1991). Histopathologic characteristics of peri-implant soft tissues in Brånemark implants with two distinct clinical and radiological patterns. *Clinical Oral Implants Research* **2**, 128–134.

Schou, S., Holmstrup, P., Stoltze, K., Hjørting-Hansen, E. & Kornman, K.S. (1993). Ligature-induced marginal inflammation around osseointegrated implants and ankylosed teeth. Clinical and radiographic observations in Cynomolgus monkeys. *Clinical Oral Implants Research* **4**, 12–22.

Türk, D. (1965). A histologic comparison of the edentulous denture and nondenture bearing tissues. *Journal of Prosthetic Dentistry* **15**, 419–434.

van Steenberge, D., Klinge, B., Lindén, U., Quirynen, M., Herrmann, I. & Garpland, C. (1993). Periodontal indices around natural titanium abutments: A longitudinal multicenter study. *Journal of Periodontology* **64**, 538–541.

Weyant, R.J. (1994). Characteristics associated with the loss and peri-implant tissue health of endosseous dental implants. *International Journal of Oral and Maxillofacial Implants* **9**, 95–102.

Weyant, R.J. & Burt, B.A. (1993). An assessment of survival rates and within-patient clustering of failures for endosseous oral implants. *Journal of Dental Research* **72**, 2–8.

Zitzmann, N.U., Berglundh, T., Marinello, C.P. & Lindhe, J. (2001). Experimental periimplant mucositis in man. *Journal of Clinical Periodontology* **28**, 517–523.

Zitzmann, N.U., Berglundh, T., Ericsson, I. & Lindhe, J. (2004). Spontaneous progression of experimentally induced peri-implantitis. *Journal of Clinical Periodontology* **31**, 845–849.

Part 8: Tissue Regeneration

Chapter 25

Concepts in Periodontal Tissue Regeneration

Thorkild Karring and Jan Lindhe

Introduction

At risk assessment in periodontal patients, the presence of sites with a residual pocket depth ≥6 mm after active treatment plays a significant role in predicting future periodontal destruction (Haffajee *et al.* 1991; Grbic & Lamster 1992; Claffey & Egelberg 1995). Thus, an important goal of periodontal therapy is to obtain a reduced pocket depth after treatment in order to prevent further disease progression. Usually, this goal can be accomplished by non-surgical therapy in patients with moderate periodontitis, whereas in severe cases, particularly in the presence of intrabony defects and furcations, the treatment must be supplemented with periodontal surgery. A fundamental objective of periodontal surgery is to provide access for proper instrumentation and cleaning of the root surface; in addition, most surgical procedures result in the elimination or the reduction of the soft tissue component of the periodontal pocket. Generally, the elimination of deep pockets is achieved by gingivectomy or apical displacement of raised tissue flaps, sometimes associated with bone contouring. In recent years, however, the use of regenerative procedures aimed at restoring the lost periodontal support has become more common.

Periodontal treatment, both surgical and non-surgical, results in recession of the gingival margin after healing (Isidor *et al.* 1984). In severe cases of periodontitis, this may lead to poor esthetics in the front areas of the dentition, in particular when applying surgical procedures including bone contouring for the eradication of bone defects. Treatment of such cases without bone contouring, on the other hand, may result in residual pockets inaccessible to proper cleaning during post-treatment maintenance. These problems can be avoided or reduced by applying regenerative surgical procedures by which the lost periodontal attachment in the bone defects can be restored. Thus, the indication of applying regenerative periodontal therapy is often based on esthetic considerations, besides the fact that the function or long-term prognosis of the treated teeth may be improved.

Localized gingival recession and root exposure may represent an esthetic problem to the patient, and it is often associated with root sensitivity. Such a situation is an indication to apply regenerative periodontal therapy to obtain root coverage in order to improve esthetics and reduce root sensitivity. Successful root coverage implies regeneration of the attachment apparatus on the exposed root surface including cementum with inserting collagen fibers, as well as an esthetically acceptable restoration of the anatomy of the mucogingival complex.

Another indication for regenerative periodontal therapy is furcation-involved teeth. The furcation area is often inaccessible to adequate instrumentation and frequently the roots present concavities and furrows which make proper cleaning of the area after resective surgery impossible. Considering the long-term results and complications reported following treatment of furcation involvements by traditional resective therapy (Hamp *et al.* 1975; Bühler 1988), it is reasonable to anticipate that the long-term prognosis of furcation-involved teeth can be improved considerably by successful regenerative periodontal therapy.

Case reports also exist demonstrating that "hopeless" teeth with deep vertical defects, increased tooth mobility or through-and-through furcations can be successfully treated with regenerative periodontal therapy (Gottlow *et al.* 1986). However, controlled clinical trials or serial case reports presenting a reasonable predictability of treating such advanced cases are not available.

Regenerative periodontal surgery

Regenerative periodontal therapy comprises procedures which are specially designed to restore those parts of the tooth-supporting apparatus which have been lost due to periodontitis. Regeneration is defined as a reproduction or reconstruction of a lost or injured part in such a way that the architecture and function of the lost or injured tissues are completely restored (Glossary of Periodontal Terms, 1992). This means that the attachment of the tooth has been regenerated when new cementum with inserting collagen fibers has formed on the detached root surface, while regeneration of the periodontal supporting apparatus (periodontium) also includes re-growth of the alveolar bone. Procedures aimed at restoring lost periodontal support have also been described as "reattachment" or "new attachment" procedures.

The term "reattachment" was used to describe the regeneration of a fibrous attachment to a root surface surgically or mechanically deprived of its periodontal ligament tissue, whereas the term "new attachment" was preferred in the situation where the fibrous attachment was restored on a root surface deprived of its connective tissue attachment due to the progression of periodontitis. Research findings, however, indicate that there is no difference regarding the possibility of restoring a connective tissue attachment, whether this has been lost because of periodontal disease or mechanically removed (Nyman *et al.* 1982; Isidor *et al.* 1985). Therefore, it was suggested that the term "new attachment" should be used to describe the formation of new cementum with inserting collagen fibers on a root surface deprived of its periodontal ligament tissue, whether or not this has occurred because of periodontal disease or by mechanical means, and that the term "reattachment" should be confined to describing the reunion of surrounding soft tissue and a root surface with preserved periodontal ligament tissue (Isidor *et al.* 1985).

Periodontal regeneration has been reported following a variety of surgical approaches involving root surface biomodification, often combined with coronally advanced flap procedures, the placement of bone grafts or bone substitute implants, or the use of organic or synthetic barrier membranes (guided tissue regeneration). However, many cases that clinically are considered successful, including cases with significant regrowth of alveolar bone, may histologically show an epithelial lining along the treated root surface instead of deposition of new cementum (Listgarten & Rosenberg 1979).

Successful regeneration is assessed by periodontal probing, radiographic analysis, direct measurements of new bone, and histology. Although histology remains the ultimative standard in assessing true periodontal regeneration, periodontal probing, direct bone measurements, and radiographic measurements of osseous changes are used in the majority of studies of regenerative therapy (Reddy & Jeffcoat 1999).

At the American Academy of Periodontology World Workshop in Periodontics in 1996, the fulfillment of the following criteria was required in order for a periodontal regenerative procedure to be considered as a therapy which can encourage regeneration:

- Human histologic specimens demonstrating formation of new cementum, periodontal ligament, and bone coronal to a notch indicating the apical extension of the periodontitis-affected root surface.
- Controlled human clinical trials demonstrating improved clinical probing attachment and bone.
- Controlled animal histologic studies demonstrating formation of new cementum, periodontal ligament, and bone.

In addition, however, it seems reasonable to require that a regenerative procedure is based on a biological concept which can explain why the treatment results in periodontal regeneration on the basis of current knowledge about periodontal wound healing.

Periodontal wound healing

Regeneration of the periodontium must include the formation of new cementum with inserting collagen fibers on the previously periodontitis-involved root surfaces and the regrowth of the alveolar bone. However, whether regrowth of alveolar bone should always be considered a requirement for success following regenerative periodontal surgery is a matter of discussion. The basis for this discussion is that a fibrous attachment may exist without opposing bone in a normal dentition, not affected by periodontitis, in the presence of bone dehiscenses and fenestrations (see Fig. 1-74).

In 1976, Melcher suggested in a review paper that the type of cell which repopulates the root surface after periodontal surgery determines the nature of the attachment that will form. After flap surgery the curetted root surface may be repopulated by four different types of cell (Fig. 25-1):

1. Epithelial cells
2. Cells derived from the gingival connective tissue
3. Cells derived from the bone
4. Cells derived from the periodontal ligament.

Previously, in most attempts to restore lost tooth support, particular attention was directed towards the regeneration of the alveolar bone. An investigation was carried out in dogs in order to examine the relationship between the re-establishment of a connective tissue attachment to the root surface and the regrowth of alveolar bone (Nyman & Karring 1979). After elevation of mucoperiostal flaps, the marginal 5–7 mm of the buccal alveolar bone of each experimental tooth was removed (Fig. 25-2). During this procedure, care was taken to minimize the mechanical injury to the connective tissue attachment on the root surface. Prior to flap closure, a notch, serving as a landmark for the histologic measurements, was prepared in the root surface at the level of the surgically reduced bone crest. After 8 months of healing, the animals were sacrificed. Histologic analysis demonstrated that although a connective tissue attachment was re-established consistently on the roots, the amount of bone regeneration varied widely. In some roots, bone regrowth was negligible (Fig. 25-3), whereas in others the bone had regenerated to its normal level. These results demonstrated that the amount of bone regrowth is unrelated to the re-establishment of a connective tissue attachment.

Another experiment was carried out in monkeys (Lindhe *et al.* 1984), in order to examine whether the presence of bone may stimulate the formation of a new connective tissue attachment. Mandibular and maxillary incisors were extracted and re-implanted

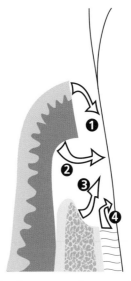

Fig. 25-1 Following flap surgery, the curetted root surface may be repopulated by (1) epithelial cells, (2) gingival connective tissue cells, (3) bone cells, or (4) periodontal ligament cells.

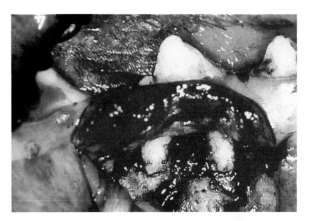

Fig. 25-2 Following flap elevation, the buccal bone, including a part of the inter-radicular and interproximal alveolar bone, is removed without injuring the connective tissue attachment on the root surface.

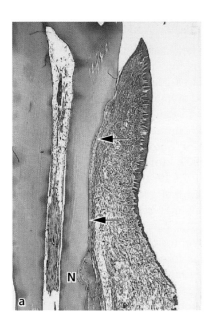

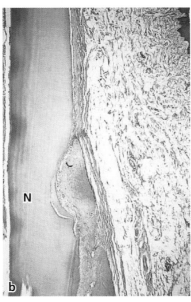

Fig. 25-3 (a) Microphotograph of specimen 8 months following bone removal. A connective tissue attachment is re-established (arrows). Bone regeneration is negligible and is confined to the notch (N) in the root surface. (b) Higher magnification of the newly formed bone in the notch area (N).

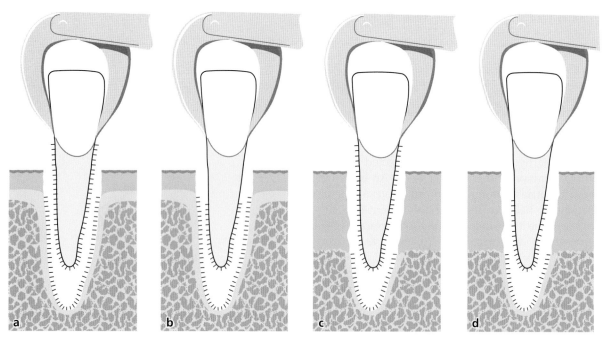

Fig. 25-4 Schematic drawing showing the four experimental conditions (a–d) under which experimental teeth were extracted and re-implanted in their own sockets.

in their own sockets under the following four experimental conditions (Fig. 25-4):

1. Non-root-planed teeth were re-implanted into sockets with normal bone height.
2. Teeth, root planed in their coronal portion, were re-implanted into sockets with normal bone height.
3. Non-root-planed teeth were re-implanted into sockets with a reduced bone height.
4. Teeth, root planed in their coronal portion, were re-implanted into sockets with reduced bone height.

Histologic examination after 6 months of healing revealed that a fibrous reunion was established in areas where the periodontal connective tissue attachment was retained at the time of re-implantation. However, in areas, where the periodontal ligament tissue was removed, the epithelium had always migrated to the apical extension of root instrumentation (Fig. 25-5). These results of healing occurred irrespective of the presence or absence of bone, indicating that the establishment of a connective tissue attachment is unrelated to the presence of alveolar bone.

Using orthodontic appliances, Karring *et al.* (1982) tilted maxillary second and third incisors in labial direction in dogs. Subsequently, these teeth were moved back to their original position. During the same period the contralateral incisors were moved to a labially deviated position. The orthodontic appliances were then used to retain the teeth in these positions for a period of 5 months before sacrifice of the animals. Histologic analysis demonstrated that in all experimental teeth, the apical termination of the

junctional epithelium was at the cemento-enamel junction. In the teeth which were retained in their labially displaced position, the level of the alveolar bone was reduced to a position about 4.5 mm apical to the cemento-enamel junction (Fig. 25-6a), while in the teeth which were moved back to their original position, the alveolar bone crest was located at a normal level relative to the cemento-enamel junction (Fig. 25-6b). This experiment demonstrated that bone resorption or bone regeneration may be induced by orthodontic forces on teeth with a pristine connective tissue attachment. The experiments described above indicate that the re-establishment of a connective tissue attachment to the root surface and the regeneration of the alveolar bone are not related to each other.

The use of bone grafts in regenerative periodontal therapy is based on the assumption that the promotion of bone regrowth may also induce cells in the bone to produce a new cementum layer with inserting collagen fibers on previously periodontitis-involved root surfaces. However, histologic studies in both humans and animals have demonstrated that grafting procedures often result in healing with a long junctional epithelium rather than a new connective tissue attachment (Caton & Zander 1976; Listgarten & Rosenberg 1979; Moscow *et al.* 1979).

Ellegaard *et al.* (1973, 1974, 1975, 1976) and Nielsen *et al.* (1980) reported that grafting materials in periodontal bony defects may be:

1. Osteoproliferative (osteogenetic), which means that new bone is formed by bone-forming cells contained in the grafted material.
2. Osteoconductive, which means that the grafted material does not contribute to new bone forma-

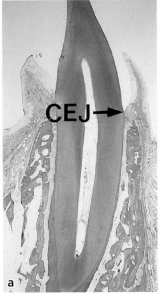
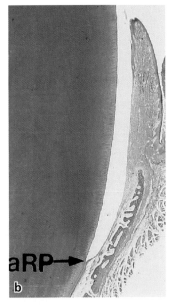
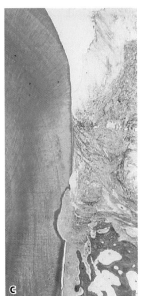
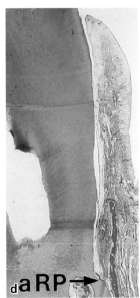

Fig. 25-5 Microphotographs showing the histological features after 6 months of healing, under the four experimental conditions (a–d) illustrated in Fig. 25-4. The teeth in (b) and (d) are those root planed in their coronal portion, and the teeth (a) and (b) are those re-implanted in sockets with normal bone height. A fibrous reunion was established in areas where the connective tissue attachment was retained (a and c) while the epithelium has migrated to the apical extension of root instrumentation (a RP) where the attachment was removed (b and d). CEJ = cemento-enamel junction.

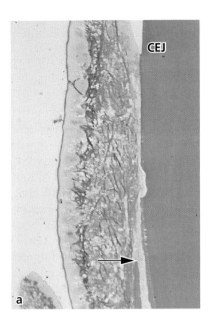
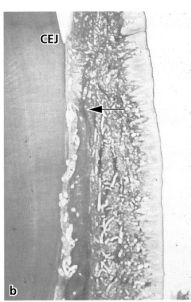

Fig. 25-6 Microphotograph of a tooth retained in its labially displaced position (a) and a tooth (b) moved back to its original position. The level of alveolar bone (arrow) is reduced in (a) while it has regenerated to its normal level (arrow) in (b). The apical termination of the junctional epithelium is at the cemento-enamel junction (CEJ) in both situations.

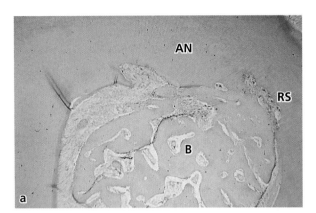

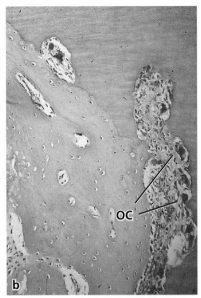

Fig. 25-7 (a) Microphotograph of furcation 6 weeks after grafting with iliac crest marrow. The furcation is completely filled with bone (B), but ankylosis (AN) and root resorption (RS) can be seen. (b) Higher magnification of the area in (a) showing ankylosis and resorption. OC = osteoclasts.

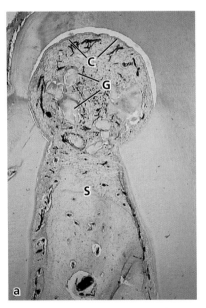

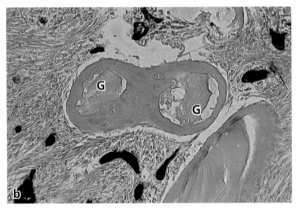

Fig. 25-8 (a) Microphotograph of a healed bifurcation defect following transplantation of non-vital bone grafts. The grafts (G) have not been reached by bone formation from the interradicular septum (S), but occur as isolated particles surrounded by "cementum". Cementum (C) and new connective tissue attachment formation have taken place along the entire circumference of the bifurcation. (b) High magnification of isolated bone grafts (G) with newly formed "cementum" on the surface.

tion *per se* but serves as scaffold for bone formation originating from adjacent host bone.

3. Osteoinductive, which means that bone formation is induced in the surrounding soft tissue immediately adjacent to the grafted material.

These studies, where various types of bone graft were placed in intrabony defects or inter-radicular lesions, revealed that cells survived transplantation only in iliac bone marrow grafts. Transplantation of iliac bone marrow grafts almost consistently resulted in bone fill in the experimental defects, but healing

was frequently accompanied by ankylosis and root resorption (Fig. 25-7). The iliac bone marrow grafts exerted an osteogeneic effect, and it was suggested that this was responsible for the induction of root resorption (Ellegaard *et al.* 1973, 1974). Jaw bone grafts and xenografts did not actively contribute to bone formation but served as a scaffold for bone regeneration (i.e. osteoconductive effect). Often, however, these bone grafts were not reached by the new bone growing out from the host bone, but occurred as isolated particles surrounded by a bone-like or cementum-like substance (Fig. 25-8). It was found that the treated bifurcation defects became filled mainly with granulation tissue derived from the periodontal ligament (Fig. 25-9). The authors (Nielsen *et al.* 1980) suggested that this invasion of ligament tissue inhibited bone formation and that the new cementum on the root surface in the bifurcation defects, including the cementum-like substance observed around the implanted bone particles, was formed by periodontal ligament cells (Fig. 25-8). Thus, it appeared from these studies that the key cells in periodontal regeneration are periodontal ligament cells rather than bone cells.

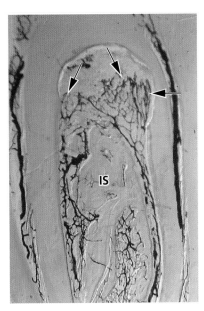

Fig. 25-9 Cleared specimen from a 1-week-old bifurcation defect treated with bone grafts. Judged from the course of the blood vessels, the granulation tissue in the defect has developed mainly from the periodontal ligament (arrows) and only to a minor extent from the inter-radicular septum (IS).

Regenerative capacity of bone cells

The ability of newly formed tissue originating from bone to produce a new connective tissue attachment was examined in a study by Karring *et al.* (1980). Roots of periodontitis-affected teeth were extracted and placed in surgically created sockets in edentulous areas of dogs. The implanted roots were covered with tissue flaps (submerged) and the results of healing were examined histologically after 3 months. A periodontal ligament was re-established in the apical portion of the re-implanted roots where, at the time of implantation, remnants of periodontal ligament tissue were preserved. In the coronal portion of the roots which were previously exposed to periodontitis and then scaled and planed, healing had consistently resulted in ankylosis and root resorption (Fig. 25-10). On the basis of this finding, it was concluded that tissue derived from bone lacks cells with the potential to produce a new connective tissue attachment.

Regenerative capacity of gingival connective tissue cells

Another experiment (Nyman *et al.* 1980) was carried out in order to examine the potential of gingival connective tissue to produce a new connective tissue attachment. The teeth were treated as described in the experiment above but were not transplanted into sockets. Instead they were placed in bone concavities prepared on the buccal aspect of the jaw and subsequently covered by tissue flaps. Thus, half the circumference of the roots was in contact with bone while the remaining part was facing the gingival connective tissue at the subsurface of the flaps. Histologic examination after 3 months of healing showed areas with periodontal ligament in the apical portion of the roots where, at the time of implantation,

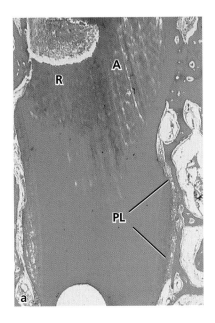
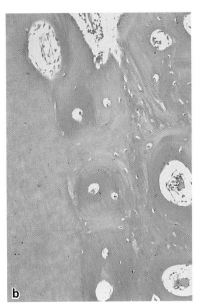

Fig. 25-10 (a) Microphotograph of a re-implanted root after 3 months of healing. A periodontal ligament (PL) has become re-established in the apical portion of the root whereas ankylosis (A) and root resorption (R) is the predominant feature in the coronal portion. (b) High magnification of the ankylosis seen in (a).

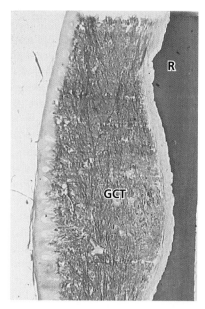

Fig. 25-11 Microphotograph of root (R) which has been re-implanted with its surface facing the gingival connective tissue (GCT). The surface exhibits extensive resorption.

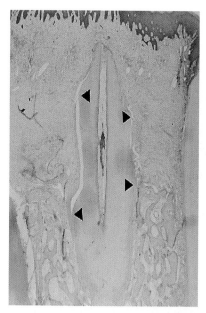

Fig. 25-12 Microphotograph showing new attachment formation (between the arrows) on a submerged root with a non-impaired periodontal ligament. Coronal to the cementum, root resorption is the predominant feature.

periodontal ligament tissue was preserved. In the coronal, previously exposed part of the roots, no signs of new connective tissue attachment were present. The root portion located in contact with gingival connective tissue demonstrated a connective tissue with fibers oriented parallel to the root surface and without attachment to the root. However, root resorption occurred at the majority of the surfaces (Fig. 25-11). On the basis of this result it was concluded that gingival connective tissue also lacks cells with the potential to produce a new connective tissue attachment.

Regenerative capacity of periodontal ligament cells

In the experiments described above, root resorption was also observed occasionally in the apical portion of the extracted and re-implanted roots (Karring *et al.* 1980; Nyman *et al.* 1980). It was suggested that this occurred because the periodontal ligament tissue retained on this part of the root had become injured during extraction, thereby allowing bone or gingival connective tissue to contact the root surface during healing and induce resorption. It was assumed that this damage of the retained periodontal ligament tissue had also restricted its potential of proliferating in the coronal direction along the root surface. Indeed, in a later study (Karring *et al.* 1985), where periodontitis-involved roots were retained in their sockets and subsequently submerged, significant amounts of new connective tissue attachment formed on the coronal portion of the roots (Fig. 25-12). The finding of new attachment only on the roots with a non-impaired periodontal ligament, but never on the extracted and re-implanted roots with an impaired ligament, indi-

cates that periodontal ligament tissue contains cells with the potential to form a new connective tissue attachment on a detached root surface.

Active root resorption occurred consistently at the root surfaces above the coronal extension of new attachment (Fig. 25-12). It was suggested that this resorption was induced by gingival connective tissue which had proliferated apically from the covering tissue flap. Thus, only cells in the periodontal ligament seem capable of regenerating lost periodontal attachment.

The final evidence that the progenitor cells for new attachment formation reside in the periodontal ligament was provided in studies in which titanium dental implants were placed in contact with retained root tips whose periodontal ligament served as a source for cells which could populate the implant surface during healing (Buser *et al.* 1990a,b; Warrer *et al.* 1993). Microscopic analysis revealed that a distinct layer of cementum with inserting collagen fibers had formed on the surfaces of the implants (Fig. 25-13a), and that these fibers, often oriented perpendicularly to the surface, were embedded in the opposite bone (Fig. 25-13b). Control implants (Fig. 25-14) placed without contact with retained roots healed with the characteristic features of osseointegration (i.e. direct contact between bone and the implant surface).

Further proof of the ability of periodontal ligament cells to produce a new connective tissue attachment was recently provided by Parlar *et al.* (2005) using a novel and unique experimental model in dogs. After resection of the crowns of the canine teeth in the dogs, the roots were hollowed to a depth of 5 mm. leaving a thin dentinal wall. Slits were then

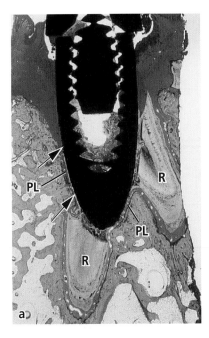
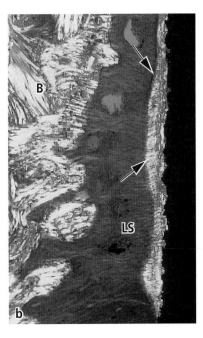

Fig. 25-13 (a) Microphotograph of a titanium implant placed in contact with retained root tips. A distinct cementum layer (arrows) and periodontal ligament (PL) in continuity with that on the roots (R) is visible on the implant surface. (b) High magnification in polarized light of the periodontal ligament formed around the implant seen in (a). A cementum layer (arrows) with Sharpey's fibers is present at the implant surface. Principal fibers, oriented perpendicular to the surface, are running across the ligament space (LS) and are inserting in the opposing bone (B) as in natural teeth (see Fig. 1-71).

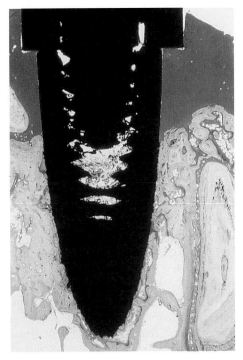

Fig. 25-14 Microphotograph of a titanium implant placed without contact with retained roots (control). This implant has healed with a direct contact between the bone and the implant surface (osseointegration).

prepared in the cavity wall to create passages from this chamber to the surrounding periodontal ligament. A titanium implant was placed into the center of each chamber, and finally a collagen barrier was placed over the chamber before the roots were submerged. Histologic analysis after 4 months of healing revealed that a periodontal ligament, bone, and root cementum had formed between the implant and the dentinal wall of the chamber. Due to the invasion of periodontal ligament tissue through the slits into the chamber, cementum had formed on the implant as well as the dentinal wall, and a periodontal ligament was consistently interposed between the implant and the bone and between the bone and the dentinal wall. Thus, there is strong evidence that the progenitor cells for periodontal attachment formation reside in the periodontal ligament and not in the alveolar bone as previously assumed (Melcher *et al.* 1987).

Role of epithelium in periodontal wound healing

Some of the roots in the experiment described above (Karring *et al.* 1985) penetrated the covering mucosa at early stages of healing, thereby allowing the epithelium to grow apically along the root surface. The amount of new connective tissue attachment on these roots was considerably smaller than that formed on the roots which remained submerged throughout the study. This finding and those of other investigators (Moscow 1964; Kon *et al.* 1969; Proye & Polson 1982) indicate that the apical migration of epithelium reduces the coronal gain of attachment, evidently by preventing periodontal ligament cells from repopulating the root surface (Fig. 25-15).

Downgrowth of epithelium into the periodontal lesion has most likely occurred to a varying extent during healing following most flap and grafting procedures applied in regenerative periodontal therapy, which may explain the varying results reported. This view is supported by the results of the monkey study by Caton *et al.* (1980). These investigators examined healing in ligature-induced periodontal lesions following treatment with four different modalities of regenerative surgical procedures:

1. Root planing and soft tissue curettage
2. Widman flap surgery without bone grafting

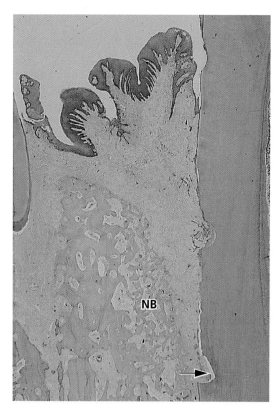

Fig. 25-15 Microphotograph illustrating an intrabony defect after regenerative treatment. New bone (NB) has formed in the defect but epithelium has migrated apically along the root surface to the notch (arrow) in the root surface indicating the bottom of the defect before treatment.

3. Widman flap surgery with the placement of frozen autogeneous red bone marrow and cancellous bone
4. Beta-tricalcium phosphate in intrabony defects.

Healing following all treatment modalities resulted in the formation of a long junctional epithelium extending to or close to the same level as before treatment.

Root resorption

In the experimental studies described previously, granulation tissue, derived from gingival connective tissue or bone, produced root resorption when contacting the curetted root surface during healing following surgery (Karring *et al.* 1980, 1985; Nyman *et al.* 1980). It should be expected, therefore, that this phenomenon would occur as a frequent complication to periodontal surgery, particularly following those procedures which include the placement of grafting materials to stimulate bone formation. The reason why root resorption is rarely seen is most likely that post-operatively, the dentogingival epithelium migrates apically along the root surface, forming a protective barrier towards the root surface (Fig. 25-15). This view is supported by the results of an experimental study in monkeys (Karring *et al.* 1984) in which roots, which previously had been subjected

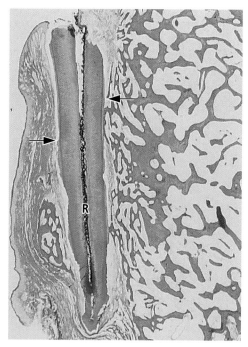

Fig. 25-16 Microphotograph of an implanted root (R) where epithelium was allowed to migrate into the wound after 2 weeks. The epithelium has migrated along the coronal, previously periodontitis-involved root surfaces down to the level indicated by the arrows. In the areas covered by epithelium, there are no signs of resorption. Apical to this level the root surfaces demonstrate root resorption.

to ligature-induced periodontitis, were extracted and re-implanted in contact with bone and connective tissue and covered with a tissue flap (submerged). After varying time intervals the submerged roots were exposed to the oral cavity by a second incision (wounding) through the covering mucosa, thereby permitting the epithelium to migrate into the wound. In specimens where the wounding occurred within 2 weeks (Fig. 25-16), the previously diseased part of the roots was covered by epithelium and showed no signs of resorption. With increasing intervals between implantation of the roots and the wounding, a steadily diminishing part of the diseased root surface was covered by epithelium, and root resorption and ankylosis became progressively pronounced (Fig. 25-17). This observation concurs with results presented by Björn *et al.* (1965) who treated 11 periodontally diseased teeth in seven human volunteers, using the submerging technique which prevented apical migration of the dentogingival epithelium. The authors reported that root resorption was indeed a common complication following this kind of therapy.

Regenerative concepts

One of the first methods used in attempts to obtain new attachment was scaling and root planing combined with soft tissue curettage (i.e. mechanical removal of the diseased root cementum and the pocket epithelium). Studies in humans (e.g. McCall 1926; Orban 1948; Beube 1952; Waerhaug 1952;

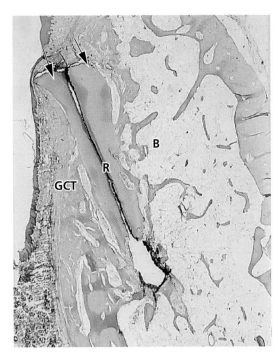

Fig. 25-17 Microphotograph of an implanted root (R) where epithelium was allowed to migrate into the wound after 4 weeks. The epithelium (arrows) covers only the coronal cut root surface. Extensive resorption is seen on the surface facing the gingival connective tissue (GCT) and resorption and ankylosis are seen on the surface facing the bone tissue (B).

Schaffer & Zander 1953; Carranza 1954, 1960) and in animals (e.g. Beube 1947; Ramfjord 1951; Kon *et al.* 1969) showed that this type of periodontal therapy resulted not only in the establishment of gingival health but also in a reduction of the initially recorded pocket depth. This decrease in the depth of the periodontal pocket was assumed to be partly the result of shrinkage of the initially inflamed gingiva, but partly also the effect of the formation of a new connective tissue attachment in the apical part of the pocket.

The possibility of obtaining new attachment became widely accepted with the work of Prichard (1957a,b), in which new attachment formation in intrabony periodontal lesions was reported as a predictable outcome of treatment. Seventeen cases were presented out of which four were subjected to a re-entry surgical procedure, revealing that these defects were filled with bone. The technique of Prichard (1957b, 1960) was only used for the treatment of three-wall intrabony defects, and the results obtained suggested that the morphology of the periodontal bony defect was essential for the establishment of a predictable prognosis. Goldman and Cohen (1958) introduced a classification of periodontal intrabony defects which was based on the number of osseous walls surrounding the defect, being either three-wall, two-wall or one-wall defects or a combination of such situations (Fig. 25-18).

The technique of Prichard (1957a,b, 1960) included the elevation of tissue flaps in order to get access to the defect. All granulation tissue in the defect was removed and the root surface was scaled and planed. In order to enhance regeneration of bone, small perforations were made with a bur at several sites of the bone walls. The flaps were sutured to accomplish complete coverage of the defect. Many clinical investigators have claimed that new attachment resulted following this type of treatment but there is little quantitative or qualitative documentation (Patur & Glickmann 1962; Wade 1962, 1966; Ellegaard & Löe 1971). Patur and Glickmann (1962) reported a clinical study including 24 intrabony defects treated according to the Prichard technique (1957a,b). The outcome was evaluated by comparing pre-operative and post-operative radiographs, measurements of the alveolar bone level adjacent to the root and study casts taken during operation and post-operatively after reflecting buccal and lingual flaps. The authors reported that new attachment had occurred in two-wall and three-wall intrabony defects but not in one-wall defects. Results from a study by Ellegaard and Löe (1971) comprising 191 defects in 24 patients with periodontal disease indicated that complete regeneration, determined radiographically and by periodontal probing, had occurred in around 70% of the three-wall defects, in 40% of the combined two-wall and three-wall defects, and in 45% of the two-wall defects.

In a later study by Rosling *et al.* (1976), 124 intrabony defects in 12 patients were treated by means of the modified Widman flap procedure (Ramfjord & Nissle 1974). Following treatment the patients were recalled twice per month for professional tooth cleaning. Re-examination performed clinically and on radiographs 2 years after therapy demonstrated bone fill-in of two-wall as well as three-wall defects. The authors suggested that this regrowth of bone was also associated with the formation of new connective tissue attachment and ascribed the successful healing mainly to the optimal standard of oral hygiene which was maintained in all patients during healing. A clinical study with almost identical results was presented by Polson & Heijl (1978). The results of several histologic studies in animals and humans, on the other hand, indicate that formation of new periodontal attachment is by no means predictable following subgingival curettage or flap surgery (Listgarten & Rosenberg 1979; Caton & Nyman 1980; Caton *et al.* 1980; Steiner *et al.* 1981; Stahl *et al.* 1983; Bowers *et al.* 1989a).

Grafting procedures

In a number of clinical trials and animal experiments, the flap approach was combined with the placement of bone grafts or implant materials into the curetted bony defects with the aim of stimulating periodontal regeneration. The various graft and

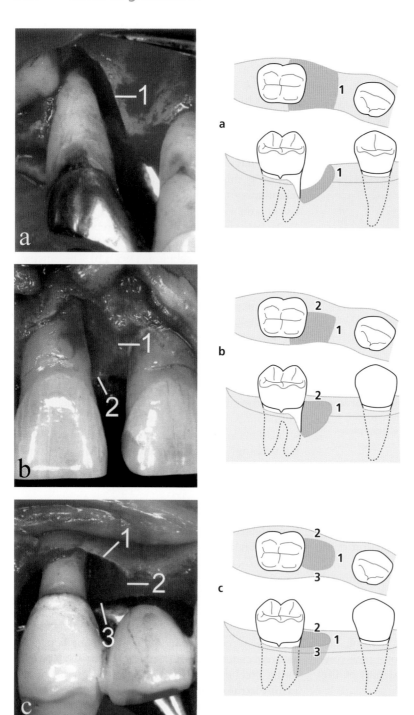

Fig. 25-18 Progression of periodontitis at a different rate on neighboring tooth surfaces results in the development of intrabony defects. Based on the number of surrounding bone walls such defects are classified as one-wall (a), two-wall (b) or three-wall (c) defects.

implant materials used so far can be placed into four categories:

1. *Autogenous grafts*: grafts transferred from one position to another within the same individual. This type of graft comprises (i) cortical bone or (ii) cancellous bone and marrow, and is harvested either from intraoral or extraoral donor sites.
2. *Allogeneic grafts*: grafts transferred between genetically dissimilar members of the same species. (i) Frozen cancellous bone and marrow, and (ii) freeze-dried bone have been used.
3. *Xenogeneic grafts*: grafts taken from a donor of another species.

4. *Alloplastic materials*: synthetic or inorganic implant materials which are used as substitutes for bone grafts.

The rationale behind the use of bone grafts or alloplastic materials is the assumption that both the regrowth of alveolar bone and the formation of new attachment would be stimulated because these materials may either (1) contain bone-forming cells (osteogenesis), or (2) serve as a scaffold for bone formation (osteoconduction), or because (3) the matrix of the bone grafts contains bone-inducing substances (osteoinduction) (Urist 1980; Brunsvold & Mellonig 1993). Such complete regeneration of the periodontal attachment apparatus following grafting procedures would imply, however, that cells derived from bone possess the ability to form new cementum with inserting collagen fibers on a previously periodontitis-involved root surface (Melcher *et al.* 1987). This assumption is in conflict with current knowledge about the biology of periodontal wound healing, that repopulation of the detached root surface with cells from the periodontal ligament is the prerequisite for new attachment formation. This means that all therapeutic procedures involving the placement of bone grafts or bone substitute implants are based on a biologic concept which cannot explain how such treatment should result in regeneration of the periodontium.

The effect of using bone grafts or alloplastic materials for periodontal regeneration has mainly been examined in case reports, while histologic evidence of new attachment and controlled clinical studies is limited. The results from such reports vary and the documentation presented usually consists of pre-operative and post-operative probing attachment levels, radiographic interpretations or re-entry procedures.

Autogenous grafts

Autogenous grafts (autografts) may retain some cell viability and are considered to promote bone healing mainly through osteogenesis and/or osteoconduction. They are gradually resorbed and replaced by new viable bone. In addition, potential problems of histocompatibility and disease transmission are eliminated with autogenous grafts. Autogenous grafts can be harvested from intraoral or extraoral sites.

Intraoral autogenous grafts
Intraoral autogenous grafts obtained from edentulous areas of the jaw, healing extraction sites, maxillary tuberosities or the mandibular retromolar area were commonly used in periodontal regenerative surgery (Mann 1964; Ellegaard & Löe 1971; Rosenberg 1971a,b; Dragoo & Sullivan 1973a,b; Hiatt & Schallhorn 1973; Froum *et al.* 1983; Stahl *et al.* 1983). Generally cancellous bone is preferred as graft material but cortical bone, applied as small chips (Rosenberg *et al.* 1979), or mixed with blood prior to the placement in the defects (Robinson 1969; Froum *et al.* 1976), was also reported to be effective in producing regeneration in periodontal intrabony defects.

The effect of intraoral autogenous grafts has been evaluated in both animals and humans. In a study in monkeys, Rivault *et al.* (1971) observed that intrabony defects filled with intraoral autogenous bone chips mixed with blood (osseous coagulum) healed with new bone formation, but no more bone was found in such experimental defects than was observed in similar control defects treated with surgical curettage. Other studies in monkeys and dogs also failed to demonstrate significant differences in bone formation between grafted and non-grafted intrabony or

furcation defects (Ellegaard *et al.* 1974; Coverly *et al.* 1975; Nilveus *et al.* 1978).

In clinical case series where intraoral autogenous grafts were used for the treatment of intrabony periodontal defects, a mean bone fill ranging from 3.0–3.5 mm was reported (Nabers & O'Leary 1965; Robinson 1969; Hiatt & Schallhorn 1973; Froum *et al.* 1975). Hiatt and Schallhorn (1973) treated 166 intrabony lesions with intraoral autogenous cancellous bone. They reported a mean increase in bone height of 3.5 mm, evaluated by clinical measurements. One-wall, two-wall, and three-wall defects were included, and the largest bone fill was observed in defects with the highest number of bone walls. A block section obtained from a patient treated in this study presented histologic evidence of new cementum, bone, and periodontal ligament formation. In controlled clinical studies, intraoral autogenous grafts were found superior to surgical debridement alone in terms of bone fill (Froum *et al.* 1976), or probing attachment (PAL) gain (Carraro *et al.* 1976) in two-wall defects. However, there are controlled studies that demonstrate more modest results regarding bone fill or PAL gain after intraoral grafting when compared to ungrafted controls (Ellegaard & Löe 1971; Renvert *et al.* 1985).

Ross and Cohen (1968) reported new bone and cementum formation in a human histologic specimen from an intrabony defect retrieved 8 months following debridement and placement of intraoral autogenous grafts. They also found that the grafts were without osteocytes and that the deposition of new alveolar bone had taken place around the grafts. Nabers *et al.* (1972) observed that new cementum and functionally oriented periodontal ligament fibers were present in half the length of a defect which was biopsied about 4.5 years after treatment with intraoral autogenous bone grafts. In other human histologic reports, bone fill and new attachment were observed coronal to reference notches placed on the treated roots at the apical termination of root planing (Hiatt *et al.* 1978) or at the most apical level of previously existing calculus (Froum *et al.* 1983; Stahl *et al.* 1983). Other investigators, however, observed an epithelial lining which occupied a varying portion of the previously diseased part of the root (Hawley & Miller 1975; Listgarten & Rosenberg 1979; Moscow *et al.* 1979). The results from these studies and those from a recent meta-analysis (Trombelli 2005) indicate that the treatment of periodontal osseous defects with intraoral bone grafts may result in periodontal regeneration, but not predictably.

Extraoral autogenous grafts
Schallhorn (1967, 1968) introduced the use of autogeneous hip marrow grafts (iliac crest marrow) in the treatment of furcation and intrabony defects. Later several studies were published demonstrating the osteogenic potentials of this material (Schallhorn *et al.* 1970; Schallhorn & Hiatt 1972; Patur 1974; Froum

et al. 1975), and as much as 3–4 mm gain in crestal bone was reported following the treatment of intrabony defects with hip marrow grafts. The effect of iliac crest marrow and of intraoral cancellous bone grafts in one-wall, two-wall, and three-wall bony defects in humans was evaluated by Patur (1974). He reported that bone fill occurred to a varying extent with both types of graft. The amount of bone fill in one-wall bony defects was larger with iliac crest marrow than with cancellous bone or when no grafts were used. Some defects within all three groups showed bone fill, and no difference was observed between the control defects and those treated with intraoral cancellous bone grafts. The author stated that even with fresh iliac crest marrow, bone regeneration is variable and unpredictable.

Healing of inter-radicular and intrabony lesions following placement of iliac crest marrow was evaluated in monkeys by Ellegaard *et al.* (1973, 1974). Regeneration occurred more frequently with the use of grafts, but iliac crest marrow frequently resulted in ankylosis and root resorption (Fig. 25-19).

Histologic evidence of periodontal regeneration in humans following the use of iliac crest marrow grafts was provided by Dragoo and Sullivan (1973a,b). At 8 months following therapy a mature periodontal

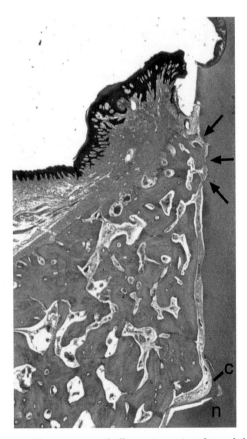

Fig. 25-19 Photomicrograph illustrating an intrabony defect 2 months following grafting with iliac crest marrow. The defect is completely filled with bone, but new cementum (c) is lacking on the root surface except for the most apical part (n) of the defect. Note that ankylosis and root resorption (arrows) are occurring in the coronal part of the defect.

ligament was present at the grafted sites and about 2 mm supracrestal new attachment had also formed. Clinical evidence of root resorption was noted in seven of the 250 grafted sites.

Due to the morbidity associated with the donor site and the fact that root resorption sometimes results, iliac crest marrow grafts are not used in regenerative periodontal therapy today.

Allogeneic grafts

Allogeneic grafts (allografts) were utilized in attempts to stimulate bone formation in intrabony defects in order to avoid the additional surgical insult associated with the use of autogenous grafts. However, the use of allogeneic grafts involves a certain risk regarding antigenicity, although the grafts are usually pretreated by freezing, radiation or chemicals in order to suppress foreign body reactions.

The types of allogeneic grafts used are frozen iliac cancellous bone and marrow, mineralized freeze-dried bone allogeneic grafts (FDBA), and decalcified freeze-dried alogeneic bone grafts (DFDBA). The need for cross matching to decrease the likelihood of graft rejection as well as the risk of disease transmission virtually eliminated the use of frozen iliac allogeneic grafts in periodontics.

FDBA is a mineralized bone graft, which loses cell viability through the manufacturing process and, therefore, is supposed to promote bone regeneration through osteoconduction/osteoinduction (Goldberg & Stevenson 1987). The freeze drying also markedly reduces the antigenicity of the material (Turner & Mellonig 1981; Quattlebaum *et al.* 1988). The efficacy of FDBA was evaluated in a study which included 89 clinicians (Mellonig 1991). At re-entry surgery it was found that 67% of the sites treated with FDBA alone and 78% of the sites treated with FDBA plus autogenous bone grafts demonstrated complete or more than 50% bone fill. Thus, FDBA plus autogenous bone appeared more effective than FDBA alone. In split-mouth studies where FDBA was combined with autogenous grafts or tetracycline powder (Sanders *et al.* 1983; Mabry *et al.* 1985), a defect fill of 60% and 80% of the initial lesion was reported. In a split-mouth study it was also shown that FDBA implantation had a similar effect on defect resolution as that achieved by DFDBA (Rummelhart *et al.* 1989) or granular porous hydroxyapatite (Barnett *et al.* 1989). However, the only controlled clinical trial comparing treatment of intrabony defects with FDBA implantation versus flap surgery failed to demonstrate any difference in terms of clinical attachment gain and bone fill between test and control sites at 1 year re-entry examination (Altiere *et al.* 1979). In addition, human histologic specimens demonstrated that implantation of FDBA in intrabony defects yielded no periodontal regeneration but resulted in a long epithelial attachment on the previously diseased root surface (Dragoo & Kaldahl 1983).

Several animal studies suggested that demineralization of a cortical bone allograft (DFDBA) enhances its osteogenic potential by exposing bone morphogenic proteins (BMPs) which presumably have the ability to induce host cells to differentiate into osteoblasts (Urist & Strates 1970; Mellonig *et al.* 1981). Several case reports presented clinical improvements and bone fill after implantation of DFDBA into intrabony defects (Quintero *et al.* 1982; Werbitt 1987; Fucini *et al.* 1993; Francis *et al.* 1995), and controlled clinical studies documented considerable gain of attachment and bone fill in sites treated with DFDBA as compared with non-grafted sites (Pearson *et al.* 1981; Mellonig 1984; Meadows *et al.* 1993). However, no statistical differences regarding attachment level changes and bone fill were found when comparing sites treated with FDBA and sites treated with DFDBA (Rummelhart *et al.* 1989).

Histologic evidence of regeneration following grafting with DFDBA was provided by Bowers *et al.* (1989b,c). Complete regeneration with new cementum, periodontal ligament, and bone amounting to 80% of the original defect depth was reported at sites treated with DFDBA, which was considerably more than that observed in defects treated with surgical debridement alone. However, animal experiments failed to confirm the regenerative potential of DFDBA grafting (Sonis *et al.* 1985; Caplanis *et al.* 1998).

The controversial results regarding the effect of DFDBA on the regeneration of periodontal intraosseous defects along with great differences in the osteoinductive potential (ranging from high to no osteoinductive effect) of commercially available DFDBA (Becker *et al.* 1994, 1995; Shigeyama *et al.* 1995; Schwartz *et al.* 1996; Garraway *et al.* 1998), and the (although minute) risk for disease transmission have raised concern about the clinical applicability of DFDBA. In EU countries, commercially available DFDBA is not granted a CE mark permitting distribution of the material within the community.

Xenogeneic grafts

The use of xenogeneic bone grafts (xenografts) in regenerative periodontal surgery was examined several years ago. Nielsen *et al.* (1981) treated 46 intrabony defects with Kielbone® (i.e. defatted and deproteinized ox bone) and another 46 defects with intraoral autogenous bone grafts. The results, which were evaluated by periodontal probing and radiographically, showed no difference between the amount of clinical gain of attachment and bone fill obtained in the two categories of defect. A study in monkeys also demonstrated that the two types of bone graft displayed similar histologic features and were frequently seen in the connective tissue of the healed defects as isolated bone particles surrounded by a cementum-like substance (Nielsen *et al.* 1980).

Recently, new processing and purification methods have been utilized which make it possible to remove all organic components from a bovine bone source and leave a non-organic bone matrix in an unchanged inorganic form (e.g. Bio-Oss®, Geistlich AG, Switzerland; Lubboc®/Laddec®, Ost Development SA, France; Endobone®, Biomet Inc. Dordrecht, The Netherlands; OsteoGraf®/N, DENTSPLY, Friadent Cera-Med, Lakewood, CO, USA; Cerabone®, aap Implantate AG, Berlin, Germany). However, differences in the purification and manipulation methods of the bovine bone have lead to commercially available products with different chemical properties and possibly different biologic behavior. These materials are available in different particle sizes or as block grafts.

To date, no controlled human study has compared the effect of such graft materials in periodontal defects with flap surgery alone, but a clinical study has demonstrated that implantation of Bio-Oss® resulted in pocket reduction, gain of attachment, and bone fill in periodontal defects to the same extent as that of DFDBA (Richardson *et al.* 1999). There are, on the other hand, several controlled clinical studies reporting about the outcome of treatment of periodontal intrabony defects with Bio-Oss used as an adjunct to guided tissue regeneration (GTR). In one of these studies, including 124 patients, the combined treatment had an added benefit of 0.8 mm PAL gain over that with flap surgery alone (Tonetti *et al.* 2004). However, conflicting results have been reported following the combined Bio-Oss and GTR treatment of intrabony defects versus GTR alone. In a recent study, significantly more PAL gain was found after the combined treatment than after GTR treatment with a collagen membrane (5.1 mm versus 4.0 mm) (Paolantonio 2002), while in another study, the clinical improvements obtained following the two treatments were similar (Stavropoulos *et al.* 2003b). This latter finding is in agreement with the results of a recent systematic review evaluating various bone grafts and bone graft substitutes as adjuncts to GTR (Murphy & Gunsolley 2003). Studies in experimental animals have also failed to show an added effect of Bio-Oss combined with GTR (Carmagnola *et al.* 2002, 2003). However, human histology (Camelo *et al.* 1998; Nevins *et al.* 2003; Sculean *et al.* 2003) and a study in dogs (Clergeau *et al.* 1996) have suggested that the placement of bovine bone-derived biomaterials in periodontal bone defects may enhance both the regeneration of a new connective tissue attachment and bone. The results of several experimental studies in animals, on the other hand, have questioned whether Bio-Oss encourages bone formation (Stavropoulos *et al.* 2001, 2003a, 2004; Aghaloo *et al.* 2004; Cardaropoli *et al.* 2005). In fact, the results of some of these studies suggest that grafting of Bio-Oss may compromise bone formation.

The use of coral skeleton as a bone graft substitute was proposed some decades ago (Holmes 1979; Guillemin *et al.* 1987). Depending on the pretreatment procedure, the natural coral turns into non-resorbable porous hydroxyapatite (e.g. Interpore 200, Interpore International, Irvine, US) or to a resorbable calcium carbonate (e.g. Biocoral, Inoteb, St Gonnery, France) skeleton (Nasr *et al.* 1999). Implantation of coralline porous hydroxyapatite in intrabony periodontal defects in humans produced more probing pocket depth reduction, clinical attachment gain, and defect fill than non-grafting (Kenney *et al.* 1985; Krejci *et al.* 1987; Yukna 1994; Mora & Ouhayoun 1995; Yukna & Yukna 1998), and similar results were found when compared with grafting of FDBA (Barnett *et al.* 1989). When porous hydroxyapatite was compared with DFDBA for the treatment of intraosseous defects, similar results were also obtained (Bowen *et al.* 1989), but another study reported clinical results in favor of this material (Oreamuno *et al.* 1990). However, both animal (West & Brustein 1985; Ettel *et al.* 1989) and human studies (Carranza *et al.* 1987; Stahl & Froum 1987) have provided only vague histologic evidence that grafting of natural coral may enhance the formation of true new attachment. In most cases, the graft particles were embedded in connective tissue with minimal bone formation.

Alloplastic materials

Alloplastic materials are synthetic, inorganic, biocompatible and/or bioactive bone graft substitutes which are claimed to promote bone healing through osteoconduction. There are four kinds of alloplastic materials, which are frequently used in regenerative periodontal surgery: hydroxyapatite (HA), beta-tricalcium phosphate (β-TCP), polymers, and bioactive glasses (bio-glasses).

Hydroxyapatite

The HA products used in periodontology are of two forms: a particulate non-resorbable ceramic form (e.g. Periograf®, Miter Inc., Warsaw, IN, US; Calcitite®, Calcitek Inc., San Diego, US) and a particulate, resorbable non-ceramic form (e.g. OsteoGraf/LD®, CeraMed Dental, Lakewood, CO, US). In controlled clinical studies, grafting of intrabony periodontal lesions with HA resulted in a PAL gain of 1.1–3.3 mm and also in a greater bone defect fill as compared with non-grafted surgically debrided controls (Meffert *et al.* 1985; Yukna *et al.* 1985, 1986, 1989; Galgut *et al.* 1992). In these studies, improvement of clinical parameters (i.e. PPD reduction and PAL gain) was more evident in the grafted sites than in the sites treated only with debridement, especially for initially deep defects. However, animal studies (Barney *et al.* 1986; Minabe *et al.* 1988; Wilson & Low 1992) and human histologic data (Froum *et al.* 1982; Moskow & Lubarr 1983; Ganeles *et al.* 1986; Sapkos 1986) showed that bone formation was limited and that a true new attachment was not formed consistently after grafting of intrabony periodontal defects with HA. The majority of the HA particles were embedded in connective tissue and new bone was only observed occasionally around particles in close proximity to host bone. A junctional epithelium lined the major part of the roots.

Beta-tricalcium phosphate (β-TCP)

β-TCP ($Ca_3(PO_4)_2$) (e.g. Synthograft®, Johnson and Johnson, New Brunswick, NJ, US) has been used in a series of case reports for the treatment of periodontal osseous lesions (Nery & Lynch 1978; Strub *et al.* 1979; Snyder *et al.* 1984; Baldock *et al.* 1985). After variable time intervals, a significant gain of bone was observed by means of re-entry or radiographs. However, there is no controlled study comparing the result of β-TCP grafting with that of open-flap debridement, and histologic data from animal (Levin *et al.* 1974; Barney *et al.* 1986) and human studies (Dragoo & Kaldahl 1983; Baldock *et al.* 1985; Bowers *et al.* 1986; Stahl & Froum 1986; Froum & Stahl 1987; Saffar *et al.* 1990) showed that β-TCP is rapidly resorbed or encapsulated by connective tissue, with minimal bone formation and no periodontal regeneration.

Polymers

There are two polymer materials that have been used as bone graft substitutes in the treatment of periodontal defects: a non-resorbable, calcium hydroxide coated co-polymer of polymethylmethacrylate (PMMA) and polyhydroxylethylmethacrylate (PHEMA), which is often referred to as HTR (hard tissue replacement) (e.g. HTR™, Bioplant Inc., New York, NY, US), and a resorbable polylactic acid (PLA) polymer (Driloc®, Osmed Corp., Costa Mesa, CA, US).

In controlled clinical studies, implantation of HTR polymer grafts in intrabony defects resulted in a defect fill of approximately 2 mm, representing about 60% of the initial defect depth, but the improved clinical response with grafting was not significantly better than that following solely flap operation (Yukna 1990; Shahmiri *et al.* 1992). Human histologic data from an experimental study (Plotzke *et al.* 1993), and from two case reports (Stahl *et al.* 1990b; Froum 1996) also revealed that grafting of osseous periodontal defects with HTR does not promote periodontal regeneration. The HTR particles were most frequently encapsulated by connective tissue with only scarce evidence of bone formation. Healing resulted in a long junctional epithelium along the root surface, and true new attachment formation was not observed.

When PLA particles were implanted into intrabony defects in humans and compared with DFDBA or surgically debrided controls, it was found that the healing results were less favorable than after flap operation alone, both in terms of clinical parameters (PPD and PAL gain), and in terms of bone fill (Meadows *et al.* 1993).

Bioactive glasses (bio-glasses)

Bio-glasses are composed of SiO_2, Na_2O, P_2O_5 and are resorbable or not resorbable depending on the relative proportion of these components. When bio-glasses are exposed to tissue fluids, a double layer of silica gel and calcium phosphate is formed on their surface. Through this layer the material promotes absorption and concentration of proteins used by osteoblasts to form extracellular bone matrix which theoretically may promote bone formation (Hench *et al.* 1972). Commercially available bio-glasses in particulate form, and theoretically resorbable, have been proposed for periodontal treatment (e.g. PerioGlass®, US Biomaterials Corp., Alachua, FL, US; BioGran®, Orthovita, Malvern, PA, US).

A human case report demonstrated that implantation of bio-glass in periodontal osseous defects resulted in a gain of clinical attachment of 2.0–5.3 mm and a radiographic bone fill of 3.5 mm, and in a controlled study, the treatment of intrabony defects with bio-glass also resulted in greater clinical improvements than surgical debridement alone (Froum *et al.* 1998). However, other controlled studies (Zamet *et al.* 1997) and split-mouth studies on grafting of intrabony defects with bio-glass (Ong *et al.* 1998) failed to demonstrate statistically significant better clinical results than surgery alone or DFDBA grafting (Lovelace *et al.* 1998). Although experimental studies in monkeys have suggested that bio-glass grafting of periodontal intrabony defects (Karatzas *et al.* 1999) may favor new cementum formation and inhibit epithelial downgrowth, there is no histologic evidence in humans that bio-glass may promote true periodontal regeneration. In a histologic evaluation of bio-glass implanted in intrabony defects in humans it was observed that, although clinically satisfactory results were produced, healing had most frequently occurred with a junctional epithelium along the previously diseased part of the root, and new cementum with inserting collagen fibers was found in only one out of five treated teeth. Bone formation was limited in all specimens (Nevins *et al.* 2000).

Evaluation of alloplastic materials

There are no controlled clinical studies demonstrating that grafting with tricalcium phosphate or polymers results in significant clinical improvements beyond that of flap surgery, whereas several reports have indicated that grafting with hydroxyapatite or bioactive glasses may produce more gain of attachment than open-flap debridement (Galgut *et al.* 1992; Zamet *et al.* 1997; Froum *et al.* 1998) or a gain similar to that obtained following grafting with DFDBA (Lovelace *et al.* 1998). Histologic evidence that the use of alloplastic or synthetic graft materials may lead to periodontal regeneration in humans is lacking, and animal experiments have failed to demonstrate regeneration of a functional periodontium following implantation of hydroxyapatite, tricalcium phosphate or polymers in periodontal lesions (Barney

et al. 1986; Shahmiri *et al.* 1992). It was reported, however, that treatment with bioactive glasses in experimental animals produced significantly more bone fill and new attachment compared with that in non-grafted controls (Fetner *et al.* 1994; Karatzas *et al.* 1999) or in sites grafted with hydroxyapatite or tricalcium phosphate (Wilson & Low 1992). Although some bone formation has been reported following the use of alloplastic materials, there is no evidence that these materials may stimulate the formation of new cementum with inserting collagen fibers. At the 1996 American Academy of Periodontology World Workshop, it was concluded that synthetic graft materials function primarily as defect fillers.

Root surface biomodification

Much research has been directed to altering the periodontitis-involved root surface in a manner that will promote the formation of a new connective tissue attachment. Removal of bacterial deposits, calculus, and endotoxins from the cementum is generally considered essential for the formation of a new connective attachment (Garrett 1977). However, it was suggested by Stahl *et al.* (1972) that demineralization of the root surface, exposing the collagen of the dentin, would facilitate the deposition of cementum by inducing mesenchymal cells in the adjacent tissue to differentiate into cementoblasts. The biologic concept is that exposure of collagen fibers of the dentin matrix may facilitate adhesion of the blood clot to the root surface and thereby favor migration of the fibroblasts. However, it is doubtful whether this concept is in accordance with current knowledge about periodontal wound healing since there is no evidence that the exposure of collagen fibers of the dentin matrix may facilitate repopulation of the root surface with cells derived from the periodontal ligament. As mentioned previously, periodontal ligament cells are required for the accomplishment of a new connective tissue attachment.

Several studies using various animal models demonstrated an improved healing response histologically following citric acid and tetracycline root surface demineralization (Register & Burdick 1976; Crigger *et al.* 1978; Polson & Proye 1982; Claffey *et al.* 1987). However, in a study in dogs where naturally occurring furcations were treated with citric acid, several specimens demonstrated ankylosis and root resorption (Bogle *et al.* 1981). This finding corroborates that of Magnusson *et al.* (1985) in monkeys, where citric acid conditioning was evaluated in combination with coronally displaced tissue flaps after 6 months. These investigators found root resorption on 28 out of 40 surfaces examined and 21 of these also presented ankylosis.

New connective tissue attachment following citric acid demineralization of root surfaces has been demonstrated histologically in humans (Cole *et al.* 1980; Frank *et al.* 1983; Stahl *et al.* 1983; Stahl & Froum

1991a). Cole *et al.* (1980) showed histologic evidence of a new connective tissue attachment and bone formation coronal to reference notches placed in the apical extent of calculus identified on the root surface at the time of surgery. However, despite histologic evidence of regeneration following root surface biomodification with citric acid, results of controlled clinical trials failed to show any improvements in clinical conditions compared to controls not treated with acid (Moore *et al.* 1987; Fuentes *et al.* 1993).

In recent years, biomodification of the root surface with enamel matrix proteins (Emdogain®) during surgery and following demineralization with EDTA has been introduced to encourage periodontal regeneration. The biologic concept is that the application of enamel matrix proteins (amelogenins) may promote periodontal regeneration because it mimics events that took place during the development of the periodontal tissues (Hammarström 1997; Gestrelius *et al.* 2000). This view is based on the finding that the cells of the Hertwigs epithelial root sheath deposit enamel matrix proteins on the root surface prior to cementum formation and that these proteins are the initiating factor for the formation of cementum. The commercially available product, Emdogain®, a purified acid extract of porcine origin, contains enamel matrix derivatives (EMD), supposed to be able to promote periodontal regeneration. However, it is not quite clear how this concept is in accordance with current knowledge about periodontal wound healing since no evidence has been provided that it is cells derived from the periodontal ligament that are encouraged to repopulate the root surface after treatment. In fact, a study in dogs (Araùjo *et al.* 2003) where re-implanted roots that had been extracted and deprived of vital cementoblasts and subsequently treated with EMD failed to prevent ankylosis and root resorption, indicating that the root surfaces did not become repopulated with cells with the capacity to form cementum. A recent study in vitro has also failed to confirm that EMD has any significant effect on periodontal ligament cell proliferation (Chong *et al.* 2006).

In case series reports, 4–4.5 mm gain of clinical attachment, and about 70% bone fill in intrabony defects were reported following treatment with EMD (Heden *et al.* 1999; Heden 2000). In a multicenter clinical study involving 33 subjects with 34 paired intrabony defects, application of EMD resulted in larger amounts of PAL gain (2.2 mm) and statistically significantly more bone gain (2.6 mm) than open-flap debridement after 36 months, evaluated clinically and radiographically (Heijl *et al.* 1997). Similar results were reported in another split-mouth clinical trial (23 patients) published more recently (Froum *et al.* 2001). In that study a PPD reduction of 4.9 mm, a PAL gain of 4.3, and a bone gain of 3.8 mm (evaluated by re-entry surgery) were observed after EMD application in 53 intrabony defects. These values were statistically significantly larger than those obtained by flap

surgery (2.2 mm, 2.7 mm, and 1.5 mm, respectively, in 31 defects).

In a more recent prospective multicenter randomized controlled clinical trial, the clinical outcomes of papilla preservation flap surgery (simplified papilla preservation flap, SPPF) with or without the application of enamel matrix proteins, were compared (Tonetti *et al.* 2002). A total of 83 test and 83 control patients with similar baseline periodontal conditions and defect characteristics were treated with either SPPF and Emdogain® or with SPPF alone. The test defects exhibited significantly more clinical attachment level (CAL) gain than the controls (3.1 ± 1.5 mm and 2.5 ± 1.5 mm, respectively).

When application of EMD was compared with GTR treatment, it was found that similar clinical improvements were obtained. In a randomized controlled clinical study, Pontoriero *et al.* (1999) compared EMD application with GTR with resorbable (two kinds: Guidor and Resolut) and non-resorbable (e-PTFE) membranes in intrabony defects. After 12 months, there were no significant differences among the groups, and EMD application resulted in a PPD reduction of 4.4 mm and a PAL gain of 2.9 mm, while the corresponding values from the membrane-treated sites (both GTR groups combined) were 4.5 mm and 3.1 mm, respectively. Silvestri *et al.* (2000) reported a PPD reduction of 4.8 mm and a PAL gain of 4.5 mm after EMD application in intrabony defects versus 5.9 mm and 4.8 mm, respectively, after GTR with non-resorbable membranes. Similar results were reported by other investigators (Sculean *et al.* 1999a,b; Silvestri *et al.* 2003; Sanz *et al.* 2004). There are studies indicating that following the application EMD in intrabony defects, clinical improvements can be achieved by the additional use of some bone graft materials (Zucchelli *et al.* 2003; Gurinsky *et al.* 2004; Trombelli *et al.* 2006), although others have failed to demonstrate a beneficial effect of this combined treatment (Sculean *et al.* 2005).

Histologic evidence of new cementum formation with inserting collagen fibers on a previously periodontitis-affected root surface and the formation of new alveolar bone in human specimens have been demonstrated following EMD treatment (Mellonig 1999; Sculean *et al.* 1999b). However, while in the study of Mellonig (1999) healing had occurred with acellular cementum on the root surface, the newly formed cementum in the study of Sculean *et al.* (1999b) displayed a predominantly cellular character. The ability of EMD to produce regeneration has been confirmed in controlled animal experiments (Fig. 25-20), following the treatment of intrabony, furcation, and dehiscence defects (Hammarström *et al.* 1997; Araújo & Lindhe 1998; Sculean *et al.* 2000). In a later study it was shown in monkeys that the combined application of EMD and autogenous bone grafts may improve periodontal regeneration in periodontal defects compared to flap surgery alone (Cochran *et al.* 2003).

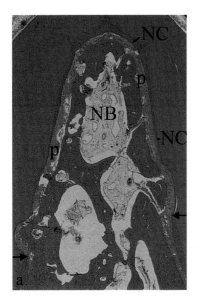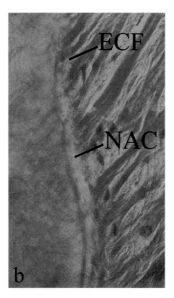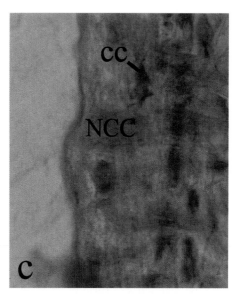

Fig. 25-20 (a) Photomicrograph of a grade III furcation defect in a dog following root surface biomodification with enamel matrix proteins and subsequently covered with a resorbable membrane. The defect has healed completely with bone (NB), a periodontal ligament (p) and new cementum (NC). The arrows indicate the apical extension of the lesion. (b) The cementum (NAC) formed on the root surface in the apical portion of the defect was acellular with inserting extrinsic collagen fibers (ECF) while (c) new cellular cementum (NCC) had formed in the coronal portion. cc = cells.

Growth regulatory factors for periodontal regeneration

Growth factor is a general term to denote a class of polypeptide hormones that stimulate a wide variety of cellular events such as proliferation, chemotaxis, differentiation, and production of extracellular matrix proteins (Terranova & Wikesjö 1987). Proliferation and migration of periodontal ligament cells and synthesis of extracellular matrix as well as differentiation of cementoblasts and osteoblasts is a prerequisite for obtaining periodontal regeneration. Therefore, it is conceivable that growth factors may represent a potential aid in attempts to encourage regeneration of the periodontium.

The effects of various growth factors were studied *in vitro*, and a significant regeneration potential of growth factors was also demonstrated in animal models. Lynch *et al.* (1989, 1991) examined the effect of placing a combination of platelet-derived growth factors (PDGF) and insulin-like growth factors (IGF) in naturally occurring periodontal defects in dogs. The control sites treated without growth factors healed with a long junctional epithelium and no new cementum or bone formation, while regeneration of a periodontal attachment apparatus occurred at the sites treated with growth factors. Similar results were reported by other investigators following application of a combination of PDGF and IGF in experimentally induced periodontal lesions in monkeys (Rutherford *et al.* 1992; Giannobile *et al.* 1994, 1996). One study examined the effect of PDGF and IGF in periodontal intrabony defects and grade II furcations in humans (Howell *et al.* 1997). At re-entry after 9 months, significantly increased bone fill was only observed at the furcation sites treated with growth factors. Consider-

able clinical improvements were also observed following a combined treatment of grade II furcations with GTR, a bone graft substitute and PDGF compared to open-flap debridement (Lekovic *et al.* 2003). It can be concluded that growth factors seem to have a positive effect on periodontal regeneration, but several important questions need to be resolved before this type of regenerative treatment can be used in humans (Graves & Cochran 1994).

Bone morphogenetic proteins (BMPs) are osteoinductive factors that may have the potential to stimulate mesenchymal cells to differentiate into bone-forming cells (Wozney *et al.* 1988). Sigurdsson *et al.* (1995) evaluated bone and cementum formation following regenerative periodontal surgery using recombinant human BMP in surgically created supra-alveolar defects in dogs. Following application of BMP the flaps were advanced to submerge the teeth and sutured. Histologic analysis showed significantly more cementum formation and regrowth of alveolar bone on BMP-treated sites as compared to the controls. Significant amounts of bone regeneration in periodontal defects have also been reported by other investigators following application of BMPs combined with various carrier systems or space-providing devices in different animal models (Ripamonti *et al.* 1994; Selvig *et al.* 2002; Wikesjö *et al.* 2003a,b). Further experimentation is needed to evaluate a possible role of BMP in periodontal regeneration.

Guided tissue regeneration (GTR)

The experimental studies (Karring *et al.* 1980; Nyman *et al.* 1980; Buser *et al.* 1990a,b; Warrer *et al.* 1993) described previously have documented that the progenitor cells for the formation of a new connective tissue attachment reside in the periodontal ligament. Consequently, it should be expected that a new connective tissue attachment would be predictably achieved if such cells populate the root surface during healing. This view was confirmed in a study in monkeys in which both gingival connective tissue and gingival epithelium were prevented from contacting the root surface during healing by the use of a barrier membrane (Gottlow *et al*. 1984). After reduction of the supporting tissues around selected experimental teeth, the root surfaces were exposed to plaque accumulation for 6 months. Soft tissue flaps were then raised and the exposed root surfaces were curetted. The crowns of the teeth were resected and the roots were submerged. However, prior to complete closure of the wound, a membrane was placed over the curetted root surfaces on one side of the jaws in order (1) to prevent gingival connective tissue contacting the root surface during healing, and (2) to provide a space for in-growth of periodontal ligament tissue. No membranes were placed over the contralateral roots. The histologic analysis after 3 months of healing demonstrated that the roots covered with membranes exhibited considerably more new attachment than the non-covered roots (Fig. 25-21). In four of the nine test roots, new cementum covered the entire length of the root. In all control specimens, the surface coronal to the newly formed cementum presented multinucleated cells and resorption cavities. In one control specimen virtually half the root was resorbed. Coronal regrowth of alveolar bone had occurred to a varying extent in test and control roots, and no relationship was found

between the amount of new cementum formation and the degree of bone regrowth. The results of this study strongly suggested that the exclusion of epithelial and gingival connective tissue cells from the healing area by the use of a physical barrier may allow (guide) periodontal ligament cells to repopulate the detached root surface. This observation provided the basis for the clinical application of the treatment principle termed "guided tissue regeneration" (GTR). Thus. GTR treatment involves the placement of a physical barrier to ensure that the previous periodontitis-affected root surface becomes repopulated with cells from the periodontal ligament (Fig. 25-22).

Treatment of the first human tooth with GTR was reported by Nyman *et al*. (1982). Due to extensive periodontal destruction, the tooth was scheduled for extraction. This offered the possibility of obtaining histologic documentation of the result of the treatment. Following elevation of full thickness flaps, scaling of the root surface, and removal of all granulation tissue, an 11 mm deep periodontal lesion was ascertained. Prior to flap closure, a membrane was adjusted to cover parts of the detached root surfaces, the osseous defect, and parts of the surrounding bone. Histologic analysis after 3 months of healing revealed that new cementum with inserting collagen fibers had formed on the previously exposed root surface (Fig. 25-23). In a later study (Gottlow *et al*. 1986), 12 cases treated with GTR were evaluated clinically, and in five of these cases histologic documentation was also presented. The results showed that considerable but varying amounts of new connective tissue attachment had formed on the treated

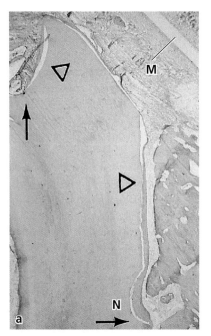 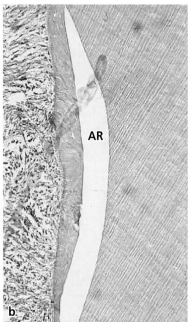 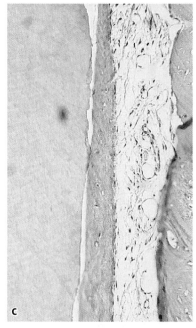

Fig. 25-21 (a) Microphotograph of membrane (M) covered root. Newly formed cementum is visible on the entire length of the buccal root surface coronal to the notch (N) and also on part of the coronal cut surface (arrow). (b, c) Higher magnifications of the areas at the upper and lower triangles in (a), showing that collagen fibers are inserted into the newly formed cementum. AR = artifact.

teeth. Frequently, however, bone formation was incomplete. The varying results were ascribed to factors such as the amount of remaining periodontal ligament, the morphology of the treated defect, technical difficulties regarding membrane placement, gingival recession, and bacterial contamination of the membrane and the wound during healing.

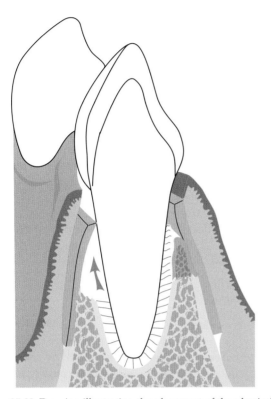

Fig. 25-22 Drawing illustrating the placement of the physical barrier which prevents the epithelium and gingival connective tissue from contacting the root surface during healing. At the same time the membrane allows cells from the periodontal ligament (arrow) to repopulate the previously periodontitis-involved root surface.

In the last decades, GTR has been applied in a number of clinical trials for the treatment of various periodontal defects such as intrabony defects (for review see Cortellini & Bowers 1995), furcation involvements (for review see Machtei & Schallhorn 1995; Karring & Cortellini 1999), and localized gingival recession defects (Pini-Prato *et al.* 1996). The efficiency of GTR in producing periodontal regeneration in these defects has been documented in animal studies (Gottlow *et al.* 1990; Araùjo *et al.* 1998; Laurell *et al.* 2006) and in several controlled clinical trials (see Chapter 43).

The clinical outcomes of GTR are most frequently evaluated by changes in clinical attachment levels (CAL), bone levels (BL), probing pocket depths (PPD), and the position of the gingival margin. In some of the studies on grade II and III furcations, horizontal changes in clinical attachment, bone level, and pocket depth were also measured. However, evidence of true regeneration of periodontal attachment can only be provided by histologic means.

Assessment of periodontal regeneration

In most studies on the effect of regenerative periodontal surgery, the outcomes are evaluated by probing attachment level measurements, radiographic analysis or re-entry operations. However, such methods do not provide proof of a true gain of attachment (i.e. formation of cementum with inserting collagen fibers coronal to the attachment level before treatment).

Periodontal probing

The inability of periodontal probing to determine accurately the coronal level of the connective tissue

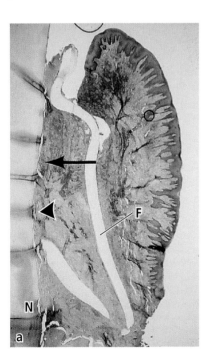

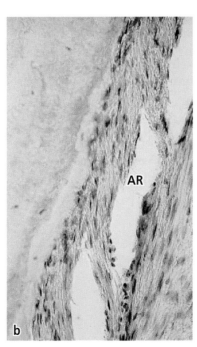

Fig. 25-23 (a) Microphotograph of a human tooth 3 months following GTR treatment using a Millipore filter (F). New cementum with inserting collagen fibers (about 5 mm) has formed from the notch (N) to the level of the arrow. Bone formation underneath the filter is lacking, probably due to the inflammatory infiltrate seen in the tissues adjacent to the filter. (b) Higher magnification of the area indicated by the arrowhead in (a) showing newly formed cementum with inserting collagen fibers. AR = artifact.

attachment has been demonstrated by several investigators (Listgarten *et al.* 1976; Armitage *et al.* 1977; Van der Velden & de Vries 1978). It is known from these studies that, in the inflamed periodontium, the probe does not stop precisely at the coronal level of the connective tissue attachment. Usually it penetrates 0.5 mm or more into the connective tissue, surpassing the transition between the apical extension of the dentogingival epithelium and the coronal level of connective tissue attachment. After therapy, when the inflammatory lesion is resolved, the probe tip tends to stop coronal to the apical termination of the epithelium. Following treatment of intrabony defects, new bone may form so close to the tooth surface that the probe cannot penetrate (Caton & Zander 1976). Thus, a gain of probing attachment level (PAL) following therapy does not necessarily mean that a true gain of connective tissue attachment was accomplished. More likely it is a reflection of improved health of the surrounding soft tissues which offer increased resistance to probe penetration.

Radiographic analysis and re-entry operations

Healing of intrabony defects following regenerative surgery is often documented by measurements made on radiographs obtained in a standardized and reproducible manner and/or assessed in conjunction with a re-entry operation. Analysis of radiographs before and after therapy and inspection of the treated area during a re-entry operation can certainly provide evidence of new bone formation. However, such "bone fill" does not prove formation of new root cementum with inserting collagen fibers (i.e. a new periodontal ligament). In fact, it was demonstrated by Caton and-Zander (1976) and Moscow *et al.* (1979) that despite the fact that bone regeneration had occurred adjacent to the root in intrabony defects, a junctional epithelium was interposed between the newly formed bone and the curetted root surface. This means that radiographic analysis and assessments of bone formation by re-entry operations are unreliable methods for the documentation of new attachment formation.

Histologic methods

In several studies healing is analyzed in histologic sections of block biopsies obtained after various forms of regenerative periodontal therapy. Histologic

analysis is the only valid method to assess the formation of a true new attachment, but it requires that the location of the attachment level prior to therapy can be assessed with a reasonable accuracy. In a few studies histologic reference notches were placed in the apical extent of calculus deposits, identified on the root surface at the time of surgery (Cole *et al.* 1980; Bowers *et al.* 1989b,c). Usually, however, a reference is obtained by producing a notch in the root surface at the level of the reduced bone height. Although such a notch may not reflect the exact extent of the periodontitis-involved root surface prior to treatment, it is considered an adequate landmark for the assessment of new attachment (Isidor *et al.* 1985). It was also suggested that clinical signs of probing attachment gain and bone fill can be accepted as evidence of periodontal regeneration in the evaluation of GTR procedures (Lindhe & Echeverria 1994). This suggestion was based on evidence of a new attachment apparatus in histologic specimens from human biopsies harvested following GTR treatment (Nyman *et al.* 1982; Gottlow *et al.* 1986; Becker *et al.* 1987; Stahl *et al.* 1990a; Cortellini *et al.* 1993) and on the biologic concept of GTR (Karring *et al.* 1980, 1985, 1993; Nyman *et al.* 1980; Gottlow *et al.* 1984).

Conclusions

There is evidence that the progenitor cells for reformation of lost periodontal attachment are present in the periodontal ligament. Consequently, a periodontal regenerative procedure needs to encourage repopulation of the previous periodontitis-affected root surface with cells from the periodontal ligament.

GTR and conditioning of the root surface with enamel matrix proteins represent the best documented regenerative procedures for obtaining periodontal regeneration in periodontal lesions, although there is some uncertainty whether enamel matrix proteins in fact stimulate the proliferation of periodontal ligament cells.

Placement of bone grafts or bone substitute implants are based on a biologic concept which cannot explain how such treatment should result in regeneration of the periodontium. There are some studies indicating that bone grafting in periodontal intrabony defects may produce clinical improvements beyond that achieved with only flap surgery, but generally bone grafts or bone substitute implants are considered as primarily defect filler materials.

References

Aghaloo, T.L., Moy, P.K. & Freymiller, E.G. (2004). Evaluation of platelet-rich plasma in combination with anorganic bovine bone in the rabbit cranium: a pilot study. *International Journal of Oral and Maxillofacial Implants* **19**, 59–65.

Altiere, E., Reeve, C. & Sheridan, P. (1979). Lyophilized bone allografts in periodontal osseous defects. *Journal of Periodontology* **50**, 510–519.

Araùjo, M. & Lindhe, J. (1998). GTR treatment of degree III furcation defects following application of enamel matrix proteins. An experimental study in dogs. *Journal of Clinical Periodontology* **25**, 524–530.

Araùjo, M., Berglundh, T. & Lindhe, J. (1998). GTR treatment of degree III furcation defects with 2 different resorbable barriers. An experimental study in dogs. *Journal of Clinical Periodontology* **25**, 253–259.

Araùjo, M., Hayacibara, R., Sonohara, M., Cardaropoli, G. & Lindhe, J. (2003). Effect of enamel matrix proteins (Emdogain®), on healing after re-implantation of periodontally compromised roots. An experimental study in the dog. *Journal of Clinical Periodontology* **30**, 855–861.

Armitage, G.C., Svanberg, G.K. & Löe, H. (1977). Microscopic evaluation of clinical measurements of connective tissue attachment levels. *Journal of Clinical Periodontology* **4**, 173–190.

Baldock, W.T., Hutchens, L.H. Jr., McFall, W.T. Jr. & Simpson, D.M. (1985). An evaluation of tricalcium phosphate implants in human periodontal osseous defects of two patients. *Journal of Periodontology* **56**, 1–7.

Barnett, J.D., Mellonig, J.T., Gray, J.L. & Towle, H.J. (1989). Comparison of freeze-dried bone allograft and porous hydroxyapatite in human periodontal defects. *Journal of Periodontology* **60**, 231–237.

Barney, V.C., Levin, M.P. & Adams, D.F. (1986). Bioceramical implants in surgical periodontal defects. A comparison study. *Journal of Periodontology* **57**, 764–770.

Becker, W., Becker, B.E. & Caffesse, R. (1994). A comparison of demineralized freeze-dried bone and autologous bone to induce bone formation in human extraction sockets. *Journal of Periodontology* **65**, 1128–1133.

Becker, W., Becker, B.E., Prichard, J.F., Caffesse, R., Rosenberg, E. & Gian-Grasso, J. (1987). Root isolation for new attachment procedures. A surgical and suturing method: three case reports. *Journal of Periodontology* **58**, 819–825.

Becker, W., Urist, M.R., Tucker, L.M., Becker, B.E. & Ochsenbein, C. (1995). Human demineralized freeze-dried bone: inadequate induced bone formation in athymic mice. A preliminary report. *Journal of Periodontology* **66**, 822–828.

Beube, F.E. (1947). A study of reattachment of the supporting structures of teeth. *Journal of Periodontology* **18**, 55–56.

Beube, F.E. (1952). A radiograhic and histologic study on reattachment. *Journal of Periodontology* **23**, 158–164.

Björn H., Hollender, L. & Lindhe, J. (1965). Tissue regeneration in patients with periodontal disease. *Odontologisk Revy* **16**, 317–326.

Bogle, G., Adams, D., Crigger, M., Klinge, B. & Egelberg, J. (1981). New attachment after surgical treatment and acid conditioning of roots in naturally occurring periodontal disease in dogs. *Journal of Periodontal Research* **16**, 130–133.

Bowen, J.A., Mellonig, J.T., Gray, J.L. & Towle, H.T. (1989). Comparison of decalcified freeze-dried bone allograft and porous particulate hydroxyapatite in human periodontal osseous defects. *Journal of Periodontology* **60**, 647–654.

Bowers, G.M., Chadroff, B., Carnevale, R., Mellonig, J., Corio, R., Emerson, J., Stevens, M. & Romberg, E. (1989a). Histologic evaluation of new attachment apparatus formation in humans. Part I. *Journal of Periodontology* **60**, 664–674.

Bowers, G.M., Chadroff, B., Carnevale, R., Mellonig, J., Corio, R., Emerson, J., Stevens, M. & Romberg, E. (1989b). Histologic evaluation of new human attachment apparatus formation in humans. Part II. *Journal of Periodontology* **60**, 675–682.

Bowers, G.M., Chadroff, B., Carnevale, R., Mellonig, J., Corio, R., Emerson, J., Stevens, M. & Romberg, E. (1989c). Histologic evaluation of a new attachment apparatus formation in humans. Part III. *Journal of Periodontology* **60**, 683–693.

Bowers, G.M., Vargo, J.W., Lerg, B., Emerson, J.R. & Bergquist, J.J. (1986). Histologic observations following the placement of tricalcium phosphate implants in human intrabony defects. *Journal of Periodontology* **57**, 286–287.

Brunsvold, M.A. & Mellonig, J. (1993). Bone grafts and periodontal regeneration. *Periodontology 2000* **1**, 80–91.

Buser, D., Warrer, K. & Karring, T. (1990a). Formation of a periodontal ligament around titanium implants. *Journal of Periodontology* **61**, 597–601.

Buser, D., Warrer, K., Karring, T. & Stich, H. (1990b). Titanium implants with a true periodontal ligament. An alternative to osseointegrated implants. *International Journal of Oral and Maxillofacial Implants* **5**, 113–116.

Bühler, H. (1988). Evaluation of root-resected teeth. Results after 10 years. *Journal of Periodontology* **59**, 805–810.

Camelo, M., Nevins, M., Schenk, R., Simion, M., Rasperini, C., Lynch, S. & Nevins, M. (1998). Clinical radiographic, and histologic evaluation of human periodontal defects treated with Bio-Oss® and Bio-Gide. *International Journal of Periodontics and Restorative Dentistry* **18**, 321–331.

Caplanis, N., Lee, M.B., Zimmerman, G.J., Selvig, K.A. & Wikesjö, U.M. (1998). Effect of allogeneic freeze-dried demineralized bone matrix on regeneration of alveolar bone and periodontal attachment in dogs. *Journal of Clinical Periodontology* **25**, 801–806.

Cardaropoli, G., Araùjo, M., Hayacibara, R., Sukekava, F. & Lindhe J. (2005). Healing of extraction sockets and surgically produced – augmented and non-augmented – defects in the alveolar ridge. An experimental study in the dog. *Journal of Clinical Periodontology* **32**, 435–440.

Carmagnola, D., Adrians, P., & Berglundh, T. (2003). Healing of human extraction sockets filled with Bio-Oss. *Clinical Oral Implants Research* **14**, 137–143.

Carmagnola, D., Berglundh, T. & Lindhe, J. (2002). The effect of a fibrin glue on the integration of Bio-Oss with bone tissue. An experimental study in Labrador dogs. *Journal of Clinical Periodontology* **29**, 377–383.

Carranza, F.A. (1954). A technique for reattachment. *Journal of Periodontology* **25**, 272–277.

Carranza, F.A. (1960). A technique for treating infrabony pockets so as to obtain reattachment. *Dental Clinics of North America* **5**, 75–83.

Carranza, F.A., Kenney, E.B., Lekovic, V., Talamante, E., Valencia, J. & Dimitrijevic, B. (1987). Histologic study of healing of human periodontal defects after placement of porous hydrozylapatite implants. *Journal of Periodontology* **58**, 682–688.

Carraro, J.J., Sznajder, N. & Alonso, C.A. (1976). Intraoral cancellous bone autografts in the treatment of infrabony pockets. *Journal of Clinical Periodontology* **3**, 104–109.

Caton J. & Nyman, S. (1980). Histometric evaluation of periodontal surgery. I. The modified Widman flap procedure. *Journal of Clinical Periodontology* **7**, 212–223.

Caton, J., Nyman, S. & Zander, H. (1980). Histometric evaluation of periodontal surgery. II. Connective tissue attachment levels after four regenerative procedures. *Journal of Clinical Periodontology* **7**, 224–231.

Caton, J. & Zander, H.A. (1976). Osseous repair of an infrabony pocket without new attachment of connective tissue. *Journal of Clinical Periodontology* **3**, 54–58.

Chong, C.H., Carnes, D.L., Moritz, A.J., Oates, T., Ryu, O.H., Simmer, J. & Cochran, D.L. (2006). Human periodontal fibroblast response to enamel matrix derivative, amelogenin, and platelet-derived growth factor-BB. *Journal of Periodontology* **77**, 1242–1252.

Claffey, N., Bogle, G., Bjorvatn, K., Selvig, K. & Egelberg, J. (1987). Topical application of tetracycline in regenerative periodontal surgery in beagles. *Acta Odontologica Scandinavica* **45**, 141–146.

Claffey, N. & Egelberg, J. (1995). Clinical indicators of probing attachment loss following initial periodontal treatment in advanced periodontitis patients. *Journal of Clinical Periodontology* **22**, 690–696.

Clergeau, L.P., Danan, M., Clergeau-Guerithault, S. & Brion, M. (1996). Healing response to anorganic bone implantation in periodontal intrabony defects in dogs. Part I. Bone regeneration. A microradiographic study. *Journal of Periodontology* **67**, 140–149.

Cochran, D.L., Jones, A., Heijl, L., Mellonig, J.T., Schoolfield, J. & King, G.N. (2003). Periodontal regeneration with a combination of enamel matrix proteins and autogenous bone grafting. *Journal of Periodontology* **74**, 1269–1281.

Cole, R.T., Crigger, M., Bogle, G., Egelberg, J. & Selvig, K.A. (1980). Connective tissue regeneration to periodontally diseased teeth. A histological study. *Journal of Periodontal Research* **15**, 1–9.

Cortellini, P. & Bowers, G. (1995). Periodontal regeneration of intrabony defects: an evidence based treatment approach. *International Journal of Periodontics and Restorative Dentistry* **15**, 129–145.

Cortellini, P., Clauser, C. & Pini Prato, G. (1993). Histologic assessment of new attachment following the treatment of a human buccal recession by means of a guided tissue regeneration procedure. *Journal of Periodontology* **64**, 387–391.

Coverly, L., Toto, P.D. & Gargiulo, A.W. (1975). Osseous coagulum. A histologic evaluation. *Journal of Periodontology* **46**, 596–606.

Crigger, M., Bogle, G., Nilveus, R., Egelberg, J. & Selvig, K.A. (1978). The effect of topical citric acid application on the healing of experimental furcation defects in dogs. *Journal of Periodontal Research* **13**, 538–549.

Dragoo, M.R. & Kaldahl, W.B. (1983). Clinical and histological evaluation of alloplasts and allografts in regenerative periodontal surgery in humans. *International Journal of Periodontics and Restorative Dentistry* **3**, 8–29.

Dragoo, M.R. & Sullivan, H.C. (1973a). A clinical and histological evaluation of autogenous iliac bone grafts in humans. I. Wound healing 2 to 8 months. *Journal of Periodontology* **44**, 599–613.

Dragoo, M.R. & Sullivan H.C. (1973b). A clinical and histological evaluation of autogenous iliac bone grafts in humans. II. External root resorption. *Journal of Periodontology* **44**, 614–625.

Ellegaard, B., Karring, T., Davies, R. & Löe, H. (1974). New attachment after treatment of intrabony defects in monkeys. *Journal of Periodontology* **45**, 368–377.

Ellegaard, B., Karring, T., Listgarten, M. & Löe, H. (1973). New attachment after treatment of interradicular lesions. *Journal of Periodontology* **44**, 209–217.

Ellegaard, B., Karring, T. & Löe, H. (1975). The fate of vital and devitalized bone grafts on the healing of interradicular lesion. *Journal of Periodontal Research* **10**, 88–97.

Ellegaard, B. & Löe, H. (1971). New attachment of periodontal tissues after treatment of intrabony lesions. *Journal of Periodontology* **42**, 648–652.

Ellegaard, B., Nielsen, I.M. & Karring, T. (1976). Composite jaw and iliac cancellous bone grafts in intrabony defects in monkeys. *Journal of Periodontal Research* **11**, 299–310.

Ettel, R.G., Schaffer, E.M., Holpuch, R.C. & Brandt, C.L. (1989). Porous hydroxyapatite grafts in chronic subcrestal periodontal defects in rhesus monkeys: a histological investigation. *Journal of Periodontology* **60**, 342–351.

Fetner, A.E., Hartigan, M.S. & Low, S.B. (1994). Periodontal repair using PerioGlas in non-human primates: clinical and histologic observations. *Compendium* **15**, 932–935.

Francis, J.R., Brunsvold, M.A., Prewett, A.B. & Mellonig, J.T. (1995). Clinical evaluation of an allogenic bone matrix in the treatment of periodontal osseous defects. *Journal of Periodontology* **66**, 1074–1079.

Frank, R.M., Fiore-Donno, G. & Cimasoni, G. (1983). Cementogenesis and soft tissue attachment after citric acid treatment in a human. An electron microscopic study. *Journal of Periodontology* **54**, 389–401.

Froum, S. (1996). Human histologic evaluation of HTR polymer and freeze-dried bone allografts. A case report. *Journal of Clinical Periodontology* **23**, 615–620.

Froum, S.J., Kushnek, L., Scopp, I.W. & Stahl, S.S. (1982). Human clinical and histologic responses to durapatite in intraosseous lesions. Case reports. *Journal of Periodontology* **53**, 719–729.

Froum, S.J., Kushnek, L., Scopp, I.W. & Stahl, S.S. (1983). Healing responses of human intraosseous lesions following the use of debridement, grafting and citric acid root treat-

ment. I. Clinical and histologic observations six months postsurgery. *Journal of Periodontology* **54**, 67–76.

Froum, S.J., Ortiz, M., Witkin, R.T., Thaler, R., Scopp, I.W. & Stahl, S.S. (1976). Osseous autografts. III. Comparison of osseous coagulum-bone blend implant with open curettage. *Journal of Periodontology* **47**, 287–294.

Froum, S. & Stahl, S.S. (1987). Human intraosseous healing responses to the placement of tricalcium phosphate ceramic implants. II. 13 to 18 months. *Journal of Periodontology* **58**, 103–109.

Froum, S.J., Thaler, R., Scopp, I.W. & Stahl, S.S. (1975). Osseous autografts. I. Clinical responses to bone blend or hip marrow grafts. *Journal of Periodontology* **46**, 515–521.

Froum, S.J., Weinberg, M.A., Rosenberg, E. & Tarnow, D. (2001). A comparative study utilizing open flap debridement with and without enamel matrix derivate in the treatment of periodontal intrabony defects: a 12 month re-entry study. *Journal of Periodontology* **72**, 25–34.

Froum, S.J., Weinberg, M.A. & Tarnov, D. (1998). Comparison of bioactive glass, synthetic bone graft particles and open debridement in the treatment of human periodontal defects. A clinical study. *Journal of Periodontology* **69**, 698–709.

Fucini, S.E., Quintero, G., Gher, M.E., Black, B.S. & Richardson, A.C. (1993). Small versus large particles of demineralized freeze-dried bone allografts in human intrabony periodontal defects. *Journal of Periodontology* **64**, 844–847.

Fuentes, P., Garrett, S., Nilveus, R. & Egelberg, J. (1993). Treatment of periodontal furcation defects. Coronally positioned flaps with or without citric acid root conditioning in Class II defects. *Journal of Clinical Periodontology* **20**, 425–430.

Galgut, P.N., Waite, I.M., Brookshaw, J.D. & Kingston, C.P. (1992). A 4-year controlled clinical study into the use of a ceramic hydroxyapatite implant material for the treatment of periodontal bone defects. *Journal of Clinical Periodontology* **19**, 570–577.

Ganeles, J., Listgarten, M.A. & Evian, C.I. (1986). Ultrastructure of durapatite periodontal tissue interface in human intrabony defects. *Journal of Periodontology* **57**, 133–140.

Garraway, R., Young, W.G., Daley, T., Harbrow, D. & Bartold, P.M. (1998). An assessment of the osteoinductive potential of commercial demineralized freeze-dried bone in the murine thigh muscle implantation model. *Journal of Periodontology* **69**, 1325–1336.

Garrett, S. (1977). Root planing: a perspective. *Journal of Periodontology* **48**, 553–557.

Gestrelius, S., Lyngstadaas, S.P. & Hammarström, L. (2000). Emdogain – periodontal regeneration based on biomimicry. *Clinical Oral Investigations* **2**, 120–125.

Giannobile, W.V., Finkelman, R.D. & Lynch, S.E. (1994). Comparison of canine and non-human primate animal models for periodontal regenerative therapy: results following a single administration of PDGF/IGF-I. *Journal of Periodontology* **65**, 1158–1168.

Giannobile, W.V., Hernandez, R.A., Finkelman, R.D., Ryan, S., Kinitsy, C.P., D'Andrea, M. & Lynch, S.E. (1996). Comparative effects of platelet-derived growth factor-BB and insulin-like growth factor-I, individually and in combination, on periodontal regeneration in Macaca fascicularis. *Journal of Periodontal Research* **31**, 301–312.

Glossary of Periodontal Terms (1992). 3rd edn. Chicago: The American Academy of Periodontology.

Goldberg, V.M. & Stevenson, S. (1987). The natural history of autografts and allografts. *Clinical Orthopaedics* **225**, 7–16.

Goldman, H. & Cohen, W. (1958). The infrabony pocket: classification and treatment. *Journal of Periodontology* **29**, 272–291.

Gottlow, J., Nyman, S., Karring, T. & Lindhe, J. (1984). New attachment formation as the result of controlled tissue regeneration. *Journal of Clinical Periodontology* **11**, 494–503.

Gottlow, J., Nyman, S., Lindhe, J., Karring, T. & Wennström, J. (1986). New attachment formation in the human periodontium by guided tissue regeneration. *Journal of Clinical Periodontology* **13**, 604–616.

Gottlow, J., Karring, T. & Nyman, S. (1990). Guided tissue regeneration following treatment of recession type defects in the monkey. *Journal of Periodontology* **61**, 680–685.

Graves, D.T. & Cochran, D.L. (1994). Periodontal regeneration with polypeptide growth factors. In: Williams, R.C., Yukna, R.A. & Newman, M.G., eds. *Current Opinion in Periodontology*. Philadelphia: Current Science, pp. 178–186.

Grbic, J.T. & Lamster, I.B. (1992). Risk indicators for future clinical attachment loss in adult periodontitis. Tooth and site variables. *Journal of Periodontology* **63**, 262–269.

Guillemin, G., Patat, J.L., Fournie, J. & Chetail, M. (1987). The use of coral as a bone graft substitute. *Journal of Biomedical Materials Research* **21**, 557–567.

Gurinsky, B.S., Mills, M.P. & Mellonig, J.T. (2004). Clinical evaluation of demineralized freeze-dried bone allografts and enamel matrix derivative versus enamel matrix derivative alone for the treatment of periodontal osseous defects in humans. *Journal of Periodontology* **75**, 1309–1318.

Haffajee, A.D., Socransky, S.S., Lindhe, J., Kent, R.L., Okamoto, H. & Yoneyama, T. (1991). Clinical risk indicators for periodontal attachment loss. *Journal of Clinical Periodontology* **18**, 117–125.

Hammarström, L. (1997). Enamel matrix, cementum development and regeneration. *Journal of Clinical Periodontology* **24**, 658–668.

Hammarström, L., Heijl, L. & Gestrelius, S. (1997). Periodontal regeneration in a buccal dehiscence model in monkeys after application of enamel matrix proteins. *Journal of Clinical Periodontology* **24**, 669–677.

Hamp, S.E., Nyman, S. & Lindhe, J. (1975). Periodontal treatment of multirooted teeth after 5 years. *Journal of Clinical Periodontology* **2**, 126–135.

Hawley, C.E. & Miller, J. (1975). A histologic examination of a free osseous autograft. *Journal of Periodontology* **46**, 289–293.

Heden, G. (2000). A case report study of 72 consecutive Emdogain-treated intrabony periodontal defects: clinical and radiographic findings after 1 year. *International Journal of Periodontics and Restorative Dentistry* **20**, 127–139.

Heden, G., Wennström, J. & Lindhe, J. (1999). Periodontal tissue alterations following Emdogain treatment of periodontal sites with angular bone defects. A series of case reports. *Journal of Clinical Periodontology* **26**, 855–860.

Heijl, L., Heden, G., Svärdström, C. & Ostgren, A. (1997). Enamel matrix derivate (EMDOGAIN®) in the treatment of intrabony periodontal defects. *Journal of Clinical Periodontology* **24**, 705–714.

Hench, L.L., Splinter, R.J., Allen, W.C. & Greenlee, T.K. (1972). Bonding mechanism at the interface of ceramic prosthetic materials. *Journal of Biomedical Materials Research* **2**, 117–141.

Hiatt, W.H. & Schallhorn, R.G. (1973). Intraoral transplants of cancellous bone and marrow in periodontal lesions. *Journal of Periodontology* **44**, 194–208.

Hiatt, W.H., Schallhorn, R.G. & Aaronian, A.J. (1978). The induction of new bone and cementum formation. IV. Microscopic examination of the periodontium following human bone and marrow allograft, autograft and non-graft periodontal regenerative procedures. *Journal of Periodontology* **49**, 495–512.

Holmes, R.E. (1979). Bone regeneration within a corraline hydroxyapatite implant. *Journal of Plastic and Reconstructive Surgery* **63**, 626–633.

Howell, T.H., Fiorellini, J.P., Paquette, D.W., Offenbacher, S., Giannobile, W.V. & Lynch, S. (1997). A phase I/II clinical trial to evaluate a combination of recombinant human platelet-derived growth factor-BB and recombinant human insulin-like growth factor-I in patients with periodontal disease. *Journal of Periodontology* **68**, 1186–1193.

Isidor, F., Karring, T. & Attström, R. (1984). The effect of root planing as compared to that of surgical treatment. *Journal of Clinical Periodontology* **11**, 669–681.

Isidor, F., Karring, T., Nyman, S. & Lindhe, J. (1985). New attachment-reattachment following reconstructive periodontal surgery. *Journal of Clinical Periodontology* **12**, 728–735.

Karatzas, S., Zavras, A., Greenspan, D. & Amar, S. (1999). Histologic observations of periodontal wound healing after treatment with PerioGlass in non-human primates. *International Journal of Periodontics and Restorative Dentistry* **19**, 489–499.

Karring, T. & Cortellini, P. (1999). Regenerative therapy: furcation defects. *Periodontology 2000* **19**, 115–137.

Karring, T., Isidor, F., Nyman, S. & Lindhe, J. (1985). New attachment formation on teeth with a reduced but healthy periodontal ligament. *Journal of Clinical Periodontology* **12**, 51–60.

Karring, T., Nyman, S., Gottlow, J. & Laurell, L. (1993). Development of the biological concept of guided tissue regeneration-animal and human studies. *Periodontology 2000* **1**, 26–35.

Karring, T., Nyman, S. & Lindhe, J. (1980). Healing following implantation of periodontitis affected roots into bone tissue. *Journal of Clinical Periodontology* **7**, 96–105.

Karring, T., Nyman, S., Lindhe, J. & Sirirat, M. (1984). Potentials for root resorption during periodontal healing. *Journal of Clinical Periodontology* **11**, 41–52.

Karring, T., Nyman, S., Thilander, B. & Magnusson, I. (1982). Bone regeneration in orthodontically produced alveolar bone dehiscences. *Journal of Periodontal Research* **17**, 309–315.

Kenney, E.B., Lekovic, V., Han, T., Carranza, F.A. & Demitrijevic, B. (1985). The use of porous hydroxylapatite implant in periodontal defects. I. Clinical results after six months. *Journal of Periodontology* **56**, 82–88.

Kon, S., Novaes, A.B., Ruben, M.P. & Goldman, H.M. (1969). Visualization of microvascularization of the healing periodontal wound II. Curettage. *Journal of Periodontology* **40**, 96–105.

Krejci, C.B., Bissada, N.F., Farah, C. & Greenwell, H. (1987). Clinical evaluation of porous and nonporous hydroxyapatite in the treatment of human periodontal bony defects. *Journal of Periodontology* **58**, 521–528.

Laurell, L., Bose, M., Graziani, F., Tonetti, M. & Berglundh, T. (2006). The structure of periodontal tissues formed following guided tissue regeneration therapy of intra-bone defects in the monkey. *Journal of Clinical Periodontology* **33**, 596–603.

Lekovic, V., Camargo, P.M., Weinlaender, M., Vasilic, N., Aleksic, Z. & Kenney, E.B. (2003). Effectiveness of a combination of platelet-rich plasma, bovine porous bone mineral and guided tissue regeneration in the treatment of mandibular grade II molar furcations in humans. *Journal of Clinical Periodontology* **30**, 746–751.

Levin, M.P., Getter, L., Adrian, J. & Cutright, D.E. (1974). Healing of periodontal defects with ceramic implants. *Journal of Clinical Periodontology* **1**, 197–205.

Lindhe, J. & Echeverria, J. (1994). Consensus report of session II. In: Lang, N.P. & Karring, T., eds. *Proceedings of the 1st European Workshop on Periodontology*. London: Quintessence Publishing Co. Ltd., pp. 210–214.

Lindhe, J., Nyman, S. & Karring, T. (1984). Connective tissue attachment as related to presence or absence of alveolar bone. *Journal of Clinical Periodontology* **11**, 33–40.

Listgarten, M.A., Moa, R. & Robinson, P.J. (1976). Periodontal probing and the relationship of the probe to the periodontal tissues. *Journal of Periodontology* **47**, 511–513.

Listgarten, M.A. & Rosenberg, M.M. (1979). Histological study of repair following new attachment procedures in human periodontal lesions. *Journal of Periodontology* **50**, 333–344.

Lovelace, T.B., Mellonig, J.T., Meffert, R.M., Jones, A.A., Nummikoski, P.V. & Cochran, D.L. (1998). Clinical evaluation of bioactive glass in the treatment of periodontal osseous defects in humans. *Journal of Periodontology* **69**, 1027–1035.

Lynch, S.E., deCustilla, G.R., Williams, R.C., Kinitsy, C.P., Howell, H., Reddy, M.S. & Antoniades, H.N. (1991). The effects of short-term application of a combination of platelet derived and insulin like growth factors on periodontal wound healing. *Journal of Periodontology* **62**, 458–467.

Lynch, S.E., Williams, R.C., Polson, A.M., Howell, T.H., Reddy, M.S., Zappa, U.E. & Antoniades, H.N. (1989). A combination of platelet derived and insulin like growth factors enhances periodontal regeneration. *Journal of Clinical Periodontology* **16**, 545–548.

Mabry, T.W., Yukna, R.A. & Sepe, W.W. (1985). Freeze-dried bone allografts combined with tetracycline in the treatment of juvenile periodontitis. *Journal of Periodontology* **56**, 74–81.

Machtei, E. & Schallhorn, R.G. (1995). Successful regeneration of mandibular class II furcation defects. An evidence-based treatment approach. *International Journal of Periodontics and Restorative Dentistry* **15**, 146–167.

Magnusson, I., Claffey, N., Bogle, S., Garrett, S. & Egelberg, J. (1985). Root resorption following periodontal flap procedures in monkeys. *Journal of Periodontal Research* **20**, 79–85.

Mann, W. (1964). Autogenous transplant in the treatment of an infrabony pocket. *Periodontics* **2**, 205–208.

McCall, J.O. (1926). An improved method of inducing reattachment of the gingival tissue in periodontoclasia. *Dental Items of Interest* **48**, 342–358.

Meadows, C.L., Gher, M.E., Quintero, G. & Lafferty, T.A. (1993). A comparison of polylactic acid granules and decalcified freeze-dried bone allograft in human periodontal osseous defects. *Journal of Periodontology* **64**, 103–109.

Meffert, R.M., Thomas, J.R., Hamilton, K.M. & Brownstein, C.R. (1985). Hydroxylapatite as an alloplastic graft in the treatment of human periodontal osseous defects. *Journal of Periodontology* **56**, 63–73.

Melcher, A.H. (1976). On the repair potential of periodontal tissues. *Journal of Periodontology* **47**, 256–260.

Melcher, A.H., McCulloch, C.A.G., Cheong, T., Nemeth, E. & Shiga, A. (1987). Cells from bone synthesize cementum like and bone like tissue in vitro and may migrate into periodontal ligament in vivo. *Journal of Periodontal Research* **22**, 246–247.

Mellonig, J.T. (1984). Decalcified freeze-dried bone allografts as an implant material in human periodontal defects. *International Journal of Periodontics and Restorative Dentistry* **4**, 41–55.

Mellonig, J.T. (1991). Freeze-dried bone allografts in periodontal reconstructive surgery. *Dental Clinics of North America* **35**, 505–520.

Mellonig, J.T. (1999). Enamel matrix derivate for periodontal reconstructive surgery: Technique and clinical and histologic case report. *International Journal of Periodontics and Restorative Dentistry* **19**, 9–19.

Mellonig, J.T., Bowers, G. & Bully, R. (1981). Comparison of bone graft materials. I. New bone formation with autografts and allografts determined by strontium-85. *Journal of Periodontology* **52**, 291–296.

Minabe, M., Sugaya, A., Satou, H., Tamara, T., Ogawa, Y., Huri, T. & Watanabe, Y. (1988). Histologic study of the hydroxyapatite-collagen complex implants in periodontal osseous defects in dogs. *Journal of Periodontology* **59**, 671–678.

Moore, J.A., Ashley, F.P. & Watermann, C.A. (1987). The effect on healing of the application of citric acid during replaced flap surgery. *Journal of Clinical Periodontology* **14**, 130–135.

Mora, F. & Ouhayoun, J.P. (1995). Clinical evaluation of natural coral and porous hydroxyapatite implants in periodontal bone lesions: results of a 1-year follow-up. *Journal of Clinical Periodontology* **22**, 877–884.

Moscow, B.S. (1964). The response of the gingival sulcus to instrumentation: A histological investigation. *Journal of Periodontology* **35**, 112–126.

Moscow, B.S., Karsh, F. & Stein, S.D. (1979). Histological assessment of autogenous bone graft. A case report and critical evaluation. *Journal of Periodontology* **6**, 291–300.

Moscow, B.S. & Lubarr, A. (1983). Histological assessment of human periodontal defects after durapatite ceramic implant. *Journal of Periodontology* **51**, 455–464.

Murphy, K.G. & Gunsolley, J.C. (2003). Guided tissue regeneration for the treatment of periodontal intrabony and furcation defects. A systematic review. *Annals of Periodontology* **8**, 266–302.

Nabers, C.L. & O'Leary, T.J. (1965). Autogenous bone transplant in the treatment of osseous defects. *Journal of Periodontology* **36**, 5–14.

Nabers, C.L., Reed, O.M. & Hamner, J.E. (1972). Gross and histologic evaluation of an autogenous bone graft 57 months postoperatively. *Journal of Periodontology* **43**, 702–704.

Nasr, H.F., Aichelmann-Reidy, M.E. & Yukna, R.A. (1999). Bone and bone substitutes. *Periodontology 2000* **19**, 74–86.

Nery, E.B. & Lynch, K.L. (1978). Preliminary clinical studies of bioceramic in periodontal osseous defects. *Journal of Periodontology* **49**, 523–527.

Nery, E.M., Lynch, K.L., Hirthe, W.M. & Mueller, B.H. (1975). Bioceramic implants in surgically produced infrabony defects. *Journal of Periodontology* **46**, 328–347.

Nevins, M.L., Camelo, M., Lynch, S.E., Schenk, R.K. & Nevins, M. (2003). Evaluation of periodontal regeneration following grafting of intrabony defects with Bio-Oss collagen: a human histologic report. *International Journal of Periodontics and Restorative Dentistry* **23**, 9–17.

Nevins, M.L., Camelo, M., Nevins, M., King, C.J., Oringer, R.J., Schenk, R.K. & Fiorellini, J.P. (2000). Human histologic evaluation of bioactive ceramic in the treatment of periodontal osseous defects. *International Journal of Periodontics and Restorative Dentistry* **20**, 458–467.

Nielsen, I.M., Ellegaard, B. & Karring, T. (1980). Kielbone® in healing interradicular lesions in monkeys. *Journal of Periodontal Research* **15**, 328–337.

Nielsen, I.M., Ellegaard, B. & Karring, T. (1981). Kielbone® in new attachment attempts in humans. *Journal of Periodontology* **52**, 723–728.

Nilveus, R., Johansson, O. & Egelberg, J. (1978). The effect of autogenous cancellous bone grafts on healing of experimental furcation defects in dogs. *Journal of Periodontal Research* **13**, 532–537.

Nyman, S. & Karring, T. (1979). Regeneration of surgically removed buccal alveolar bone in dogs. *Journal of Periodontal Research* **14**, 86–92.

Nyman, S., Karring, T., Lindhe, J. & Planten, S. (1980). Healing following implantation of periodontitis-affected roots into gingival connective tissue. *Journal of Clinical Periodontology* **7**, 394–401.

Nyman, S., Lindhe, J., Karring, T. & Rylander, H. (1982). New attachment following surgical treatment of human periodontal disease. *Journal of Clinical Periodontology* **9**, 290–296.

Ong, M.M., Eber, R.M., Korsnes, M.I., MacNeil, R.L., Glickman, G.R., Shyr, Y. & Wang, H.L. (1998). Evaluation of bioactive glass alloplast in treating periodontal intrabony defects. *Journal of Periodontology* **69**, 1346–1354.

Orban, B. (1948). Pocket elimination or reattachment? *New York Dental Journal* **14**, 227–232.

Oreamuno, S., Lekovic, V., Kenney, E.B., Carranza, F.A. Jr., Takei, H.H. & Prokic, B. (1990). Comparative clinical study of porous hydroxyapatite and decalcified freeze-dried bone in human periodontal defects. *Journal of Periodontology* **61**, 399–404.

Paolantonio, M. (2002). Combined periodontal regenerative technique in human intrabony defects by collagen membranes and anorganic bovine bone. A controlled clinical study. *Journal of Periodontology* **31**, 770–776.

Parlar, A., Bosshardt, D.D., Unsal, B., Cetiner, D., Haytac, C. & Lang, N.P. (2005). New formation of periodontal tissues around titanium implants in a novel dentin chamber model. *Clinical Oral Implants Research* **16**, 259–267.

Patur, B. (1974). Osseous defects. Evaluation, diagnostic and treatment methods. *Journal of Periodontology* **45**, 523–541.

Patur, B. & Glickman, I. (1962). Clinical and roentgenographic evaluation of the post-treatment healing of infrabony pockets. *Journal of Periodontology* **33**, 164–171.

Pearson, G.E., Rosen, S. & Deporter, D.A. (1981). Preliminary observations on the usefulness of decalcified freeze-dried cancellous bone allograft material in periodontal surgery. *Journal of Periodontology* **52**, 55–59.

Pini-Prato, G., Clauser, C., Tonetti, M.S. & Cortellini, P. (1996). Guided tissue regeneration in gingival recessions. *Periodontology 2000* **11**, 49–57.

Plotzke, A.E., Barbosa, S., Nasjleti, C.E., Morrison, E.C. & Caffesse, R.G. (1993). Histologic and histometric responses to polymeric composite grafts. *Journal of Periodontology* **64**, 343–348.

Polson, A. M. & Heijl, L. (1978). Osseous repair in infrabony defects. *Journal of Clinical Periodontology* **5**, 13–23.

Polson, A.M. & Proye, M.P. (1982). Effect of root surface alterations on periodontal healing. II. Citric acid treatment of the denuded root. *Journal of Clinical Periodontology* **9**, 441–454.

Pontoriero, R., Wennström, J. & Lindhe, J. (1999). The use of barrier membranes and enamel matrix proteins in the treatment of angular bone defects. A prospective controlled clinical study. *Journal of Clinical Periodontology* **26**, 833–840.

Prichard, J. (1957a). Regeneration of bone following periodontal therapy. *Oral Surgery* **10**, 247–252.

Prichard, J. (1957b). The infrabony technique as a predictable procedure. *Journal of Periodontology* **28**, 202–216.

Prichard, J. (1960). A technique for treating infrabony pockets based on alveolar process morphology. *Dental Clinics of North America* **4**, 85–105.

Proye, M. & Polson, A.M. (1982). Effect of root surface alterations on periodontal healing. I. Surgical denudation. *Journal of Clinical Periodontology* **9**, 428–440.

Quattlebaum, J.B., Mellonig, J.T. & Hensel, N.F. (1988). Antigenicity of freeze-dried cortical bone allograft in human periodontal osseous defects. *Journal of Periodontology* **59**, 394–397.

Quintero, G., Mellonig, J.T., Gambill, V.M. & Pelleu, G.B. Jr. (1982). A six-month clinical evaluation of decalcified freeze-dried bone allografts in periodontal osseous defects. *Journal of Periodontology* **53**, 726–730.

Ramfjord, S.P. (1951). Experimental periodontal reattachment in Rhesus monkeys. *Journal of Periodontology* **22**, 67–77.

Ramfjord, S.P. & Nissle, R.R. (1974). The modified Widman flap. *Journal of Periodontology* **45**, 601–607.

Reddy, M.S. & Jeffcoat, H.K. (1999). Methods of assessing periodontal regeneration. *Periodontology 2000* **19**, 87–103.

Register, A.A. & Burdick, F.A. (1976). Accelerated reattachment with cementogenesis to dentin, demineralized in situ. II. Defect repair. *Journal of Periodontology* **47**, 497–505.

Renvert, S., Garrett, S., Schallhorn, R.G. & Egelberg, J. (1985). Healing after treatment of periodontal intraosseous defects. III. Effect of osseous grafting and citric acid conditioning. *Journal of Clinical Periodontology* **12**, 441–455.

Richardson, C.R., Mellonig, J.T., Brunsvold, M.A., McDonnell, H.T. & Cochran, D.L. (1999). Clinical evaluation of Bio-Oss: a bovine-derived xenograft for the treatment of periodontal osseous defects in humans. *Journal of Clinical Periodontology* **26**, 421–428.

Ripamonti, U., Heliotis, M., van der Heerer, B. & Reddi, A.H. (1994). Bone morphogenetic proteins induce periodontal regeneration in the baboon (papio ursinus). *Journal of Periodontal Research* **29**, 439–445.

Rivault, A.F., Toto, P.D., Levy, S. & Gargiulo, A.W. (1971). Autogenous bone grafts: osseous coagulum and osseous retrograde procedures in primates. *Journal of Periodontology* **42**, 787–788.

Robinson, R.E. (1969). Osseous coagulum for bone induction. *Journal of Periodontology* **40**, 503–510.

Rosenberg, M.M. (1971a). Free osseous tissue autografts as a predictable procedure. *Journal of Periodontology* **42**, 195–209.

Rosenberg, M.M. (1971b). Re-entry of an osseous defect treated by a bone implant after a long duration. *Journal of Periodontology* **42**, 360–363.

Rosenberg, E.S., Garber, D.A. & Abrams, B. (1979). Repair of bony defects using an intraoral exostosis as a donor site. A case report. *Journal of Periodontology* **50**, 476–478.

Rosling, B., Nyman, S. & Lindhe, J. (1976). The effect of systematic plaque control on bone regeneration in infrabony pockets. *Journal of Clinical Periodontology* **3**, 38–53.

Ross, S. & Cohen, W. (1968). The fate of an osseous tissue autograft. A clinical and histologic case report. *Periodontics* **6**, 145–151.

Rummelhart, J.M., Mellonig, J.T., Gray, J.L. & Towle, H.J. (1989). A comparison of freeze-dried bone allograft and demineralized freeze-dried bone allograft in human periodontal osseous defects. *Journal of Periodontology* **60**, 655–663.

Rutherford, R.B., Niekrash, C.E., Kennedy, J.E. & Charette, M.F. (1992). Platelet-derived and insulin-like growth factors stimulate regeneration of periodontal attachment in monkeys. *Journal of Periodontal Research* **27**, 285–290.

Saffar, J.L., Colombier, M.L. & Detienville, R. (1990). Bone formation in tricalcium phosphate-filled periodontal intrabony lesions. Histological observations in humans. *Journal of Periodontology* **61**, 209–216.

Sanders, J.J., Sepe, W.W., Bowers, G.M., Koch, R.W., Williams, J.E., Lekas, J.S., Mellonig, J.T., Pelleu, G.B. Jr. & Gambill, V. (1983). Clinical evaluation of freeze-dried bone allografts in periodontal osseous defects. Part III. Composite freeze-dried bone allografts with and without autogenous bone grafts. *Journal of Periodontology* **54**, 1–8.

Sanz, M., Tonetti, M.S., Zabalegui, I., Sicilia, A., Blanco, J., Rebelo, H., Rasperini, G., Merli, M., Cortellini, P. & Suvan, J.E. (2004). Treatment of intrabony defects with enamel matrix proteins or barrier membranes. Results from a multicenter practice-based clinical trial. *Journal of Periodontology* **75**, 726–733.

Sapkos, S.W. (1986). The use of periograft in periodontal defects. Histologic findings. *Journal of Periodontology* **57**, 7–13.

Schaffer, E.M. & Zander, H.A. (1953). Histological evidence of reattachment of periodontal pockets. *Parodontologie* **7**, 101–107.

Schallhorn, R.G. (1967). Eradication of bifurcation defects utilizing frozen autogenous hip marrow implants. *Periodontal Abstracts* **15**, 101–105.

Schallhorn, R.G. (1968). The use of autogenous hip marrow biopsy implants for bony crater defects. *Journal of Periodontology* **39**, 145–147.

Schallhorn, R.G. & Hiatt, W.H. (1972). Human allografts of iliac cancellous bone and marrow in periodontal osseous defects. II. Clinical observations. *Journal of Periodontology* **43**, 67–81.

Schallhorn, R.G., Hiatt, W.H. & Boyce, W. (1970). Iliac transplants in periodontal therapy. *Journal of Periodontology* **41**, 566–580.

Schwartz, Z., Mellonig, J.T., Carnes, D.L. Jr., de la Fontaine, J., Cochran, D.L., Dean, D.D. & Boyan, B.D. (1996). Ability of commercial demineralized freeze-dried bone allograft to induce new bone formation. *Journal of Periodontology* **67**, 918–926.

Sculean, A., Pietruska, M., Schwartz, F., Willershausen, B., Arweiler, N.B., & Auschill, T.M. (2005). Healing of human intrabony defects following treatment with enamel matrix protein derivative alone or combined with a bioactive glass. A controlled clinical study. *Journal of Clinical Periodontology* **32**, 111–117.

Sculean, A., Windisch, P., Keglevich, T., Chiantella, G.C., Gera, I. & Donos, N. (2003). Clinical and histologic evaluation of human intrabony defects treated with an enamel matrix protein derivative combined with a bovine-derived xenograft. *International Journal of Periodontics and Restorative Dentistry* **23**, 47–55.

Sculean, A., Donos, N., Brecx, M., Reich, E. & Karring, T. (2000). Treatment of intrabony defects with guided tissue regeneration and enamel-matrix proteins. An experimental study in monkeys. *Journal of Clinical Periodontology* **27**, 466–472.

Sculean, A., Donos, N., Chiantella, G.C., Windisch, P., Reich, E. & Brecx, M. (1999a). GTR with bioresorbable membranes in the treatment of intrabony defects: a clinical and histologic study. *International Journal of Periodontics and Restorative Dentistry* **19**, 501–509.

Sculean, A., Donos, N., Windisch, P., Brecx, M., Gera, I., Reich, E. & Karring, T. (1999b). Healing of human intrabony defects following treatment with enamel matrix proteins or guided tissue regeneration. *Journal of Periodontal Research* **34**, 310–322.

Selvig, K.A., Sorensen,R.G., Wozney, J.M. & Wikesjö U.M. (2002). Ultrastructure of tissue repair following rh-BMP-2 stimulated periodontal regeneration. *Journal of Periodontology* **73**, 1020–1029.

Shahmiri, S., Singh, I.J. & Stahl, S.S. (1992). Clinical response to the use of the HTR polymer implant in human intrabony lesions. *International Journal of Periodontics and Restorative Dentistry* **12**, 294–299.

Shigeyama, Y., D'Errico, J.A., Stone, R. & Somerman, M.J. (1995). Commercially-prepared allograft material has biological activity in vitro. *Journal of Periodontology* **66**, 478–487.

Sigurdsson, T.J., Lee, M.B., Kubota, K., Turek, T.J., Wazney, J.M. & Wikesjö, U.M.E. (1995). Periodontal repair in dogs: Recombinant human bone morphogenetic protein-2 significantly enhances periodontal regeneration. *Journal of Periodontology* **66**, 131–138.

Silvestri, M., Sartori, S. Rasperini, G., Ricci, G., Rota, C. & Cattaneo, V. (2003). Comparison of intrabony defects treated with enamel matrix derivative versus guided tissue regeneration with a nonresorbable membrane. A multicenter controlled clinical trial. *Journal of Clinical Periodontology* **30**, 386–393.

Silvestri, M., Ricci, G., Rasperini, G., Sartori, S. & Cattaneo, V. (2000). Comparison of treatments of infrabony defects with enamel matrix derivate, guided tissue regeneration with a nonresorbable membrane and Widman modified flap. A pilot study. *Journal of Clinical Periodontology* **27**, 603–610.

Snyder, A.J., Levin, M.P. & Cutright, D.E. (1984). Alloplastic implants of tricalcium phosphate ceramic in human periodontal osseous defects. *Journal of Periodontology* **55**, 273–277.

Sonis, S.T., Williams, R.C., Jeffcoat, M.K., Black, R. & Shklar, G. (1985). Healing of spontaneous periodontal defects in dogs treated with xenogeneic demineralized bone. *Journal of Periodontology* **56**, 470–479.

Stahl, S. & Froum, S. (1986). Histologic evaluation of human intraosseous healing responses to the placement of tricalcium phosphate ceramic implants. I. Three to eight months. *Journal of Periodontology* **57**, 211–217.

Stahl, S. & Froum, S. (1987). Histologic and clinical responses to porous hydroxylapatite implants in human periodontal defects. Three to twelve months postimplantation. *Journal of Periodontology* **58**, 689–695.

Stahl, S. & Froum, S. (1991a). Human suprabony healing responses following root demineralization and coronal flap anchorage. Histologic responses in seven sites. *Journal of Clinical Periodontology* **18**, 685–689.

Stahl, S. & Froum, S. (1991b). Healing of human suprabony lesions treated with guided tissue regeneration and coronally anchored flaps. Case reports. *Journal of Clinical Periodontology* **18**, 69–74.

Stahl, S., Froum, S. & Kushner, L. (1983). Healing responses of human teeth following the use of debridement grafting and citric acid root conditioning. II. Clinical and histologic observations: One year post-surgery. *Journal of Periodontology* **54**, 325–338.

Stahl, S., Froum, S. & Tarnow, D. (1990a). Human histologic responses to the placement of guided tissue regenerative techniques in intrabony lesions. Case reports on nine sites. *Journal of Clinical Periodontology* **17**, 191–198.

Stahl, S., Froum, S. & Tarnow, D. (1990b). Human clinical and histologic responses to the placement of HTR polymer particles in 11 intrabony lesions. *Journal of Periodontology* **61**, 269–274.

Stahl, S., Slavkin, H.C., Yamada, L. & Levine, S. (1972). Speculations about gingival repair. *Journal of Periodontology* **43**, 395–402.

Stavropoulos, A., Kostopoulos, L., Nyengaard, J.R. & Karring, T. (2004). Fate of bone formed by guided tissue regeneration with or without grafting of Bio-Oss or Biogran: an experimental study in the rat. *Journal of Clinical Periodontology* **31**, 30–39.

Stavropoulos, A., Kostopoulos, L., Nyengaard, J.R. & Karring, T. (2003a). Deproteinized bovine bone (Bio-Oss) and bioactive glass (Biogran) arrest bone formation when used as an adjunct to guided tissue regeneration (GTR): an experimental study in the rat. *Journal of Clinical Periodontology* **30**, 636–643.

Stavropoulos, A., Karring, E.S., Kostopoulos, L. & Karring T. (2003b). Deproteinized bovine bone and gentamycin as an adjunct to GTR in the treatment of intrabony defects. A randomized controlled clinical study. *Journal of Clinical Periodontology* **30**, 486–495.

Stavropoulos, A., Kostopoulos, L., Mardas, N., Nyengaard, J.R. & Karring, T. (2001) Deproteinized bovine bone used as an adjunct to guided bone augmentation: an experimental study in the rat. *Clinical Journal of Implant and Dental Related Research* **3**, 156–165.

Steiner, S.S., Crigger, M. & Egelberg, J. (1981). Connective tissue regeneration to periodontal diseased teeth. II. Histologic observation of cases following replaced flap surgery. *Journal of Periodontal Research* **16**, 109–116.

Strub, J.R., Gaberthüel, T.W. & Firestone A.R. (1979). Comparison of tricalcium phosphate and frozen allogenic bone implants in man. *Journal of Periodontology* **50**, 624–629.

Terranova, V. & Wikesjö, U.M.E. (1987). Extracellular matrices and polypeptide growth factors as mediators of functions of cells of the periodontium. *Journal of Periodontology* **58**, 371–380.

Tonetti, M., Cortellini, P., Lang, N.P., Suvan, J.E., Adrians, P., Dubravec, D., Fonzar, A., Fourmosis, I., Rasperini, G., Rossi, R., Silvestri, M., Topoll, H., Waallkamm, B. & Zybutz, M. (2004). Clinical outcomes following treatment of human intrabony defects with GTR/bone replacement material or access flap alone. A multicenter randomized controlled clinical trial. *Journal of Clinical Periodontology* **31**, 770–776.

Tonetti, M., Lang, N.P., Cortellini, P., Suvan, J.E., Adriaens, P., Dubravec, D.. Fonzar, A., Fourmosis. I., Mayfield, L.J.A., Rossi, R., Silvestri, M., Tiedemann, C., Topoll, H., Vangsted, T. & Wallkamm, B. (2002). Enamel matrix proteins in the regenerative therapy of deep intrabony defects. A multicentre randomized controlled clinical trial. *Journal of Clinical Periodontology* **29**, 317–325.

Trombelli, L., Annunziata, M., Belardo, S., Farina, R., Scabbia, A. & Guida, L. (2006). Autogenous bone graft in combination with enamel matrix derivative in the treatment of deep intra-osseous defects: a report of 13 consecutively treated patients. *Journal of Clinical Periodontology* **33**, 69–75.

Trombelli, L. (2005). Which reconstructive procedures are effective for treating the periodontal intraosseous defect. *Periodontology 2000* **37**, 88–105.

Turner, D.W. & Mellonig, J.T. (1981). Antigenicity of freeze-dried bone allograft in periodontal osseous defects. *Journal of Periodontal Research* **16**, 89–99.

Urist, M.R. (1980). *Fundamental and Clinical Bone Physiology*. Philadelphia: J.B. Lippincott Co. pp. 348–353.

Urist, M.R. & Strates, B. (1970). Bone formation in implants of partially and wholly demineralized bone matrix. *Journal of Clinical Orthopedics* **71**, 271–278.

Van der Velden, U. & de Vries, J.H. (1978). Introduction of a new periodontal probe: the pressure probe. *Journal of Clinical Periodontology* **5**, 188–197.

Wade, A.B. (1962). An assessment of the flap operation. *Dental Practitioner and Dental Records* **13**, 11–20.

Wade, A.B. (1966). The flap operation. *Journal of Periodontology* **37**, 95–99.

Waerhaug, J. (1952). The gingival pocket. *Odontologisk Tidsskrift* **60**, Suppl. 1.

Warrer, K., Karring, T. & Gotfredsen, K. (1993). Periodontal ligament formation around different types of dental titanium implants. I. The selftapping screw type implant system. *Journal of Periodontology* **64**, 29–34.

Werbitt, M. (1987). Decalcified freeze-dried bone allografts: a successful procedure in the reduction of intrabony defects. *International Journal of Periodontics and Restorative Dentistry* **7**, 56–63.

West, T.L. & Brustein, D.D. (1985). Freeze-dried bone and coralline implants compared in the dog. *Journal of Periodontology* **56**, 348–351.

Wilson, J. & Low, S.B. (1992). Bioactive ceramics for periodontal treatment: comparative studies in the Patus monkey. *Journal of Applied Biomaterials* **3**, 123–129.

Wikesjö, U.M., Xiropaidis, A.V., Thomson, R.C., Cook, A.D., Selvig, K.A. & Hardwick, W.R. (2003a). Periodontal repair in dogs: space-providing ePTFE devices increase rhBMP-2ACS-induced bone formation. *Journal of Clinical Periodontology* **30**, 715–725.

Wikesjö, U.M., Xiropaidis, A.V., Thomson, R.C., Cook, A.D., Selvig, K A. & Hardwick, W.R. (2003b). Periodontal repair in dogs: rhBMP-2 significantly enhances bone formation under provisions for guided tissue regeneration. *Journal of Clinical Periodontology* **30**, 705–714.

World Workshop in Periodontology (1996). The American Academy of Periodontology. *Annals of Periodontology* **1**, 618–670.

Wozney, J.M., Rosen, V.B., Celeste, A.J., Mitsock, L.M., Whitters, M.J., Kriz, R.W., Hewick, R.M. & Wang, E.M. (1988). Novel regulators of bone formation: molecular clones and activities. *Science* **243**, 1528–1534.

Yukna, R. (1990). HTR polymer grafts in human periodontal osseous defects. I. 6-month clinical results. *Journal of Periodontology* **61**, 633–642.

Yukna, R. (1994). Clinical evaluation of coralline calcium carbonate as a bone replacement graft material in human periodontal osseous defects. *Journal of Periodontology* **65**, 177–185.

Yukna, R., Cassingham, R.J., Caudill, R.F., Evans, G.F., Miller, S., Mayer, E.T. & Simon, J.F. (1986). Six month evaluation of Calcitite (hydroxyapatite ceramics) in periodontal osseous defects. *International Journal of Periodontics and Restorative Dentistry* **6**, 34–45.

Yukna, R., Harrison, B.G., Caudill, R.F., Evans, G.H., Mayer, E.T. & Miller, S. (1985). Evaluation of durapatite as an alloplastic implant in periodontal osseous defects. II. Twelve month re-entry results. *Journal of Periodontology* **56**, 540–547.

Yukna, R., Mayer, E.T. & Amos, S.M. (1989). 5-year evaluation of durapatite ceramic alloplastic implants in periodontal osseous defects. *Journal of Periodontology* **60**, 544–551.

Yukna, R. & Yukna, C.N. (1998). A 5-year follow-up of 16 patients treated with coralline calcium carbonate (BIO-CORAL) bone replacement grafts in infrabony defects. *Journal of Clinical Periodontology* **25**, 1036–1040.

Zamet, J.S., Darbar, U.R., Griffiths, G.S., Bulman, J.S., Brägger, U., Burgin, W. & Newman, H.N. (1997). Particulate bioglass as a grafting material in the treatment of periodontal intrabony defects. *Journal of Clinical Periodontology* **24**, 410–418.

Zucchelli, G., Amore, C., Montebugnoli, L. & De Sanctis, M. (2003). Enamel matrix proteins and bovine porous bone mineral in the treatment of intrabony defects: a comparative controlled clinical trial. *Journal of Periodontology* **74**, 1725–1735.

Index

esthetics (*continued*)
single-tooth problem 683, *684–5*
treatment goal 655
treatment modality review 1148
estradiol 312
estriol 312
estrogen 312
bone resorption treatment *91*
chronic periodontitis 425
gingival disease 408
hormonal contraceptives 316
pregnancy 313–14
smokers 315
tissue response 316
ethnicity *see* race/ethnicity
Eubacterium 224
exopeptidases 295
exopolysaccharides 227
Extent and Severity Index (ESI) 130–1,
135
extraction of teeth
cortical plasticity 121
neuroplasticity 121
periodontal ligament receptors 108–9,
113, 116, *117*
phantom tooth phenomenon 121
sensory amputation 119–20
sensory nerve damage 120
extravascular circulation 46, *47*

facial artery 43, 44
factor VIIc 316
factor XIIc 316
famciclovir 379
familial aggregation, aggressive
periodontitis 447, 449
Fc gamma receptors (FcγR) gene
polymorphisms 336, *337*, 338
FcγRIIa polymorphisms 336, *337*, 338
fetal growth restriction, *Campylobacter
rectus* 482
fetal–placental unit 481
fetor hepaticus 1327
fever, necrotizing periodontal
disease 463
fiberotomy
forced tooth eruption 1005, *1006*
with orthodontic treatment 1274
fibrin 104
fibrinogen 479
fibroblast growth factor (FGF) 87
alveolar bone healing 89
ridge augmentation 1093
fibroblasts 19, 33
dental pulp infection 515
smoking effects 321
fibroplasia 60
osseointegration 104, *105*
fish malodor syndrome 1334
fixed partial dentures (FPD) 676–7, 679–
80, 683, 1208–18
abutments 1223–4
fractures 1224
avoidance with implants 1177
cantilever pontics 1213–15
cantilever units 588, *590*, 1182–3, *1184*
cantilevered 588, *590*
cast post 1223
cement-retained 1233
complete-arch fixed complete
denture *1210*, 1211
complications 1211, 1222–4, 1235
diagnostic waxing 1212
dowels 1223
forces during function 1211–12
full-arch tooth replacement 1210–11
high risk 1177, **1178**
implant-supported 676–7, 679–80,
683, 1181, 1182
biomechanical risk reduction 1212

clinical success assessment 1215–16
immediate provisionalization 1215
success/survival rate 1234–5
implant-to-implant supported 1208,
1211–16
long-term success 1223–4
partially edentulous tooth
replacement therapy 1211–16
patient assessment 1208–9
prosthesis design 1210–16
retention loss 1224
screw-retained 1213, 1233
splinted metal–ceramic 1186
straight 683
success/survival rate 1234–5
support with implant and natural
teeth combination 1183–4
survival rate 1223–4
tooth-implant supported 1208,
1216–18
complications 1217, 1218
implant loss risk 1217
maintenance 1218
natural tooth intrusion 1217–18
tooth-supported 1125–36, 1175–6,
1179
treatment planning 1209–11
flap handling instruments 805
flap margin recession *842*
flap procedures 786–93
apically positioned 1000, *1001*, 1002,
1003
ectopic tooth eruption 1006, 1008
apically repositioned 788–9, 813–14
beveled 789, *790*
clinical outcomes 931–2, **933**
coronally advanced flaps *985*, 986,
988, **990**
envelope flap 987, *989*, 1014, *1015*
hard tissue pockets 807–8
healing 813–14
implants 1054–5
modified operation 787–8
mucoperiosteal flaps 786, 787, 788,
1073
maxillary anterior single-tooth
replacement 1157
maxillary sinus floor elevation
1102
operation with/without osseous
surgery 806
rotational **990**
soft tissue lesion excision 817
soft tissue pockets 806, *807*
suturing 808–11
tension elimination 992
flexible spiral wire (FSW) retainer *1245,
1246*, 1248–9, *1250–1*
floss holders 715
flossing 714–15
instruction 725
traumatic lesions 396, *397*
fluoride
anticaries action 736
chlorhexidine synergism 753
crystals in woodsticks 715
halitosis treatment 1336
plaque control 746
toothpaste 741
foam brushes 718
foods, allergic reactions 394
forced tooth eruption 1002, 1003–5,
1006
with fiberotomy 1005, *1006*
procedure 596
foreign body
impaction 497
reactions 398
formaldehyde dehydrogenase 229
formaldehyde lyase 229

free graft procedures, edentulous
ridge 1013–17, *1018–19*, 1020,
1021–3
free soft tissue graft procedures
epithelialized **990**
gingival augmentation 966, *967*
healing 995–6
interpositional grafts 1014, *1015, 1016*
pouch graft procedures 1013–14
ridge augmentation 1013–17, *1018–
19*, 1020, *1021–3*
root coverage 972, 982, *984*, 985–7,
988–9, 990, **990**, 991–2
thickness 992
freeze-dried bone allogeneic grafts
(FDBA) 554–5
frenectomy 1274–5
frenotomy with orthodontic
treatment 1274–5
fungal infection
chlorhexidine activity 748
gingival disease 380–3
linear gingival erythema 382
see also Candida albicans (candidiasis)
furcated region 823
furcation
definition 823
incisors 826
mandibular molars 825–6
mandibular premolars 826, *827*
maxillary molars 824, *825*
maxillary premolars 825
probing 828
furcation defects
degree III 936–7
guided tissue regeneration 904
mandibular degree II 933–6, 942
maxillary degree II 936
regenerative therapy 840–3, *844*, 904,
932–7
techniques 942
furcation entrance 823, *824*
exposure *842*
molars 828
furcation fornix 823, *824*
furcation involvement
aggressive periodontitis 657–67
anatomy 824–6
assessment 580–3
automated probing systems 580
barrier membranes 906, *908*, 932–7
basic periodontal examination 657
chronic periodontitis *575*, 667, *668*,
669–73
classification 827
degree 582
diagnosis 826–8, *829*
differential diagnosis 829–30
extraction of tooth 843
guided tissue regeneration 840–3, 913
implant planning 682–3
molar uprighting 1262–3
occlusal interference 353, 829–30
orthodontic treatment 1262–3
papilla preservation flaps 916, *917*
prognosis 843, 845–6
radiography 828, *829*, 830
regeneration of defects 840–3, 903
regenerative procedures 541–2
barrier membranes 932–7
risk assessment 1309
root debridement 773
root separation and resection 832–5,
836, 837–8, *839*, 840, **845**
root surface biomodification 557
terminology 823–4
trauma from occlusion 353
treatment 823–46
goal 655
tunnel preparation 832

gingival recession (*continued*)
 treatment comparison 817–18
 see also root coverage
gingival sulcus 17
 subgingival plaque 194
Gingival Sulcus Bleeding Index 130
gingivectomy
 beveled 1000, *1001*
  internal 805, *806*
 healing 812–13
 with orthodontic treatment 1275,
  1276
 procedures 784–6
 surgical technique 805, *806*
gingivitis
 artefacta 397
 bacterial flora 408
 chronic 735
 chronic periodontitis risk 422
 clinical signs/symptoms 408
 collagen loss 290, 292
 control agents **743**
 dento-gingival epithelium 290, *291*
 diabetes mellitus-associated 411
 diagnosis 583–4
 epithelial cells 289–90, *291*, 292, *293*
 experimental studies 756–7
 foreign body 398
 histopathological features 287, *288*,
  289
 hormonal contraceptive use 316
 immune reactions 286–7
 index systems 574–5
 inflammation 289
 inflammatory reaction 286–7
 lesions 289–90, *291*, 292, *293–4*
 leukemia-associated 411–12
 lymphocytes 289
 menstrual cycle-associated 409
 microbiology 145–6, *147–8*, 148
 necrotizing 459
  acute form 463–4
  chronic form 463–4
  diagnosis 464–5
  histopathology 465–6
  host response 468
  interproximal craters 461–2
  lesion development 460–1
  recurrent 464
  traumatic ulcerative gingival lesion
   differential diagnosis 396–7
  treatment 472
  ulcerative 413–14, 426
 neutrophils 286, *288*, 293
 oral contraceptive-associated 411
 periodontitis in adults 133, 134
 plaque removal 710
 plaque-induced 406, **407**, 407–8, 422,
  1298
 plasma cells 292, *293*
 polymorphonuclear leukocytes 289
 pregnancy 313, 314, 409–10
 prevalence 738, 739
 prevention in periodontitis
  prevention 426
 progression to periodontal
  disease 414–15
 puberty-associated 312, 408–9
 smoking 319
 spectrum of disease 405
 spirochetes 221
 supportive periodontal therapy 1302
 supragingival plaque
  accumulation 735, 736
 susceptibility 423
 treatment goal 655
 see also acute necrotizing ulcerative
  gingivitis (ANUG)
gingivoplasty 805
 soft tissue sculpting 1020, *1021–3*

gingivostomatitis, herpetic
 necrotizing periodontal disease
  differential diagnosis 463, 464–5
 primary 378–9, 464–5
glucose intolerance 153
 see also diabetes mellitus
glucose oxidase, plaque control 744
glutathione 311
glycoprotein pellicle 188
glycoproteins 23
glycosaminoglycans 23
glycosyl-phosphatidyl-inositol
 (GPI) *337*
Good Clinical Practice Guidelines 757–8
Gore Tex Periodontal Material® 928
grafting procedures
 free gingival 1008
 gingival augmentation 966–7
 interpositional 1014, *1015*, *1016*
  combined with onlay grafts 1020
 maxillary sinus floor
  elevation 1107–8
 onlay grafts 1015–17, *1018–19*, 1020,
  1021–3
  combined with interpositional
   grafts 1020
 roll flap procedure 1011–13
 soft tissue for ridge defects 1010–11,
  1089
 see also free soft tissue graft
  procedures; pedicle graft
  procedures
granulation tissue
 interpositional grafts 1014
 peripheral inflammatory root
  resorption 869, 870
 tooth socket healing 55, *56*, 57, *58*, 60
growth factors 559
 alveolar bone healing 88–9
 delivery systems 1093
 osteoinductive/osteopromotive 87
 ridge augmentation 1093
 tooth socket healing 57, 60
growth hormone (GH) 88
guided bone regeneration (GBR) 1083–5
 augmentation materials 1085–7
 bone grafts 1084–5, 1086–7
 bone morphology 1084–5
 bone substitute materials 1084–5,
  1086–7
 clinical concepts 1088–92
 long-term results 1087–8
 patient selection 1084
 soft tissue morphology 1085
guided tissue regeneration (GTR) 555,
 559–61, 793
 aggressive periodontitis 661, *663*
 attachment 1260
 barrier membranes 905–7
 bioabsorbable materials 930
 citric acid demineralization
  combination 942–3
 clinical outcomes 931–2, **933**
 combined procedures 940, *941*, 942–3
 with demineralized freeze-dried bone
  allograft 940, **941**, 942
 enamel matrix derivative
  comparison 558
 evaluation 562
 furcation
  defect regeneration 840–3, *844*, 904,
   932–7
  involvement 913
 healing 914
 intrabony defects 903, 905, *906*, *907*,
  910
  membranes 930–2
 oral hygiene 1261
 orthodontic tooth movement 1261–2
 pedicle soft tissue graft with barrier

 membrane for root
  coverage 980–1, *983*
 peripheral inflammatory root
  resorption 871
 post-operative morbidity 926–8
 root coverage **990**, 992
  healing 995
gum-wing profile 997

Halimeter™ 1329, *1331*, *1332*
halitophobia 1332, 1333
 therapy 1333–4
halitosis
 blood-borne 1327, 1334
 chlorhexidine use for oral
  malodor 753
 classification 1333
 confidant use 1337
 control 1325–37
 diagnosis 1328–30, *1331–2*, 1333
 drug-induced 1334
 epidemiology 1325–6
 extraoral 1327, **1328**, 1334–5, 1337
 instructions for patient 1328, *1330*
 intraoral 1326–7, 1335–7
 morning 1334
 odor characteristics 1326
 oral inspection 1330, *1332*, *1333*
 organoleptic evaluation *1331*
 organoleptic measurements 1328
 pathogenesis 1326–7, **1328**
 pathologic 1335
 practice flowchart 1328, *1329*
 prevalence 1325–6
 questionnaire 1328, *1331*
 sulfide monitor 1329–30, *1331*, *1332*
 temporary 1333, 1334
 treatment 1333–7
  adjustment 1337
  planning 1334–5, 1335–7
hand instruments, root
 debridement 768–70, *771*
hard tissue
 replacement 556
 resorption mechanisms 865–6
 see also alveolar bone; bone
Haversian canals 38, 39, *40*, 41
health education 695–6
health survivor effect 141
heart disease, postmenopausal
 women 315
heat necrosis, implants 614–15
hematologic disorders
 chronic periodontitis 425
 gingival manifestations 395–6
 implant patient 644
 surgery contraindication 800
hemidesmosomes 12–13, 14, 16, 18
 epithelial cell rests 30, *31*
 junctional epithelium attachment 19
hemiseptal defects 901–2
hemoglobin, glycated (HbA1c) 162
hemostasis, local 801
hepatitis, dental team protection 687
hepatitis B infection, chlorhexidine
 activity 748
herb extracts, plaque control 745–6
hereditary gingival fibromatosis 383–4,
 413
herpes simplex virus (HSV)
 dental team protection 687
 erythema multiforme 390
 gingival disease 378–9
 periodontal infection 225
herpes virus infections 378–80
 primary gingivostomatitis 463, 464–5
herpes zoster 379–80
Hertwig's epithelial root sheath 4
 fragmentation 32
 remnants 30